NEW DIMENSIONS IN OTORHINOLARYNGOLOGY
—
HEAD AND NECK SURGERY

Volume 2

NEW DIMENSIONS IN OTORHINOLARYNGOLOGY — HEAD AND NECK SURGERY

Volume 2

Proceedings of the XIIIth World Congress,
Miami Beach, FL, 26–31 May 1985

Editor:

Eugene N. Myers

Department of Otolaryngology
University of Pittsburgh School of Medicine,
Eye and Ear Hospital, Pittsburgh, PA, U.S.A

1985

EXCERPTA MEDICA, Amsterdam–New York–Oxford

International Congress Series No. 680
ISBN 0 444 80730 6

Published by:
Elsevier Science Publishers B.V. (Biomedical Division)
P.O. Box 211
1000 AE Amsterdam
The Netherlands

Sole distributors for the USA and Canada:
Elsevier Science Publishing Company Inc.
52 Vanderbilt Avenue
New York, NY 10017
USA

Library of Congress Cataloging-in-Publication Data

World Congress of Otorhinolaryngology. (13th : 1985 :
Miami Beach, Fla.)
New dimensions in ORL and head and neck surgery.
(International congress series ; no. 680)
Includes indexes.
1. Otolaryngology--Congresses. 2. Head--Surgery--Congresses. 3. Neck--Surgery--Congresses. I. Myers, Eugene N., 1933- . II. Title. III. Series.
[DNLM: 1. Head--surgery--congresses. 2. Neck--surgery--congresses. 3. Otolaryngology--congresses.
4. Otorhinolaryngologic Diseases--surgery--congresses.
W3 EX89 no. 680 / WV 100 W927 1985n]
RF16.W67 1985 617'.51 85-25258
ISBN 0-444-80729-2 (Elsevier Science Pub. Co. : v. 1)
ISBN 0-444-80730-6 (Elsevier Science Pub. Co. : v. 2)

Printed in The Netherlands

New dimensions in otorhinolaryngology - head and neck surgery, vol. 2.
E. Myers, editor

THE SIGNIFICANCE OF LANGERHANS CELLS IN CHOLESTEATOMA

BJÖRN ÅBERG (1), GUY HEYDEN (2), MATS JONTELL (2), STAFFAN EDSTRÖM (1), ANDERS TJELLSTRÖM (1)

Departments of Otorhinolaryngology (1) and Oral Pathology (2), University of Göteborg, Sweden

INTRODUCTION

The reason for bone resorption in cholesteatoma has not been sufficiently elucidated. Recently, Langerhans cells[1,2,3] have been suggested to be involved in this process. Langerhans cells have the capacity of recognizing and presenting antigen to the cell-mediated immune system and possibly release bone resorption factors[1,2,4].

The aim of this study was to investigate the occurrence rate of Langerhans cells in the keratinizing epithelia in cholesteatoma and to evaluate their pathologic significance.

MATERIALS AND METHODS

Cholesteatoma specimens from thirteen patients undergoing cholesteatoma surgery were studied. Eight female, 5 male. Age 14 - 77 years. The patients were subjected to combined approach tympanoplasty or radical mastoidectomy under general anesthesia. Eight patients were operated for the first time and 5 were reoperated because of recurring cholesteatoma after previous surgery. There was no sign of infection in any of the ears immediately prior to the surgery, and no steroid treatment had been administered which otherwise might have influenced the results.

During the surgical procedure the cholesteatoma specimens were taken in big pieces with adjacent epithelium from the ear canal and tympanic membrane. Four specimens of epithelium obtained from the ear canal of patients undergoing stapedectomy served as controls. Also ear canal skin infected by aspergillus fungus, a well known cell-mediated immune reactive antigen, was used for comparative reasons.

The specimens were immunohistochemically[5] investigated. Monoclonal antibodies were used as immunological markers (anti-HLA-DR, anti-LEU 6, anti-LEU 4) in order to demonstrate Langerhans cells, T-lymphocytes and activated epithelial cells.

RESULTS

No HLA-DR antigens were found on the epithelial cells in cholesteatoma nor on ear canal epithelia from patients undergoing stapedectomy. In fungus-infected ear canal epithelia an intense activation of lymphocytes and epithelial cells was found. In cholesteatoma tissue no increase of Langerhans cells was found when compared to normal ear canal skin and tympanic membrane. Presence of HLA-DR expressing cells (activated T- and B-lymphocytes) in cholesteatoma were occasionally found.

CONSLUSION

The pathogenesis of cholesteatoma and bone resorption cannot be explained by cell-mediated immune response.

ACKNOWLEDGEMENTS

Grants were received from the Gothenburg Medical Society.

REFERENCES

1. Veldman JE, Visser CE, Schuurman H-J, de Groot JCMJ, Huizing EH (1984) Otolaryngology - Head and Neck Surgery 92:1-6
2. Gantz BJ (1984) Ann Otol Rhinol Laryngol 93:150-156
3. Rowden GR (1980) J Invest Dermatol 75:22-31
4. Abramson M, Moriyama H, Huant CC (1984) Acta Otolaryngol (Stockh) 97:437-442
5. Sloberg K, Jonsson R, Jontell M (1984) J Oral Pathol 13:516-524

© 1985 Elsevier Science Publishers B.V. (Biomedical Division)
New dimensions in otorhinolaryngology - head and neck surgery, vol. 2.
E. Myers, editor

SUBPERIOSTEAL ABSCESS COMPLICATING CHRONIC OTITIS MEDIA

S.M.AHMADIZADEH, M.D., FACS.
Simetry St., Ahwaz, IRAN

INTRODUCTION

Mastoid air cells, being a part of middle ear cleft, may be widely expanded or ivory sclerotic with hypocellular and diploetic variation in between.

Whether these variations influence the behavior of middle ear mucosa in response to infection or unique factor(s) govern the type of mastoid as well as behavior of middle ear mucosa is a matter of theortical dispute.

The commonest abcesses resulting from mastoid disease form in the postauricular region, which occur usually in children with acute mastoiditis.[1]

MATERIAL AND METHODS

This study consisted of a group of patients presented at Ahwaz University hospitals between 1978-1984.

Chronic ear discharge, postauricular swelling and pain with or without postauricular fistula were the presenting symptoms.

There were 45 cases in this group, 26 males and 19 females.

The age of patients was between 6-40 years with the following distribution:

6-10 years	12 cases
10-20 years	29 cases
25-40 years	4 cases

History of ear discharge varied from 2 months to many years.

Seven patients suffered from postauricular fistula with intermittent periods of discharge at the time of admission.

The main operative finding in 37 cases including all who had postauricular fistula was cholesteatoma.

In this latter group cholesteatoma was very extensive--more extensive than preoperative x-ray evaluation.

OPERATION

Radical mastoidectomy in most cases was performed either at one session or two weeks following primary incision.

Comparison between these two methods is not meant here.

It is to be mentioned that during the same period of study 18 operations of cortical mastoidectomy have been performed for the reason of acute mastoiditis associated with subperiosteal abcess.

This figure shows significant overwhelming numbers of chronic over acute cases with subperiosteal abcess.

DISCUSSION

Destruction of lateral wall of the antrum has already been shown to be due to cholesteatoma.[2]

In this study subperiosteal abcess has been added to the clinical picture.

CONCLUSIONS:

1) With antibiotic armamentarium subperiosteal abcess occurs more frequently in chronic than in acute otitis media.

2) Every case of subperiosteal abcess associated with chronic otitis media should be regarded to have underlying cholesteatoma unless proven otherwise. More so cases with postauricular fistula.

3) Proper management of ear infection in youngsters should be strongly emphasized.

REFERENCES

1. Saunders and Paparella (1971) Atlas of Ear Surgery, Second Edition, C. V. Mosby Co.

2. Shambaugh and Glosscock (1981) Surgery of the Ear, Third Edition, Saunders

New dimensions in otorhinolaryngology – head and neck surgery, vol. 2.
E. Myers, editor

OTOMYCOSIS IN KARACHI

M. H. A. BEG, A. T. BUKHARI
K. V. Social Security Site Hospital,
Manghopir Road, Karachi

INTRODUCTION

Fungal infections of the ear's external meatus are found world wide,[1] being more common in tropics where fungi flourish in the heat & humidity. Spores which are freely available in atmosphere, Settle in the ear and mycelia invade the skin. Very little data is available about this probelm from tropics and the aim of present study was to observe fungal disease clinically & on culture. This study was done between March 1980 to Feb 1981.

MATERIAL & METHODS

There is fairly high humidity in Karachi all year round and patients have been seen throughout the year. The ears of 80 patients were examined. Direct Microscopy was carried out in some cases. Culture on Sabound dextrose agar was used. The centre of plate was inoculated at one or two places. Positive cultures were obtained in three to five days. The plates were kept for 10 days before any cultures were declared negative.

Results.

Seventy four cultures showed positive growth of fungi. Fifty two of these patients were males and 22 females. Aspergillus was the commonest fungus in the series with 51 positive cultures of which A. niger was found in 35 cases, A. fumigatus in 5 cases & indentified Aspergillus in 11 cases, (Table I). Other fungi including penicillium Sp., Candida Sp. were also isolated.

Discussion.

Yamashita[2] has isolated 48 genera of fungi from 2880 patients. Normally they do not cause problem until suitable growing conditions occur. These include water in the ear, wax which has become soft, otitis externa & otitis media. Environmental & atmospheric humidity may enable fungi to flourish. It is a unilateral disease[3], as were our 64 cases. It is also more common in younger age group[4].

It is inadvisable to syringe out the fungus, suction or dry mopping is the treatment of choice, local application of fungicide is advisable & we have used Zinc Undecylenate 8% cream for local application in the ear canal twice a week & have found it as good as any other antifungal agent.

Candida is more commonly isolated in Europe, but have formed only 2.5% of our isolates.

Table I
Fungi isolated in Otomycosis

Fungi	No of cases		Percentage
Aspergillus			
niger	35 ()	51	69
funigatus	5 ()		
unidentified	11		
Penicillum Sp	11		15
Mucor Sp	8		11
candida Sp	2		2.5
Aspergillus/Penicillium	2		2.5
	74		100

REFERENCES

1. Friedman, I., (1974) Otomycosis in Pathology of the Ear, Blackwell Scientific Publications, Oxford, P 27.

2. YAMASHITA, K. (1963) Fungal Flora in the ear, nose, throat and mouth of man, Japan Journal of Medical Mycology 4, 136-149.

3. EMMONS, C. W., BINFORD, C. H., UTZ, J. P., KWON-CHUNG, K. J., Otomycosis in Medical Mycology (1977), Lea & Febiger, Philadelphia p483-454.

4. YASSIN, A., MOSTAFA, M. A. and MOAWAD, M. K. (1964) Fungus infection of the Ear (Clinical and Cultural Studies), Journal of Laryngology 78, 591-602.

New dimensions in otorhinolaryngology – head and neck surgery, vol. 2.
E. Myers, editor

NONSPECIFIC NECROTIZING PETROSITIS IN CHILDREN

ALDO CASSOL STAMM AND JOSÉ ANTONIO PINTO
Research and Study Center of Ibirapuera Hospital,Sao Paulo-SP
Av. Ruben Berta 3350 -C4074,BRASIL

INTRODUCTION

We have described a disease,wich is an unusual form of chronic otitis media in very young children,that progressed silently to cause irreversible facial paralysis and deafness.We have called this rare form of the disease Nonspecific Necrotizing Petrositis[1].

Many etiologies may produce granulation tissue and bone destruction in the temporal bone,and some times a definitive diagnosis is impossible [1,2].

In our patients the pathological findings were nonspecific necrotizing osteitis.The culture shows the presence of gram-negative organisms such as:Pseudomonas aeruginosas,Proteus mirabilis and Klebsiella sp.

It's our purpose to present six children with Nonspecific Necrotizing Petrositis to call attention,for the facial paralysis and deafness in young children with chronic otitis media.

MATERIAL AND METHODS

Our six cases,were children with two and three years old.The clinical feature common to all cases was otorrhea,beginning at the first months of life,with silent evolution to a complete peripheral facial paralysis and deafness.In one case the disease was bilateral.

The physical examination was similar in all cases.A mucopurulent secretion and exuberant granulation tissue filled the external canal and middle ear.It contained sequestered osseous fragments of the otic capsule.

Radiology showed bony destruction of the lateral epitympanic wall, disappearance of the ossicles and severe destruction of the otic capsule,involving the facial nerve with areas of osseous sequestrum.

Therewas no hearing on the affected side.

Eletrical tests of the facial nerve function were inexcitable and the electromyography reveled fibrillation potentials.

The treatment applied was surgical(Subtotal Petrosectomy)[1].Findings were similar in all six cases.We removed bloody granulation tissue with osseous fragments,free and sequestered,that were pieces

pieces from the cochlea and semicircular canals(otic capsule).

The facial nerve was destroyed in almost its total lenght in the Fallopian canal,making treatment difficult.Although this disease was aggressive,the intradural structures remained intact.

The surgical cavity extended as far as the apex of the petrous pyramid and was bordered by the meninges of the middle and posterior fossae.We identified the proximal stumps of the facial nerve in only two cases.In these,we used a graft of the great auricular nerve.In the others we perfomed a hipoglossal-facial nerve anastomosis.In one a muscle transposition was indicated and the other one died due to fulminant meningites by Klebsiella sp.

Pathology report was an inflammatory process characterized by histiocytary proliferation,infiltration of lymphocytes and plasma cells.The facial nerve was degenerated and invaded by inflammatory tissue.The bone tissue was devitalized,looking like sequestered.

Table I shows the treatment and results of the six chlidren with Nonspecific Necrotizing Petrositis.

TABLE I
MANAGEMENT OF NONSPECIFIC NECROTIZING PETROSITIS IN CHILDREN

CASE	AGE YEARS	SIDE	TREATMENT	INFECTIOUS PROCESS	RECOVERY OF FACIAL PARALYSIS
1	2	R	STP-HFNA	HEALED	FAIR
2	3	R	STP-GRAFT	HEALED	GOOD
3	2	BIL.	BIL.STP	HEALED	POOR
4	3	R	STP-GRAFT	......	DEATH
5	2	L	STP-HFNA	HEALED	GOOD
6	2	R	STP HFNA	HEALED	FAIR

STP-Subtotal Petrosectomy,HFNA Hypoglossal-Facial Nerve Anastomosis

REFERENCES

1.Stamm,A.C.,Pinto.J.A.,Coser,P.L. and Marigo,C.:Nonspecific Necrotizing Petrositis:An unusual Complication of Otitis in Children. Laryngoscope.,94:1218-1222,1984.

2.Stamm,A.C.,Pinto,J.A. and De La Cruz,A.:Facial Nerve Paralysis Secondary to Chronic Petrositis in Children.In:M. Portmann. Proceedings of the Vth Internacional Symposium on the Facial Nerve-Bordeaux-France.Publisher Masson S.A.-Paris.Publication date June,1985.

New dimensions in otorhinolaryngolcgy - head and neck surgery, vol. 2.
E. Myers, editor

AUTORADIOGRAPHIC STUDIES OF MINERAL TRANSPORT FROM REGIONS OF BONE RESORPTION IN EXPERIMENTAL CHOLESTEATOMA

RICHARD A. CHOLE & STEVEN P. TINLING

Department of Otolaryngology, University of California, Davis, School of Medicine, 4301 X St., #208, Sacramento, California 95817 U.S.A.

INTRODUCTION

Contact between bone and aural cholesteatomas results in bone destruction. Anatomical studies have shown that this process is mediated by cellular elements in the subepithelial space. Although multinucleated osteoclasts are seen in human and experimental cholesteatomas,[1] some investigators have suggested that mononuclear cells may resorb bone directly or indirectly by release of enzymes.[2,3] Thompsen et al.[2] suggested that a mononuclear histiocyte may release lysosomal enzymes and cause a general release of mineral and collagen from adjacent bone. Abramson et al.[3] have concluded that both osteoclasts and macrophages resorb bone in active cholesteatomas. Chole,[1] however, found no anatomical support for non-osteoclastic bone resorption in an extensive study of human and gerbilline cholesteatomas. In this study, the mineral matrix of bone was prelabelled with radioisotopes and their fate traced autoradiographically. The underlying assumption for this experiment is that label released by non-specific enzymes will be equally dispersed throughout the periosteal space and in all cell types, whereas label released due to osteoclasts or histiocytes must first pass through these cells and thus they would exhibit higher grain densities.

MATERIAL AND METHODS

Young, growing gerbils were given ^{45}Ca or $^{3}[H]$ tetracycline (0.25mCi in divided doses) resulting in general bone labelling. Cholesteatomas were induced by surgical ligation of their external auditory canals.[4] After three months, the animals were killed and bones with attached cholesteatoma were fixed, dehydrated and embedded in Epon. Sections were coated with Kodak NTB-2 nuclear emulsion. After two months of exposure, slides were developed and counterstained. Photographs taken at 1000X were analyzed; bone, background and each cell type were studied by determining grain counts and profile areas on a Zeiss Videoplan. Grain densities were determined in each field and were expressed as a percentage of adjacent bone grain density. Grain densities were compared using the Student t-test for independent variables and the Kruskal-Wallace one-way analysis of variance.

RESULTS

For ^{45}Ca and $^{3}[H]$ tetracycline (TCN) grain density was highest over bone and background was acceptable. Grain density appeared to be highest over osteoclasts when compared to other cells (see Fig. 1). Grain density in mononuclear cells in the subepithelial space was low.

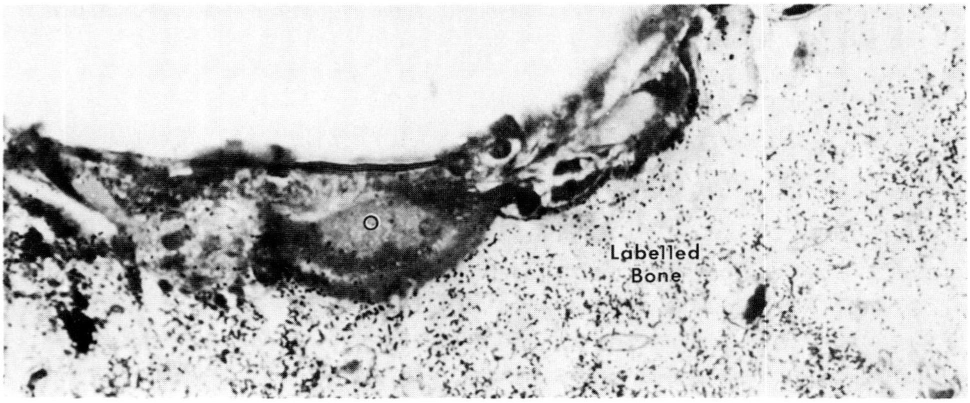

Fig. 1. A typical area of active bone erosion near a cholesteatoma. An osteoclast (O) is present with increased grain density (^{3}[H] tetracycline).

The grain density over osteoclasts was larger in both the ^{45}Ca and ^{3}[H] TCN preparations. The ^{3}[H] TCN preparation had a significantly higher grain density than other cells ($p < 0.01$) but the ^{45}Ca preparation showed no statistical difference due to higher scatter (see Fig. 2). Histiocytes had minimal labelling.

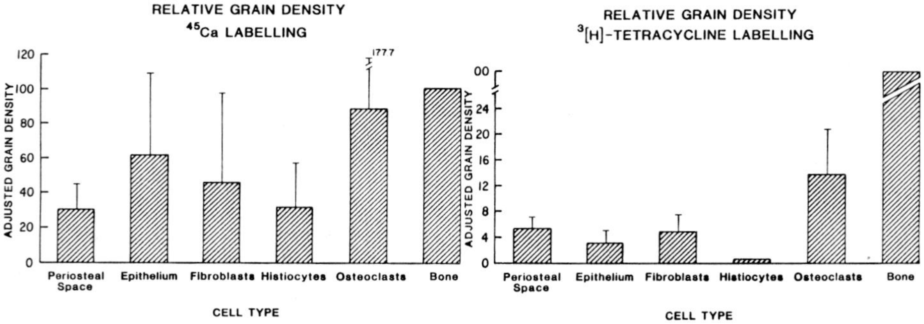

Fig. 2. A. A comparison of the grain density over each cell type ^{3}[H] TCN ($p < 0.01$). B. A comparison of the grain density over each cell type ^{45}Ca (p = ns).

CONCLUSIONS

This study supports prior anatomical studies in our laboratory, that the multinucleated osteoclast is primarily responsible for bone erosion in cholesteatoma. Histiocytes and mononuclear cells do not appear to play a direct role

REFERENCES

1. Chole RA (1984) Laryngoscope 94(1):76-95
2. Thompsen J et al. (1974) J Laryngol Otol 88:983-992
3. Abramson M, Mariyama H, Huang CC (1984) Acta Otolaryngol 97:437-442
4. McGinn MD, Chole RA, Henry KR (1982) Acta Otolaryngol 93:61-67

New dimensions in otorhinolaryngology - head and neck surgery, vol. 2.
E. Myers, editor

SENSORINEURAL HEARING LOSS IN CHRONIC OTITIS MEDIA PATIENTS TREATED TOPICALLY WITH EAR DROPS

M. FRADIS, J. BEN-DAVID, L. PODOSHIN, and B. BASHARA

Department of Otolaryngology, Haifa Medical Center (Rothschild), Faculty of Medicine, Technion, Haifa, Israel

INTRODUCTION

In 1941 Hulka (1) first reported a sensorineural hearing loss (S.N.H.L.) in patients suffering from acute otitis media (COM). The usual treatment in COM is the topical application of ear drops containing a combination of steroids, neomycin and polymixin B, the later two, known to be ototoxic when given systemly. For the first time in 1978, Smith and Myers (2) raised the question of ototoxicity of ear drops. Thus, we thought it would be of interest to investigate the connection between the ear drops and the S.N.H.L.

MATERIAL AND METHODS

150 patients suffering from COM, aged 6-65 years, were investigated and followed up for a period of 1 to 2 years. 124 were treated with ear drops containing Dexametasone (1 mg), Neomycine (5 mg) and Polymyxine B (10,000 U/ml). 26 patients treated by ear drops containing only steroids (1 mg Dexametasone) were our control group. These were excluded: 1) patients with sensorineural hearing loss due to other causes. 2) patients under 6 years of age or above 65 years of age.

RESULTS

The age distribution showed the greatest number being in the 10-19 age group (39.5% in the investigated group and 46.2% in the control group. The sex distribution of the patients was 54.7% males and 45.3% females. Regarding the type of perforation of the ear drum, outstanding are the central perforations, 41.1% in the investigated group and 61.5% in the control group. Regarding the distribution of the patients by the presence or absence of discharge was as follows: 61% in both groups of patients discharge was found, most of it being purulent. Considering the patients' complaints: there was no significant difference in both groups, except tinnitus (23.3% in the investigated patients as against 42.3% in the control group).

Considering the mean hearing theshold in all frequencies at the first and last visit, and the difference between them, the following was found: the mean difference in the sensorineural hearing theshold in the investigated group was 6.0 decibel as against -0.9 dB in the control group (P<0.025). Considering S.N.H.L. as related to the time of treatment in the follow-up period, we see that in patients that were continuously treated the mean S.N.H.L. was 10.9dB as against 3.6 dB in patients that were treated with short (3 months) inter-missions (P<0.005) and 1.8 dB in patients treated with long (6 monghs) inter-missions (P<0.001).

DISCUSSION

To-day there is no doubt that chronic otitis media causes a S.N.H.L. The question is: what is most responsible for this hearing loss - the ear drops or the disease itself. Out of 124 patients of the investigated group, 23 patients did not receive any treatment prior to their examination in our clinic, out of this number, 14 had unilateral COM during a mean period of 7.1 years. The mean hearing loss in the diseased ear was 17.8 dB as against 6.6 dB in the healthy ear (P<0.001). These facts demonstrate that the disease itself causes a S.N.H.L. The investigated 124 patients had a mean sensorineural hearing loss of 6 dB as against the control group treated by steroids alone after 1.5 years of follow-up. The difference is significant (P<0.025). This demonstrates the influence of the topical ototoxic treatment upon S.N.H.L.

If we consider these data in the investigated group during a mean of 1.5 years there was a 6 dB hearing loss, that means 4 dB a year. On the other hand, in patients who did not receive any treatment the difference between the hearing loss in the diseased ear and healthy ear was 11.2 dB (17.8 - 6.6). The mean duration of the disease in patients being 7.1 years, the mean yearly hearing loss is 1.5 dB. If we compare the former findings with these we see that the influence of the ear drops are significant and even surpass the damage done by the disease itself.

Our conclusion is: The treatment with ear drops containing neomycin and polymyxine B may cause the major part in the S.N.H.L. in chronic otitis media.

REFERENCES

1. Hulka JH (1941) Otolaryngol 33:333-350
2. Smith BM, Myers MG (1978) Paper read before the Research Forum of American Assoc of Otolaryngology and the Assoc for Research in Otolaryngology, Las Vegas

© 1985 Elsevier Science Publishers B V. (Biomedical Division)
New dimensions in otorhinolaryngology - head and neck surgery, vol. 2.
E. Myers, editor

RESULTS OF TREATMENT OF OTOSCLEROSIS WITH PLATINUM TEFLON PISTON AND PARTIAL STAPEDECTOMY

T. BRASK, M.D., Ph.D.

ENT-department, Odense University Hospital, DK-5000, Odense C, Denmark

Since Shea in 1958 introduced the stapedectomy operation for otosclerosis, this method has superseded the earlier methods. Today there are 3 main variations of stapedectomy:

1) Total stapedectomy with a prosthesis.
2) Partial stapedectomy with a prosthesis.
3) Partial stapedectomy with preservation of the posterior crus.

Until 1978 we only used total stapedectomy in my department. Though our results were satisfying compared with results from other departments, I decided to change to partial stapedectomy due to literature information and on account of theoretical considerations. The prosthesis we use now is a platinum teflon piston with a diameter of 0.6 mm (Richards). This prosthesis is used without covering the aperture in the footplate of the stapes with any sort of tissue.

The purpose of the present study was to compare the results of our partial stapedectomies with the results of our total stapedectomies and the results in the literature.

More than 400 patients have now been operated with the platinum teflon piston from Richards. To value the method basically the results of the first 100 consecutively primary operations will be given.

From an operative technical point of view the results can be expressed in a simple way by means of:

1) the postoperative air bone gap.
2) the change of the sensineural hearing loss in relation to the operation.

From the patients' point of view the results can be expressed by means of the gain of speech reception threshold (SRT).

All ear surgeons want to demonstrate their results as good as possible. They do it in different ways, so a comparison between different materials is nearly impossible. Some ear surgeons give their results as a successrate, while other ear surgeons mostly use figures calculated in different ways. It is thus usual to demonstrate the postoperative air bone gap as a mean of 500, 1000 and 2000 Hz.

Using the American Standard the postoperative air bone gap is calculated as the difference between the postoperative air conduction and the preoperative bone conduction.

We find, it is more reliable to calculate the postoperative air bone gap for each of the frequencies 500, 1000 and 2000 Hz separately and to compare with the postoperative bone conduction.

As the postoperative bone conduction improves in most cases - in our results in 87% - the postoperative mean air bone gap - when using the American Standard - will often be presented more favourable than when using the postoperative bone conduction.

It is unquestionable that the postoperative bone conduction represents the real cochlear function better than the preoperative as the cochlear mechanical system more or less has been reestablished by a technical successful operation for otosclerosis.

For further demonstration of this I have calculated the postoperative air bone gap using both the postoperative bone conduction and the preoperative bone conduction.

FIG I

RESULTS OF 100 CONSECUTIVELY PARTIAL STAPEDECTOMIES AIR-BONE GAP POSTOPERATIVE (REF. POST-OP. BC)

	500 Hz	1000 Hz	2000 Hz
MEAN	4.1 dB	3.5 dB	3.1 dB
SD	4.5 dB	4.2 dB	3.7 dB
RANGE	0→20 dB	0→20 dB	0→15 dB
≦10 dB	97%	98%	99%

FIG II

RESULTS OF 100 CONSECUTIVELY PARTIAL STAPEDECTOMIES AIR-BONE GAP POSTOPERATIVE (REF. PRE-OP. BC)

	500 Hz	1000 Hz	2000 Hz
MEAN	-1.5 dB	-3.1 dB	-4.2 dB
SD	9.9 dB	9.3 dB	9.5 dB
RANGE	-20→20 dB	-30→15 dB	-25→20 dB
≦ 0 dB	63%	72%	80%
≦10 dB	96%	96%	94%

The conclusion of the first 100 consecutively primary operations is that 100% improved concerning speech reception threshold, which is the most important result. By comparing the results of total stapedectomies with those of partial stapedectomies we found an improvement of about 4 dB concerning the SRT values and bone conductions. It was not possible to compare with the results of literature as they were calculated in different ways.

It would be very valuable if an international standard procedure concerning calculating the postoperative results could be determined. This will be the condition for a further progress.

New dimensions in otorhinolaryngology - head and neck surgery, vol. 2.
E. Myers, editor

J.Bernard CAUSSE TECHNIQUE FOR OTOSCLEROSIS SURGERY

J.B.CAUSSE,M.D. and J.R.CAUSSE, M.D.
Otology Clinic, 2 avenue Alphonse Mas, 34325 Béziers BP 4225 France

J.Bernard CAUSSE technique for otosclerosis surgery consists in performing a 0.8mm stapedotomy at the posterior third of the footplate, associated with a large veingraft interposition and a vigorous inflation of the middle ear. This technique allows the surgeon to benefit from the advantages of both the small fenestra technique without interposition (1) and of the stapedectomy with interposition (2). This procedure avoids the respective inconveniences of both techniques (that is to say the risk of fistula in case of small fenestra without interposition technique; the risk of enzymatic reactivation, and the risk of bleeding into the vestibule in case of total or anterior stapedectomy with veingraft interposition). The own advantage of this technique is to avoid the risk of rupture of the membranous labyrinth, as it locates the hole in the only area where the membranous labyrinth is not underneath the footplate (3,4). In 2% of the cases, a lack of resorption of the labyrinthine fluids induces an inflation of the saccule and utricule, which are then located very near the footplate. If the piston stands above the membranous labyrinth, in these 2% of cases where the saccule is very near the footplate, a tympanic membrane retraction may induce, by pressure of the piston onto the saccule, a change in the endolymphatic pressure, causing a rupture chiefly of the Reissner or of the basilar membrane. When such membrane is ruptured, it induces a shift in the cochlear microphonic potentials from 80 to 20 Mv, with an audiogram showing nearly no hearing left. The audiometric curve looks like a plateau-curve at the level of 70 or 80 dB. The pure tone and speech Weber test shifts towards the best ear. If the membrane does not heal, this apparently dead ear will remain. If the healing occurs, the hearing may return a very good one (Fig.1).

The combination of a large veingraft interposition and of a piston located in another area than above the membranous labyrinth, allows early and vigorous inflation of the middle ear. The inflation of the middle ear is very important as blood stagnating in the middle ear after the operation may induce adhesion tissues jamming the function of the long process of the incus. The long process of the incus has to be compared to a record-player-arm and the piston to the needle of the record-player. In contrast, in the small fenestra without interposition technique, early and vigorous inflation may induce a fistula or a dead ear by sudden pressure of the piston upon the saccule. The rupture of the membranous labyrinth is the major risk resulting in a severe cochlear drop in the postoperative follow-up of otospongiosis.

This technique has allowed J.Bernard CAUSSE to perform a series of 6,724 operations, in between the occurrence of two dead ears, at the rate of an average 1000 operations a year, and to obtain remarkable hearing improvement.

REFERENCES

1. Shea JJ (1963) The teflon-piston operation for otosclerosis. Laryngoscope 73:508-509
2. Causse JR (1965) Present problems in the surgery of otosclerosis. The J.of Laryng.Otol.79/4:265-299
3. Causse JB and Causse JR (1984) Technique for otosclerosis. The Amer.J. of Otology 5/5:392-394
4. Causse JB, Causse JR and Parahy Ch. (1985) Stapedotomy technique and results. The Amer.J.of Otology 6/1:68-71

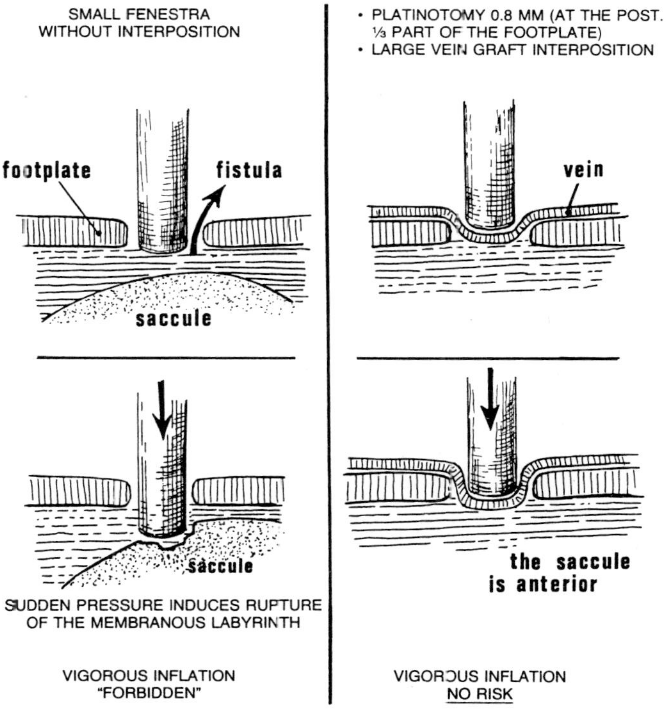

Figure 1. Sudden pressure on the membranous labyrinth.

New dimensions in otorhinolaryngology - head and neck surgery, vol. 2.
E. Myers, editor

CHANGES IN BONE CONDUCTION THRESHOLD DURING STAPEDECTOMY

V. COLLETTI - V.RICCI

Dept of Otolaringology, University of Verona, Italy.

INTRODUCTION

The present investigation deals with intraoperative bone conduction (B.C.) changes of patients undergoing surgery for otosclerosis and describes how the inner ear reacts to different surgical procedures on the footplate.

The implications of this study are twofold: (1) evaluation of the direct iatrogenic effect on the inner ear in regard to the technique utilized; and (2) indications for the procedures which minimizes damage to the inner ear function.

PATIENTS AND METHOD

Bone conduction changes in 8 otosclerotic patients undergoing stapedectomy under local anesthesia were evaluated by means Békésy audiometry.Frequency range 500 - 4000 Hz was studied ipsilateral to the ear being operated while the controlateral ear was masked. In each patients the B.C. threshold was determined after each of the following procedures: (1) elevation of the tympanomeatal flap; (2) perforation of the footplate; (3) stapedotomy (0,7-0,8 mm); (4) partial stapedectomy half anterior, half posterior; (5) total stapedectomy; (6) vein grafting (for procedure 4-5); (7) placement of the piston; (8) tympanomeatal flap in its original position.

RESULTS

Figure 1 (A,B) presents mean values of B.C. levels observed at surgery in the three conditions, total, partial stapedectomy and stapedotomy.

Significant threshold shifts are systematically recorded during surgery in the range 1 - 4 kHz, with 1.5 kHz being the most involved frequency. The degree of B.C. threshold shift is proportional to the area of the fenestrated footplate(A).

B.C. level recovers (B) when the area of the footplate is covered by the vein graft and the prosthesis is inserted. The recovery is observable only in partial stapedectomy and in stapedotomy.

The Table, adjacent to Fig. 1 (A,B), displays the statistical analysis on the data reported in the Fig.

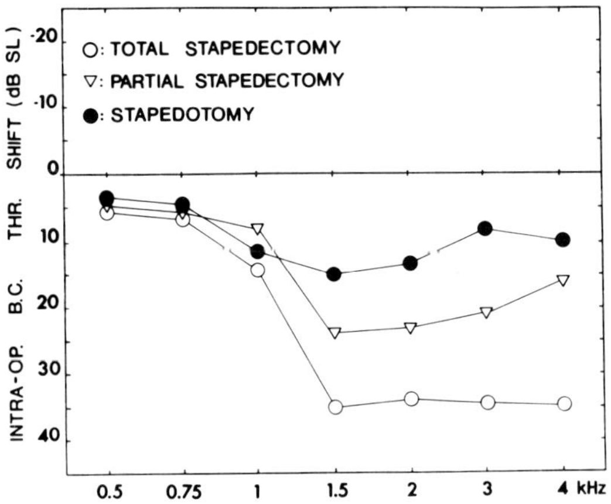

STATISTICAL ANALYSIS (Wilcoxon Test) OF DATA FROM FIGURE 1

	0.5	0.75	1	1.5	2	3	4 kHz
A	–	–	–	a,b,c	a,b,c	a,b,c	a,b,c
B	–	–	–	a,c,d	a,c,d	a,c,d	a,c,d
C	–	–	–	a,b,d	a,b,d	b,d	b,d

Legend
A, tot. stapedectomy; B, part. stapedectomy; C, stapedotomy.
Statistically significant difference ($P < 0.005$): a,b,c,d.
a, pre vs intra-op.; b, A vs C; c, A vs B; d, C vs B.

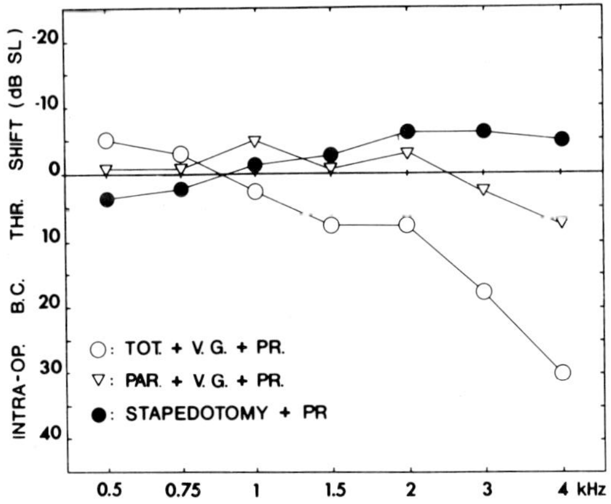

STATISTICAL ANALYSIS (Wilcoxon Test) OF DATA FROM FIGURE 2

	0.5	0.75	1	1.5	2	3	4 kHz
A	–	–	–	b	b,c	a,b,c	a,b,c
B	–	–	–	–	c	c	c,d
C	–	–	–	b	b	b	b,d

Legend
A, tot. stapedectomy, v. graft, prosthesis;
B, part. stapedectomy, v. graft, prosthesis;
C, stapedotomy, prosthesis.
Statisctically significant difference ($P < 0.005$):a, b, c,d.
a, pre vs intra-op.; b, A vs C; c, A vs B; d, B vs C.

DISCUSSION

The data of the present investigation show that (1) B.C. threshold undergoes systematic changes both in threshold and in difference limen of intensity during surgery: (2) these changes are observed mainly at mid-high frequencies and are strictly related to the surgical procedure on the footplate; (3) the degree of B.C. threshold shift is proportional to the area of the fenestrated footplate, being largest after total stapedectomy.

These observations can be interpreted in terms of B.C. physiology, recalling some of the numerous components involved in this complex mechanism: (1) the compressional B.C. component (2) inner ear fluid inertial component and (3) ossicular inertial component.

An alteration in the first two components is likely to occur for at least two reasons: 1) a decrease in perilynphatic pressure after opening the vestibule; 2) a leak or shunt with respect to the cochlear volume changes proportional to the area of the fenestrated footplate.

The prominent elevation in the B.C. responses at 1.5 kHz can be attributed to total missing of the ossicular inertial component resulting from surgery.

The significant differences observed in B.C. thresholds shifts as a function of the area of the fenestrated footplate indicate that for preservation or improvement of high frequencies stapedotomy is the technique of choice.

New dimensions in otorhinolaryngology - head and neck surgery, vol. 2.
E. Myers, editor

ALTERED BONE REMODELLING IN OTOSCLEROSIS

OTTÓ RIBÁRI and ISTVÁN SZIKLAI
Dept. of Otorhinolaryngology, Szeged University of Medical Sciences, H-6701 Szeged, Pf. 422, Hungary

INTRODUCTION

Perivascular bone remodelling occurs physiologically in the cochlea, as generally in any other bone. This takes place in an individual way: perivascular osteoblasts disappear from the primary osteons, while the matrix is disorganized. Simultaneously, changes can be seen in the opposite direction: during the matrix depolymerization, the first signs of repolymerization appear. In otosclerosis, however, the interstitial bony tissue has generally been replaced by spongiotic - hypervascularized - bone, more strictly related to the embryonal type than to the mature - secondary osteon-containing - bone. Cellular events in the otosclerotic bone have been exhaustively investigated morphologically, but the background molecular history is only currently undergoing clarification.

MATERIAL AND METHODS

Otosclerotic and normal bone samples were gained during stapedectomy operations on patients with a min. 3o dB air-bone gap. Cyclic-3',5'-adenosine monophosphate /cAMP/ and cyclic-3',5'-guanosine monophosphate /cGMP/ contents were determined with RIA KITs from Amersham /England/.

Otosclerotic stapes footplates and meatal temporal bone were cultured in Earle's MEM for 72 h /95% O_2-5% CO_2 atmosphere/. Organ cultures were pulse labelled with ^{3}H-proline /5 uCi/dish from 1o-2o Ci per mmol spec. act./. Proline incorporation into the collagenase digestible proteins /collagen/ was measured as described previously /1/. Collagenase-like peptidase activity secreted into the medium was assayed by the method of Kojima et al. /2/. Samples were treated with Ipriflavone, which was a kind gift of the Chinoin Pharm. Co., Hungary.

RESULTS AND DISCUSSION

cAMP and cGMP contents were measured as indicators of bone resorption, besides their signal processing function in the metabolism and endocrinological regulation. The otosclerotic stapes contains some 4o times more cAMP than the meatal bone, while the cGMP content is higher in the meatal bone /Table I/.

TABLE I

cGMP AND cAMP CONTENTS OF OTOSCLEROTIC AND NORMAL CORTICAL BONE

Sample	pmol cAMPxmg^{-1}bone $\bar{X} \pm$ SD	pmol cGMPxmg^{-1}bone $\bar{X} \pm$ SD
Stapes footplate	48 $\pm$ 32.8^{+}/n=7/$^{+}$	1.o4 $\pm$ o.184^{+}/n=11/
Stapes superstructure	27 $\pm$ 18.3^{+}/n=5/	o.52 $\pm$ o.195^{+}/n=7/
Meatal temporal bone	1.3 $\pm$ 1.31 /n=5/	2.63 $\pm$ 1.29o/n=5/

+P o.o1 relative to control ++P o.o5 relative to control

This means a high cellular activity, but does not explain whether collagen synthesis or collagenolysis is the primary event in otosclerosis. In our organ culture system, we have checked both these sides of the remodelling /Figs. 1-2/. The collagen biosynthesis is less extensive /not significantly/ in the otosclerotic stapes footplate than in the normal temporal bone, while Ipriflavone treatment /I_{1o} and I_{5o} = 1o and 5o umol, respectively, in Fig. 1/ elevated it much more strongly in the otosclerotic bone /Fig. 1, C: cortical bone; S: stapes footplate/. The C1-peptidase activity was slightly higher in the culture medium of the otosclerotic bone /Fig. 2, S: stapes/ than that of the cortical temporal bone /Fig. 2, C: cortical bone/. Ipriflavone increased these ac-

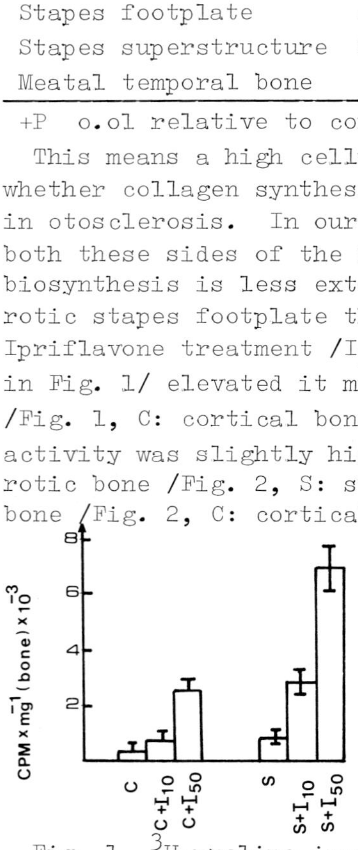

Fig. 1. ^{3}H-proline incorporation into the collagenase digestible proteins of the organ cultured bone.

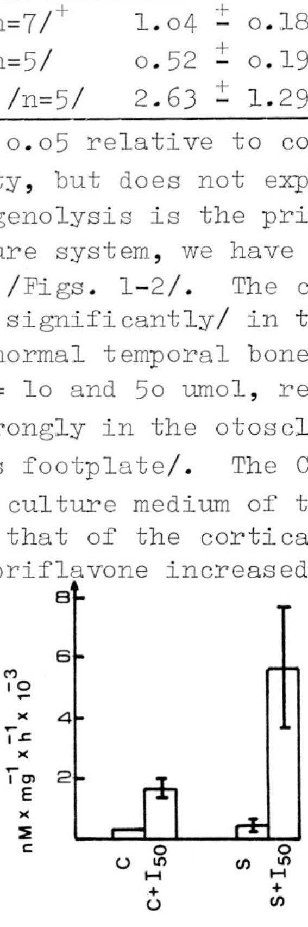

Fig. 2. C1-peptidase activity in the culture medium.

tivities. As bioflavonoids are cAMP-phosphodiesterase inhibitors, and both collagen synthesis and C1-peptidase activity are osteoblastic in origin, the primary effector in otosclerosis is the osteoblast.

REFERENCES

1. Peterkofsky, B., Diegelman, R. /1971/ Biochemistry, 1o:988-993
2. Kojima, K., Kinoshita, H. et al. /1979/Anal.Biochem., 1oo:43-5o

New dimensions in otorhinolaryngology - head and neck surgery, vol. 2.
E. Myers, editor

PARACUSIS WILLISII, TALE OR TRUE?

JOUKO SUONPÄÄ, EEVA PEKKARINEN AND ALTTI SALMIVALLI
Department of Otorhinolaryngology, University Hospital, SF-20520 Turku (Finland)

INTRODUCTION

Earlier studies by Aniansson (1) and Cohen & Keith (2) have shown the destroying effect of background noise on the word discrimination scores of subjects with sensorineural hearing impairment. On the contrary the patients with conductive hearing disorder, especially those with clinical otosclerosis, often voluntarily report their ability for better discrimination at high levels of background noise. This phenomenon - Paracusis Willisii - has little documentation in the literature.

The aim of present study was to examine the effect of increasing background noise on word discrimination in subjects with clinical otosclerosis and compare the results with a group of normal hearing subjects.

METHOD

A word list consisting of di- and trisyllables and developed for Finnish speech audiometry by T. Palva (3) was recorded by a man speaker in an anechoic room. The recordings were further treated by mixing pink noise and re-recorded through an artifical body (Kemar) in an anechoic room. Before recordings the speech level was calibrated to 60 dB SPL and 65 dB SPL respectively for free field and Kemar. The speech level was held constant and the noise level was changed in 5 dB steps. Three S/N levels were used: -13, -8 and -3 dB.

Twenty subjects with clinical otosclerosis all having bone conduction thresholds better than 30 dB were tested. The control group consisted of 20 subjects free from ear diseases. The mean age of the former group was 44 years and that of the control group was 49 years. The pure tone average (PTA) in the otosclerosis group was 47.8 dB and in the reference group it was 9.0 dB.

All audiological examinations were conducted in a soundtreater chamber. Word recognition testing was performed with speech at 30 dB above the patient´s SRT. The listeners were asked to repeat exactly the word they heard and the tester wrote the answer down.

RESULTS

The mean discrimination scores and standard deviations of the two groups are shown in table I. The discrimination scores were almost equal in quiet in both groups. When the S/N was -3 dB the mean scores decreased only 0.8 per cent in the otosclerosis group and 3 per cent in the reference group. At the higher noise levels the decrease of the discrimination scores was continuously slower in the subjects with otosclerosis. At the highest S/N level -13 dB the discrimination scores of the otosclerosis group (mean 60.2 %) were significantly (p = 0.0043) better than the scores of the reference group (47.5 %).

TABLE I
DISCRIMINATION SCORES (%) IN QUIET AND DIFFERENT S/N RATIOS

	QUIET		S/N -3 dB		S/N -8 dB		S/N -13 dB	
	MEAN	SD	MEAN	SD	MEAN	SD	MEAN	SD
Otosclerosis	97	3.7	96	3.3	84	8.2	60	15.2
Reference group	97	3.5	94	4.5	78	9.9	47	10.5

p = 0.0043

DISCUSSION

This study confirms the hypothesis that the subjects with conductive hearing loss seem to discriminate better than subjects with normal hearing at the presence of high noise. It may be assumed that a conductive hearing loss like otosclerosis, filtrates the annoying effects of the noise. The other reason for this phenomenon may be the fact that these people are used to listen very carefully because of their handicapness. However, the sensorineural hearing disorder increases the annoying effect of the noise (1). So the former hypothesis seems to be a more reliable explanation for this phenomenon. Whatever the reason of the paracusis Willisii may be, it seems to be a clinical entity.

SUMMARY

Discrimination scores of two groups, one consisting of 20 ears with clinical otosclerosis and the other reference group 20 normally hearing ears, were measured in an acoustical laboratory at varying levels of background noise (S/N -3, -8, and -13) and in quiet. By increasing noise levels the word discrimination scores of the otosclerosis group were better than the scores of the reference group. At the highest noise level tested (-13 dB) the otosclerosis group achieved significantly better scores (60 %) than the reference group (47 %).

REFERENCES

1. Aniansson G (1974) Acta Otolaryngol (Stockh) Suppl 320
2. Cohen RL, Keith RW (1976) J Speech Hear Res 19:48
3. Palva T (1955) Acta Otolaryngol (Stockh) 45:231

New dimensions in otorhinolaryngolcgy - head and neck surgery, vol. 2.
E. Myers, editor

OTOSCLEROSIS - ASSOCIATION WITH HLA BW 35

PROF DR. J.M. TATO, E.J. HAAS, E.H. RAIMONDI, L. VERRUNO

INTRODUCTION

There is a firm and solid relationship accepted internationally between HLA genotype and its tendency or resistance in acquiring different pathologies (1) (2).

In order to find an association HLA - pathology, we should take hold of population and family studies.

Family studies are applied to clearly hereditary diseases. In these groups it exists an obvious possible bond corroborated thrcugh formal analysis.

Population studies are or the contrary, done in patients with no family acquaintances.

Under these two parameters this piece of work was focused. It was done this way because of the strong family appotionment and based on the autcinmunity theory of otosclerosis pathogenesis (3) (4).

MATERIAL AND METHODS

Out of a 56 patient sample -at the moment studied-, 41 were unrelated and 15 belonged to 5 families.

We considered basal the frecuency which we published and had previously registered in the argentine population (5)

HLA antigens were determined by linfotoxicity techniques using PRICAI's RA battery: 120 seri capable of detecting specificities shown up to now.

Svejgaard's method for statistic analysis vas applied to results.

RESULTS

43,9% had HLA BW 35 antigen -from 41 unrelated patients-.

60,0% had HLA BW 35 antigen -from the 15 family related patients-, uot of which 93% were otosclerotic.

We particularly point out that 4 of the 5 families studied bore the antigen.

	Frequency of non otosclerotic	Frequency of otosclerotic	x^2
BW 35	21,3%	43,9%	4,4

DISCUSSION

The deviation found in otosclerotic patients referred to HLA BW 35, indicates there is an association between this pathology and the antigen.

It should be emphasized that the presence of HLA BW 35 in general unselected po pulation results in 2.7 relative risk of disease.

This means that a patient picked out at random and bearing the antigen, has 2.7 more chances of suffering otosclerosis than a patient who doesn't.

IN CONCLUSION

We wish to point out that of all patients up to now probed, there exists a tendency associating HLA BW 35 and Otosclerosis, even though we can't have for the moment definite conclusions.

BIBLIOGRAPHY

1. Rubinstein, Pablo, HLA - Disease Associations: In Search of Meaning. Theoretical aspects of HLA - The American Association of Blood Banks, 103/128 - 1982

2. Dausset J. Svejgaard, Mourant A.E. Dissease Association with polymorphisms other than HLA. In: A.eds and Disease. Copenhagen: Munksgaard, 1977: 12-9.

3. Yoo, T.J. et ALL. Type II Collagen - Induced Autoinmune otospongiosis. A preliminary report. Ann Otol Rhinol Larungol 92, 103-108 - 1983.

4. Yoo, T.J. Etiopathogenesis of otosclerosis: A hypothesis. Ann Otol Rhinol Laryngol 93. 28-33. 1984.

5. Haas, E y col. Frecuencia relativa de los antígenos HLA, de sus genes codificadores y de los haplotipos constituídos por ellos en la población general argentina. Premio Osvaldo Botaro. Academia Nacional de Medicina 1983.

© 1985 Elsevier Science Publishers B.V. (Biomedical Division)
New dimensions in otorhinolaryngology – head and neck surgery, vol. 2.
E. Myers, editor

INTEREST OF THE TOMOGRAPHIC STUDY OF THE VESTIBULAR AQUEDUCT

J.M. BERTRAN, M. TRUJILLO
Department of E.N.T. and Neuroradiology, Centro Ramón y Cajal, Madrid, Spain

INTRODUCTION

From the beginning of this radiological technique 17 years ago (1) multiple indications have been attributed to it. We were interested in knowing its usefulness at the present time.

MATERIAL AND METHODS

We have studied 49 patients with Menière's Disease.Since in 4 patients the process was bilateral, the study is based on 53 ears.

The fluctuating hearing loss was measured by Glycerol's Test.

We have used POSCHL's projection with tomographic cuts of 1 mm. of the whole labyrinthine block. In 20% of the cases we have used VALVASSORI and CHIESA's semiaxial projection with a 20° rotation starting from the strict lateral.

RESULTS

Visibility of the Vestibular Aqueduct (A.V.) according to GADO and ARENBERG's classification (2): Type I=5 (9.43%) Type II=14 (26.41%) and Type IV/V=34 (64.15%).

Periaqueductal and perilabyrinthine pneumatization according to STAHLE and WILBRAND's classification (3): Type 1=5 (9.43%), Type 2=11 (20.75%) and Type 3=37 (69.81%).

Glycerol's Test was not done in 13 cases because of side effects from the general point of view. In 21 ears it was positive and in 19 negative. The relation to the previous classifications was as shown in Table I.

From this series of 49 patients, 18 were treated surgically following the failure of medical treatment, using as a technique for conserving hearing, the Decompression (16) or Shunt (2) of the Endolymphatic Sac.

The evaluation of the results was done following the norms of the AAOO of 1972 (4) (Table II).

DISCUSSION

There exists a radiological picture in Menière's Disease:

1. Absence of visualization of the vestibular aqueduct (64%).
2. Absence of perilabyrinthine pneumatization (70%).

TABLE I

RELATION GLYCEROL TEST - VISIBILITY VESTIBULAR AQUEDUCT.

A.V.	Glycerol positive	Glycerol negative	Total
Type I	1 (4.76%)	4 (21.05%)	5
Type II	8 (38.09%)	3 (14.28%)	11
Type V	12 (57.14%)	12 (63.15%)	24

TABLE II

RELATION GLYCEROL TEST and A.V. - SURGERY ENDOLYMPHATIC SAC

	A + B	D
A.V. Type I/II	4	4
A.V. Type V	6	4
Glycerol positive	4	4
Glycerol negative	4	2

There is no relationship between Glycerol's Test and the tomographic study of the A.V.; it is not visible in 57% of the positive tests and in 63% of the negative ones.

A negative Glycerol Test or an A.V. not visible isn't a counterindication for the performance of surgery of the Endolymphatic Sac. In 50% and in 60% respectively of those operated successfully there appeared these conditions.

We think that the interest of this technique is double:

1. To locate the Endolymphatic Sac and supply some anatomic data of great surgical value.
2. Do away with any other pathology (Acoustic Neuroma).

REFERENCES

1. Clemis JD, Valvassori GE (1968). Otolaryngol.Clin.North Am. 1: 339-346.

2. Gado MH, Arenberg K (1975). Radiology 117: 621-626.

3. Stahle J, Wilbrand H (1974). Acta Otolaryngol. 78: 36-48.

4. Arenberg K, Brandenburg J, Sauer R, Kaemmerle A (1980). Otolaryngol. Clin. North Am. 13: 681-692.

New dimensions in otorhinolaryngology - head and neck surgery, vol. 2.
E. Myers, editor

MODIFICATION OF THE UVULOPALATOPLASTY OPERATION RESULTING IN DECREASED INCIDENCE OF VELOPHARYNGEAL INCOMPETENCE AND POSTOP RECURRENCE OF OBSTRUCTIVE SLEEP APNEA SYNDROME

HERBERT L. BAKER, M.D.

Chief of Otolaryngology, V.A. Medical Center, Portland, OR; Helmet Haas, M.D. Pulmonary Medicine, Sleep Laboratory, Oregon Health Sciences University, Portland, OR.

INTRODUCTION

A review of 50 modified Uvulopalatoplasty operations from May 1, 1982, through December, 1984, performed at the Portland V.A. Medical Center, the Oregon Health Sciences University, and Emanuel Hospital, are presented. All patients in this study had pre- and postop polysomnography. The objectives of this study are as followed:

#1. To define anatomic limitations of soft palate that is safe to remove without causing velopharyngeal insufficiency.

#2. A modification of the lateral pharyngeal wall closure technique to prevent further scarring.

Sleep apnea syndrome is characterized by an episodic obstruction with anatomic and functional alterations in the upper airway during sleep or oral pharyngeal collapse while supine. Fujita described the syndrome of obstructive sleep apnea where there is at least 10 seconds of cessation in air flow while there is normal respiratory effort and O_2 saturation fall below 85% during sleep[1].

MATERIAL AND METHODS

Two cadaver specimens were dissected by the Anatomy Department at the Oregon Health Sciences University's Dental School.

Figure 1 (on the following page) illustrates anatomical findings. Marked in red is the levator veli palatini muscle in the soft palate coronal head, as well as the connections of the palatopharyngeus and palatoglossus muscles posterior. In this figure, it is very obvious when retacting the uvula forward, there is a definite crease at the beginning of the veli palatini muscle, and if the soft palate uvula is resected to this point. Velopharyngeal insufficiency is almost completely prevented.

The second modification of the uvulopalatopharyngoplasty operation that is demonstrated on the cadaver (Figure #2) is the lateral pharyngeal wall closure technique to prevent future scarring of the soft palate. With other techniques, after trimming the redundant mucosa in the tonsil fossa, the mucosa sutured to the soft palate will cause scarring of the soft palate down to the posterior pharyngeal wall in 3-4 months. To prevent this complication, the author uses dissection of the mucosa off the tonsil fossa, trimming the redundant mucosa and the palatopharyngeus muscle, creating a deeper sulcus in the lateral pharyngeal wall. We use a two layer closure, first with two horizontal mattress sutures placed laterally in the tonsil fossa. Then second, the mucosa is closed without tension. This widens the lateral dimensions of the oral pharynx which increases the patients airway and enhances the nasopharyngeal opening with resection of the uvula.

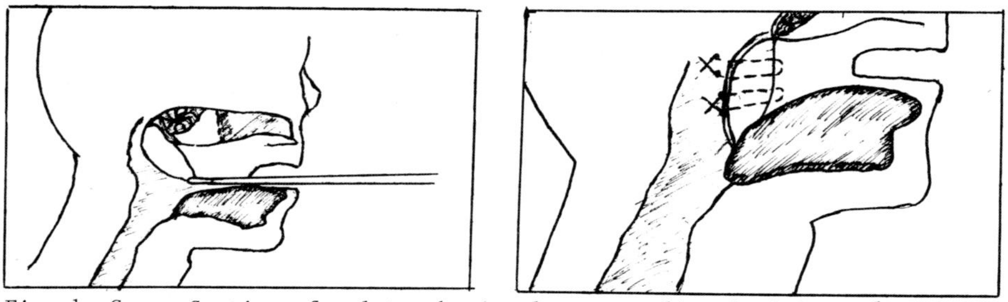

Fig. 1. Cross Section of palate showing levator veli palatini muscle.

In summary, this study illustrates that #1. A definite anatomical limit to removal of soft palate has been demonstrated through a cadaver dissection preserving the leviated veli palatini muscle. #2. A modification of the lateral pharyngeal wall closure technique has been described to allow for maximum tension to be in the tonsil fossa and not on the soft palate to prevent future scarring.

The one feared complication of velopharyngeal incompetent or voice change using the modified palatoplasty technique and with approximately 70% long term effectiveness improvement or cure of obstructive sleep apnea, as well as up to 95% cure or significant improvement of snoring was illustrated in this study. It is our feeling that the modified uvulopalatopharyngoplasty technique will improve the surgical success in treating obstructive sleep apnea when aligned with an active weight reduction and exercise program for these patients.

REFERENCES

1. Fujita, S., M.D., Conway, W., M.D., Zorick, F., M.D., Roth, T., PhD: Surgical Correction of Anatomic Abnormalities in Obstructive Sleep Apnea Syndrome: Uvulopalatopharyngoplasty. Otolaryngology Head & Neck Surgery 1981; 89:923-934.

2. Simmons, F.B., M.D., Guilleminault, C., M.D., Silvestri, R., M.D.: Snoring, and Some Obstructive Sleep Apnea Can Be Cured by Oropharyngeal Surgery. Archives of Otolaryngology, August 1983; 109:503-507.

New dimensions in otorhinolaryngology - head and neck surgery, vol. 2.
E. Myers, editor

VESTIBULAR NEURECTOMY FOR MENIERE'S DISEASE. MIDDLE FOSSA OR RETROLABYRINTHINE APPROACH?

JAVIER GAVILAN, CESAR GAVILAN, MANUEL D TOMAS
Department of Otolaryngology, La Paz Hospital, Universidad Autónoma, Madrid (Spain)

INTRODUCTION

Vestibular neurectomy is the most effective surgical treatment for Meniere's disease. Both the middle fossa (MF) approach and the retrolabyrinthine (RL) approach, are effective in relieving vertigo while preserving hearing.

PATIENTS AND METHODS

Between February 1968 and May 1973 we performed 139 middle fossa vestibular neurectomies for Meniere's disease. In 59 cases the minimum follow-up period was 10 years. There were 44 men and 15 women. Age range was 27 to 57 years, with a mean age of 43 years. Twenty-seven patients (45.8%) had surgery on the right side.

Auditory function and results were evaluated according to AAOO guidelines[1].

RESULTS

Six patients (10.2%) had a class A result; 29 patients (49.2%) had a class B result; 22 patients (37.3%) were class C, and 2 patients (3.3%) were class D results. Fifty-seven of 59 patients (96.6%) were relieved of vertigo. The two remaining patients developed Meniere's disease in the unoperated ear. A new MF vestibular neurectomy in this side definitively relieved vertigo in these patients[2]. Hearing improved or stabilized in 62.7% of the patients and tinnitus was relieved or improved in 52.5% of our patients.

Residual unsteadiness occurred postoperatively in 10 patients (16.9%). The MF vestibular neurectomy has proven a safe procedure. Transient facial paralysis appeared in 7.1% of the cases. Postoperative deafness occurred only in 3.4% of the cases. Other complications were seldom present.

DISCUSSION

The vertigo control rate in Meniere's disease for MF and RL neurectomy must be the same as in both procedures a surgical section of the vestibular nerve is achieved. Total vestibular neurectomy, no matter which surgical approach is used, must relieve vertigo in 100% of the patients with unilateral Meniere's disease. Hearing is similarly peserved in both types of neurectomy. We do not perform endolymphatic sac surgery because the results of such therapy are rather poor and may be due to the placebo effect[3].

It is when one examines the complications of the two approaches that the RL neurectomy emerges as an alternative to the MF neurectomy. The incidence of transient facial paralysis following MF neurectomy ranges from 3% to 7%,[4,5] while no facial paralysis is present with the RL technique[6,7]. Total hearing loss is present in 2.8%[8] to 9%[4] of MF neurectomies, while no complete hearing loss is reported with the RL approach. Finally, the RL neurectomy can be performed in patients of any age, while the MF approach has important disavantages in patients older than 60 years, in whom the dura is often especially adherent and fragile.

REFERENCES

1. Alford B (1972) Trans AAOO 76:1462
2. Gavilán J, Gavilán C (1984) Arch Otolaryngol 110:785
3. Thomsen J, Bretlau P, Tos M, Johnsen NJ (1981) Arch Otolaryngol 107:271
4. Glasscock ME, Kveton JF, Christiansen S (1984) Otolaryngol Head Neck Surg 92:67
5. Fisch U (1970) Adv Otorhinolaryngol 17:202
6. McElveen JT, House JW, Hitselberger WE, Brackman DE (1984) Otolaryngol Head Neck Surg 92:136
7. Silverstein H, Norrell H (1982) In: Brackmann DE (ed) Neurological Surgery of the Ear and Skull Base. Raven Press, New York, pp 303-315
8. Fisch U (1981) In: Shambaugh GE, Shea JJ (eds) Proceedings Sixth Shambaugh International Workshop on Otomicrosurgery. Strode Publs, Huntsville, pp 335-338

New dimensions in otorhinolaryngology - head and neck surgery, vol. 2.
E. Myers, editor

RETROLABYRINTHINE VESTIBULAR NEURECTOMY WITH SIMULTANEOUS MONITORING OF EIGHTH NERVE AND BRAIN STEM AUDITORY EVOKED POTENTIALS

HERBERT SILVERSTEIN, M.D., ALAN B. McDANIEL, M.D., JACK WAZEN, M.D.
HORACE NORRELL, M.D.

Ear Research Foundation, 1921 Floyd Street, Sarasota, FL 33579

INTRODUCTION

Vestibular neurectomy performed through the retrolabyrinthine approach (RVN) is an effective method to relieve inner ear vertigo while preserving hearing. It is easier, quicker, and safer than the middle fossa approach (MFVN), and results are better than the endolymphatic sac procedures. Since we introduced this procedure in October, 1978, sixty patients have undergone RVN. In 29 patients, intraoperative monitoring of direct eighth nerve potentials was performed and correlated with postoperative auditory function.

METHOD

The technique of RVN has been well described previously (1). Intraoperative monitoring of evoked potentials is performed using an ear mold and click generator placed in each ear. Brainstem responses (BAER) are recorded from skin electrodes. The cochlear promontory potential (ECoG NP) is recorded with a needle electrode placed through the facial recess and the eighth nerve action potential (8NP) is recorded using a teflon coated silver wire electrode placed on the cochlear nerve in the cerebellopontine angle (2). A Nicolet Pathfinder II computer is used to generate acoustic stimulus and record the evoked responses.

RESULTS

Of the 60 patients who underwent RVN, 55 had Meniere's Disease, three had vestibular neuronitis and two had traumatic labyrinthitis. Follow-up was from three months to six years. Vertigo was cured in 75% and markedly improved in 20%. Ninety-five percent of patients would recommend RVN for relief of vertigo.

No patient had a complete loss of hearing after surgery. Postoperatively, puretone average was maintained to within 20dB of the preoperative level in 83%, and the speech discrimination score maintained to within 20% in 80%. Pressure and fullness were improved in 18/33 (55%). Tinnitus was improved in 39% and worse in 22%. Unsteadiness was mild and occasional in 73%, a constant complaint in 22%, and did not occur in 5%.

Complications include wound infection (8), benign positional vertigo (7), CSF leak (6), and delayed, transient facial weakness (1). Five patients subsequently required transcochlear eighth nerve section for persistent vertigo (1) unsteadiness (2), and tinnitus (2), all having complete relief after eighth nerve section. No patient has required this procedure in the last 30 cases.

Intraoperative changes of 8NP latency of less than 0.3msec were associated with hearing to within 15dB of the preoperative levels. Waves I and II of the BAER apparently are generated from the cochlea and the cochlear nerve. An additional patient had total eighth nerve section for vertigo and tinnitus. The 8NP changed promptly with partial cochlear nerve section. The ECoG NP was unchanged for 25 minutes after total eighth nerve transection. Delays in display of BAER's due to averaging 1500 to 3000 clicks limits its' usefulness. The 8NP is the most rapid and sensitive technique for monitoring cochlear nerve trauma.

DISCUSSION

The results of curing or improving vertigo by RVN are equal to those from MFVN. Hearing preservation is statistically superior using the RVN (3). We hope that through the use of intraoperative monitoring of auditory evoked potentials the incidence of postoperative hearing loss will be reduced. We feel that intraoperative eighth nerve monitoring will become standard practice in the future.

REFERENCES

1. Silverstein H, Norrell H (1980) Retrolabyrinthine Surgery: A Direct Approach to the Cerebellopontine Angle. Otolaryngol Head Neck Surg, 88:462-469

2. Silverstein H, Wazen J, Norrell H, Hyman SM (1984) Retrolabyrinthine Vestibular Neurectomy with Simultaneous Monitoring of Eighth Nerve Action Potentials and Electrocochleography. Am J Otol, 5:552-555

3. De La Cruz A, McElveen JT (1984) Hearing Preservation in Vestibular Neurectomy. Laryngoscope, 94:874-877

© 1985 Elsevier Science Publishers B.V. (Biomedical Division)
New dimensions in otorhinolaryngology – head and neck surgery, vol. 2.
E. Myers, editor

RESULTS OF VESTIBULAR NERVE SECTION AND NEUROLYSIS OF THE EIGHTH CRANIAL NERVE IN MENIERE'S DISEASE

T.HAID; M.E.WIGAND and M.BERG
ENT Clinic at the University Erlangen-Nuremberg (Director:Prof.Dr.M.E. Wigand), Erlangen,FRG

INTRODUCTION

In order to eliminate the distressing attacks of vertigo,numerous patients must eventually be subjected to surgery after repeated conservative treatments have proved unsuccessful.Surgery can be based on various modalities: f.e.injection of streptomycin into the tympanic cavity (LANGE),ultrasound (ARSLAN),saccotomy (PORTMANN),shunt operation (HOUSE) and neurectomy of the vestibular nerve (HOUSE) on the affected side.We have performed with good success the section of the eighth cranial nerve as the method of choice. Moreover,we have increasingly resorted to a so-called neurolysis of the eighth cranial nerve in patients with Menière's disease (WIGAND et al.)

MATERIAL

In 70 patients affected with Menière's disease who had received conservative treatment without success,we carried out three different modes of surgery.In the first group,53 patients were subjected exclusively to neurectomy of the vestibular nerve since 1974.In the second group,11 patients had so-called neurolysis of the 8th cranial nerve since 1981 and in the third group both neurectomy of the 8th cranial nerve and neurolysis on the affected side have been carried out since 1984 on 6 patients.

METHOD

Neurectomy of the affected side consisted in dissecting both the inferior and superior vestibular nerve and vestibulo-facial anastomoses through the transtemporal route via a middle fossa approach.

In the case of the so-called neurolysis or neuro-vascular decompression after DANDY and JANETTA,the extended transtemporal access route through the middle fossa was chosen.This approach provides ample view of the fundus of the internal auditory meatus with the porus and cerebello-pontine angle.Frequently,remarkable compression-suspected contacts were found between greater arteries or veins with the 8th cranial nerve,either near the brain stem in the region of the porus acusticus internus or more laterally in the internal auditory meatus proper.Such contact points were cushioned with periosteal muscle plugs.Strangulations of the vascular-neural bundle were also seen to be caused by taut arachnoidal tissue with dislocation of the cochlear-vestibular nerve,which had to be eliminated.

RESULTS

In the first group,32 out of 53 Menière patients were no longer afflicted by vertigo after surgery.18 patients were found suffer from some vertigo attacks which,however,were distinctly reduced in frequency and intensity.Overall,in this group,surgery as a measure to eliminate vertigo had obtained an encouraging success rate of 94%.Evaluation in this group is based on long-term results of even 11 years standing.

In group 2,10 out of 11 subjects with Menière's disease experienced the intended surgical elimination of vertigo.5 patients were attacked again by fits of vertigo 1 to 2 years after neurolysis,but they were felt to be less severe than before operation.Gradual atrophy of the periosteal muscle cushions between vascular-neural bundles is seen as a likely cause of this. This prompted us 1 1/2 year ago to use silastic sponge wrapped with fascial tissue.

In the third group the success in vertigo suppression was as high as the first group.

In group 1,among 48 patients who still had a hearing ability before surgery,there were 5 (= 11%) whose tone threshold in the ear involved was found to have improved by 10dB and more.The audiometric curve,however,remained mostly unchanged.Hearing deteriorated by 10dB or more in 12 subjects.Among them the hearing loss was usually no higher than 20dB.In 3 cases,a loss of hearing was experienced in the ear operated on.These patients had a pre-operative hearing threshold of 60dB and lower.Some patients manifested fluctuating results in the audiometric control before and after surgery.It was interesting to note that in 16 Menière cases,whose hearing threshold invariably tended to impair before surgery,neurectomy managed to stop this process.Fortunately,a similar course was observed in the other two groups as well.

In slightly more than 50% of the patients making up the 2nd group,hearing remained unaffected by the operation.In 5 cases,the hearing curve was seen to deteriorate only slightly (not in excess of 20dB).

In the 3th group,the post-operative audiograms of 6 patients revealed results which were similar to those obtained in group 2.

Surgery was found to exercise a rather encouraging beneficial effect on tinnitus in group 1.The ringing in the ear either abated in intensity or disappeared altogether in the operated ear in more than 50%.As far as the other two groups are concerned,in one third of the subjects,operation influenced tinnitus positivily.

CONCLUSION

1. Neurectomy of the vestibular nerve or neurectomy combined with neurolysis,intended to stop the vertigo attacks and to restore the ability to work in patients affected with Menière's disease,has achieved a particulary high success rate.

2. The preliminary results obtained with neurolysis of the 8th cranial nerve indicate that,for some cochleo-vestibular disturbances including Menière's disease,a therapy is being developed.These pathologies have been assumed to be of cochlear or labyrinthine origin.

REFERENCES

1. ARSLAN,M.:Treatment of Menière's Syndrom by direct application of ultrasounds waves to the vestibular system,Proc.of V Congress of Oto-Rhino-Laryng.1955
2. DANDY,W.E.:Concerning the cause of trigeminal neuralgica,Ann.Surg.24,447 (1934)
3. HOUSE,W.F.:Surgical exposure of the internal auditory canal and its contents through the middle cranial fossa,Laryngoscope 71,1363 (1961)
4. JANETTA,P.J.:Neurovascular compression in cranial nerve and systemic disease,Ann.Surg.192,518 (1980)
5. LANGE,G.:Intratympanale Streptomycin-Therapie des M.Menière,Fortsch. Med. 14,609 (1971)
6. PORTMANN,M.:The saccus endolymphaticus and an operation for draining the some for the relief of vertigo,J.Laryng. 42,809 (1927)
7. WIGAND,M.E.;HAID,T.;BERG,M.;RETTINGER,G.:Otochirurgische Neurolyse des VIII.Hirnnerven bei progressiven cochleo-vestibulären Störungen,Arch. Oto-Rhino-Laryngol. 235,531 (1982)

New dimensions in otorhinolaryngology - head and neck surgery, vol. 2.
E. Myers, editor

PUPILLARY DYNAMICS IN PATIENTS WITH MENIERE'S DISEASE

HIROAKI INOUE, TAKUYA UEMURA AND KATSUYA MATSUNAGA

Dept. of Otolaryngology, Faculty of Medicine, Kyushu University, Fukuoka 812, Japan

This is the first report on a newly devised pupillograph, which can record the pupillary responses of both eyes simultaneously in the subject taking the supine position. Three cases with Meniere's disease in the attack and quasi-attack stages showed a similar abnormality of the pupillary light contraction on the affected side, compared with the unaffected side, which disappeared in the interval stage. These results are discussed with regard to the potential role as the cause of Meniere's disease.

TABLE

Maximum velocities of pupillary contraction obtained from three cases with Meniere's disease in the different stages.

	STAGE	AFFECTED SIDE		UNAFFECTED SIDE
CASE 1	ATTACK	6.69±0.63	$<$**	8.02±0.37
	QUASI-ATTACK	7.38±0.38	$<$**	8.56±0.92
	INTERVAL	8.02±0.52	=	7.81±0.56
CASE 2	ATTACK	7.62±0.35	$<$*	8.47±0.57
	INTERVAL	7.56±0.37	=	7.42±0.62
CASE 3	QUASI-ATTACK	6.35±0.24	$<$*	6.96±0.29
	INTERVAL	6.20±0.49	=	6.00±0.57

* $p<0.05$ ** $p<0.01$

REFERENCES

1. Uemura T, Itoh M, Kikuchi N (1980) Autonomic dysfunction on the affected side in Meniere's disease. Acta Otolaryngol 89:109-177.
2. Loewenfeld IE, Rosskothen HD (1974) Infrared pupil camera. A new method for mass screening and clinical use. Am J Ophthalmol 78:304-313.

Intratympanic treatment with Gentamicin for Menière's Disease

G. LANGE, Städtische HNO-Klinik Wuppertal

INTRODUCTION

We have been performing transtympanic therapy for Menière's disease with ototoxic antibiotics for 15 years on 85 patients. During 15 years of experience we developed many details, therapeutic procedures became easier an safer.

THERAPEUTIC PROCEDURE

Gentamicin (Refobacin R) is administered into the tympanic cavity via a normal ventilating tube as used for the treatment of mucoserotympanon. It is placed into the posterior part of the tympanon over the window region.In a routine case five times per day 0,3 ml Gentamicin (total 1,5 ml = 50 mg) are given into the external meatus of the diseased ear. The patient is lying flat on his back. His head must be turned halfway (45 ^{o}) to the contralateral healthy side. Using slight pressure in the external meatus (Politzer baloon) the liquid is transported into the middle ear, while the patient swallows. Gentamicin will accumulate in the niches of the windows and penetrate. Patients must keep their position for at least 0,5 h.

Our actual treating program: We begin at 7 a.m. with the first instillation. The same dose is given every 3 ^{hs} until 7 p. m. Therapy must be executed in hospital by physicians. The amount of Gentamicin given as well as intervals can be varied. Hearing is controlled daily, by audiometry. Before each instillment nystagmus reactions and vertigo are controlled. Therapy is successful as soon as the slightest inner ear reaction is observed, usually after 2 - 10 days.

INDICATIONS

The only disadvantage of this therapy is its possible influence on the hearing threshold. It should be used in unilateral cases suffering from frequent and severe attacks.

RESULTS

85 patients: 95 % in 15 years had no further attacks. Some of them had to be treated repeatedly. Attacks were much less severe in those few cases who could not be completely cured. Tinnitus is influenced in 35 %, periauricular pressure in 43 %. Hearing remained unblessed in 76 % of our cases. It sometimes even improved after attacks did not reoccur. Those who lost their hearing were frequently not even aware of this. Before a patient enters into therapy, he should know that is creates vertigo. This has nothing to do with Menière's attacks, but is caused by a reaction of inner ear to the ototoxic drug. Vertigo usually will disappear after some time. Only very few individuals - mostly elderly people - will suffer from it over a long period of time.

Prof. Dr. Gert Lange
Heusnerstraße 40
D 5600 Wuppertal 2

© 1985 Elsevier Science Publishers B.V. (Biomedical Division)
New dimensions in otorhinolaryngology - head and neck surgery, vol. 2.
E. Myers, editor

AN EPIDEMIOLOGICAL STUDY OF MENIERE'S DISEASE IN TOYAMA PREFECTURE

K.MIZUKOSHI, Y.WATANABE, N.OHASHI, H.KOBAYASHI AND H.SHOJAKU

Department of Otolaryngology, Toyama Medical & Pharmaceutical University, P.O.BOX 930-01, 2630 Sugitani, Toyama (Japan)

INTRODUCTION

In 1974, the Meniere's Disease Research Committee of Japan, which is supported by the Ministry of Health and Welfare, was founded with 17 members. In its first survey, 580 cases of definite Meniere's disease were collected by the members of the Committee during the period January 1973 to December 1974. Then between April 1975 and December 1976, the second nationwide survey was carried out by the same members(Mizukoshi et al. 1979. Watanabe et al. 1981).

In the present survey, 492 patients with Meniere's disease were diagnosed by 779 member clinics of the Toyama Medical Association in 1974, 1978 and 1982.

An epidemiological and clinical study of these patients was made in comparison with 120 patients with Meniere's disease in the Neurotological clinic of the University Hospital during 1979-1983.

MATERIAL AND METHOD

In order to collect as many of the same kind of Meniere's disease cases as possible, the Committee drafted the diagnostic criteria of the disease(Watanabe et al. 1981). In this survey the epidemiological data from the 492 patients was collected from the 779 members of the Association by using a data-processing sheet containing questionnaires, and was compared with the detailed epidemiological and clinical data of the 120 patients in the University Hospital series.

RESULTS AND COMMENTS

The characteristic epidemiological and clinical features of Meniere's disease in Toyama Prefecture were obtained from this prefecture survey as followed.

Individual Factors(Personal Factors)

Sex-ratio: In the Association survey of 492 patients, the male to female ratio was 107 males and 385 female. On the other hand, the sex-ratio of the

University series was 47 males and 73 females.

Age-Distribution: The age distribution peaked at 50-59 years for males and 60-69 years for females in the Association survey. In the University survey, the age distribution at onset peaked at 40-49 years for both males and females.

Family History: 9.2% of the 70 Meniere's patients giving family history, had a close relative who also suffered from the same disease.

Marriage: There was a higher incidence of Meniere's disease in married persons in accordance with the nationwide survey results.

Environmental Factors

Season and Time of Onset: there was a high frequency of initial vertigious attacks in the morning and in the afternoon in the University survey.

Geographical Distribution: There were more patients in the cities of east Toyama than in the rural area of west Toyama. The incidence of Meniere's disease in Toyama Prefecture was estimated as 174 per million population per year, which was a similar rate to the Japan wide one-day survey(160/1,000,000. Watababe et al. 1981).

Occupational Distribution: There was an apparently higher incidence of Meniere's disease among technicians or white-collor workers than among farmers, fishermen, laborers, and those engaged in blue-collor work.

In the University survey, the incidence of bilateral Meniere's disease was 9.2%(11/120), which was in accordance with the nationwide survey(48/520, 9.2%) (Mizukoshi et al. 1979).

From these epidemiological features in Toyama Prefecture, it was reconfirmed that the occurence of vertiginous attacks in Meniere's disease is influence a much more by individual factors than by environmental factors. However, the etiology of Meniere's disease has not yet been fully elucidated from the epidemiological point of view nor from the pathophysiologic standpoint.

REFERENCES

1. Mizukoshi K, Ino H, Ishikawa K, Watanabe Y, Yamazaki H, Kato I, Okubo J, Watanabe I(1979) Epidemiological survey of definite cases of Meniere's disease collected by the seventeen members of the Meniere's Disease Research Committee of Japan in 1975-1976. Adv. ORL 25:106-111.

2. Watanabe I, Mizukoshi K, Nakae K, Okubo J(1981) Epidemiologic studies of Meniere's disease in Japan. In: Vosteen K.H, et al.(eds) Meniere's Disease. Georg Thieme Verlag Thieme-Stratton Inc. Stuttgart, pp. 194-198.

New dimensions in otorhinolaryngology - head and neck surgery, vol. 2.
E. Myers, editor

GENTAMYCIN-TREATED MÉNIÈRE'S DISEASE EVALUATED BY ROTATORY TESTS

LARS ÖDKVIST, CLAES MÖLLER, JAN THELL, BIRGITTA LARSBY AND DAG HYDÉN
Department of Otolaryngology, University Hospital, S-581 85 Linköping(Sweden)

INTRODUCTION

Topical gentamycin treatment of patients with a disabling degree of Ménière's disease has been introduced as an alternative to vestibular neurectomy(Beck and Schmidt 1978). The present paper describes a group of patients treated with gentamycin and followed-up by rotatory tests.

MATERIAL AND METHODS

Twelve patiens suffering from unilateral Ménière's disease, having severe and frequent vertigo attacks, were treated with middle ear gentamycin installments. The mean age was 56 years (40-62). The ear to be treated had a hearing loss of 50-110 dB (mean 67 dB). Daily installments of gentamycin through the ear drum were given until first signs of destruction type of nystagmus appeared. Usually it took 4-7 installments(mean 5.5). In the follow-up was used history, clinical examination, electronystagmography, stabilometry and the broad frequency band rotatory test described by Larsby et al.(1982) and Hydén(1982). This test includes sinusoidal or pseudo-randomized oscillations in the frequency range 0.5-4.5 Hz in trials of each 40 sec. The instruction to the patient was either to fixate a stationary target on the wall or in darkness to imagine a stationary target in front of them. Eye movements were recorded by electrooculography and head movements with an angular rate sensor attached to a biteboard. Computer analyses were performed calculating the gain and phase of the eye movements.

RESULTS

An additional hearing loss in the treated ear appeared in half of the patients(Ödkvist et al. 1984). None of the patients had any vertigo attacks during the follow-up period 0.5-4 years after the treatment. Some slight unsteadiness was present in 4 of the patients. The stabilometry was normal in all cases(Tropp et al. 1985). The bithermal caloric test showed a loss of response in the treated ears. Ice water irrigation induced a few nystagmus beats in 3 patients. In the broad frequency rotatory test the patients showed some reduction in gain values during most test situations most prominent in the darkness pseudo-randomized test. In the stationary target test at the low frequency oscillations, gain was not significantly different in the treated group compared to normals. Asymmetrical responses as postulated by Ewald's second law was present in pseudo-randomized testing in darkness.

DISCUSSION

After a unilateral peripheral vestibular loss the patient after some time becomes free from symptoms thanks to the central compensation. The 12 patients with a gentamycin induced vestibular inner ear destruction followed the same pattern according to history, clinical investigation and stabilometry. The broad frequency rotatory test unveiled, however, some loss of VOR-gain and a slight asymmetry. According to sinusoidal testing in light the compensation was sufficient however. The overall results indicate that the gentamycin method could be used even in the age group up to 60.

REFERENCES

1. Beck C, Schmidt CL (1978) Ten years of experience with intratympanally applied Streptomycin(Gentamycin) in the therapy of morbus Ménière. Arch Oto-Rhino-Laryng 221:149-152
2. Hydén D (1982) Thesis. The broad frequency band rotatory test. A vestibular system study in man. Linköping University Medical Dissertations No. 152
3. Larsby B, Tomlinson RD, Schwarz DWF, Istl Y, Fredrickson JM (1982) Quantification of the vestibular ocular reflex and visual vestibular interaction for the purpose of clinical diagnosis. MBEC 20:99-117
4. Ödkvist LM, Bergholtz LM, Lundgren A (1984) Topical gentamycin treatment for disabling Ménière's disease. Acta Otolaryngol (Stockh) Suppl 412:74-76
5. Tropp H, Odenrick P, Ödkvist LM (1985) Stabilometry for study of postural control in patients with vertigo of central or peripheral origin. To be published.

ACKNOWLEDGEMENT

This study was supported by a grant from the Swedish Research Council Board.

New dimensions in otorhinolaryngology - head and neck surgery, vol. 2.
E. Myers, editor

HYPERINSULINISM ASSOCIATED WITH MIGRAINE AND MENIERE'S DISEASE

F. W. PULLEN, II, M.D. (1) RODOLFO LOW PH.D. (2) Dept. of Otolaryngology, Mercy Hospital, Miami, Florida, U.S.A., LARRY PEARCE, M.D., TODD TROOST, M.D. (3) Dept. of Neurology, BOWMAN-GRAY SCHOOL OF MEDICINE, Winston-Salem, North Carolina, U.S.A.

409 Mercy Professional Building, 3661 South Miami Avenue, Miami, Florida 33133

Recently, a relationship between high blood insulin levels and the symptoms of Meniere's and Migraine has been established. Dietary control has played a major role in the alleviation of symptoms of Migraine and, recently, Meniere's Disease.

From 1968 to 1977, Rodolfo Low, Ph.D., worked in Colombia, South America with Migraine patients and published several articles showing the behavior of refined sugar such as glucose on the production of insulin in the body.

It was theorized that large amounts of insulin started the counter regulatory catecholamines, e.g. epinephrine and norepinephrine, which in turn produce vasoconstriction and vasodilation of the cerebral arteries. The prostaglandins also played a role in this subsequent dilation of the blood vessels. He claimed that Migraine attacks could be prevented by a diet rich in unrefined carbohydrates, and not just a low carbohydrate diet as was previously thought. We studied 30 Migrainuers and corroborated this theory. Meniere's Disease can also be produced by this type of abnormal regulatory insulin mechanism, and we studied 15 patients with Meniere's, relieving symptoms in over two thirds.

Cerebral blood flow studies were also performed and have shown a relationship between hyperinsulinemia and the vasodilation and vasoconstriction which occurs immediately following a challenge glucose test in susceptible Migrainuers.

METHODS

A group of thirty patients were selected whose diagnosis of Migraine headache had been clearly established by either a neurologist or our center and all other causes of headaches had been carefully eliminated from the study. The second step was to perform a five hour glucose and insulin tolerance test at fasting and then at 15, 30, 60, 90, 120, 180, 240, and 300 minutes.

In addition to this group of thirty patients, a second group of fifteen patients was selected whose diagnosis of Meniere's Disease was also clearly established by fluctuating sensorineural hearing loss, tinnitus, and episodic vertigo. One patient with Migraine was tested for regional cerebral blood flow (rCBF) by the OMBST 133 Method. All patients were treated with a no refined sugar and no medication diet, but ample complex carbohydrates.

RESULTS

Thirty patients with Migraine, classic cluster and common type, have been treated in the past three years. Over 90% have been totally relieved. This program was also used at the Department of Neurology, Bowman-Gray School of Medicine, where 21 patients were studied with relief of cephalgia obtained in over 84% of Migrainuers.

Fifteen Meniere's patients were selected and subjected to the same insulin and glucose tolerance testing. Only one patient had normal insulin values. Eleven patients have done very well with stable hearing and no further vertigo. Three patients have had occasional relapses, but are able to relate them to being off the diet.

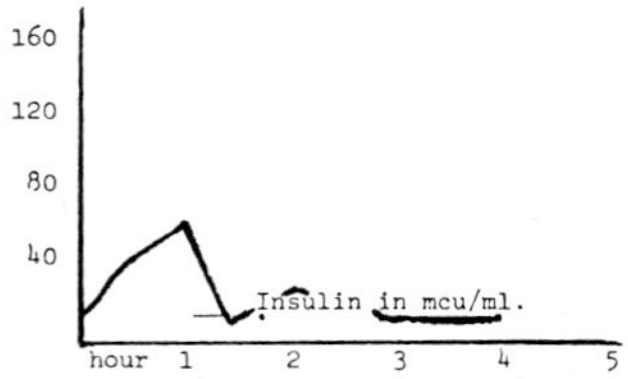

Figure 1. Average concentration of insulin in the blood plasma of 20 healthy individuals after the ingestion of 100 grams of glucose.

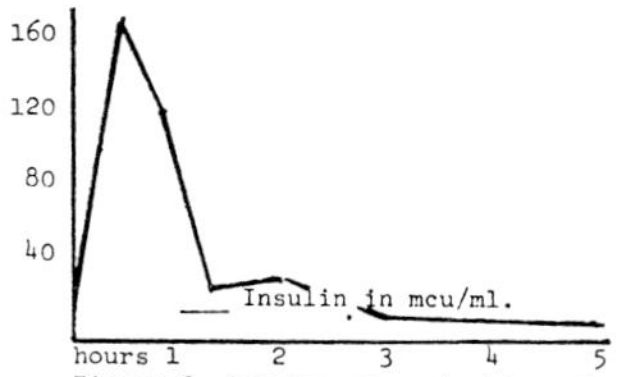

Figure 2. Average concentration of insulin in the blood plasma of eight migraine sufferers after the ingestion of 100 grams of glucose.

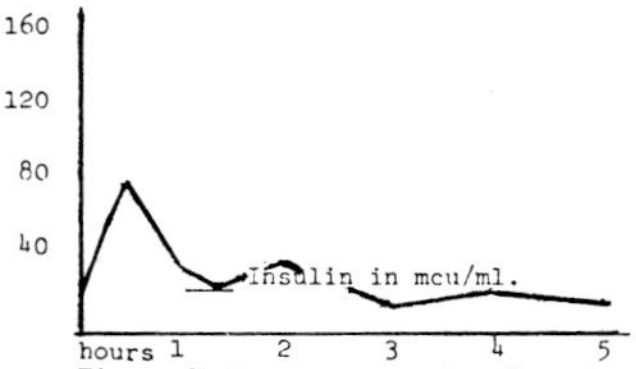

Figure 3. Average concentration of insulin in the blood plasma of eight migraine sufferers after ingesting a quantity of whole wheat bread equivalent to 100 grams of pure starch.

CONCLUSIONS

The result of our study has allowed us to postulate the following conclusions:

1. Hyperinsulinemia is the most frequent cause of Migraine and Meniere's Disease.
2. The diagnosis and treatment of Migraine and Meniere's Disease can be established on the basis of clinical history and metabolic testing including glucose tolerance testing.
3. Over 90% of patients with Migraine are relieved by a regimen high in complex carbohydrates and with no refined carbohydrates or simple sugars eaten.
4. Meniere's Disease has been shown in over 60% of the cases to be similar to Migraine with essentially the same etiology, and is controlled by dietary control. The younger Meniere's patients did better than the longer chronic cases.

REFERENCES

1. Albernaz, Mangabeira PL, Fukuda Y. Glucose, Insulin and Inner Ear Pathology, Acta Otolaryngol (Stockh) 97, 496-501.

2. Low, R. and M. Casas. (1977). Insulin response to different refined and unrefined carbohydrates. Tribuna Medica (Colombia), 652:30-32.

3. Spencer, J. (1981). Hyperlipoproteinemia, Hyperinsulinism, and Meniere's Disease, Southern Medical Journal, Vol 74, No. 10, 1194-1197.

4. Updegraff, W.R. (1979). Vertigo in diabetes patients. 60th Scientific Meeting Neurological Equilibriometric Soc, Turku.

New dimensions in otorhinolaryngology - head and neck surgery, vol. 2.
E. Myers, editor

THE USE OF HISTAMINE IN THE MANAGEMENT OF MENIERE'S DISEASE

J. SAID & AGUAYO
Departamento de Audiclogía, Servicio Otorrinolaringología, Hospital General, Centro Médico La Raza, IMSS

INTRODUCTION

In 1970 Siirala and Helgar[3] found a neurovascular disfunction related to stress. Histrochemistry[2] and electronic microscope studies by Morrison, confirmed the enzymatic regulation of the active transport of ions at the cell membrane of the endolymphatic epithelium. The Histamine[1], plays a very important role on the physiopathology of this disease because, it stimulates the H1 and H2 receptors of the blood vessels, producing vasodilation increase of permeability and reduction of the endolymphatic pressure.

MATERIAL AND METHODS

Twenty patients with Diagnosis of Meniere' Disease were selected, all of them had previously taken diurectic blockers of the laberintic system and sedatives without improvement. Four of them did not continue the study. The patient's ages varied between 12 and 56 years, the greatest incidence was found in the fourth and fifth decade of life. There was not a significant difference in sex. In all cases, complete clinical audiological and vestibular function study was made before treatment, confirming the diagnosis. The treatment was applied twice a week. We used Histamine Sulphate with three day intervales between each application. We started with a decim of mililiter and increased gradually the dosis based on the clinical response. The maximum dose used was one mililiter. The clinical response was determined by the presentation of papula of more then one centimeter of diameter, facial eritema and headache. We found a moderate reaction in just one patient. The audiologic study and vestibular function evaluations were made at 10 and 20 weeks after the beginning of the treatment.

RESULTS

Before treatment, 18.8% right ears and 12.5% left ears were classified as normal; after the treatment, the number of normal right ears increased to 43.8% and left ears to 50%. In hearing loss, the greatest change was found in the group classified as medium. The percent decreased from 50% to 25% in the right ears, and from 37% to 31.2% in the left ears. In the slight and severe groups of right ears, we did not find a difference before and after treatment. In the left ear groups, an important difference was found before and after our treatment. The treatment improved the phonemic captation in 84.6% of right ears and 85.7% of left ears. We evaluated the vestibular function, based on the Mayo Clinic Classification. The four variable that we studied were: time, intensity, frecuency and duration. 32 ears were evaluated and we found paresis in two cases (4 ears). We also studied our cases with the pendular vestibular stimulation test which confirmed our findings before and after treatment. Intense tinnítus was present in 100% of our cases, before treatment and disappeared in 31.2%, was slight in 37.5%, moderate in 18.8% and was unchanged in 12.5%. Before treatment, all patients presented vertigo, which disappeard completely in 43.8% and was notably reduced in 50%. It must be pointed out, that the vertigo was disabling in more than 65% of our patients. The results were studied by a Z Test and T Student Test and were found statistically significant.

CONCLUSIONS

The principal symptom in primary endolymphatic hydrops or Meniere's Disease is vertigo, but we must not forget the importance of the hearing loss and of the tinnítus. Most of the cases have bilateral involvement, but one ear can be affected. The ear loss damage can appear as normal in audiometric and laberinthic evaluations. So it must be stressed that a carefull evaluation in patients with "unilateral" afection must be made. The treatment with histamine controls 93.8% of vertigo cases, 68.2% of tinnítus, 90.6% in hearing loss, 85% in phonemic captation and 87.5% in vestibular function. The treatment with histamine is an alterantive to the surgical treatment of vertigo. Our results are encouring, but we need to increase our number of studied patients to get significant statistics.

REFERENCES

1. ROCHA AND SILVA M. (1978) HISTAMINE: Chemistry, Metabolism and Physiological and Pharmacological Actions. Handbuch der Experimentellen Pharmakologie. Vol. 18:1-19.
2. SCHYER R.W. (1962) Evidence that Induced Histamine is an Intrinsic Regulation of the Microcirculation System. Am J. Physiol. 202:66-72.
3. SIIRALA, U. AND GELHAR, K. (1970) Further Studies on the Relationship Between Meniere Psychosomatic Constitution and Stress. Acta Otolaringol. 70/2:142-147.

© 1985 Elsevier Science Publishers B.V. (Biomedical Division)
New dimensions in otorhinolaryngology - head and neck surgery, vol. 2.
E. Myers, editor

DISTENDED MEMBRANOUS LABYRYNTH IN CASES OF CONGENITAL ANOMALIES

HARUO SAITO, MUTSUHIRO FURUTA

Department of Otolaryngology, Kochi Medical School, Kochi, Department of Pathology, Kycto National Hospital, Kyoto (Japan)

INTRODUCTION

Histopathologic studies on temporal bones with idiopathic endolymphatic hydrops suggested that Meniere's disease would be congenitally defined entity[1].

Interest in the present paper has focused on the incidence of distended Reissner's membrane in the temporal bones acquired from patients with congenital anomalies.

MATERIALS & METHOD

Thirty six serially sectioned temporal bones acquired from various congenital anomaly syndromes were studies on distended Reissner's membrane. Nineteen normal temporal bones were served as controls.

TEMPORAL BONE HISTOPATHOLOGIC FINDINGS

Of 36 temporal bones studied, 16 demonstrated presence of distended Reissner's membrane. In the ears with distended Reissner's membrane, the vestibular aqueducts were small, short, straight, and had no funnel shaped dilatation. The epithelial lining of the rugous portion of the endolymphatic duct in those ears with distended Reissner's membrane was notably flattened and did not covered with cuboidal epithelia. Subepithelial fibrosis was not observed in those specimens.

In the temporal bones of control group, distension of Reissner's membrane was 3 out of 19 temporal bones.

DISCUSSION

In the present study, temporal bones acquired from patients with various forms of congenital anomalies were selected to investigate the possible relation between distended Reissner's membrane and congenital anomalies and the distension was more often observed among those ears, a significant level of 2.5 %.

Large area of the rugous portion of the endolymphatic duct was lined by flat cells. The finding was noted in the specimens from Meniere's disease[2-4]. The changes would be expected to impair absorptive function of the endolymphatic duct. Cases in this report may coincide with the asymptomatic and symptomatic forms of Schuknecht[5]. As there are sporadic cases which have no other severe anomalies in the other part of the body, there might be more cases of this categogy to be detected by closer observation on clinical cases of progressive sensorineural hearing loss in children.

REFERENCES

1. Sando I, Ikeda M (1984) Acta Otolaryngol 97:558
2. Shambaugh GEJr et al (1969) Arch Otolaryngol 89:38
3. Saito H et al (1977) Acta Otolaryngol 83:465
4. Schindler RA et al (1979) Laryngoscope 89:95
5. Schuknecht HF, Gulya AJ (1983) Ann Otol Rhinol Laryngol 92(Suppl 106):1

New dimensions in otorhinolaryngology – head and neck surgery, vol. 2.
E. Myers, editor

MEDICAL CARE AND TREATMENT FOR MENIERE'S DISEASE: METHOD TO EVALUATE THEIR EFFICACY

KOJI TOKUMASU, AKIRA SALTO AND SATOSHI YONEDA

Kitasato University, School of Medicine, Dept. of Otolaryngology, Sanamihara City (Japan)

INTRODUCTION

Our strategy for the treatment of Meniere's disease is to relieve patient's complaints of vertigo and cochlear signs. It is necessary to give a patient adequate advice to encourage him to do well in his daily life. The way to treat a patient and a statistical evaluation of its efficacy were presented in the cases of Kitasato University Hospital, Sagamihara City.

TREATMENT IN DIFFERENT STAGES AND FOLLOW-UP STUDY

In the acute stage, a patient feels vertigo, nausea, vomiting and strengthened tinnitus at rest. A bed rest in lateral lying position with the intact ear lowered and parenteral administration of vestibular depressants and antiemetics are necessary. In the following subacute stage, a patient is recommended to leave his bed as soon as possible since it may promote aquisition of the central compensation. In the chronic stage, endeavor for prophylaxis of recurrence of vertiginous attacks is most important. Daily cares and pharmaceutical therapies by diuretics, vasodilators and minor tranquilizera are applied. 427 cases with Meniere's disease had visited the Neurootological clinic of Kitasato University Hospital from 1971 to 1984. Number of patients, who had been free from the attacks and had left our clinic since 3,5 and 10 years ago was countered. The percentages of those cases may correspond to the rate of 3,5 and 10 % respectively (Fig 1).

STATISTICAL EVALUATION OF THE EFFICACY OF TREATMENT

The method of AAOO (1972) is too hard to be applied in cases treated pharmaceutically in order to evaluate the efficacy of the therapy. In our method, the difference between the mean interval times of attacks in the same long time course before and after the treatment was statistically evaluated. A sample aged 40 years with left Meniere's disease is shown in Fig. 2, whose vertiginous attacts had improved 2 years after the onset. ($P<0.05$)

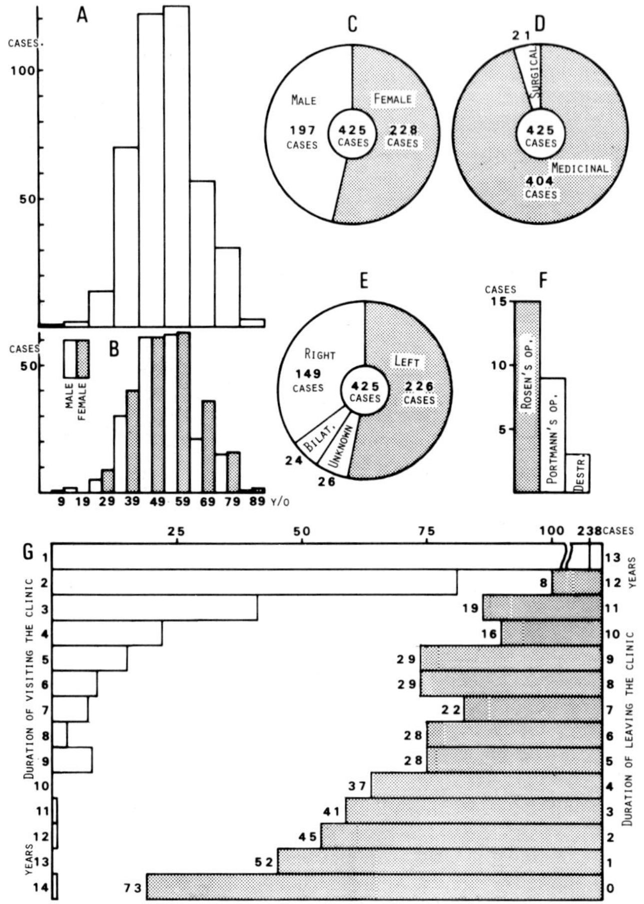

Figure 1. 427 cases with Meniere's disease in Kitasato University Hospital from 1971 to 1984

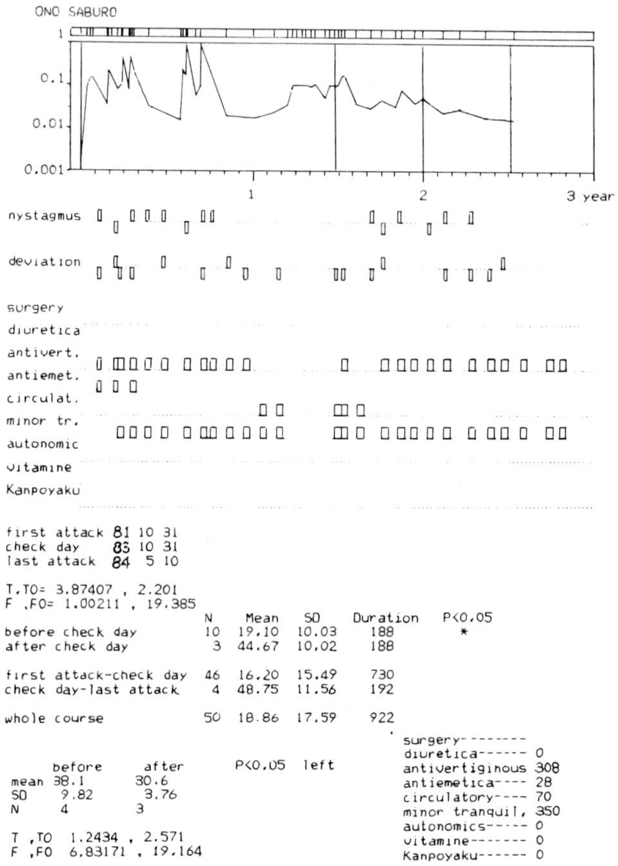

Figure 2. The time curve of the interval of two successive vertiginous attacks and its statistical evaluation. The top: the reciprocal of the internal in logarythmic scale.

© 1985 Elsevier Science Publishers B.V. (Biomedical Division)
New dimensions in otorhinolaryngclogy – head and neck surgery, vol. 2.
E. Myers, editor

PORTABLE CRANIO-CARPOGRAPHY - A NEW SCREENING METHOD FOR VERTIGO

DR.BHUTADA S.S.
Chairman & Head - Institute of Research in O.R.L. Pune 411002 INDIA

INTRODUCTION

Occupational Health in E.N.T. Speciality is a need of an Hour of our country which is making hurricane progress in all sectors of Industries. Industrial hazards in Otorhinolaryngology are not only causing Noise Induced Deafness - but many other E.N.T. diseases which are not been explored till recent days. In the survey of 10,000 workers in last 7 years from different factories, like Chemical, Textile, Agarbatti, Tobacco, Saw Mill, it has been observed that about 7% of the workers have the symptoms of Vertigo. We have fabricated a Portable Cranio-Carpography, an economic procedure which has solve this problem of screening the Industrial workers for vertigo. It is very useful method in conducting the Disease Detection Camps at the factory premises or at Public places in the programme of Community Health Services on Common Problem of O.R.L. & Occupational Health. This simple, easy procedure can be carried out in small Consulting E.N.T. Clinic in available small dark room in any factory premises.

PROCEDURE/TECHNIQUE

Cranio-Carpography (CCG) is an objective and quantitative test. In this test the head and body imbalance is recorded photographically in a very simpler and understandable procedure.

MATERIAL

I - Photographic Requirement : a) SLR - Camera with Wide Angle lens F/L 24 mm with aperture at 'B', b) Film - 100 ASA fast, Black and White, c) Cable Releaser - 50 ft. long.

II - Lighting System : Plate with 3 lights bulbs (red) are kept at distance of 10 cms from each other, one at Centre to present region Vertex other two for shoulder.

III - Sleep Mask : To close eyes visual stimulus is nullified.

IV - Equipment : Portable Tripod Stand with 4 meter height adjustable with a side bar 1 meter (long) for camera attachment.

V - Measuring Carpet : Measuring Carpet on which patient performs stepping test and it helps in measuring the ranges of Deviation and Angle of Rotation with distance walked.

C.C.G. & ITS TECHNIQUE :

A verticle, 3 meter height, tripod stand kept at centre line of measuring carpet with adjustable horizontal bar of about 1 meter long with camera at end, (with wide angle lens) facing to central line. Light System Fixed on head of patient with eyes closed by sleeping mask. Test is performed in Dark Room. Patient, on line, is asked to perform 80-100 steps on the spot in one minute. Head and Shoulder movements are caught in the Camera at 'B' aperture Controlled by cable releaser.

Length of walking distance (Normal range 38.98 cms) by patient alongwith its Angle of Deviation (Normal - Rt.side 70°-50°) & Angle of Rotation (Normal R-98°L-51.6°) at final position are measured and compared with photographic measurement except lateral sway is measured on positive film. (Normal range 17 to 20 cms).

DISCUSSION

Amongst 1100 patients from different factories and Disease Detection Camps, only 86 patients had complained of Vertigo. The analysis of investigated 70 cases is as follows : a) 37 cases showed peripheral vestibular lesion, b) 11 cases showed central lesion, c) 11 cases showed vertigo of origin other than above, d) 11 cases CCG was within normal limit.

Presenting nature of Vertigo in studied cases was varied from C/o rotation, blackout, sense of imbalance and light headedness. Symptoms such as headache, nausea, vomiting, impaired hearing, visual disorders, etc., directs us towards the causative factor and site of origin of vertigo.

Age : 44 cases were above the age of 40 and 26 cases were between 20 to 40 years. In respects that vertigo is more commonly seen in advanced age than in younger age.

Sex : Males had a predominance in our study because the data collected were from different factories where male workers were in majority. Thus, ratio does not carry any significant effect.

Occupation :

All the patient were from various industries. In many patients C/o Vertigo, no topodiagnosis is possible, hence, detail investigations were done to find out the exact site, nature and extent of lesion. Results of detail investigations are as follows :

(A) Craniocarpography, (B) Audiological Assessment,: i) Rinne Test, ii) Webers Test, iii) Pure Tone, iv) SISI, v) Tone Decay,

(C) Tympanometry : i) Compliance - Normal/Abnormal, ii) Pressure - Normal/-ve, iii) Stapecial reflex - Present/Absent, (D) Caloric Test : i) Normal, ii) Abnormal, iii) Not Done.

RESULTS

C.C.G.	No. of cases	Audiological Assessment (i)	(ii)	(iii) AC >< 20db	BC	(iv)	(v)	Tympanometry (i)	(ii)	(iii)	Caloric Test (i)	(ii)	(iii)
Peripheral:													
Cond. Deafness	18	+3 -1	Sa-15 Co-3	>15	3	-	-	Abn.	-ve	P-18	11	-	7
Cochlear lesion.	27	+22 -5	Sa-5 Op-20 Co-2	>25 <2	8 19	+12	-	N	-ve	P-13 A-9	4	Hypo 23	-
Central:													
VIII N. Lesion	3	+3	Op-3	>3	3	+3	+3	N	N	A-3	-	Hypo 3	-
Br.Stem. Lesion.	9	+9	Co-9	>9	9	-	-	N-6	N-6	P-5 A-4	6	Hypo 3	-
Temp.Lobe Lesion.	2	+2	Sa-2	>2	2	-	-	Abn	Abn	P-2	-	-	2
Other Origin.	11	+11	Co-11	>8 <3	2 9	-	-	N	N	-	11	-	-

CCG test is useful in differentiating the cases of peripheral from central lesion. 37 cases had peripheral and 11 had central lesion. In rest of the 22 cases CCG was not significant. The above diagnosis was based on Angle of Rotation & Angle of Deviation & Central Sway. Present study have similar results as with conventional methods.

CONCLUSION

(1) Portable C.C.G. is the only quickest method possible for mass screening programme in detecting lesion of vertibular apparatus, peripheral or central, (2) It helps in detecting latent cases of vertigo, (3) It is economical - saves cost & time, (4) Equipment is fabricated in India except Camera, (5) It's photographic picture is self explanatory about lesion of Neuro Vertibular tract and most informative as E.C.G. and E.E.G., (6) It's invention helps in taking 'Door Step' Health Services at remote (rural) places - An attempt to reach towards 'Health For All By 2000'.

New dimensions in otorhinolaryngology – head and neck surgery, vol. 2.
E. Myers, editor

NON-NEOPLASTIC SUPRAGLOTTIC LARYNGEAL STRICTURE OF ADULT ONSET

MICHAEL L. SCHWARTZ, M.D., HYUN T. CHO, M.D.

Department of Otolaryngology, Columbia Presbyterian Medical Center, New York City, New York

INTRODUCTION

Supraglottic stenosis is an uncommon condition. When present, it is usually caused by external trauma to the neck but also may be seen as a consequence of intubation injury or caustic substance ingestion.[1] Laryngeal stricture has also been seen as a result of certain granulomatous inflammatory disorders. Sarcoidosis has been most notable in causing pure supraglottic obstruction.[2, 3]

We wish to present four patients with progressive supraglottic stricture as a result of chronic nonspecific inflammatory disease. Despite extensive investigation including serologic and skin testing, baterial and fungal studies as well as multiple biopsies, no inciting etiologic agent or disorder could be identified. The patient profiles are presented in Table I.

Table I - PATIENT PROFILES

AGE	SEX	SYMPTOMS	SITE OF STRICTURE	BIOPSY	TREATMENT
38	M	EXERTIONAL DYSPNEA HOARSENESS	SUPRAGLOTTIC LARYNX	CHRONIC INFLAMMATION AND FIBROSIS	HEMISUPRAGLOTTIC LARYNGECTOMY
29	F	INTERMITTENT STRIDOR	SUPRAGLOTTIC LARYNX	CHRONIC INFLAMMATION	MEDICAL
54	M	PROGRESSIVE STRIDOR	SUPRAGLOTTIC LARYNX	CHRONIC INFLAMMATION AND FIBROSIS	HEMISUPRAGLOTTIC LARYNGECTOMY (ONE GRANULOMA FOUND IN SURGICAL SPECIMEN)
62	F	INTERMITTENT STRIDOR	SUPRAGLOTTIC LARYNX	CHRONIC INFLAMMATION AND FIBROSIS	HEMISUPRAGLOTTIC LARYNGECTOMY

Three patients have successfully undergone hemisupraglottic laryngectomy for relief of airway obstruction. The fourth patient has to date been able to be maintained on intermmittent steroid therapy. An etiologic diagnosis of sarcoidosis was given to one patient with a prior history of pulmonary disease in whom one non-caseating granuloma was found in the surgical specimen of his resected larynx.

DISCUSSION

Laryngeal stricture as a consequence of inflammatory disease has usually been associated with granulomatous disorders.[3] These have included infectious agents (such as tuberculosis, rhinoscleroma, fungal disease and syphilis), foreign body reaction (berylliosis), and autoimmune disorders (pemphigoid, Wegener's granulomatosis and sarcoidosis). The biopsy finding of nonspecific chronic inflammation in a patient with isolated supraglottic stenosis should prompt a thorough diagnostic evaluation for any of the abovementioned entities.[4]

We were only able to confirm a possible granulomatous etiology in one of our patients. We are suspicious that all may represent either the end stages of one of these disorders or a continued response to an unknown as yet inciting agent. This hypothesis of a nonspecific inflammatory response by the upper airway to a variety of agents to which some may be susceptible has been discussed in other reports.[5]

TREATMENT

Since the natural history of this disorder seems to be progressive over a period of years, some patients may benefit from steroids and anti-inflammatory agents early on. If the disease has progressed to fibrosis and scarring with stenosis and airway obstruction, treatment must be surgical.

Surgical treatment is designed according to the following principles: 1) the stricture is not caused by a malignant neoplastic lesion, 2) the chronic inflammatory process may continue after the surgery and restricture is possible, 3) the procedure must not interfere with the normal protective and phonatory mechanisms of the larynx.

Several authors have proposed techniques for supraglottic reconstruction.[6,7,8] We favor a technique of hemisupraglottic laryngectomy (Fig. 1) in which the epiglottis is split vertically and removed in continuity with the false cord and aryepiglottic fold of one side. The arytenoid is spared and the result is complete excision of the entire hemisupraglottis. This procedure was used on three of our patients with excellent results and minimal postoperative morbidity. Follow-up has been one, three and four years respectively.

In the setting of benign stricture of the supraglottis we feel this procedure is superior to either complete supraglottic laryngectomy or to simple epiglottectomy. The former is too radical a resection than is necessary and the latter predisposes to early recurrence of stricture.

A.

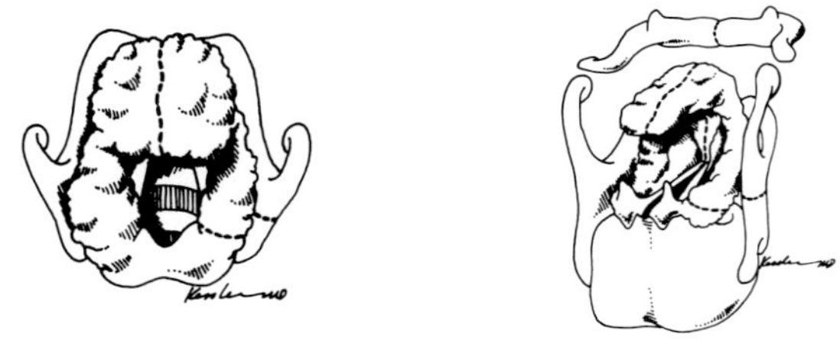

B.

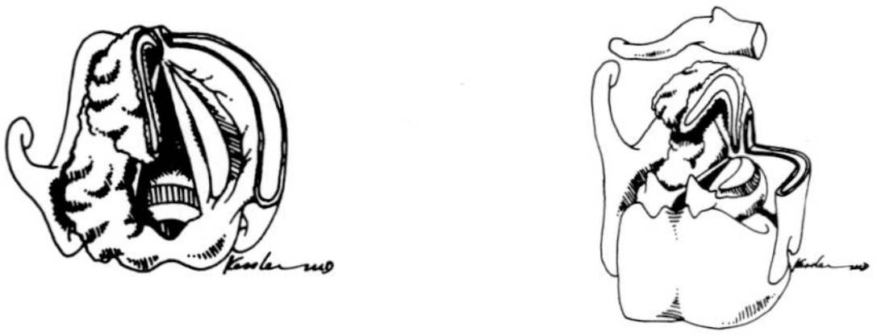

Fig. 1. Technique of hemisupraglottic laryngectomy. A. The surgical margins are outlined around the strictured supraglottis. B. Complete excision of the hemisupraglottis.

REFERENCES

1. Lucente FE, Biller HF (1979) Otol Clin N Amer 12:837-840
2. Neel HB, McDonald TJ (1982) Ann Otol Rhinol Laryngol 92:359-362
3. Haar JG, Chaudry AP, Kaplan HM and Milley PS (1980) Laryngoscope 90:1225-1229
4. Calcaterra TC (1972) Arch Otolaryngol 96:341-345
5. Maillard A, Goepfert H (1978) Arch Otolaryngol 104:197-201
6. Alonso WA (1985) In: Bailey B, Biller HF (eds) Surgery of the Larynx. WB Saunders, Philadelphia, pp 155-173
7. Ogura JH, Biller HF (1971) Ann Otol Rhinol Laryngol 80:492-510
8. Montgomery WW (1968) Ann Otol Rhinol Laryngol 77:534-547

New dimensions in otorhinolaryngology - head and neck surgery, vol. 2.
E. Myers, editor

LARYNGOTRACHEOPLASTY WITH LONG-TERM STENTING IN THE TREATMENT OF LARYNGOTRACHEAL STENOSIS

SHIANN YANN LEE

Department of Otolaryngology, National Taiwan Univ Hosp No. 1, Chang-Te Street, Taipei, Taiwan, ROC 100

INTRODUCTION

The treatment of laryngotracheal stenosis continues to challenge the otolaryngologist.

PATIENTS

This study comprises 72 patients with laryngotracheal stenosis treated by reconstructive surgery with long-term silicone T-tube stenting in the Department of Otolaryngology, National Taiwan University Hospital from 1977 to 1984.

METHODS

Laryngotracheoplasty with endo-laryngotracheal stenting

A tracheostomy was performed. Under general anesthesia, a vertical skin incision was made to expose the trachea and larynx. The trachea, cricoid and thyroid cartilages were split partly or wholly as in the procedure of laryngotracheal fissure. The cartilage incision should be kept along the anatomical midline.

All the thick, hard and stabilized intra- or extra-luminal scar tissue were fully preserved and undermined to form a pedicle-like flap which was rotated or shifted onto the cartilage-defected part or weak area of the anterior wall to cover the stent firmly.

The mucosa tenting sutures were done gently and meticulously on the entire cut edges at the intervals of 2-5 mm with 4-0 or 5-0 Dexon. The mucosal layer was laid firmly between the stent and extraluminal tissue layer. The mucosa tenting sutures were fixed to any extraluminal connective tissue layer. The author would rather call it *mucosal tenting suture* because this procedure was so unlike the classical lateropexy of the trachea.

Then the two separated points of the anterior commissure were approximated. An adequate silicone T-tube was applied. The caliber should be as wide as possible if only its lower arm could be inserted into the tracheal lumen. The endotracheal T-tube was sometimes used as an endolaryngeal stent for laryngotracheal stenosis. The T-tube might be indwelt supraglottically, glottically or subglottically.

Finally, the operative wound was closed with interrupted simple sutures of the skin, but no tissue layers between T-tube and skin were approximated. This step was special in this surgical technique because more space for the new airway could be obtained. The T-tube was usually removed after six months of stenting.

RESULTS

There was one patient who died of sepsis complicating the primary disease. In the remaining 71 patients, 64 were successfully decannulated, but 7 patients failed to be decannulated though they are now living well with good respiratory and phonatory functions carrying a T-tube. The success rate was 90.1%.

DISCUSSION

In choosing the method for the treatment of laryngotracheal stenosis, the principle should be aimed at restoration of the physiological function.

It seems that supraglottic placement of the stent might interfere with the movement of the vocal cords. Laryngostroboscopic findings, however, have revealed that despite supraglottic stenting, glottic closure and sphincteric function remain undisturbed.

A small piece of biopsy specimen taken from the reconstructed anterior wall at extubation, has shown microscopically squamous cell metaplasia on the healthy granulation tissue. The squamous cell layer is continuous with ciliated epithelium of the normal respiratory mucosa at the edge of the stenotic area. In a large defect area, re-epithelization by thick squamous cell metaplasia is found. There is a smooth mucosa surface over the stenotic region. It needs 6 months for stenting to establish such a stable and firm airway with sufficient patency.

CONCLUSION

With high success rate (90.1%), this new surgical technique of laryngotracheoplasty is performed as follows: 1. Exposure of the stenotic region by laryngofissure, cricoid splitting (anterior and/or posterior) and tracheal incision (vertical). 2. Debridement of infected soft tissue. 3. Relaxation or displacement of heavy scar tissue. 4. Tenting suture of the laryngotracheal mucosa remnants. 5. The caliber of the T-tube larger than tracheal size. 6. The operative wound closed only by full layer skin interrupted simple sutures (never approximation of the soft tissue layer). 7. Stenting for at least 6 months to ensure a patent lumen of the airway.

REFERENCES

1. Meyer R (1982): Reconstructive surgery of the trachea. Georg Thieme Verlag, Stuttgart, Thieme-Stratton, Inc., New York.
2. Montgomery WW (1980): Manual for care of the Montgomery silicone tracheal T-tube. Ann Otol Rhinol Laryngol Supp. 73, Vol. 89, No. 4, Part 5.
3. Schuller DE (1980): Long-term stenting for laryngotracheal stenosis. Ann Otol Rhinol Laryngol 89:515-519.
4. Lee SY (1978): Experimental study on laryngeal trauma. JOSROC* 13:31-34.
5. Lee SY (1983): Surgical reconstruction with long-term stenting in the treatment of chronic laryngotracheal stenosis. JOSROC* Supp. 1, Vol.18, No. 2.

* JOSROC: The Journal of Otolaryngological Society of the Republic of China.

© 1985 Elsevier Science Publishers B.V. (Biomedical Division)
New dimensions in otorhinolaryngolcgy - head and neck surgery, vol. 2.
E. Myers, editor

GLOTTOGRAPHIC MEASUREMENT OF THE EFFECTS OF LARYNGEAL PARALYSIS: A PRELIMINARY REPORT

ROM R. KARIN, M.D., DAVID G. HANSON, M.D., BRUCE R. GERRATT, PhD., PAUL H. WARD, M.D., STEVEN M.J. HUNT

Veterans Administration Medical Center and Division of Head and Neck Surgery, School of Medicine, University of California, Los Angeles, California, U.S.A.

INTRODUCTION

The dysphonias associated with unilateral vocal cord paralysis are well known. While the anatomic differences and the phonatory consequences of lesions involving the recurrent, superior, and vagus nerves have been well described (1,2), there are surprisingly few published reports of the physiological effects of these neurologic disorders. In an attempt to more clearly describe the pathophysiology of the laryngeal dysfunction in laryngeal paralysis, videolaryngoscopy and multichannel simultaneous glottography were employed.

MATERIALS AND METHODS

The subjects for this study included 12 adult males with well documented lesions causing unilateral vocal cord paralysis; four patients had recurrent laryngeal paralysis, four had vagal nerve paralysis, and four had superior laryngeal paralysis. Four age and sex matched subjects with normal voices served as controls (Table 1). The subjects were asked to sustain the vowel /i/ as long as possible at a normal conversational level of loudness and comfortable pitch. Videolaryngoscopy was performed with a laryngoscope coupled to a video camera. Photoglottography (PGG), as a measure of glottal area, was performed by passing a flexible fiberscope through the nose to a supraglottal position; the light passing through the glottis was measured using a phototransistor placed on the neck below the level of the glottis (3). Electroglottography (EGG), as a measure of vocal fold contact, was accomplished by measuring the impedence between two electrodes placed on either side of the thyroid alae (4). EGG aids in determining opening and closing points in the glottic cycle. All signals were digitized at 20 kHz and analyzed by computer. Fifty cycles were analyzed for each subject during the midportion of their sustained phonation. Speed quotient (SQ) values were calculated by dividing the duration of the opening phase by the duration of the closing phase.

	N	AGE RANGE	MEAN AGE
NORMAL	4	54-65	58
RECURRENT	4	47-67	59
VAGAL	4	51-62	58
SUPERIOR	4	36-68	55

Table 1. Number and age of subjects by diagnosis

RESULTS

The distribution of SQ values are presented in Table 2. The difference between the SQ of the normal group and each of the patient groups was tested using the Mann-Whitney U test. The mean SQ in both the recurrent paralysis group (0.57) and the vagal paralysis group (1.33) were significantly different from the normal group (0.92), and from each other ($p<0.005$). The mean SQ in the superior paralysis group (0.87) was not significantly different from normal. Figure 1 compares two representative glottic cycles obtained from a typical photoglottogram from patients with recurrent and vagal nerve paralysis and a normal subject, with their respective speed quotients.

	MEAN SPEED QUOTIENT	STANDARD DEVIATION	MANN-WHITNEY U TEST
NORMAL	0.92	0.13	
RECURRENT	0.57	0.13	$p < 0.005$
VAGAL	1.33	0.20	$p < 0.005$
SUPERIOR	0.87	0.27	$p > 0.05$

Table 2. Distribution of speed quotient values by subject group.

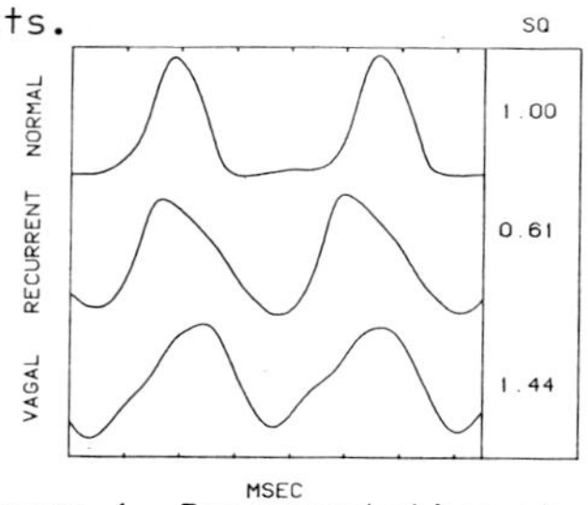

Figure 1. Representative photoglottograms of subject groups.

DISCUSSION

SQ appears to clearly differentiate recurrent from vagal vocal cord paralysis. In the photoglottograms of the recurrent paralysis patients the vocal cords open quickly and close relatively slowly. This would be expected with a flaccid vocal cord which opens easily with increasing subglottal pressure. In contrast, the waveforms of the vagal paralysis patients have a slow opening phase and a faster closing phase, suggesting a relatively stiffer vocal cord. The reasons for the increased SQ in patients with vagal paralysis are not yet fully understood. This difference implies a quite different pathophysiology of vocal cord vibration in these two types of laryngeal paralysis.

ACKNOWLEDGEMENTS

This work supported by NIH Grant NS20707.

REFERENCES

1. Ward PH, Berci G, Calcaterra TC (1977) Transactions of the American Academy of Ophthalmology and Otolaryngology 84:78-79

2. Aronson AE (1980) In: Clinical Voice Disorders, An Interdisciplinary Approach. Thieme-Stratton, Inc., New York, p. 84

3. Hanson DG, Gerratt BR, Ward PH (1983) Annals of Otology, Rhinology & Laryngology 92:413-420

4. Childers DG, Krishnamurthy AK (1985) A critical review of electroglottogrphy, in press

New dimensions in otorhinolaryngology – head and neck surgery, vol. 2.
E. Myers, editor

SILICONE INJECTION FOR THE UNILATERAL PARALYSIS OF THE VOCAL CORD

SATOSHI KITAHARA

Department of Otolaryngology, National Defense Medical College,
3-2 Namiki Tokorozawa Saitama (Japan)

INTRODUCTION

Silicone injection for vocal rehabilitation in case of unilateral recurrent laryngeal paralysis is a clinically useful therapeutic method because the manipulation of injection is not so difficult and it does not cause much pain for a patient.

It is necessary to obtain glottal closure as much as possible. In addition, it is better to obtain normal vibratory pattern even in the paralyzed vocal cord to restore normal voice. A factor of breathiness in hoarseness would be reduced by obtaining sufficient glottal closure. And a factor of roughness would be reduced by improvement of vocal vibratory pattern.

INJECTION UNDER DIRECT LARYNGOSCOPY

Generally speaking, silicone injection under direct laryngoscopy is precisely and easily performed. For anesthesia, local anesthesia using 4% xylocain is prefered. In case of difficulty to perform it under local anesthesia, neurolept-analgesia is applied because a patient can phonate.

Two types of silicone are used in our clinic. One is fluid type and the other is silastic type. Fluid type, set in a specially made cartrige beforehand, can not be vulcanized after injection. Even without vulcanization, it is effective for not so severe case. Silastic, phycon 6500, is vulcanized by use of catalyst after injection. Therefore this type of silicone is said more effective and recommendable to use for a severe case.

For injection, the laryngoscope is inserted deeply in order to push the false vocal cord laterally. An injection needle must be injected as laterally as possible on the surface of the vocal cord. The eye of the needle should be faced to the lateral. The depth of injection must be 3-4 mm. After injection the laryngoscope is pulled out a little to let a patient phonate. If the result is not satisfactory, an additional injection is performed. A vibratory pattern of the vocal cords is observed by use of a laryngostroboscope during an operation. This procedure is effective as an operation monitor. An excellent vibration of the paralyzed vocal cord is observed immediately after injection, post operative voice would be normally restored.

INJECTION UNDER INDIRECT LARYNGOSCOPY

When silicone injection under a direct laryngoscope can not be carried out, injection under an indirect laryngoscope is performed.

The indications of silicone injection under an indirect laryngoscope are as follows;

1. Inducing dyspnea by inserting direct laryngoscope
2. Heart lesion or it's postoperation
3. Aneurysm or it's postoperation
4. Hypertension

Fig. 1 shows the instrument of indirect injection. It's main structure was made similar to the Frenkel type laryngeal forceps. A guide was built in the center of the body. The needle has a stopper at 3-4 mm from the tip. An operator manuplates an indirect laryngoscope by the left hand, and a grip of the injector by the right hand. Therefore, a co-worker doctor has push the piston of the injector. The length of needles are 30 cm and 60 cm. Anesthesia is lacal.

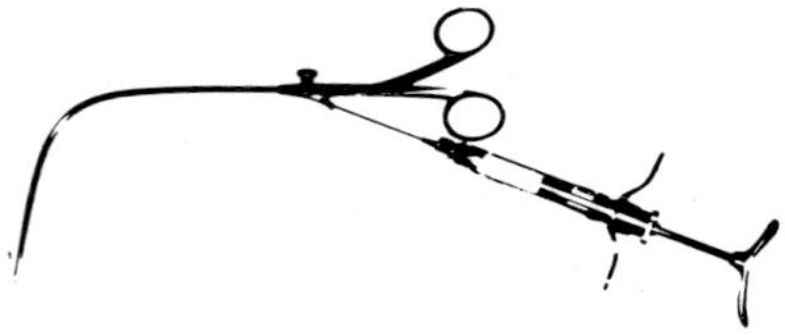

Fig.1. Injector under indirect laryngoscopy

CONCLUSION

Improvement of voice after injection is influenced by many factors. Among them, the condition of a paralyzed vocal cord before injection might influence on the post operative result. To obtain excellent result,

1. There is not remarkable atrophic change in the paralyzed vocal cord
2. There is not remarkable insufficient glottal closure
3. There is not remarkable difference between the levels of the both vocal cords

REFERENCE

1. KITAHARA S (1975) J Jap Bronchoesophagol 25:7-21

© 1985 Elsevier Science Publishers B.V. (Biomedical Division)
New dimensions in otorhinolaryngology - head and neck surgery, vol. 2.
E. Myers, editor

A NEW CLASSIFICATION OF UPPER AIRWAY STENOSIS

H LACCOURREYE MD, J LACAU ST GUILY MD, D BRASNU MD, F CHABOLLE MD, A. FABRE MD
Hopital Laennec, 42 rue de sèvres 75007 Paris, France.

Laryngotracheal stenoses are usually classified as either laryngeal (glottic, subglottic and supraglottic) stenosis or tracheal and laryngotracheal stenosis. These classifications correspond to the anatomical division of the upper airway but do not provide an accurate description of the stenosis.

A new classification is proposed, based on cartilages involved and laryngeal mobility. Anatomically, stenosis involves specifically the cricoid, the arytenoid cartilages and the tracheal rings. Cricoid and tracheal rings are fixed cartilages ; arytenoids are mobile. If the stenosis extends to the arytenoids, arytenoid mobility and consequently laryngeal mobility are impaired. That is why we subdivide laryngotracheal stenoses into two types according to laryngeal mobility. Table presents the new classification compared with the usual classification

NEW CLASSIFICATION	**USUAL CLASSIFICATION**	
	Normal laryngeal mobility	impaired laryngeal mobility
glottic stenosis	anterior glottic st	arytenoid st
glotto sub glottic st	-	cricoarytenoid st
subglottic stenosis	cricoid st	-
tracheal stenosis	tracheal st	-
laryngotracheal st	cricotracheal st	arytenocricotrach st arytenotracheal st

Laryngeal immobility occurs only when the stenosis involves arytenoid cartilage, whereas mobility is normal when the arytenoids are not involved. Glottic stenosis are defined as anterior glottic stenosis and classified as mobile. Arytenoid stenosis cannot be anatomically considered to be glottic stenosis.

The stenotic arytenoid lesions are periarthritis, ankylosis, luxation of the cricoarytenoid joint, interarytenoid fibrosis and synechia between the vocal processes. In case of isolated arytenoid stenosis, laryngoscopy and tomograms are usually normal. The most common cause of arytenoid involvement is intubation : post intubation laryngeal immobility may be caused by either paralysis of the recurrent nerve or arytenoid stenosis, but seems to be, in our experience, most often due to arytenoid stenosis. A medial thyrotomy is always necessary in post-intubation laryngeal immobility ; it provides a direct visualization of the arytenoid area.

The arytenoid involvement can be associated with cricoid, cricotracheal or tracheal lesions

We have used this classification to classify 200 cases of stenosis with respiratory impairement which were treated at Laennec Hospital from 1965 through 1984.

165 stenoses were easily classified. Most of them (143) were iatrogenic (post intubation and/or tracheotomy).

- In 110 patients, laryngeal mobility was normal. The distribution of the stenosis types was as following : cricoid stenosis N = 7, tracheal stenosis N = 73, cricotracheal stenosis N = 28, anterior glottic stenosis N = 2.
- Arytenoid cartilages were involved in 55 patients : in 22 patients the arytenoid involvement was isolated. In 33 patients, it was associated as following : cricoarytenoid stenosis N = 20, arytenocricotracheal stenosis N = 12, arytenotracheal stenosis N = 1

35 stenoses were less easily classified. 21 were secondary to external injury or ingestion of caustic substances. 30 had been previously operated. They have been described as "complex" stenoses because they were extensive and associated with multicartilagineous involvement (including thyroid cartilage or epiglottic lesion), recurrent nerve paralysis, vestibular (supraglottic) lesions, oesopharyngeal lesions. Nevertheless, even in these complex stenoses the importance of laryngeal mobility and cartilage lesions location must be emphasized.

This classification allows for more accurate description of the anatomical lesions and facilitates the choice of operative procedure.

REFERENCES

1. Laccourreye H, Beutter P, Bodard B, Bessède JP, Lacau st guily J, Pichancourt P (1980). Les sténoses laryngotracheales. Indications et résultats. A propos de 59 cas. Ann. Otolaryng.(Paris), 97 : 691-702

2. Laccourreye H, Brasnu D, Lacau st guily J, Chabolle F (1984). Classification des stenoses laryngotracheales de l'adulte. Ann. Otolaryng. (Paris), 101 : 31 - 34

3. Laccourreye H, Chabolle F, Brasnu D, Lacau st guily J (1984) Immobilités laryngées postintubation. Ann. Otolaryng (Paris) 101 : 253-259.

© 1985 Elsevier Science Publishers B.V. (Biomedical Division)
New dimensions in otorhinolaryngology - head and neck surgery, vol. 2.
E. Myers, editor

NON-STEROIDAL ANTI-INFLAMMATORY DRUGS IN OTITIS MEDIA WITH EFFUSION

S.J. ABRAMOVICH, J. O'GRADY, A. FULLER, R. LAVELLE AND M. MacKINNON
ENT Department and Department of Clinical Pharmacology,
St Bartholomew's Hospital, London, EC1

INTRODUCTION

A potential role for prostaglandins in the inflammation and bone resorbtion in otitis media with effusion has been suggested together with the possibility of benefit from treatment with non-steroidal anti-inflammatory (NSA) drugs.[1] Prostaglandins mediate hyperalgesia, oedema, erythema, bone resorbtion and NSA1 drugs act by inhibiting synthesis of prostaglandins.

PATIENTS AND METHODS

The levels of prostaglandin E_2 (PGE_2) were measured in therapeutic aspirates of the effusion fluid from 13 children suffering from secretory otitis media. The aspirate samples were diluted 1:1 with buffer and the concentration of PGE_2 determined by direct radioimmunoassay.[2] The lower limit of detection for the assay was PGE_2 1ng/ml. The effect of non-steroidal anti-inflammatory agent Naproxen 5mg/kg. twice daily for eight weeks on the condition were studied on 24 children in a placebo controlled double-blind trial.

The patient fulfilled following criteria: children aged 4-10 years, history of being hard of hearing and/or recurrent otalgia with otological signs of middle ear effusion, conductive hearing loss of 20 dBnHL or greater at three or more frequecnies (250, 500, 1000 and 2000Hz) on audiogram, low compliance and type B tympanogram (flat curve).

After eight weeks treatment the children were reassessed. Statistical analysis of otalgia and hearing loss was carried out on the change of scores using Mann-Witney U test, parametric tests were not appropriate to non-normally distributed data.

RESULTS

Nineteen middle ear aspirates from 13 children, 6 of whom had bilateral aspirations were examined. Detectable levels of PGE_2 (greater than 1.0ng per mil) were present in 7 aspirates from 7 children and ranged from PGE_2 1.0 to 14.4ng per ml. In 4 of the 6 patients who had bilateral aspirations, PGE_2 was detectable in the aspirate from one ear but not the other. However, the severity of otalgia and hearing loss was almost identical in the ears with detectable level of PGE_2 and those without. The lack of correlation between the levels of PGE_2 and the otalgia and hearing loss in these patients with bilateral effusions suggests that the accumulation of PGE_2 is a secondary phenomenon.

In a separate trial of Naproxen , 11 patients received active drug and 13 received placebo. Naproxen had no significant effect on otalgia or hearing loss compared to placebo. However, there was some tendency of resolution of otalgia in Naproxen group (6 out of 7) compared to placebo group (8 out of 11). The absence of any effect of Naproxen, compared to placebo provides evidence against an important role of prostaglandins in the disease process. These findings albeit relatively small numbers suggest that it is unlikely that non-steroidal anti-inflammatory drugs will be of considerable therapeutic benefit in secretory otitis media.

REFERENCES

1. Jung TTK, Smith DM, Juhn SK, Gerrard JM (1980)
Effect of prostaglandin on the composition of chinchilla middle ear effusion. Annals of Otology, Rhinology & Laryngology 89: suppl. 68 153-160.

2. Salmon J.A. (1978) A radio-immunoassay for 6 Keto PGF_1.
Prostaglandins 15/3: 387-97.

New dimensions in otorhinolaryngology - head and neck surgery, vol. 2.
E. Myers, editor

ELECTROCOCHLEOGRAPHY AND BRAIN STEM POTENTIALS IN HERPES ZOSTER (RAMSAY-HUNT SYNDROME)

S.J. ABRAMOVICH (1) and D.K. PRASHER (2)
(1) ENT Department, St. Bartholomew's Hospital, London, EC1
(2) Medical Research Council Neuro-Otology Unit, Institute of Neurology, National Hospital, Queen Square, London, WC1N 3BG

INTRODUCTION

Herpetic infection of the geniculate ganglion was the explanation given by Ramsay Hunt in 1907 for cases in which vesicular eruption is found in the external ear; spread of infection invariably leading to facial paralysis. The VIII nerve may also be involved resulting in hearing loss and vestibular disturbances. The histological studies of aural herpes zoster were limited to temporal bones and indicated that the Organ of Corti, the ganglia in the modiolus and the VII and VIII nerves can be affected (Friedman, 1974). Head and Campbell in 1900, however, reported some degeneration in the gasserian ganglion, the sensory root of the trigeminal nerve and through the pons.

In our study audiometric investigations and electrophysiological recordings of cochlear and brain stem potentials were done in order to elucidate further the type of hearing disorder in patients with accepted diagnosis of Ramsay Hunt syndrome.

PATIENTS AND METHODS

Thirteen patients with Ramsay Hunt syndrome (9 males and 4 females) were investigated. Their ages ranged from 21 to 73 years with the mean of 49 years. The diagnosis was supported by the detection of raised varicella virus antibodies. All patients presented with vesicular eruption; 8 patients had a complete facial palsy whilst the other 5 had a partial palsy; 11 patients had a unilateral hearing loss and 2 had normal hearing; 10 patients complained of tinnitus, one of whom had normal hearing; 11 patients complained of vertigo.

Auditory and vestibular function were assessed. Transtympanic electrocochleography (ECochG) was done and summating potential (SP) and action potential (AP) ratio SP/AP was assessed. Enhanced SP was suggestive of endolymphatic hydrops (Gibson, 1982). Brain stem auditory evoked potentials (BAEP) were recorded. The latencies and morphology of waves I, III and V was assessed which represent electrical activity generated in the cochlear nerve, pons and midbrain respectively.

RESULTS

The hearing loss was worse at high frequencies with a mean of 57 dB nHL at 4000 Hz. The loudness discomfort levels were measured in 10 patients and in all revealed a reduction in the dynamic range indicating the presence of loudness recruitment. Tone decay was measured in 6 patients, 4 of whom revealed a significant abnormal adaptation. The caloric test was done in 9 patients, all of whom had a canal paresis.

ECochG was done in five patients and showed a normal pattern of AP. The input/output curve indicated the presence of recruitment. The SP was not enhanced and the mean SP/AP ratio was of 21%. There was no indication of any secondary endolymphatic hydrops. BAEP were clearly abnormal in 7 out of 13 patients on the affected side. In another patient it was not possible to record any responses due to severe hearing loss. Wave I was within normal limits in all 7 patients, but latencies of wave III and V were prolonged and in one case deranged. One patient with abnormally delayed latencies of wave III and V had normal hearing.

From our results it is clear that there is no correlation between the hearing loss and abnormality of brain stem responses. Cochlear pathology invariably results in normal brain stem responses. There was a slight tendency for greater abnormalities of the BAEP in patients with complete facial paralysis. With the small number of patients tested, it was not possible to establish any significant difference in patients with normal and abnormal BAEP in terms of recovery or the effect of treatment with steroids. Abnormalities of BAEP detected in patients with aural herpes zoster may reflect brain stem involvement, however, it is not clear how a distorted input from the nerve to the brain stem may affect the subsequent component generators.

In conclusion, it is possible on the basis of the BAEP findings, to suggest that in Ramsay Hunt syndrome both cochlear and retrocochlear involvement may occur.

REFERENCES

1. HUNT JR (1907) Herpetic inflammations of the geniculate ganglion: A new syndrome and its complications. J. Nerve Ment. Dis. 34 : 73 - 96

2. FRIEDMAN I (1974) Herpes Zoster Oticus. In Pathology of the Ear. Blackwell Scientific Publications. Oxford. pp 442 - 448

3. HEAD H, CAMPBELL AW (1900) The Pathology of Herpes Zoster and its bearing on sensory localization. Brain 23 : 353 - 523

4. GIBSON WPR, PRASHER DK, KILKENNY G (1982) Diagnostic significance of transtympanic electrocochleography in Meniere's disease. Ann. Otol. 92 : 155 - 159

New dimensions in otorhinolaryngology – head and neck surgery, vol. 2.
E. Myers, editor

ANATOMICAL FACTORS THAT AFFECT THE CONGENITAL CHOLESTEATOMA OF A FETUS TEMPORAL BONE

KENJI AIMI, M.D.

Otolaryngology-Head and Neck Surgery University of Illinois

College of Medicine, Chicago IL.

Introduction

Congenital cholesteatomas occur commonly in the middle ear, but also appear in the petrous pyramid and the diploic portion of the skull. Because of their appearance in those diverse locations, source of the ectodermal tissue is considered nonspecific and the cause of migration is generally viewed as random developmental anomaly.

In 1983 I have published a theory regarding the congenital middle ear cholesteatoma embryogenesis. (1) This theory was based on my embryological observations concerning the tympanic membrane formation. Through this study it was postulated that the growth of the meatal plate ectoderm which failed to be contained at the annular plane, may produce overgrowth into the mesenchyme of the vicinity of the tympanic annulus. This migrated ectodermal nest will be the source of congenital cholesteatomas.

Initially this theory was applied only to the middle ear cholesteatomas, but by subsequent observations it was concluded that the same theory is applicable to the petrous as well as diploic cholesteatomas.

Wide anatomical separation of those cholesteatomas from the tympanic annulus to the petrous pyramid or a diploic portion of the skull are well explained when the developmental position shift of the migrated epidermoid is taken into account.

Considering the position of the tympanic ring relative to the petrous bone, in the early stage of tympanic membrane formation, the meatal plate arrived at the annular plane can place migrated epidermoid into the petro-occipital mesenchyme.

A migrated epidermoid in the mesenchyme, as shown in the illustration, next to the tympanic ring of a fetus of this age, may belong either to the posterolateral fontanel or to the petro-occipital suture. (Fig. 1) Growth of the mastoid and the petrous pyramid is expected to shift the epidermoid into two separate directions.

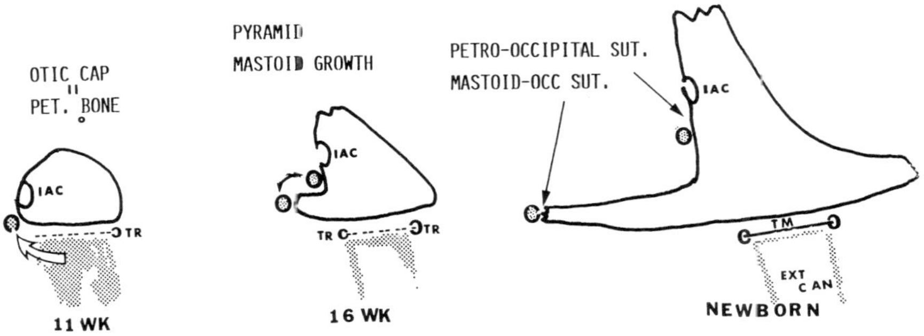

From those observations I have speculated that meatal plate ectodermal migration can be the source the diploic as well as the petrous cholesteatomas.

Summary

The meatal plate overgrowth and sequestration by the tympanic ring during the tympanic membrane formation was proposed as an embryogenesis of a congenital cholesteatoma. When the developmental posisiton shift is taken into account, petrous pyramid cholesteatomas as well a diploic cholesteatomas can be explained in the same manner as the middle ear cholesteatomas.

References

1. Aimi K. (1983) Role of the tympanic ring in the pathogenesis of congenital cholesteatoma. Laryngoscope 93: 1140-1145.

New dimensions in otorhinolaryngology – head and neck surgery, vol. 2.
E. Myers, editor

PSYCHOLOGICAL ASPECTS OF LABYRINTHINE PATIENTS

ANA MARIA BACCARI KUHN

Assistent Professor of Escola Paulista de Medicina, Rua Botucatu nº 834 - 04023 - Sao Paulo - Brazil

INTRODUCTION

The role of emotional factors in patients with vertigo has been widely debated. Because of this, several studies have attempted to establisch the extent to which emotional factors are envolved in those patients.

The presente work is a study of a psychological analisis in forty patients with peripheral vestibular syndromes. For that,we used the psychological interview to evaluate the symptomatology and etiological factors; and also the Color Pyramid Test (CPT) to evaluate the personality in both its manifest and latent levels.

MATERIAL AND METHOD

The present study took place at the Otoneurology Sector of the Otorhinolaryngologic Clinic of Escola Paulista de Medicina.

The material consisted of forty patients whose ages ranged from 25 to 76 years and who were submitted to otoneurological evaluation and psychological tests.

The otoneurological evaluation was performed according to Mangabeira Albernaz et alii (1983).

The psychological evaluation was composed by psychological interview and the Color Pyramid Test, according to Schaie & Heiss (1964).

RESULTS

By using the psychological interview and the C.P.T. this study has been divided in three groups: a) predominantly psychogenic; b) predominantly organic and c)both psychogenic and organic.

1) As to group of patients with predominantly psychogenic factor, we could find out Achromatic syndrome lowered at manifest level (70%) and wide range choise (75%) at manifest level and at latent (70%);showing an insufficiency of defensive mechanism and an intense receptivity related to affective emotional stimulation.

As to the formal aspect to the pyramid type-C-carpet estructure was noted at both levels manifest (53.3%) and latent (76.7%).

2) As to the group of patients with predominantly organic factor we were able to find a significantly Achromatic syndromes lowered at manifest level (100%),concurrently a Wide flexible chromatic formula was observed at latent level (57.1%),

and wide range choise increased at manifest level (71.4%) and (85.7%) at latent level.

Such results shown us a pseudonormality condition which was characterized by the ability of selecting the emotional affective stimulii. However the inner rebound upon those stimulii has shown the inability of demonstrating their instinctive emotional needs. As to the formal aspect to the pyramid,type-C-carpet structure was noted at both levels manifest (47.8%) and latent (85.7%),and also we could noted type-L-Layer structure (47.8%) at manifest level,pointing out psychologic resources of defensive and stereotyped nature.

3) As to the group of patients with predominantly psychogenic and organic factors,we could find out a significantly Achromatic syndrome lowered (100%) at manifest level and (53.8%) at latent level.

Concurrently a Wide chromatic constant formula, predominance was noted only at manifest level (53.8%),while a Wide range choice was noted a both levels (69.2%).

Such results showed an intense receptivity related to affective emotional stimulation,together with constriction attempts concerning the psychological field.

Type-C-Carpet structure predominance was noted at both levels (76.9%) manifest and (71.8%) at latent levels.

CONCLUSION

By the psychological interview and the Color Pyramid Test, we can arrive to the following conclusions: a) the emotional imaturity was the common predominant aspect; b) the predominantly psychogenic factor was greater than the predominantly organic ones.

REFERENCES

1. Mangabeira Albernaz,PL; Ganança,MM; Caovilla,HH; Ito,YI; Castro,HD Atlas de Vectoeletronistagmografia. Aché, São Paulo, 1984.
2. Schaie,KW & Heiss,R Color and personality, Has Huber, Berna, 1964.

New dimensions in otorhinolaryngology – head and neck surgery, vol. 2.
E. Myers, editor

AUTOGRAFT AND HOMOGRAFT TORP AND PORP IN THE RESTORATION OF THE MIDDLE EAR *

In a period of 7 years we have tried to restore the transmission system of the middle ear, combining autograft and homograft with TORP and PORP. A few years before, I had negated any kind of synthetical material for the restoration of the transmission system of the ear. Influenced by the enormous success of some famous ear surgeons, we have tried the use of TORP and PORP made of poroplast, plastipore and organic glass- ceramics to reconstruct the secure connection between the tympanic membrane or graft to the inner fluids. However, we were confronted with the same problems as in using only autograft and homograft. We are convinced that once we had a middle ear condition in which only partial destruction has taken place:

1) dry middle ear
2) functioning tube
3) pathologically no changed mucosa of the tympanic cavity
4) partially intact tympanic membrane and ossicular chain
5) surgeons are experienced and skillful,

the restoration of the middle ear can be reached very easily with auto- and homograft, or also with synthetic material.

However, if those factors are not satisfactorially present, we have a middle ear condition in which the the total tympanic membrane and ossicular chain up to the footplate are absent and also in conditions of spontaneous radical operations or conditions after radical operation, the restoration of the middle ear conductive system is extremely difficult, particularly when a big surgical cavity is existing and the medial wall of the tympanic cavity is covered with thick fibrous and granulation tissue forming the surrounding of the widows and the tympanic ostium of the tube.
Here we are also faced with important problems:

1) the restoration of the posterior canal wall and removal of the big surgical cavity,
2) rebuilding of a new tympanic membrane and and physiologically normal cavity,
3) free windows and tympanic ostium of the tube.

I would like to present a table from which the functional results at 66 patients , who were operated by using auto-homograft, TORP and

PORP are to be seen.

Improvement was observed as follows:

- more than 30 dB at 18 patients, that is 27.3%
- between 20 and 30 dB - 24 patients, that is 36.4%
- between 10 and 20 dB - 16 patients, that is 24.2%
- no improvement at 8 patients, that is 12.1%.

This table has been prepared at the basis of functional results up to 3 months after the cperation.

Two years after the operation the percentage of hearing gain are under 50%. This fact shows, that TORP and PORP are not materials which are able to bring a revolutionary change in ear surgery at a condition after redical operation, when the total tympanic membrane and ossicles are absent, up to the footplate.

In conclusion, the restoration of the middle ear after spontaneous or radical operation is a problem which is not yet solved satisfactorially. Many surgeons have reached good healing and functional results but up to now, no reliable general technique has been developed.

Our long experiences with homograft en bloc, more than 25 years, and less longer with TORP (poroplast, plastipore and ceramics) have shown that the best healing and functional results would be reached by a precise restoration of the conductive systemof the middle ear by combinations between homograft en bloc and TORP and PORP, because with the homograft transplantation en bloc we are able to restore a stable tympanic membrane and a normal tympanic cavity. The most difficult problem is the elimination of adhesions at the oval window and eustachian tube.

Finally, I am convinced, that a perfect surgical technique in connetion with the cooperation of the patient will bring the restoration of the middle ear to success.

* Prof.Dr.med. Christian Betow, Berlin - F.R.G.

© 1985 Elsevier Science Publishers B.V. (Biomedical Division)
New dimensions in otorhinolaryngology – head and neck surgery, vol. 2.
E. Myers, editor

OTITIS MEDIA WITH EFFUSION, DIAGNOSTIC AND THERAPEUTIC ELEMENTS*

Otitis media with effusion has increased in incidence in the last decade, particularly in children; it has becoma the principal Illness in pediatric otology. A large amuont of publications in recent time has been dealing with the presence of fluids in the middle ear, the main etiological factors are known, but their exact role in the development and evolvement of the disease and their interrelationship are partially unknown, or contradictory. In this paper I would like to concentrate on the value of diagnostical methods and on the surgical therapy of the disease. This mainly statistical report has the purpose to summorize the experience of the Free University of Berlin with the disease. The cases of 1000 patients operated at the Charlottenburg University Clinic were studied, 250 were invited to a re- examination; this re- examination consisted of the usual diagnostic procedure, oto- and rhinoscopy, audiology and impedance tympanometry.

The results already show a slight decrease in the incidence of operations due to otitis media with effusion. The frequency of operations due to this disease has decreased consistently from 361 cases in 1981, over 305 cases in 1982, to 235 in 1983. This progressive and substantial decrease in incidence over 3 years probably is due to the increased attention of the physicians to this disease, its diagnosis and treatment.

Like stated by many authors, the disease in this study also appeared more often in male patients, most of the cases appearing between 3 and 5 year olds, a seasonal dependance could not be established in this study. Regarding the therapy, the percentage of tubulations and grommet insertions was very low (5.5%). The reasons for the rare intrusions probably were complications and injuries to the tympanic membrane, which in most of the cases is still growing, as well as foreign body rections. Tubulations were only performed on few and complicated cases, resistant to other kinds of therapy, or continuously recurring. At patients over 20 years tubulation prevailed (57%). The main therapy of the whole group of patients consisted of adenoidectomy with contemporaneous paracenthesis and suction of the effusion (53%), this method also showed the highest rates of normalization at the re- examination 1 to 3 years after surgery (79%), while only 46.2% of the patients tubulated presented normal findings.

250 patients were re- examined in 1984, in order to show the progress of the disease, diagnostical predictability, and long term results of the therapy. The audiograms performed show a higher hearing loss in young children and infants. 54% of the patients aged 1 to 4 had hearing threasholds over 40 dB, while only 26.1% of the 8 to 12 year olds presented hearing losses at this level. This fact also shows the extreme danger of the disease in early childhood. Audiology reached a sensitivity of 74%. Especially in infants it is not very reliable, and too little specific for this disease. In spite of that, it offers valuable information on the hearing decrease and the evolvement of the illness.

Impedance tympanometry did not reveal significant diferences of types at various age groups. Type B or flat tympanograms were found in 79% of the cases, only 6.2% had the normal type A curve. The high sensitivity of 93.8% and the specifity of 91% show, that impedance tympanometry is the most reliable diagnostic procedure. Stapedial muscle reflex controls were not performed, because of their low predictability and specifity. They could be of importance however, when audiology and tympanometry show unclear or contradictory findings.

Another diagnostical procedure of utmost importance, otoscopy, was omitted in these statistics, since it depends to great extents of the subjective opinion of the examiner. It should be an indispensable element in the series of diagnostical procedures, along with audiology and tympanometry.

A better consideration of middle ear effusions at childrens or infants controls and within scholastic controls would reduce further the incidence of this disease, which has already been falling in the last years.

* W. Betow, Berlin - F.R.G.

New dimensions in otorhinolaryngology - head and neck surgery, vol. 2.
E. Myers, editor

REVERSIBLE UNILATERAL SUDDEN HEARING LOSS IN ACQUIRED LATENT SYPHILIS

M. HARELL and M. ENGLENDER
Department of Otolaryngology, E. Wolfson Hospital, Holon 58100, Israel

INTRODUCTION

The turn of the century brought important discoveries in the battle against syphilis. Later, in the 1940's, penicillin became the drug of choice in the cure of syphilis (1).

Syphilis, both congenital and acquired, may cause sensorineural hearing loss (2). Congenital syphilis is transmitted transplacentally by the infected mother to the child. The late lesions of congenital lues develop after the second year of life and include the triad of Deafness, Interstitial Keratitis and Hutchinson's Teeth. In acquired syphilis, deafness frequently occurs in the tertiary phase as a result of luetic meningo-encephalitis.

The occurence of sudden sensorineural hearing loss (SHL) in the latent phase of acquired syphilis is less frequently recognized. It is our purpose to call attention to this potentially reversible cause of SHL.

CASE REPORT

A 39 year old woman was admitted to our department with a left SHL, accompanied by severe vertigo and vomiting (Fig. 1). Physical examination and routine blood tests were normal and so were skull and temporal bone X-rays. According to our SHL protocol, the patient was put on I.V. lidocaine, 600 mg t.i.d. Ten days later no improvement in hearing was noted, although vertigo, nausea and vomiting had ceased. At that time a positive VDRL result was obtained. FTA-abs and TPI confirmed the already suspected diagnosis of otosyphilis. On further interrogation the patient admitted having contracted syphilis 20 years before. We put her on a three months therapy consisting of penicillin and steroids. Her hearing improved dramatically and toward the end of treatment became almost normal (Fig. 2). It has remained such for two years.

DISCUSSION

Hearing loss in congenital syphilis without other stigmata is rare or nonexistent (2). Early (infantile) congenital syphilitic hearing loss is usually overshadowed by the often fatal multisystem involvement. Late (tardive) congenital syphilis (3,4) has been most extensively described by Hutchinson. However, it is not well appreciated that acquired syphilis can cause deafness. The clinical picture of acquired syphilitic involvement of the inner ear includes both vestibular and auditory symptoms and is usually bilateral. Unilateral SHL in latent acquired syphilis is very rare. Occasional cases of SHL have been reported, usually in the tertiary phase, due to neurosyphilis (5). In our patient's case, deafness occured in the late latent phase, without central nervous system involvement, with excellent response to treatment.

In view of the rising incidence of acquired lues, one should keep in mind that otosyphilis may appear during the latent stage, unrelated to neurosyphilis.

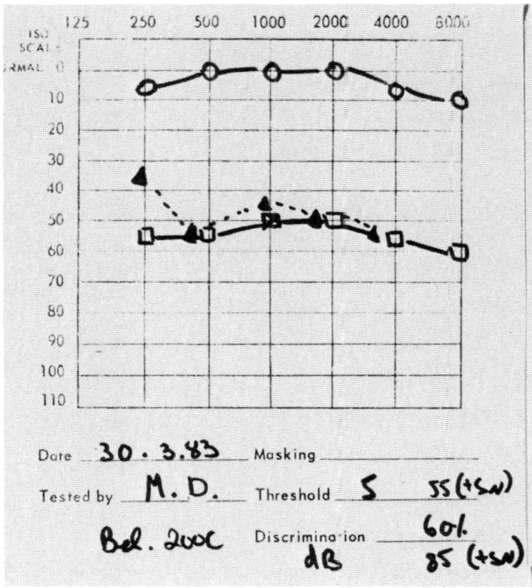

Fig. 1. Initial Audiogram

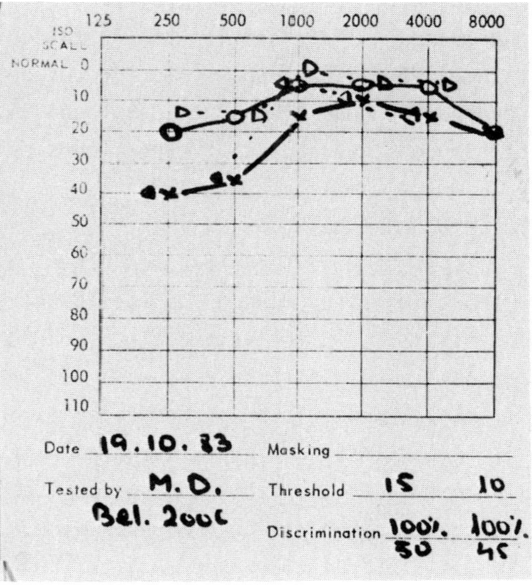

Fig. 2. Final Audiogram

REFERENCES

1. Becker GD (1979) Laryngoscope 89: 1273-1286
2. Nadol JB (1975) Laryngoscope 85: 1888-1897
3. Kerr AG, Smith GDL, Cinnamond MJ (1973) J Laryngol & Otol 87: 1-12
4. Adams DA, Kerr AG, Smith GDL, Cinnamond MJ (1983) J Laryngol & Otol 97: 399-404
5. Clemis JD (1977) Tex Med 73: 60-65

© 1985 Elsevier Science Publishers B.V. (Biomedical Division)
New dimensions in otorhinolaryngology - head and neck surgery, vol. 2.
E. Myers, editor

TECHNIQUE FOR EVALUATING THE INSTALLATION AND ACUTE COCHLEAR INJURY FROM ELECTRODE INSERTION IN HUMAN TEMPORAL BONE PREPARATIONS

P.A. BURGIO
Otologic Products/Life Science Sector, 3M Center, St. Paul, MN 55144

INTRODUCTION

Studies have shown that electrodes inserted greater than 10 mm into the cochlea can cause damage to cochlear tissues.[1-3] This damage results in sensorineural degeneration and formation of fibrous tissue and new bone.[4] The tissues formed in response to the damage can occlude scala tympani. This report describes techniques developed to view the installation of cochlear implants and the results of experiments using these techniques.

MATERIALS AND METHODS

The first experiment was conducted to evaluate the possibility of mechanical disruption of the osseous spiral lamina and the basilar membrane during insertion of a 6 mm electrode through the round window and 6 mm into scala tympani. The electrode used was the 3M Cochlear Implant System/House Design. Six otolaryngologists inexperienced in installing cochlear implants placed the electrodes in the prepared temporal bone. (See Figure 1.)

The second experiment evaluated a specific technique for installing and securing a round window electrode wire. This experiment also evaluated the stability of the electrode in both the niche and on the round window membrane when the wire on the squama was moved. The ball-tipped wire electrodes used in the 3M Cochlear Implant System/Vienna Deisgn were installed in the round window using the mastoid facial recess approach by three otolaryngologists. After installation, a one inch diameter cylinder was rolled over the electrode on the surface of the skull with a force of 2000 grams. This rolling action was designed to simulate some common types of force the wire could be exposed to in clinical situations. (See Figures 2 and 3.)

Both the intracochlear experiments and the extracochlear experiments were recorded on video tape. Each installation was viewed and scored according to a set criteria by a team of three evaluators knowledgeable in cochlear anatomy.

RESULTS

In the first experiment, a clear video image of the insertion was recorded. Any injury to the tissues could be readily observed. The results showed that 100% of the insertions were safe with respect to the basilar membrane and associated organ of Corti. Ninety-six percent of the insertions were safe for

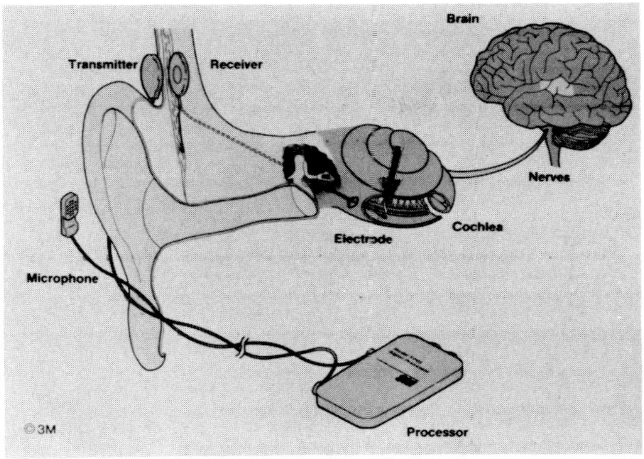

FIGURE 1: The model used in this experiment was a formalin-fixed human temporal bone in which the mastoid and facial recesses were opened by standard surgical procedure and two microscopes with video equipment. The arrow shows the view of the video equipped microscope.

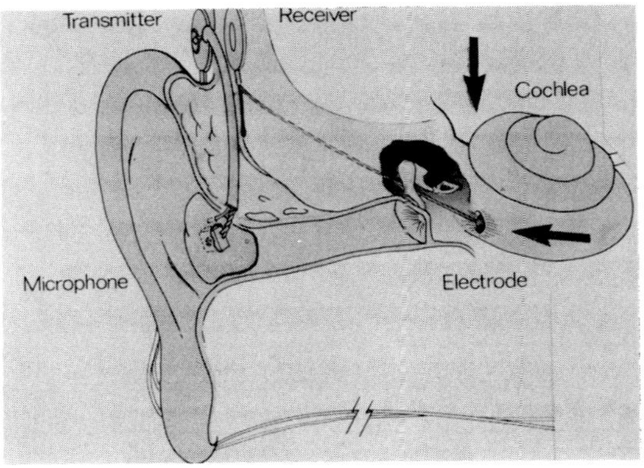

FIGURE 2: The model used in this experiment was a formalin-fixed human temporal bone opened to the round window with standard surgical technique. The electrode was photographed in the round window by one video equipped microscope. Another video equipped microscope focused down scala tympani, viewing the electrode ball in contact with the round window membrane. Arrows show the views of the video equipped microscopes.

the osseous spiral lamina.

The results of the extracochlear electrode installation show that in 100% of the cases (N=15), the electrode was installed so that the ball of the electrode was in the round window niche and in contact with the round window membrane. The study also showed that the electrode was securely held in contact with the membrane even when the portion of the wire on the squama was moved.

DISCUSSION

These procedures, involving specially prepared human temporal bones, microscopes equipped with video cameras, video recorders, and monitors, provide a way to evaluate methods for securing an electrode in place. The procedures also allow evaluation of acute cochlear injury resulting from electrode insertion.

The results of the intracochlear implant experiments demonstrate that the 6 mm 3M Cochlear Implant System/House Design electrode can be installed with a high level of safety to the cochlear tissues. Mechanical damage of the cochlear duct or the osseous spiral lamina is known to cause sensorineural degeneration, and formation of fibrous tissue and new bone. Long electrodes that do cause damage to cochlear tissues should not be used since they can limit the future insertion of new electrode styles. Thus, electrodes which minimize damage during installation help preserve the remaining nerve fibers and prevent occlusion of the scala due to formation of new tissue.

The evaluation of the extracochlear implants indicates that the electrode of the 3M Cochlear Implant System/Vienna Design can be properly installed 100% of the time so the ball of the electrode is in direct contact with the round window membrane. In addition, the specified method for suturing the electrode holds the ball securely in place, even if the wire near the receiver is exposed to forces similar to those possible *in situ*.

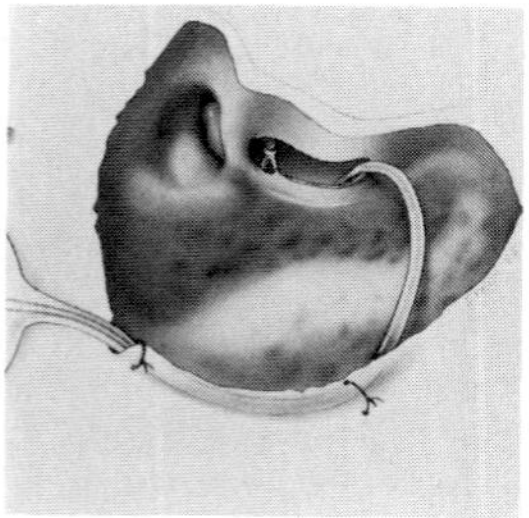

FIGURE 3: The electrode lead was installed by placing the ball tip at the round window and the wire under the lip of the undercut area of the mastoid cortex. The wire was held in place by sutures.

REFERENCES

1. Galey FR (1984) Acta Otolaryngol (Stockh) Suppl 411, pp 38-44
2. Johnsson L-G, House WF, Linthicum FH (1982) In: Cochlear Implants: Progress Perspectives. Ann Otol Rhinol Laryngol, pp 74-89
3. Sheppard RK, Clark GM, Pyman BC, Webb RL (1985) Ann Otol Rhinol Laryngol 94: 55-59
4. Spoendlin H (1984) Ann Otol Rhinol Laryngol (Suppl) 112: 76-82

© 1985 Elsevier Science Publishers B.V. (Biomedical Division)
New dimensions in otorhinolaryngology - head and neck surgery, vol. 2.
E. Myers, editor

OFFICE MANAGEMENT OF MALIGNANT OTITIS EXTERNA

IRWIN HARRIS, M.D., F.A.C.S.

Assoc. Clin. Prof., Div. Head & Neck Surgery, Rm.31-24 Rehabilitation Ctr.
UCLA School of Medicine, Los Angeles, Ca. 90024 U.S.A.

In 1968 Chandler[1] proposed the term "malignant external otitis" to indicate the seriousness of necrotizing external otitis due to Pseudomonas Aeroginosa in elderly diabetic patients. It is a most appropriate descriptive term, for Dorlands Medical Dictionary defines malignant as "virulent, and tending to go from bad to worse." Six of Chandlers' patients had facial palsy and seven died. These infections tend to involve skin, cartilage, and bone. They may extend to adjacent underlying tissues involving the cranial nerves VII through X, meningitis and ultimate death. He stated "the infection is resistant to ordinary methods of treatment", and he described in-hospital management with weeks of parenteral antibiotic therapy, and the surgical removal of disease tissue.

The purpose of this paper is to stress our experience that early aggressive and intensive local therapy of malignant external otitis in the office can prevent the more invasive forms of this disease and effect a cure.

Nadol[2] described the histopathology of malignant external otitis starting in the external auditory canal and spreading to the retromandibular fossa, probably along the tympanomandibular suture.

Awareness of the predilection for Pseudomonas to spread along vascular and fascial planes rather than pneumatized tracts is extremely important in following the pathways of progression of malignant external otitis (as differentiated from that of sub-acute or chronic mastoiditis). Computerized axial tomography and magnetic resonance imaging added to standard radiographic techniques can help trace soft tissue involvement and bone destruction.

CASE REPORT

A.L., Caucasian male, age 61, was first seen on 10/24/83 with a chief complaint of pain and swelling of the right ear associated with diminished hearing. One week previously he had been treated by his family doctor because his ear was blocked and he had trouble with his balance. To remove wax, the ear was irrigated, which caused a roaring sensation and then the ear became painful and swollen. Previously this right ear had drained intermittently and the hearing had been impaired for almost 40 years.

His insulin dependent diabetes (70 U daily) was out of control.

Fifteen years previously he had a severe syncopal reaction to penicillin requiring resuscitation.

The right war was markedly edematous with visible granulation tissue, and a culture revealed Pseudomonas. A CAT scan of the temporal bones was reported as showing hypodevelopment and chronic mastoiditis on the right.

The patient was hospitalized and placed on parenteral tobramycin, 120 mg every 8 hours, colistin packs were placed in the ear and his diabetes was controlled. After one week he left the hospital against advice, the ear canal still markedly edematous, suppurating and eardrum not yet visible. He agreed to office treatments, 7 days a week, consisting of irrigating the abscess pockets deep in the canal with gentamycin through a 17 gauge canula using a Zeiss microscope. After 2 weeks of treatment a 6x3 mm cartilage sequestrum was removed from the anterior abscess cavity. The ear drum was first visible on 12/23/83 (2 months after the first visit) and the ear was dry and healed one month later (1/20/84) and has remained so for the past 1½ years.

SUMMARY

A case of progressive necrotizing, malignant, virulent Pseudomonas otitis externa in a 61 year old diabetic male is reported to emphasize that an effective cure can be obtained by daily office therapy with gentamycin if hospitalization is refused by a patient.

Early recognition and intensive daily therapy may contribute to the cure of this disease by preventing the complications of mastoiditis, cranial nerve involvement, meningitis and high risk of fatality.

In order to obtain early and intensive therapy for this disease it is necessary that such information continue to be disseminated to our colleagues in primary care, as well as in otolaryngology.

REFERENCES

1. Chandler JR (1977) Ann Otol Rhinol Laryngol 86:417-429

2. Nadol JB (1980) Am J Otolaryng 1:359-371

© 1985 Elsevier Science Publishers B.V. (Biomedical Division)
New dimensions in otorhinolaryngology – head and neck surgery, vol. 2.
E. Myers, editor

POSSIBLE UTILITY OF 40 Hz EVENT RELATED POTENTIAL IN ELECTRIC RESPONSE AUDIOMETRY

MASARU AOYAGI, MASASHI YOKOTA and JIRO HARADA
Department of Otolaryngology, Yamagata university, School of Medicine, Yamagata 990-23 (Japan)

INTRODUCTION

Though electric response audiometry has made great progress by means of auditory evoked brain stem response, it is still difficult to obtain trustworthy measurements of low and middle frequency hearing thresholds in young children. The aims of the present paper are to verify the reliabilty of the 40 Hz evevt related potential (40 Hz-ERP) in response to low and middle frequency tone pips, and to assess the clinical utility of the 40 Hz-ERP in the estimation of hearing sensitivity in young children.

MATERIALS AND METHODS

As normal subjects, 21 adults aged 21 to 32 years, and 9 children aged 4 to 7 years were studied. Furthermore, 16 adults with impaired hearing aged 23 to 65 years and 24 children with impaired hearing aged 3 to 7 years were examined. The adults hearing was previously tested useing standard pure tone audiometry, and the children were tested mainly by play audiometry. Audiograms of the subjects with impaired hearing indicated various types and degrees of disorders.

The acoustic stimuli were 0.5, 1 and 2 kHz tone pips, each having 2 periods of rise and fall and 2 plateaus. They were applied through headphones at a repetition rate of 40 Hz. Recording electrodes were placed at the vertex and ipsilateral ear lobe, with a ground electrode on the forehead. The amplifier cut off frequencies were 8 Hz and ´20 Hz. A total of 1000 responses were averaged with a sweep time of 50 msec. At each acoustic stimulus, two responses were averaged. All adults were examined during awake states, and children were sedated by oral administration of triclofos during examination.

The main criteria for detecting a response were (1) general morphology of wave form, (2) replicability and (3) peak latency When the judgment of a wave form was difficult, power spectrum analysis and digital filtering by means of FFT algorithm were carried out in additon to the analog filtering.

RESULTS

(1) Normal subjects

There was a significant difference between the detectability of the response in adults and in children at 0.5 kHz, but no significant differences were detected at 1 and 2 kHz. At all frequencies, the mean thresholds were less than 15 dB, and standard deviations were less than 10 dB in adults. In children, however, both values were higher than those in adults, except at 2 kHz. One reason for this finding might be the fact that children were examined while asleep.

(2) Subjects with impaired hearing

The correlations between the 40 Hz-ERP and behavioral thresholds in patients were analysed. The correlation coefficients in adults were higher than those of children in each stimulus frequency. However, no significant differences were observed between 0.5 and 1 kHz in both groups. At 2 kHz, the correlations were almost same as the other frequencies.

Table 1 shows the mean differences and standard deviations between the 40 Hz-ERP and behavioral thresholds in patients with impaired hearing. The mean differences in adults were smaller than in children at all frequencies.

TABLE 1 : Difference between 40 Hz-ERP and behavioral thresholds

		Adults	Children
0.5 kHz	Mean	5.0 dB	23.1 dB
	S.D.	13.3	16.7
1 kHz	Mean	6.5	12.3
	S.D.	16.5	18.2
2 kHz	Mean	10.8	12.8
	S.D.	17.5	20.7

DISCUSSION

From these results, it may be assumed that the test reliability of the 40 Hz-ERP is not good enough for predicting accurate behavioral hearing thresholds in low and middle frequency ranges in young children who should be sedated during examination.

On the other hand, the 40 Hz-ERP is useful for the objective estimation of hearing thresholds in adults, especially at low and middle frequencies. But,even in adults, the reliability of the 40 Hz-ERP in the assessment of hearing sensitivity is lower than the auditory evoked brain stem responses with low and middle frequency tone pips.

© 1985 Elsevier Science Publishers B.V. (Biomedical Division)
New dimensions in otorhinolaryngology - head and neck surgery, vol. 2.
E. Myers, editor

SYNAPTIC ALTERATIONS IN THE ACOUSTIC CORTEX OF THE RAT FOLLOWING INSULIN INDUCED HYPOGLYCHEMIA

S.J. BALOYANNIS, T.C. THEOHARIDES, L.S. MANOLIDES

Department of O.R.L., Laboratory of Neuropathology-Otohistopathology, Aristotelian University of Thessaloniki, Thessaloniki (Greece)

INTRODUCTION

Electron microscopic studies of hypoglychemic alterations of cortical and subcortical neurons in experimental animals revealed that in some areas of the brain, having a selective vulnerability, the principal morphological changes consist of vacuolization of neurons, mitochondrial swelling and internal disorganization of the mitochondria[2,3,4]. In an attempt to define the early stages of synaptic changes due to uncomplicated hypoglychemia in the rat, we induced hypoglychemia by intraarterial injections of insulin and studied several cortical and subcortical areas, including the acoustic area of the temporal cortex, the CA-I region of hippocampus, the tectum, the corpora striata and the cerebellar cortex. The present work concentrates upon morphological and morphometric alterations of neuronal synapses in the acoustic area of the rat's brain, following uncomplicated hypoglychemia.

MATERIAL AND METHODS

Ten male Lewis rats of 325gr mean body were subjected to hypoglychemia by intracarotid infusion of insulin. Arterial gas tensions, blood pH, acid base status, blood pressure, rectal temperature and plasma glycose concentration was monitored before and after insulin administration

Sixty minutes after insulin administration, the plasma glycose level was decline to 1/2mg% and remained between 42mg% and 45mg% for 30 minutes. Subsequently, the animals were sacrified and the brains were processed for electron microscopy.

RESULTS

Most of the presynaptic terminals in the acoustic cortex contained large number of polymorphic synaptic vesicles, some of them been dilated. In a large number of synapses the vesicles were loosely filling the entire profile of the terminal and only few of them were accumulated in the "active zone" of the synapses. Perforated synapses were not unfrequently seen especially in the superfical layer of the acoustic cortex. Some presynaptic profiles contained numerous vesicles which were clumped into dense masses located in the center of the terminal. Some of the presynaptic terminals were enlarged and contained few dilated synaptic vesicles, dilated cisternae of smooth endoplasmic reticulum, fibrils and mitochondria exhibiting internal disorganization. Most of those synapses were attached to dilated postsynaptic terminals containing few cisternae of smooth endoplasmic reticulum and loosely dispersed fibrillary material. A substantial number of presynaptic terminals attached to the smooth surface of dendritic profiles, demonstrated enormous dilatation and contained large cavities lined by membraneous profiles. The same cortical area demonstrated extensive dilatation of the postsynaptic terminals which included few polymorphic vesicles. In most of the synapses the synaptic cleft was dilated and contained fibrillary material.

The curvature of a large number of synapses was neutral, namely both the pre- and postsynaptic membranes been flat. Some of the synapses demonstrated a positive curvature, the postsynaptic membrane been protruded into presynaptic terminal, whereas a limited number of synapses demonstrated a negative curvature, the presynaptic membrane been protruded into postsynaptic terminal.

The morphometric study revealed a substantial decrease of the total number of the synaptic vesicles in the "active zone" of the synapses after hypoglychemia in correlation with normal controls. In normal controls the mean number of the synaptic vesicles in the "active zone" was 270 ± 40 whereas after hypoglychemia the number droped to 70 ± 40.

The acoustic areas of the cortex seem to be extremely sensitive to hypoglychemia probably due to highly specialezed neuronal function involving sensitive neurotransmitter systems. From the morphological point of view, the perforated synapses which are frequently seen in the acoustic cortex of the experimental animals and the human brain[1] suggest the high functional significance of that cortical area as well as the plasticity of the synaptic development and consequently explains the selective vulnerability of that area to hypoglychemia.

REFERENCES

1. Baloyannis S.J., Manolides L.S. (1985) In: Perforated Synapses in the Acoustic Area of the Human Brain. Acta Otolaryngol., Stockholm, Suppl. in Press

2. Brown A.W., Brierley J.B. (1973) In: The earliest Alterations in the Rat Neurons after Anoxia-Ischemia. Acta Neuropath., Berlin, 23:9-22

3. Brown A.W., Brierley J.B. (1972) In: Anoxic ischemic Cell Change in Rat Brain. Light Microscopie and fine Structures Observations. J. Neurol. Soc., 16:59-84

4. McGee-Russel S.M., Brown A.W., Brierley J.B. (1970) In: A combined light and electron microscopic Study of early anoxic ischemic Cell Change in Rat Brain. Brain. Res. 20:193-200

© 1985 Elsevier Science Publishers B.V. (Biomedical Division)
New dimensions in otorhinolaryngology - head and neck surgery, vol. 2.
E. Myers, editor

FIRST DIALYSIS' BEDSIDE RECORDING OF BRAINSTEM AUDITORY EVOKED RESPONSES (BAERs)

A. BATTISTELLA, B. DI PAOLO*, T. DI MARCO*, G. DEL ROSSO*, M. EVANGELISTA*
Institutes of Otorhinolaryngology and Nephrology*, SS. Annunziata University Hospital, 66100 Chieti (Italy)

INTRODUCTION

The clinical manifestations of neurological dysfunctions could appear during the first hemodialysis and at most times during the last hours or just afterwards. They are documentable through the use of evoked potentials and became more altered as uremia progresses (1). Frequently symptoms such as headache, nausea, vomiting, muscular cramps, appearing during the first dialytic settings reveal an osmotic gradient between the intra-extracerebral compartments with a "shift" of water into the brain inducing cerebral "edema" or "swelling".

The purpose of this study is to document the relationship with the different phases of dialysis and obtain a meaningful explanation of the physiopathology of the disequilibrium syndrome induced by first dialysis sessions.

MATERIAL AND METHODS

Ten fully informed patients took part in our study (7 ♂, 3 ♀, mean age 38.50 ± 10.20 yrs, range 16-68 yrs); they were affected by chronic renal failure for 54.3 ± 13.50 months. The patients started the dialytic treatment (not urgently); each recording was performed in a partially sound isolated room used for the dialytic treatment of a single patient. Active Ag/AgCl disk electrodes fixed at the vertex with collodion (C_z of the International System 10-20) and referred to the examined ear lobe, while the contralateral ear was used as ground. We measured a wide spectrum of clicks of alternating polarity, lasting 100 usec with an intensity of 70 dB above the subjects threshold at 11 cycles/sec (TDH-49, Amplaid Stimulator MK 10). The signal was filtered through a passing-band of 500-2000 Hz. Each tracing was the average of 2000 artifact-free relevations.

RESULTS

On ten patients repeatedly analyzed before undergoing the first dialysis the interpeak I-V was at higher normal values; 3 hours afterwards it resulted increased but still within the normal limits of variability (from 3.87 msec for males and from 3.86 msec for females); after the 26th hour post-dialysis it became significantly short. When 3 patients were again examined during the 14th hemodialysis, the abovementioned pre- and post-dialysis variations did not appear significant. Wave I remained at values of about 1.8-2.0 msec in more than 70% of the cases; wave III in most cases (80%) appears as a big complex of long duration which almost englobed even the I wave, most times it is not evidenced certainly; at times waves I and V appeared fused into one; rarely we visualize waves VI and VII. Noteworthy, the extreme "structural disorder" of the evoked morphogram has induced us to have great difficulty in identifying and recognizing the morphology.

CONCLUSIONS

Chemical-physical variations induced by the first few dialytic setting, could cause disequilibrium of the cerebral grey matter, of the cerebrospinal fluid, of the ocular tone and of the inner ear. It is normal that these alterations shall be amplified as the nervous impulse travels towards the acoustic pathways; when trasmitted the acoustic potential becomes distorted, the resulting BAER tracing can therefore appear in a great variability. During hemodialysis it is possible that we cause a modification of the osmotic equilibrium of the inner ear and subsequently a labirinthic "hidrops", the decongestion of which induces the latency's and amplitude's changes. These should be functional as demonstrated by the obscillation of latencies of all the waves: the interpeaks/ratio is unconstant and a total subversion of the normal morphology is the characterizing aspect.

Some pathologic mechanisms interact in a complex manner: the decrease in axonal conduction velocity, the space-time disorganization of the neuronal recruitment and the possible, intermittent and disorganized activation of parallel neurons with increased or decreased conduction velocity.

REFERENCES

1. Albertazzi A, Di Paolo B, Del Rosso G, Gambi D, Rossini PM (1981) Neurophysiological abnormalities in uremic encephalopathy. Proc XVIII Congr EDTA, Parigi, pp 652-657

© 1985 Elsevier Science Publishers B.V. (Biomedical Division)
New dimensions in otorhinolaryngology - head and neck surgery, vol. 2.
E. Myers, editor

CLINICAL AND EXPERIMENTAL STUDIES IN SECRETORY OTITIS MEDIA

JAMSHEED A. KHAN

E.N.T. Surgeon, 26 Preston Drive Wanstead, London, Ell (United Kingdom)

INTRODUCTION

There has been considerable disagreement concerning the aetiology of this disease and its medico-surgical management. Effectiveness of the use of grommet is associated with possible complications (Editorial, British Medical Journal 1981).

Various pharmaco-therapeutics agents such as urea surface tension lowering agents, antibiotics, steriods, and proteolytic enzymes have been investigated in the past decade, but have not proved effective, convenient and safe in reducing the viscosity of middle ear effusions (Bauer 1968, Hagan 1977).
Carbocisteine on the other hand has been suggested to have a beneficial effect (Taylor & Dareshani 1975).

The purpose of this study was to investigate a) whether radio labelled ^{35}S-carbocisteine appears or concentrates in the middle ear space; b) whether short-term treatment with cold carbocisteine is effective; c) whether carbocisteine is a useful adjunct to surgical myringotomy in childhood secretory otitis.

MATERIAL AND METHODS

Animal studies of the distribution of ^{35}S-Carbocisteine in guinea pigs with eustachian tube occlusion.

Twenty one healthy male albino guinea pigs (300-450 g) were used in this study. Experimental effusions were obtained by blocking the pharyngeal orifice of the eustachian tube transpalatally using a polytef plug (Kahn and Campbell, 1981). A polythene cannula was inserted and ^{35}S-carbocisteine (200 uci per animal; 40-60 mg/kg) was introduced. Ear perfusates, using 0.15 to 0.2 ml. saline were obtained from the operated and control ears. Nine animals were killed 0.5 hours after dosing (Group I), seven at three hours (Group 2) and five at 24 hours (Group 3). Tissue samples were stored at -10°C and homogenized and counted within a maximum period of one week. Whole blood was collected in harparinized tubes and stored at -4°C.

Studies on the prophylactic and therapeutic effects of carbocisteine in a guinae pig model of middle ear effusion

Forty six healthy albino guinea pigs (300-500 g) were selected for this study. Animals were allocated to four groups and were dosed daily orally with Carbocisteine (30 mg./Kg body weight), according to study protocol (Table I).

Animals were sacrificed by exsanguination and temporal bullae were fixed in neutral formal saline solution (10 per cent - V/V) for histological examination. Pathological findings were assessed by independent observers. Fischer's exact test was used for analysis of the findings Table 2

Human studies (c) A Double Blind Study

In this study, carbocisteine syrup (Berk-Pharmaceuticals Limited) was compared with placebo and with Elixir containing bronmpheramine, phenylephrine and phenylpropanolamine (BPP). 58 children with secretory otitis media completed a double blind trial which studied the speed of resolution of middle ear

Group	Number of animals completing study	TREATMENT	
		Phase I (Days 1 - 14)	Phase II (Days 15 - 28)
1	10	A	A
2	10	B	A
3	12	A	B
4	10	B	B

Treatment schedule for each group of guinea pigs.

Treatment A : carbocisteine 30mg/kg in cerculia base.

Treatment B : cerculia base alone.

TABLE 1

Pathological Finding Under Consideration	Group or Groups Compared	No with Pathology	No without Pathology	Total No of Animals	Significance level (p value)
Submucosal	1 (active treatment throughout)	3	7	10	)
	4 (base alone throughout)	8	2	10	) p = 0.10
	1 + 2 (active treatment) (days 15-28)	7	13	20	)
	3 + 4 (base alone days 15-28)	16	6	22	) p = 0.05
Mucoperiosteal Reaction	1 (active treatment throughout)	2	8	10	)
	4 (base alone throughout)	7	3	10	) p = 0.10
	1 + 2 (active treatment) (days 15-28)	4	16	20	)
	3 + 4 (base alone days 15-28)	12	10	22	) p = 0.05
New Bone Formation	1 (active treatment throughout)	1	9	10	)
	4 (base alone throughout)	6	4	10	) p = 0.10
	1 + 2 (active treatment) (days 15-28	2	18	20	)
	3 + 4 (base alone days 15-28)	10	12	22	(p = 0.05

Statistical analysis of pathological findings in operated ears.
Fishers exact test on above 2 x 2 tables.

TABLE 2

Sample	TIME AFTER DOSING (HOURS)		
	0.5 (n = 9)	3.0 (n = 7)	24.0 (n = 5)
Brain	3.7 ± 5.5	0.8 ± 0.2	0.4 ± 0.2
Heart	4.6 ± 2.4	3.2 ± 2.0	0.2 ± 0.1
Kidney	704 ± 158	112 ± 26	1.0 ± 0.6
Liver	38.7 ± 3.1	48.8 ± 13.1	0.7 ± 0.4
Lung	13.2 ± 4.5	9.0 ± 4.4	0.5 ± 0.3
Spleen	11.4 ± 5.1	3.1 ± 0.7	0.7 ± 0.5
Blood	60 ± 51	74 ± 46	1.7 ± 1.0

n = No of animals

Distribution of ^{35}S in tissues (% dose/mg tissue x 10^5) and body fluids (% dose/l) following I.V. injection of ^{35}S-carbocisteine (Mean ± Standard Deviation)

TABLE 3

Sample	TIME AFTER DOSING (HOURS) 0.5 (n = 5)	3.0 (n = 2)	24.0 (n = 5)
Eustachian tube mucosa:			
Operated ear	5.1 ± 3.2		3.2 ± 2.9
Control ear	4.55 ± 2.1		0.9 ± 0.5
Middle ear mucosa:			
Operated ear	5.5 ± 2.9	12.2	0.8 ± 0.6
Control ear	5.1 ± 2.8	6.4	0.8 ± 0.5
Tympanic bullae bone:			
Operated ear	1.0 ± 0.5	3.5	0.2 ± 0.1
Control ear	1.2 ± 0.6	2.7	0.3 ± 0.2
Ear perfusates (% dose/litre):			
Diseased ear)	6.4 ± 10.0	1.0 ± 0.8	0.9 ± 0.5
Control ear)		0.9 ± 0.9	0.4 ± 0.5
Overall means ± SD	6.4 ± 10.0	1.0 ± 0.8	0.6 ± 0.5

The numbers of animals used in this Table are less than those in Table 3 because it proved technically difficult in some animals to have ^{35}S concentration measured separately in normal and diseased ears.

Concentrations of ^{35}S (% dose/mg tissue x 10^5 in the middle ear cleft following I.V. injection of ^{35}S-carbocisteine (Mean ± Standard Deviation)

TABLE 4

Group	No of animals completing study	No of effusions in operated ears	Time of appearance of effusions (days) Phase I	Phase II	No of effusions in control ears
1	10	2	1 x 7	1 x 21	0
2	10	3	2 x 14	1 x 21	0
3	12	7	1 x 7 4 x 14	2 x 21	1
4	10	8	4 x 14	4 x 21	0

Incidence and time of appearance of middle ear effusion (confirmed by myringotomy) according to treatment group

TABLE 5

Time period under consideration	Group or Groups Compared	No with effusion	No without effusion	Total no of animals	Significance level (p level)
Days 1-28	1 (active treatment throughout)	2	8	10	)
	4 (base alone throughout)	8	2	10	) p = 0.05
	1 + 2 (both active treatment) (days 15-28)	5	15	20	)
	3 + 4 (base alone days 15-28)	15	7	22	) p = 0.05
Days 1-14	1 + 3 (active treatment)	6	16	22	)
	2 + 4 (base alone)	6	13	20	) N.S.
New effusions days 15-28 (Animals developing) (effusion days) (1-14)	1 + 2 (active treatment)	2	13	15	)
	3 + 4 (base alone)	6	9	15	) N.S.

Statistical analysis of middle ear effusions in operated ears.
Fishers exact test on above 2 x 2 tables.

TABLE 6

SEVERITY OF PATHOLOGICAL LESION

GROUP	Mild = 1	Moderate = 2	Severe = 3	Very Severe = 4	Total Score
1 (n = 10)	3	4	2	0	17
2 (n = 10)	3	2	1	0	10
3 (n = 12)	3	5	3	0	22
4 (n = 10)	3	2	3	2	24

Arbitrary scores for the severity of the pathological lesions in each treatment group. Animals with pathological findings judged to lie in an intermediate category, e.g. moderate - severe have been allocated to both categories.

The total score derives from multiplying the number in each category by the score (1-4) of that category and summing the result.

TABLE 7

effusions after myringotomy and insertion of grommet, assessment being made by pure tone audiometry. For assessment of the effect of carbocisteine on the various measure of auditory performance analysis of variance was followed by Duncan's multiple Comparison Test.

RESULTS

a) The present study showed that significant concentration of radiolabelled material was detected in middle ear cleft, blood samples and ear body fluids following IV ^{35}S-carbocisteine administration in guinae pigs induced with serous otitis media (Table 3,4). The single dose 40-60 mg/kg is comparable to total human dosage, given over 24 hours (10 mg.tids) nevertheless it is difficult to compare ^{35}S-carbocisteine levels to that in man.

b) Of the animals in Group I receiving active treatment only two out of 10 developed an effusion compared with eight out of ten animals treated with base alone (Table 5,6). This difference was significant P=0.05. It is also possible to make assessment of efficacy of the treatment from consideration of number of effusions becoming apparent during Phase 1 (14 days) and Phase 2 (the last 14 days). Severity of pathological lesions have also been assessed by combining Groups 1 & 2 & 3 (Table 7). Results of this study suggest that Carbocisteine might have a possible therapeutic effect if otitis media is established though it does not seem to have any prophylactic action in preventing the development of tympanic effusions.

c) The results of clinical trial were calculated by comparing the mean change in hearing thresholds at various frequencies at the initial assessment and at the end of trial. Fig. 1 shows that the effect of Carbocisteine on air condiction is superior to that of placebo and BPP in the range of 1-4KHz. Audiometric improvement seemed to be correlate well with normalization of the appearnace of the tympanic membrane on regular otoscopic examination.

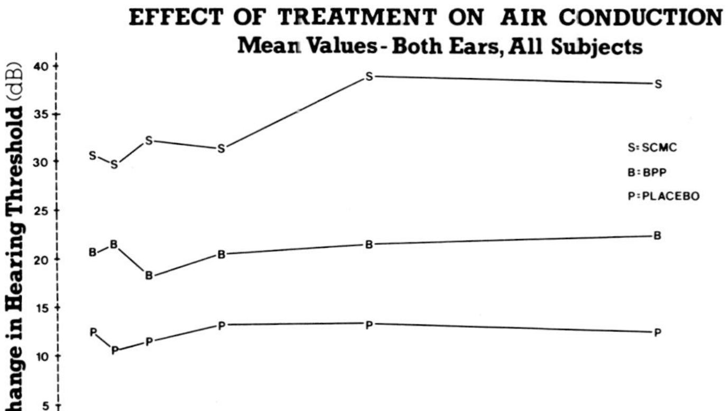

CONCLUSIONS

From my study I concluded that: 1) Carbocisteine is preferential retained in middle ear space, 2) Carbocesteine might have a possible therapeutic benefit if otitis media with effusion is established and has no prophylactic action on the development of tympanic effusions.

While unable to study ^{35}S-Carbocisteine distribution in man or its effect on middle ear histology to the same degree the results of clinical trial here reported point to an efficiency in human disease equivalent to that seen in the animal model. Carbocisteine has potential use in their management. I suggest that Carbocisteine is a useful adjunct to surgical management of secretory otitis media and that it be further studied as an alternative to myringotomy.

REFERENCES

Bauer, F. (1968) Treatment of 'Glue Ear" by intratympanic injection of urea. Journal of Laryncgology and Otology, 82: 717-722.

British Medical Journal (1981) Editorial-Secretory otitis media and grommets 282:5Ø1-5Ø2.

Hagan, W. E. (1977) Surface tension lowering substance in eustachian tube function. Laryngoscope, 87:1Ø33-1Ø45.

Khan, J. A., and Campbell, J. C. (1981) Studies on the production of middle ear effusion in the experimental animal. Journal of Laryngology and Otology, 95:987-993.

Taylor, P. H., and Dareshani, N. (1975) S-Carboxy-methyl-cysteine syrup in secretory otitis media. British Journal of Clinical Practice, 29: 177-18Ø.

© 1985 Elsevier Science Publishers B.V. (Biomedical Division)
New dimensions in otorhinolaryngology - head and neck surgery, vol. 2.
E. Myers, editor

HEARING EVALUATION WITH THE COMBINATION OF TRANSTYMPANIC ELECTROCHOCLEOGRAPHY AND BRAIN STEM RESPONSES AUDIOMETRY

PEDRO LUIZ COSER AND MARIA JOSE SANTOS COSER

Universidade Federal de Santa Maria, Santa Maria (Brasil)
Rua Duque de Caxias, 1668/304, 97100, Santa Maria, Rio Grande do Sul (Brasil)

We had studied 2000 consecutive patients from 1978 to 1983, 1320 were children with communicative disorders and 680 were adults with a variety of neurotological conditions.

The examinations were performed with the AMPLAID MEDELEC ERA MK III EQUIPMENT with the amplification filters set at 16/3200 Hz.

The electrodes were placed at promontory, mastoid and forehead (active, reference and ground) for EChoG and at the forehead, ipsi-lateral mastoid and controlateral mastoid (Active, reference and ground) for BSRA examinations.

The main stimulus used was the 100 us Click and in some cases the 1 and 2 KHz (2 sine waves) were also used at the presentation rate of 10 pps when doing morphological and latency studies and at 20 pps when looking for threshold.

The following findings were considered abnormal in EChoG: 1) AP Waveform broad, diphasic and "abnormal"; 2) III-V intermal larger than 2.2 ms at 85 dBHL; 3) Absence of wave V with III present; 4) Absence of waves III and V with I present; 5) Absence of all waves with AP absent (Choclear lesion) or with AP present (retrochoclear lesion); 6) V-V interval larger than 0.2, 0.3, or 0.4 ms in cases of PURE SENSORYNEURAL hearing loss on one side of no more than 45, 55, or 65 cBHL at the frequency of 4 KHz. 7) AP-V interval larger than 4.5 ms at 85 dBHL; 8) Threshold of wave V Higher than 20 dBHL; 9) Latency of wave V larger than 6 ms at 85 dBHL; 10) latency of wave V smaller than 6.8 ms at threshold.

The above criteria are valid only for click stimulation responses.

The anesthesia we used to do EChog in adults was the application of a very small amount of phenol onto the tympanic membrane; in babies we used general inhalatory anesthesia and in children Ketamine without one complication because of the anesthesia or of the electrode placement.

The EChog is up to ten times faster than BSRA to be done.

THe Inner Ear evaluation is very much better done by EChoG than with BSRA. EChoG includes information of Hydrops presence (because of the summating potential) and BSRA suggested choclear disfunction in cases of severe nerve or Brain Stem lesions when the waves I,III and V could not be demonstrated despite of normal functioning chocleas.

The Brain Stem pathways could be only evaluated by BSRA.

The reproducibility of the responses of EChoG were better than with BSRA because of the better signal to noise ratio in EChoG.

In our experience we have found that BSRA can be used alone only in cases of evaluation of babies as a screening procedure and in the evaluation of adults with normal hearing.

The remaining cases will be better evaluated with EChoG looking for Threshold and hydrops alterations and in sequence with BSRA at 85 cBHL looking for qualitative alterations.

New dimensions in otorhinolaryngology - head and neck surgery, vol. 2.
E. Myers, editor

CHANGES OF STAPEDIUS REFLEX PARAMETERS DURING CONTROLLED STIMULATION

S. SCIUTO, P. GRACILI and M. POERIO

Dept. of Otolaryngology, Ospedale S. Giovanni Evangelista, Tivoli, Roma, Italy

INTRODUCTION

The value of the stapedius reflex (SR) for protection from noise-induced hearing damage has been disputed. One of the main arguments against SR function in that respect has concerned its decay during long-lasting acoustic stimulation.

It is known that changes in the acoustic stimulus signal counteract the reflex decay (1,2). Moreover it has been demonstrated that very short pauses in the acoustic stimulus reactivate the reflex response (3).

Purpose of this study is to evaluate the modifications of the SR during a long-lasting acoustic stimulation periodically interrupted by short pauses.

This kind of stimulation was intended to cause the rhytmic contraction-relaxation of the stapedius muscle (SM) avoiding the SR decay. The avoidance of the decay phenomenon made it possible to verify whether any modification of the SR could be referred specifically to the SM fatigue.

METHODS

The experiments were performed on 40 normoacoustic subjects, and on 31 subjects with sensorineural hearing loss over 35 dB from 2000 to 8000 Hz bilaterally.

1 KHz tone bursts with an amplitude equal to the stapedius reflex treshold (SRT) + 10 dB were administered at 300 msec pause interval. This rhythm of stimulation was chosen to permit complete SM relaxation between the stimuli and to avoid the SR decay. The acoustic stimulation was maintained for 15 min. and the SR was recorded at 1, 3, 5, 10 and 15 minutes. Moreover the some kind of testing was performed using 500 and 2000 Hz tone bursts respectively on 5 and 7 healtly subjects. A tympanometer with an X-Y plotter were used for response measuring and recording.

To make data amenable to statistical comparisons the figures of the SR amplitude at 3, 5, 10 and 15 minutes were calculated relatively to the SR amplitude at 1 minute which was considered equal to 10.

RESULTS

The amplitude of the SR consistently decreased under stimulation. This decrease occurred invariably and was directly related to the stimulation time. After 15 min. the SR amplitude was about 50 % of its 1 minute value.

No significant differences in this respect were observed between normoacusic and ipoacusic subjects. Similar results were also observed at 500 and 2000 Hz.

DISCUSSION

According to our observations, the SM contraction amplitude tend to decrease after repeated raise of the SR over a long-lasting time span.

We suggest that this phenomenon depends on incomplete relaxation and not on inadequate contraction of the SM. The muscle maintains a tonic contraction during the after-bursts pause so that the following stimulus induce a contraction of lesser amplitude. The stifness of stape would remain high notwithstanding the decrease in compliance variation which is detected by impedentiometry. The change in compliance on suspending the acoustic stimulation confirms this hypo tesis. Infact the SM completely relax after the last stimulus and the recording steeply attains to the starting baseline.

The observed phenomenon is clearly distinguishable from the SR decay as it looks dependent on muscle performance and not on the cochlear system or the afferent auditory pathway. Infact : - no differences were observed between normoacusic and ipoacusic subjects; - no differences were observed at 500,1000 and 2000 Hz.

CONCLUSIONS

Our observations confirm the effectiveness of the SR for protection from noise-induced hearing damage. Infact, during long-lasting acoustic stimulation the SM maintains a partial contracture also when the sound intensity lowers under the SRT. Consequently the rise time of the SR is shortened and the protection mechanism is improved.

REFERENCES

1. Lutman, N.E., Martin, N. (1978) J Sound Vib 56:137
2. Borg, E., Odman, B. (1979) Acta Otolaryngol (Stockh), 87:421
3. Borg, E. (1980) Acta Otolaryngol 90: 1-5

New dimensions in otorhinolaryngology - head and neck surgery, vol. 2.
E. Myers, editor

THE ACOUSTIC FUNCTION OF THE TRAGUS

MANABU HONDA, SUSUMU TSUKAHARA, IWAO OHTANI, JIN OUCHI
Fukushima Medical College, Fukushima 960 (Japan)

INTRODUCTION

The human tragus overhangs anterior to the external auditory canal. Thus it should be considered that the tragus is related to the acoustic function of the external ear. In these facts, we experimented on the acoustic function of the tragus.

EXPERIMENTAL APARATUS

In the present work, the sound source was used a loudspeaker driven by a signal generator (TECTRONIXS FG 504) and the frequency of the sound was modulated by linear ascending pulses repeatedly (frequency range was from 0.1 kHz to 10 kHZ). The sound pressure was measured by a very small electret condenser microphone (RION EU-22), so that it was able to placed in the external auditory canal. And obtained response were averaged and analyzed by a Analyzing Recorder (YEW MODEL 3655).

METHODS AND RESULTS

I.This experiment(Fig.1) was performed in a patient, who was resected of the tragus surgically. In this patient, an artificial tragus was applied to measure what influences the tragus gives on the acoustic function of the external ear. After addition of artificial tragus(Fig.1-b), the peak appeared at 2 to 3kHz ,shifted towards low frequency area by about 200Hz, and the gain in 4 to 8kHz increased by about 5dB. Moreover the response was made a flat response.

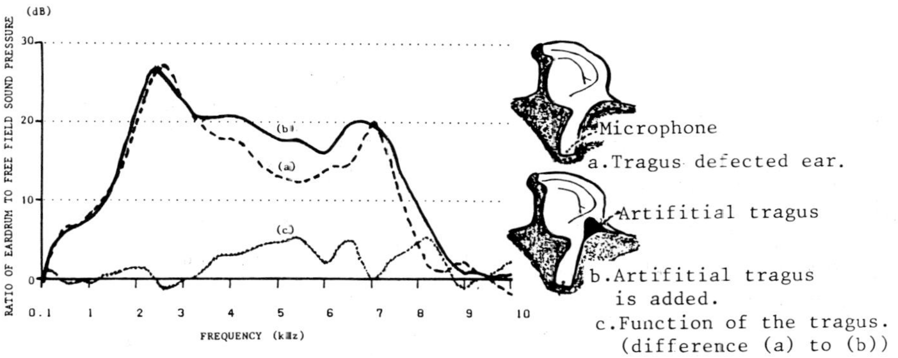

Fig.1 Response of the tragus defected ear, a-tragus defected ear, b-artifitial tragus is added and c-tragus effect.

II.This experiment was performed in 10 normal ears. These ears were made into the experimentally tragus defected ears by deflection of the tragus, and measured the function of the tragus. Similar to the previous experiment, according to presence or absence of the tragus the peak in the range of 2 to 3 kHz was shifted and the gain in the range up to 3 kHz was changed.

III.This experiment was used a silcon model (KOKEN LM#7 1202). This tragus was defected to measure function of the tragus. Similar to the results obtained from experiments in humans, according to presence or absence of the tragus the peak shifted and the gain increased.

IV.In order to measure what influences the tragus gives on various parts of the external ear, this experiment(Fig.2) was used a model of external auditory canal (plastic), concha (clay) and tragus (clay). The model of external auditory canal showed a single resonance at about 3.5kHz (Fig.2-a). When a model of concha was added to this canal model, the peak at 3.5 kHz was shifted towards the lower range slightly. And the second peak at 8 to 9 kHz was appeared(Fig.2-b). Then a tragus model was added to this model, and the peak observed at 3.5 kHz shifted further towards the lower range of about 3 kHz. In association with this change, the second peak and the gain showed elevation and shift. The gain in the range of 4 kHz to 6 kHz also, was increased and flatted (Fig.2-c).

These findings indicated as follows.

1.The tragus increased the acoustic length of the external auditory canal, and lowering the frequency of the canal resonance.

2.The tragus helped the acoustic function of the auricle, and it raised the acoustic response of 4 kHz to 8 kHz up to about 5 to 7dB.

3.The tragus formed part of horn shape of external ear, and it caused the acoustic response of the horn under 8 kHz to be a flat response.

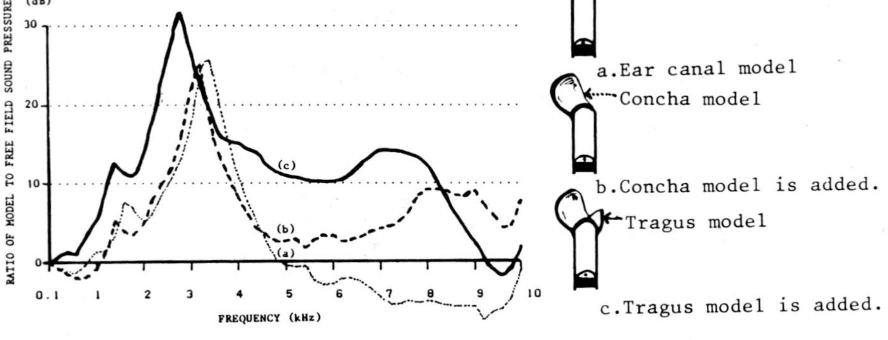

Fig.2 Response of the external ear model; a-ear canal model(plastic), b-concha model is added(clay) and c-tragus model is added.

New dimensions in otorhinolaryngology - head and neck surgery, vol. 2.
E. Myers, editor

SIMULTANEOUS MULTIFREQUENCY TYMPANOMETRY USING FOURIER TRANSFORMS OF BROAD-BAND NOISE

VERNON D. LARSON (1), DANIEL M. SCHWARTZ (2), J. DOUGLAS HARMON (3)

VA Medical Center (1,3), Augusta, GA 30910, USA; University of Pennsylvania School of Medicine (2), Philadelphia, PA, USA; and Medical College of Georgia, Augusta, GA, USA (1,3)

INTRODUCTION

A difference in static pressure across the tympanic membrane alters the primary resonance of the middle ear which, for the normal ear, occurs in the frequency region of 1200 Hertz. Colletti's (1,2,3) research demonstrated that the study of tympanometric data in the frequency region of the resonance often yields more diagnostic information than data derived from a single low frequency probe tone. The purpose of this paper is to describe tympanometric results obtained using a method by which as many as 400 tympanograms may be recorded simultaneously by analyzing the spectrum of a broad band noise.

MATERIALS AND METHODS

A white noise was delivered to ears using a standard admittance probe assembly (Grason Stadler, 1722) under static pressure conditions from -400 to +200 daPa. The noise was monitored using a miniature microphone in the assembly and was directed to analysis equipment which performed a Fast Fourier transform (B&K, Model 2033 Signal Analyzer). The digitized data were passed to a computer (Hewlett Packard, Model 1000F) for storage and conversion to tympanometric form. Up to 400 tympanograms could be made available by the computer for sequential viewing in a standard two-dimensional format. As an option, a series of tympanograms could be arrayed in three-dimensional form.

Eighteen normal adult subjects (9 males and 9 females) were studied. Each had hearing levels less than 15 dB from 250 to 8000 Hz and had normal, standard tympanograms and eardrum immittance. Each had middle ear pressures between -10 and +10 daPa. Six patients having a diagnosis of otosclerosis were also studied.

RESULTS

Figure 1 shows the mean tympanometric data for the group of 18 normal subjects presented in three-dimensional form. In general, and in agreement with previous observations (1,2,3), the curves (plotted for 31 frequencies in the range from 250 to 4000 Hz) show distinct pattern changes as a function of frequency. Specifically, for the low frequencies, the typical V-shaped configuration was recorded. Above 1200 Hertz, the curves assumed an inverted and V shape. At 3000 Hz, the tympanograms flattened. In the region of 2375 Hz, a trough was observed at the intersect of the +200 daPa condition. An analysis of the male and female data separately showed that the depth of this trough occurred at frequencies of 2250 and 2600 Hz for the males and females respectively. In addition, the bandwidth of this trough was narrower for the males (125 Hz) than for the females (375 Hz).

The six otosclerotic ears differed primarily and remarkably from the normals in the frequency at which the inverted V tympanogram occurred. In each case, the inverted V was established clearly at a much higher frequency (3000 Hz). More importantly, relatively flat tympanograms were observed over a broad frequency region between 1000 Hz to 3000 Hz.

This procedure appears to provide the same information as discrete high frequency tympanometry and offers the advantage of providing greater frequency resolution in a very short period of time (less than ten minutes per subject). The female - male differences may necessitate the establishment of normative data for each sex in order to differentiate accurately the pathologic ear. Studies to this end as well as studies of false negative and false positive rates associated with high frequency tympanometry are being conducted in our laboratories.

ACKNOWLEDGES

This work was supported by funding provided by the U.S. Veterans Administration Office of Rehabilitation Research and Development.

REFERENCES

1. Colletti V (1975) Acta Otolaryngol 80:54-60
2. Colletti V (1976) Audiology 15:106-119
3. Colletti V (1977) Audiology 16:278-287

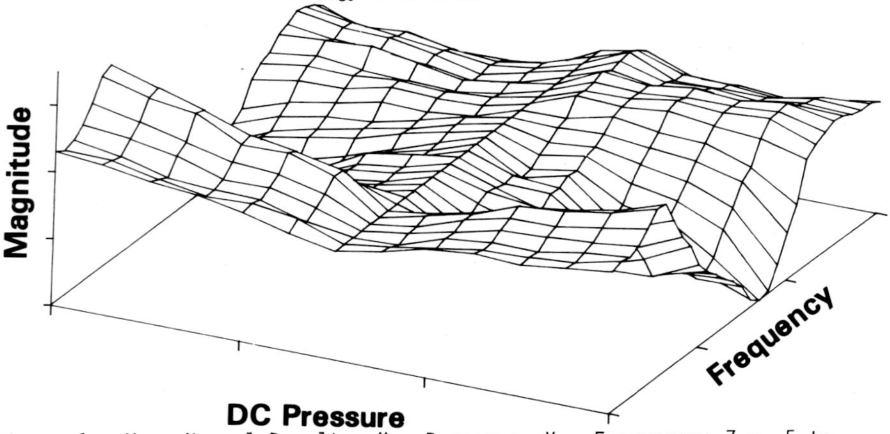

Figure 1. Mean Normal Result. X = Pressure; Y = Frequency; Z = -5 to +5 Decibels

New dimensions in otorhinolaryngology - head and neck surgery, vol. 2.
E. Myers, editor

AUDITORY BRAINSTEM RESPONSE RECOVERY FUNCTIONS IN MULTIPLE SCLEROSIS

JAMES F. LEFFINGWELL, M.D. AND STEVEN J. KRAMER, PH.D.

Department of Otolaryngology, University of Texas Medical Branch, Galveston, Texas 77550 U.S.A.

INTRODUCTION

In other evoked potential investigations of multiple sclerosis (MS), some patients have shown normal conventional auditory brainstem responses (ABR); however, by using other more "stressful" stimulus paradigms, such as fast repetition rates, these patients have indicated an abnormality in neural conduction, thus increasing the sensitivity of the ABR evaluation (1-2). In the present study, a non-conventional stimulus paradigm (forward masking) was used to measure how the response to one particular sound was affected by another preceeding sound as a function of the time delay between the 2 sounds (3). The purpose was to develop a means of temporally "stressing" the auditory system in order to provide a more sensitive measure of possible subtle neurological involvement in MS patients than conventional ABR.

SUBJECTS AND METHODS

Eight patients (mean age = 34 years) with normal otologic histories, normal hearing, and definite MS according to the criteria of McAlpine et al (4) and 27 normal control subjects (18 to 33 years of age) were studied. The probe stimuli used to evoke the ABRs were 0.1 msec broadband clicks presented at 50 dB HL. The masking stimuli were short-duration (60 ms) wideband noise-bursts with 10 ms rise-fall times. The noise-burst preceded the probe click by varying delay times ΔT. The values to ΔT used were 0, 5, 25, and 100 ms. Two responses at each ΔT, as well as unmasked responses, were obtained. Response averaging was done using a Nicolet CA1000. Mean latency shifts, relative to unmasked control, were analyzed using a repeated measures analysis of variance. Individual data for the MS patients were compared to the normal mean data and considered abnormal when greater than two standard deviations from the mean.

RESULTS

Compared to the control group, all 8 MS subjects had normal unmasked wave I latencies and 6 (75%) had normal unmasked wave V latencies. Thus only 25% of the clinical group had abnormal conventionally obtained ABR responses. Forward masking produced mean latency shifts for wave I and V in MS patients that were greater than those produced in controls. (Fig. 1) All latencies for all ΔTs for wave V were statistically significant at the 0.05 level of confidence. The wave I latencies were not statistically significant from normative data. Only one of the MS patients had an abnormal latency shift for wave I, when compared to normals, for temporally masked ABRs. However, 6 patients (75%) were abnormal, i.e., outside 2 S.D. of normal latency shifts at one or more ΔTs for wave V. (Fig. 2)

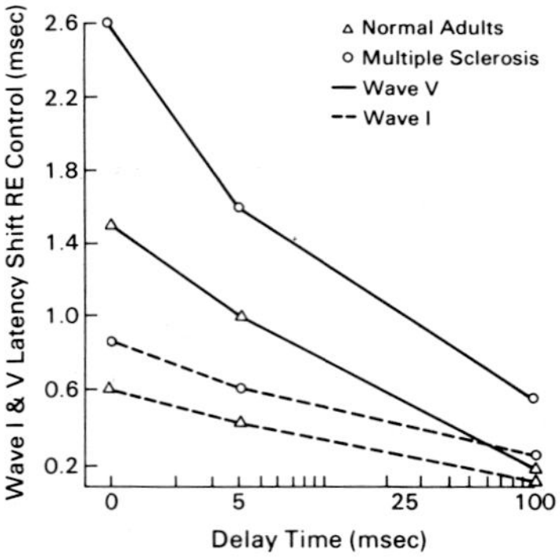

Fig. 1 Mean Latency Shifts

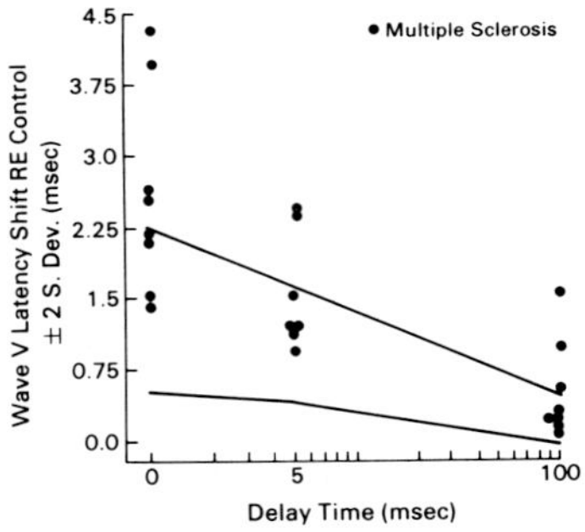

Fig. 2 Latency Shifts for MS Patients

COMMENTS

Intergroup comparisons disclose a distinct tendency for greater wave V forward masking latency shifts in patients with MS compared with normal control subjects, i.e., 4 additional patients (50%) were demonstrated to have subtle auditory impairment that could not be detected by conventional stimulus paradigms (unmasked responses). Moreover, the 2 patients who failed even the conventional ABR continued to fail using the more "stressful" auditory stimulus.

Demyelination produces an inability to transmit high-frequency trains of impulses throug nerve fibers because of an unusually prolonged refractory period, reduces an axon's maximu firing frequency, and results in temporal dispersion and desynchrony of neural impulses (6). Demyelination of the central (brainstem) auditory pathway could interfere with the precise neural timing relations that are necessary for ABR recordings. By "stressing" the temporal responding capabilities of the auditory pathways using forward masking, the neur synchrony is further disrupted and can enhance the sensitivity of the ABR to detect such deficits.

REFERENCES

1. Robinson, K. and Rudge, P.: Abnormalities of the auditory evoked potentials in patie with multiple sclerosis. Brain 100: 19-40 (1977).

2. Shanon, E; Gold, S.; Himelfarb, M.: Assessment of functional integrity of brainstem auditory pathways by stimulus stress. Audiology 20: 65-71 (1981).

3. Kramer, S. and Teas, D.: Forward masking of auditory nerve (N_1) and brainstem (wa V) responses in humans. J. Acoust. Soc. Am. 72: 795-803 (1982).[1]

4. McAlpine, D.; Lumsden, C.E.; Acheson, E.D.: Multiple Sclerosis: A Reappraisal, ed 2. New York. Churchill Livingston, 1972.

5. Waxman, S.G.: Membranes, myelin, and the pathophysiology of multiple sclerosis. New Engl. J. Med. 306: 1529-1533 (1982).

© 1985 Elsevier Science Publishers B.V. (Biomedical Division)
New dimensions in otorhinolaryngology - head and neck surgery, vol. 2.
E. Myers, editor

HIGH-FREQUENCY AUDIOMETRY IN CLINICAL PRACTICE

I. W. S. MAIR, E. LAUKLI

Department of Otorhinolaryngology, University of Tromsø, 9000 Tromsø (Norway)

INTRODUCTION

The conventional audiometric frequencies are at octave intervals from 0.125 to 8 kHz. The upper limit of the auditory range in man is around 20 kHz, at least in younger individuals, and is processed at the basal end of the cochlea.

Bredberg (1) has demonstrated a greater degree of inner hair cell degeneration in the basal coil of the human cochlea with increasing age. Contributing factors are: cochlear mechanics which ensure that this region of the basilar membrane will be activated irrespective of the stimulus frequency; the nearness of both the oval and round windows which results in an increased possibility of damage from excessive pressure fluctuations at the stapedial foot-plate or spread of infection through the round window, and the less well-developed vascular supply in this region (2).

METHODS AND RESULTS

Although high-frequency (HF) hearing was first tested in the nineteenth century, clinical interest has first arisen after the introduction of a commercial HF audiometer (3). We have used this instrument during the past three years, and first investigated the range of HF thresholds in young, otologically normal individuals. It became apparent that establishment of a zero dB hearing level is not meaningfull for these frequencies. Threshold reproducibility was next studied and proved to be of the same order of magnitude as for the conventional audiometric frequencies.

HF sensitivity becomes progressively poorer with increasing age, with lowering of the upper frequency limit of hearing, although individual variability is considerable.

We have studied 300 noise-exposed workers in addition to a number of subjects following impulse trauma. The latter produces threshold elevation throughout the HF range, while steady-state noise-induced hearing loss (NIHL) is characterised by the typical symmetrical dip at 3-6 kHz, and relative threshold preservation at the higher frequencies. We have not been able to reproduce the HF steady-state NIHL reported by others, and agree with Osterhammel's (4) conclusion that HF audiometry cannot be used as an early indicator of individual susceptibility to steady-state NIHL.

It is not possible with this instrument to differentiate between middle ear transmission effects on HF thresholds and the possible sensorineural results of inner ear involvement. A solution to this problem may be provided by the recently introduced electric transduction audiometer (5).

The effects of surgery have also been studied. Traumatic tympanic membrane rupture from fireworks may produce threshold elevation at all frequencies, which is restored to normal values in the lower frequencies after successful myringoplasty, but remains unchanged in the HF range, presumably indicating an impulse NIHL. Following stapedectomy for otosclerosis, threshold improvement is also found by conventional audiometry, while deterioration is typical in the higher frequencies. A comparison was therefore made of threshold changes throughout the frequency range 0.25-20 kHz following stapedectomy (n=28) and myringoplasty (n=36). Threshold improvement was significantly greater at the frequencies 0.25-4 kHz following stapedectomy, while post-operative hearing loss was less in the 8-20 kHz range after myringoplasty.

This is the first report in which pre- and post-operative threshold comparisons have been extended into the HF range, and confirms the greater risk of inner ear trauma following oval window surgery. HF audiometry may be useful as a monitor of surgical techniques.

REFERENCES

1. Bredberg G (1968) Acta Otolaryngol Suppl 236: 1-135
2. Axelsson A (1968) Acta Otolaryngol Suppl 243: 1-134
3. Fausti SA, Frey RH, Erickson DA, Rappaport BZ, Cleary EJ (1979) J Acoust Soc Am 66: 1713-1718
4. Osterhammel D (1979) Scand Audiol 8: 85-90
5. Tonndorf J, Kurman B (1984) Ann Otol Rhinol Laryngol 93: 576-582

© 1985 Elsevier Science Publishers B.V. (Biomedical Division)
New dimensions in otorhinolaryngology – head and neck surgery, vol. 2.
E. Myers, editor

CLINICAL APPLICATION OF SUMMATING POTENTIAL IN THE DIAGNOSIS OF INNER EAR DISEASES

TORU OHASHI, NOBUO YOSHIE, KAZUTO SHIMADA
Dept. Otolaryngology, Institute of Clinical Medicine, University of Tsukuba, Ibaraki (Japan)

INTRODUCTION

It has been made clear that a study of the SP in electrocochleogram can provide diagnostically the useful information about inner ear pathology. However, a variability of the absolute SP amplitude among subjects has become a kind of problem for the clinical application of the SP. In an attempt to reduce this variability, the measure of the SP/AP ratio is expected to become a useful diagnostic indicator. This study aimed to examine the diagnostic efficiency of the SP/AP ratio and the SP amplitude in inner ear diseases.

METHODS

Transtympanic electrocochleography was performed on 23 normal ears, 24 ears affected by clinically defined Ménière's disease and 25 ears affected by hair cell destruction without any evidence of endolymphatic hydrops. Tonebursts having 2 wave rise-fall time and 8 msec duration for the frequencies of 2, 4, 6, 8 kHz were used as acoustic stimuli.

RESULTS

1) The changes of the SP/AP ratio were observed as a function of toneburst frequency in normal ears. It became clear that the SP/AP ratio at 2 kHz, 4 kHz toneburst stimulation showed the larger values measurable with certainty and that the SP/AP ratio at 6 kHz, 8 kHz toneburst stimulation was highly variable among subjects including both the negative and the positive SP/AP ratio. The SP/AP ratio at the latter stimulation was considered to be clinically less useful.

2) As for the effect of interstimulus interval (ISI) upon the SP/AP ratio, it almost unchanged at the ISI of higher than 100 msec, while it increased remarkably at the ISI of lower than 80 msec.

3) The SP/AP ratio and the SP amplitude were measured as a function of stimulus intensity for 4 kHz toneburst at 30 msec ISI between two pathclogical ears groups. Fig 1 demonstrates the measure of the SP/AP ratio. The indivisual curves were judged to be abnormal if they fell outside ± 2 SD (Standard Deviation) normal limits indicated by dark area in this fig. 75% of the curves appeared above normal limits in Ménière ears group, while in hair cell loss ears group most curves (77%) were in normal limits. Fig 2 shows the input-output curves of the

SP amplitudes superimposed on ± 1 SD normal limits (dark area in this fig). 58% of the curves were in normal limits in Ménière ears group, while 79% of the curves appeared below normal limits in the hair cell loss ears group.

CONCLUSION

Our results made it clear that the SP/AP ratio could serve as an efficient diagnostic indicator to separate the Ménière ears and the hair cell loss ears but that it could not differenciate the hair cell loss ears from the normal ears. The SP amplitude was a useful indicator to differentiate the hair cell loss ears from the normal ears.

Fig. 1

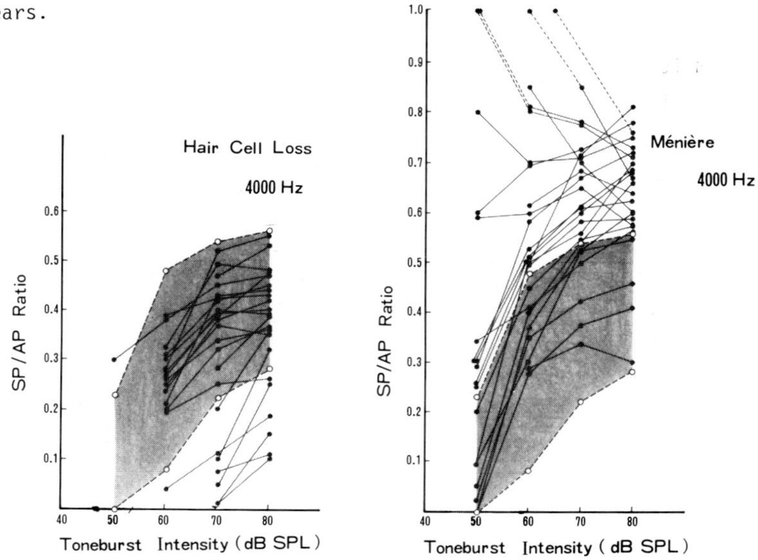

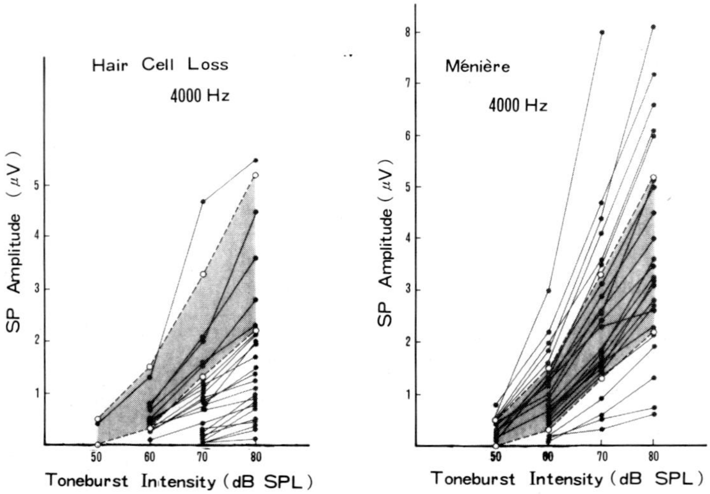

Fig. 2

New dimensions in otorhinolaryngology - head and neck surgery, vol. 2.
E. Myers, editor

DUST PRODUCED DEAFNESS - AN ENTITY IN THE INDUSTRIAL COMPLEX IN COMPARISON TO NOISE INDUCED DEAFNESS

DR.S.S.BHUTADA
Chairman & Head - Institute of Research in ORL, Pune 411002, INDIA

INTRODUCTION

Hearing and Sight vital gifted senses to human being carries tremendous importance in the modern life. Ambient noise includes all sounds present in an environment. Usually not acceptable, has proved more dangerous and is increasing with industrial growth leads to deafness. When deafness is considered with Industrial Noise Induced Deafness is the one which strikes to our mind and Dust Produced Deafness comes with Question? What is it? Is it ever possible? Dust Produced Deafness is an hearing impairment found in workers, farmers working in dusty zones - or dust polluted area of factories. Dust is evolved in many factories. Amongst the few which we have studied were Chemical, Textile, Snuff (Tobacco Powder), Paprika, Saw, Agarbatti, etc. Threshold level values are crossed in many such Industries beyond our imagination at the work place. It is needless to say that it carries definate impact on the organ exposed to it. The question is to what extent ?

Every Individual on this earth inhales approx. 10,000 to 12,000 litres of air per day. Workers at polluted working place working at least 8 hours a day inhales the dust to what extent can be measured with the specific formula. Dust particles are airborn and settles only under the influence of gravity - inertia - sedimentation and diffusion. Deposition of dust in upper respiratory tract is the result of physical laws and patterns of Anatomical structure of nose, throat and ear and diameter and density of the particulate. More than 5 to 15 diameter particles gets deposited in Nasal x Pharyngelary. Dust loading subject depends on its mean level & duration of service.

Varieties of dust - gases, fumes, smokes evolved during production comes in contact with upper respiratory mucosa as it is first area to bear the brunt of effects of such material from industries. Till recently effects of URT region is neglected to the great extent and it carries more importance as important organ like Ear, Nose and Throat lies in this area. Hence it is time to realise and recognise the importance of E.N.T. in Occupational Health.

Mechanism : Patho-Physiological changes in U.R.T. Release due to industrial dust.

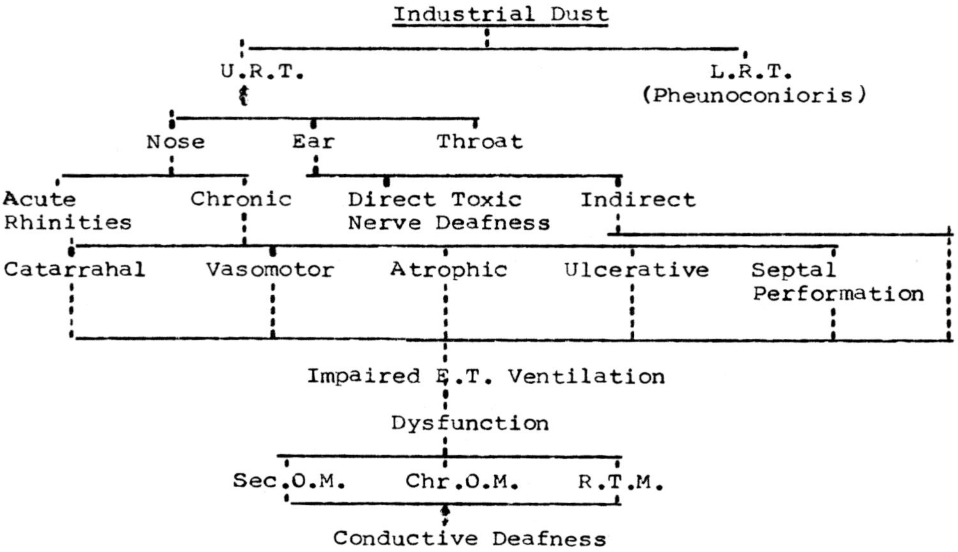

Methodology of Study : (1) Clinical Examination, (2) Histopathology, (3) Pathological Routine Investigations, (4) Ultra Microscopy.

Demographic Aspect : Results of Clinical Observations :-
Total Workers : 2150 from Dusty Zones, Factories : a) Chemical-750, b) Textile-400, c) Snuff-500, d) Others-500.
Age : 18 to 50 years, Sex : Male 96%, Female 4%
Low Socio-Economic Group : Income Rs.40-60/Capita, Duration of Exposure to dust - 5 years to 35 years, (a) H/o Smallpox - 0.1%, (B) H/o Smoking - 83% (Tobacco Chewing 63%).
Symptoms : (1) Loss of Hearing - 74%, (2) Rhinorrhea Sneezing - 60%, (3) Nasal Obst. - 54%, (4) Blocking of Ears - 39%, (5) Tinnitus-24%, (6) Otorrhea - 10%, (7) Cough - 18%, (8) Non-Nasal Sympt.-30%, (9) H/o Attacks of VMR - 20%, (10) Irritable Throat or Maggoty Sensation - 30% : a) Chemical-16, b) Textile-34, c) Snuff-86,d)Eng-4

Results of Clinical Observations : Lab Investigation :-
1) Mild Anaemia Hb 124 m% - 38%, 2) Eosinopilia - 68% (Court Rise 6 to 34%), 3) V.D.R.L. - +2%, 4) Evidence of other E.B., Leprosy ETC-2%, 5) X-Rays Sinuses Bil Maxillary : i) Sinusitis-36%, ii) Unil(R) 20%, iii) Unil (L)- 3%, 6) X-Ray Chest Pneumonitis - 32 (Textile 18%) 7) Urine - ALB +2%, Sugar + 2.5%, 8) X-Ray Mastoid : Chr.Mastoidities (UNI)-10%, 9) Microchrome Test - XE.

<u>Sputum Exam</u> : Exfoliative Cytology of Workers : a) Industrial Chemical - 23% Metaplasia c̄ Atypia, b) Snuff - 10% Metaplasia c̄ Atypia
Nasal Smear : a) Chemical - 13% Metaplasia c̄ Atypia.
b) Snuff - Eosinophilia - 18%.

<u>Types of Deafness in Industries</u> :
(1) Conductive, (2) Sensori neural, (3) Mixed

CONCLUSIONS

1) Dust Produced Deafness in workers is found in factories where dust is evolved and beyond T.L.V. values.
2) Clinical Examination of Ear - Ear drum with the help of magnification is must to know the pathological status of Middle Ear & will be a differentiating point from Noise Induced Deafness.
3) Audiometric Examination is must and reveals the type of Deafness. Tympanometry reveals middle ear functional status will be a diagnostic feature.
4) Pre-employment ENT & Audiological checkup will be useful as a diagnostic feature in doubtful cases.
5) Noise Induced Deafness is permanent entity and not curable while Dust Produced Deafness is curable.
6) Early detection by periodic examination of High Risk worker will be a major step towards prevention of Dust Produced Deafness.
7) Protection of High Risk Workers from dust by : (A) 1. Education of use of Dust Mask, 2. Good House Keeping in factories.
(B) Reduction dust evolution : i) by redesigning of machines,
ii) by good ventilation system of work places.
8) Efficient Glowing Health of worker is key towards gain of High Production.

REFERENCES

1. Dr.Bhutada S.S. - Study of Effects of Chemical Dust in ENT Region - Jr. Indian Assoc. of Occup. Health - Nov/Dec 1978.
2. Bhutada S.S. - 'Effects of Snuff Tobacco Powder on URT Mucosa'.
3. A Cuschier & Baker - Introduction to Research in Medical Science - 1978.
4. T.Egami, I.Lande & J.Sobel - 'Noise Induced Hearing Loss' - A human temporal bone case report. Jr.of Occup.Med.Vol.21/No.7/ July 1979.
5. L.E.Humes & H.F.Bess : Noise & Hearing, Jr. of Occup. Medicine Vol.21/No.7/July 1979.
6. D.R.R.Muir - Clinical Aspects of Inhaled Particles - Page 8 to 12

New dimensions in otorhinolaryngology - head and neck surgery, vol. 2.
E. Myers, editor

PREVENTION OF SENSORINEURAL DEAFNESS

D.Dimov T.Shirov

ENT Research Institute,Medical Academy,

Sofia,Bulgaria

Hearing in people has an important socil function.A loss of hearing causes severe,irreversible changes in an individual's psychology and behaviour,and badly damages his social capabilities. Sensorineural deafness is a poliethiological ilness.A detailed knowledge of its causes allows us to minimise these of them we can influence and in this way to reduce the number of suffers.Hence in this work we aim to select those ethiological moments which we can influence and in this way to construct a systematic programme for the prevention of this illness.

Materials and Metods.

The investigation was conducted on 1500 patients with sensorineural hearing damage who we have been examining over the last ten years in the otoneurological and audiological department of the ENT Research Institute of the Medical Academy,Sofia,Bulgaria. The average age those investigated was 36 years old ranging from 3 to 58.We noticed that the majority of sufferers were men with the man-woman ratio of 1,56:1.This corresponds with the findings of Oda (1980) who reports a ratio of 1,47:1.

We started our investigations with detailed case histories. We took particular interest in the age at which deafness set in, and in the causes for such occurrences.In case of hereditary deafness we looked in addition into family histories for the detection of similar cases.We made medico-genetic investigationes into some of them in order to proove family predisposition to such illnesses.

Objective investigation consisted of a thorough otolaryngological examination to find out the exact state of these organs. Hearing examinations included tonal theshold audiometry on all the patients and when necessary we employed evoked response audiometry (ERA) and the SISI-test.

For the detection and detailing of the ethiological moments we made some additional investigations-virusological, rentgenological, toxicologocal, REG etc.

Results.

According to the age when deafness occured the results are as follows: up to 1 yearold-550 (37%), up to 2 years-275 (18%), up to 3 years-230 (15%), up to 5 years-135 (9%), up to 10 years-110 (7%), up to 20 years-75 (5%) and over 20 years-125 (9%).

The most common cause for hearing loss was infectional-toxicologocal. For example we observed sudden loss of hearing during viral infections in 146 cases (9%) and during infectious diseases in 270 cases (18%). Examples of the latter kind of disease included meningitis-110 patients, measles-58 patients, scarlet fever-45 patients, pertusis-27 patients and parotitis-30 patients. The average percentage of above-mentioned diseases was 27%.

Vascular causes accounted for 330 patients (22%). We have observed hearing impairments during hipertonic and hipotonic illnesses and also in vertebro-basilar insuffitiency.

Toxic agents played a part in 275 patients (18%). These are most often ototoxic drugs like antibiotics Neomycin, Streptomycin, Gentamycin, Collimycin, Kanamycin, Monomycin; antitumor drugs-Bleomycin, Vancomycin etc. In two cases the onset of the illness was coused by the taking of salicilates and in the three other couses-furosemid.

In 12%-180 patients impairment of hearing was caused by acute and chronic inflammations of the middle ear. Otogenic intracranial complicationsas a rule also caused hearing loss.

In 195 patients (13%) trauma was observed.8% of our patients suffered hearing ioss after head injuries and 3%-after acute noise trauma.

In 1% of cases we discovered a tumor-neurinoma nervus stato-acusticus.

In 2% one or both parents had hearing problems.

In 15%-195 patients we couldn't discover the exact reson for hearing disorder.

In 675 patients (45%) there was total deafness e.g.hearing threshold over 90 dB.,while in 825 patients (55%) we detected residual hearing in the range of 60-90 dB.

Discussion.

As we can see from the results above,hearing in childhood is more vulnerable than in adulthood.In the first three years of life about 70% of our patients lost their hearing.This can be explained by the more damaging course of the infectious disease at this age and the weaker resistance of the child's organism.Hence we have to put all our efforts into taking proper precautions with pregnant women and with young children.It is necessary to minimise the taking of drugs during the first three months of pregnancy and in particular to avoid completely all ototoxic drugs.Prgnant women have to be removed immidiately from work-places in when the following agents can be found-some chemical substances,gasses,radioactiv substances etc.In the cases of deaf parents or relations we have to make medico-genetic investigations.Alcohol and cigarette-smoking should be discouraged,and all infectious diseases should be properly treated during the period of pregnancy.

In early childhood it is necessary to prescribe antibiotics only in individual cases and with strict controls.Regular vaccination and immunisation reduces the severity of the most common infectious diseases.We must take special care of the newly-born child of deaf parents in whom we might suspect heriditary problems.The same care must be taken of these children whose mothers suffered damaging effects during pregnancy.We have to provide antiviral profilaxy during viral epidemics.It is important to treat in good time all naso-pharyngeal diseases and to do all we can to prevent ear inflammation.

In adults the effect of infectious diseases decreases ang the influence of vascular,toxic and proffesional factors increases.We must regularly give hearing test to those patients taking certain antibiotics,antitumor drugs and also those having undergone radiotherapy.We must treat in a good time all middle ear inflammations and also prevent as early as possible vascular diseases of the CNS. It is futhermore essential to treat systematicaly and in good time all chronic cardio-vascular diseses diabetes and hipertonia.Special attention must be payd to hearing impairment during viral epydemics. Excessive noise should be eleminated and traumatism and occupational injuries should be reduced.

The systematic and purposeful application of such precautions in all levels of the medical service should reduce the relative number of these severe,crippling illnesses.

© 1985 Elsevier Science Publishers B.V. (Biomedical Division)
New dimensions in otorhinolaryngology – head and neck surgery, vol. 2.
E. Myers, editor

THE UNDERSTANDING OF RUNNING SPEECH WITHOUT LIPREADING BY MULTI-CHANNEL COCHLEAR PROSTHESIS PATIENTS

T.J. REDHEAD, R.C. DOWELL, G.M. CLARK, A.M. BROWN, B.C. PYMAN and R.L. WEBB

Department of Otolaryngology, University of Melbourne, Parkville, Victoria, 3052, Australia

INTRODUCTION

The aim of the University of Melbourne cochlear implant project is to enable patients to communicate not only with the aid of lipreading but with auditory input alone. This paper describes studies aimed at assessing this ability in a series of patients. The patients were 14 profoundly postlingually deaf patients who obtained no significant benefit from conventional hearing aids. They were the first 14 patients to receive the 22-channel prosthesis which has been developed by the University of Melbourne and Cochlear Corporation. The engineering of the prosthesis (1), the biological safety issues (2), and the surgical technique (3) have been addressed elsewhere.

METHOD

Patients were assessed postoperatively using the speech tracking technique (4) under conditions of lipreading alone, lipreading with the prosthesis and, for four patients, prosthesis alone. These four had shown good ability to understand speech without lipreading. Patients were also assessed using the open set CID everyday sentence test (5).

RESULTS

Table 1 shows the speech tracking results for two groups of patients: Group A who were able to perform very well with prosthesis alone, and Group B who were only tested with lipreading. For both groups, a highly significant improvement is seen when the prosthesis is combined with lipreading ($p < 0.001$). The Group A patients perform better with the prosthesis alone than with lipreading alone.

TABLE 1
SPEECH TRACKING (WORDS/MIN)

GROUP	LIPREADING ALONE	LIPREADING PROSTHESIS	PROSTHESIS ALONE
A	15.9	53.2	21.5
B	18.3	42.1	–

The mean scores for open set sentence testing using untrained material are given in Table 2 for preoperative, three-month postoperative and twelve-month postoperative testing. All patients were able to recognize some of this material with the prosthesis alone. The Group A patients performed significantly better ($p < 0.01$) and both groups improved significantly from three to twelve months postoperatively ($p < 0.01$).

TABLE 2
OPEN SET CID SENTENCE TEST (%)

GROUP	PREOPERATIVE	3 MONTHS	6 MONTHS
A	0	38.5	71.5
B	0	6.2	22.0

DISCUSSION

It is clear that a proportion of deaf patients using the multi-channel cochlear prosthesis are able to understand running speech without lipreading. These patients perform significantly better on most of the speech tests. They do not differ significantly in age from the others, but their mean length of profound deafness is significantly less than the rest of the patients, and this may be a factor affecting the performance. The cochlear prosthesis allows the four best patients to carry out interactive conversations on the telephone. Most of the other patients can also use the telephone, but need a highly contextual situation. It is apparent that the multi-channel cochlear prosthesis can be seen as more than an aid to lipreading, particularly for recently deafened patients.

REFERENCES

1. Money, D.K. (1984) Adv. Audiol. 2: 145-147.
2. Shepherd, R.K., Clark, G.M., and Black, R.C. (1983) Acta Otolaryngol. Suppl. 399: 19-31.
3. Clark, G.M., Pyman, B.C., Webb, R.L., Bailey, Q.E. and Shepherd, R.K. (1984) Ann. Otol. Rhinol. Laryngol. 93(3): 204-207.
4. De Filippo, C.L. and Scott, B.L. (1978) J. Acoust. Soc. Am. 63: 1186-1192.
5. Davis, H. and Silverman, S.R. (1970) In: Hearing and Deafness. Holt, Rhinhart and Winston, New York.

© 1985 Elsevier Science Publishers B.V. (Biomedical Division)
New dimensions in otorhinolaryngology – head and neck surgery, vol. 2.
E. Myers, editor

DIFFERENTIAL DIAGNOSIS OF SENSORY-NEURAL HEARING LOSS

DR. L. H. HIRANANDANI

Madam Cama Road, Bombey 400 039 INDIA

DISCUSSION

There are two aspects to this: 1) to identify the causative agent, and 2) to locate the site of lesion. Is it in the end organ, the eighth nerve or the pons and midbrain?

The patients are subdivided into age groups: 6 months, 6 years, 14 years, 30-40 years.

Six Month Olds

In most cases only when the child is 6 months old, the mother finally discovers that the baby cannot hear. A brainstem evoked response is performed and diagnosis is confirmed.

In order to identify the causative agent, the following is investigated: the mother's health during pregnancy; history of birth trauma, and of deep jaundice soon after birth.

If all of these prove normal, the diagnosis is genetic disorder. History of consanguenous marriage or other children born deaf is helpful. Finally, the genetic specialist studies the problem to pinpoint the actual defect.

Six Year Olds

The majority of our Indian patients are first seen at this age. There is a history of infection which may be viral and bacteria, such as different types of meningitis, tuberculosis, typhoid, measles and many others.

History shows that the child could hear and talk until the age of 2 years, but became deaf following infection.

Fifteen Year Olds

At age 15 years, the cause is again infection; the child could have developed unilateral deafness due to land noise from firecrackers. The other cause is mumps; the unilateral deafness is accidentally detected because the hearing in one ear was lost at the age of two and was due to mumps.

Thirty to Forty Year Olds

Between ages 30 and 40 it is due to Meniere's disease or eighth nerve tumor. The differentiating points are known to otologists.

Over Forty

Above 40 the cause is vascular pathology. Presbycusis is known. We have come to the conclusion that it could be spasm and/or thrombosis of the internal auditory artery. This can be compared to the coronary artery. Such patients may be hypertensive, diabetic, over-weight and have high blood lipids.

Syphilis as the cause must be excluded. Other causes due to ototoxic drugs and noise should also be investigated.

Temporary deafness with or without giddiness could be attributed to serotonin deficiency as in cases of migraine. Three such patients, suffering from migraine for several years, with a history of aura affecting the cerebrum, such as amblyopia, now have temporary deafness, tinnitus and giddiness followed by headache. The author feels that the site of action due to serotonin deficiency has shifted from the cerebral vessels to the internal auditory artery. This needs biochemical research.

The author considers this to be a new observation which, to their knowledge, has not been reported in the literature.

© 1985 Elsevier Science Publishers B.V. (Biomedical Division)
New dimensions in otorhinolaryngology - head and neck surgery, vol. 2.
E. Myers, editor

TOPOGRAPHIC RECORDING OF AUDITORY BRAINSTEM RESPONSE

KAZUHITO SHIMADA, TORU OHASHI AND NOBUO YOSHIE

Department of Otorhinolaryngology, University of Tsukuba School of Medicine, Sakura-mura, Ibaraki 305 (Japan)

INTRODUCTION

Recent advances in technology have made it possible to collect abundant ABR information at one time with multi-channel recording. With the purpose of clarifying the nature of scalp distribution of ABR in mind, computer maps (topograms) based on reference-invariant recordings were composed in this study.

MATERIALS AND METHODS

Simultaneous, 16-channel ABR recordings of 14 adults with normal hearing were studied. Acoustic clicks with an intensity of 70 dBnHL were presented monaurally and binaurally through headphones. Scalp electrodes were located according to the 10-20 system (Fig.5). A non-cephalic reference was placed at the laryngeal prominence. An aluminum foil strip with ECG paste was wound around the neck to bypass ECG and EMG noise currents. Each set of sixteen Jewett wave V peak amplitudes was mapped by computer.

RESULTS

The laryngeal prominence reference was contaminated with noise; however, the metal neck belt was effective in reducing it (Fig.1). Topograms in Fig.2 are based on wave V amplitudes averaged over the 14 normal subjects. Note the difference between Fig.2A and Fig.3; source derivation delineates details of the distribution. Fig.4 is an example of a peak latency topogram.

DISCUSSION

Since the origins of ABR components are deeply seated in the volume conductor of the brain and the skull, careful consideration is essential for the interpretation of an ABR topogram. The techniques employed in this study suggest a plausible methodological approach. It was revealed that the topograms are similar for monaural stimulation in either side, though there is slight asymmetry; bilateral stimulation is a somewhat different case.

The use of ABR topography as a clinical neurophysiological tool however, still leaves much room for improvement.

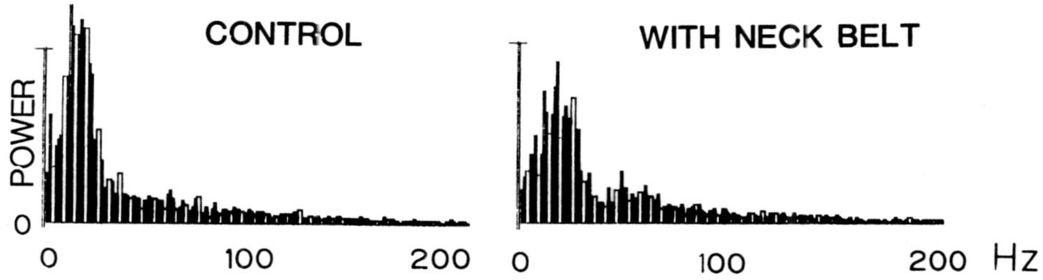

Fig. 1. Power spectra of background noise.

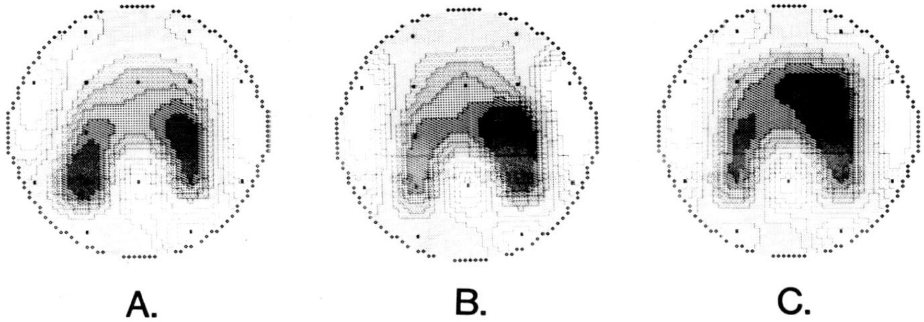

Fig. 2. Source derivation topogram of wave V.
A: Right ear stimulation. B: Left ear stimu. C: Bilateral ear stimu.

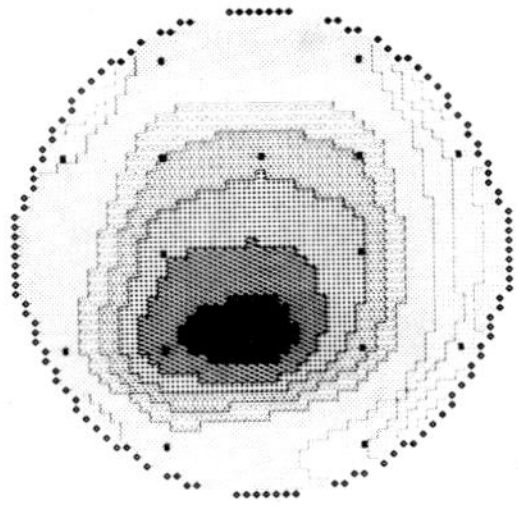

Fig. 3. Average potential reference topogram of wave V; from the same data as Fig. 2A.

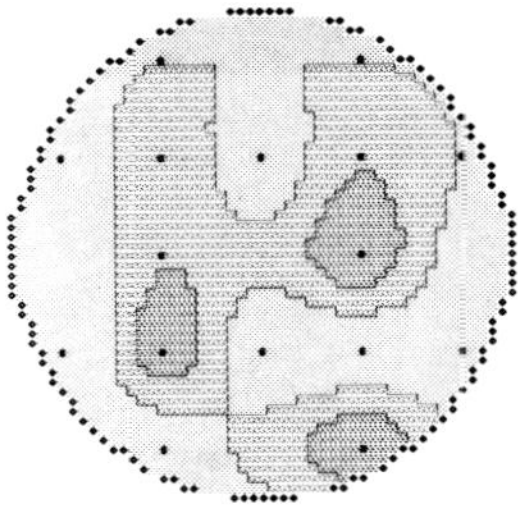

Fig. 4. Peak latency topogram of wave V.
Pz = 0 μs
48 μs/contour

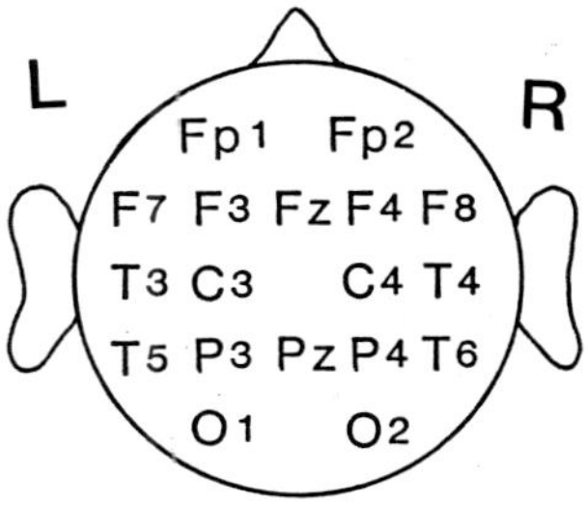

Fig. 5. Montage.

© 1985 Elsevier Science Publishers B.V. (Biomedical Division)
New dimensions in otorhinolaryngology – head and neck surgery, vol. 2.
E. Myers, editor

RELATIONSHIP BETWEEN AUDITORY BRAINSTEM RESPONSE ABNORMALITIES AND PURE-TONE AUDIOMETRY

TOSHIAKI YAGI.,SHUNKICHI BABA.,YUZURU KOBAYASHI., & HIDEYUKI AOKI
Department of Otolaryngology, Nippon Medical School
1-1-5 Sendagi, Bunkyo-ku Tokyo 113 (Japan)

INTRODUCTION

The auditory brainstem response (ABR) is one of the response that can be evoked from the auditory nerve and successive brainstem auditory structures by sound stimuli. There have been many reports on the relationship between the pure-tone threshold and ABR threshold, and close values of the threshold of these two tests have been demonstrated. Regarding the pure-tone audiometry in patients with ABR wave abnormalities, however, there have been few investigations, except for a report presenting several pure-tone audiograms in cases that showed ABR abnormalities. In this study, we are trying to analyze and clarify the relationship between ABR abnormalities, which are partial wave disappearance (only wave I response, wave I-III responses, and wave I-IV responses) and marked prolongation of the interwave latency, and the results of pure-tone audiometry.

MATERIALS AND METHODS

The subjects of the study were 43 ears in 30 patients who showed partial wave disappearance or marked interwave latency prolongation of wave I to V of their ABRs in the unilateral or bilateral ears. In all of these patients, relaibale results of standard pure-tone audiometry were obtained.

Eighteen patients had lesions in the cerebellopontine angle. They comprised acoustic tumor, epidermoid tumor, facial neuroms, meningioma, and stenosis of the internal auditory meatus. The others were pontine gloma, degenerative disease, vascular lesions, sphenoid ridge meningioma and unknown origin.

RESULTS

Patients with only wave I response

Wave I response alone was observed in 14 ears of 12 cases. Among them, there were several subjects who showed wave I and II responses. We classified these as only wave I response, since, even in normal subjects wave II could not be recorded frequently. Thus we thought that, in this study, it was meaningless to separate these conditions as different categories of response. The pure-tone threshold of these ears exhibited various degrees from almost normal to total loss. The mean and SD of the average hearing level of five frequencies (250-4000 Hz) were 52.2±25.1 dB.

Patients with waves I-III responses

There were only four ears in four patients showed wave I through III. The hearing level of these cases was almost normal. The mean and SD of average hearing level were 26.8±12.9 dB.

Patients with waves I-IV responses

Ten ears in nine patients exhibited wave I through IV responses. The hearing level of these patients was almost normal. The mean and SD of average hearing level were 14.4±4.0 dB.

Patients with marked interwave latency prolongation

Obious prolongation of the interwave latency was observed 15 ears in 12 cases. In this study, a response showing more than 4.5 ms in the interwave latency of I to V was categorized as marked interwave latency prolongation. The audiogram resembled that of the only wave I response, that is, hearing level in this group ranged from normal to showing profound hearing loss. The mean and SD of the average hearing level were 38.5±30.7 dB.

DISCUSSION

Click-evoked ABR is the sum of the neural activity of the auditory nerve and/or the brainstem auditory pathways synchronized with click stimuli. The number of neurons which synchronized with click stimuli, decreased gradually towards the higher hierachy of brainstem auditory structures. This means that neurons compose ABR wave form were part of the auditory neurons. Thus, if these neurons are damaged by some reason, other auditory neurons remain intact. Therefore, it is understandable that there should be pathological conditions that show normal audiogram with abnormal ABR wave form.

The pure-tone threshold in cases with waves I-III and I-IV were almost normal. On the other hand, that in cases with only wave I and marked I-V latency prolongation were in a wide range. Among them, subjects with internal auditory canal pathology showed moderate to profound hearing loss. Thus, cases with ABR abnormalties, partial wave disappearance and marked interwave latency prolongation, commonly exhibited a normal pure-tone audiogram, except for those with internal auditory canal pathclogy.

New dimensions in otorhinolaryngology - head and neck surgery, vol. 2.
E. Myers, editor

PRESENCE OF IMMUNOGLOBULINS (IgA, IgG) AND SECRETORY COMPONENT IN THE HUMAN ENDOLYMPHATIC SAC

W.J. ARNOLD[1] and H.J. ALTERMATT[2]

Depts. of Otolaryngology[1] and Pathology[2], Kantonsspital, CH-6000 Lucerne, Switzerland

INTRODUCTION

A few experiments have been figured out to prove the existence of a local inner ear system capable of autonomous immune reactions. Thus, the inner ear of the guinea pig appears to be capable of a specific, autonomous humoral immune response, as shown by Harris [2,3]. The site of antibody production, however, is unknown. Therefore, we have looked for the three main immunoglobulin classes (IgA,IgG,IgM) and for the secretory component (SC) of IgA in the human endolymphatic sac by two different immunohistochemical methods.

MATERIALS AND METHODS

Endolymphatic sacs of adult persons without known diseases of middle or inner ear were removed at autopsy and fixed for 3 h (formaldehyd 40%, 10ml; mercuric-(II)-chloride, 6g; glacial acetic acid, 5ml; distilled water, to a total volume of 100ml), rinsed for 21 h in ethyl alcohol (70%), and processed for conventional histology. Deparaffinized sections were stained for IgA, IgG, IgM and SC by two different methods. (1) Direct method with a 1:100 dilution of antisera (rabbit anti-human sera, Dakopatts, Copenhagen, Denmark) and fluorescein isothiocyanate as fluorochrome. (2) The indirect PAP (peroxidase-antiperoidase) method with a 1:1,1000 antiserum dilution. The usual positive and negative controls were included at each examination.

RESULTS

Both immunohistochemical stains reveal the presence of IgA and SC (Fig.1) at identical locations, namely in the epithelial layer and in the lumen of the endolymphatic sac, particularly of the proximal part. There are plasma cells with cytoplasmic IgA in the perisaccular region. A marked IgG-positivity appears in several perisaccular cells, in the nùmerous lymph- vessels, in the vicinity of the basement membrane of the epithelium, and in epithelial cells, mainly of the distal endolymphatic sac. The stains for IgM are negativ.

DISCUSSION

The presence of IgA and of SC in epithelial cells and in the lumen of the endolymphatic sac strongly suggests an active secretion of IgA into the endolymph, as demonstrated by two different methods. The IgG found in lymph vessels and in the epithelium of the endolymphatic sac may be of systemic origin. The synthesis of SC by epithelial cells such as those of digestive, respiratory and female reproductive tract has extensively been demonstrated, mainly by immunohistochemical methods, including ultrastructural studies [1]. The existence of a similar secretory process within the endolymphatic sac is the most likely explanation of our immunohistochemical findings. We are not aware of previous studies demonstrating the presence of secretory IgA in the endolymph in man. IgA, presumably derived from perisaccular cells, would thus be secreted into the endolymph. Among the functions attributed to secretory immunity, the neutralization of toxins and viruses, the prevention of absorption of antigens ("immune exclusion"), and the inhibition of bacterial adherence [4] might contribute to the defence of the inner ear against infections and antigenic challenges. Recent studies [5] support the immunologic active function of the endolymphatic sac: The total amount of an experimentally induced antibody concentration within the endolymph is dramatically decreased following destruction of the endolymphatic sac.

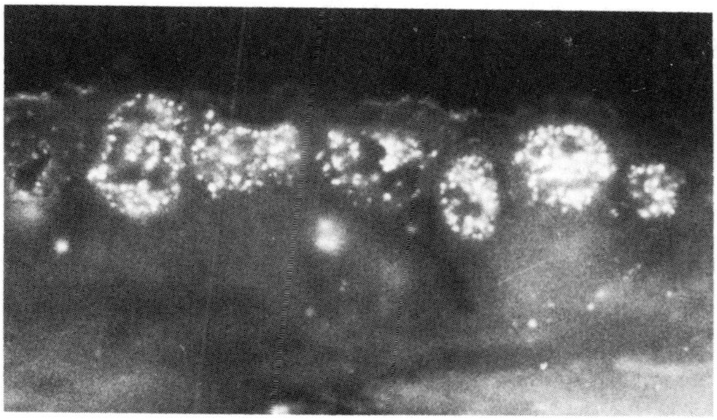

Fig. 1. Intracytoplasmic secretory component in epithelia of the human endolymphatic sac (fluorescein isothiocyanate) x480.

ACKNOWLEDGEMENTS

We thank Miss M. Economou and Miss I. Trachsel for her excellent technical assistance.

REFERENCES

1. Bienenstock J, Befus AD (1980) Mucosal immunology. Immunology 41: 249-270
2. Harris JP (1983) Immunology of the inner ear: response of the inner ear to antigen challenge. Head Neck Surg 91: 18-23
3. Harris JP (1984) Immunology of the inner ear: evidence of local antibody production. Ann Otol Rhinol Lar 93: 157-162
4. Mc Nabb PC, Tomasi Tb (1981) Host defence mechanisms at the mucosal surface. A Rev Microbiol 35: 477-486
5. Morgenstern C (1984) Antibody production in experimental endo lymphatic hydrops. Results presented on invitation of the International Collegium Oto-Rhino-Laryngologicum Amicitiae Sacrum, Corfu, Sept. 9-12, 1984

© 1985 Elsevier Science Publishers B.V. (Biomedical Division)
New dimensions in otorhinolaryngology – head and neck surgery, vol. 2.
E. Myers, editor

ASSESSMENT OF THE VESTIBULAR FUNCTION IN EXPERIMENTAL ANIMALS BY THE RECORDING OF SHORT LATENCY VESTIBULAR EVOKED RESPONSE

JOSEF ELIDAN, M.D.; JOHN LIN, M.D.; VICENTE HONRUBIA, M.D.
Div. of Head & Neck Surgery, UCLA School of Medicine, Los Angeles California, U.S.A.

INTRODUCTION

Over the past few years a method has been developed for the induction and the recording of short latency vestibular evoked response (VsER) to brief angular acceleration stimuli in experimental animals (1,2). The response waveform, latency and amplitude have been described in intact animals and following unilateral or bilateral labyrinthectomy (1,2). The purpose of the present paper is to summarize the known response characteristics, to document new data which were obtained by using a new, more powerful stimulation system and to demonstrate the usefulnes of this method for the evaluation of the vestibular system and its response to various drugs and conditions.

MATERIAL AND METHODS

The details of the technique for the induction and recording of VsER have been described in the previous publications (1,2). The present study was conducted on 25 cats of 2-3.5 Kg body weight. Impulsive angular acceleration stimuli, 20,000°/sec^2 peak intensity (measured directly on the animal's head) and 2-3 msec rise time, were used to activate the horizontal or the vertical semicircular canals. The averaged response was presented vertex positive upward and recorded by an x-y plotter.

RESULTS

The normal VsER (Fig.1A) consists of 6-8 waves, a few microvolts in amplitude and 1-2 msec in duration. The latency of the first wave-P1 (vertex positive) is 1.5-2 msec with respect to the start of the head acceleration. It depends on the peak value and on the rise time of the stimuli. The response was not affected by white noise of 100 dB SPL close to the animal's ear, nor by paralysis of the animal induced by succynilcholin. Bilateral labyrinthectomy or the animal's death caused complete disappearance of the response, whereas reversible disappearance was obtained by briefly induced anoxia or by local application of lidocain (4%) directly in the perilymphatic space. Unilateral labyrinthectomy resulted in asymmetric responses whereby excitatory angular acceleration stimuli produced larger and shorter latency potentials than did inhibitory stimuli (Fig.1B). Ethacrynic acid (EA), either 20-100 mg/kg I.V., or 0.1-0.25% solution applied locally in the perilymphatic space, was found to have only minimal effect on the VsER.

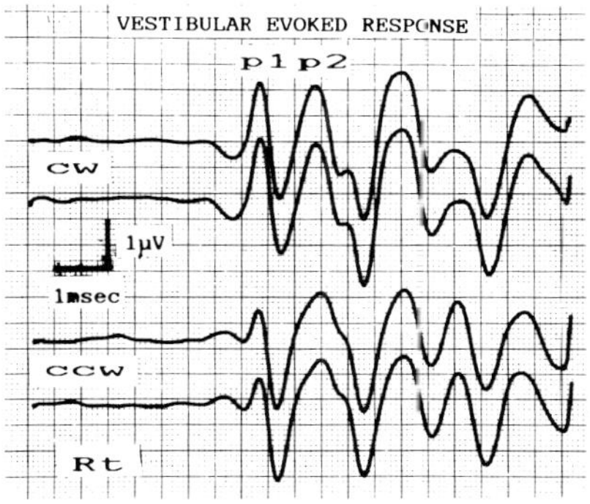

Fig.1A. A typical VsER recorded from a cat with clockwise (CW) and counterclockwise (CCW) acceleration stimuli.

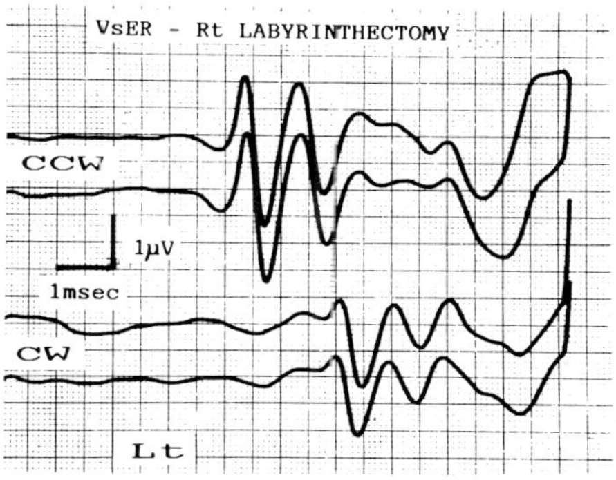

Fig.1B. After Rt labyrinthectomy CCW stimuli which are excitatory to the LT SCC evoked larger and shorter latency response than did CW stimuli.

DISCUSSION

This study demonstrates short latency VsERs which were evoked by much stronger stimuli than used previously, improving the signal to noise ratio and shortening the latency of the response. The recording of the acceleration directly on the animal's head made it possible to determine the true biological latency of the response. The results of local application of anesthetic, anoxia and labyrinthectomy proved the inner ear origin of this potential. The differential effect of EA on the responses to acoustic and acceleration stimuli supports the vestibular origin of this response.

REFEENCES

1. Elidan J, Sohmer H, Nitzan M (1982) Recording of short latency vestibular evoked potentials to acceleration in rats by means of skin electrodes. EEG Clin. Neurophysiol. 53:501-505
2. Elidan J, Sohmer H. Lev S, Gay I (1984) Short latency vestibular evoked response to acceleration stimuli in cats recorded by skin electrodes. Ann. Otol. 93:257-261

Supported by the Silbert International Scholars Program and the National Institute of Health (NS09823, NS08335).

© 1985 Elsevier Science Publishers B.V. (Biomedical Division)
New dimensions in otorhinolaryngology – head and neck surgery, vol. 2.
E. Myers, editor

INDIVIDUAL PROJECTIONS OF THE SEMICIRCULAR CANAL CRISTAE IN THE VESTIBULAR NUCLEI OF THE FROG

VICENTE HONRUBIA, M.D., ALEXANDER KURUVILLA, M.D., CARLOS SUAREZ, M.D. and STEFAN SITKO
Div. of Head and Neck Surgery, UCLA School of Medicine, Los Angeles, CA 90024.

The projections of primary afferent fibers from each semicircular canal in the vestibular nuclei of the frog have been demonstrated with the aid of horseradish-peroxidase labeling of individual nerve branches.[1] Fig. 1 summarizes the differential pattern of innervation from the three cristae: anterior (ANT), horizontal (HOR) and posterior (POST) in each of the vestibular nuclei: cerebellar (C), superior (S), ventral (V), descending (D) and medial (M). The filled circles represent a greater density of innervation than do the empty circles; crosses indicate absence of innervation. The location of nerve terminals is separated to indicate ventral, central and dorsal (VCD) or rostral, middle and caudal (RMC) positions in each nucleus. Fibers from each crista predominate in certain areas, such as the horizontal crista in the central part of the ventral nucleus. In the medial nucleus, however, inputs from different cristae completely overlap. This nucleus is innervated only by the very thin fibers which have the more regular spontaneous activity but are more insensitive. The different patterns of innervation in different nuclei suggest that the vestibular nuclear complex may subserve two different functions. The medial nucleus seems better equipped to sustain tonic influences than to signal changes in activity produced by quick natural head movements. The thin fibers to this nucleus provide the physiologic background for the maintenance of vestibular tonus. The other nuclei are better equipped to channel information from a given receptor independently. Interestingly, they are innervated by thick, irregular, more sensitive fibers. The possible reflex action of these connections was evaluated for the case of physiologic stimulation of the horizontal semicircular canal. The theoretically expected contraction of the individual ocular muscles derived from well established receptor-nucleus connections is illustrated in Fig. 2. Stimulation of the horizontal semicircular canals through a connection in the ventral (or superior) nucleus activates the ipsilateral medial and contralateral lateral recti. The excitation of these canal fibers, which overlap with fibers from the anterior semicircular canal in the ventral part of the nucleus, activates the neurons connected to the ipsilateral superior rectus and the contralateral inferior oblique muscles. Likewise, they activate the neurons connected to the posterior semicircular canal in the dorsal aspect of the nucleus, leading to the contraction of the ipsilateral superior oblique and contralateral inferior rectus muscles. The contractions of these two pairs of antagonistic vertical muscles do not induce vertical motion since they cancel each other out; instead, they restrain the eye, providing greater stability in the vertical plane. Under the influence of the medial and lateral recti, the eye continues to rotate in the horizontal vector, as expected. A similar effect could be demonstrated during vertical head movements. Thus, it appears that the central connections, while complex, remain complementary.

NUCLEI

RECEPTORS		C	S	V	D	M	
ANT.		●●●	●○○	●○○	●○○	●●●	R
		●●●	●○○	●○○	○○○	xxx	M
		●●●	●○○	●○○	●○○	●●●	C
HOR.		●●●	○●○	○●○	○●○	●●●	R
		●●●	○●○	○●○	○○○	xxx	M
		●●●	○●○	○●○	●●○	●●●	C
POST.		●●●	○○●	○○●	○○●	●●●	R
		●●●	○○●	○○●	○○○	xxx	M
		●●●	○○●	○○●	●●●	●●●	C
		VCD	VCD	VCD	VCD	VCD	

FIG 1. The relative density of innervation in the vestibular nuclei from the cristae.

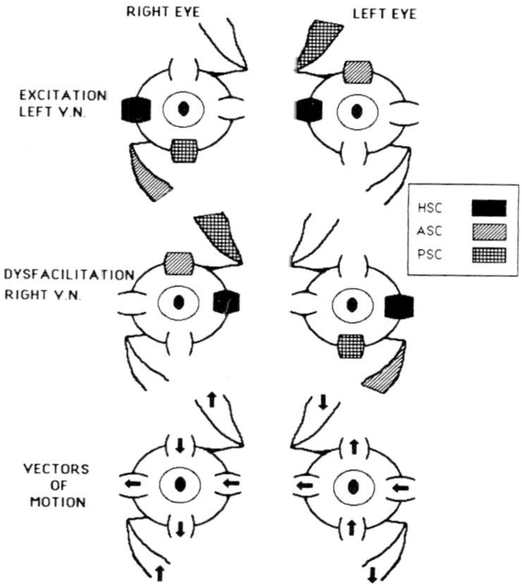

FIG. 2. The muscles activated (top) or inhibited (middle) during stimulation of the horizontal canals by a counterclockwise rotation. Bottom: Arrows indicate the expected direction of motion by each nucleus.

ACKNOWLEDGEMENTS

This work was supported by NIH grants NS07059, NS08335 and NS09823.

REFERENCE

1. Suarez C, Honrubia V, Kuruvilla A, Sitko S, Schwartz IR (1985) Central projections of primary vestibular fibers in the bullfrog. II. Nerve branches from individual receptors. Laryngoscope (in press).

© 1985 Elsevier Science Publishers B.V. (Biomedical Division)
New dimensions in otorhinolaryngology - head and neck surgery, vol. 2.
E. Myers, editor

THE EFFECT OF ASPIRIN ON THE CONCENTRATIONS OF PROSTAGLANDINS IN THE PERILYMPH

T.T.K. JUNG, M.D., PH.D.,[1] S.K. JUHN, M.D.,[1] T. MORIZONO, M.D.,[1] J. EDLIN, B.S.,[1] D. HWANG, PH.D.[2]

[1]Department of Otolaryngology, University of Minnesota Medical School, Minneapolis, Minnesota 55455 (U.S.A.)

[2]Department of Nutrition, Louisiana State University, Baton Rouge, Louisiana 70810 (U.S.A.)

INTRODUCTION

The salicylate ototoxicity has been known for almost a century. Several case reports on aspirin-induced hearing loss, tinnitus and vertigo were reported in the 1940s. McCabe and Day (1965) reported hearing loss after aspirin-treatment in five normal volunteers.[1] Myers and Berstein (1965) reported 20-40 dB hearing loss after aspirin treatment which was reversible in 24-72 hours.[2] The exact cause of salicylate ototoxicity is not known. Possible causes suggested over the years included hydrops of the labyrinthine fluids, intracochlear metabolic disturbance or mechanical displacement of structures,[1] morpholic changes, and alteration of biochemical or enzymatic activity.[3] More recent studies of histopathology of cochlea after aspirin-treatment failed to show any morphological changes.[4]

We suspected prostaglandins (PGs) might be the cause of salicylate ototoxicity since aspirin is an inhibitor of PG-producing cyclooxygenase. Our preliminary findings on PG levels in chinchilla perilymph showed higher levels of 6-keto-$PGF_{1\alpha}$ in perilymph compared to CSF and marked decrease after indomethacin or aspirin-treatment.[5] Recently, PG-levels in guinea pig perilymph three hours and three days after aspirin-treatment were reported.[6]

The purpose of this study was to assess the effect of aspirin on the threshold of hearing and on the levels of PGs in the perilymph, CSF and acqueous humor in chinchillas.

MATERIALS AND METHODS

Normal chinchillas weighing between 400-600g were used in this study. Under ketamine anesthesia (20 mg/kg), samples of serum, perilymph, CSF and acqueous humor were taken. Aspirin (300 mg/kg) was administered intraperitoneally (IP). Salicylate levels were determined by a calorimetric method. Hearing threshold was measured by compound action potential. PG was measured by radioimmunoassy (RIA) using more sensitive (^{125}I) RIA kits (New England Nuclear, Boston, MA).

RESULTS AND DISCUSSION

The concentration (Mean ± stand error) of 6-keto-$PGF_{1\alpha}$ in normal perilymph was 2.1 ± 0.6 ng/ml which was four times higher than CSF (0.52 ± 0.16 ng/ml) and 30 times higher than aqueous humor (0.07 ± 0.04 ng/ml). After aspirin injection, levels of 6-keto-$PGF_{1\alpha}$ in perilymph decreased by 1/2 of normal levels (1.16 ± 0.12 ng/ml) in two hours and by 1/3 (0.62 ± 0.55 ng/ml) in 24 hours. Levels of 6-keto-$PGF_{1\alpha}$ in CSF also decreased by 1/6 of normal levels (0.087 ± 0.026 ng/ml) in two hours and by 1/7 (0.068 ± 0.034 ng/ml) in 24 hours. Levels in aqueous humor dropped about 1/2 (0.04 ± 0.02 ng/ml) in two hours then returned to normal level in 24 hours.

The concentrations of PGE_2 in normal perilymph (43.7 ± 19.6 pg/ml) was not significantly different from normal CSF (46.3 ± 34.4 pg/ml), whereas the level in aqueous humor (65.3 ± 38 pg/ml) was slightly higher. There was a slight decrease in the levels of PGF_2 in perilymph and in CSF 24 hours after aspirin injection (31.9 ± 10.8 pg/ml and 16.4 ± 8.7 pg/ml respectively), whereas there was essentially no change in aqueous humor (57.3 ± 21.3 pg/ml).

From the known biological action of PGs, action of PGs in the inner ear can be speculated. PGs probably act as humoral mediators of the cochlear microcirculation homeostasis by balancing vasodilation (PGE_2, PGI_2, PGD_2) and vasoconstriction ($PGF_{2\alpha}$). They may affect inner ear fluid dynamics by stimulating adenylate cyclase and affecting transmembrane ion transport. PGI_2, measured as 6-keto-$PGF_{1\alpha}$, seems to be the principal PG in the perilymph. Aspirin ototoxicity could be due to microvascular constriction and hypoxia and abnormal transmembrane ion transport secondary to decreased levels of PGI_2 in the inner ear tissue as reflected by levels in perilymph.

ACKNOWLEDGEMENT

This study was supported by the Deafness Research Foundation.

REFERENCES

1. McCabe PA, Dey FL (1965) Effect of aspirin upon auditory sensitivity. Ann Otol Rhinol Laryngol 74:312-325

2. Myers EN, Bernstein JM (1965) Salicylate ototoxicity: A clinical and experimental study Arch Otolaryngol 82:483-493

3. Silverstein H, Berstein JM, Davies DG (1967) Salicylate ototoxicity: A biochemical and electrophysiological study Ann Otol Rhinol Laryngol 76:118-128

4. Deer BC, Hunter-Duvar I (1982) Salicylate ototoxicity in the chinchilla: A behavioral and electron microscopy study J Otolaryngol 11:260-264

5. Jung TTK, Juhn SK (1984) Prostaglandins in the perilymph Abstract of ARO Midwinter Research Meeting 7:107

6. Escoubet B, Amsallem P, Ferrary E, TranBuHuy P (1985) Prostaglandin synthesis by the cochlea of the guinea pig: Influence of aspirin, gentamycin and acoustic stimulation Prostaglandins 29:589-599

© 1985 Elsevier Science Publishers B.V. (Biomedical Division)
New dimensions in otorhinolaryngology – head and neck surgery, vol. 2.
E. Myers, editor

STAPHYLOCOCCI IN ACUTE OTITIS MEDIA

PEKKA KARMA, TAPIO VIRTANEN, PAUL GRÖNROOS, ELJA HERVA
Department of Otolaryngology, University of Tampere, SF-33520 Tampere, Finland

Introduction. The role of staphylococci in acute otitis media (AOM) is unclear. Although possibly a contaminant of middle ear fluid (MEF) specimens, S. aureus (Sta) is also thought to be a pathogen (1,2), and even coagulase negative staphylococcus (Stn) to have some active role in MEFs of otitis media (3,4). This paper aims to analyse the occurrence and possible role of staphylococci in clinically different types of AOM.

Material and methods. We analysed 5217 MEFs of 1203 children, 3 months to 6 years old. 3497 MEFs were obtained from ears with AOM and 1720 from ears without acute symptoms and signs during postacute control visits. The recruitment of children, the clinical classification of ear attacks, their treatment, as well as sampling, processing and analysing of MEF specimens have been described earlier (5,6). Acute visits during antimicrobial treatment or within less than 2 weeks apart were excluded.

Only staphylococcal bacteriology is here reported. Sta was identified by its ability to produce coagulase. Stn species were not further identified. Beta-lactamase producibility of staphylococci was tested with the clover leaf or the chromogenic cephalosporin method.

Results. The occurrence of staphylococci in different clinical subgroups is presented in the following Table I.

Table I	AOM, all		Primary^{x} AOM		Recurrent^{xx} AOM		Postacute OM	
	Attacks	MEFs	Attacks	MEFs	Attacks	MEFs	Attacks	MEFs
Total No.	2400	3497	467	685	1933	2812	1186	1720
% with Sta	4.4^{a}	3.4^{a}	3.9^{b}	3.1^{b}	4.5^{c}	3.5^{c}	7.7^{abc}	6.3^{abc}
% with Stn	12.7^{b}	9.7^{d}	18.4^{ac}	14.3^{ac}	11.3^{ac}	8.6^{a}	9.4^{bc}	7.4^{cd}

^{x}=the very first, ^{xx}all except primary, $^{a,c}p < .001$, $^{b}p < .01$, $^{d}p < .05$

The incidence of staphylococci in ears with acute otorrhea through spontaneously perforated drum was about twice as high as in unperforated AOM ears. However, their number was so small that the incidence difference between all and unperforated AOM ears (<1% unit) was not significant. As Table I shows, Sta occurred with the same frequency in primary and recurrent AOM. Further, in non-acute attacks the frequency of Sta was significantly higher but that of Stn significantly lower than in AOM. On the other hand, during the first few years of life, the occurrence of both staphylococcal groups in acute MEFs distinctly decreased, and from 4 years on they were both rare (Table II).

Table II. Staphylococci in MEF cultures of acute otitis media according to age

MEFs	Age 6-11 months	12-23 months	2-3 years	4-6 years
Total No.	1238	1916	269	67
% with Sta	4.9^{ab}	2.9^{ab}	1.1^{b}	0
% with Stn	11.3^{c}	9.3^{d}	7.8	1.5^{de}

$^{a,b}p < .01$, $^{c,d}p < .05$

Sta grew pure in 69 % of acute MEFs with Sta. For Stn the respective figure was 65 %. If MEFs with staphylococci were excluded, pure cultures were found significantly more often, in 89 %. Sta was isolated bilaterally in 17 % of all attacks with Sta and Stn in 27 % of all attacks with Stn. Both findings became rarer with increasing age.

The proportions of beta-lactamase producing strains of all otitis-strains tested in three successive periods from 1977 to 1983 did not much vary, and were 81 % to 87 % for Sta and 54 % to 61 % for Stn.

Discussion. This study showed the incidence of Sta and Stn to be of the order of 3 to 4 % and 7 to 9 % in children in recent years in Finland. The increase of the incidences in draining ears, and the decrease of incidence with increasing age might suggest that bacteria were ear canal skin contaminants. However, neither these findings nor the decreasing proportion of bilateral Sta or Stn findings with increasing age proves this, and may also be due to e.g. the virulence or host-resistance related factors. On the other hand, the finding that 2/3 of both bacteria grew in pure culture, and that their incidence figures in clinically different cases showed different patterns, suggest that at least part of MEF-staphylococci are more than contaminants.

1. Klein JO (1980) Ann Otol Rhinol Laryngol 89: Suppl 68:98
2. Sugita R, Kawamura S, Ichikawa G et al. (1983) Int J Ped Otorhinolaryngol 6:135
3. Feigin RD, Schackelford PG, Campbell J et al. (1973) Pediatrics 52:569
4. Bernstein JM, Myers D, Kosinski D et al. (1980) Ann Otol Rhinol Laryngol 89: Suppl: 68:104
5. Karma P, Virtanen T, Pukander J et al. (1985) Acta Otolaryngol (Stockh) 99:285
6. Luotonen J, Herva E, Karma P et al. (1981) Scand J Infect Dis 13:1977

© 1985 Elsevier Science Publishers B.V. (Biomedical Division)
New dimensions in otorhinolaryngology – head and neck surgery, vol. 2.
E. Myers, editor

HISTOPATHOLOGIC STUDY OF POLYVALENT PSEUDOMONAS VACCINE ON EXPERIMENTAL PSEUDOMONAS OTITIS MEDIA.

CHONG SUN KIM, KYUNG KYUN OH, MAN KEE PAIK

Department of Otolaryngology, College of Medicine, Seoul National University
Seoul (Korea)

INTRODUCTION

It has been known that one of the most common organisms in chronic otitis media is pseudomonas aeruginosa, sometimes very resistant to antimicrobial therapy especially in elderly or immunosuppressed patients(1). The pseudomas vaccine has been used in experimental animals and in some other human conditions (2-3). It is our purpose to study the histopathologic produced by the pseudomonas vaccine in the development of otitis media by pseudomonas aeruginosa in rats. An animal model of experimental pseudomonas otitis media was used to development of otitis media induced by one type of pseudomonas aeruginosa.

MATERIALS AND METHODS

The vaccine was prepared from heat killed whole cells of 10 representative serotypes of pseudomonas aeruginosa. Pseudomonas otitis media was developed in rats. Following ether anesthesia and ear canal cleansing with betadine solution, transtympanic inoculation of 0.05ml of bacterial suspension containing 10^9 organisms per ml was done. Two groups of animal models were developed by inocualtion of one serostype of pseudomonas aeruginosa in non-vaccinated and vaccinated rats. In the non-vaccinated group, animals were sacrificed and vaccinated rats. In the non-vaccinated group, animals were sacrificed on the 3rd day, on the 7th day. And on the 14th day following inoculation of bacteria. In the vaccinated group vaccine I was injeded intraperitoneally on the day 0 and on the 4th day, and vaccine II was injected on the 2nd day and on the 6th day. On the 10th day, pseudomonas was inocualted into the bulla, and the animalls were sacrificed on the 3rd day, on the 7th day, and on the 14th day after inocualtion of bacteria. The protective effect of the polyvalent vaccine was evaluated by histopathologic evaluation of mucoperiosteum of the promontory area of rat's temporal bones under H&N staining.

RESULTS

The histopathological findings in the non-vaccinated group showed mild inflammatory changes with infiltration of polymorphonuclear leukocytes (PMNs) in the subepithelial layer in 3 day animals. One week animal showed epithelial metaplasia to cuboidal cells and subepithelial space was thickened with heavy inflammatory of polymorphonuclear leukocytes. Two week animal showed prominent epithelial metaplasia with progressive fibrosis in the subepithelial space accompanied infiltration of PMNs, lympocytes and plasma cells. In the vaccinated group, 3 day animal showed mild thickening of the subepithelial space with PMNs and occasional lymphocytic infiltration. In one week animal, no significant evidence of epithelial metaplasia was seen. The subepithelial space was slightly thickened with infiltration of PMNs lymphocytes, macrophages, and plasma cells. Two week animal showed no progression of epithelial changes, and mild fibrosis in subepithelial space was noted accompanied by occasional clumping of histiocytes.

SUMMARY

Epithelial changes were significant in the non-vaccinated animals, however it was minimal in the vaccinated animals. Epithelial changes in the non-vaccinated animals were remarkable with cuboidal or ciliated columnar cells and goblet cell formation at one week and two weeks. However, the changes were minimal in the vaccinated animals at these same intervals. In the subepithelial space, cellular changes were signifcant in the non-vaccinated animals with marked infiltration of neutrophilis in one week and two week animals, and lymphocytic infiltration in two week animals. However, these changes were found to be minimal in the vaccinated animals.

CONCLUSION

The results suggest that heat killed whole cell polyvalent pseudomonas accine seems to have protective effect against middle ear infection of rats induced by pseudomonas aeruginosa (Pa.13). The mechanisms of protective effect of the vaccine remains to be determined.

REFERENCES

1. Meyerhoff, W.F., Gates, G.A., Montalbo, P.J. : Pseudomonas mastoiditis. Laryngoscope 87 : 483-492, 1977
2. Pennington, J.E. : Preliminary investigation of Pseudomonas aeruginosa vaccine in patients with leukemia and cystic fibrosis. J. Infect. Dis., 130 : 159-162, 1974
3. Millican, R.C., Evans, G., Markley, K. : Susceptibility of burned mice to Pseudomonas aeruginosa and protection by vaccination. Ann. Surg. 163 : 603-610, 1966

New dimensions in otorhinolaryngology - head and neck surgery, vol. 2.
E. Myers, editor

MAST CELL DEGRANULATION MAY CAUSE NEURONAL DEGENERATION

T.C. THEOHARIDES (1), S.J. BALOYANNIS (2) AND L.S. MANOLIDES (2)
Department of Biochemistry and Pharmacology, Tufts University School of Medicine, Boston, MA, U.S.A. - (1) and Department of O.R.L., Laboratory of Neuropathology - Otohistopathology, Aristotelian University School of Health Sciences, Thessaloniki, Greece (2)

INTRODUCTION

Mast cells are plentiful at interfaces with the body's exterior, and are known to secrete numerous mediators in response mostly to allergenic stimuli (1-4). They have also been identified in the central nervous system where they are plentiful around the meninges and in bifurcation of vessels, and their numbers are increased during the development of the organism (50). Mast cells contain a variety of powerful mediators, such as histamine, prostaglandins, leukotrienes and kinins (1-4), all of which could have profound effects on CNS pathophysiology, especially the degree of vasodilatation, the integrity of the blood-brain barrier and the functional status of the neuronal circuitry. Furthermore, mast cells have been shown to be the richest source of proteolytic enzymes in the body (10), making them possible candidates for participation in degenerative diseases of the CNS. It is important to note that many neuropeptides are capable of degranulating mast cells (11) and they, along with other mast cell mediators, are suspected of playing an important role in CNS function (12). In spite of this mounting indirect evidence of the potential mast cell role in CNS pathophysiology, however, there has been precious little work on their biochemistry and pharmacology. Indeed, in recent reviews on the heterogeneity of human mast cells, there was no mention of CNS mast cells (13). Here we report that degranulated mast cells are associated with neuronal demyelination.

MATERIALS AND METHODS

Mast cells were collected from peritoneal cavities of male Sprague-Dawley rats (300 g from Charles River Labs) and were added to short-term cultures of brain slices of allogeneic rats. Peritoneal mast cell degranulation was induced by addition of 1.0 µg/ml of the classic non-immunologic, secretagogue compound 48/80 for 10 min at 37°C; the effect of 48/80 on brain mast cells was tested at 10 µg/ml. Controls included neuronal tissue with culture medium, mast cells or 48/80 alone, and the supernatant fluid from mast cells which had secreted in response to 1 µg/ml 48/80 for 5 min at 37°C elsewhere. All cultures were transferred following treatment, and were examined for 10 days after H & E, Golgi-Cox and myelin stains, as well as with phase contrast and electron microscopy.

RESULTS

Those brain sections co-cultured with degranulated peritoneal mast cells or with medium from mast cells previously induced to secrete, both times with 1 µg/ml 48/80, showed extensive demyelination and neuronal degeneration. Control cultures showed normal neuronal architecture with no mast cell involvement. Brain sections cultured in the presence of 1 0 µg/ml 48/80 also showed extensive demyelination and such areas were associated with accumulations of mast cells with altered granule architecture. Most importantly, these brain mast cells showed <u>no degranulation</u> while they contained numerous empty-looking secretory granules.

It appears that repetitive or extensive release of CNS mast cell secretory products may participate in neuronal degeneration, including such direct central sensory endings as those of the olfactory or acoustic nerves. Furthermore, the release of secretory products from CNS mast cells appears to occur without the degranulation classically seen with peritoneal mast cells.

REFERENCES

1. Metcalfe, D.D., Kaliner, M.A. and Donlon, M.A. (1981) The mast cell. CRC Crit. Rev. Immunol. 3:23-74.

2. Foreman, J.C. (1981) The pharmacological control of immediate hypersensitivity. Ann. Rev. Pharmacol. Toxicol. 21: 63-81.

3. Bach, M.K. (1982) Mediators of amaphylaxis and inflammation. Am. Rev. Microbiol. 36: 371-413.

4. Lagunoff, D. and Martin, T.W. (1983) Agents that release histamine from mast cells. Am. Rev. Pharmacol. Toxicol. 23: 331-351.

5. Baloyannis, S.J. and Theoharides, T.C. (1981) Mast cells in the central nervous system, Mat. Med. Greca 9: 142-150.

6. Goldschmidt, R.C., Hough, L.B., Glick, S.D. and Padawer, J. (1984) Mast cells in rat thalamus: nuclear localization, sex difference and left-right assymetry. Brain Res. 323: 209-217.

7. Panula, P., Yang, H.Y.T. and Costa, E. (1984) Histamine containing neurons in the rat hypothalamus. Proc. Natl. Acad. Sci. (USA) 81: 2575-2576.

8. Orr, E.L. (1984) Dural mast cells: source of contaminating histamine in analyses of mouse brain histamine levels. J. Neuro Chem. 43: 1497-1499.

9. Mokhtarian, F. and Griffin, P.E. (1984) The role of mast cells in virus-induced inflammation in the murine central nervous system. Cell. Immunol. 86: 491-500.

10. Theoharides, T.C. (1981) Mast cells and precursor protein molecules. Persp. Biol. Med. 24: 499-502.

11. Theoharides, T.C. and Douglas, W.W. (1981) Mast cell histamine secretion in response to somatostatin analogues. Structural considerations. Eur. J. Pharmacol. 73: 131-136.

12. Theoharides, T.C. (1983) Mast cells and migraines. Persp. Biol. Med. 26: 672-675.

13. Austen, K.F. (1984) The heterogeneity of mast cell populations and products. Hosp. Pract. 19: 135-146.

New dimensions in otorhinolaryngology - head and neck surgery, vol. 2.
E. Myers, editor

PAGET´S DISEASE OF THE TEMPORAL BONE

GLORIA MORELLO-CASTRO,MD

Visiting fellow,massachusetts Eye and Ear Infirmary.Harvard Medical School,Mass USA.;INCS and Delfos Medical Center.Av Hospital Militar 151.Barna,Cat,Spain

INTRODUCTION

A mixed type(sensorineural and conductive) hearing loss is a common complication of Paget´s disease of the skull.The pathological bases for the hearing losses have not been demostrated.In an attempt to answer these questions, histological studies were performed on 24 temporal bones from 15 subjects who had Paget´s disease.The findings in eight of these temporal bones from four patients were previously reported by Davies.In the material are nine temporal bones from five subjects on whom audiometric data is available.

These specimens were selected for graphic reconstruction of the cochleae to enhance the probability of correlating pathological changes with sensorineural hearing loss.

MATERIAL AND METHODS

The temporal bones were prepared for light microscopic study in the routine manner of the Massachusetts Eye and Ear Infirmary.The cochlea of the nine temporal bones with audiometric data were graphically reconstructed as described by Guild (1921) and Schuknecht(1953) with measurements made from the basal ends of the cochleae.

For each millimeter segment a judgment was made of the percentage of hair cells missing.The magnitude of loss (atrophy) of the striae vasculares was estimated in 10% increments for each millimeter along the cochlear ducts.The spiral ganglia were reconstructed in a manner similar to that of the organ of Corti .The counts were multiplied by 10 because only every tenth section was prepared for histological study and by a correction factor of 0.9 to account for nuclei bisected at the interface of sections,Otte and Schuknecht(1978).

The counts were converted to percentages of normal by using the normative related data of Otte and Schuknecht(1978).

The frecuencies of the auditory spectrum were arranged on the abcisa of the graph in accordance with the location of their points of maximun displacement along the basilar membrane.The Koening scale was used by which frequencies above 900Hz are plotted on the logarithmic scales and those below 900 Hz on the arithmetic scale.This plotting method by which frequency and pathology are parallel coordinates takes into account their spatial distribution.

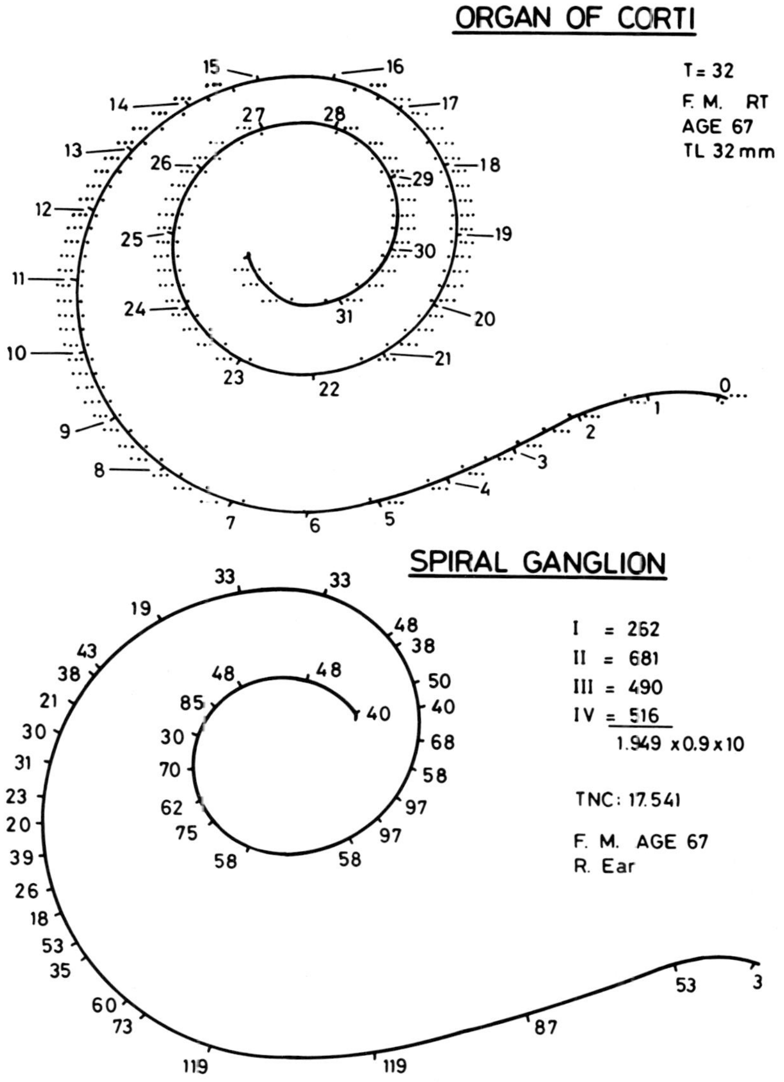

Fig 1 .(case 1;right ear).Reconstruction of the organ of Corti of average(length 32 mm) and spiral ganglion showing the total populations in each segment.The larger digits outside the drawn spiral indicate the number of ganglion cells counted in that location.The total number of of ganglion cells was estimated as 1949x0.9x10=17541.

Cytocochleograms and audiogram for the cases report appear in the following Figures.

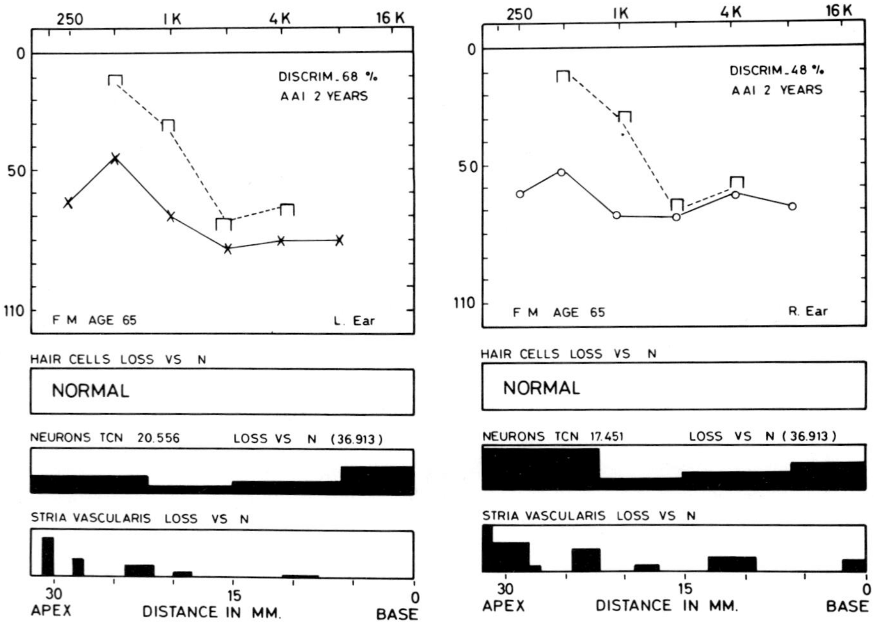

Fig 2 (case 1)This patient with known generalized Paget ´s disease first noted a handicapping hearing loss at the age of 55.He died at the age of 67 of renal failure and congestive heart disease.The AAI (audiogram to autopsy interval)was two years.Speech discrimination is 48% on the right and 68% on the left.The organ of Corti is normal. The total neuronal population are 17541,and 20556 in the right and left ears respectively and over 2358,6129,4410,and 4644 in segments I,II, III,IV in the right ear and 2322,7740,4923,and 5571 in segment I,II, III,IV in the left ear.When compared to congenital normal, the cochlear neural loss is 53% on the right and 44% on the left.The stria vascularis shows mild patchy atrophy.

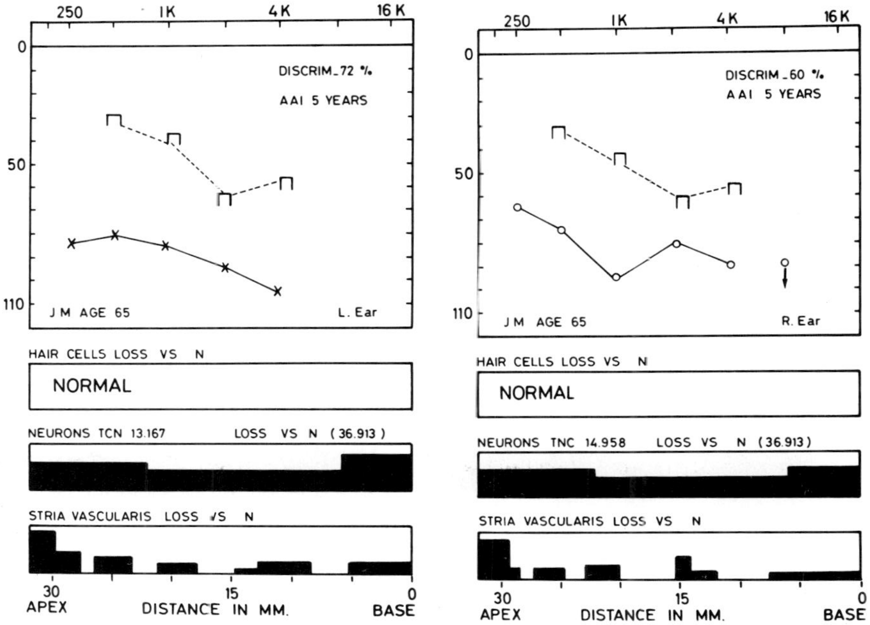

Fig 3 (case2).This patient was first noted to have Paget´s disease at the age of 23.He died at the age of 70 years of multiple organ failure following fracture of a femur.The AAI (audiogram to autopsy interval) was five years.Speech discrim is 60% on the right and 72% on the left.The hair cells populations of the organ of Corti are normal. The total neural populations are 14958 and 13167 in the right and left ears respectively and over 1989,6120,3384,3465 in segments I,II,III, and IV in the right and 1134, 5382, 3177,3474 in the left.When compared to congenital normal, the neural loss is 50% on the right and 64% on the left.There is a patchy atrophy of the stria vascularis.

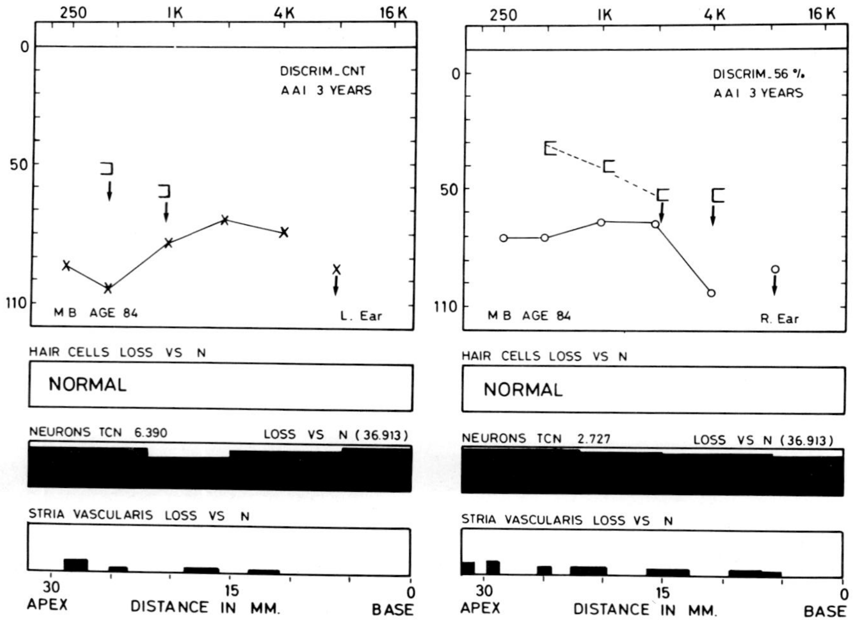

Fig.4 (case3) At the age of 80 the patient complained of hearing loss. At the age of 84 a diagnosis of Paget's disease of the skull was made by radiography. At the age of 87 she had a cerebral infart and died. The AAI was 3 years. Speech discrimination is 56% on the right and CNT on the left. The hair cells populations are normal in both ears. The total neuronal populations are 2727 and 6390 in the right and left ears respectively and over 810,1215,432, and 270 in segments I,II,III,and IV and 306,2844,2034,1206 in segments I,II,III and IV in the left ear. The cochlear neural losses, compared to congenital normal are 92% on the right and 82% on the left. There is scattered mild atrophy of the stria vascularis.

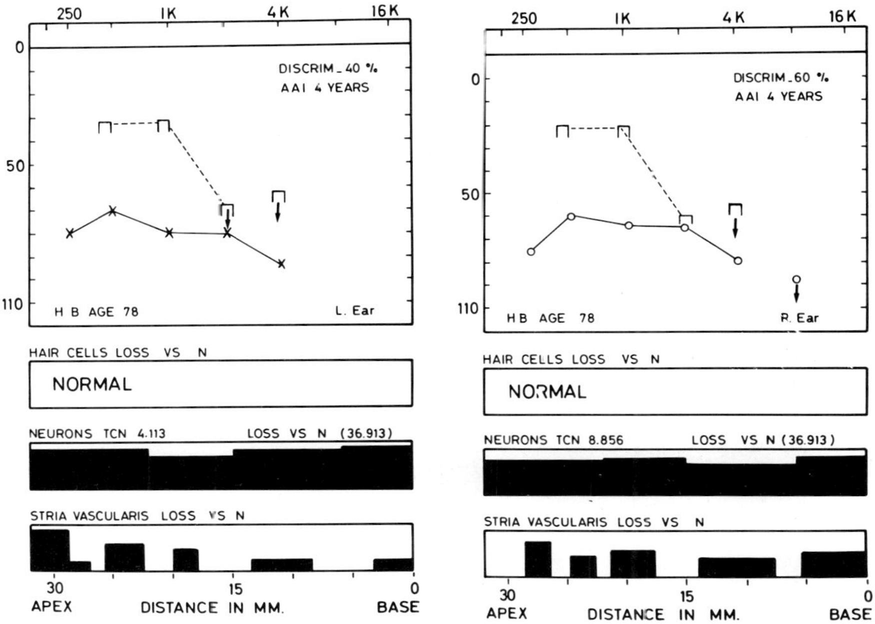

Fig 5 (case 4).This patient was diagnosed as having Paget's disease at the age of 83 .He first complained of hearing loss at the age of 78.He died nine months later of unrelated causes.The AAI interval was 5 years.Speech discrimination is 60% on the right and over 50% on the left.The organ of Corti appears normal.The total neural populations is 8856 and 4113 on the right and left ears respectively and over 1755 in segment IV in the right ear and 792 in segment IV in the left ear. The cochlear neuronal loss compared to congenital normal is 76% on the right and 89% on the left.There is moderately severe patchy atrophy of the stria vascularis.

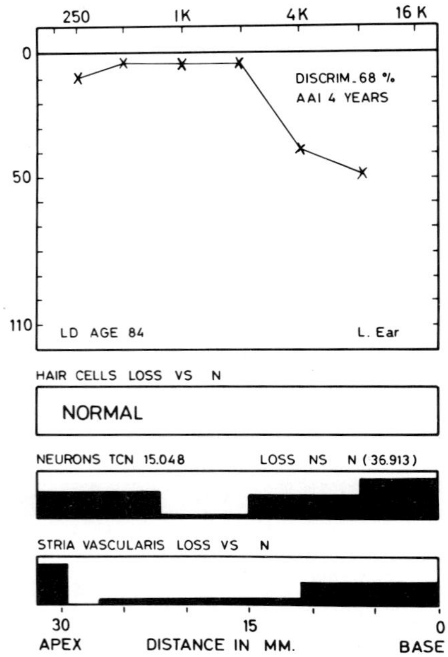

Fig 6 (case5).He died at the age of 53 years of coronary thrombosis and both temporal bones were removed for histological study.The AAI is 4 years.The speech discrim is 68% .Only the left temporal bone shows pagetoid changes which involve principally the posterior wall of the petrous bone but not the bony labyrinth.The organ of Corti is normal. The total neuronal populations is 15.o48, on the left ear and over 999, 4905,5634,and 3510 in segments I,II,III, and IV respectively.

RESULTS

Eight of the nine ears selected for graphic reconstruction show the classical mixed type of deaffness.The threshold patters are descending for bone conduction and flat for air conduction ,thus the bone conduction and air conduction curves approximate each other at the high frecuencies.There is therefore a progressively decreasing magnitude of conductive loss from low to high frequencies which is characteristic of stiffness lesions(as opposed to mass lesions)of the sound transmission system.

In all ears, the tympanic membranes and ossicles appeared to be intact.There was no evidence of fixation or ankylosis.Even when the petros bones were markedly enlarged by the Pagetoid process,the ossicles were not encroached upon by pagetoid bone.In most specimens the internal auditory canals were slightly narrowed but not enough to compress the enclosed nerve trunks.Most specimens show an increase in the number of microfisures.In general the ears showed good hair cell populations but a loss of neural populations in excess of that expected for age.The studies did not yield a clear explanation for the conductive and sensorineural hearing losses.It is postulated that the conductive losses may be based on subtle mechanical influences of the Pagetoid bone on the sound transmission system and that the sensorineural loss is due to an interference with the motion mechanics of the cochlear duct, possibly by changes in the physical properties of the basilar membrane.

ACKNOWLEDGEMENTS

Grant(number):EE83/2-73.C.I.R.I.T.,was received for the study which led to the preparation of this paper, and I´m greatly indebted to Dr Harold F Schuknecht for giving me the opportunity and the the facilities to carry out these investigations.

REFERENCES

1. Davies,D.G.,1969:Paget´s Disease of the temporal bone.Acta Oto-Laryngol. suppl 242.
2. Guild,S.R.,1921 :A graphic reconstruction method for the study of the organ of Corti.Anat Rec ;22:141-57.
3. Koenig,W.,1949:A New Frequency Scale for Acoustic Measurements.Bell.Lab Rec ,p299,August.
4. Otte,J.,Schuknecht,H.F.,and Kerr,A.C.,1978:Ganglion cells populations in normal and pathological human cochleae.Implications for cochlear implantation,Laryngoscope,88:1231-46.
5. Schuknecht,H.F.,1958:Techniques for study of cochlear function and pathology in experimentals animals .Arch.Otolaryngol,58:377-397.

New dimensions in otorhinolaryngology - head and neck surgery, vol. 2.
E. Myers, editor

THE FIBRINOLYTIC ENZYME IN CARRAGEENIN-INDUCED OTITIS MEDIA OF GUINEA PIG

H. NAKAYOSHI[1)], Y. NODA[1)], M. NAKAMURA[2)], T. KOSUGI[2)]
Departments of Otorhinolaryngology[1)] and Physiology[2)], School of Medicine, University of the Ryukyus, Okinawa, Japan

INTRODUCTION

It has been known that the fibrinolytic enzyme was related to the process of inflammation[1)]. Especially, it was clarified that the plasminogen activator of fibrinolytic enzymes played an important role on relating to the initiation and prolongation of inflammation[2),3)]. The role and pathophysiological significance of the fibrinolytic enzyme in inflammatory process of otitis media was not well known until present time. In this paper, the role and significance of the fibrinolytic enzyme originated from mucous membrane of tympanic cavity was studied in carrageenin-induced otitis media of guinea pig.

MATERIALS AND METHODS

Fibrinolytic activity of mucous membrane of tympanic cavity in various animals was determined by means of fibrin plate. That is, mucous membrane of tympanic cavity from 4 to 5 animals was summated and this collected mucous membrane was dissected into small pieces. These small pieces were homogenized and the homogenate, then, was sonicated by ultrasonic cell disruptor. Finally, after centrifugating at 10000 r.p.m. for 10 minutes, the fibrinolytic activity of the supernatant was determined by means of fibrin plate. In order to induce an experimental otitis media, the administration of carrageenin solution (1 %) was procedured to the tympanic cavity of guinea pigs. On the following 3 hours to 3 weeks, macroscopic and histopathological findings was observed on the degree of inflammatory response. Furthermore, the fibrinolytic activity of mucous membrane in tympanic cavity with carrageenin-induced otitis media was determined.

RESULTS

1) Fibrinolytic activity of mucous membrane in tympanic cavity of various animal with non-inflammation.

As shown in Figure 1, fibrinolytic activity in dog was stronger than that in guinea pig and rabbit. Furthermore, the fibrinolytic activity of mucous membrane in tympanic cavity was inhibited by t-AMCHA.

2) Macroscopic findings of the middle ear.

After the injection of carrageenin into tympanic cavity, at 12 hours marked edema and retention of exudate was observed. After the injection of carrageenin, at one week inflammatory response was subsided (Table 1).

3) Fibrinolytic activity of mucous membrane in tympanic cavity with otitis media induced by carrageenin.

After induced otitis media, at 7 days the fibrinolytic activity was increased, compared with the activity of non-treated mucous membrane and at 3 days after the injection (Fig. 2).

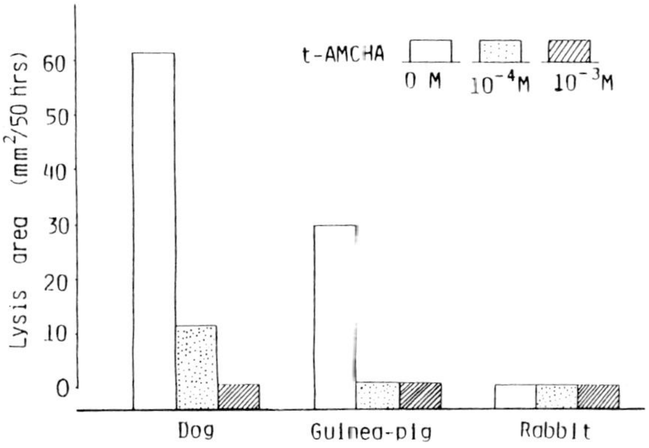

Fig. 1. Fibrinolytic activity of mucous membrane in tympanic cavity of various animals. After incubating at 37°C, 50 hours, the lysis area was measured. t-AMCHA indicates synthetic antiplasminic reagent, tranexamic acid. Open column in this figure indicates the lysis area of fibrin plate without t-AMCHA. Dotted column indicates the lysis area of fibrin plate including t-AMCHA (final concentration 10^{-4} M). Shaded column indicats the lysis area of fibrin plate including t-AMCHA (final concentration 10^{-5} M).

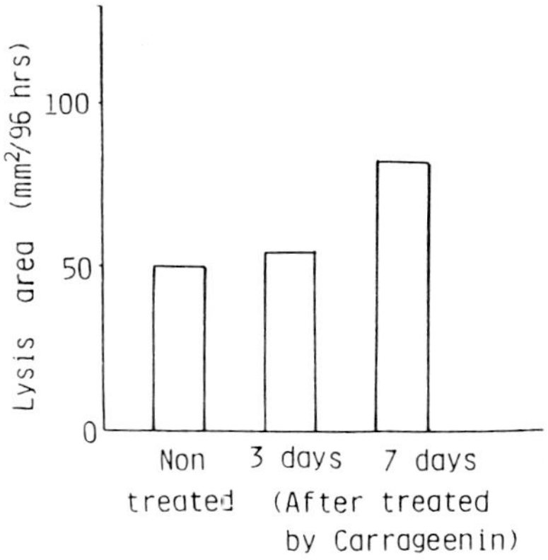

Fig. 2. Fibrinolytic activity of mucous membrane in tympanic cavity with otitis media of guinea pig induced by carrageenin. Mucous membranes from 4 to 5 guinea pigs were summated and homogenized. Extract was spotted to fibrin plate and after incubating at 37°C, for 96 hours lysis area was estimated.

TABLE 1

MACROSCOPIC FINDINGES IN TYMPANIC CAVITY AFTER THE INJECTION OF CARRAGEENIN.

Guinea-pig No.	Edema of mucous membrane.	Exudate	Time after the injection
1	±	+	3 hrs
2	−	++	
3	±	−	6 hrs
4	+	+	
5	++	++	12 hrs
6	+	++	
7	+	++	1 day
8	+	++	
9	+	++	2 days
10	+	++	
11	±	+	3 days
12	±	+	
13	+	−	1 week
14	−	−	
15	+	−	2 weeks
16	−	−	
17	+	−	3 weeks
18	−	−	

++ : remarkable ± : slight

\+ : moderate − : unchanged

DISCUSSION

In order to study on relationship between fibrinolytic enzyme and inflammatory process of otitis media, it was clarified that the guinea pig was most useful from the view point of anatomical characteristics and the fibrinolytic activity of mucous membrane in tympanic cavity. It was suggested that the increased fibrinolytic activity at the late stage of experimental otitis media played an important role to repair the inflammatory locus. Although data on microscopic findings of mucous membrane was not shown in this paper, it was observed that the regeneration of cell lining mucous membrane in tympanic cavity started at 5-7 days after the injection of carrageenin. From these results, it was suggested that the changeable fibrinolytic activity of mucous membrane was related to the process of otitis media.

REFERENCES

1. Kosugi T, Morimitsu T, Matsuo O, Mihara H (1980) Arthus tonsillitis in the rabbit -Histological findings and fibrinolytic activity in blood- Acta Oto-Laryng 9(3,4):309-315
2. Kosugi T, Kinjo K, Takagi I, Matsuo O, Mihara H, Nishikaze O (1981) Antiplasmin activity in carrageenin-induced inflammation of rats. Int J Tiss Reac Ⅲ(3-4):173-176
3. Kosugi T, Takagi I, Kinjo K, Nakagawa S, Noda Y, Mihara H. (1983) Control of Arthus tonsillitis by the administration of antiplasminic agent. Int J Tiss Reac V(2):205-215

New dimensions in otorhinolaryngology - head and neck surgery, vol. 2.
E. Myers, editor

EXPERIMENTAL STUDIES ON THE AMPLITUDE MODULATED ELECTRICAL STIMULATION OF THE EAR IN CATS

KWAN TAEK NOH, SOON JAE HWANG, SUN O CHANG, DUK HWAN LIM
Department of Otolaryngology, College of Medicine, Seoul National Unviersity
Seoul (Korea)

INTRODUCTION

Cochlear implant is the most recent advance in the treatment of cochlear deafness. It is well known that the proper selection of the electrical stimulus is perhaps the most important component of gaining optimum results with an electronic cochlear prosthesis. To this end, we compared amplitude modulated electrical stimulus to conventional electrical stimulus by measuring two parameters; brainstem evoked response and poststimulus time histogram of a single auditory nerve fiber.

MATERIAL AND METHODS

We utilized 10 cats for our study, 5 in the first phase and 5 in the second phase. Cats weighing 3-3.5Kg with good Preyer's reflex were anesthetized with pentothal sodium injected intraperitoneally. Cochlear deafness was induced by sucking out perilymph via the round window. In the first phase with brainstem evoked response, four types of stimulation were utilized; 1. acoustic stimualtion as control, 2. conventional electrical stimulation with monopolar electrode, 3. conventional electrical stimulation with bipolar electrode, 4. 50KHz amplitude modulated electrical stimulation with bipolar electrode. Acoustic stimulations to the test ear were given. 90dB SPL logon at 2, 4 and 6KHz through ear canal receiver. The electrodes were implanted 5mm via the scala tympani. Acosutic stimuli were converted into electrical currents of 0.2mA, 0.6V of 2, 4 and 6KHz respectively. And the conventional electrical stimuli were amplitude modulated into 50KHz currents. These stimulations were applied at twenty times per second, totally 1024 stimulations per test.

In the second phase with PST histogram of a single auditory nerve fiber, we measured directly a single auditory nerve fiber response to three different stimuli; 1.acoustic stimualtion as control, 2. conventional electrical stimulation with bipolar electrode, 3. 50KHz amplitude modulated electrical stimulation with bipolar electrode.

RESULTS

Normal cat's brainstem evoked responses to acoustic stimulation as a control group demonstrate that all waveforms are well formed and present. The conventional electrical stimulation with monopolar electrode produces only waves I & V, and other waveforms are not well seen. The conventional electrical stimulation with bipolar electrode produces all waveforms but are not distinctly formed. But 50KHz amplitude modulated electrical stimualtion reveals all waveforms distinctly as is the case in the acoustic control group. Analysis of average wave V latencies throughout all frequencies tested reveals that the amplitude modulated electrical stimulation more closely resembles that of the acoustic control gorup.

The poststimulus time histogram of each unit shows that the response of amplilude modulated electrical stimulation closely resembles that of the normal acoustic stimualtion in its latency of preferred phase and its enveloping shape of response as well. But the conventional electrical stimulation response curve and its preferred phase latency do not approximate the acoustic group.

CONCLUSION

We have found that the 50KHz amplitude modulated electrical stimulation more closely resembles the normal acoustic system than the conventional electrical stimulation. Therefore amplitude modulated electrical stimulation should provide more optimum results in generating sound perception to cochlear deaf patients.

REFERENCES

1. Brackmann, D.E. : The cochlear implant: Basic principles. Laryngoscope 86 : 373-388, 1976
2. Evans, E.F. : The frequency response and other properties of single fibers in the guinea pig cochlear nerve. J. Physiol. 226 : 263-287, 1972
3. House, W.F., Berliner, K.I. : The cochlear implant. Otolaryngol. Clin. N. Am.: 15 (4) : 917-924, 1982
4. Kiang, N.Y., Moxon, E.C. : Physiologic considerations in artificial stimulation of the inner ear. Ann. Otol. Rhinol. Laryngol. 81 : 714-730, 1972
5. Merzenich, M.M. et al : Neural encoding of the sound sensation evoked by electrical stimulation of the acoustic nerve. Ann. Otol. Rhinol. Laryngol. 82 : 486, 1973
6. Simmon, F.B., and Glatike, T.J. : Comparison of electrical and acoustical stimulation of the cat ear. Ann. Otol. 81 : 731-738, 1972

© 1985 Elsevier Science Publishers B.V. (Biomedical Division)
New dimensions in otorhinolaryngology - head and neck surgery, vol. 2.
E. Myers, editor

SOME CONSIDERATIONS ON THE PATHOPHYSIOLOGY OF MÉNIÈRE'S DESEASE-ON THE RELATIONS BETWEEN THE CLINICAL EXPERIENCES AND THE RESULTS OF THE EXPERIMENTAL ENDOLYMPHATIC HYDROPS

NOZUE, M., MINETA, H., SERIZAWA, Y., FUJIKAWA, K., MORI, Y., AND KIKAWADA, T.
Dept. of Otolaryngology, Hamamatsu University School of Medicine, Hamamatsu, Japan

INTRODUCTION

According to our clinical experiences, in typical Ménière's disease, spontaneous nystagmus is usually observed during the attack of vertigo. Furthermore, in long standing cases, the threshold of hearing level rises and the caloric responses are strongly reduced even after the improvement of vertigo.

On the other hand, many papers report that the pathology of Ménière's desease is endolymphatic hydrops.

To observe the relations between the clinical and experimental findings, endolymphatic hydrops were induced in guinea pigs by obliteration of the endolymphatic sac.

MATERIALS AND METHODS

Thirty three guinea pigs were used. By opening the occipital head bone, the endolymphatic sac was exposed, and the endolymphatic sac and duct were obliterated by bone dust and wax. After observation of spontaneous nystagmus and caloric response, the animals were sacrificed.

RESULTS

1) Endolymphatic hydrops were successfully produced in 26 out of 33 guinea pigs (78.8%).
2) The spontaneous nystagmus was observed in only 2 out of 26 cases (7.7%). Furthermore, these spontaneous nystagmus were observed in association with labyrinthitis.
3) Endolymphatic hydrops were more marked when the animals were kept alive longer after operation.
4) The cases with severe endolymphatic hydrops tended to show markedly decreased caloric response to cold water stimuli.

CONCLUSIONS

From these results, we presume that the endolymphatic hydrops itself may not always produce such spontaneous nystagmus as we usually see in Ménière's disease. So, in addition to endolymphatic hydrops, some other factors may be necessary to produce attacks of vertigo and spontaneous nystagmus. On the other hand, the findings of caloric nystagmus may show the same pathophysiology as Ménière's disease.

TABLE 1

RELATIONS BETWEEN THE TIME AND THE DEGREE OF ENDOLYMPHATIC HYDROPS

(w: week, m: month)

	none	mild	moderate	severe
0 - 1w	3	3	0	2
2 - 1m	1	0	3	2
2 - 3m	0	1	3	1
4 - 6m	0	1	1	3
7m-	2	1	0	3

TABLE 2

RELATIONS BETWEEN THE RESPONSE TO THE COLD WATER STIMULI AND THE DEGREE OF ENDOLYMPHATIC HYDROPS

	mild	moderate	severe
no response	1	5	7
decreased	0	1	2
normal	4	1	2

REFERENCES

1) Kimura RS and SchuKnecht HF (1965): Membranous hydrops in the inner ear of the guinea pig after obliteration of the endolymphatic sac. Pract. Oto-Rhino-Laryng. 27: pp 343-354

2) Kimura RS (1967): Experimental blockage of the endolymphatic duct and its effect on the inner ear of the guinea pig. A study on endolymphatic hydrops. Ann. Otol. 76: pp 664-688

3) Stahle J and Bergman B (1967): The caloric reaction in Ménière's disease. Laryngoscope 77: pp 1629-1643

4) Paparella MM, Goyocoolea MV, Meyerhoff WL et al (1979): Endolymphatic hydrops and otitis media. Laryngoscope 89: pp 43-54

5) Mineta H (1984): The study on the experimental endolymphatic hydrops. J. of Otolaryng. of Japan 87: pp 956-968

New dimensions in otorhinolaryngology - head and neck surgery, vol. 2.
E. Myers, editor

A STUDY USING THE ABR TEST IN GUINEA PIGS WITH INNER EAR MEMBRANE LYMPHATIC HYDROPS

WANG QI (1), *Director. K.J. LEE.(2)*
Deartment of Otolaryngology, Wuhan Medical College, Second Hospital People's Republic of China

(This research was completed at the education and research center, Director, Dr. K. J. Lee of St. Raphael Hospital, from Sept. 1982-April 1984)

The auditory brainstem response (ABR) testing device is an objective auditory function test which has proved to be very helpful in the assessment of the auditory system and various neurological disorders. It has become an important diagnostic method in the field of otolaryngology. However, the explanation of auditory brainstem response testing has not been satisfactory.

This experiment was done according to Professor Kimura's method using an endolymphatic sac obliteration operation on 40 guinea pigs. Postoperatively, 23 cases agreed with the research demands: continuing survival, no distirct nystagmus, and abnormal ABR wave changes.

MATERIAL AND METHODS

The Synap I and Nicolet were used to measure cochlea potential. Adult albino guinea pigs, weighing between 340 g to 766 g, were used in this study, the right ear of each animal was operated on whereas the left ear remained as a control.

The operation were performed under sterile and anesthetic conditions using a Zeiss operating microscope. The operative approach was from the posterior cranial fossa, which is the position of the intermediate portion of the endolymphatic sac destruction. To achieve this, a fine burr drill was used to pass through the vestibular aqueduct. The bone wax was then used to seal off the duct orifice.

RESULTS

The ABR testing results show that all the cases have the same data preoperatively. However, upon weekly postoperative follow-up, 5 cases developed increased wave I latency, prolongation of the intrapeak latency I-III, I-V, and II-III is normal on the operative lateral ear; In another set of the study, all of the 10 cases studies also were obviously changed, No. 300002, on the second postoperative day wave I appeared distinctly changed. The wave I latency is obviously prolonged. Due to death from postoperative complications the remaining 8 cases could

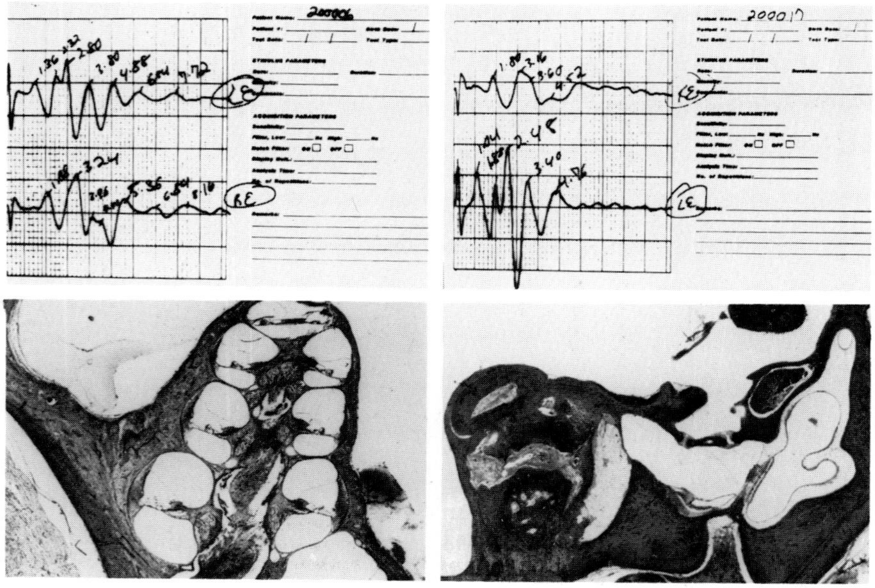

Figure. The ABR typical waves and pathologic specimens change.

not be evaluated. An interesting case showed the existence of a fibrous pathological change and new ostosis in the cochlea, but the vestibule's outward appearance is collapsed saccule and epithelial cell atrophy.

CONCLUSION

This study showed that ABR testing could effectively measure the amplitude and latency changes in wave I generated from the cochlea of guinea pigs. Pathological ABR changes resulted in decreased amplitude and prolonged latency of wave I in guinea pigs with inner ear endolymphatic hydrops.

REFERENCE

R.S. Kimura and H.F. Schuknecht (1965): Membranous Hydrops in the Inner Ear of the Guinea Pig after Obliteration of the Endolymphatic sac. Pract. Oto-rhinolaryng. 27:243-254.

New dimensions in otorhinolaryngology - head and neck surgery, vol. 2.
E. Myers, editor

THE EFFECT OF LABYRINTHECTOMY ON THE STRUCTURE OF THE ENDOLYMPHATIC SAC

HELGE RASK-ANDERSEN, ULLA FRIBERG
Department of Otolaryngology, University Hospital, S-751 85 Uppsala (Sweden)

INTRODUCTION

The exact role of the endolymphatic sac (ES) in the inner ear is still unclear. Different functions have been proposed:

1. Resorption of endolymph[1,2]
2. Secretion of endolymph[3]
3. Pressure regulation of the labyrinth[4]
4. Phagocytic and immunodefensive function in the inner ear[1,5,6]

This investigation was undertaken to obtain more information about the possible secretory role of the ES in the inner ear.

MATERIAL AND METHODS

Twenty albino mice underwent a left-sided surgical labyrinthectomy, leaving the right ear as control. The animals were killed 2, 7 and 14 days after surgery. The temporal bones were processed for transmission electron microscopy.

RESULTS

Two days after labyrinthectomy the sac lumen had collapsed. The light epithelial cells showed vesiculation of cytoplasm and the width of the lateral intercellular spaces (LIS) was increased. The dark cells appeared metabolically hyperactive, with increased electron density of cytoplasm and nuclear chromatin. Dark cells were often seen to displace light cells and to partially take over their contact with the lumen.

Seven days after labyrinthectomy the lumen of ES was distended and contained a homogeneous substance. The sac had doubled its volume as compared with the normal control ear. The normally wide LIS were collapsed and generally the light cells no longer faced the luminal space. The cytoplasm of the dark cells contained numerous polyribosomes and extensive rough endoplasmic reticulum together with a number of membrane-bound granules. The delimiting membrane of these granules frequently appeared to fuse with the apical cell membrane, thereby apparently releasing the granular content directly into the luminal space. The nature of this material corresponds with the homogeneous substance of the sac lumen.

CONCLUSIONS

The present findings seem to suggest that the ES in the mouse has a secretory capacity. It is believed that this secretion is accomplished by the dark cells.

The light cells are believed to have an absorptive function.

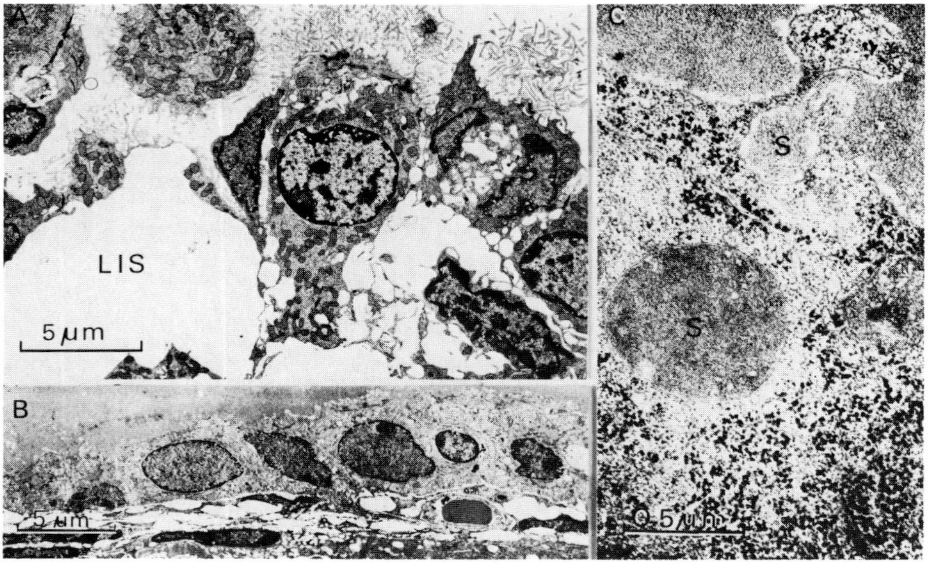

Fig. 1 A. Epithelial outline of endolymphatic sac in control ear. Note the wide lateral intercellular spaces (LIS). Both light (microvilli- or mitochondriarich) and dark cells surround the LIS. B. Epithelial outline of endolymphatic sac 7 days after labyrinthectomy. The LIS are collapsed and the dark cells have replaced the light cells. The content of the lumen is darkly stained. Presumably secretory granules are seen in the apical cytoplasm of the dark cells. C. The apical cytoplasm of a dark cell 14 days after labyrinthectomy at higher magnification. The delimiting membrane of a granule has merged with the apical cell membrane, apparently discharging the granular contents into the sac. S: secretory granule.

ACKNOWLEDGEMENTS

This study was supported by grants from the Swedish Medical Research Council (project No. 03908). We are grateful to Mrs Birgitta Jansson for skilful technical assistance.

REFERENCES

1. Lundquist (1965) Acta Otolaryngol Suppl 201
2. Kimura RS, Schuknecht HF (1965) Pract Otorhinolaryng 27:343-355
3. Seymour JC (1954) J Laryngol 68:698-711
4. Secretan JP (1944) Acta Otolaryngol 32:119-163
5. Guild SR (1927) Am J Anat 39:1-56
6. Rask-Andersen H, Stahle J (1980) Acta Otolaryngol 89:283-294

© 1985 Elsevier Science Publishers B.V. (Biomedical Division)
New dimensions in otorhinolaryngology - head and neck surgery, vol. 2.
E. Myers, editor

A microanalysis study on human auditory ossicles

JM Sánchez-Fernández, JM Rivera and JA Zubillaga

Departments of Otolaryngology, Pathology and Physics, University of Basque Country and Basurto Civil Hospital, Bilbao, Spain

INTRODUCTION

The normal human middle ear ossicles development usually have been studied by histological procedures. Nowadays, to acquiere a complete chemical and structural data from a bone may be used bio-histo and immunochemical studies, as well as electron microscopy techniques (TEM, SEM).

The purpose of the present paper is to establish by microanalysis the normal pattern of human auditory ossicles.

MATERIAL AND METHODS

For this study we have employed two groups of material. The components of the first group were: one fetus of 2oo mm c.r.l. Two male newborns, the first of 34o c.r.l. , from a diabetic mother, presenting eye and mandibular malformations, however the appearance of his middle ear ossicles was normal. The second of 23o mm c.r.l. has an achondroplastic skull, shorth limbs with fingers of the same lenght, external ears normal but with malformations of his middle ear ossicles. His dead was by a respiratory failure. Two male infants of 8 months old, one dead by hearth failure and the other by a respiratory disease. Two adults men, 30 to 40 years old, one dead by traffic accident and the other by a respiratory disease. The components of the second group were: a male newborn, a male infant and a male man 30 years old. They were dead by respiratory diseases and traffic accident respectively. The specimens of the first group were fixed by immersion in a 2% solution of glutaraldehyde (2 hours) in phosphate buffer at pH 7.4. Dehydrated in acetone and dried by the critical point method. In the second group the material was freezed in liquid nitrogen at -190ºC. The preparations were examined without coating in a JEOL SR 32 SEM microscope with a X-ray detector model LINK SR2-2oo. The analysis conditions were always the same that is: 20Kv. Spectrum lenght 1024. The total counting time was 200 secs. The magnification x1000. In order to calibrate our instrument we have established a window line of Calcium and Phosphorus following the peaks obtained with a standard samples of Monetite. Two kinds of spectra were taken: one of the outer layer (periosteal bone surface), and the other on the inner layer (endosteal matrix), after drilling away the periphery of the malleus head and incus body. All the spectra were obtained from the center to the periphery of malleus head and incus body.

RESULTS

In this paper we only present the results corresponding to the malleus and incus. In all these specimens, the mean value of the Ca/P molar ratio corresponding to the endosteal layer of the malleus head ranges from o.88 to 1.14 and in the incus body from 0.89 to 1.07,unless the malleus head (2) and incus body (1.5) from infant 3 and adult 3 cryofixed.Malleus and incus have an homogeneous distribution of Ca/P molar ratio in three of our specimens (newborn 1,adult 1 and infant 1). In the adult 3 and infant 3 cryofixed a significant difference appears in the Ca/P molar ratio between the malleus head and incus body.In the fetus ,the malleus and incus Ca/P molar ratio (0.93 and 0.89) is below adult and infant mean values. In our specimens the Ca/P molar ratio diminishes from the center to the periphery in the malleus head and incus body.Finally,we have detected alterations in Ca/P molar ratio(0.5) in the malleus head of the newborn l(diabetic specimen), even though he has a normal appearing ossicles,while in the newborn 2 (achondroplastic specimen) with a malleus malformation ,we didn´t find any significant alteration in his Ca/P molar ratio.

DISCUSSION

Landis et al [1,2],and Landis & Glimcher[3] have shown that bone tissue preparation by anhidrous treatment with ethylene glycol and with dry ultracryomicrotomy prevent the artifacts attributable to aqueous solvents fixation which cause mineral phase transformation of calcium and phosphorus.In the present work,bone tissue was prepared with fixation in aqueous glutaraldehyde solution and by cryofixation,but we didn´t find any significant difference in our results between the two methods. The Ca/P molar ratio represent the principal value in the labile mineral phases of diverse calcium phosphate solid components.In our findings the average endosteal value of the Ca/P molar ratio corresponding to the endosteal layer of the malleus head ranges from 0.88 to 1.14 and in the incus body from 0.89 to 1.07.These values are according with that of Landis & Glimcher[3], and probably correspond to monetite or brushite.

In the future we shall present the normal stapes microanalysis and the results in another pathological conditions.

REFERENCES

1. Landis WJ,Paine MC,Glimcher MJ.(1977).Electron microscopic observations of bone tissue prepared anhydrously in organic solvents.J Ultrastruct Res 59:1-30
2. Landis WJ,Hauschka BT,Rogerson CA, Glimcher MJ(1977).Electron microscopic observations of bone tissue prepared by ultracryomicrotomy.J Ultrastruct Res 59:185-206
3. Landis WJ,Glimcher MJ (1978).Electron diffraction and electron probe microanalysis of the mineral phase of bone tissue prepared by anhydrous techniques. J Ultrastruct Res 63:188-223

© 1985 Elsevier Science Publishers B.V. (Biomedical Division)
New dimensions in otorhinolaryngology - head and neck surgery, vol. 2.
E. Myers, editor

THE MORPHOLOGY OF THE NORMAL OSSICLES

L. Z. SZABO

ENT Clinic of the Postgraduate Medical School, Budapest (Hungary)

My experience was that normal human ossicles differed greatly from each other individually in their tissue structure. The ossicles were removed from the cadavers of 56 healthy people who died in accidents and series of sections at 8 mm thickness were prepared. Each 10th section was examined. The sections were projected on microscopic screen and margins of the bones, lumens of vessels and areas of marrow cavity were marked and bony lacunas and alive osteocytes cells counted. The areas were measured by planimetry and put into proportion which enabled me to calculate the dimensions of volume since each other section represented a thickness of 80 microns. The prepared ossicle material was evenly distributed between the ages of 4.5 months to 87 years.

It became obvious that the individual differences between the ossicles are determined by age. In the section of a 4.5 months old newborn's incus the 98% of the bony lacunes contains alive osteocytes. From the age 1 year the saturation with osteocytes is around 90% up to the age of 35 years. After 35 years the number of the bony cells decreases. By the age of 40 the filling of the bony lacunes is only 70%. Between the ages 40 and 50 the osteocytes gradually disappear from the ossicles. Over the age of 50 I have never found living osteocytes in any of the ossicles. Despite this fact the ossicles are present in the human body unchanged in their shape. It is a unique situation, that the tissue lacking cells does not absorbe. The metabolism of the intercellulare tissue in the ossicles was entablished with Tetracycline-technique.

What's the reason of the destruction of bony cells? Examination of blood vessel system of the ossicles answers this question. In the ossicles of the newborn the proportion of the blood vessels is 4%. By the age of 1 year this is being reduced to 2.8% In the meantime the number of osteocytes decreases from 100% to 90%. This is physiologic postnatal change. Until the age of 35 the volume of blood vessels is unchanged. Then again it begins to diminish, and by the age of 50 it is only 2%. The reduced blood consumption is not enough to keep bony cells alive, and so they necrotise.

The bony tissue after having lost its cells begins to

degenerate. This is marked by the gradual dilatation of the marrow cavities. While from the time of birth to the age of 40 to 45 the ossicles become more compact, and the marrow cavities get narrow, during the later years they due to reabsorption. The external configuration however remains unchanged, the ossicle preserves its function.

New dimensions in otorhinolaryngology - head and neck surgery, vol. 2.
E. Myers, editor

SCANNING ELECTRON MICROSCOPY OF COCHLEAR BLOOD VESSELS

TETSUYA TONO, TOMOYUKI NAGAI and TAMOTSU MORIMITSU
Department of Otolaryngology, Miyazaki Medical College, Miyazaki, Japan

INTRODUCTION

Recent technical advances in scanning electron microscopy allow us to visualize covered surfaces of tissues and cells by selective removal of connective tissue components. The overall structure of periendothelial cells has been described in several organs with the use of enzymatic digestion and HCl hydrolysis (1,2), The purpose of this paper is to demonstrate the results of scanning electron microscopic observations on periendothelial cells and perivascular autonomic nerve fibers fully disclosed in the cochlea from the arterial to the venous side.

MATERIALS AND METHODS

White guinea pigs, weight 250 g to 350 g, with good Preyer's reflex were used. Two techniques were employed to remove perivascular connective tissues:

(1) HCl hydrolysis with or without prior trypsin digestion

Cochleae removed were separated into the modiolus, the spiral lamina and the external wall. They were immersed in phosphate-buffered Ringer's solution containing 2.5 mg/ml trypsin (DIFCO 1:250) for 0-30 minutes at 37°C. After fixation in 3% phosphate-buffered glutaraldehyde, they were hydrolized with 8 N HCl for 10-20 minutes at 60°C.

(2) Combination of resin-injection and HCl hydrolysis

Following blood washout with heparinized Ringer's solution, the animal was perfused with 3% phosphate-buffered glutaraldehyde, then, Mercox-resin was injected into the ascending aorta. Cochleae removed were immersed in the same fixative. After using fine forceps under a stereo-light microscope to expose objective vessels filled with Mercox-resin, the vessels were hydrolized with 8 N HCl for 20-30 minutes at 60°C.

RESULTS AND DISCUSSION

HCl hydrolysis with or without prior trypsin digestion successfully removed the covering connective tissues and the basal lamina, exposing the adventitial surfaces of periendothelial cells. However, since this method deforms the angioarchirecture, the combination of resin-injection and HCl hydrolysis was also used, allowing visualization of periendothelial cells with their angioarchitecture relatively intact.

The shape and arrangement of periendothelial cells vary remarkably along the vessels. Six types of vascular segments were classified according to the overall morphology of periendothelial cells: (1) arteries with compact elongated smooth muscle cells oriented transversely; (2) arterioles with compact spindle-shaped smooth muscle cells arranged in circular fashion; (3) precapillary arterioles with less compact branched smooth muscle cells and helically oriented processes; (4) capillaries with widely scattered pericytes and longitudinally oriented primary processes which branch out fine processes in succession; (5) postcapillary venules with scattered spidery pericytes and radially oriented processes; (6) venules and veins with scattered polygonal pericytes and irregularly oriented processes. All the vascular segments are found in the modiolus, but only precapillary arterioles, capillaries and postcapillary venules are found in the spiral lamina and the external wall.

Such morphological differences suggest that each vascular segment has a different role in the cochlear vascular system. Periendothelial cells of arteries and arterioles have a structure adapted to narrowing the vascular lumen upon constriction. Those of precapillary arteioles which locate between the arterioles in the modiolus and all the capillary areas in the cochlea appear to have less power, but they may still exert delicate control over capillary blood flow distribution. A characteristic feature of capillary pericytes in the cochlea is the coral-like branching of cytoplasmic processes. These fine processes are prominent in the spiral capillary and the strial capillary. Such structures seem adventageous for the maintenance of constant blood flow of these capillaries even in the presence of mechanical vibration. Periendothelial cells of venous side vessels do not appear to have much power to narrow the vescular lumen. But many processes of periendothelial cells which overlap and interconnect with each other are presumed to be involved in preventing an excessive loss of blood elements.

In spite of no information about histochemical categories of autonomic nerves, present SEM techniques also provide information as to the innervation pattern of vascular segments. The artery and the arterioles are always innervated either densely or sparsely. But nerve fibers do not always reach to the precapillary arterioles, The prevalence of the autonomic nervous system as a control mediator on the precapillary arterioles seemingly depends on the area where they are found in the cochlea. The frequency of innervated precapillary arterioles decreases from the modiolus, to the spiral lamina, with disappearance in the external wall. Innervated capillaries are seen in the modiolus and the spiral lamina. But they are rare and their functional significance remains uncertain. On the venous side, no nerve fibers are observed in association with the vessels.

REFERENCES

1. Nagai, M., Nagai, T. and Morimitsu, T. 1982. Scanning electron microscopy of the nasal glands and vessels. Arch Otorhinolaryngol 237:67.
2. Fujiwara, T. and Uehara, Y. 1984. The cytoarchitecture of the wall and innervation pattern of the microvessels in the rat mammary gland: A scanning electron microscopic observation. Am J Anat 170:39.

New dimensions in otorhinolaryngology - head and neck surgery, vol. 2.
E. Myers, editor

THE EFFECT OF HEMODILUTION BY DEXTRAN ON THE COCHLEAR BLOOD FLOW.

E.HULTCRANTZ (1), A.F. NUTTALL (2), F.SCHEIBE (3), J.M. MILLER (2)
Inst of Otolaryngology, University of Uppsala, (Sweden) (1).
Kresge Hearing Research Inst, University of Michigan, AnnArbor,(2)
ENT-Clinic (Charité) Humboldt University, Berlin (DDR) (3)

INTRODUCTION

A viral disease or a vascular accident are among the most commonly accepted theories explaining Sudden Deafness. These two theories are not completely contradictory as a viral disease could directly influencethe cochlear blood vessels or increase the platelets adhesivness thereby causing "sludging" and reduction of the cochlear blood flow.

Low molecular weight dextran, Dextran 40 (MW 40000) is commonly used in the treatment of Sudden Deafness. Dextran 40 increases capillary blood flow in general by hypervolemic hemodilution and by decreasing factor VIII (I), but a clinical effect by the drug on Sudden Deafness has been difficult to prove.

The purpose of the present study was to investigate whether and how a slow infusion of Dextran 40 influenced the cochlear blood flow and study the effect of hemodilution by Dextran 40 and Dextran 75 (MW 75000) on the cochlear blood flow.

MATERIAL AND METHODS

Guinea pigs, anaesthetised and tracheotomised, were used. The left bulla was opened ventrally and a Laser doppler probe (Medpacific, L-D 5000) was placed over the second turn of the cochlea to measure the cochlear blood flow. A second Laser probe (Perimed, Periflux) was attached to the abdominal skin. The right carotid artery was cannulated for blood pressure measurements and one jugular vein was cannulated for infusions and blood withdrawal. Compound Action Potentials (CAP:S) were registered from a round window electrode during click-sound stimulation. Five of the animals got infusions of Dextran 40 (10% in Saline),10 ml/kg bwt/h for about I hour Three of them were also hemodiluted using Dextran 40 and Saline to replace the blood. Six other animals were normovolemic hemodiluted with Dextran 75 (6% in Saline). 2.5ml blood was withdrawn every 10 min and replaced by Dextran 75. Three of them were exposed to Carbogen intermittently during the experiments.

RESULTS

The cochlear blood flow (CBF) rose by 75% during the Dextran 40 infusion, but reached a steady state early and began to fall as soon as the infusion ended. The Htc fell from 41-26% due to the infusion. The normovolemic hemodiluation increased the CBF by 100% when the Htc was around 17% without regard to whether. Dextran 75 were used. The CAP:s initially improved during the hemodilution, but declined when the Htc dropped below 20%. In one case it was possible to improve the CAP:s at Htc 16% by letting the animal breath Carbogen. The skin flow increased much more than the CBF during the hyper- and normovolemic hemodilution and reacted more readily on changes in blood pressure, indicating a higher degree of autoregulation in the cochlea.

DISCUSSION AND CONCLUSION

Dextran 40 is hyperoncotic and draws extracellular fluid into the blood vessels, which increases the blood volume and decreases blood viscosity, resulting in increased Cardiac Output and tissue blood flow. If the cochlea, however, has the same strong autoregulation as the brain (2) the CBF should not increase and that might be a reason for a poor clinical effect in some patients with Sudden Deafness. This was not the case, but the effect on CBF was lesser than on skin blood flow. Dextran 40 has a half-life of 5 h in the circulation and dextran with higher MW stays proportionally longer. As blood viscosity is related to Htc the registered effect on CBF could be expected to be about the same with Dextran 40 infusion and normovolemic hemodilution. This was the case. One clinical study by Dauman et al 1983(3) has shown promising results using hemodilution with Dextran 60 in patients with Sudden Deafness. As normovolemic hemodilution with Dextran 75 is a much lesser strain on the circulatory system and has a more longlasting effect than Dextran40 infusion, it should be considered in the treatment of Sudden Deafness.

REFERENCES

1. Åberg M, Hedner U, & Bergentz S-E. 1979. Effect of dextran on factor VIII. Ann Surg 189:243

2 Wood JH, Simeone Fa, Kron RE. 1982. Rheological aspects of experimental hypervolemic hemodilution with low molecular weight dextran. Neurosurgery 11:739

3 Dauman R, Cros A.M., Mehsen M. and Cazals Y. 1983. Hemodilution in Sudden Deafness: First Results. Arch Otorhinolaryngol 238:97

New dimensions in otorhinolaryngology - head and neck surgery, vol. 2.
E. Myers, editor

EFFECT OF VANADATE ON COCHLEA AND ITS DISTRIBUTION

TAKAYUKI NAKANO, TAMOTSU MORIMITSU AND MINORU IDE
Department of Otolaryngology, Miyazaki Medical College, Miyazaki, Japan

INTRODUCTION

Vanadium, a transition metalic element, is generally well known as a toxic element together with cadmium, arsenic and chromium. It is distributed broadly in vivo as a trace element. Recently, it has been disclosed that oxides of vanadium, especially vanadic acid of oxidation with the number of 5, inhibit various ATPases. The inhibition coefficiency against Na, K-ATPase is equal to that of ouabain, a powerful inhibitor to this enzyme.

Therefore, we have studied electrophysiologically, the effect on the inner ear of vanadate. Moreover, because vanadate may possibly accumulate in the cochlea in such a condition, X-ray micro-analysis was attempted afterwards.

MATERIALS AND METHODS

(1) Electrophysiological experiment

Guinea pigs (weighing 250 to 300g), having good Pryers' reflex, were employed for the experiments. The perfusion liquid for use was prepared by dissolving o-sodium vanadate in the Tris saline buffer and further by adjusting to a pH of 7.4. After opening a small hole in the scala vestibuli and the scala tympani and inserting a glass pipet with an approximately 50 u tip. The perfusion was carried out at a flow rate of 5 ul/min.

(2) X-ray micro-analysis

The subjects for experiments were the same guinea pigs that had been used for electrophysiological experimentation. The specimen was immediately fixed with glutar, and treated according to the method for the preparation of transmission electron micro-scopic samples. As to metal evapration, Al-evaporation was carried out using a compact coater CC-50 and the X-ray micro-analyzer EPM-810Q of the Shimazu wave-length dispersion model was used.

The results of measurement were treated with a computer using the color mapping method featuring the system and indicated in color on CRT. The measurements were made with 3 elements, vanadium, sulfur and magnesium.

RESULTS AND DISCUSSION

In the case of perfusion with 1mM vanadate, the transient over-shoot persisted for approximately 10min, followed by falling EP together with a fall of the CM.

About 30min after starting the perfusion, the EP value was 52mV and the CM fell down to about 20%. In order to investigate the effect on the EP of different levels of vanadate, a liquid was perfused at each level of 1,5 and 10mM. The similar transient over-shoot was noted, followed by a gradual fall of the EP. The degree of its fall was in the order of the concentration. When anoxia was performed after about 60min, generation of the -EP was noted, but the value was smaller than normal. As to the fall of the EP noted after 20min due to the perfusion at each the levels, the EP values obtained at 1, 5 and 10mM were 67, 58 and 42mV respective falling degrees of 16, 27 and 46%. Although performance of anoxia during perfusion with 10 mM vanadate generated -EP, the -EP value was -20mV when anoxia was perfomed after 20 min of perfusion, whereas the -EP was generated only up to as low as -10mV when anoxia was again performed approximately 50 min later. This fact suggests that the -EP decreases with increasing time of perfusion.

In X-ray microanalysis, compaired the control group with the perfusion group, although nearly no vanadium was noted in the spiral ligament, spiral prominence and Reisners' membrane, the stria vascuralis region indicated more vanadium than normal. Regarded as the sulfur, nearly no difference was noted between the normal group and the treated group in the same sample. In addition the Mg distribution also noted nearly no difference between them. In another sample, accumulation of vanadium was obviously noted the stria vascuralis region.

Next, the organ of Corti was investigated after perfusion with vanadate, vanadium was scarcely noted in Henssens' cells, Deiters' cells and the tectorial membrane, but its accumulation was noted to coincide with hair cells. Further, it was noted also in the limbs and the osseus spiral lamina.

As to the distribution of Mg in the same regions, revealing much Mg in the osseus spiral lamina.

The experiments were carried out not using specific agents such as furosemide and ouabain but using a vanadium compuond being usually present in vivo though minor in quantity. The results disclosed that perilymphatic perfusion with the compound lowered EP that was present like a battery source when induced potential was generated in the inner ear, followed by lowered CM.

Further, it was noted that changes appeared in the -EP value depending on perfusion time.

Moreover the investigation of the distribution of vanadium by a new technique termed EPMA provided data, well coinciding with the results of the electrophysiological study.

In view of the specific accumulation of vanadium as a result of EPMA analysis together with the electrophysiological results, the vanadate probably affected at first the stria vascularis and then the hair cells.

© 1985 Elsevier Science Publishers B.V. (Biomedical Division)
New dimensions in otorhinolaryngology - head and neck surgery, vol. 2.
E. Myers, editor

ON THE USE OF HOMOGRAFT TREATING OZENA - Prof. Dr. med. Christian Betow

Aims of the treatment of ozena are:
- restoral of the mucous secretion
- restoral of the smelling capability
- elimination of cacosmia
- removal of headache
- revitalization of the strongly atrophic nasal mucosa

Medical as well as surgical methods were suggested. I would like to indicate a few of the medicamentous and surgical methods of treatment:

Medicamentous treatment:
. nose irrigation (1 teaspoon Na Cl for 1 l. water), LUGOL solution
. GOTTSTEIN-screw tamponade
. snuffing Dextropur (as unguent or powder)
. giving vitamins (vit. A,B,C, pantotenic acid, D,F (VEIDS)
. stellate block (BEICKERT), novocain (SHARMA, HIBLER, JANNOULIS)
. serotherapy and vaccine therapy- probably with additional therapy (STERNBERG, MARSCHIK)
. nose drops in the following composition: vitamin A 30.000 IE, Menthol 0,05, 0,1 oliv. of 30 ml. drops to be installed in the morning and evening).

Surgical treatment:
surgical methods of treatment have the purpose to narrow the wide nasal cavity in order to reach a better humidity and to act against the incrustation and exsiccation of the nose.

1. Blockage of the ductus parotideus "physiological operation" and constant supply of humidity for the nose (that means rhinorrhea, also when eating).
2. Implantation of tissue
   a) porous beef-bone (ECKERT-MÖBIUS)
   b) iliac bone as an autograft (UNTERBERGER)
   c) artificial implants and cartilage chips
   d) silicone chips (HUIZING 1969), umbelical implants.
3. Radical operation of the maxillary sinus and reposition of the maxillary sinus (B. GAAHNE). Both interventions easily lead to exsication of the nose and the pharynx mucosa.

After experimental examinations on animals in 1959, we were able to perform the first homograft transplantation en bloc in middle ear surgery. Our experience regarding the homograft tissue, preserved in Cialit 1 : 5000, enabled us to preserve different kinds of homologous tissue and a sufficient supply for our tissue bank. From this we used most successfully preserved costal cartilage to correct the saddle nose and to treat the ozena.

Implanting homograft cartilage, the following technique was used: in local or insufflation anesthesia, a mucous incision was made from the upper crista of the labial foldto the frenulum and laterally until the level of the canine tooth. After removal of the periostium to the anterior, inferior, and lateral border of the apertura piriformis a part of the bony edge of the apertura is removed by drill or chisel as far as to achieve a free access into the anterior, inferior and lateral nose canal. Then the mucous periostium is to be mobilized at the base of the lower nasal canal, the lateral nose wall and in difficult cases also at the middle lateral nose wall and the septum. Now the implantation of the bone cartilage can take place. The icised wound is sewn with 2 or 3 sutures.

According to our observations the results are as follows: a hyperintensive reaction of the host's organism leads to a bluish-red coloration of the transplant. The red change in colour is caused by rushing in of the vessels. The reactive inflammation enhances the revitalisation of the strongly atrophic mucosa.

The advantage of homograft implantation is constant disposal of desired quantities of preserved costal cartilage. Therefore, a patient is not exposed to the danger of a surgical trauma or to complications which might occur taking autogenous cartilage from the ribs. The incidence of infections can nearly be excluded, as in consequence of the preservation in Cialit solution the cartilage is not sensible to bacterial growth.
This disease is quite seldom in Germany, in the course of 20 years only 12 of the 32 operated patients could be re-examined. In one case the result was satisfactory, all other results were good.

Seeing the good late results, this surgical procedure of homograft cartilage implantation has proved to be one of the possibilities treating ozena.

New dimensions in otorhinolaryngology - head and neck surgery, vol. 2.
E. Myers, editor

EPISTAXIS: ASSOCIATION OF METHODS IN POSTERIOR TAMPONEMENT

SYDNEY CASTAGNO,MD,PhD
ROGER L. CASTAGNO,MD,PhD
LUCIO A. CASTAGNO,MD
Department of Otolaryngology,Federal University of Pelotas School of Medicine.
Rua General Osorio,1585. Pelotas,96100,Brazil

INTRODUCTION

Posterior epistaxis treatment has been changing in the last decade.Several techniques are described with distincts applications and results.Most of them are sophisticated procedures and depend on a well structured ard equiped medical services.

This paper however is addressed to those doctors who have to work with poor facilities and use the combined anterior-posterior nasal packing.The classical posterior tamponement of Bellocq is in our experience more traumatic and less confortable for the patient than the posterior nasal packing with balloons. Moreover,nasal packing with balloons are easier to perform.

Considering the absence of low cost national material adequate to the treatment of posterior epistaxis we developed a balloon prepared with unexpensive and easy-to-find materials,which will be presented now.

MATERIAL AND METHODS

We have used: a) 20 cm latex tube; b) 2 cm of extremity of a surgical glove finger; c) 1.5 cm of a plastic tube (the inside tube of a ball-point pen); d) approximately 50 cm of resistent string (figure 1: A to D).

The 1.5 cm plastic tube is put inside the 20 cm latex tube,as the plastic tube prevents the colabation of the latex one.The surgical glove finger is tied to the latex tube with a resitent string loose about 20 cm long (figure 1: E-F).

The balloon is put through the nasal floor inside the nasopharynx and filled with 10 ml of water.Then the anterior nasal packing is done.The two loose strings from the balloon are exteriorized through the nostril and tied on the anterior nasal pack: *this is an important complement that holds both tamponements in place* (figure 2).

RESULTS

Between 1973-84 we have treated 240 patients with posterior epistaxis using the above described technique,most of them on an ambulatorial basis.In just 4 (1.7%) patients the epistaxis remained out of control and we had to do the classical posterior tamponement of Bellocq.

Most of our patients had epistaxis secundary to hypertension (87%).Sex distribution indicates 67% males and 33% females and there was a marked prevalence of epistaxis over the 50 years (85%).

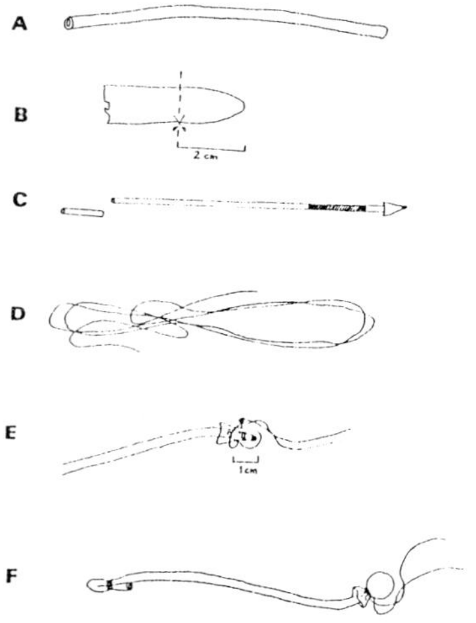

Fig. 1. Material used to make the balloon: A- 20 cm latex tube; B- 2 cm of extremity of a surgical glove finger; C- 1.5 cm of a plastic tube; D- resistent string.

D- Making the balloon.
E- Balloon filled.*Attention to the loose strings.*

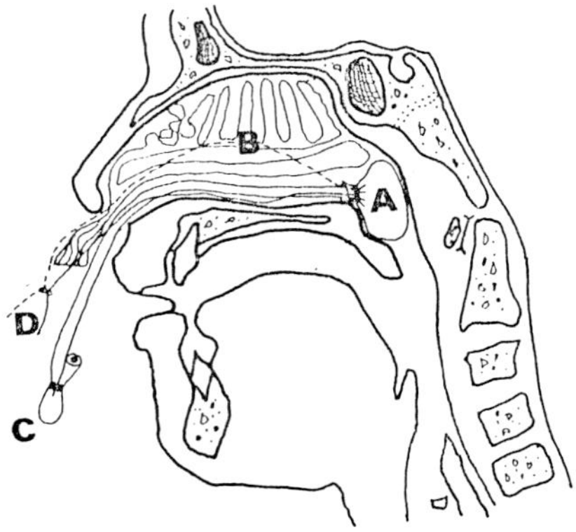

Fig. 2. Association of anterior-posterior nasal packing: A- balloon inside the nasopharynx; B- anterior nasal packing; C- 20 cm latex tube; D- *two strings that hold both tamponements in place.*

DISCUSSION

Even though several new techniques and some serious complications with posterior nasal packing have been described we believe that this is a highly useful procedure for the otorhinolaryngologist who has to work with poor facilities. None of our patiets had serious complications.This balloon is specially indicated to countries where doctors need to conjugate effective and low cost technique.

REFERENCES

1. Hicks J, Norrius J (1983) Laryngoscope 93:876-879.
2. McDonald T, Pearson B (1980) Arch Otolaryngol 106:635-638.
3. Merland J et al (1980) Laryngoscope 90:1694-1704.
4. Rosnagle R at al (1980) Arch Otolaryngol 106:137-142.
5. Wang L, Vogel D (1981) Otolaryngol Head Neck Surg 89:1001-1006.

© 1985 Elsevier Science Publishers B.V. (Biomedical Division)
New dimensions in otorhinolaryngology - head and neck surgery, vol. 2.
E. Myers, editor

VALVE PHENOMENON IN NASAL OBSTRUCTION

GONZALO CORVERA M.D., JORGE CORVERA M.D. and CARLOS S. CASTILLO M.D.
Gabinete de Fisiologia Nasal, Mexico City

INTRODUCTION

Bridger (1) defines the nasal valve as a collapsible flow limiting segment in the nose, acting as a Starling resistor, that above certain values keeps the nasal air flow constant in spite of a further increase in respiratory effort. The purpose of this paper is to detect the possible role that a unidirectional flow limiting structure ("valve", VP) could play in the cause of nasal obstruction.

METHODS

An active anterior rhinomanometry (RMM) was made in 200 consecutive patients with nasal obstruction. Tumors and infection cases were excluded. The values were computer processed and expressed in two graphs. In the first, P values are plotted in the y axis, and F values in the x axis. To study the resistance as a function of flow, the second graph plots nasal resistance (NR) in the y axis and flow in the x axis. To evidentiate the "valve phenomenon", the NR values of inspiration and expiration were compared.

RESULTS

The RMM diagnoses made are shown in table 1. We define "nasal obstruction" when the nasal resistance is found consistently greater than 1.5 DPa/l/sec.

TABLE 1. TYPES OF NASAL OBSTRUCTION FOUND

	BILATERAL	RIGHT FOSSA	LEFT FOSSA	TOTAL
Structural	32	14	17	63
Functional	25	9	3	37
Structural + functional	-	-	-	14
Direct valvular	4	2	2	8
Combined direct valvular	-	-	-	30
Inverse valvular	1	1	-	2
Combined inverse valvular	-	-	-	20

In "structural obstruction", the resistance does not drop below 1.5 after vasoconstriction, and in "functional obstruction" it does. A VP was defined when the NR values were different for expiration and inspiration. When inspiratory NR was greater, a "direct valve" (DVP) was considered and an "inverse valve" (IVP) when expiratory NR was greater. The DVP was diagnosed in 35.6% of the obstructed patients and the IVP in 17.8%. After vasoconstriction, there was a considerable reduction of the patients that exhibited the valve phenomenon, 16.1% and 5.7% respectively. These cases were studied to determine the behavior of the valve phenomenon at different flow rates. The results are expressed in figure 1.

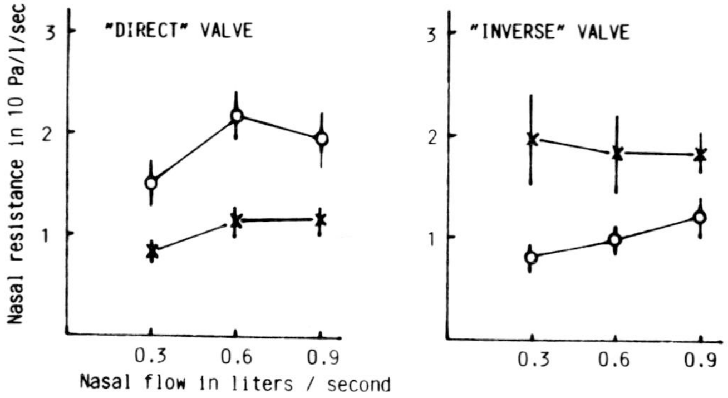

Fig. 1. Nasal resistance at different flow rates in valve phenomenon.

In DVP the average inspiratory NR is twice as high as the expiratory NR, this ratio remains constant at the different flow rates. In IVP the expiratory NR values remain constant at the flow rates studied, but the inspiratory NR values increase with the higher flow rates.

We did not find evidence of the nasal valve maintaining a constant flow through the nose, as had been previously reported (1). Our findings suggest that it is the resistance that remains constant while the pressure increases, producing an increment in the flow rate, at least in the range tested.

We have found a high prevalence of a unilateral flow limiting phenomenon in patients that complain of nasal obstruction, suggesting that it plays an important part in producing the symptom. Its frequent association with other types of obstruction compared to its relatively rare occurrence by itself (18% vs 4%) could indicate that this "valve" is part of the normal anatomy of the nose, producing obstruction in the presence of aggravating factors. We did not find any reason to suppose that it plays another, more "physiological" role in regulating air flow through the nose.

REFERENCE

1. Bridger GP: Physiology of the Nasal Valve. Arch Otolaryng 92:543-553, 1970.

New dimensions in otorhinolaryngology – head and neck surgery, vol. 2.
E. Myers, editor

ELECTRON MICROSCOPIC STUDY OF SCLEROMA IN INDIA

DR. MRS. SANDRA DESASCUZA. DR. A.R. CHITALE
Jaslok Hospital & Research Centre, 15 G. Deshmukh Marg, Bombay - 400 026

INTRODUCTION

Scleroma a chronic indolent granulomatous disease has three overlapping clinical stages, Catarrhal, granulomatous and sclerotic, and three corresponding microscopic phases, the first of chronic inflammatory infiltration, the second of a plasmacytic infiltrate with the appearance of a characteristic foamy Mikulicz cel s containing the K. Rhinoscleromaticus bacilli and third of fibrosis with distortion. As the Frisch bacillus is often difficult to stain and impossible to see in the third phase of fibrosis ultrastructural studies were carried out in 20 cases using a 100 S Jeol Electron Microscope.

RESULTS OF ELECTRON MICROSCOPY.

In patients in stage I plasma cells and histiocytes containing vesicles with degenerating bacilli were seen. In stage II and III plasma cells

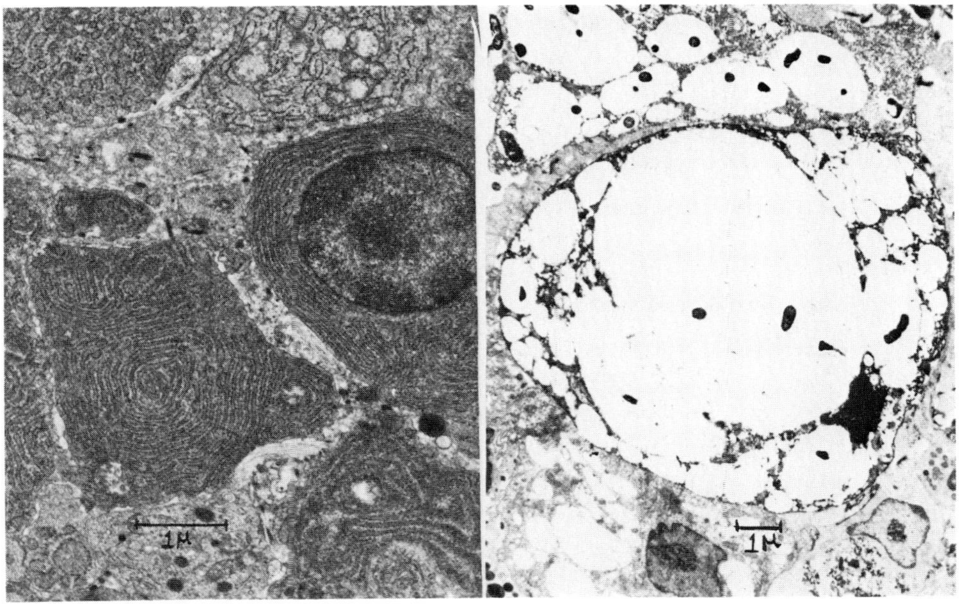

Fig. 1a) Plasma cells with characteristic concentric RER. Fig 1b) Foam cells rich in osmiophilic bacilli.

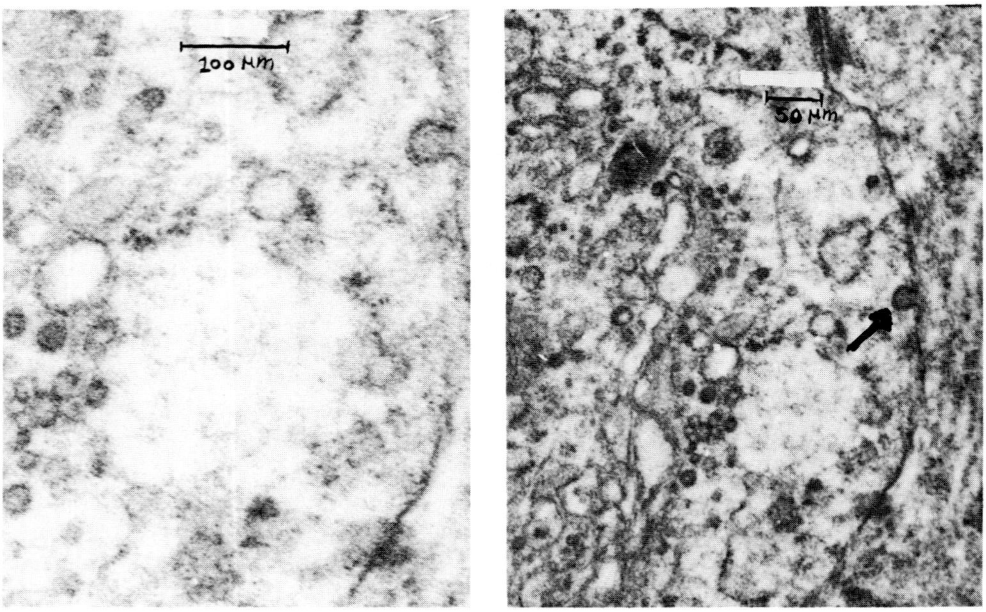

Fig 2a) Non foamy histiocyte containing virions Fig 2b) The budding virion is enlarged.

with characteristic endoplasmic reticulum (fig 1a), foam cells with vacuoles containing bacilli, and bacilli in various stages of development and degeneration could be studied. In late stage II and stage III cases dilated rough endoplasmic reticulum filled with grey material representing previrus particles, virions in clusters (fig 2a) and a budding virion (fig 2b) were observed.

CONCLUSION

EM in Scleroma facilitates ultrastructural observations of Mikulicz and plasma cells, demonstration of bacilli in the later stages and demonstration of virions and virus like particles. From this study although preliminary we concluded that : a) Scleroma was most responsive to treatment in earlier stages from EM findings before and after treatment. b) Virus like particles were demonstrated in EM only in later stages c) Response to treatment was best in cases where only bacilli were demonstrated and poorest where only the virus was seen. It may be therefore the appearance of the virus which makes the disease intractable, and further study will certainly open more avenues on offering an advanced case better treatment.

New dimensions in otorhinolaryngology - head and neck surgery, vol. 2.
E. Myers, editor

MICROSURGICAL TREATMENT FOR POSTERIOR EPISTAXIS

V.DIAMANTE, I.LAZARO, L.BARBON AND G. HAEDO
Pasteur 740 - Buenos Aires - Argentina

INTRODUCTION

The purpose of this work is to describe a simple microsurgical procedure to deal with all kinds of posterior nasal epistaxis.

MATERIAL AND METHODS

Technique

Patient's position: flat on his back, the head slightly flexed and turned towards the surgeon.

Surgeon's position: seated on the contralateral side.

Assistant's position: to the surgeon's right.

Location of the microscope: facing the surgeon. Ocular lenses were 12.5; 200 mm objective lenses with 6x magnification or 300 mm with 10z were used.

Anesthesia

As a rule, it was general, with intubation and an inflatable bulb, to avoid blood and clot aspiration. When contraindicated, local anesthesia may be given after previous sedation.

Surgical procedure

The bivalve speculum is placed in the nostril; the lower turbinal is fractured downwards and outwards and the middle turbinal, upwards and inwards. The speculum is then inserted in the middle meatus to support the fractured turbinals.

Having gained a good exposure, the thin bony wall separating the nose from the sinus is transfixed with the surgical knife to identify the posterior wall of the maxilar sinus. A transversal incision is made in the nasal mucosa, from the middle turbinal's root to the lower's. The mucoperiosteum is detached and a posterior flap made, exposing the vertical portion of the palatine bone.

Working on, the sphenopalatine notch is usually found at the top end of the incision, just below the middle turbinal's root. Releasing the artery from its sheath, electrocautery is performed by mono- or bi-polar technique, as far as possible from the notch. The flap is replaced and the turbinals relocated in their original position, tamping the nostril with vaseline=coated gauze.

RESULTS

In our series of 120 cases of microsurgical endonasal electrocautery of the sphenopalatine artery we have only had two failures. One was due to detachment of the scab, most likely because of deficient electrocautery technique. The other one was an unfortunate location error in a referred patient. Though not bleeding at the time of surgery, his sphenopalatine artery was electrocauterized, but blee ding recurred postoperatively, as the etmoidal artery was actually affected.

CONCLUSIONS

The procedure described offers several advantages, outlined below:

- Simple and fast technique.
- The artery is fully exposed.
- Local anesthesia may be used.
- Surgical trauma is minimal.
- No postoperative complications.
- Hospitalization is brief.
- Lengthy tamping, both painful and risky, is avoided.

However, there are three situations where surgery is contraindicated:

- Severe nasal deformity is present.
- Neoplasias are present at the site.
- Lack of training in microsurgery on the surgeon's part.

To sum up, the authors believe that the endonasal approach to the sphenopalati ne artery is the treatment of choice for all forms of posterior epistaxis.

© 1985 Elsevier Science Publishers B.V. (Biomedical Division)
New dimensions in otorhinolaryngology - head and neck surgery, vol. 2.
E. Myers, editor

NEW CONCEPTS IN SCLEROMA MANAGEMENT

M.E. EL MALLAH (1), A.A. HAROON (2), S.H.. EL-TAYEB (3), R.Y. KHALIL (4).
Departments of Otolaryngology (1), Microbiology and Immunology (2,4) and Clinical Pathology (3)
AL-AZHAR (1,3) and AIN-SHAMS (2,4) UNIVERSITIES.
CAIRO, EGYPT

INTRODUCTION

Cellular immune (C.I.) deficiency in scleroma was revealed by the authers.(1) It is bimodal in nature; needed to develop the disease and is aggravated by it. Its degree determines the histopathologic and clinical pictures.

Kl. Rhinoscleromatis was proved to be the causative agent experimentally in nude mice.(2)

Normal phagocytosis and impaired killing function of leucocytes was found in scleroma patients.(3)

As a result, scleroma management was revised and new concepts emerged.

Is depressed C.I. through hyperactivity of "suppressor" cells, whence immunosuppressive agents are indicated; or through hypoactivity of "helper" cells, thence an immunorestorative is needed.

Impaired killing function of leucocytes combined with depressed C.I. lengthen the course of treatment (trt.) required and necessitates the use of bactericidal antibiotics in alternating courses to reduce drug toxicity and emergence of resistant strains.

Surgery has to be done early, rather than late to remove as much granuloma with its content of intracellular organisms, reducing greatly those left behind rendering them more accessible to antibiotic local and systemic. Surgery, also decreases the factor inhibiting C.I. and leaves no granuloma to fibrose, eliminates nasal obstruction and replaces the metaplastic epithelium with healthy one with better functional and cosmetic results, more gained if done early.

This work aims to scrutinize a plan of trt., and to look for a reliable end point for trt. rather than clinical judgement alone.

MATERIAL AND METHODS

34 patients were studied clinically, histopathologically, bacteriologically and immunologically before, during and after trt., using E-rosetting, total and active as non specific in vitro tests for C.I.(4) and L-migration inhibition using scleroma antigen as a specific in vitro test(5). Tuberculin testing was used as in vivo test because B.C.G. vaccination is a routine in our country. The regimen, followed was medical

based on levamisole, an immuno-restorative[6] and antibiotics chosen through an antibiogram not imperically. Bactericidal ones were selected, two at a time, preferably one by injection, changing in alternate courses, continued until clinical and pathological healing supportive and local measures were advised with levamisole until immunological recovery. Surgery was done 5-7 D after onset of medical trt.

RESULTS

Patients were regardedcured after clinical and histopathologic healing as well as immunologic recovery. It took about 3 m to attain cure, yet it varies with the stage, extent and duration of the disease.

This regimen was found excellent, when followed precisely. Yet relapses do occur if trt. was stopped early or local cleansing was neglected, to improve when resumed again.

No antibiotic of choice exists. Strains resistant to streptomycin and tetracyclines were encountered.

Convergence of tuberculin testing from negativity to positivity was found a reliable end point for trt., as an office test. Yet cases remaining negative inspite of clinical healing should have other laboratory immunologic tests to be done.

C.I. impairment can be safely attributed to hypoactivity of "helper" cells. Thus all immunosuppressives as antimitotics and carticosteroids and preferably irradiation have to be avoided.

REFERENCES

1. El-Mallah, M.E.; Haroun, A.A.; Khalil, R.Y. and Abdel-Razik, I. (1984): Scleroma: Clinico-histopathologic and immunologic studies. The Egyptian Journal of Otolaryngology 1, 53.

2. Haroun, A.A.; Abdel Razik, I. and El-Mallah,M.E. (1985): Experimental Study in scleroma The Journal of the Egyptian Public Health Association 60,1-2.

3. Haroun, A.A.; Soliman, L. and Nassar, M. (1982): Phagocytosis and intracellular killing in scleroma Procedings of the 5th Annual Ain Shams Medical Congress Abstract 61, p 33. (5-8 March).

4. Felsburg, P.J.; Edelmann, R. and Robert, H. (1976): The active erythrocyte rosette test: Correlation with delayed cutaneous hypersensitivity. Journal of Immunology, 116, 1116.

5. Falk, R.E. and Zabriskie, J.B. (1970): "The capillary technique for measurement of inhibition of leucocytic migration as assessment of cellular mediated immunity in" In vitro Methods in Cellular Mediated Immunity" 1st ed. Edited by Bloom, B.R. andGlade, G.R. p 301 Academic Press, N.Y.

6. Asquith, P. (1980): "The clinical use of leramisole - a critical review". In "Recent Advances in Clinical Immunology" edited by Thompson, R.A. Number two. Churchill Livingstone. Edinburgh, London and New York.

Senior Auther, 59 Ramsis St., Cairo, Egypt.

© 1985 Elsevier Science Publishers B.V. (Biomedical Division)
New dimensions in otorhinolaryngology - head and neck surgery, vol. 2.
E. Myers, editor

AN ENVIRONMENTAL STUDY IN RHINOSCLEROMA

D.K. GOSAVI, VIVEK GOSAVI & A.G. BHAVTHANKAR
Miraj, Maharashtra (India)

Rhinoscleroma still remains an enigma and a challenge to Otolaryngologists, Microbiologists and Epidemiologists. Though uncommon in developed countries, it still poses a problem in underdeveloped areas of the world. In fact, Muzyka & Gubina (1971) on surveying 9,721 cases of scleroma notified between 1945-1961 in all endemic foci throughout the world reported that the incidence of rhinoscleroma is rising in recent years and it had made appearance in many countries where it had never been previously recorded. In 2 years, since this project was undertaken, we have seen 84 cases. All these cases have been from the border areas of Maharashtra & Karnataka (India). This large number as compared to only 289 in Asia as reported by Muzyka & Gubina during 16 years, makes us feel that cases are not reported properly and we need a thorough epidemiological survey of rhinoscleroma in Asia & India in particular.

It is now generally agreed that the causative organism in rhinoscleroma is *Klebsiella rhinoscleromatis* and that in most patients there is a poor standard of domestic hygiene. We have, therefore, tried to investigate into the various possible factors in the environment of this so called 'unhygienic' domestic living of these patients and their families with a view to find:

i) Occurance of *K. rhinoscleromatis* in nature outside the human nose.

ii) In the noses of family members of the patients.

iii) Its possible mode of transfer or implantation.

iv) Its association with 'Rhinoscleroma' granuloma.

MATERIAL AND METHODS

The work is done by a team of medical and paramedical personnel. By visiting 12 localities from where scleroma patients had come, 274 samples were collected for culturing from various sites eg. different anatomical sites of cattle dust, cattle-dung, compost etc. The material was cultured on Blood agar &

MaCconkey's medium in the laboratory. Identification of the organisms was done by

i) Characteristic colonies of *Klebsiella* group

ii) Morphological characters of the organisms under light microscopy

iii) Biochemical and Enzymatic reactions on their subcultures for a) Lactose b) Glucose c) Malonate d) Lycine e) V.P. f) M.R. g) Citrate h) Urease

The organisms detected by above methods were as follows:

ENVIRONMENTAL SAMPLES - 274

1.	*K. rhinoscleromatis*	Nil
2.	*K.pneumoniae*	29%
3.	*Staphylococci*	74.5%
4.	*E.coli*	43%
5.	*Pseudomona*	2.5%
6.	Others: *Strepto, Citrobactor, B.Subtilis,* etc.	14.5%
7.	No growth	Nil

DISCUSSION

K.rhinoscleromatis was detected in 17 out of 84 patients ie. in 20.24% of proved cases. None of the samples from the cattle, environmental material and the relatives of the patients revealed *K. rhinoscleromatis* any time. However, *K.pneumoniae* was detected in 29% samples such as various anatomical sites of domesticated cattle, cattle-sheds, dung-hills and compost. *K.pneumoniae* have also been isolated from the nasal swabs of nine patients ie. 14.29% who have a proved scleroma granuloma of typical histopathology, where we expected *K.rhinoscleromatis.* These observations lead us to following conclusions:

1. *K.rhinoscleromatis* is not an inhabitant of normal nose.
2. Rhinoscleroma granuloma may be caused by *K.pneumoniae* also.
3. It is possible that some strains of *K.pneumoniae* become converted or mutated into *K.rhinosclaromatis* after long incubation in the micro-environment of the nose inside the cell, which has constraintive effect on the biochemical expression of organisms.

© 1985 Elsevier Science Publishers B.V. (Biomedical Division)
New dimensions in otorhinolaryngology - head and neck surgery, vol. 2.
E. Myers, editor

CERAMICS IN RECONSTRUCTIVE SURGERY OF THE ANTERIOR SKULL BASE AND THE FACIAL BONES

KLAUS JAHNKE
Dept. of Otorhinolaryngology, University of Tübingen (Germany)

Six years experience with aluminium oxide ceramic and porous tricalcium phosphate ceramic in surgery of the anterior skull base and the facial bones are reported. The indications for their use are defects following severe trauma, radical frontal sinus surgery, tumour resection and malformations.

In extensive animal experiment, pure aluminium oxide ceramic has been shown to be outstandingly biocompatible. Our experiences in reconstruction of the ossicular chain were similarly encouraging (Jahnke and Plester, 1981).

In facial and skull base surgery, we have used perforated aluminium oxide ceramic plates to reconstruct, in particular, the entire anterior skull base after severe trauma or tumour resection to reduce the risk of dural prolapse and its consequences or, in selected cases, the walls of the paranasal sinuses, for example the posterior wall of the frontal sinus. Even when these plates have a supporting function, their biomechanical properties are not as important as their excellent biocompatibility because they are usuallly coming in contact with sinus mucosa. According to the principle of extradural reconstruction (Jahnke, 1980) more stable relationships and mucosal covering of the implant are achieved.

An extensive defect in the frontal bone was closed by wiring in place a large, relatively thick plate of bio-inert ceramic. Perforated ceramic sheets were used in only a small number of cases to reconstruct orbital walls after tumour resection or extensive trauma to the orbital floor.

Porous tricalcium phosphate ceramic (TCP) was first tested in extensive animal experiments in guinea pigs, rabbits, the pneumatised areas of the hen's humerus and in the mastoid of domestic pigs exhibiting excellent biocompatibility; macropores: 100µm-1mm; micropores: 1-20µm.

The animal experiments showed, as did the subsequent clinical experience, that porous TCP implanted into suitable bony sites is partially or completely resorbable and can be replaced by the body's own bone, depending on the following factors: 1. degree of porosity

2. crystalline structure 3. size of the implant 4. site of implantation (e.g. over or under periosteum) 5. recipient (e.g. age).
We obtain the ceramic in fragile sheets, 1 or 2 mm thick. They are shaped with either a bone nippler or a diamond burr. Some of the material we pulverized.

Bacteriological investigations with commonly cultured pathogens such as Haemophilus influencae and various streptococci showed neither a bacteriostatic effect of porous TCP nor any facilitation of bacterial growth. The ceramic was generally soaked in gentamicin solution and thus functioned as an antibiotic depot. Usually, it was then coated with human fibrin glue after implantation.

In the forehead, we have used TCP ceramics mainly to fill in bony defects resulting from severe trauma or very occasionally after a Riedel's radical operation on the frontal sinus. Before the implant was used within the frontal sinus, we first removed all the mucosa and smoothed the bone. Good results were achieved when there was a large area of contact between the ceramic and the posterior sinus wall and when the frontal sinus was shallow. Even then the ceramic was only gradually replaced by bone, the process lasting up to several years, depending on the size of the implant. We thought it important - as in the obliteration of mastoid cavity - to seal off the implant from the nasal cavity with vital tissue, e.g. a galea and periosteal flap or bradytrophic tissue like cartilage and perichondrium.

In one case, we were able, at a second-stage operation to further reconstruct a completely shattered nose, to obtain implanted material for histological examination 2 years after surgery. Near normal, newly-formed bone we found highly vascular connective tissue and remnants of crystalline ceramic. No macrophages or foreign body giant cells could be demonstrated.

In two cases, we used this material successfully to reduce the size of defects following resection of tumours of the nose and sinuses where it could be placed submucosally with wide contact with the floor of the nose. TCP ceramic is definitely not suited for implantation in soft tissue, i.e. in wide defects in the forehead because resorption will take place without bony replacement.

REFERENCES

1. Jahnke K, Plester D (1981) Ann Otol Rhinol Laryngol 90: 640-642
2. Jahnke K (1980) Laryngol Rhinol 59: 111-115

© 1985 Elsevier Science Publishers B.V. (Biomedical Division)
New dimensions in otorhinolaryngology - head and neck surgery, vol. 2.
E. Myers, editor

INTRANASAL SURGERY WITH THE CARBON DIOXIDE LASER

RONALD ALLEN KIRSCHNER, Bernard C. McDonnell, Robert F. Giuliano

The Institute For Applied Laser Surgery

Suite IL-17, Two Bala Plaza, Bala Cynwyd, Pa. 19004, U.S.A.

The Carbon Dioxide Laser has proven itself to be an excellent tool for intranasal surgery. This laser modality serves as an excellent cutter and a fair coagulator. It can be used with the aid of a micromanipulator mounted on an operating microscope or freehand in what we call the " machro mode."

We have utilized the laser in the macro mode when dealing with anterior nasal problems. In the posterior aspects where the access is limited we are currently using the microscope and the micromanipulator.

Specialized nasal speculae for laser surgery of the nose have been developed. The hand-held specula are right and left handed. They have asymetric length blades. The longer blade is used to protect the septum from inadvertent damage when the turbinates are being treated. These are available with a medium blade length and with a longer blade. A self retaining model is available as well. These speculae are sandblasted and anodized to minimize reflection. Each has a built in channel for smoke evacuation.

A number of nasal problems have been dealt with effectively with the Carbon Dioxide Laser. Externall, these include: a paring type technique for Rhinophyma, use as an ablating tool, use as a cutting tool for minor and major excisions. and for treating telangiectasia and other vascular problems. Intranasally, the conditions that have been amenable to treatment include: Ablation of vascular lesions such as hemangiomas and Rendu Osler Weber Syndrome, and other conditions such as vasomotor rhinitis, polyps, polypoid degeneration, adenomata and others.

For treatment of Vasomotor Rhinitis and hypertrophy of the inferior turbinate bodies, the patient is usually placed in the sitting position in an E.N.T. treatment chair. The nose is topically anesthetized with 10% topical cocaine which is applied via applicator. The patient's eyes are then protected by eye pads that are soaked in saline. The remaining areas of the face are protected with wet towels. The inferior turbinate bodies are then treated with the laser at low settings of less than 10 watts, single pulse mode. The resection is followed by the use of intranasal beclamethasone (Beconase-Glaxo). This regimen has proven to be very successful in patients that have been treated with other modalities previously.

With most cases of intranasal surgery with the laser we have been able to eliminate nasal packing following the procedure. The patient has much less pain following the procedure. This is possible due to the fact that the nerve endings are seales as well as well as the small vessels.

We expect to shortly be able to report the use of a new optical system that will allow the use of the laser in more inaccessable areas of the nose and the sinus cavities.

We are quite certain that there will be many additional intranasal and paranasal applications for the Carbon Dioxide Laser in the near future.

The inherent properties of the Carbon Dioxide Laser have allowed us to perform a number of these procedures on a short procedure or office basis. This has a significant impact on overall medical costs.

New dimensions in otorhinolaryngology - head and neck surgery, vol. 2.
E. Myers, editor

A MORPHOLOGIC AND IMMUNOHISTOCHEMICAL STUDY ON THE EFFECT OF PARASYMPATHETIC FIBER NEURECTOMY ON NASAL MUCOSA

V.DIAMANTE, L.BARBON, C.FALASCA, I.LAZARO, E.MARESO AND S.MONTES
Pasteur 740 - Buenos Aires - Argentina

INTRODUCTION

There has been considerable controversy over the value of parasympathetic neurectomy for cholinergic and allergic rhinitis. As from 1980, in a series of 200 patients, we started to carry out surgery at the most proximal aspect of these fibers, particularly the branches innervating the nostrils. This work was performed for three main purposes: to confirm differential clinical diagnosis of cholinergic vs.allergic rhinitis; to demonstrate that pre or post ganglionar parasympathetic fiber neurectomy leads to immunohistochemical and morphologic changes, restoring normal nasal mucosa function; and to insure that no alterations in mucosal cell structures occur postsurgery.

MATERIAL AND METHODS

Our series comprised a total of 200 patients plus 10 controls (normal apparently healthy individuals). Ten patients had a clinical diagnosis of cholinergic rhinitis and underwent sphenopalatine neurovascular surgical section. The other 10 had a diagnosis of allergic rhinitis which had progressed to recurrent nasoetmoidal polyposis, the vidian nerve was severed. By light microscopy, the various mucosal layers were observed, and by electron microscopy (EM) ultraestructural morphology was recognized. Besides, histochemical identification of Igs G, M, A and E was also performed by standar methods.

RESULTS

Controls. Plentiful intercellular filaments; Igs M, A and G in superficial mucus, chorion plasmatic cells and glandular pockets; Ig E in superficial mucus, mastocytes and glandular pockets.

Cholinergic rhinitis patients. Pre.op: stratified plane epithelium, highly vascularized chorion and edematous endothelium; moderate inflammation. Plentiful hypertrophic, hyperplasic glands no significant cellular alterations; Igs M and A minimal, IgG abundant in superficial mucus; Ig E readily detected in chorion mastocytes.

Post.op: chorion much less vascularized with collagen homogeneization; reduction in glandular hyperplasia, no cellular changes at EM, Ig G levels much lower in all cells; Ig E hardly detectable in chorion and mucus.

Allergic Rhinitis patients. Superficial epithelium pseudostratified; chorion severely edematous; decrease in intercellular filaments at EM; Igs G and A in superficial mucus and plasmocytes; Ig M minimal; Ig E plentiful in mastocytes. In patients with vidian nerve section: pseudostratified epithelium; moderate chorion edema; no significant structural changes at EM; Ig G scanty in mucus and plasmocytes, Ig M levels higher in plasmocytes, Ig A and Ig E much lower both groups of patients that underwent surgery achieved edema and superficial capillary reduction, with collagen condensation. There was a decrease in the number of glands in the cholinergic group; Igs E and A levels in mucus and chorion mastocytes dropped noticeably, particularly in the allergic group. Obstruction clearance in the cholinergic group was 94%, with 4% persistence and 2% recurrence. Rhinorrhea, improvement was 85% with 5% persistence and 10% recurrence. Recurrent nasoetmoidal polyposis was cleared in 84%; it reappeared in 16%; 6% had hypolacrimation as a complication.

CONCLUSIONS.

- Our immunohistochemical and morphologic data enabled confirmation of clinical differential diagnosis.
- Parasympathetic fiber neurectomy, vidian or sphenopalatine, leads to a marked reduction in cellular alterations of nasal mucosa, reflected in significant clinical improvement.
- The absence of structural changes is further supported, for either surgical mode, by electron microscopy.
- Vidian nerve section is only indicated for recurrent nasoetmoidal polyposis.
- The resection of sphenopalatine fibers is recommended for cholinergic rhinitis.
- The endonasal approach was adopted throughout and seems particularly suitable for these pathologies.

© 1985 Elsevier Science Publishers B.V. (Biomedical Division)
New dimensions in otorhinolaryngology - head and neck surgery, vol. 2.
E. Myers, editor

NASAL CRYOTHERAPY WITH CARBON DIOXIDE

EDMIR AMÉRICO LOURENÇO, M.D.; CLEMENTE ISNARD RIBEIRO DE ALMEIDA, Ph.D.
Department of Otorhinolaryngology of the Medical School in Jundiaí - São Paulo, BRAZIL

INTRODUCTION

Since freezing began to be utilized in Medicine, several applications have been tested in Otorhinolaryngology. Nasal cryotherapy in the treatment of chronic rhinitis has been tested with several kinds of apparatus, using different gases and probes.

The present paper intends to demonstrate the advantages of the nasal cryotherapy in the cases of chronic rhinitis, allergic, vasomotor or drug induced, utilizing CO_2 (carbon dioxide).

MATERIAL AND METHODS

We submitted 44 patients, all suffering from nasal obstruction due to hypertrophy of the turbinal mucous membranes, including allergic, vasomotor and drug induced rhinitis, to one single therapic procedure. The results were observed for a period of 30 to 90 days (see Table 1).

All of the above mentioned patients had already been submitted to clinical, topical and sistemic treatments without improvement in their condition.

Topic anesthesia of the nasal mucous membranes was used in 40 patients. In four of the other mentioned patients, only topic vasoconstrictor was used and none of the patients, including a boy with only 11 years old, complained about pain.

The apparatus and the probe were plained and constructed under our supervision. It was utilized pressurized CO_2, which produced low temperatures, up to -70 to -80 ºC.

We did not register any cases of hemorrhages, septum perforation, sinusitis, serous otitis, turbinal bone necrosis, fever or chronic headaches in the post-therapy phase. All these complications usually occur with liquid nitrogen. The only post-therapy symptoms observed were rhinorrhea varying between 12 and 14 hours and sometimes an increase in the number of sneezes.

RESULTS

The improvement or total absence of the nasal obstruction was quite evident, and could be noticed in all patients, as can be verified in Table 1.

TABLE 1

NASAL OBSTRUCTION 30 TO 90 DAYS AFTER THE CRYOTHERAPY

	Assymptomatic	Improvement	Unaltered	Total
N	18	26	0	44
%	41	59	0	100

All other symptoms decreased in various percentages, depending on the patient.

COMMENTS

At present observation, we concluded that cryotherapy with CO_2 is a very effective procedure, less agressive to the mucous membrane and consequently to its phisiology. Aditional advantages have been observed as the following: it is more acceptable by the patient than any surgery or nasal cauterization; topical anesthesia is enough to avoid pain, beeing supportable even without anesthesia; do not cause bleeding; it forms only a fibrin membrane instead of forming crusts; do not produce scars or synechia, septum perforation, sinusitis, serous otitis, turbinal bone necrosis, fever, headache.

REFERENCES

1. Leden, Hans Von: Criocirugia de la cabeza e cuello. Acta ORL. Iber - Amer. XXII, 3: 275-290, 1971.
2. Leite, F. A. e col.: Criocirurgia em Otorrinolaringologia. Revista Brasileira de ORL., 43: 224-229, 1977.
3. Moore, J. R. M. and Bicknell, P. G.: A comparison of cryosurgery and submucous diathermy in vasomotor rhinitis. The Journal of Laryngology and Otology, 94: 1411-1413, Dec. 1980.
4. Ozenberger, J. M.: Cryosurgery in chronic rhinitis. Presented at the Meeting of the Eastern Section of the American Laryngological, Rhinological and Otological Society, Inc., Boston, Mass., jan. 7, 1970.
5. Principato, J.: Chronic vasomotor rhinitis: Cryogenic and other surgical modes of treatment. The Laryngoscope, 89: 619-638, 1979.

New dimensions in otorhinolaryngology - head and neck surgery, vol. 2.
E. Myers, editor

CRYOSURGERY : A NEW THERAPY FOR RHINOSCLEROMA

A. MAHER. S. ZAKI and S.M. HAMMAM
Professors of Otolaryngology, Microbiology and Pathology, Faculty of Medicine, Alexandria, Egypt

INTRODUCTION

Otolaryngologists are well aware of the resistance of rhinoscleroma to treatment. Until now, there is no definite, universally-accepted line of therapy resulting in definite cure. X-Ray treatment, radium therapy, autogenous vaccines, diathermy excision and antibiotics have succeeded only in restricting the evolutive activity of the disease and mitigating its symptoms [1]. In the past two decades, cryosurgery has been developed into a therapeutic tool in many fields of surgery for its controlled lethal effect on living cells [2]. The aim of this work is the assessment of its effect on the clinicopathologic and bacteriologic picture of rhinoscleroma.

MATERIAL AND METHODS

The study material comprised forty volunteer rhinoscleroma patients from both sexes and different age groups, not subjected to previous treatment of any form.

A punch biopsy specimen taken from each nostril under surface anaesthesia was preserved in 10% formaldehyde, processed and stained by haematoxylin-eosin, the rest was in cubated on blood agar and Mac-Conkey's agar for 24 hours at 37°c. Subcultures were prepared to obtain pure colonies and the agglutination test was used for identification.

Punch biopsies from the cryo-cauterized tissues immediately, and at weekly intervals, after each cryoapplication were examined histopathologically and bacteriologically. Simultaneous biopsies from the unoperated nasal cavities served as controls.

RESULTS

A- Histopathologic: biopsies immediately after the first cryoapplication showed loosening and separation of surface epithelium cells, oedema and swelling of subepithelial zone and granulomatous lesions with intracellular vacuolations.

Two weeks later, hydropic changes affected the Mickulicz cells, accompanied by extensive haemorrhagic and necrotic areas. Inflammatory cells and new capillaries appeared near the necrozed zones and remaining rhinoscleroma foci.

Two weeks after the second cryoapplication, biopsies revealed hemorrhagic areas with considerably disintegrated granuloma, cells new healthy granulation tissue and collagen fibers.

After the third cryoapplication, two more weeks later, dense fibrous tissue and collagen fibers replaced the lesions. Few foci of necrosis and hemorrhage persisted.

B- Bacteriologic: results are shown in tables I & II.

Table 1. Percentage cure of patients related to frequency of cryoapplication.

No. of applications	No. of cures	%
I	-	0
II	4	10
III	26	65
IV	10	25
Total	20	100

Table 2. Lethal effect on Klebsiella rhinoscleromatis immediately-and one week-after cryoapplication.

No. of applications	Immediate culture		Culture after one week	
	+ve	-ve	+ve	-ve
I	2	38	40	-
II	-	40	36	4
III	-	36	10	26
IV	-	10	-	10

C- Clinically: a sharp zone of demarcation and minimal inflammation followed cryocautery. Necrosis followed and sloughs separated leaving a clean granulation base. No bleeding occured. Regression of granulomatous mass improved the airway considerably. Healing was almost complete without adhesions and no recurrences were detected for 6 months.

DISCUSSION

Mickulicz cells contain viable bacilli killed by protracted bactericidal antibiotic therapy (with toxic side-effects).

Rinoscleroma is immunosuppressive and irradiation induces fibrosis with further immuno-suppression. Surgery and diathermy are limited to the obstructive sequelae. Cryosurgery ruptures Mickulicz cells, liberates and kills intracellular bacilli. Moreover it renders tissues antigenic eliciting an auto-immune reaction which extends destruction further.

Cryosurgery avoids hazards, limitations and side-effects of other therapies by a simple, safe and painless outpatient procedure with relative anaesthesia and no bleeding.

REFERENCES

1- Curkovic,M.: Streptomycin in treatment of scleroma. Arch Otolaryngol 1950; 52 : 253.

2- Miller, D.: Cryosurgery as a therapeutic modality in treatment of tumours of head and neck. Proc Roy Soc Med 1974 ; 67:69.

New dimensions in otorhinolaryngology – head and neck surgery, vol. 2.
E. Myers, editor

OSTEOPLASTIC WIDENING OF THE NASAL PASSAGES

SHARAD S. PARULEKAR, M.D. M.S. F.R.C.S. F.A.C.S.
Hearing Heights, P. O. Box 1244, Corbin, Kentucky 40701, U.S.A.

Chronic nasal obstruction may be devastating and pose as a complex and challenging problem and its improvement may lead to a happy and thankful patient. Even with adequate, hitherto well known treatments, there do remain stubborn cases where natural narrow boney nasal cavities seem to be the contributing etiology.

MATERIAL AND METHODS

The present study comprises an experience on fifty patients with developmental narrow nasal passages who were treated in Corbin from 1980-85 by Osteoplastic Widening alongwith other nasal procedures when required. They underwent pre- and post-operative nasal scopic, manometric, radiologic and subjective evaluations and these were compared.

ANALYSIS AND RESULTS

There were 29 males and 21 females. The lowest age was 17 years, the highest was 72 and the mean was 38. Six patients had a trans-antral approach and 44 had an intranasal one. Bilateral widening was done in 46 patients and unilateral in 4 and septoplasty in 42. Eight were previous rhinosurgical failures with persistent obstruction. Submucous resection of turbinates (SMRT) was done in 14. Two had nasal adhesions and widening alongwith internal splinting helped to seperate the lysed raw areas during healing. Surgery may be done under general or local anesthesia as in or outpatient procedure depending upon the patient's emotional makeup. Blood regurgitation through the lacrimal punctum and stubborn bleeding from the descending palatine occured each in one patient and caused concern, but no long term problems. Severe nasal pressure and headaches may be immediate problems, but seem amenable to medication and definitely to removal of the packs in 48 hours. With narrow nasal passages, septoplasty rarely gives complete relief unless combined with some corrective lateral wall procedures. Maximum relief is obtained when widening is combined with SMRT. This has the super-added effect of the combination and maximum lateralisation allowed by breaking the anterior anchoring bone. The results were excellent in almost all the patients.

DISCUSSION

Rhinostenosis was considered a serious problem by the early rhinologists and its importance still remains. The nasal obstruction may be unilateral or bilateral and may lead to smell disturbances, rhinolalia clausa, sniffing, uncomfortable osculation, snoring or problems of the Eustachian tubes. The three prime functions of the nose are humidification, warming and filtration of the inspired air and these are adversely affected in obstruction or destructive nasal operations to the detriment of the lungs. Airflow is proportional to the fourth power of the radius. Slight changes in the diameter lead to profound changes in the ability to convey air. The Bernoulli phenomenon and the venturi effect are brought into play. Narrowness of the nasal passage leads to increased velocity of the airflow and negative pressure which is readily transferred onwards.[1] It can be safely predicted there would be a profound favourable effect with corrective treatment to the nose.

Several procedures have been described, but somehow fail to relieve a certain class of patients. It seems logical to surgically expand the nasal passages and this encroachment into the maxillary sinuses seems not to have any after effects. The nasoantral party wall gets its major blood supply from above and there is no risk of necrosis with a superior based osteoplastic lateralisation with inferior osteotomy cuts. Trans-antral widening was first performed in Zambia in 1967 followed by 35 and later by 55 cases with good results.[2] Williams in 1975 described a similar operation in 8 cases where he incised the septal mucosa and excised the party wall bone.[3] The contra-indications to the Parulekar operation are acute infection, atrophic rhinitis, adverse healing or previous maxillary artery clipping. The approach is intra-nasal for simplicity, but transantral, sublabial and direct when the party wall bone is thick. Topical cocaine dissolved in oxymetazoline minimizes bleeding. An inferior meatus nasal antrostomy is first made. The inferior border of the naso-antral wall is osteotomized posteriorly. Intra-nasal lateralwards pressure follows to fracture, shift and bring on the desired surgical improvement. Intra-muscular dexamethasone decreases swelling and internal plastic splints prevent syneche. Terramycin vaseline nasal packing for upto 5 days holds the wall in the desired position during the healing process.[4]

A systematic approach is essential and this includes a correct deduction of the etiological diagnosis. Corrective surgery is done after trial of medical therapy. Osteoplastic widening is time-tested and propounded as a superior technique when indicated. A planned logical approach would be richly beneficial.

REFERENCES

1. Gray LP (1967) J. Laryng & Otol 81:953-986
2. Parulekar S (1970) J Indian Medical Profession 17:7502-7511
3. Williams RG (1975) J Laryngol & Otology 89:527-530
4. Parulekar SS (1984) Chronic Nasal Obstruction, Letter to the Editor, accepted for publication, Ear Nose & Throat Journal.

New dimensions in otorhinolaryngology - head and neck surgery, vol. 2.
E. Myers, editor

RHINOSCLEROMA: "CONTRIBUTICNS TO ITS TREATMENT"

FRANCISCO SALAVERRY (1) and HERMANN DIAZ (2)
Otorhinolaringology Service "Dos de Mayo" Hospital, Lima - PERU

SUMMARY

From 1981 to 1984 we have diagnosed and treated five patients with "Rhinoscleroma" from different Peruvian regions. In all cases the diagnosis was made by the clinical picture, Biopsy, and Investigation of Klebsiella Rhinoscleromatis in the nasal secretion.

Our contribution to the treatment of this disease has been the use of RIFAMPICIN and Corticosteroids not reported in the Latin American Medical literature before.

Surgery was done to remove granulomatous tissue resulted from the natural healing or from the treatment. We have also done Microsurgery in Larynx, tracheotomy, and applied Acrylic Prothesis in nose in three of our patients.

MATERIAL AND METHODS

The following elements should be taken off for the diagnosis: Patients' origin, living conditions, and the clinical picture which comprises three phases:

- First Phase or Atrophic, clinically corresponds to an atrophic rhinitis or non-specific chronical catarhal process.
- Second Phase or Hypertrophic, it is characterized by the appearance of granulomatous tissue in the nose causing a nasal obstruction. It also appears in the oropharynx, soft palate, and tonsils. There is also a laryngeal affection which shows as dysphonia.
- Third Phase or Cicatricial, there is a transformation of the granulomatous tissue into a cicatricial one, clinically there is a dyspnea which may be asphyxiant, and the laryngeal affection is more intense.

Biopsy showed the histopathological damage, and it should be taken from places showing more activity, such as nodules and hypertrophic congested zones.

The"Klebsiella Rhinoscleromatis" investigation must be performed on the secretion taken from the nose and pharyns. It can also be performed on the secretion from the laryngeal mucosa or from the bronchial washing.

Treatment

Antibiotherapy. "RIFAMPICIN", the reasons that led us to use this antibiotic were the following:

- Its effectiveness against Gram - negative bacterias.
- The great similarity between Klebsiella Rhinoscleromatis (Friedlander's bacillus) and the Klebsiella Rhinoscleromatis.
- It does not have the Ototoxic effect of the Streptomycin (selected antibiotic

for the treatment of Rhinoscleroma).
- Easy handling by patients.

Corticosteroids. We use them to:
- Reduce the inflamation.
- Lessen the fibrous transformation.
- We prefer "DEXAMETASONA" because it is mostly known and approachable to the patient in our country.

Surgery. Consisting of:
- Removal of the granulomatous or cicatricial tissue.
- Tracheotomy in the event of air blocking of higher tract.
- Microsurgery in larynx.

Prothesis. Made out of acrylic, which we place in nose to prevent blocking after surgery.

Therapeutic Scheme. It varies in accordance with the phase in which the Rhinoscleroma is treated:
- Whether the illness is in the first phase.

RIFAMPICIN 300 mg., three times a day for three weeks; twice a day during the fourth and fifth weeks, and from the sixth week on and for a period of four months or more, one capsule of Rifampicin during the even weeks, and two capsules during the odd weeks.

DEXAMETASONA 4 mg., two times a day for one month.

VITAMINE "A", as per the physician's criteria.
- Whether the illness is in the second or third phase.

RIFAMPICIN 300 mg., four times a day during ten days; from the eleventh day to the third month, three times a day; from the fourth month and for a year, two capsules a day.

SURGERY, it varies according to the patient.

VITAMINE "A", as per the physician's criteria.

CONCLUSIONS

With the above-mentioned treatment, we have erradicated the disease 100 percent. The symptomatology improved in all patients except of two cases where the larynx (dysphonia) manifestations persisted.

ACKNOWLEDGEMENTS

Our thanks to Head and Neck Surgery Service of our Hospital for their cooperation, Dr. Elbio Flores Cevallos and Dr. Adolfo Merino Martijena who prepared the acrylic prothesis.

REFERENCES

1. Valentin Thompson and col., (1984) "Rhinoscleroma in Argentina"

2. Dow Chemical Company, (1981) "The Rifampicin"

3. Lidio Granato and col., (1977) Rhinoscleroma: "Considerations of a case"; Brazilian Magazine of Otorhinolaringology.

4. Chevallier Jackson, (1942) Rhinoscleroma: "Diseases and Injuries of the Larynx"

5. Luiz Rogerio Pires and Liacyr Ribeiro, (1972) Rhinoscleroma: "Surgical treatment" - Sep. of the XXI Brazilian Congress of Otorinolaringology.

6. Ortiz, "Rhinoscleroma in Peru", (1965), (Thesis work) - U.N.M.S.M.

New dimensions in otorhinolaryngology – head and neck surgery, vol. 2.
E. Myers, editor

OSTEOLYTIC SINUSITIS AND PNEUMOMEDIASTINUM: DECEPTIVE OTOLARYNGOLOGIC COMPLICATIONS OF COCAINE ABUSE

VANESSA G. SCHWEITZER, M.D.

Department of Otolaryngology--Head and Neck Surgery, Henry Ford Hospital, Detroit, Michigan U.S.A.

Cocaine, a benzoylmethylecgonine ($C_{17}H_{21}NO_4HCl$), is a psychologically disruptive and powerful dependence inducing central and sympathetic nervous system stimulant extracted from the waxy leaves of the coca plant Erythoxylon coca.[1] The socially disaffiliated, those already experimenting with heroine and other illicit drugs, and the young and immature are all poor candidates for the recreational use of cocaine (trade names: snow, gold dust, nose candy, "Bolivian marching powder").

Recreational cocaine abuse via intranasal "snorting", "free-base" smoking, "body-packing", or intravenous injection can be lethal with acute overdosage precipitating hypertensive crisis, ventricular arrhythmias, hyperpyrexia, clonic-tonic convulsions, and cardiorespiratory arrest. Chronic abuse can cause septicemia with endocarditis and hepatitis, lung damage, and psychiatric disturbances including dysphoric agitation, post-use depression, hallucinations, and paranoid psychosis.[2] Furthermore, the street drug cocaine can be laced with numerous adulterants including mannitol, dextrose, sucrose, lactose, Inositol, lidocaine, amphetamines, quinine, heroin, Epsom salts, and plaster of Paris, which not only decrease the purity and street value, but in some cases, exacerbate the local and systemic drug toxicity.[3]

The routes of administration (or transport) of cocaine are 1)intranasal ("snorting"), 2)"free-base" smoking, 3)intravenous injection, 4)"body-packing", and 5)oral ingestion (mixed with cocktails). The most common route is intranasal "snorting", inducing the transient euphorigenic effects within 3 minutes.[2] Increasing illicit use of cocaine and the misuse of licit over-the-counter drugs are known causative agents of nasal septal perforation with loss of smell and taste. Although 2-3 mg/kg is the recommended maximum dose for topical nasal anesthesia, cocaine snorters may use 1000 mg or more daily on a "run". The actual incidence of cocaine induced nasal and sinus complications is probably higher than the 4.8% reported in the 1960's due to the ease of drug availability, the increasing trend setting misuse of cocaine among the affluent, and the relative infrequency of intranasal exam of patients evaluated for common cold and allergy-like nasal symptoms.[4] Etiologic factors in cocaine-induced nasal septal perforation include mechanical disruption of the intact mucosa by drug particles, chronic vasoconstriction producing reduction in blood flow and tissue oxygenation with end stage mucosal atrophy and necrosis, and ciliary paralysis with compensatory mucosal hypertrophy of the paranasal sinus lining. Rebound or "paradoxical" nasal stuffiness following acute "runs" of snorting are further exacerbated by topical OTC intranasal phenylephrine, oxymetazoline, beclomethasone diproprionate and flunisolide. Moreover, the newer administrative route of smoking the volatile alkaline "free-base" residue of the adulterated street drug provides a plasma concentration in 7 seconds with the same physiological and subjective effects of intravenous cocaine.[1,3] Excessive intrathoracic pressure generated on Valsalva maneuver, rapidly disseminates the smoked "free-base" cocaine but can precipitate spontaneous pneumothorax, pneumomediastinum, and pneumopericardium due to rupture of the tracheobronchial tree or intrapulmonary blebs.

Presented are two cases demonstrating unusual complications of cocaine abuse: 1)nasal septal bony and cartilaginous necrosis with saddle-nose deformity and osteolytic sinusitis secondary to chronic intranasal "snorting" and 2)tracheobronchial rupture with pneumomediastinum and subcutaneous emphysema secondary to smoking "free-base" cocaine.

CASE HISTORY I

A 23 year old male presented with sudden onset of hoarseness, shortness of breath, chest pain, and a stiff neck following a "binge" of "free-base" smoking implementing the Valsalva maneuver. Clinical and radiologic evaluation demonstrated cervical subcutaneous emphysema, bilateral apical pneumothoraces, pneumopericardium, and pneumomediastinum (Figure 1). Symptoms and radiologic abnormalities resolved on conservative medical management of bedrest, pulmonary toilet, and 50% oxygen.

CASE HISTORY II

A 29 year old female presented with halitosis, rhinitis, chronic facial fullness, intermittent epistaxis, despite several years of antihistamine, decongestant, steroid nasal spray, and antibiotic therapy. Head and neck examination demonstrated complete bony and cartilaginous necrosis of the nasal septum, erosion of the medial walls of the maxillary sinuses, saddle-nose deformity, rhinolalia, and buckling of the lower lateral cartilages in the dome area of the nose. Axial CT scan of the paranasal sinuses showed bony destruction of the medial walls of the ethmoid and maxillary sinuses with concomitant sinus opacification (Figure 2). The patient admitted to snorting 1-3.5 grams of cocaine daily. Following drug detoxification, surgical therapy included bilateral Caldwell-Luc antrostomies and auricular cartilage implants to the nasal dorsum and alae.

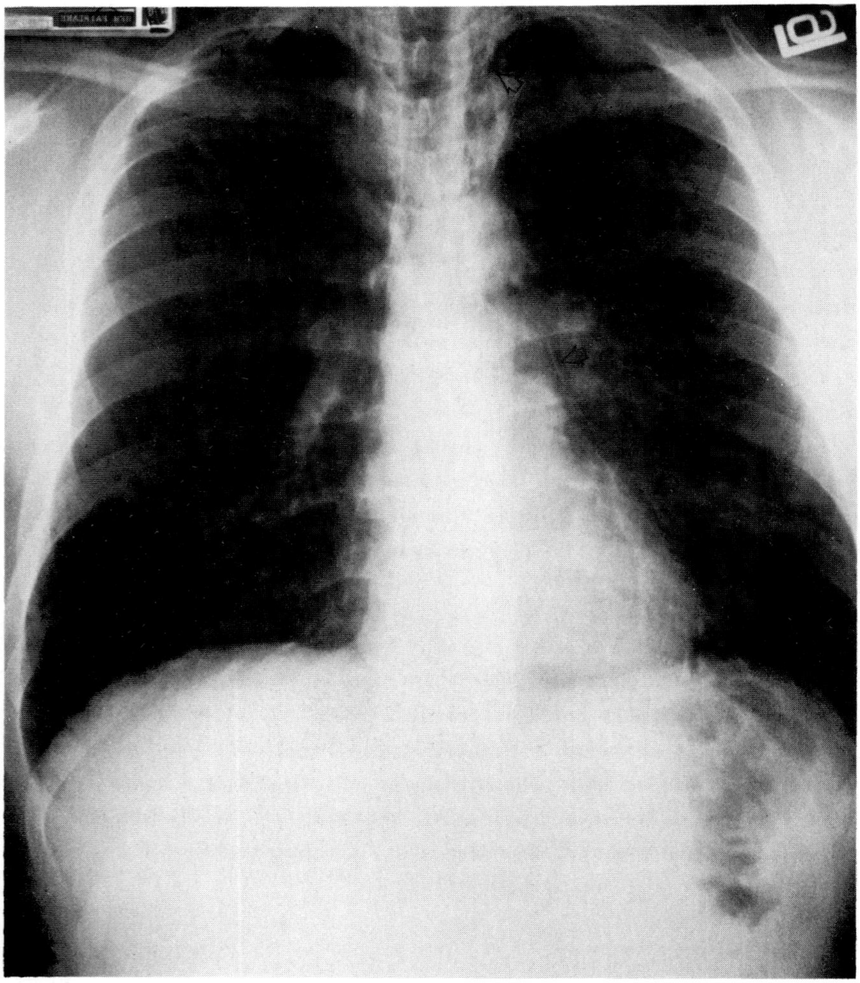

Figure 1 Chest x-ray demonstrates bilateral apical pneumothoraces, pneumopericardium, and pneumomediastinum caused by increased intrathoracic pressure generated on Valsalva maneuver while smoking "free-base" cocaine (arrows).

REFERENCES

1. Goodman and Gillman. The Pharmacological Basis of Therapeutics, Sixth Edition McMillan Publishing Co. Inc., pp. 307-308, 553-557, 1981.

2. Adverse Effects of Cocaine Abuse. The Medical Letter on Drugs and Therapeutics. 26(662):51-52, May 25, 1984.

3. Cocaine: Consumer's Handbook. David Lee, And/OR Press, Berkeley, CA, 1976.

4. Messinger E: Narcotic Septal Perforations Due to Drug Addiction. JAMA 179(12):126-127, March 24, 1962.

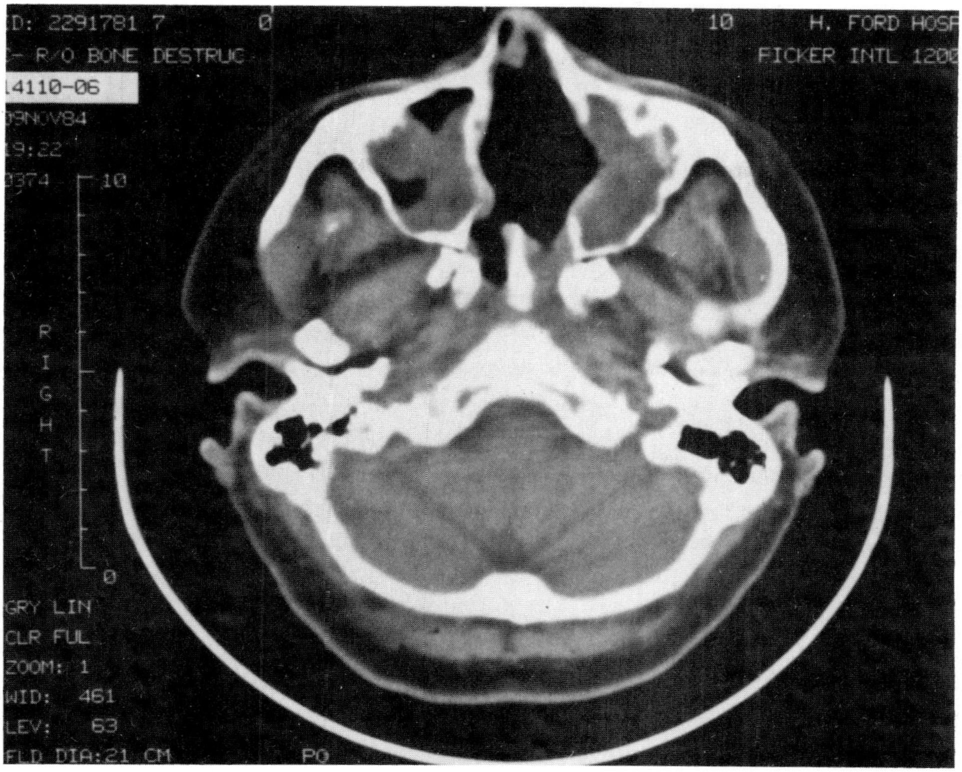

Figure 2 Axial CT scan of the paranasal sinuses demonstrates bony erosion of the medial walls of the maxillary and ethmoid sinuses with sinus opacification secondary to chronic intranasal cocaine "snorting".

REFERENCES (continued)

5. Miller FF: Occurrence of nasal septal perforations with the use of intranasal dexamethasone aerosol. Ann Allergy 34:107-109, 1975.

6. Vilensky W: Illicit and Licit Drugs Causing Perforation of the Nasal Septum: Case Report. J Forensic Sciences 27(4):958-962, Oct 1982.

7. Soderbert-Warner ML: Nasal septal perforation associated with topical corticosteroid therapy. J Pediatrics 105:840-841, 1984.

8. Schoelzel E, Menzel M: Nasal Sprays and Perforation of the Nasal Septum. JAMA 253(14), April 12, 1985.

New dimensions in otorhinolaryngology - head and neck surgery, vol. 2.
E. Myers, editor

EPIDEMIOLOGIC, CLINICAL AND HISTOLOGICAL STUDY OF RHINOSCLEROMA

SUAREZ GUTIERREZ, SAUL

From the Department of Otolaryngology of the Regional Medical Center of National University of Trujillo-Peru

INTRODUCTION

Rhinoscleroma is a rare chronic granulomatous disease predominately of the nasal passages but commonly affecting other areas of the respiratory tract as well.

Findings on physical examination of patients with rhinoscleroma differ depending on clinical stage of the disease and the anatomical localizations.

Although Rhinoscleroma is a endemic disease of the tropical regions, some cases have been found in Trujillo-Peru, located in the subropical region. There is a lack of scientific reports of local cases, largely due to the difficulty in diagnosis.

For this reason, we have decided to investigate Rhinoscleroma; its epidemiology, and its clinical and histological findings.

MATERIAL AND METHODS

The study was done in 14 patients with clinical and histopathologic diagnosis of Rhinoscleroma. These patients attended the Regional Medical Center, from March 15, 1982 to March 15, 1984.

RESULTS

Epidemiological studies have shown that from 12,448 patiens treated in the outpatient office of the hospital during two years, 14 were diagnosed with Rhinoscleroma, with an incidence of 0.1%. The age range was 10 to 50 years with a high incidence between 30-39 years (28.6%).

However, if referring to Holinger P.H., who reports about patients that may have symptoms for over 10 years prior to diagnosis, we can deduce that Rhinoscleroma may occur before the age of 10.

In reard to sex it attacks men and women equally; in our study 8 men and 6 women were diagnosed.

Out of 14 patients: 12 (85.7%) came from the subtropical region (the northern coast of Peru) while the other two came from a tropical region (the Peruvian jungle). The subtropical region has an average temperature of 21ºC with a 65% humidity and no rain, because of the Andean mountain and the polar Humbolt stream.

The 85.7% of affected patients with this disease belong to the lower class who live in poor living conditions including malnutrition and crowed living quarters, it is spread not only by these factors but also due to prolonged exposure to a contaminated person. This makes advisable for all family members living with the contaminated person to be examined.

All patients were found to have nasal involvement, with this being the only site of disease in 50% of the cases. The other affected areas where as follows: nasopharyngeal 28.6%, oral cavity and pharynx 14.3% and larynx 7.1%. The prognosis and complication are in direct relation with the spread of the disease so when it involves the lower respiratory tract it can cause such a serious respiratory insufficiency than it may provoke death.

The clinical picture is characterized by an obstructive nasal stenosis, hard granulomatous nodules in the nasal cavities and with less frecuency crust and cicatrization.

The diagnosis of the 14 patients was based on the symptoms and histopathological confirmation characterized by large vacuolated histiocytes (Mikulicz), though these cells typify Rhinoscleroma, their presence is not necessarily pathognomic.

However, some of these cases received different treatment initially, because Rhinoscleroma was not the original diagnosis.

Two therapeutic schemes were used. They are as follows: the first group was treated with streptomycin 2 gr/d the first week continuing with oral oxytetracycline 2 gr/d for approximately three months. The second group received streptomycin 2 gr/d the first week continuing with 80 mg of trimethropin + 400 mg of sulfamethoxazole 2 tablets every 12 hours, also for three months. The first group showed better therapeutic response.

We state that individual consideration must be given to patients of different age, sex and socio-economic condition as well as a long-term follow-up.

REFERENCES

1. Caldarelli, D.D., Friedberg, S.A. and Harris A.A.: Medical and Surgical Aspects of the Granulomatous Diseases of the Larinx. Otolaringol Clin North Am., Vol 12; 4: 774-776, 1979.
2. Holinger, P.H., Gelman, H.K. and Wolfe, C.K.: Rhinoscleroma of the Lower Respiratory Tract. Laryngoscope, 87: 1-9, 1977.
3. Shum, T.K., Whitaker, C.W. and Meyer, P.R.: Clinical Update on Rhinoscleroma. Laryngoscope, 92: 1102-1153, 1982.
4. Simposium: Escleroma, XIX Congreso Nacional de Otorrinolaringologi̍a. Mazatlan, Mexico, 1970: 77-114.
5. Stiernberg, Ch.M. and Clark, W.D.: Rhinoscleroma - A Diagnostic Challenge. Laryngoscope 93: 866-870, 1983.

New dimensions in otorhinolaryngology – head and neck surgery, vol. 2.
E. Myers, editor

TREATMENT OF ALLERGIC AND VASOMOTOR RHINITIS BY BILATERAL PARTIAL INFERIOR TURBINECTOMY

KB BHARGAVA, GN SHIRALI, US ABHYANKAR AND KC GADRE
Dept. of Otorhinolaryngology, LTMG Hospital and LTMM College, Bombay, India

ABSTRACT

A new indication for the simple old operation of bilateral excision of the anterior one-third of the inferior turbinates has been presented for the effective treatment of allergic and vasomotor rhinitis. It was performed on the assumption that the anterior ends of the inferior turbinates act as 'trigger zones' for allergic and vasomotor rhinitis. This assumption is based on the observation that most of the local treatments of allergic and vasomotor rhinitis are applied to this area. Only patients having more than 30 sneezes in a day during an attack were selected in this series. Turbinectomy was effective in 88.9% of cases.

INTRODUCTION

Many local treatments have been described for allergic and vasomotor rhinitis. Local cautery of the anterior ends of both inferior turbinates and the nasal septum with 15% silver nitrate was carried out by Bhargava et al (1) and was found to be a simple and effective treatment in 68.3% of patients, with good relief from sneezing and rhinorrhea. Gill (2) gave intraturbinate injections of hydrocortisone with good relief in 84% of cases.

Since the treatments mentioned above were successfully applied to the anterior ends of the inferior turbinates, these areas appear to be 'trigger zones' for allergic or vasomotor rhinitis. Based on this assumption, bilateral excision of the anterior one-third of the inferior turbinates was carried out.

Usually surgical management for sneezing is not recommended. Goldingwood (3) performed Vidian neurectomy in 242 cases with good relief from rhinorrhea, but substantial bouts of sneezing persisted. Quite a few patients experienced complications.

Most of the surgeons usually excise posterior one-third of the turbinates or carry out unilateral turbinectomy, hence there is no relief from sneezing. In this series, the relief from sneezing is obtained because the anterior ends of the inferior turbinates, which are the trigger zones for sneezing, are excised on both sides. With unilateral turbinectomy, the trigger zone on the other side can continue to cause sneezing.

MATERIAL AND METHODS

Turbinectomy was performed in 30 cases, and 27 patients reported for follow up. No attempt was made to distinguish between allergic rhinitis and vasomotor rhinitis, but only patients who sneezed at least 30 times a day during an attack were selected. 15 patients were males while 12 were females. The age of 77.8% of cases was between 16 and 30 years.

Turbinectomy was carried out under local anaesthesia after sedating the patient. Use of adrenaline minimized the bleeding during turbinectomy to a great extent. On both sides, anterior one-thirds of the inferior turbinates were excised (Fig.1). The nose was then packed with vaseline ribbon gauze for 48 hours.

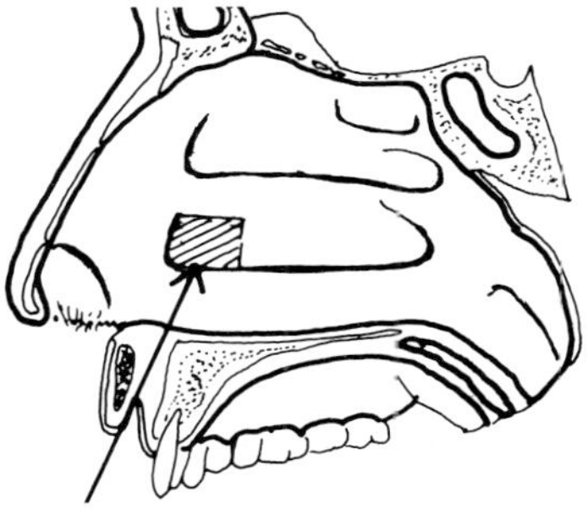

Figure 1 - The arrow points to the anterior one-third of the inferior turbinate which is to be excised.

RESULTS

The treatment was considered to be effective when patients obtained good or fair relief. Cases with 0 to 5 sneezes a day during an attack were classified as having good results. Those with 6 to 10 sneezes a day during an attack were grouped under fair results. A poor relief meant persistence of more than 10 sneezes a day(Table I).

TABLE I - Results of symptomatic relief, in 27 cases

Symptoms	Cases	Good	Fair	Poor	P-value
Sneezing	27	77.8%	11.1%	11.1%	<0.001
Rhinorrhea	25	68%	20%	12%	<0.001
Blocking	16	81.2%	6.3%	12.5%	<0.001

One case developed synechia, while 3 out of 27 patients complained of temporal headache for 2 months on exposure to cold air. None of them developed atrophic rhinitis. Out of 24 patients having good or fair results, 4 cases (16.7%) have shown partial or total recurrence of symptoms over a period of 3 years. One has to wait for long term results.

REFERENCES

1. Bhargava KB, Abhyankar US, Shah TM (1980) J Laryngol Otol 94 : 1025-36
2. Gill BS (1966) J Laryngol Otol 80 : 506-10
3. Goldingwood PH (1973) Laryngoscope 87 : 1673-83

New dimensions in otorhinolaryngology - head and neck surgery, vol. 2.
E. Myers, editor

A DOUBLE-BLIND, COMPARATIVE EFFICACY AND SAFETY STUDY OF TAZIFYLLINE, CLEMASTINE AND PLACEBO IN PATIENTS WITH SEASONAL ALLERGIC RHINITIS; A TWO-CENTRE STUDY

EINO HOLOPAINEN, BERTEL GRAHNE, HENRIK MALMBERG, YRJÖ ALLAS, MARTTI SORRI AND PEKKA SIPILÄ

Dept. of Otolaryngology, University of Helsinki, Helsinki, and Dept. of Otolaryngology, University of Oulu, Oulu, Finland

INTRODUCTION

Tazifylline is a new potent H_1-receptor antagonist, shown to be without central nervous system activity in animal experiments[+]. This report describes a clinical trial, performed in May-June, 1984, to compare efficacy and safety of tazifylline, clemastine, and placebo in patients with seasonal allergic rhinitis.

PATIENTS AND METHODS

83 patients, 40 males and 43 females, aged 16-61 years, were admitted to the study. All had had rhinitis symptoms from pollen during 2 or more previous seasons, and pollen allergy had been confirmed by history, skin tests and RAST.

The study was performed as a parallel, double-blind trial with random allocation of patients to 3 therapy groups: tazifylline (27 patients), clemastine (28), and placebo (28). The groups were well matched as to mean age, sex ratio, physical examination, skin tests, and chronicity and severity of symptoms. Throughout the 6-week trial the patients daily recorded nasal and ocular symptoms on a 0-4 scale, and measured nasal resistance with peak-flow meters. To obtain baseline values, the patients used placebo for 2 weeks prior to the anticipated start of symptoms. After this wash-in period, the antihistamine, at a daily dose of 20 mg of tazifylline or 2 mg of clemastine, divided into 2 doses, or placebo (2 lactose capsules) was taken for 4 weeks. Clinical examinations were carried out at 0, 2, 4 and 6 weeks and efficacy evaluation at 4 and 6 weeks. Laboratory safety tests (hemogram, blood chemistries, urinalysis) were performed at the start and at the end of the trial.

In the statistical analysis the Kruskal-Wallis test and parametric analysis of variance were used for group comparison and the Friedman Rank Sum test for changes within each treatment group.

+ Syntex Research Centre 1983, Edinburgh (Scotland).

RESULTS

13 patients (3 on tazifylline, 7 on clemastine, and 3 on placebo) were excluded from all analyses because of non-compliance in record-keeping or drug usage.

The mean weekly scores for total nasal symptoms (sneezing, rhinorrhea, blockage) did not reveal significant differences between the 3 treatment groups, although the placebo group clearly had more nasal symptoms. Nasal symptom scores did not show a significant increase from baseline values in any of the groups, presumably because pollination was exceptionally poor in the early season of 1984 (below 50 grains/m^3 on 24 of 28 therapy days) Eye symptom scores showed the same trends as nasal scores. The reduction of symptoms towards the end of the trial was greatest in the tazifylline group.

In the patients' evaluation of treatment efficacy only tazifylline was significantly more effective than placebo. Table I shows the investigators' evaluation of efficacy.

TABLE I

FINAL EVALUATION OF TREATMENT EFFICACY BY INVESTIGATORS

	% of patients		
Control of symptoms	Tazifylline	Clemastine	Placebo
Total control	20.9	20	9.1
Substantial control	62.5	40	31.8
Minor control	8.3	35	45.5
Aggravated symptoms	8.3	5	13.6

P value (antihistamines vs placebo) < 0.05

Differences between the two antihistamines were not significant.

Adverse events

Sedation was reported by 24% in the tazifylline group, 33% in the clemastine group, and by 10% in the placebo group. Only one patient in the tazifylline group experienced severe tiredness. Other side-effects were infrequent; of the 5 patients reporting G.I. system events, 2 used placebo, and of the 2 patients reporting dryness of the mouth, one used placebo and the other clemastine. Laboratory safety tests demonstrated no abnormalities.

New dimensions in otorhinolaryngology – head and neck surgery, vol. 2.
E. Myers, editor

EFFECT OF IN VIVO TREATMENT WITH GAMMAGLOBULIN-HISTAMINE IN SENSITIZED GUINEA PIGS

MORIHIRO IRIFUNE, TAMOTSU HARADA, SATOSHI OGINO, ICHIRO OKAWACHI AND TORU MATSUNAGA
Dept. of Otolaryngology, Osaka University Medical School Osaka, Japan

INTRODUCTION

In order to assess in a multilateral manner the effect of G-H* treatment on nasal allergy. We studied its influence in actively sensitized animals.

MATERIAL AND METHODS

After a sensitizing application of 10% TDI** to the noses of fifteen guinea pigs, we confirmed sensitizations by applicating 5% TDI. The eitht sensitized guinea pigs received a subcutaneous injections of: Guinea pig G-H for the treated guoup(A) and saline for the control group(B). The seven nonsensitezed animals received, a subcutaneus injections of:Guinea pig G-H for the preventively treated group(C) and saline for the control group(D).

Symptom score was made by observing the clinical symptom and the therapeutic effect was assessed in accordance with the change. Furthermore, after these challenge in animals, study was made centering around the histamine which is considered to participate in the onset of nasal allergy as chemical mediater in blood, the mucous membrane of the noses and the lungs.

RESULTS

Effectivity is shown in the table 1 in terms of the improvement of clinical symptoms. The change in mean values of symptom score for G-H treated group and saline one in each weeks is shown in the Figure 1. "Effective" group treated with G-H has a trend of higher quantity of histamine in each tissues in comparison with "no change" group receiving saline.

---

*G-H: Gammaglobulin-Histamine conjugate
**TDI: toluene diisocyanate

Group	Drug administered	Sensi-tization	(卄) Remarkably effective	(+) Effective	(±) No change	(−) Worse	Total
A	G-H	(+)	2	3	2	0	7
C	〃	(−)	0	0	1	1	2
B	Saline	(+)	0	0	1	0	1
D	〃	(−)	0	0	2	3	5

Table 1. Effectivity of each group

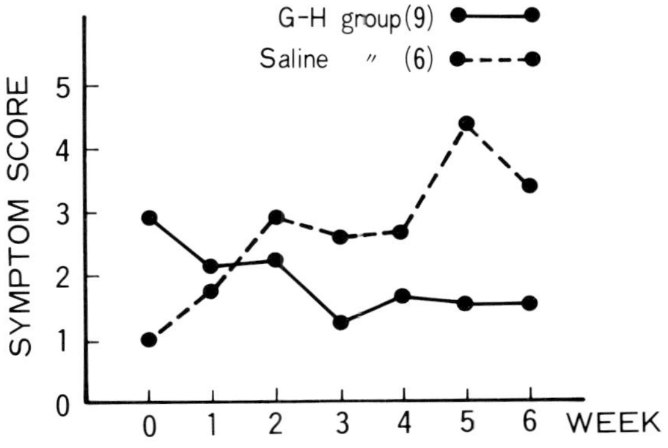

Fig.1. Change of average symptom score

COMMENT

This experiment distined to the model animals with nasal allergy verifed the safety and a manifest therapeutic effect of clinical symptoms by use G-H. After comparison made on the tissue histamine contents, it is suggested that the effectivity of G-H has a close relation with histamine release.

REFERENCES

1. Parrot, J.L, et Laborde, C.(1954): The histamine-fixing power of blood serum. J. physiol., Paris, 46:492-495

2. Ishikawa T, Shimada T, Kessok N, Kiyoi M(1979): Inhibition of rat mast cell degranulation and histamine release by histamine-rat Gammaglobuline conjugate. Int. Arch. Allergy Appl. Immunol. 59:403-407

New dimensions in otorhinolaryngology - head and neck surgery, vol. 2.
E. Myers, editor

A STUDY OF ALLERGENS IN NASOBRONCHIAL ALLERGY

S.N.JAIN

Medical Mycology & Allergy Research Centre,
Mahavir Hospital, Hyderabad - 500 004,
Andhra Pradesh, India

INTRODUCTION

Nasobronchial Allergy forms one of the major respiratory disorders. Allergens responsible for causing allergy differ from region to region with the variations in eco-geographic and climatic conditions[1]. In the present study, the profile of allergens and their seasonal variations in causing Naso-bronchial allergy was determined by intradermal skin testing in 250 patients at Mahavir Hospital in Hyderabad during October 1982 and September 1983.

MATERIAL AND METHOD

Selection of antigens was made based on the clinical history, the seasonal occurance of the symptoms and the presence of pollen and fungal spores from the regional calender prepared by operating air-samplers for a period of two years preceeding the study. The antigens tested were House Dust Mite (HDM), Dusts, Pollen, Fungi, Danders and Ingestants. On the basis of the seasonal manifestation of the symptoms, patients were classified into five groups (Table I)

On an average 18-20 antigens were tested in each case. The antigens (0.01 to 0.02 c.c.) were injected in a concentration of 1:500 except for HDM, which was given in a concentration of 1:5000. Buffered saline was used as control. The reactions (wheal & erythema) were read after 15 to 20 minutes.

RESULTS AND DISCUSSION

Only 11 patients showed negative skin test reactions to all the antigens and the remaining were positive to one or more than one antigen. Skin test positivity showed seasonal variations. The positive reactions obtained for individual allergens within their respective groups are given in Table I.

Table 1.

POSITIVITY OF SKIN TEST REACTIONS (PERCENT VALUE) DURING DIFFERENT SEASONS.

	Summer	Rains	Winter	Rain & Winter	Perinneal
HDM	50	80	67	71	75
Dusts	38	63	51	64	68
Pollen	24	39	41	47	42
Fungi	24	43	26	21	37
Danders	33	17	53	40	28
Ingestants	-	28	26	8	24

HDM was the predominant allergen as has been reported by Hendrick et al[2]. Dusts formed the next common allergens in which prevalence of House Dust was highest. This is in concurrence with the study of other workers[2,3]. Pollens as a cause of allergy was third in the order. The predominant allergenic pollens are Cyperus rotandus, Amaranthus spinosus, Cassia occidentalis, Ricinus communis, Argemone mexicana, Brassica campestris, Parthenium hysterophorus. Similarly Candida albicans, Asperqillus flavus, Asperqillus fumigatus, Helminthosporium and Alternaria are the predominant allergenic fungal spores.

The study demostrated the spectrum of allergens responsible for causing Nasobronchial Allergy in Hyderabad. In most of the cases skin test reaction was reflecting the behaviour of the disease either as a perinneal or as seasonal disorders. The allergens as determined by skin testing correlates with the atmospheric data of Hyderabad.

REFERENCES

1. Anand P, Agashe SN (1984) Immunological approaches to extra mural environmental Naso-bronchial allergy. Ind J Otolaryo 30 : 39-44
2. Hendrick DJ, Davies FJ, D' Souza MF, Pepys J (1975) An analysis of skin prick test reactions in 656 asthmatic patients. Thorax 30 : 2-7
3. Sarasfield JK (1974) Role of house dust mite in childhood asthma. Arch Dis Child 49 : 711-715

New dimensions in otorhinolaryngology – head and neck surgery, vol. 2.
E. Myers, editor

DYNAMICS OF MAST CELLS IN HUMAN ALLERGIC NASAL EPITHELIAL LAYER AFTER PROVOCATION WITH ALLERGEN

SHINICHI KAWABORI, MINORU OKUDA* AND TOKUJI UNNO

Department of Otolaryngology, Asahikawa Medical College, Asahikawa, 078-11, *: Department of Otolaryngology, Nippon Medical School, Tokyo, (Japan)

INTRODUCTION

Recently evidence has accumulated supporting the theory that mast cells in the nasal epithelial layer play an important role in onset of nasal allergic symptom.

According to our clinical experience, natural attacks of nasal allergy occur consecutively many times a day, and that, repeated nasal provocation with allergen can cause repeated symptoms as early as a few hours after provocation.

The purpose of this study is to elucidate whether or not mast cells migrate in a short time to the nasal epithelial layer in patients with nasal allergy.

MATERIAL AND METHODS

Subjects

Patients having typical perennial symptoms of nasal allergy, nasal eosinophilia , positive skin test and positive provocation test to house dust, were selected for the present study. They were divided into three group according to the different observations of the study. The number of case examined were 10, 25 and 5 respectively in group 1, 2 and 3.

All nasal epithelial layers were gently scraped with a blunt ear currete from the anterior part of the unilateral inferior turbinate after removal of nasal secretion by both nasal blowing and suction.

In group 1, scrapings were collected at the same time from three different sites, i.e., upper, middle and lower sites and used for histamine assay.

In group 2, the nasal epithelial layers were first obtained from the upper site . And the middle and lower sites were provoked with house dust discs. Patients had nasal allergic symptoms for 5 minutes and scrapings were collected 10 minutes and one hour after provocation respectively from each of the middle and lower sites. The specimens were used for histamine assay.

Histamine assay was performed by the modified Shore's method. 20 mast cells or more were observed each ten minutes and one hour after provocation in all five patients under electron microscope. Structural changes in the granules of degranulating mast cells were assessed by the criteria descrived elsewhere(*). Degranulation rate is number of changed granules/ number of total granules in every mast cell.

*: Kawabori S et al. (1983) Nasal allergy, 13:181-189

RESULTS

1. Site difference of histamine content in the anteror part of inferior turbinates

Significant difference was not statistically revealed among differnt sites using a paired t-test.

2. Time course variation of histamine content after provocation

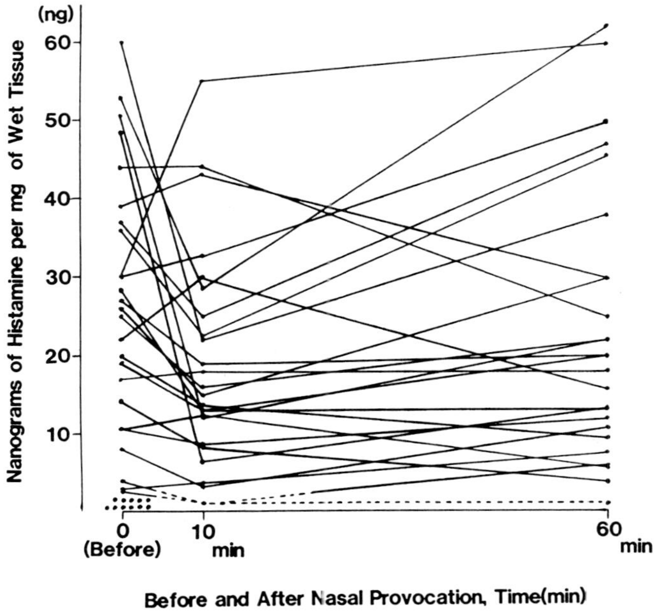

Left figure shows the results. Histamine content ten minute after provocation significantly decreased compared with before provocation ($p < 0.05$) using a paired t-test. When histamine content was compared between ten minutes and one hour after provocation, statistical significant difference was not revealed, but a tendency to increase was shown($P < 0.1$). Significant difference was not statistically revealed between before and one hour after provocation.

3. Electron microscopic study

In the nasal epithelial layers, 230 basophilic cells were observed both 10 minute and one hour after provocation. One cell was thought to be basophil and all remaining cells were judged to be mast cells. One of 5 patients showed decrease of degranulation rate after one hour compared with 10 minutes($p < 0.05$) and another one patients showed a tendency to decrease($p < o.1$).

SUMMARY

The results suggested that the histamine content of nasal mast cells in the epithelial layer decreased 10 minutes after provocation and showed a tendency to recover again one hour after provocation. We thought that some mast cells begin to the epithelial layer in a short time.

New dimensions in otorhinolaryngology - head and neck surgery, vol. 2.
E. Myers, editor

SURVEY OF AIRBORNE ALLERGIC POLLENS IN NORTH CHINA

Li Wu-kung and Wang Chang-sheng

Shanxi Medical College First Hospital, Taiyuan, Shanxi Province, People's Republic of China

This is a survey of airborne allergic pollens in North China, based on the research which was started by the establishment of an allergy clinic and allergy surveying group for studying the geographical distribution of airborne allergic pollen in North China, which aimed at studying the relation between allergic diseases and airborne allergic pollen distribution in Taiyuan, the capital of Shanxi Province.

MATERIAL AND METHODS

Collection of airborne pollen was undertaken in the usual way with the Durham type samplar, and stained with Calberla's stain. The pollen were identified and counted.

Observation of Results:

Types of pollen (occurrence in order of a given year):

Ulmus L., Populus L., Acer L., Salix L., Fraxinus Juglandaceae, Quercus L., Betula L., Biota Orientalis, Pinus L., Chenopodiaceae, Humulus L., Cannabis Sativa L., Ricinus Communis L., Artemisia L., Amaranthaceae, Plantago L., Compositae, Leguminosae, Umbelliferae, Graminecae, Cyperaceae.

STUDY 1. Survey of allergic airborne pollens at Taiyuan beginning from 1 March 1975 to 28 February 1986.

1. Material and Methods: As described earlier.

2. Observation of Results: Number of pollen grains of various prominent plant in spring and late summer-autumn is as follows: (1) spring - Ulmus 116 grains; Populus 556; Salix 2904; Acer 16; Fraxinus 8; (2) summer-autumn - Artermisia 6302; Chenopodiaceae 204.

3. Results of pollen curves in a year: There are usually two peaks in a given year: in April, the total pollen grains being 3326, of which elm, poplar and willow form the chief component; in the August-September curve, Artemisia forms the chief component.

4. Appearance of the peaks of various pollens: Ulmus pollen appears in the middle of March, poplar pollen peak on 6 April, the willow pollen peak on 8-9 April, the Artemisia peak on 30 August to 5 September.

STUDY 2. Survey of airborne pollen in 5 districts of Shanxi Province, beginning from 1 March 1977 to 28 February 1978.

Geography: the 5 districts are Datung, Yuanping, Xinxien, Xixien and Changchih.

Climate: Datung is situated in the North of Shanxi; the temperature during a

severe cold spell, may fall to -28°C or to -30°C. Xinxien and Taiyuan are in the middle of the province; Taiyuan during a severe cold spell, experiences -16°C to -20°C. Datung is situated in the latitude of 40°15'; Taiyuan: 37°52'N, Changchih 36°15'N. Some of them are near 112°30'.
Results of the survey in 5 districts of Shanxi Province: The two peaks during a year are also noted but the pollination periods of various plants are diffent due to the difference of latitude in which the 5 districts are situated. The total number of pollen of various plants in April varied in the 5 districts; e.g. Datung 7832 grains; Yuanping 2211; Changchih 3921; Xixien 5120; Xinxien 249. The chief components of the two peaks being pollen of elm, poplar and willow in April, but during August-September Artemisia is the chief component from 30 August to 5 September. The appearance of maximum amount of some chief pollen grains is in relation with the latitude.

Pollination of elm appears first but the amount is not abundant. From the viewpoint of latitude, in the north of Shanxi, the pollination of elm was delayed about one month in Datung and Yuanping than in the middle part of Shanxi, such as Taiyuan, where the peak of pollination of elm is in the middle of March, i.e. the northward we progress the later pollination appears.

Pollination of populus in Datung was on 16 April. The maximum amount of pollen grains was 5135; at Changchih, on 2 April, the number of pollen was 384. The pollination of Salix: In Datung the peak was on 20 April; in the middlepart of Shanxi such as Taiyuan the peak was on 6-7 April. Among summer-autumn pollen the number of the pollen grains of Artemisia was abundant, its pollination date in various districts varied as mentioned above.
STUDY 3. Survey of the airborne pollen at Laiyang of Shandong province was conducted between 14 March 1980 to 13 March 1981.
Geographically, Laiyang is situated in the latitude of 37°N and in the longitude of 120°. Climate: the temperature, when severely cold, falls to -20°C.
Appearance of various chief pollens: Two peaks are also present, total grains of March being 1166; the components of the spring peak are elm, poplar and willow while those of the summer-autumn are Artemisia and Cannabis Sativa. Pollination of poplar was in March with a total of 308 grains and the peak of Salix was on 17-18 April; the peak of Artemisia on 18 August.
STUDY 4. Survey of airborne pollens at Huohot, capital of Inner Mongolia Autonomous Region and Lanzhou, capital of Gansu Province.
Collection of airborne pollen was conducted between April 1983 and 31 March 1984 at Huohot, capital of Inner Mongolia Autonomous Region and also between 2 March 1983 and 1 March 1984 at Lanzhou, capital of Gansu province.
Geography: Huohot is situated in the latitude of 40°47'N and longitude 111°41'; Lanzhou is in the latitude 36°N and longitude 104°.

Climate: At Huohot, lowest temperature may reach -24.7°C while in Lanzhou it may fall to -18°C to -20°C.

Results of airborne allergic pollen in the districts of Lanzhou and Huohot: Two peaks were also observed. The total number of pollen grains in April were: Lanzhou 2504, Huohot 4278. The chief components of the peak in spring were elm, poplar and willow, but in this peak Biota Orientalis dominated at Lanzhou and at Huohot Ulmus dominated; in the summer-autumn peak Artemisia was also the chief component.

Appearance of the chief pollen: At Lanzhou in the spring Biote Orientalis had 1498 grains; at Huohot in the spring Ulmus 3522 grains.

Pollination of poplar in Datung was on 16 April, the maximum amount of pollen grains was 5135; in Changchih it was 2 April with the number of pollen being 384.

SUMMARY AND CONCLUSION

This paper presents the survey of 9 districts in North China. As a rule, there are two curves present, as is shown elsewhere. The components of the peaks of the curves in spring are nearly the same, they are usually formed of Ulmus, Populus and Salix; but excepting that, in the spring curve of Lanzhou, Biota Orientalis dominates, and in that of Huohot, Ulmus dominates.

In contradistinction to Artmisia, there are two exceptions such as in south China: (1) In Shanghai, Ricinus and Humulus are found to be the major offender instead of Artemisia, and (2) at Kwangzhou, Kwangdong province Wood Ephedra, Wild Amaranth are also found to be major offenders instead of Artemisia.

In addition to the major offender, Artemisia which was said to be dominant in Shenyang (Moukden) of Laoning province. Ragweed (the three split-leaved plant) was first discovered at Shenyang (and Tehling, Fushuen and Dandong) by Dr Xia Fengyuen. A question is raised "How it came to China". Preventive measures must be taken to eradicate it; otherwise, it will certainly spread all over China. Check its growth before it is too late.

New dimensions in otorhinolaryngology - head and neck surgery, vol. 2.
E. Myers, editor

COMPARATIVE STUDY OF STANDARD X-RAY, SINUSCOPY AND B-MODE ECHOGRAPHY IN THE DIAGNOSIS OF THE MAXILLARY SINUSITIS (ABOUT 270 SINUSES)

B. BERTRAND (ENT Dept.) and J.P. TRIGAUX (Dept. of Radiology)
University of Louvain, Cliniques Universitaires de Mont-Godinne, B-5180 Yvoir, (Belgium)

INTRODUCTION

The aim of this paper is the comparison of three paraclinical examinations : standard X-Ray, sinuscopy, and B-mode echography, in diagnosis of the lesions in chronic maxillary sinusitis. Sinuscopy will serve as reference for the two non-surgical examinations.

MATERIAL AND METHODS

This study includes 135 patients of all ages and both sexes, suffering from chronic maxillary sinusitis over a period of more than 3 months. Breakdown by age group shows a high proportion of children and young people, with 37 subjects less than 10 years old and 27 subjects aged from 10 to 20 years (Table I). Thus 270 maxillary sinuses were explored. The 3 examinations were performed in a period that did not exceed 20 hours.

TABLE I
AGE GROUPS (135 subjects)

Years	0-10	10-20	20-30	30-40	40-50	50-60	60-70	70-80
N	37	27	12	17	13	11	14	4

We suggest four distinct radiographic, sinuscopic and echographic categories (Class 1 to 4) according to the gravity of the lesions observed. The findings of this study are summarized in the table II (number of cases and percentage).

TABLE II
REPARTITION OF THE MATERIAL

Class	X-Ray	Sinuscopy	B-mode echo
1	53 (19.62 %)	15 (8.47 %)	106 (39.25 %)
2	77 (28.51 %)	53 (29.94 %)	54 (20.00 %)
3	55 (20.37 %)	68 (38.41 %)	51 (18.88 %)
4	85 (31.48 %)	41 (23.16 %)	59 (21.85 %)
Total	270 (100 %)	177 (100 %)	270 (100 %)

X-Ray

The X-Ray "WATERS" technique, or nose-chin view, was chosen in a routine examination.

Class 1 : normal radiographic image.

Class 2 : minor radiographic lesions; isolated polypoid formations, or a surrounding homogenous mucosal thickening of less than 4 mm.

Class 3 : lesions of medium severity; several, possibly confluent, polypoid formations or a surrounding mucosal thickening exceeds 4 mm, while still leaving some sinusal lumen.

Class 4 : major radiographic lesions.

Sinuscopy

Sinuscopy is performed by puncture through the inferior meatus, under local anesthetic for adults and general anesthetic for children less than 14 years old.

Class 1 : normal appearance, fine and transparent mucosa.

Class 2 : minor gravity lesions; hyperplastic and congestive mucosa, isolated polypoid formations tolerated.

Class 3 : medium severity lesions; several confluent polypoid formations reduce notably the antral lumen.

Class 4 : severe sinuscopic lesions; very extensive polypoid formations and abundant mucopurulent secretions.

B-mode echography

The emitting probe (Philips 3.5 Mega Hz, 6 mm) is placed on the canine fossa and the sinusal cavity is scanned with a compound movement.

Class 1 : the sound wave stops immediately beyond the soft tissues of the face. That can happen in two circumstances : either the sinus is normal and the air contained in the sinus cavity does not propagate the sound wave, or else the bony wall is too thick and it stops the sound wave.

Class 2 : slight mucosal thickening, situated anteriorly.

Class 3 : obvious echogenic zone anteriorly, sometimes of polypoid aspect.

Class 4 : very marked passage deeper by the ultrasonic beam, most often with strengthening posteriorly. This image corresponds to a sinusal cavity filled with inflammatory tissues or secretions.

RESULTS

The results were compared class by class for the 3 examinations.

X-Ray vs sinuscopy

As we demonstrated in a previous paper, there does exist a good overall correspondence between the 2 examinations : since there is concordance of 59.8 % between the equivalent classes, and this increases to 92.6 % if a divergence of 1 class is considered to be acceptable.

B-mode echography vs sinuscopy

Once again, we find a relatively good correlation reaching 46.8 % for the equivalent classes, and 86.44 % if a divergence of 1 class is accepted. This is due to the echography technique itself. In the cases included in class 1 for sinuscopy and in that for echography, the ultrasonic beam is halted by the intrasinusal air. In those cases classified 2, 3 and 4 for sinuscopy but 1 for echography, it must be conceded that the ultrasonic beam is thrown back by the bony wall. When setting aside from the total number of examinations, the number of failures of the method due to the thickness of the bony wall, we then obtain 61 % of correlation for the equivalent classes, and 94.8 % of correlations where there is divergence of 1 class between the two examinations. Thus the results are comparable with the findings by radiography with a 2.2 % advantage in favor of echography.

X-Ray vs B-mode echography

The scores are respectively of 58.51 % and 88.5 %. When leaving aside the echography class 1 that correspond to X-Ray class 2, 3 and 4 for the same reasons as those mentionned before, we obtain a correlation of about 73 % rising to 97.22 % by admitting a divergence of one class.

CONCLUSIONS

B-mode echography appears to give an efficient performance that is fully comparable to standard X-Ray if one leave aside those cases where the sound wave is not transmitted. Moreover, repetition of B-mode echography, for the diagnosis and follow-up of chronic maxillary sinusitis, does not subject patients and particularly children, to cumulative doses of roentgen radiation.

REFERENCES

1. Bertrand B, Robillard Th (1985) Comparative study of standard radiology, sinuscopy and sinusomanometry in the maxillary sinus of the adult (about 465 maxillary sinuses). Rhinology 23 : 169-180 (in press).
2. Bockmann P, Andreasson L, Holmer NG, Jannert M, Lorine P (1982) Ultrasonic versus radiologic investigation of the paranasal sinuses. Rhinology 20 : 111-117.
3. Friedrich JP et al (1979) L'ultrasonographie sinusale maxillaire : corrélation avec la sinusoscopie. Société de Broncho-Oesophagologie de langue française, Marseille, 12 mai.
4. Jannert M, Andreasson L, Holmer HG, Lorine P (1982) Ultrasonic examination of the paranasal sinuses. Acta Oto-laryngol (Stockholm), suppl 389.
5. Mann W (1979) Diagnostic ultrasonography in paranasal sinus disease : a 5-years review. ORL 4 : 168.
6. Trigaux JP, Bertrand B, Remacle M, Robillard Th, de Fays F (1984) Usefulness and limitations of sinus echography in the child. Acta ORL Belgica 38 : 321-330.

© 1985 Elsevier Science Publishers B.V. (Biomedical Division)
New dimensions in otorhinolaryngology - head and neck surgery, vol. 2.
E. Myers, editor

EXPERIMENTAL ACUTE PNEUMOCOCCAL SINUSITIS IN RABBITS - A NEW WAY FOR RESEARCH IN SINUSITIS.

B DRETTNER, P JOHANSSON, J KUMLIEN and H SCHIRATZKI

Department of Otolaryngology, University Hospital, S-141 86 Huddinge, Sweden

INTRODUCTION

Pathophysiological factors involved in the development of sinusitis are not completely understood. An animal model makes it possible to study each particular factor involved.

METHODS

Since Streptococcus Pneumoniae is the most common finding in acute sinusitis we decided to use clinical isolates of pneumococci. They were isolated from nasopharyngeal cultures from outward patients with otitis media acuta. They were mixed and inoculated in the rabbit maxillary sinus. Pneumococcus type 6 was used.

The superior parts of the rabbit maxillary sinuses were exposed through holes drilled through the dorsal wall of the sinus. Under an operating microscope the maxillary ostium on one side was blocked with Histoacryl. The other sinus served as a control.

Skin insicions were sutured with Dexon. The following day a challenge dose of 10^9 colony forming units of Streptococcus pneumoniae capsular type 6 was injected into the blocked sinus. A sterile intramuscular syringe was used.

RESULTS

All rabbits developed unilateral nasal discharge, sneezing and in some cases swelling of the nose on the affected side. The experiment was terminated on day 5 and the affected sinus was in all cases filled with purulent discharge. The mucosa was thick and reddish. The control side was macroscopically normal. Rutine histology showed a marked thickening of the mucosa with infiltration of granulocytes, lymphocytes. Smears obtained from the purulent discharge showed predominance of granulocytes, most of them in various stages of disintegration.

Among seven rabbits infected with pneumococci the same bacterial strain was re-isolated from the sinus in five rabbits.

During these experiments blood flow measurements of the sinus mucosa have also been performed, using two kinds of methods, microspheres labelled with Sn^{113} representing a non-diffusable tracer and $Rubidium^{86}$ chloride representing a diffusable tracer. The same methods have been used earlier in normal rabbits and those with chronic sinusitis and the results obtained in those did not differ significantly from each other.

In the acute model of maxillary sinusitis using $Rubidium^{86}$ the mucosal blood flow was 0.57 ml x min^{-1} x g^{-1} in the inflamed sinus mucosa and did not differ significantly from the control sinus. However, in these series a high content of radioactivity in the sinus secretion was found. This probably reflects an increased vascular and mucosal permability. In order to study this possibility microsperes labelled with Sn^{113}, e.g. a non-diffusable tracer, was used. In this series of experiments eight rabbits were used. The mean blood flow in the inflamed rabbit sinus mucosa was 1.03 ml x min^{-1} x g^{-1} and on the control side 0.79 ml x min^{-1} x g^{-1}. No radioactivity was found in secretion. This difference is statistically significant ($p = 0.01$).

New dimensions in otorhinolaryngology - head and neck surgery, vol. 2.
E. Myers, editor

SINUSITIS IN A GROUP OF ORGAN TRANSPLANT RECIPIENTS

HARRIS SD, PETERS GE, COPELAND SK

The Division of Otorhinolaryngology, Dept. of Surgery, The University of Alabama at Birmingham, Birmingham, Alabama, U. S. A.

INTRODUCTION

Recipients of organ transplants have increased susceptibility to infections due to their immunocompromised status. Our study reports the incidence and clinical course of sinusitis in a large group of transplant patients.

MATERIAL AND METHODS

The records of 1223 patients receiving organ transplantation at the University of Alabama at Birmingham between 1970 and 1984 were reviewed. This group included patients receiving renal, cardiac, liver and bone marrow transplantation. Twenty-four patients were found who had been diagnosed as developing sinusitis following transplant surgery. Eighteen patients out of the 24 had radiographic evidence of sinusitis, and these 18 were selected for further study. The information collected on these 18 patients included the presenting symptoms, physical examination results, radiographic findings, laboratory studies, methods of treatment used and results of treatment.

RESULTS

Incidence Rates of Sinusitis. The incidence of sinusitis in the renal transplant group was 14 of 1177 patients, or 1.1%. Average onset of sinusitis was two years after transplantation. In the cardiac transplant group, 2 of 44 patients developed sinusitis, or 4.5%. Average onset was 6.5 months following surgery. The single liver transplant patient and single bone marrow transplant patient surviving 30 days after surgery both developed sinusitis.

Presenting Signs and Symptoms. Ten of the 18 patients with sinusitis complained of headache. Nine patients complained of nasal drainage, 2 of congestion, and one patient noted anorexia. Seven patients had purulent nasal discharge. Six patients had temperature elevations above 100° F. and 4 had antral tenderness.

Radiographic Studies. Eighteen patients in our study had radiographic evidence of sinusitis. Eleven patients had opacification of at least one sinus, and seven patients had air fluid levels. Three patients had mucosal thickening in addition to their other findings. Thirteen patients had involvement limited to the maxillary sinus, 8 with unilateral and 5 with bilateral disease. Four patients had unilateral pansinusitis, while one patient had frontal sinusitis alone.

Laboratory Studies. Culture results were available from either antral irrigation or open surgical intervention in 6 patients. Pseudomonas was isolated in 4 of these patients, Haemophilus influenza in 3 patients, and Streptococcus viridans in 2.

Treatment and Results. Fifteen of the 18 patients were treated initially with antibiotics. Ampicillin, Ceclor, and erythromycin were used most often, with medication changes made according to culture results when necessary. Seven patients resolved with antibiotic treatment alone. Five of the 8 patients who did not respond to antibiotics underwent antral irrigation, and one of these patients resolved. One patient resolved following antral irrigation alone and 2 patients resolved without treatment. The 7 patients who had not responded to either antibiotic therapy or antral irrigations underwent open surgical intervention. In 6 of these 7 patients surgery consisted of Caldwell Lucs with nasal antral windows, and in the seventh patient frontal sinus trephination was performed. Fifteen patients had resolution of sinusitis, 2 patients had residual chronic sinusitis following surgery, and one patient expired from causes unrelated to sinusitis several months after surgery.

CONCLUSIONS

Our findings suggest that although sinusitis is not a common complication in the organ transplant recipient, sinus infections that do occur are often due to uncommon pathogens, and a large percentage of these cases require open surgical intervention for adequate treatment.

INTRANASAL MICROSURGERY OF ALL PARANASAL SINUSES, THE SEPTUM AND THE LACRIMAL SAC IN HYPOTENSION - 25 YEARS EXPERIENCE.

Joachim, HEERMANN, Krupp Hospital, 43 Essen, West Germany

The introduction of the binocular microscope in ear surgery (Holmgren 1923) was developed 35 years before the intranasal microsurgery (HEERMANN, H. 1958). Hypotension is very important to achieve good results (Flunitrazepam, Chlorpromazine Isoflurane, Nitroglycerine). The microscope in a balanced movable position can be focused by head motions of the surgeon on a patient in a Semi-sitting-Fowler position. An adjustable headrest is guided by a nurse.

In 98% of patients requiring removal of pathology from the maxillary sinus the external Caldwell-Luc approach could be spared. Not included are cases with malignancies and oro-antral fistulas. Extensive large inferior and in some cases also superior fenestrations (HEERMANN, J. 1974) of the maxillary sinus are necessary with removal of the naso-antral ridge. This allows complete removal of the sinus contents under binocular and endoscopic vision with aid of angulated ear curettes, ear forceps, punch and chissels. Finally the sinus cavity is packed with gelfoam saturated with antibiotics and antifungal solutions for 3 weeks. Performing yearly ca. 2897 (1983) intranasal operations (1983: maxillary sinus 206, ethmoid sinus 183, frontal sinus 42, tear sac 98) we had only 1 mortality in 1960 two weeks after a purulent ethmoidal reoperation because of metastatic brain abscesses. Using routinely antibiotics we have not seen a postoperative meningitis for more than twenty years. We have not had in 25 years a persisting disturbance of the visus or ocular mobility and under binocular vision our iatrogenic cerebrospinal fluid leakage rate in more than 4000 ethmoid operations is up today 0%. Binocular microsurgery is safer than monocular endoscopic surgery.

The external Toti approach in lacrimal sac surgery leaves the patient with a visible scar, partial resection of the palpebral ligament and partial removal of the bony frame of the horizontal tear ducts (secondary canaliculus stenosis). In intranasal surgery only the medial half of the sac is removed. In cases of

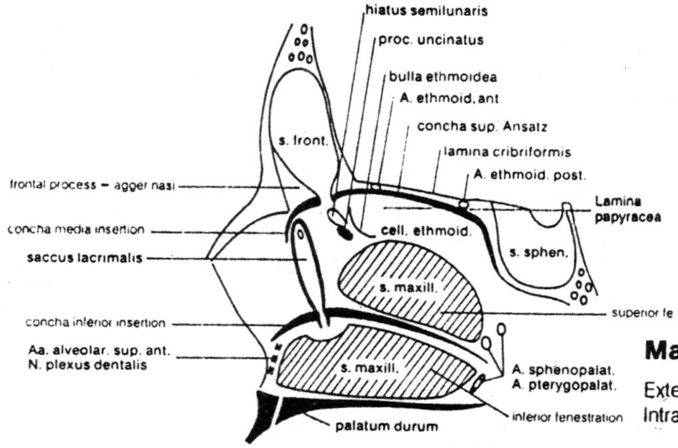

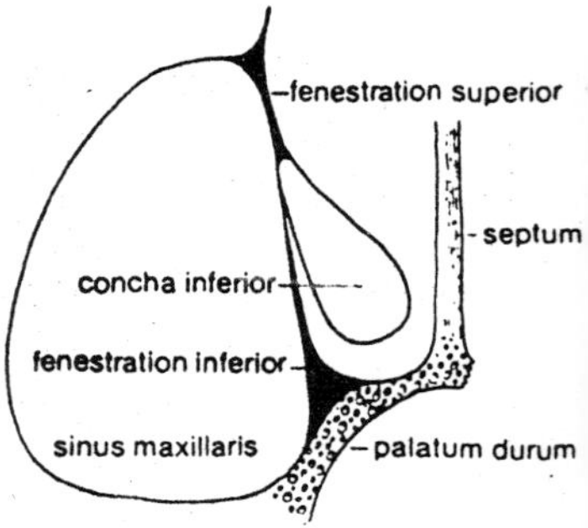

Maxillary sinus surgery:	1981	1982
External Caldwell-Luc approach	2	1
Intranasal microsurgical approach	170	204

aplasia or stenosis of the horizontal ducts, Heermann, J. Sen. used a glass prosthesis in 1923 (Jones 1962) and Heermann, H. introduced a stainless steel prosthesis in 1930. Since 1966, we prefer a selfmade polyaethylen prosthesis. During the last 5 years we used only 8 tubes (4 cases with congenital aplasia).

Surgery of the ethmoidal sinuses:

Indications in 183 intranasal operations 1983
1) Chronic suppurative disease, empyema, mucocele.
Acute infection with severe exophthalmus.
2) Polyposis
3) Tumor
4) Orbital decompression via lamina papyracea.
Sphenoid sinus surgery
Frontal sinus surgery
Maxillary sinus surgery
Osteoplastic frontal sinus surgery
Pituitary gland surgery
Optic nerve decompression
Cerebrospinal fluid leak

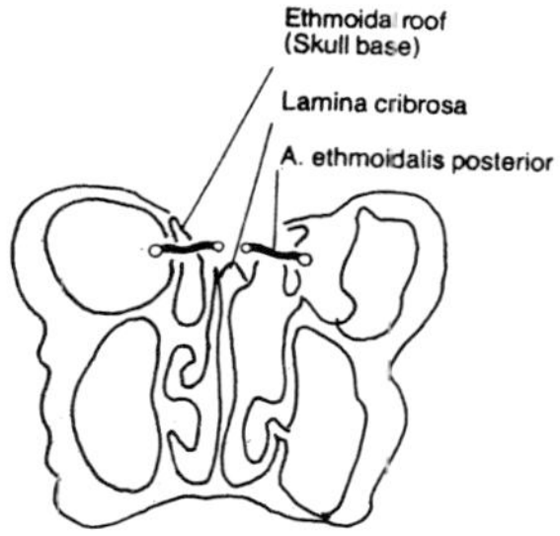

Frontal sinus surgery:	1982	1983
External osteoplastic approach	5	15
Intranasal microsurgical approach	39	42

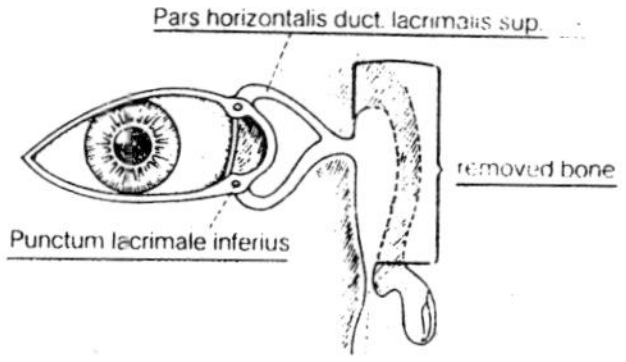

REFERENCES:

1. HEERMANN, H.: Endonasal surgery with the use of the binocular microscope. Arch. Ohr Nas. Kehlk. hk. 1958, 171:295.

2. HEERMANN, J. Jr.: Endonasal microsurgical resection of mucosa from the maxillary sinus. Z. Laryngol. Rhinol. 1974, 53:938.

3. HEERMAN, J. Jr.: Tunnel-polyaethylen-prosthesis in stenosis of the horizontal lacrimal duct after endonasal tear sac operation. Laryng. Rhinol. (Stuttg.) 1966. 45:842.

4. HEERMANN, J. Jr.: Endonasal microsurgery of the ethmoid sinus on a patient in a semi-(sitting)-Fowler position with hypotension. HNO 1982, 30:180.

5. HEERMANN, J. Sen.: Permanent connection of the tear ducts and the nose after failure of Toti and West operation or tuberculosis. Klin. Mol. Augenheilk. 1925, 74:±92.

6. HEERMANN, J. Sen.: Glass-prosthesis of the inferior lacrimal duct-7 years experience. Z. HNO 1930, 27:574.

7. Messerklinger, W.: Tecnnik und Möglichkeiten der Nasenendoskopie. HNO (Berl.) 1972, 20:133

8. Wigand, M.E., Steiner, W.: Endonasale Kieferhöhlenoperation mit endoskopischer Kontrolle. Laryngol. Rhinol. Otol. (Stuttg.) 1977, 56:421.

New dimensions in otorhinolaryngology - head and neck surgery, vol. 2.
E. Myers, editor

MODIFIED INTRANASAL ANTROSTOMY

DR. KIRAN K. SHARAN

Nema Mansion, Exhibition Road, Patna-800001, Bihar (India)

SUMMARY

Modified Intranasal Antrostomy has minimised the indications of "Cald Well Luc" operation. This procedure can be successfully utilized in empyema, haemorrhagic fluid, antral foreign body, mucosal thickening, polypoidal mass in the antrum and recurrent antrochoanal polyp.

In cases of recurrence of antrochoanal polyp, this surgical procedure was of particular advantage, as there is no procedure of preventing recurrence of antrochoanal polyp below the age of ossification of maxilla. The present procedure has been utilized in 600 different conditions of maxillary antrum in three year duration (1979-1982).

INTRODUCTION

In this procedure opening in inferior meatus (lateral wall) is sufficiently enlarged and then angled scoup is introduced in the antrum through this opening, and pathological conditions of maxillary antrum are scraped out thoroughly. By modifying "intranasal antrostomy", the additional approach of making opening at cannine fossa on gingivolabial fold could be avoided obtaining the results of Cald Well Luc Operation.

MATERIAL AND METHOD

The cases were from Ear, Nose and Throat Department of Nalanda Medical College Hospital and my private clinic during 1979 to 1982. The diagnosis was established by history, clinical examination and investigations. The emphasis was on radiological examination. After proper investigation patients were prepared for operation. Most of the cases were operated under local anaesthesia; but some of smaller age groups and apprehensive patients were operated under general anaesthesia.

For local anaesthesia patients were given Diazepam (10 mgm) orally one and half hour before operation and then Fortwin (30 mgm) and Phenergan (50 mgm) were administered by intramuscular injection about 45 minutes before operation.

The patient lies on the operation table supine keeping the head end elevated to 30°. After draping, with good illumination the nasal cavity was properly inspected. 2% xylocain was locally infiltrated in the region of inferior meatus. A vertical incision was given in the lateral wall of inferior meatus. The mucosa was then elevated and underlying bone was exposed. Then opening was made in lateral wall of inferior meatus. The opening was sufficiently enlarged. The angled scoup was then introduced in the antrum through this opening and the pathological lesions were scraped out. This was followed by suction.

In recurrent antrochoanal polpy, the mass was removed either through nasal or oral route; and then modified intranasal antrostomy was done. Since the mucosa is scraped completely no chance of recurrence is left.

The antral cavity was then packed with antibiotic ointment applied packing gauge. The nasal cavity was not packed thereby leaving airway patent. Post-operatively, pack was removed after 24 hours and antral wash on 5th day.

OBSERVATION

From 1979 to 1982, this procedure was utilized in following 600 different cases:

	CASES	PERCENTAGES(%)
1) Recurrent antrochoanal polpy	30	5
2) Empyema of maxillary antrum	55	9.2
3) Haemorrhagic fluid in maxillary antrum	88	14.7
4) Mucosal thickening (generalized)	382	63.6
5) Mucosal thickening (localized)	45	7.5
	600	100%

Recurrent Antrochoanal polpy

Out of 30 operated cases, 25 cases were cured and 5 cases did not turn up for follow up (between 6 months to 2 years). So, there was 100% cure rate.

Antral empyema

Out of 55 cases, 38 or 84.4% were cured. Recurrence was observed in 7 cases or 15.6 %; whereas 10 cases did not turn up for follow up.

Generalized mucosal thickening of maxillary antrum

Out of 88 cases, 60 turned up for follow up. 56 operated cases or 93.3 % were cured. And only 4 cases or 6.7% had infection.

Generalized mucosal thickening of maxillary antrum

Out of 382 cases operated cases, 290 turned up for follow up and 240 cases or 82.7 % were found to be cured. Recurrence was observed in 50 cases or 17.3%.

Localized mucosal thickening and small polypoidal mass in antrum

Out of 45 operations, 35 cases turned up for follow up. Out of these 33 cases or 94.3% were cured and recurrence was observed in 2 cases or 5.7%.

DISCUSSION

Pondey Maingot (1937) advocated that intranasal antrostomy provides satisfactory results. There is no interference with infra-orbital nerve, and there is avoidance of antrobuceal fistula. But, there is no mention of scouping out the diseased mucosa.

Harper & Row (1973) stated that during intranasal antrostomy, cysts within the antrum are often obliterated by the passage of any curved instrument. But, here the technique has been further advanced by scraping the pathological lesions by introducing angled scoup.

Hall & Colman (1975) further suggested that in intranasal antrostomy the second dentition in children is less vulnerable. But there is no mention of eradication of antral disease by scouping the mucosa which was adopted by author.

The literature is rich in the presentation of the technique of "intranasal antrostomy" but there is no mention regarding the modification which has been adopted here.

REFERENCES

Maingot Pondey (1973) - Medical Publications Ltd. (London), Post-graduate Surgery,3:4756.

Hampstead, Be (1939) - End results of Intranasal opening for maxsinusitis, Arch. Otolaryngology - 30:11

Harper & Row (1973) - Walter H. Maloney - 3:19

Hall, S. Colman, B.M. (1975) - ELBS - 11th Ed. Edinburgh - Diseases of the Nose, Throat & Ear, Chapter 11:78.

New dimensions in otorhinolaryngology – head and neck surgery, vol. 2.
E. Myers, editor

ASPECTS OF PRONASE TREATMENT ON CHRONIC SINUSITIS
— III PENETRATION INTO SINUS TISSUE OF ORALLY ADMINISTERED PRONASE —

M. ISHIDA(1), H. UDA(2), S. FUJISAKI(3), K.SAITO(3) AND T. NAKAMURA(3)
(1) Department of Otorhinolaryngology, Suita Municipal Hospital, Osaka, JAPAN
(2) Department of Pathology, Kagawa Medical College, Kagawa, JAPAN
(3) Department of Pharmacological Research, KAKEN Pharmacological Co., Osaka, JAPAN

INTRODUCTION

About twenty years have passed since the chemotherapeutic application, in Japan, of orally administered Streptomycetes protease G. Since then, Fujisuki, speculating that orally administered proteases or their inhibitors might play an important role in modifying the inflammatory process. Using PAP, we studied the effects and distribution of pronase in mucous membranes surgically removed from twenty patients.

METHOD

The study involved twenty patients undergoing surgical treatment for chronic maxillary sinusitis. For seven of the twenty patients, the mucous membranes were first excised from the right maxillary sinus, after which pronase was administered orally to the patient for one week prior to removal of the mucous membranes from the left maxillary sinus. Eleven patients were given pronase for one week prior to removal of membranes from one sinus only, and the two remaining patients were given no pronase at all prior to surgery.

Mucosal specimens from all twenty patients were examined immunohistologically for the presence of exogenous pronase after first being fixed in a 10% formalin solution and embedded in parafin. A peroxidase/antiperoxidase staining method, utilizing antisera from rabbits containing antibodies specific for pronase

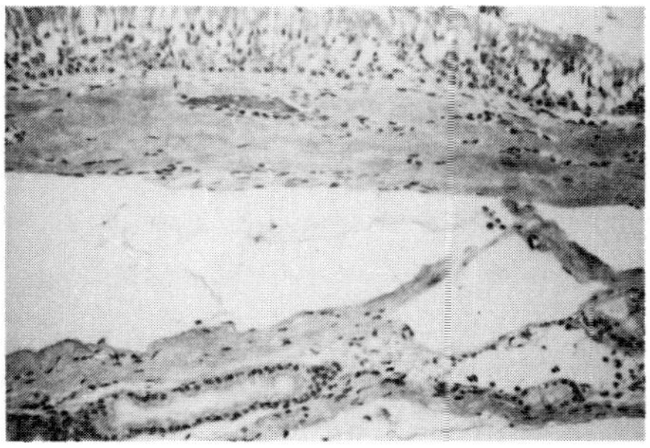

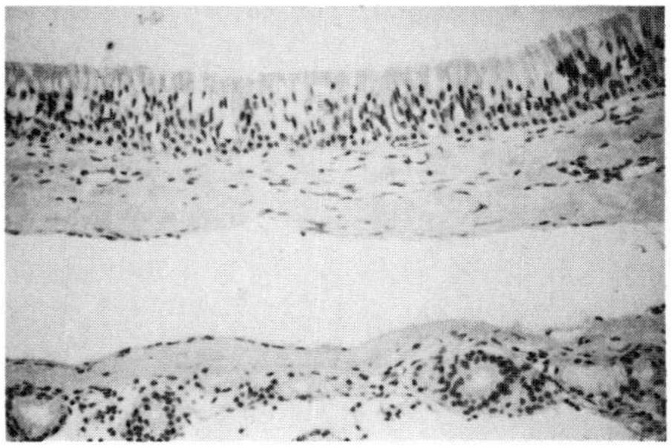

fractions A and B, was used. Hemotoxylin counterstaining provided excellent contrast.

We chose the 32 fold dilution for this study.

RESULTS

The tissue sample was treated with rabbit antisera to pronase fraction B and stained using the PAP method. Staining of the surfaces of pseudostratified ciliated epithelium and serous epithelium, the interstitial spaces and the lumen of the vessels indicate that the test is positive for pronase. (Photo I)

To confirm the validity of the test in revealing the presence of pronase, this photo shows a sample of the maxillary sinus membrane removed from the same patient, also after pronase administration. This specimen, however, was treated only with normal rabbit sera before PAP staining. Although the tissue contains pronase, absence of stain shows the test to be negative for the pronase antigen-antibody complexes demonstrated in the previous slide, thus confirming the test's specificity. (Photo 2)

A histopathological comparison of tissues removed from patients after receiving pronase therapy with those removed from patients prior to or receiving no therapy revealed: [1]. inhibition of membrane edema; [2]. increased fibrin deposition; [3]. diminished eosinophile and lymphocyte infiltration; and, [4]. proliferation of mucous glands within the mucosa.

Strong positive PAP staining after pronase administration demonstrated pronase deposits in: [1]. the stroma; [2]. the epithelium and seromucous glands; [3]. the lumen of the vessels; and, [4]. the neutrophiles and macrophages removed from the tissues.

DISCUSSION

The work of other researchers in this area have shown that small amounts of proteolytic enzyme are absorbed after oral administration, and are detectable in the serum bound to α_2 macroglobulin. Our study demonstrated that the exogenous proteolytic enzyme, pronase, concentrates in the nasal mucosa, and apparently works in combination with endogenous enzyme promoting an acute inflammatory process that assists healing. We believe this conclusion is supported by our findings, which suggest the destruction of mediators involved in the inflammatory process, and a decrease in the number of bacteria present as a result of enzymatically induced tissue necrosis and sloughing.

© 1985 Elsevier Science Publishers B.V. (Biomedical Division)
New dimensions in otorhinolaryngology – head and neck surgery, vol. 2
E. Myers, editor

RADICALLY OPERATED SINUSITIS OF THE SPHENOIDAL SINUS

OLOF PALMGREN, M.D. AND BERTEL GRAHNE, M.D.
Dept. of Otolaryngology, University of Helsinki and Koskela Hospital
Helsinki (Finland)

Nine patients underwent radical surgery for sphenoidal sinusitis at the Department of Otolaryngology,University of Helsinki, during the period 1975-1985. Six patients aged 35-75 were female and three patients aged 43-70 were male. The mean age was 52 years.

SYMPTOMS

All these patients had experienced headache, one patient for two years, two patients for half a year and the remainder for at least one month. The headache was in some cases continuous, in others paroxysmal (1). Two patients experienced sight disturbances and in one of the the left eye first and then the right getting gradually blind.

DIAGNOSIS

Although sphenoidal sinusitis is a rare disease, there is reason to remember that such cases occur (2). Upon taking an X-ray of the paranasal sinuses one a-p view is not enough (3). A minimum of three projections should always be taken, one of them a lateral view, since sphenoidal sinusitis may be present even though all other sinuses are clear. The examination may be complemented by tomography and computer tomography. An ORL examination can be negative and in general no reliable evidence is obtained from blood specimens. Careful history-taking and exact X-rays are important.

TREATMENT

The operation is performed under general anesthesia and the surgitechnique is as follows. The lower and the middle portions of the nasal columella are detached, turned upwards and attached to the back of the nose. This block includes the anterior portion of the septal cartilage. A wide septum resection is made. The anterior wall of the sphenoidal sinus is removed and bacterial, fungal and histological speciments are taken from the contents of the sphenoidal cavity. The thick mucosa of the latter is removed entirely, leaving a wide opening. In this way the sphenoidal cavity is connected with one of the nasal cavities. Crushed pieces of bone and cartilage are interposed between the septal blades. The wound is closed with catgut sutures and skin is sutured with synthetic material. A long moistened gauze tampon is left in the sphenoidal cavity and the nasal cavities are tamponaded for some days.

OPERATIVE FINDINGS

In 8 cases the opened sphenoidal cavity showed a thickened mucosa. In 3 cases the cavity was filled with a greenish-yellow caseous mass which proved to be aspergilloma. In one of them the tumorous mass had grown through the base of the skull into the brain. In 2 cases the mucosa was polypous,in 2 cases a mucocele and in one case a large cyst was found. Histological changes indicative of chronic infection were present in all cases, and in three cases Aspergillus mycelium was found. In these cases the diagnosis was made on the basis of the histological findings. Fungal culture was unsuccesful, which is a common experience (4). Cultures on the specimens obtained from the sphenoidal cavity were positive for Haemophilus infl. in 3 cases for E. coli in one case and for Staphylococcus epid. in one case. In the remaining cases cultures were negative.

AFTER-TREATMENT

The patients stayed in the hospital for 3-11 days. The patient who showed aspergilloma extending into the brain died. In all other cases the result was good and so far there have been no recurrences. The follow-up time ranges from three months to 9 years and 8 months, the average being 4 years and 5 months.

REFERENCES

1. Benton JS,Siu K (1975) Chronic inflammatory lesions of the sphenoid sinus. Surg Neurol 4:333.
2. Levine H (1978) The sphenoid sinus, the negleted nasal sinus. Arch Otolaryngol 104:585
3. Dale BAB,Mackenzie IJ (1983) The complications of sphenoid sinusitis. J Larynol Otol 97:661.
4. Grahne B, Paavolainen M, Mäkinen J, Hyrske J (1981) Aspergillosis of the sphenoid and maxillary sinuses. Rhinology Suppl 1:187.

New dimensions in otorhinolaryngology - head and neck surgery, vol. 2.
E. Myers, editor

MODIFIED AND CODIFIED SONOTUBOMETRY

BO FRIBERG BSc, INGEMAR MELÉN MD, LARS OLÉN MD
ENT-department, Kärnsjukhuset, S-541 85 Skövde (Sweden)

INTRODUCTION

The muscular opening function of the Eustachian tube (ET) is considered important for the normal function of the middle ear. No simple method is available which is suitable for the doctor's examination room and at the same time reliable for the assessment of the ET function. The idea underlying STM is to provide a straight forward method for the qualitative evaluation of the ET opening function. STM has however been critizised as it is believed that false positive sound recordings may take place because of noise of muscular or mucosal origin.

AIM

The aim has been to design a modified method of STM which can eliminate every "false" sound recording i e all sound artefacts should be separated from "true" signals.

METHOD AND PROCEDURE

The equipment has basically been identical with that described by Virtanen. The original signal given by the sound source in the nostril has been marked or coded by the computer in order to be able to identify it. The recorded sound in the external ear canal is sent back to the computer for identification and is then checked by the computer for the degree of probability. The coded signals given are pure sinus tones at 5 kHz, 6.3 kHz, 8 kHz and 10 kHz. The microphone probe, airtightly attached to the external ear, has a hole drilled which is connected to a pressure transducer. During the tests the subject was asked to swallow sips of water four times and to swallow empty four times. Every deglutition was made only on command. After the initial test the subject was asked to make a Valsalva manoeuvre or a Toynbee manoeuvre to create an overpressure or an underpressure in the middle ear. The test procedure was then repeated, the pressure changes and the sounds were recorded simultaneously. Some of the subjects tested had the ability to voluntarily open the ET and also keep the tube open for some time. Only subjects with healthy middle ears were studied. Altogether 25 grown ups were included in the study, 16 men and 9 women.

DISCUSSION AND CONCLUSION

The present coded sonotubometric method (CSTM) can guarantee that no false positive openings are recorded in the ear canal. If other sounds compete, e g another tone with the same frequency as the coded one, this will be disclosed. With this method it is still not possible to quantitatively evaluate the muscular opening function of the ET. The test is purely qualitative and a positive recording means for certain that the ET can open. In contrast to recordings of the ET function by pressure chamber technique or by using a tympanometer CSTM offers a possibility to study the ET function when there is no pressure difference between the middle ear and the pharynx. Simultaneous registration of pressure equilibration and CSTM shows that a positive recording implies a true air- and soundpassage. In order to reduce problems with standing waves and to get more uniform spreading of sound in the human body the test signal used in CSTM should preferably be white noise.

Clinically CSTM can be used to study pharmacological effects on the ET.

Another application of the method is the analysis of mechanisms for the equilibration of under- and overpressures in the middle ear. Thus the method could be used in studies in a pressure chamber to reveal a possible peristalsis of the ET. The combination of tympanometry and CSTM is believed to serve as a clinical method for assessment of the ET function in the doctor's examination room.

REFERENCES

1. Andreasson L, Ivarsson A, Luttrup S, Möllerström B, Tjernström Ö: Eustachian tube function measured as pressure equilibration and sound transmission capacity. A comparison in healthy ears. ORL I Otorhinolaryngol Relat Spec 1984; 46(2):74-83

2. Holmquist J, Olén L: Measurment of eustachian tube function. J Otolaryngol 1980; 94,16

3. Virtanen H: Eustachian tube sound conduction. Helsinki 1977

© 1985 Elsevier Science Publishers B.V. (Biomedical Division)
New dimensions in otorhinolaryngology - head and neck surgery, vol. 2.
E. Myers, editor

TOPICAL USE OF TOBRAMYCIN, GENTAMICIN, NEOMYCIN + POLYMYXIN B, DEXAMETHASONE AND LIDOCAINE IN THE TREATMENT OF OTITIS

MAURICIO MALAVASI GANANÇA, PEDRO LUIZ MANGABEIRA ALBERNAZ

E.N.T. Department of Escola Paulista de Medicina, Rua Botucatū 834, 04023 - São Paulo, Brazil

INTRODUCTION

Diffuse external otitis and otitis media are the most routinely observed ear inflammations in the pediatric and otorhinolaryngologic clinics.

Knowledge of anti-inflammatory, anti-allergic, anti-hipersensitizing clinical experiences suggest that the use of corticosteroids, combined or not with antibiotics, formulated as otic solutions are of great value for the topical treatment of otitis externa and media.[1,2]

The most topically used antibiotics for the therapy of otitis are neomycin, polymyxin B, chloramphenicol and rifamycin. Because of the crescent increase in resistance by microbial strains to these antibiotics, the topical usefulness of aminoglycoside antibiotics such as gentamicin and tobramycin have been studied.[1,2]

When administered parenterally, neomycin, polymyxin B, gentamicin and tobramycin are potencially ototoxic for humans. The topical use of these antibiotics for the treatment of middle ear infections has increased markdely in humans, with great success, and so far there has not been clinically observed ototoxic reactions. However, there are laboratory animals susceptible to topical applications of aminoglycosides and other antibiotics. Results of these studies cannot be clinically extrapolated to humans, due to inter-species sensitivity differences. Due to the deleteric action of ototoxic agents it is hypothesized that the hypertrophic inflammation of the mucosa during otitis media is a protection factor for the cochlear and vestibular ducts.[1,2]

MATERIAL AND METHODS

Thirty patients with diffuse external otitis and a hundred and eighty patients suffering from acute or reacuted chronic middle ear infection were selected.

Diagnosis was based on the patient's history, E.N.T. examination and bacteriological cultures.

The external otitis group was treated by means of dexamethasone only. The otitis media group was treated by means of one of the following preparations : 1) neomycin + polymyxin B + lidocaine ; 2) neomycin + polymyxin B + dexamethasone; 3) gentamicin; 4) gentamicin + dexamethasone; 5) tobramycin; and 6) tobramycin + dexamethasone.

For each solution the treatment dosage was four drops, three times a day, during seven consecutive days.

The evaluation criteria were based upon symptomatology, otoscopic findings, audiological examination and bacteriological culture results, before and after the treatment. At the last day of the therapy the patients were classified as cured, improved or inaltered.

The chi square test (x^2) was used to analyse the data with the assumed standard error $\leq$ 5.0 % to evaluate statistical differences of the therapies.

RESULTS

Concerning the otitis media group treated by means of dexamethasone, the therapeutic results (87.2 % of cured and improved patients) were judged to be good.

Related to the otitis media group, the clinical responses are shown in Table 1.

TABLE 1.
TREATMENT RESULTS.

Drugs	% of cured and improved patients
Tobramycin + Dexamethasone	93.3
Tobramycin	86.7
Gentamicin + Dexamethasone	80.0
Gentamicin	73.3
Neomycin + Polymyxin B + Dexamethasone	70.0
Neomycin + Polymyxin B + Lidocaine	56.7

Tobramycin + dexamethasone, tobramycin and gentamicin + dexamethasone have proved to be more efficient than neomycin + polymyxin B + dexamethasone or lidocaine. Dexamethasone was considered to be useful whereas lidocaine wasn't.

There was no clinically significant adverse or side effects, and audiogram results didn't show any ototoxic reaction with the topical use of these solutions.

REFERENCES

1. MANGABEIRA ALBERNAZ PL, GANANÇA MM, RISKALLA PE, FISCHER AR (1970) Otites externas difusas : antibiotico-corticoterapia local. Rev. Otorrinolaring. (Chile) 30:60-62

2. MITTELMAN H (1972) Ototoxicity of ototopical antibiotics : past, present and future. Transactions of the American Academy of Ophtalmology and Otolaryngology 76:1432-1443

New dimensions in otorhinolaryngology - head and neck surgery, vol. 2.
E. Myers, editor

COCHLEO-VESTIBULAR FINDINGS IN THE FAMILIAL LATERAL AMYOTROPHIC SCLEROSIS (VAN LAERE'S DISEASE)

CIRÍACO CRISTÓVÃO T. ATHERINO, JAMES P. MATTOS, THEODOCIO ATHERINO
Serviço ORL, Hospital de Ipanema, INAMPS, and Instituto de Neurologia Deolindo Couto, UFRJ, Rio de Janeiro, Brasil

The familial LAS with cochleo-vestibular involvement is an uncommon pattern of the disease and it is also known as Van Laere's disease (progressive chronic familial bulbo-pontine palsy). Three brothers have been evaluated regarding the otoneurological findings.

The eldest (case nº 1), a 19-year-old woman with a severe neurological involvement (facial dyplegia, dysphagia, generalized muscular weakness and fasciculations, amyotrophy of the tongue, paravertebral muscles and upper extremities) has presented a marked impairment of the cochleo-vestibular function: a severe bilateral sensorineural hearing loss with very poor discrimination scores; pathological decay of the stapedius reflex in 500 and 1000 Hz bilaterally; asymmetry of the horizontal optokinetic nystagmus, and bilaterally absent responses in rotatory and caloric vestibular tests.

The 2nd brother (case nº 2), a 15-year-old man, only reported an 1-year history of progressive bilateral hearing loss. The otoneurological examination revealed a bilateral moderate sensorineural hearing loss with good discrimination scores only with image tests; absence of stapedius reflexes bilaterally; and bilaterally reduced responses in the bithermal irrigations.

The 3rd sister (case nº 3), a 12-year-old girl, had no complaints. Her hearing was within the normal limits; presence of the stapedius reflexes but with a pathological decay in 1000 Hz left ear; during the caloric irrigations she has not presented nystagmus with the eyes closed but only with the eyes opened, except in the cold irrigation of the right ear.

COMMENTS

As Van Laere[1] has pointed out, the disease has a progressive pattern in its familial involvement: the pathologic findings are much more pronounced in the eldest than in the 2nd brother, and in the latter more than in the 3rd patient. Patients nº 1 and 2 reported the hearing loss as the 1st manifestation of the disease. The poor monosylabic discrimination scores associated with a moderate sensorineural hearing loss as in case nº 2 has a retrocochlear signification[2,3,4]. In case nº 1 the stapedius reflexes were present despite of the facial dyplegia, but with a marked decay; we didn't find any explanation to this, only a hypothesis of a stapedius muscle amyotrophy. In case nº 2 the reflexes were absent characterizing a decruitment, a retrocochlear finding[2,3,5]. In case nº 3 the hearing and the reflexes were within the normal range, but in 1000 Hz left ear there was a reflex decay. Hirsch (1983)[5] has noted that, in brain stem lesions, there were no reflex decay and suggested that this finding would be directly related to VIII nerve lesions. However, his patients had a hearing loss of 60 dB or less, which is not the case of patient nº 1 whose hearing loss was beyond this level. Case nº 3 is also out of these criteria because we don't do routinely reflex tests in normal hearing patients.

The vestibular examination of case nº 1 showed an asymmetry of the horizontal optokinetic nystagmus which, in the absence of spontaneous nystagmus, suggested a central lesion[2,6,7], frequently supratentorial[3]. The absence of responses at the rotatory swing test must be analysed with caution because of the common cortical inhibition[3], but with other signals has a complementary value as a central feature. The caloric test showed no responses even with iced water. The 2nd brother presented a marked bilateral vestibular weakness, while the youngst sister, asymptomatic, showed no eye fixation nystagmus supression, suggesting a retrolabyrinthine lesion[3,6].

When we analysed these findings we had a general view of the audiovestibular evolution of this disease. We also pointed out the importance of the familial otoneurological examination in cases of suspicion of LAS with auditory and/or vestibular involvement as a diagnostic clue.

REFERENCES

1. Van Laere (1966) Rev Neurologie (Paris) 115:289-295.
2. Kosoy J (1977) Acta Oto-Laryngol, supp.343:36-65.
3. Mangabeira-Albernaz PL, Ganança MM (1976) Vertigem. Ed. Moderna, São Paulo, pp.82-109.
4. Mattos JP et al (1982) Arq Neuro-Psiq (S.Paulo) 40:201-207.
5. Hirsch A (1983) Audiology 22:463-470.
6. Padovan I et al (1975) Acta Oto-Laryngol 79:319-324.
7. Uemura T et al (1979) Examen Otoneurologico. Ed.Medica Panamericana, Buenos Aires, pp.55-115.

New dimensions in otorhinolaryngology - head and neck surgery, vol. 2.
E. Myers, editor

RECONSTRUCTION OF THE MIDDLE-EAR WITH HYDROXYAPATITE IMPLANTS

JAN J. GROTE
University Hospital Leiden, ENT-Department, Rijnsburgerweg 10,
2333 AA Leiden (The Netherlands)

For the reconstruction of the middle ear with alloplastic implants, the main interest is focussed on material criteria in order to find the ideal implant material for the middle ear. For a successful use of alloplasts a combination of good material criteria and surgical criteria is necessary. Even in the middle ear different materials may be needed. The criteria for the reconstruction of a posterior canal wall differ from those of the reconstruction of the middle-ear chain. The last ten years we have tested different new implant materials in extensive long-term in vitro and in vivo studies and since 1978 we are using hydroxyapatite, which is the main constituant of living bone tissue. The advantage of hydroxyapatite ceramic is the possibility of the fabrication of two different types, a dense form and a porous form. The porous form will be remodelled in living bone tissue, whereas the dense form with its bio-active surface will be integrated in the middle ear without resorption. The bone of the host grows into the pores or on the surface of the implant as normal living bone. The epithelium on top of the implant is as the normal middle-ear lining. We have tested this material not only in non-infected but also in infected middle ears in long-term studies. The implant is regarded as bone tissue and is remodelled as normal living bone.

Essential for the reconstruction, especially in cholesteatoma surgery, is the total eradication. Open technique with the removal of all the diseased tissue with safe margins is the first aim. For the reconstruction procedure three aims are essential. The conduction system, being the mobile middle-ear chain, and its suspension, being drummembrane and canal wall, must be regarded as a monobloc. This is comparable with homologous total implants and essential for a good lasting function and prevention of extrusion. The conduction must be equivalent to normal, so the pre-fabricated implants must be tested not only with regard to biocompatibility, but also to its biomechanical qualities. The suspension, being the canal wall and the drummembrane, must be integrated in the host.

In all cases a retroauricular incision is made. A cranial based periosteal flap is mobilized and the epithelium of the posterior canal wall or the cavity is preserved as much as possible. The posterior canal wall is reconstructed with a canal wall prosthesis of porous hydroxyapatite, placed into two grooves, one anteriorly in the zygomaroot, and one posteriorly along the facial ridge. The prosthesis can be burred easily with a diamond burr like normal living bone. Essential is the preservation of the soft tissues on top of the new canal wall. The cranial based periosteal flap is placed inside the new canal wall and a fasciagraft underneath the remnants of drummembrane and preserved canal wall skin. A wide aereated middle ear, continuous with the mastoid cavity is created. In this study 30 canal wall prostheses are evaluated. The control period is from two to seven years. No canal wall prosthesis was extruded. Especially in the beginning in three patients defects in the skin of the canal wall were present, although there was a small lining on top of the implant. One of the drummembranes showed a dry postoperative perforation. In three patients a retraction pocket occurred. There was no recurrent cholesteatoma. In those patients, in which a re-inspection was done, a biopsy showed remodelling in living bone tissue.

For the reconstruction of the middle-ear chain the assembly method was prefered. In case of a missing incus, an incus prosthesis of dense hydroxyapatite guaranteed a simple procedure. The prosthesis is placed between the head of the stapes and the handle of the malleus underneath the drummembrane. For the individual distance between stapes and handle of the malleus three steps are present. Mostly part of the first step has to be removed. The corpus of the incus prosthesis has a niche for the adjustment to the stapeshead. The bioactive surface of the prosthesis gives a good integration in the middle-ear chain. In a study of 60 incus prostheses, with an average follow-up period of three years and a minimal follow-up period of one year, no extrusion occurred. In one patient the prosthesis showed a displacement after the operation and in one patient the incus prosthesis was removed because of a post-operative infection and perforation. In this series of patients the air bone gap closure according to the Fl. index was 86.6% within 20 dB, 66.6% within 10 dB and 5% showed no improvement. More important was that the hearinggain stayed constant over the whole control period.

For the reconstruction of a missing stapes and incus an incus/stapes prosthesis is still in development, whereas in case of a total empty middle ear a drummembrane/malleus prosthesis in combination with the incus/stapes prosthesis and the canal wall prosthesis forms a total alloplastic middle ear. Ten patients are now evaluated with a total alloplastic middle ear. Hydroxyapatite implants have shown in long-term animal and clinical studies to be very successful. The material is the anorganic basis of living bone tissue and as such not regarded as an alloplastic implant, and integrated in the body.

© 1985 Elsevier Science Publishers B.V. (Biomedical Division)
New dimensions in otorhinolaryngology - head and neck surgery, vol. 2.
E. Myers, editor

CHOLESTEATOMA IN CHRONIC SUPPURATIVE OTITIS MEDIA WITH CENTRAL PERFORATION

M.N. JAMAL, M.D.
Assist. Prof. Faculty of Medicine, Jordan University, Jordan

INTRODUCTION

Cholesteatoma is known to be associated with attic and marginal types of perforation. However, its presence with the central types in chronic suppurative otitis media (C.O.S.M.) was reported[1,2]

MATERIAL AND METHODS

One hundred and eighty three patients with (C.O.S.M.) were investigated during 1978-1983. Diagnosis was established by history taking, relavant clinical examination including otomicroscopy and suction clearance on some occasion. Investigations included pure tone audiogram, plain x-ray of mastoid and culture swabs from the ears.

Thirty five patients (19%) proved to have cholesteatoma with the central type of perforation and they constitute the material of this study.

RESULTS

Age and sex distribution: 22 patients were males and 13 were females, the youngest and the oldest were 9 and 65 years respectively with an average age of 24 years and the majority (54%) were below 20.

Ear discharge was present for less than 5 years in 57% of the patient.

Clinical examination revealed the presence of cholesteatoma in 28 patients while 7 needed suction clearance for its detection. Perforation was subtotal in 33 patients and small in 2. The contralateral ear showed central perforation with no cholesteatoma in 5 cases, central perforation and cholesteatoma in 4 and in 2 a posterior marginal perforation in 1 and a mastoid cavity in the other.

Complications included lateral sinus thrombosis (2), meningitis (2) and facial nerve paresis (1).

Surgery was done on 31 patients, radical mastoidectomy (24), modified radical mastoidectomy (5) and CAT (2). The choice of operation depended on the findings at exploration and table 1 shows condition of the ossicles at operation.

Table 1

Condition of ossicles	No. of patients	%
Erosion of stapes & incus	14	45
All Eroded	6	19.3
Incus alone	5	16.2
Stapes alone	4	12.9
All intact	2	6.4
Total	31*	100

*Number of operated cases were 31

DISCUSSION

The marked difference between our incidence of cholesteatoma (19%) and what had been reported (37-72)[1,2] seems to be due to the selection in the latter group of operated cases only, compared to the inclusion of all clinical cases in our series. Besides we agree that only an epidermoid sac would qualify for the definition of a cholesteatoma.[3] Neither the duration of discharge nor nasal or throat pathology seem to have played a role in its formation.

Different explanations were suggested for the presence of cholesteatoma in the young age group.[4,5] The large percentage of young patients in this series (54%) support the belief that cholesteatoma with the central type of perforation can be of congenital origin or a sequel of secretory otitis media.

In conclusion, because of dangerous complications and extensive bone destruction, we conclude that central perforation with cholesteatoma should be considered as "unsafe" and should be treated accordingly.

REFERENCES

1. Ruggle RL, Koconis CA (1966) Laryngoscope 77:337-340.
2. Rice DH (1975) Arch Otolaryngol, Vol. 101:626-627.
3. Sade J (1978) Journal Royal Society of Medicine Vol. 71: 716-732.
4. Gremank (1982) Acta Otolaryngol 94/Suppl. 386 (68-69).
5. McDonald TJ, Cody DTR and Ryan RE (1984) Ann Otol. Rhinol Laryngol 93:637-640.

New dimensions in otorhinolaryngology - head and neck surgery, vol. 2.
E. Myers, editor

RECURRENT CHOLESTEATOMA OF THE INFRATEMPORAL FOSSA

R.T. YUKO M.D., DON BLAKESLEE M.D.

Department of ENT, Fitzsimons Army Medical Center, Aurora, Colorado, 80045 (USA)

INTRODUCTION

The clinical presentation and surgical management of cholesteatoma within the confines of the middle ear and mastoid process are well known to the practicing otolaryngologist. The purpose of this paper will be to review the extra-aural spread of cholesteatoma as exemplified by two case reports. Inherent to the problem of extra-aural cholesteatoma are specific surgical and management problems, which will be discussed.

GENERAL BACKGROUND

The extra-aural spread of cholesteatoma from the middle ear and mastoid areas is a well recognized complication. However, there are few reported cases in the literature. The common sites of erosion out of the mastoid and middle ear spaces include the middle fossa plate, sigmoid sinus, petrous apex, post-auricular soft tissue, posterior cranial fossa, and the mastoid tip. This erosion arises as a direct extension of inflamed cholesteatoma. Marked bony destruction and expansion occurs secondary to the osteolytic effect of the inflamed cholesteatoma.

A review of the literature reveals two case reports by Kreutzar and DeBlanc, who presented the direct extension of inflamed cholesteatoma from the mastoid and external auditory canal respectively. Of note is that their second case initially presented as a temporal fossa mass. In 1979 Luetje reported two cases of extension into the sternocludomastoid muscle. One by direct extension, and the other by iatrogenic implantation.

Within the past two years at Fitzsimons Army Medical Center, two 25 year old males have presented with suspected infratemporal fossa abscesses. However, in both cases this was proven to be an unsuspected manifestation of extra-aural cholesteatoma.

CASE 1

The first case is that of a 25 year old male who initially presented with a tender, left preauricular swelling. A suspected abscess was confirmed by CT scan and further delineated to lie within the infratemporal fossa. The initial incision and drainage revealed an unsuspected cholesteatoma matrix. Further examination by CT scan and re-exploration demonstrated a defect of the bony and cartilaginous external canal with extension of the cholesteatoma into the temporal and infratemporal fossae. There was also extension into the middle cranial fossae through a tegmen defect.

CASE 2

The second case is that of a 25 year old male who presented with pain and swelling of the right temporal region. Again, an abcess was suspected, with a CT scan confirming its presence and further delineating its position in the infratemporal fossa. The diagnosis of extra-aural cholesteatoma was made on initial incision and drainage. The definitive surgical procedure revealed a well defined cholesteatoma sac extending from a postauricular sinus opening, though the substance of the temporalis muscle, below the zygomatic arch, and into the infratemporal fossa.

DISCUSSION

This first case exemplifies the destructive potential of inflamed cholesteatoma, allowing for direct extension into the infratemporal and middle cranial fossae. The patient had undergone a tympanomastoid procedure for cholesteatoma as a child, and this recurrence likely represents an acquired cholesteatoma. The management problem in this case lies in the difficulty in exteriorizing the cholesteatoma sac. Despite what was felt to be an adequate surgical removal of the lesion, the patient has undergone two additional procedures for recurrence or persistence of the cholesteatoma.

Whereas the first case demonstrated an obvious extension from an acquired cholesteatoma, the failure in the 2nd case to demonstrate any middle ear or mastoid disease, with no apparent connection to the well defined sac leads one to consider this a congenital cholesteatoma. Of note is that there was no obvious defect of the zygomatic root, a potential site of pneumatization and congenital cholesteatoma. Also of note is that the CT scan failed to define the limits of the cholesteatoma sac, although it clearly demonstrated the extension into the infratemporal fossa. The auriculo-temporal incision used compromised the vascular pedicle to the auricle, resulting in sacrosis of a portion of the superior helical rim - despite haparin therapy. As with the first case, exteriorizing the sac was difficult, as the patient has since presented with persistence or recurrence of the cholesteatoma.

The treatment approach in all cases of cholesteatoma emphasizes a fundamental rule, as put forth by Portmann. This is the knowledge that "a stable biological equilibrium of a squamous epithelial surface depends on the relationship between the volume of air circulating on its surface and the surface area of the skin in contact with the circulating air." Failure to achieve adequate ventilation leads to desquamation, maceration, and hyperplasia of deep layers; that is the development of cholesteatoma. The difficulty in achieving this end-point is evident in the cases presented, with the potential for recurrence and/or persistence obvious.

CONCLUSION

In conclusion, the following points can be made:

Two cases have been discussed which demonstrate an unusual presentation of extra-aural cholesteatoma which may mislead the unwary physician;

The need for a complete neuro-otologic work-up is essential for pre-operative planning and post-operative follow-up;

The infratemporal fossa is an area infrequently visited by the otolaryngologist and necessitates an inovative surgical approach;

Total extirpation and exteriorization of cholesteatoma involving the temporal, infratemporal, and middle cranial fossa is difficult at best;

Due to the underlying pathophysiology of the disease process, persistence and/or recurrence is likely;

Routine follow-up is mandatory for a potentially life--long and life-threatening disease process.

REFERENCES

1. Kreutzer & DeBalnd, Arch OTO Vol. 108, May, 1982, p. 320

2. Luetje, Laryngoscope 89: 1979, p. 1755

3. Portmann M., The Middle Ear and Temporal Bone

New dimensions in otorhinolaryngology - head and neck surgery, vol. 2.
E. Myers, editor

"BACTERIOLOGY OF CHOLESTEATOMA" - MARK J. LEVENSON, M.D., SIMON C. PARISIER, M.D., WARREN ZELMAN, M.D., MANHATTAN EYE, EAR & THROAT HOSPITAL, 210 E. 64th STREET, NEW YORK, NEW YORK 10021

INTRODUCTION:

Considerable controversy exists as to whether organisms cultured from the external auditory canal of patients with chronic otitis media are truly reflective of bacteriologic conditions within the mastoid. If the organisms cultured from the external auditory canal are contaminants or saprophytes, then these cultures could be misleading, and result in inappropriate antibiotic therapy. We have not encountered a previous study in the antibiotic era comparing pre-operative cultures taken from the external auditory canal, or middle ear space, when perforation is present, with cultures taken intra-operatively from the mastoid cavity in the same patient with cholesteatoma. In order to test the hypothesis of whether identity exists between organisms cultured from the two sites, we undertook a pilot study of sixteen consecutive patients operated on for cholesteatoma over a three month period.

Methods:

Sixteen consecutive patients, four children, twelve adults with previously unoperated ears and the clinical diagnosis of chronic otitis media with cholesteatoma were studied bacteriologically. Cultures were obtained from the middle ear space if a perforation was present, or from the external auditory canal. Cholesteatoma matrix was plated directly onto culture medium intraoperatively. Pre-operative and intraoperative cultures were then compared.

Results:

Pseudomonas aeruginosa, staphlococcus aureus, and staphlococcus epidermidis were by far the most frequently encountered organisms in pre and intraoperative cultures. Significant identity existed between pre and intraoperative cultures (81% of cases). The bacteriologic results are summarized in Table 1.

Table 1: Cultures of 16 patients with cholesteatoma:

	PRE-OP	INTRAOP
AEROBES:		
P. AERUGINOSA	50%	43%
S. EPIDERMIDIS	31%	25%
S. AUREUS	25%	12%
P. VULGARIS	12%	-
ENTEROCOCCUS	6%	6%
E. COLI	6%	6%
B-HEMOLYTIC STREPTOCCI	6%	6%
NO GROWTH	12%	18%
MULTIPLE ORGANISMS	25%	12%

Discussion:

Significant identity appears to exist between aerobic organisms cultured preoperatively from the middle ear or external auditory canal, and intraoperative cultures obtained from the mastoid cavity in cases of cholesteatoma.[1] In cases of reduced host immunity or impending intratemporal or extratemporal complications, carefully obtained cultures from the external auditory canal may serve as a meaningful method of determining initial antibiotic therapy.

The question still remains whether anaerobic organisms demonstrated within the mastoid cavity in up to 76% of cases of chronic otitis media by Brook, are significant in thepathogenesis of chronic supprative otitis media.[2,3] Anaerobes have been shown to protect aerobes in vitro from the effects of antibiotics by the production of penicillinases, etc.,and may behave synergistically in the infectious process. Fortunately, many anaerobes are also sensitive to peniccillins (carbenicillin, ticarcillin, etc.); however, in those patients unresponsive to conventional treatment, especially when there is no aerobic growth in culture, anaerobes should be sought with appropriate microbiologic techniques.

References:

1. Levenson MJ, Parisier SC, (1985) Infections in Surgery 4: No. 4 pp.260-267
2. Neu HC,(1984) Otolaryng. Clinics North Amer. 17:No. 4 pp 745-751
3. Brook I, (1983) Anaerobic Infections in Childhood, G.K. Hall Publishers, Boston pp. 142-145

New dimensions in otorhinolaryngology - head and neck surgery, vol. 2.
E. Myers, editor

CLINICAL RESULTS WITH BONE-ANCHORED HEARING AIDS

GUNNAR LIDÉN,[1,2] ANDERS TJELLSTRÖM,[1] NORMAN BERLINGER[2]
Departments of Otorhinolaryngology, (1) Sahlgren's Hospital, University of Gothenburg, Sweden and (2) University Hospital, University of Minnesota, Minneapolis, USA

Although the objective of surgery or medical treatment for middle ear disease and conductive hearing loss is to get a dry ear with satisfactory hearing, we know that this goal cannot always be reached. Some patients are in need of a hearing aid, but are unable to use a conventional air-conduction instrument because the ear starts to drain when it is obstructed by a mold. These patients may benefit from a conventional bone-conduction hearing aid. Such an instrument has many disadvantages. The bone-anchored hearing aid provides a new and better type of amplification through direct bone conduction for these patients. The bone-anchored hearing aid is attached to a skin-penetrating abutment which is internally fixated to a titanium screw sitting in the temporal bone (1). In the Department of Otolaryngology of Sahlgren's Hospital, Gothenburg, we started to use the titanium implants in the temporal bone as a new approach to wearing bone conduction hearing aids in 1977. The surgical procedures are generally performed under local anesthesia and consist of two stages. During the first step, a 4 mm long titanium screw is gently inserted into the temporal bone. After about four months, when the titanium fixture is stable, a skin-penetrating titanium abutment is attached to the implant. By means of a coupling element, a newly developed vibrator adapted to the impedance of the skull is directly connected to the fixture.

The *indications* for using a bone-anchored hearing aid are:
- Any patient who uses a conventional bone conduction hearing aid
- Any patient who uses air conduction hearing aids with chronically draining ears
- Any patient who needs amplification but conventional air-conduction hearing aids cannot be used because of chronic ear disease. Medically, these patients will be diagnosed as including those with:
- Congenital atresia in whom surgery is contraindicated,
- Operated congenital atresia with hearing loss but the ear drains if mold is used,
- Chronic otitis media, operated or non-operated, with conductive or mixed hearing loss,
- Radical mastoidectomy and meatoplasty experiencing uncontrollable feedback when using air conduction amplification,
- Chronic conductive loss in one ear and an unaidable sensorineural loss in the opposite ear.

Contraindications for using bone-anchored hearing aids include:
- Mixed hearing loss in which air conduction thresholds are worse than 80 dB H.L. (average 0.5-2.0 kHz) and bone conduction thresholds worse than 50 dB H.L.
- Speech discrimination below 60 percent.
- Pure sensorineural hearing loss.
- Emotionally unstable or developmentally delayed patients.

RESULTS

Titanium implants have been osteointegrated in the temporal bone and found to remain stable. Since 1977, 129 patients have received titanium implants for attachment of 87 bone-anchored hearing aids and in cases of malformed external ears or missing pinnas, attachment of 42 auricular prostheses. Only three fixtures of a total of 201 implanted and used fixtures (1.5%) have failed to integrate with the bone. Four of the skin-penetrating abutments of a total of 201 (2%) have been disconnected because of infections. The performance of the bone-anchored hearing aids in comparions with the conventional bone conduction aids has been tested with Békésy audiometry and a test for identification of sentences in speech noise (2, 3). The tone thresholds improved 10-20 dB in the frequency range 600-6000 Hz. The test for identification of synthetic sentences in speech noise showed that the signal-to-noise ratio which gave 50% intelligibility of the sentences improved an average of 3.3 dB. This corresponds to an average improvement in intelligibility of 25% when the bone-anchored aid was used.

The patients' subjective evaluation of the bone-anchored hearing aid correlated very well with the gain in discrimination accomplished and showed superior wearing comfort, improved quality of sound, favorable aesthetic appearance, improved intelligibility of speech, and reduced consumption of batteries.

REFERENCES

1. Tjellström A, Lindström J, Hallén O, Albrektsson T, Brånemark PI (1981) Amer J Otol 2:304
2. Håkansson B, Tjellström A, Rosenhall U (1984) Scand Audiol 13:3
3. Carlsson P, Håkansson B, Rosenhall U, Tjellström A. In preparation.

New dimensions in otorhinolaryngology - head and neck surgery, vol. 2.
E. Myers, editor

STAGING OF CHOLESTEATOMA

CHIANG-FENG LIEN
Dept.of Otolaryngology,Veterans General Hospital,Taipei,Taiwan,R.O.C.

INTRODUCTION

Cholesteatoma is a disease of middle ear cleft. Some small attic cholesteatoma occupies only at part of attic with partial destruction of malleus head, but the pars tensa is intact and mesotympanum is well aerated. Other large cholesteatoma may occupy all the middle ear cleft with destruction of all the ossicles except the footplate and the mesotympanum is completely atelectatic. Without description of the extent of destruction of the middle ear cleft, the results of surgery are hard to compare. Cholesteatoma has been subgrouped according to its extension in the middle ear cleft by Palva et al (1). Atelectasis is to some extent correlated to retraction pocket and cholesteatoma (2). Aeration of the middle ear is important to hearing restoration and recurrence of cholesteatoma. Destruction of the ossicles indicates the severity of cholesteatoma, also directly affects hearing restoration. Therefore a staging system of cholesteatoma considering the extension of cholesteatoma, atelectasis and destruction of the ossicles is recommended.

MATERIAL AND METHODS

From April 1981 to Oct. 1984, 151 ears of cholesteatoma were operated and staged according to the CAO system developed by the author.

"C" represents the extension of cholesteatoma in the middle ear cleft. "A" represents the degree of atelectasis. "O" represents the number of ossicles destroyed by cholesteatoma. Each of C,A and O is scored as 1,2,3 according to the degree of the severity (Table I). For example, a case of C2A2O1 represents a cholesteatoma occupying two areas in the middle ear cleft with moderate atelectasis and destruction of one ossicle. The total score of C,A and O ranges from 3 to 9. Among them, score 3 and 4 represent early stage of cholesteatoma. Score 5 and 6 represent moderate stage and score 7,8 and 9 represent advanced stage.

RESULTS

The staging of 151 ears of cholesteatoma are listed in Table II. There were 14 early cases (9%), 45 moderate stage cases (30%),and 92 advanced cases (61%).

The various combinations of CAO shown in Table II indicate the complexity of manifestation of cholesteatoma and the importance of considering all C,A and O factors in staging of cholesteatoma.

TABLE I

CAO STAGING SYSTEM OF CHOLESTEATOMA

Score	C (Cholesteatoma)	A (Atelectasis)	O (Ossicle)
1	at one area of middle ear cleft*	normal or Grade I atelectasis	normal or destruction of one ossicle
2	at two areas of middle ear cleft	Grade II or III,but anterior half of mesotympanum is still aerated.**	destruction of two ossicles
3	at three or more areas of middle ear cleft	Grade IV,more than posterior half of mesotympanum is unaerated.***	destruction of three ossicles

* Five areas of middle ear cleft are tympanic cavity, attic, aditus, antrum and mastoid air cells.
** In case of tympanic membrane perforation, less than half of the middle ear mucosa is destroyed.
***In case of tympanic membrane perforation, more than half of the middle ear mucosa is destroyed.

TABLE II

STAGES AND VARIOUS COMBINATIONS OF CAO SYSTEM

Stage	Total Score	Various Combination	Number	Total Number
Early	3	C1A1O1	9	14
	4	C1A1O2,C2A1O1	5	
Moderate	5	C1A2O2,C1A3O1,C2A1O2, C2A2O1,C3A1O1	21	45
	6	C1A3O2,C2A2O2,C2A3O1, C3A1O2,C3A2O1	24	
Advanced	7	C1A3O3,C2A3O2,C3A1O3, C3A2O2,C3A3O1	19	92
	8	C2A3O3,C3A2O3,C3A3O2	37	
	9	C3A3O3	36	

REFERENCES

1. Palva A, Karma P, Karja J (1977) Cholesteatoma in children.Arch Otolaryngol 103:74-77
2. Sade J, Avraham S, Brown M (1981) Atelectasis,retraction pocket and cholesteatoma. Acta Otolaryngol 92:501-512

© 1985 Elsevier Science Publishers B.V. (Biomedical Division)
New dimensions in otorhinolaryngology – head and neck surgery, vol. 2.
E. Myers, editor

A COMPARATIVE STUDY OF PRESSURE EQUILIZING TUBES

EDUARDO MADIEDO, JR., M.D.
San Antonio, Texas, USA

INTRODUCTION

Secretory Otitis Media is one of the most common problems in the pediatric population of the United States. It is the main cause of hearing loss in children. In spite of all the clinical research over the past few years, a clear etiology is not known. At the present, we continue to treat this entity in a symptomatic fashion. Several different tubes have been designed and at the present time, there are more than fifty types on the market. However, we still do not have the ideal tube which stays in the tympanic membrane enough time to solve the problem without getting obstructed or causing a complication. This prospective study was designed to compare the efficacy of the short term Shepard grommet teflon tube and the long term Goode T tube. Each patient served as his own control. A Goode-T tube was inserted in the left ear and Shepard grommet tube in the right ear. This study, in one thousand patients, began in June of 1979 and the consecutive myringotomies with insertion of pressure equilizing tubes were completed in September of 1984.

MATERIAL AND METHODS

The age of the patients ranged from six months to eighty four years. All of the patients underwent pre-operative audiological evaluation. All the patients had a medical management trial before the surgical procedure with antimicrobial therapy and oral decongestants. There were 602 males and 398 females. The most common indication for the insertion of pressure equilizing tubes was secretory otitis media. Insertion of pressure equilizing tubes as a single procedure amounted to 198 cases and the remainder had a combined procedure with adenoidectomy in 506 patients and with T&A in 296 patients. Radiological evidence of sinusitis was present in 304 patients. All the procedures were performed under general anesthesia in the operating room of the hospital. A Goode T tube, 1mm inside diameter, 12mm long and with 4mm flanges, was inserted in the left ear and a Shepard grommet teflon PE tube, 1mm inside diameter with wire, was inserted in the right ear. The follow up of the patients was every three months or PRN according to pain, sensation of pressure or discharge. From the 1000 patients (2000 insertions of PE tubes), 721 patients or 1442 insertions of PE tubes were followed-up. The data were processed by an NCR computer 8210. The criteria used to remove the tubes were absence of episodes of episodes of otitis media, normal appearance of the tympanic membranes and normal hearing 1 1/2 years after the insertion of the pressure equilizing tubes. There is no established criteria for removal of pressure equilizing tubes. Several tubes had to be removed due to persistent drainage which did not respond to the routine management. The most common organism found was Pseudomonas aeruginosa. 87 patients had nultiple insertions of pressure equilizing tube, up to 8 times. In three cases, a cholesteotoma was present. Perforations which appeared to be dry with no recurrence of the otitis media were repaired with a transcanal tympanoplasty with medial fascial graft. All the patients in this study were restricted from aquatic sprots and they were advised to use a cotton ball with Vaseline on the outside in both ears while taking a shower or shampooing their hair.

DISCUSSION

There is no statistically significant difference regarding quadrant of insertion of type of anesthetic. From the 652 patients who had the Shepard tube extruded, we found that only 113 (17.33%) of the patients had the Goode T tube extruded. However, we found that in 206 (45.04%) of the cases, the T tube was plugged and in some cases had to be removed because it was not possible to unplug it. Alson, a permanent perforation was left in 23 cases for the T tube (20.35%) and in 12 cases for the Shepard grommet (1.84%), which appeared less traumatic. Infections were most common for the T tube in 232 (32.17%) of the 721 follow-up patients. For the ears with the Shepard tube, only 80 (11.09%) of the patients had infection. Psuedomonas aeruginosa was the most common organism by culture. A criteria for the removal of PE tubes should be established.

SUMMARY

A comparative prospective study between the Goode T tube and the Shepard grommet tube was performed and the advantage of each tube has been discussed. The author considers that the Goode T tube can be used for most of the cases. The T tube can be cut in order to shorten the length of the flanges at the time of surgery in patients where a short term PE tube is indicated. There in no ideal tube which fulfills all the needs of patients with secretory otitis media. Future research is still in need.

BIBLIOGRAPHY

1. Armstrong, B.W.: What Your Colleagues Think of Tympanostomy Tubes. The Laryngoscope, 78:1303-1313, 1968.

2. Goode, R.L.: Advantages of the T-Tube for Short and Long-Term Middle Ear Ventilation. The Laryngoscope., 93:376-378, 1983.

3. Leopold, D.A. and McCabe, B.F.: Factors Influencing Tympanostomy Tube Function and Extrusion: A Study of 1,127 Ears. Otolaryngol. Head Neck Surg., 88:447-454, 1980.

4. Miller, G.F.: Eustachian Tubal Function in Normal and Diseased Ears. Arch. of Otolaryngol. 81:41-48, 1965.

© 1985 Elsevier Science Publishers B.V. (Biomedical Division)
New dimensions in otorhinolaryngology - head and neck surgery, vol. 2.
E. Myers, editor

T-TUBE FOR LONG-TERM MIDDLE EAR VENTILATION

LARS HOLME NIELSEN and GITTE HESSEL-ANDERSEN
Department of Otorhinolaryngology, Central County Hospital
DK 34oo Hilleroed (Denmark).

INTRODUCTION

The effectiveness of ventilation tube treatment in cases of middle ear effusion has been substantiated through prospective,randomized studies (1). The duration of the tube function period is important in the problem-prone group of patients with recurring secretory SOM. The T-tube (TT) was designed for cases requiring long-term ventilation (2).

This is a retrospective, consecutive study of the course, complications and sequelae of treatment with the T-tube.

MATERIAL AND METHODS

56 consecutive patients were treated with TT tubulation for SOM from October 198o through April 1984(fig.1). A total of 11o tubulations were performed. 15 ears were reintubated once and 2 ears had been treated 3 times. The procedure was bilateral in 35 patients. The distribution on the sides was equal. The sex ratio was 2.3: 1 (males/females).

The median age at (first) TT tubulation was 7 years (range 1 - 33 years). Previous tubulation with a grommet had been performed between 0 and 11 times (mean: 3.4 grommets per ear).

There were 6 patients with cleft palates (11%).

RESULTS

Hearing. Audiometry was performed with determination of SRT and PTA. The influence of TT-tubulation on the hearing loss is documented in fig. 2.,the postoperative values defined as the best within 3 months of the operation.

Duration. By using the life-tabel-method we noted an approximate rectilinear extrusion rate with a half-life value of 17-18 months (fig.3).

Complications

During treatment. 17 TT's were plugged once. while one tube was occluded at 2 and another at 3 occations. Discharge occurred in 29 cases, 2 of these several times. Peritubal granulation was found in 3 ears but it subsided without active treatment. There were no episodes necessitating extubation.

Late complications. At the termination of the study the TT had been extruded or

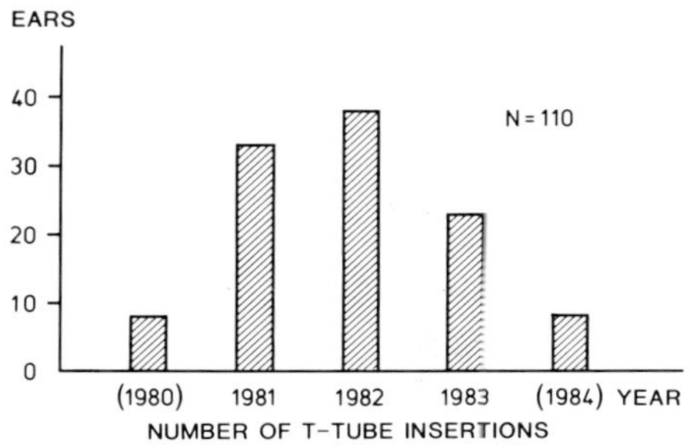

Fig. 1

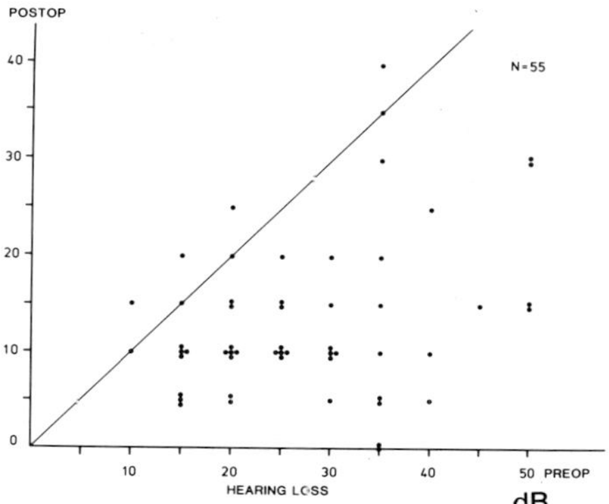

Fig. 2

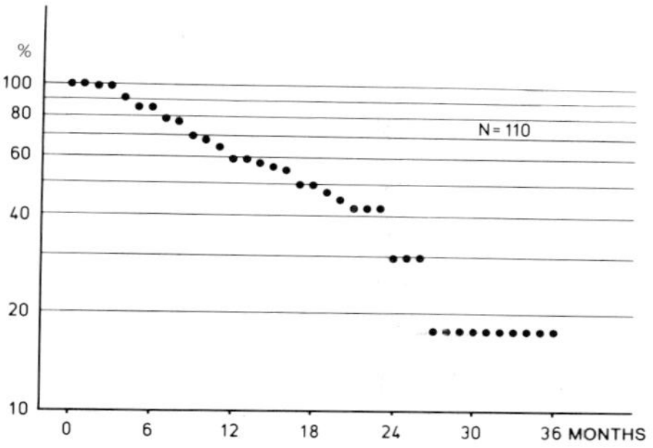

Fig. 3

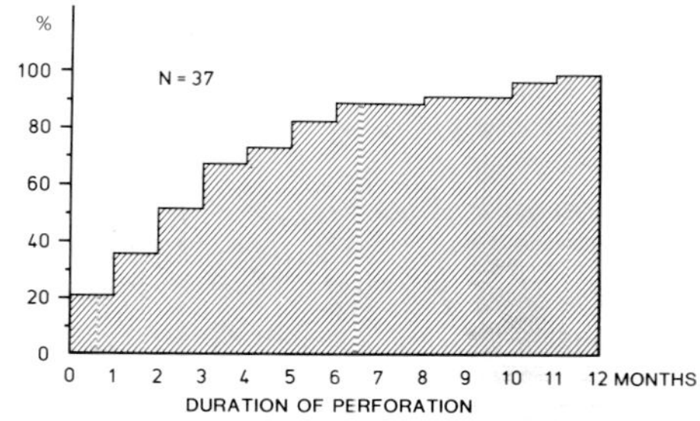

Fig. 4

extubated in 43 ears. 37 healed uneventfully, while 6 still had a perforation in the tympanic membrane. Fig. 4 demonstrates how long it took for the closure to become evident. 2 of the 6 patients were extubated shortly before termination of the study. The remaining 4 patients had post-removal perforation of 4-37 months standing.

DISCUSSION

It is our opinion that the amount and nature of complications during and after TT treatment are tolerable.

TT may be considered in case of:

1) long-term ventilation need is anticipated, independent of the presence of atrophy of the drum or middle ear atelectasis,

2) pre-term extrusion of previous grommets,

3) postponement of (final) surgery in juvenile patients.

REFERENCES

1. Lildholdt T (1983) Acta Otolaryngol Suppl. 398
2. Goode RL (1983) Laryngoscope 93: 376-378

© 1985 Elsevier Science Publishers B.V. (Biomedical Division)
New dimensions in otorhinolaryngology – head and neck surgery, vol. 2.
E. Myers, editor

DEEP NECK ABSCESS OF OTOGENIC ORIGIN: BEZOLD'S ABSCESS REVISITED

E. SMOUHA, M.D., V.K. ANAND, M.D., M.J. LEVENSON, M.D., M.D.F.DECK, M.D., S.C.PARISIER, M.D. Departments of Otolaryngology and Radiology, Manhattan Eye, Ear & Throat Hospital, New York, New York (U.S.A.)

Bezold's abscess is an uncommon complication of suppurative mastoiditis in the post-antibiotic era. In this paper, we review five cases of deep neck abscess of otogenic origin which presented to our hospital in the last three years, and contrast these with Bezold's original description. The early administration of antibiotics for otitis media has certainly influenced the incidence, pathogenesis, and bacteriology of this complication. All our cases required early surgery, and all had favorable outcomes. Computerized tomography (CT) has been a valuable tool for preoperative assessment of the anatomic spread of the abscess.

Bezold[1] originally described an entity in which large air cells in the mastoid tip fill with pus. Perforation of the thin plate of bone near the digastric ridge allows pus to track into the neck. An abscess forms medial to the sternocleidomastoid muscle that may extend along the sheath of the great vessels to enter the retropharyngeal space, larynx, or mediastinum. Fluctuance is not a predominant finding. Pneumococcus was the most frequent causative organism.

Our first case exemplifies Bezold's description. This 20 year old woman developed acute otitis media with purulent otorrhea. Despite conventional antibiotic treatment, she presented after two weeks with fever, facial weakness, dysphagia, and a tender swelling in the neck. Examination revealed a draining ear, unilateral facial paralysis, a large tense mass in the neck, and medial displacement of the lateral pharyngeal wall. At surgery, a deep neck abscess was drained which involved the parapharyngeal, pretracheal, and retropharyngeal spaces. A simple mastoidectomy was performed; granulation tissue and erosion of the mastoid tip were found. A preoperative CT scan was helpful in demonstrating the anatomic extent of the neck infection. Operative cultures yielded Streptococcus intermedius from the mastoid and Peptostreptococcus from the neck. The infection resolved with appropriate antibiotic therapy.

Our second patient was a 50 year old male who neglected an acutely draining ear and presented after three weeks with a painful necrotic eschar over his sternocleidomastoid muscle. Surgical exploration revealed suppurative mastoiditis with perforation of the bony cortex near the posterior canal wall, and abscess formation within the body of the muscle. Cultures grew Staphylococcus epidermidis from the mastoid, and Staphylococcus aureus from the neck. Prolonged wound care and antibiotics were necessary to effect resolution.

Two further cases exemplified abscess formation in the setting of chronic mastoiditis. Both patients had undergone radical mastoidectomies for cholesteatoma years before. After a long period without intervening problems, each presented with fever, purulent aural drainage, and a tender mass in the upper neck. At surgery, both patients had recurrent cholesteatomas. In both, the suppuration eroded through the mastoid tip at the digastric ridge to form an abscess medial to the sternocleidomastoid muscle.

The last case was an elderly diabetic male who developed a necrotizing pseudomonas external otitis. Despite prolonged in-hospital antibiotic treatment, he developed facial paresis and a tender, erythematous swelling in the postauricular area. CT scan revealed clouded mastoid air cells, erosion of the bony cortex of the mastoid tip, and a cystic mass inferomedial to the tip. At surgery, there was granulation tissue in the mastoid, necrosis and osteitis of the tip, and abscess formation in the soft tissues of the neck deep to the sternocleidomastoid insertion. Cultures yielded Pseudomonas aeruginosa.

Our cases of deep neck abscess of otogenic origin presented in a variety of clinical settings. In two patients, a neck abscess evolved from an acute suppurative mastoiditis. One of these developed rapidly, while the other was more indolent. Two patients developed neck abscesses from chronic mastoiditis with recurrent cholesteatoma. In both of these cases, infection migrated to the neck after erosion of the tip, conforming to Bezold's original description. In the final case, abscess formation occurred as a sequela of necrotizing external otitis.

Both aerobes and anaerobes and gram-positive organisms were cultured, and the neck and mastoid yielded different organisms in three cases. These diverse bacteriologic findings were certainly influenced by the early administration of broad-spectrum antibiotics.

CT scan was valuable in accurately delineating the path of spread of neck infection in four of our cases. In two cases, extension of the mastoiditis to the neck was diagnosed by CT. We advocate preoperative CT in the diagnosis and surgical planning of neck abscess of otogenic origin.

References:

1. Bezold F, Siebenmann F (1908) Textbook of Otology, E.H. Cosgrove & Co., Chicago.
2. Endicott JN, Nelson RJ, Saraceno CA (1982) Laryngoscope 92:630-633

New dimensions in otorhinolaryngology – head and neck surgery, vol. 2.
E. Myers, editor

CHOLESTEATOMA - AN EPIDEMIOLOGICAL STUDY AMONG MEMBERS OF KIBBUTZIM IN NORTHERN ISRAEL

L. PODOSHIN, M. FRADIS, Y. BEN-DAVID*, A. MARGALIT, A. TAMIR and L. EPSTEIN**

Dept. of Otolaryngology,* Haifa Medical Center (Rothschild), and Dept. of Family and Community Health,** Faculty of Medicine, Technion, Haifa, and Kupat Holim, Health Insurance Institute of General Federation of Labour, Israel

INTRODUCTION

Cholesteatoma (C) is a middle ear lesion of obscure origin. It behaves like an uncontrolled growing tumor, with the capability of destroying both the soft and hard tissues surrounding it. The epidemiological information about C is scarce. Genetic, ethnic, socio-economic and climatic factors were seldom the issue in the study of C. There is a great deal of uncertainty about the etiology and pathophysiology of C, thus enhancing the need for an epidemiological study. The purpose of this study was to determine the rate of Chronic Otitis Media (COM) and C among members of kibbutzim. The kibbutz is a collective settlement in which there is joint sharing of responsibility for all activities and services including health.

MATERIAL AND METHODS

Three groups were studied. They were defined according to the height above and below sea level of the kibbutz: a) in a plateau area about 225 m above sea level; b) in the Lake Kinneret area - 212 m below sea level; c) in the Mount Carmel area - 400 m above sea level. The people examined were more than 10 years old and many of them were born outside Israel. All of them live in the same socioeconomic environment, eat similar food and receive the same level of medical care and treatment. Every subject was examined by an otolaryngologist with a pneumatic otoscope. C was diagnosed on histological examination of tissue that had been removed from an affected ear. A subject who met the criteria of COM or C was treated and followed-up in hospital.

RESULTS

3056 subjects - 1664 women and 1392 men were examined. 29 (0.95%) were found to have COM. 12 of them were found to suffer from C as well (0.4% of overall). Unilateral COM was found in 9 patients (26.5%), bilateral COM was found in 11 patients (32.4%), unilateral C was found in 11 patients (32.4%). Bilateral C was found in one patient. The prevalence rate of COM was found to be 0.95% and of C 0.4%. 41% of the patients who had COM suffered from C as well. In addition to demographic factors, the influence of altitude was investigated but the differences were not found to be significant. The highest age group prevalence of C was 21-30 years, COM was more prevalent in males than females (0.02>P>0.01), in Ashkenasi than Sepharadi* (0.05>P>0.02) and in industrial and agricultural workers (0.05>P>0.02) as compared to others (Table I). Among C patients a family history was found in 64%. In 71% of patients, their illness began in infancy. 20% of the patients did not know of their disease till they were examined in this study.

TABLE I

PREVALENCE (%) OF COM AND CHOLESTEATOMA BY ETHNIC ORIGIN IN THE EXAMINED POPULATION

Ethnic Origin	n	COM		Cholesteatoma	
		No.	%	No.	%
Ashkenazi	2246	27	1.20	12	0.53
Sepharadi	684	2	0.29	0	-
Total	2930	29		12	

DISCUSSION

Few epidemiological studies have dealt with the prevalence of C in the general population. The results of these studies were very different each from the other (1-4). We reviewed members of kibbutz which is a society of Jews living at the same socioeconomic level. Our results are similar to those found in surveys of white Caucasians, French and English in Canada (Ratnesar, 1976). They found COM in 1.5% as against 0.95% in our study. The results of this study emphasize the need for performing more extensive studies in an attempt to determine the rate of C in the general population. The necessity for preventive ear examinations, earlier diagnosis and treatment of C is emphasized as well.

REFERENCES

1. Sade J (1982) Cholesteatoma and Mastoid Surgery. Kugler Publishers, Amsterdam
2. Baxter J, Ling D (1974) Canad J Otolaryng 3:110-111
3. McCabe BF, Sade D, Abramson M (1977) Cholesteatoma First International Conference. Aesculapuis Publication Company, Birmingham, Alabama, USA
4. Ratnesar P (1976) J Otolaryng 5(2):121-125

---

* Ashkenazi refers to Jews whose origin is largely from Europe; Sepharadi refers usually to Jews whose family originated in Africa and Asia.

New dimensions in otorhinolaryngology - head and neck surgery, vol. 2.
E. Myers, editor

EAR DISEASE IN THE AUSTRALIAN ABORIGINE

A B N RAO
Royal Darwin Hospital, PO Box 41326, Casuarina N.T. 5792, AUSTRALIA

INTRODUCTION

About 40,000 years ago in the Glacial period people from South East Asia reached the shores of Australia. The Dutch and finally the British were the late settlers and the colonisation began in 1788. Before the arrival of Europeans, Aboriginals occupied the entire continent including Tasmania and their number at that time was 300,000. There were numerous conflicts between the Aboriginals and the new comers which have resulted in many Aboriginals being killed and very few full blooded are still in existence.

Economic backwardness, dispossession of land and isolation has resulted in the worst kind of living conditions, leading to chronic ill health, wide spread malnutrition, infant mortality, trachoma and chronic suppurative otitis media. This situation is now rectified by the recent state and federal legislation which provides special health facilities and financial assistance on a priority basis. The majority of the population are now living in the Northern Territory and they constitute 25% of the population. And as per information released by the Australian Bureau of Statistics in 1981 the following are the details:

1. Australian Population = 14,926,800
2. Australian Aboriginal Population = 208,000
3. Northern Territory Population = 124,500
4. (a) Northern Territory Aboriginal Population = 27,840
   (b) The growth rate is 1.8%
   (c) Hearing impairment in Aboriginal children is 157 per 1,000 (National average is 16 per 1,000).
   (d) There are approximately 2,500 cases of CSOM and nearly half of them need assistance in hearing.

In a typical case the tympanic membrane shows a huge central perforation mainly involving the anterior portion and exposing the handle of malleus and the eustachian orifice. Negroid type of nose with wide nasal cavities and mucoid nasal discharge is quite common.

DISCUSSION

The ear problem is aggravated due to heat and humidity and hence the proportion of discharging ears is more in coastal communities like Bathurst Island, where almost every infant had otitis media before the age of 3/12 to 4/12 and it is interesting to note the lack of usual symptoms of acute O.M. There is no history of any pain or pyrexia. Only a discharging ear which appears to be due to a severe necrotic type of infection. At this stage these children are treated with a course of antibiotics. In 50% to 60% the discharge continues for many years.

We are not sure whether we are dealing with the problem of lack of resistance, genetic problems, protein calorie deficiency or is there any abnormality in the Collagen and the middle layers of the tympanic membrane.

Accordingly, some of the possibilities to be considered are:-

1. Should we give Gamma-globulin for recurrent otitis media?
2. Should we change the regime of triple antigen in these children?
3. Should we administer long term antibiotics in the at risk population?
4. Should we try to raise their immunity by using immuno-potentiating drug (e.g. Levamisole)?

A proposed clinical trial of the immuno-potentiating drug Levamisole on 50 Bathurst Island infants aged 2 to 12 months has had to be abandoned due to adverse publicity. This population group would have been ideal because almost 100% of all children born there in the last 9 years developed bilateral ear discharge before 15 months old. There are about 60 children born each year.

No complication of CSOM or cholesteatoma is noted. In chronic cases treatment consists of cleaning the ears, insufflating with Acid Boracic in Iodoform powder, and supplying the hearing aids as all of them developed profound conductive deafness. In most of the schools FM radio amplification is used to communicate with the children in the classrooms and this seem to be more successful than the conventional method. At the age of 13 or 14 discharge usually stops and Myringoplasty is undertaken. In about 75% we are able to close the perforations and in all the cases we may not achieve normal hearing but still we feel myringoplasty and tympanoplasty are justified to prevent the recurring infection as all these children would like to swim due to hot tropical climate.

At present research is in progress to identify the aetiology and in particular to find out whether Chlamydia is responsible for this chronic disease.

ACKNOWLEDGEMENTS

My grateful thanks are due to the N.T. Government and the NH & MRC for their financial assistance, Dr Gurd, Dr Keith Fleming and Dr Wilson for their encouragement to study this problem and finally to Sister Giles and Erlinda for professional and secretarial assistance..

New dimensions in otorhinolaryngology – head and neck surgery, vol. 2.
E. Myers, editor

ATHANIKAR'S HYPOTHETICAL MODIFICATION OF FACIAL NERVE DECOMPRESSION BASED ON RETICULOMETRY

DR. MRS. K. A. ATHANIKAR

Professor and Head of the E.N.T. Department, B.J. Medical College, Pune 411 001 Maharashtra, INDIA

INTRODUCTION

Bell's facial paralysis is serious not as it endangers life but because the person affected loses "The language of facial expression". It takes away the personality of the patient and poses great social and functional problems. This unique nerve is travelling through tight bony canal which is the main hurdle in speedy recovery. About 10 to 18% of patients have complete paralysis with all fibres destined to degeneration and require active surgical intervention.

Present study aims to do **RETICULOMETRY** - microscopic measurement of the surface area of vertical part of the fallopian canal to know whether this study adds to the knowledge of the otologist attempting to offer full and final recovery.

MATERIAL AND METHODS

25 fresh cadaveric adult temporal bones were obtained and washed with normal saline. Radical mastoidectomy was done and fallopian canals were dissected out. Dissected canals were fixed, decalcified, and dehydrated serially in 70%, 80% and 90% alcohol. Transverse sections of 7μ were taken with the help of microtome. About 1956 H & E stained slides were studied with reticule. Reticule - occular micrometer is having 1 sq.cm. area which is devided into 400 small squares of 0.25 sq.mm. area each. Total number of squares were counted over the entire fallopian canal. Difference between the squares out side the circle of the canal and inside the circle were counted and area in sq. mm. is calculated.

OBSERVATION TABLE

SHOWING TOTAL NUMBER OF SQUARES AND SURFACE AREA IN SQ.MM.

	Total No. of Sqs.	Total area in sq.mm.	Sq. outside circle	Area in sq.mm.	diff. in squres	Area in sq.mm.
Avg.	120	30	80	20	40	10

DISCUSSION

Reticulometric observations reveal that fallopian canal is not circular but is ovoid. It also indicates that the fallopian canal is narrower by 1.0 mm to 1.5 mm. adjacent to the sinus tympani for about 2 mm.

10 sq.mm. area of the fallopian canal is out side the radius of the circle of the fallopian canal. According to bio-physical law of pressure, pressure is inversly proportional to the surface area. Pressure of the oedema fluid remaining constant, nerve fibres and blood vessels in area 'AEBC' of the fallopian canal will have to sustain more pressure effects as surface area is less. Blood supply of the facial nerve is in in longitudinal fashion and is incorporated in periosteum. Blood vessels also behave as end arteries. By routine method of facial cecompression, facial nerve is exposed and sheath insion is taken. But in order to achieve the ultimate goal of decompression, the nerve should be gently dislodged in the canal itself to let the oedema fluid come out from the area 'AEBC' taking care not to disturb chorda tympani and stapedial vessels. The area (about 2 mm.) adjacent to the sinus tympani should be completely drilled away through posterior tympanotomy and particular attention should be given to this area of the fallopian canal.

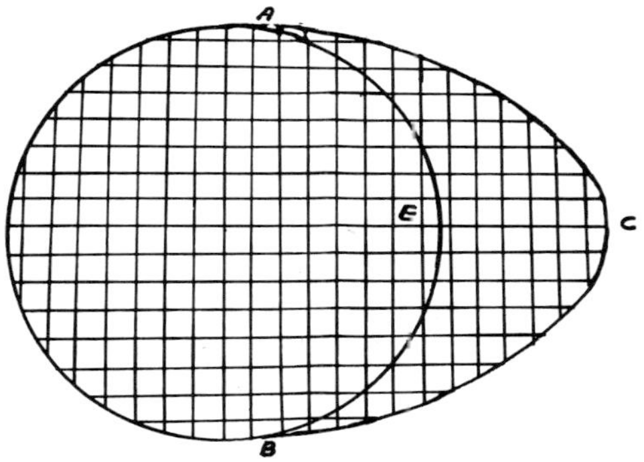

Line drawing showing area 'AEBC' sustaining more pressure effects.

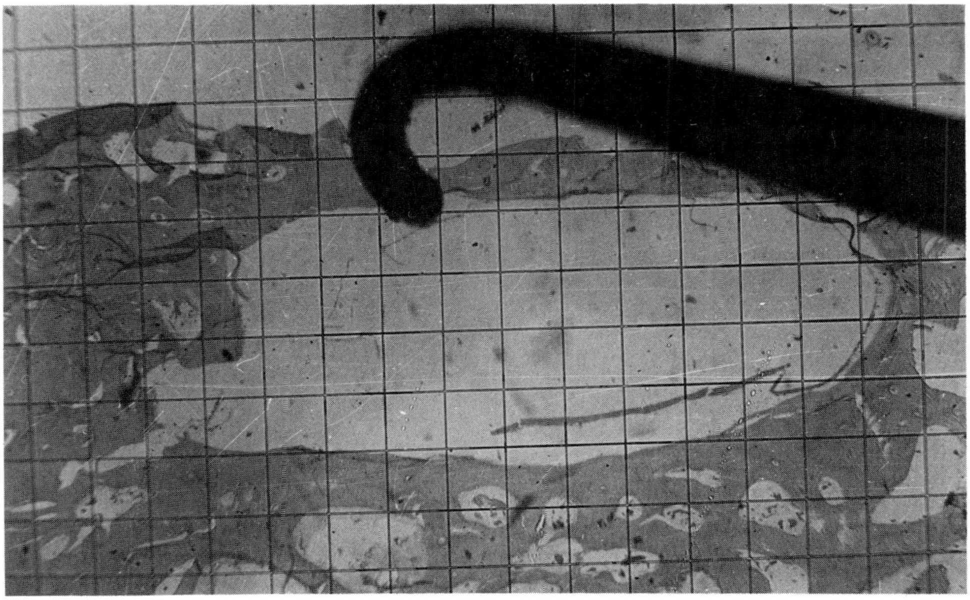

Photo-micrograph of Fallopian Canal viewed through reticule alongwith facial nerve dislodger.

© 1985 Elsevier Science Publishers B.V. (Biomedical Division)
New dimensions in otorhinolaryngology - head and neck surgery, vol. 2.
E. Myers, editor

CRANIAL NERVES ALTERATIONS DURING BELL'S PALSY

R.F.Bento; A.Miniti; A.J.Tedesco-Marchese. Facial Nerve Group, Depts of Otolaryngology, Neurology and Neurosurgery, University of Sao Paulo, Medical School, Sao Paulo, Brazil

INTRODUCTION

In the last years, some authors was suggesting that some cases of Bell's Palsy may be part of a clinical picture of a cranial polyneurophaty. (Nieuwmeyer P.A.; Hendrix R.A.; Adour K.K.).

In order to evaluate this involvment we've studied 107 consecutive cases of Idiophatic Facial Paralysis cared for at the Facial Paralysis Group of our University.

MATERIAL AND METHODS

107 consecutive patients with Facial Paralysis in wich the following diagnosis resources didn't show a definite etiology. Age average 32 years, between 15 and 71 years.

Diagnosis resources:

a) History and physical ENT examination
b) Laboratorial exams: Glucose Test, Syphilis Tests (FTA-ABS) and Mantoux Test
c) Site diagnose exams: Shirmer Test, Stapedial Reflex, Chemical Gustometry
d) Electric Tests (Hilger and Electromyography)
e) Audiogram and Impedance Tests
f) Temporal Bone Multidirecional Tomography

These cases was submited to a Otoneurologic examination according the routine estabilished by Miniti and Col. (3) that we use in our clinic:

I Cranial Nerve (Olphatory) - Discrimination and perception of garlic, coffee and anissed smell.

Ocular system evaluation by the Oftalmologic Department.

V Cranial Nerve (Trigeminal)

a) Sensibility tactil and thermal
b) Eye-lid reflexes
c) Jaw motricity
d) Temporal and Masseter muscles tonus

VIII Cranial Nerve (Cocleo-Vestybular) - Audiometric and Vestybular Tests.

IX and X Cranial Nerves (Vagus and Glossopharingeal)

a) Palate simetry, motricity
b) Vocal cords motricity
c) Nausea reflex of the pharinx
d) Taste of the posterior tongue

XI Cranial Nerve (Spinal)

a) Shoulders inspection

b) Sternocleido and Trapesius muscles tonus and motricity

XII Cranial Nerve (Hipoglossus) - Tongue movimentation, Facyculation and tonus.

Besides these cases we performed in healthy adults between 20 and 30 years, all the above tests, and we called control group.

RESULTS

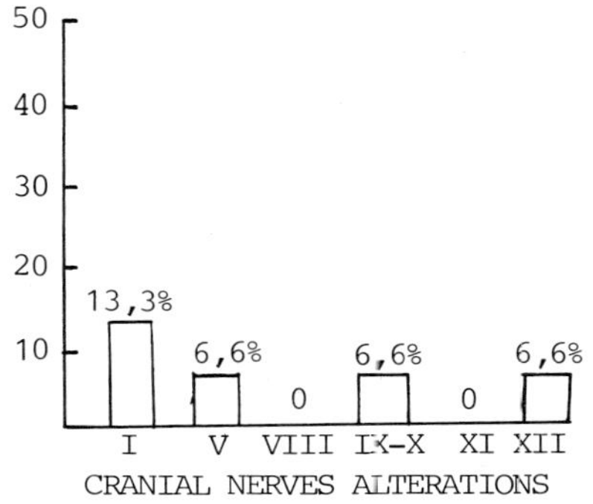

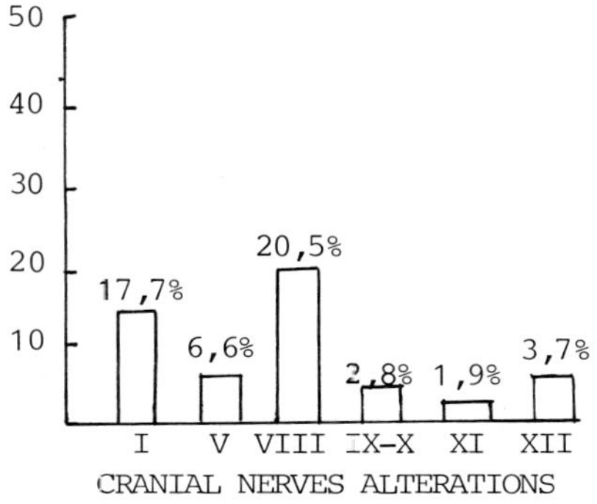

FIGs. 1 and 2 - The graphic nº 1 represente the alteration of the tests in the control Group. And nº 2 the alterations in the Bell's Palsy patients. The Oftalmologic evaluation in all cases do not demonstrate any alteration of the cranial nerves.

DISCUSSION AND CONCLUSION

We didn't found a significant diference between the control group and the 107 patients tested.

The Idiophatic Facial Palsy was a isolate pathology in the great majority of the cases.

If occur some involvment in other cranial nerve, it was sub-clinical.

REFERENCES

1) Adour K.K.:(1976) Cranial Polyneuritis and Bell Palsy. Arch. Otolaryngol. 102:262-264.

2) Hendrix R.A.; Melnick W.: (1983) Auditory Brain Stem Response and Audiologic tests in Idiophatic Facial Nerve Paralysis. Otolaryngol. Head Neck Surg. 91:686-690.

3) Miniti A.; Formigoni L.G.; Caldas A.C.G.; Leite M.A.F.; Marone S.A.M.; Sampaio P.L.: Sequencia no estudo otoneurológico. Lab. UPJOHN, Sao Paulo 1980.

4) Nieuwmeyer P.A.; Koch P.A.M.; Visser S.L.; Feenstra L.: (1982) Bell's Palsy: A Polyneurophaty. Clin. Otolaryngol. 7:293-298.

New dimensions in otorhinolaryngology – head and neck surgery, vol. 2.
E. Myers, editor

FACIAL NERVE TUMORS

OSVALDO GOMES DE SOUZA
Department of Otolaryngology, Hospital Felicio Rocho, Felice Rosso Foundation
Av. Contorno, 9155 5º andar 30.000 Belo Horizonte M.G. (Brasil)

ABSTRACT
Intratemporal tumors involving the facial nerve are uncommom. Both diagnosis and treatment are challenging. Twenty-one different types of tumors involving the facial nerve were seen by the author from 1972-1984, representing 7% of palsies treated in his department, 14 (66.66%) benign (TABLE I). Five were females and 9 males, from 3 to 64 years old, mean 35. Nine tumors were left and 5 right. Seven malign which will not be discussed. The facial nerve paralysis caused by cerebellum ponthine angle neuromas were not included, either.

TABLE I
SUMMARY OF CASES

Cases	Age	Sex	Tumor Type	Site	Approaches	Rehabilitation	Results
1.MAF	59	F	F.Neuroma	gg-Labyrinth	FM*	Graft	Poor
2.RFC	15	M	F.Neuroma	gg-Parotid	TL**	Graft	Good
3.RON	15	M	F.Neuroma	Tympanic	TM***	Graft	Excellent
4.JVS	26	M	F.Neuroma	Tympanic	TM	Graft	Poor
5.MCF	35	F	F.Neuroma	Meatal	TL	T.Removal	Poor
6.WSM	20	M	Neuroma UO******	Meatal	TL	T.Removal	Good
7.NTR	61	F	Neuroma UO	Meatal	TL	T.Removal	Good
8.DEC	32	M	Glomus Tumor	T.Mastoid	TM	T.Removal	Poor
9.MESS	64	F	Glomus Tumor	g-Jugularis	Surgical	Treatment Refusal	
10.MSP	59	M	Glomus Tumor	g-Tynpanic	TM	T.Removal	Good
11.MGS	3	F	Eos.Granuloma	Mastoid	TM	T.Removal	Good
12.AGV	29	M	Congenital Chol.	ggLabyrinth	FM	Graft	Poor
13.JMO	19	M	Meningioma	gg-Meatal	SO****	Plastic	Poor
14.JSP	64	M	Plasmacytoma	Mast.Meatal	IL*****	Graft	Poor

*Middle Fossa ** Translabyrinthine *** Transmastoid **** Suboccipital
***** Infralabyrinthine ****** Undetermined Origin.

MORE DETAILED REPORT OF CASES 1 AND 14.

MAF, a 59-year-old female complained of sudden facial nerve paralysis for one year, on left side, without any recovery at present time. Labeled Bell's palsy.

Ph. examination: ear, nose, and throat were normal. Total facial nerve palsy and absence of tearing on left side. Audiogram was normal and symmetric. ENG: symmetric hyporeaction. Tympanometry: A type curves with no stapedial reflex on left . RX: erosion in medial portion of superior semicircular canal, just superior to internal auditory canal. CT: erosion in antero-superior part of pyramid. Surgery: through the middle cranial fossa approach, a tumor mass of 2.5 x 2cm was totally removed from labyrinth and geniculate segments of facial nerve, plus homograft (sural nerve) from meatal to tympanic portions (AP: facial neuroma) 30% facial function recovered after one year.

JPS, a 64-year-old white man, complained of intermittent discharge, otalgia, and hearing loss on left side for one year and progressive facial nerve paralysis 3 months ago. Ph. examination: total facial nerve palsy 20% decrease of lacrimation on same side. Audiogram: total hearing loss on left. Otoscopy: polyp filling external auditory and pathologic study revealed non-specific cronic inflammatory process. RX: great erosion involving middle ear and whole otic capsule. CT:normal. Left carotid arteriography: normal. Surgery: through infralabyrinthine approach and after identification of internal carotid artery, tumor of 2.5 x 2cm was totally removed. It was impossible to separate nerve from tumor. Removal was in block from mastoid to meatal segments. Tumor eroded whole middle ear, ossicles, coclea, lateral and superior canals. Sural nerve graft was carried out between stumps from mastoid to meatal segments using 10-0 mononylon for suture.(AP: plasmacytoma). Comment: Complete evaluation for multiple myeloma was done later.

SUMMARY

Fourteen cases of benign tumors with facial nerve involvement were presented. Even though thorough evaluations, at different times, were carried out in all cases, the definite diagnosis only could be established, in most cases, after surgery. The roentegenograms and more recently the CT scanner among all test, were the most helpful. If one complete evaluation is performed or total dissection indicated in those cases in which facial palsies did not recover after six months, we can find facial tumors more frequently. We managed tumors from all different segments of facial nerve. Different approaches such as transmastoid , translabyrinthine, transtemporal (MF), and infralabyrinthine were used to treat the related tumors.

REFERENCES

1. Fisch, U. et al.Pathology of intratemporal tumors involving the facial nerve. Facial Nerve Surgery- KUGER MEDICAL PUBLICATIOS BV, 448 - 56, 1977.
2. Pulec, J. L. Facial nerve tumors. ANN: OTOL, 86: 962 - 32, 1969.
3. Pulec, J. L. Facial nerve tumors. LARYNGOSCOPE,82: 1160 - 76 jun. 1972.

New dimensions in otorhinolaryngology - head and neck surgery, vol. 2.
E. Myers, editor

CLINICAL EVIDENCE OF CNS INVOLVEMENT IN BELL'S PALSY

P. HANNER, O. ANDERSEN, L. FRISEN, U. ROSENHALL and S. EDSTRÖM
Depts of Audiology, Neurology, Ophthalmology and Otolaryngology, University of Göteborg, Göteborg, Sweden

Twentyeight patients with acute facial palsy were clinically investigated with special reference to CNS involvement. The mean age was 41.6 years (range 14-76 years). The male-female ratio was 10/18. 43 per cent of the patients were classified as solitary facial nerve dysfunctions while the remaining part showed evidence of brainstem impairment or cranial poly-neuropathy. The most frequent finding was an abnormal corneal reflex. Three patients showed evidence of brainstem migrating disorder which means an initial affection of taste accompanied or followed by dysesthesia corresponding to the lingual branch of the trigeminal nerve. Another patient showed symptoms consistent with a multifocal disease as shown as paresthesia in the legs and bilateral positive Babinski signs. Five patients had abnormal brainstem audiometry. Four patients had pathological optokinetic nystagmus which could be demonstrated as an eye motility disorder indicating brainstem impairment. Four patients had optic neuropathy which is a retrobulbar demyelinating process of the optic nerve. Secondary manifestations develop in the retinal nerve fibre layer with degeneration of the axons. Funduscopic differencies are seen between the normal, slightly opaque nerve fibre layer and the slit like defects representing the atrofied axons. It is concluded that Bell's palsy is a designation of different neuropathologic conditions which have the facial nerve in common.

© 1985 Elsevier Science Publishers B.V. (Biomedical Division)
New dimensions in otorhinolaryngology – head and neck surgery, vol. 2.
E. Myers, editor

SURGICAL ANATOMY OF THE FACIAL NERVE
IDENTIFICATION TECHNIQUES FOR AVOIDING ITS LESION

MIGUEL A. LACOUR, GLORIA BALDISSEROTTO AND VALENTIN THOMPSON
Division of Otorynolaryngology of the Pirovano County Hospital
Buenos Aires, Argentina

The fundamental condition for avoiding facial paralysis during surgery, is a thorough knowledge of the anatomy of the facial nerve. It is also necessary to know which are the exact sites in which lesions of the nerve usually occur, according to the type of otologic surgery being performed and thus develop a systematic and routinary technique for identifying the nerve.

1. Anatomic Investigation of the Facial Nerve from the surgical point of view (2nd and 3rd portions).

Dissections were performed in 40 temporal bones. The measurement of the angling between the facial nerve and other anatomical elements was carried out in two ways: a) Directly, with millimetric calibre.
b) Radioanatomic method, placing radio-opaque substance in the facial canal and obtaining x-rays in vertical, sagittal and profile views.

2. Lesion Topography: The sites where facial lesions most consistently and frequently occurred are described for each type of surgery. For this, the results of 16 re-operations performed between 1962 and 1984, were studied.

	CASES
A. MASTOIDECTOMY	2
B. STAPEDECTOMY	2
C. MIDDLE EAR RADICAL	4
D. TYMPANOPLASTIES	6
E. AURICULAR DYSGENESIS	2

3. Techniques for the Identification of the Facial Nerve.

RESULTS

1. Anatomic Investigation
   a) The nerve presents great variations in its course. These variations are more significant along its 3rd portion, than in its 2nd portion.
   b) The otologic surgeon can observe that the shortest distance is seen between the posterosuperior part of the tympanic annulus and the posterior third of the 2nd portion of the facial nerve. This is the relationship which consistently is most permanent between both structures.
   c) The 3rd portion of the facial nerve generally crosses the plane of the tympanic annulus at its lower third, but it may pass completely inside it, or rarely, outside it.

2. Lesion Topography

The sites where lesions of the nerve are typical and consistent or at least most frequent. for each type of surgical operation:

A. Mastoidectomy. Lesion of the nerve is generally produced at the level of the outlet of the corda tympani.

B. Stapedectomy. The lesion is currently highly unlikely, but when it does happen, it 's at the level of the 2nd portion. It 's possible when a facial nerve is dehiscent, an anatomical circumstance which occurs much more frequently in the posterior half of the 2nd portion of the nerve. This is also likely to occur in cases of stapedial artery hemorrhage or an exaggerated outflow of perilymphatic fluid.

C. Middle Ear Radical. The site where lesions generally occur is at the angle of the nerve, between the 2nd and 3rd portions, or a bit lower at the beginning of the 3rd (at the level of the pyramid), when reducing the wall of the facial, which must be resected if a dry cavity is desired.

D. Tympanoplasty. The typical site for the lesion is the angle between the 2nd and 3rd portions. When a Posterior Tympanotomy is performed a lesion of the nerve at the level of the pyramid of the stapes muscle is also likely, when cases with highly sclerotic mastoid process are operated. The cleansing of the facial and tympanic sinus is particularly hazardous in the case of large cholesteatomas, which affect the posterior tympanic wall.

E. Auricular Dysgenesis. The nerve crosses obliquely (at 60°) rathe than taking a horizontal course (at 90°) coming out through the stylomastoid foramen, as is habitual. The facial nerve is often dehiscent (35% of the cases) while the aberrant direction of the same is proven in 20% of the cases. The abnormal course of pair VII appears to be most frequent when there is a mayor facial deformity associated.
The lesion can be produced practically anywhere, but when it is confirmed during surgery it is necessary to totally decompress the nerve, from the geniculate ganglion to the site where it emerges from the temporal bone, in order to prevent a permanent facial paralysis.

3. Identification of the Facial Nerve

It is necessary to develop a systematic and routinary surgical technique, in order to avoid lesion of the nerve. The three techniques we generally use, for identifying the nerve are:

I. First Technique. In the mastoid process (identify the upper third of the 3rd portion of the nerve). It is the most frequently used and is especially important in those surgical cases which offer the greatest difficulties (Laberintectomy, Decompression of the endolymphatic sac, or resection of large cholesteatomas, that affect tympanic and facial sinus). For the systematic identification of the facial nerve we always try to approach the middle ear performing a mastoidectomy, as a first Tympanoplastic instance.

II. Second Technique. In the mastoid process (identify the lower third of the 3rd portion of the nerve, near the stylomastoid foramen).
This technique is useful, especially in those cases where it is difficult to identify the facial nerve at the level of the upper third of the 3rd portion, because of severe otic pathology, mainly in tumors of the middle ear.
The zone of the torus digastricus must be opened, which indicates the insertion of the sternocleydomastoid and the stylomastoid muscles.
Once the stylomastoid foramen has been identified, the facial nerve should be followed upward.

III. Third Technique. In the mastoid process and tympanic cavity.
It is generally used when the pair VII is being decompressed. It is begun following the first technique described (I). Afterwards, an orderly assessment of the following structures is made:

1. The corda tympani
2. The 2nd portion of the facial nerve
3. The stapes
4. The stapes muscle
5. The cochleariformis process

The facial nerve must be identified at its 2nd portion, at the level of the cochleariformis process, since the incus and the stapes are neither reliable nor fixed points, for this identification.

BIBLIOGRAFY

1. Anson, B.J.; Bast, T.H. Related Structures of the Ear in Man. American Academy Meeting.
2. Sheehy, J.L. and Crabtree, J.A.: Tympanoplasty: Staging the operation. Laryngoscope, 83:1594, 1973.
3. Farrior, J.B.: Systematized approach to surgery for cholesteatoma. Arch. Otolaryngol. 97:188,1973.
4. Portmann, M.:"Open" or "closed" Technique in surgery of the middle ear. Ann. Otol. Rhinol. Laryngol. 77:927,1968.
5. Snow, J.B. Controversy in Otolaryngology. W.B. Saunders Company. 1980.
6. Portman, M. The Ear and Temporal Bone. Masson Publishing U.S.A. 1979.

New dimensions in otorhinolaryngology – head and neck surgery, vol. 2.
E. Myers, editor

SUB MANDIBULAR SALIVARY GLAND SCAN: A PROGNOSTIC INDICATOR OF BELL'S PALSY A PRELIMINARY REPORT

G. ROSEN, I.Y. VERED, I. GARTY
Department of Otolaryngology and Department of Nuclear Medicine, Central Emek Hospital, Afula, Israel

INTRODUCTION

The ultimate outcome of peripheral facial nerve paralysis is difficult to predict. Therapeutic efforts should be directed toward patients in whom bad prognosis is anticipated. Once irreversible pathological changes occur and neurolysis develop, treatment will not alter the natural course of Bell's palsy. Up to now there is no one single prognostic test which can predict accurately the outcome of the disease, and in this presentation it is not proposed to present one.

Magielsky and Blatt (1958) described sub-mandibular salivary flow as a test to aid in the foretelling of the outcome of facial nerve paralysis. May et al. (1976) found that the salivary flow test was the most valuable in predicting the prognosis of facial paralysis. On the involved side, salivary flow rates diminished earlier than the response to maximal stimulation or nerve excitability tests. (Delay of 2 days between paralysis onset and flow changes in comparison with 3-14 days delay in electrical tests).

MATERIAL AND METHODS

We started collecting the saliva but were unhappy with the technical side of the procedure. As the idea was sound we looked for a simpler way to gain the same results and decided to perform the sub mandibular salivary gland scan as a prognostic test.

Fifty patients who underwent brain scan for possible cerebral lesions were screened as to the uptake of the radio isotope in the sub mandibular salivary glands. The patients had no known salivary gland lesion, or facial nerve lesion for that matter. The uptake proved to be symmetrical in the sub mandibular salivary glands. Then 40 consecutive patients with early unilateral peripheral facial nerve paralysis of unknown origin had salivary gland scans. The scan was part of a complete facial paralysis workup that included auditory, vestibular, lacrimal, stapedius reflex and electrical tests. The patients had no history of salivary gland disease. Scans were preferably done in 4 days after the onset of Bell's palsy.

An Elsint Dymax-C-E1 Gamma camera was used. Patients were seated facing the camera and 10 mCi of 99m-Tc pertechnetate were injected I.V. Photographs were

Photographs were then taken for the first 5 minutes only with a sequence of 30 sec per frame. Two regions of interest were focused over the sub mandibular salivary glands and the concentration of the Tc-99m in the glands was obtained in kilo counts (Figures 1 and 2).

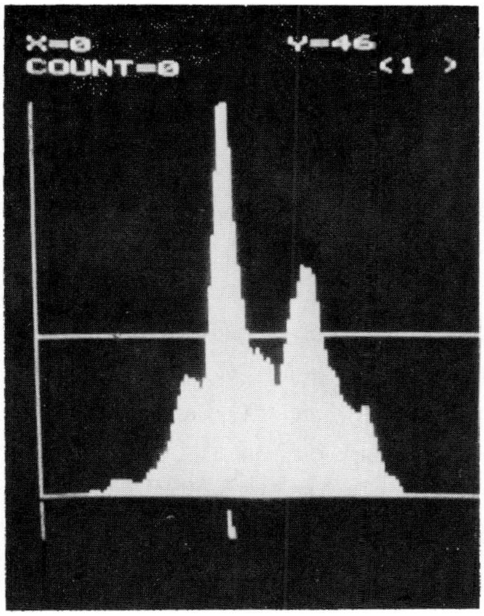

Fig. 1. Graph of kilo count and the comparison between left and right sides.

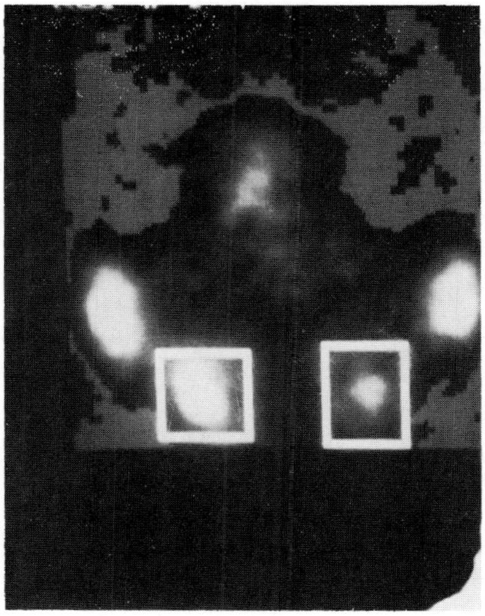

Fig. 2. Sub mandibular salivary gland scan region of interest and difference between the two sides.

The relative uptake of each gland was calculated in percentages. The whole test lasted about 6 minutes, radiation dose was low - 10m rad per examination - and the cost reasonable. Salivary scan may be performed in all ages. No special coopėration is necessary.

RESULTS

The results of 40 patients with unilateral Bell's palsy who had the sub mandibular salivary gland scan are summarized in Table 1.

TABLE I

SUB MANDIBULAR SALIVARY GLAND SCAN: A PROGNOSTIC INDICATOR OF BELL'S PALSY

RESULTS OF 40 CONSECUTIVE CASES

	No. of Patients	Complete Recovery	Partial Recovery	Complete Paralysis
Symetrical Normal Scan	21	19	2	0
Diminished on the Involved Side	19	7	10	2
Diminished on the Normal Side	0	0	0	0

Several topognostic tests are routinely performed in cases of peripheral facial paralysis of unknown origin. May et al. (1976) states that if these patients are followed right from the onset of the paralysis, loss of taste and salivary flow are observed first. The salivary flow test has not attained much popularity, though. Various reasons can be listed:

1) It usually cannot be done in children;
2) The insertion of polethylene tubing into Wharton's duct openings may be difficult or unpleasant to the patient;
3) Once the result is in error, repetition of the test may be hampered by edema of the ducts;
4) Pressure or kinking of the tubing may lead to an unreliable count of the drops.

As one can see from the results the validity of the test shown here is no better than other time honoured tests. With our test we did not get any break-through in the prognostic tests of facial palsy. But, if you believe in the salivary collecting test, then we suggest that you try our method.

© 1985 Elsevier Science Publishers B.V. (Biomedical Division)
New dimensions in otorhinolaryngology – head and neck surgery, vol. 2.
E. Myers, editor

THE FACIAL MOTOR NUCLEUS SOMATOTOPY IS RESTORED AFTER FACIAL NERVE REGENERATION IN NEONATAL BUT NOT ADULT RATS

LARS THOMANDER* and HÅKAN ALDSKOGIUS**

*Dept. of Otolaryngology, Uppsala University, S-751 85 Uppsala (Sweden) and
**Dept. of Anatomy, Karolinska Institutet, S-104 01 Stockholm (Sweden)

INTRODUCTION

Despite the use of modern microsurgical techniques for the treatment of peripheral nerve injuries, functional recovery after complete nerve transection in adult mammals is usually poor. Functional recovery after corresponding nerve injuries in very young mammals is usually excellent (for review see Selzer[1]).

In the present study, the horseradish peroxidase (HRP) technique was used to compare to what extent the somatotopical organization is restored after motor nerve injury in the adult and neonatal period.

MATERIAL AND METHODS

The facial nerve was transected in adult (n=10) and newborn (n=19) rats. The nerve stumps were approximated with epineural sutures in the adults. In the newborn rats, the stumps were prevented from separating by retaining a piece of the epineurium. Several months later, one of two separate facial nerve branches was transected bilaterally, and the proximal stump exposed to HRP. Furthermore, in five animals, axotomized when newborn, wheat germ agglutinin-HRP conjugate was injected into the whisker follicle muscles of row A bilaterally.

One to two days later the animals were perfused, and serial brain stem sections processed for the visualization of HRP-labeled neurons (cf. Thomander[2]).

RESULTS

In the adult rats, labeled nerve cell bodies were found in a well defined compact group in the facial motor nucleus (FMN) on the control side. On the operated side, however, the labeled cells were widely scattered throughout the FMN. An average of about 45% of the labeled neurons on the regenerated side were located outside the normal pool. The total number of labeled neurons did not differ significantly between the two sides, (cf. Thomander[2]).

In the newborn, labeled neurons were found in well defined groups on both control (Fig. 1 A, C) and operated sides (Fig. 1 B, D). The number of labeled neurons was significantly lower on the regenerated side, Table I.

CONCLUSION

The results show that normal FMN somatotopy is not restored in adult rats, but is completely restored in rats operated on when newborn. Furthermore, there is no significant loss of motor neurons in the adults. In the newborn, however, a significantly smaller number is observed on the regenerated side.

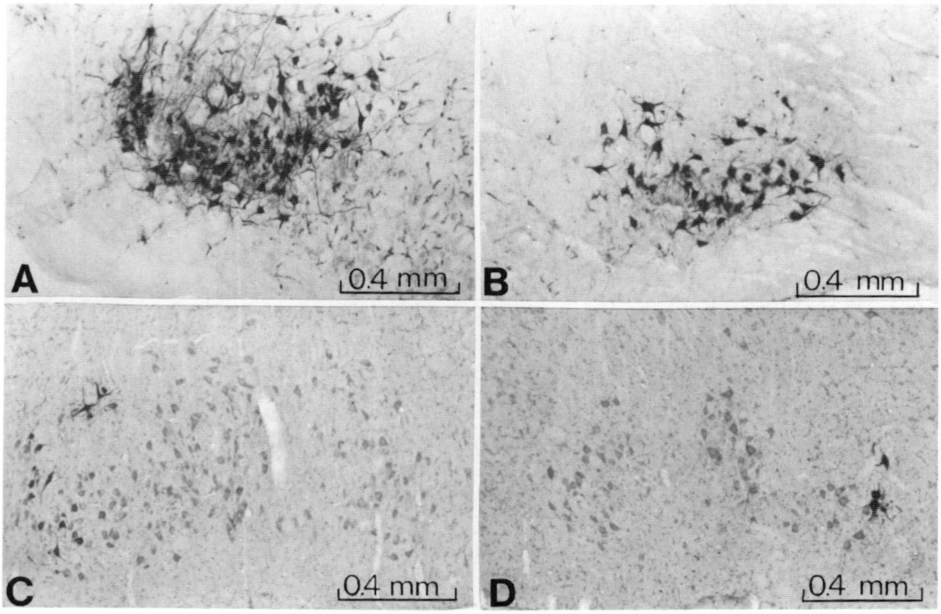

Fig. 1. HRP-labeled neurons in FMN after application to superior buccal ramus, A and B after injection to whisker row A, C and D. Control sides left and axotomized sides right. Medial is to the middle. Neutral red.

TABLE 1

Number of HRP labeled neurons in FMN (mean ± SD)

Nerve branch	Control side	Operated side	Number of Animals
r. buccalis superior	549 ± 66	140 ± 122	7
r. buccalis inferior	594 ± 56	82 ± 71	7

ACKNOWLEDGEMENTS

Supported by the Swedish Medical Research Council (project no. 07503).

REFERENCES

1. Selzer FE (1980) In: Sumner AS (ed) The physiology of peripheral nerve disease. W.B. Saunders Company, London, Toronto, Philadelphia, pp 358-431
2. Thomander L (1984) Acta Otolaryngol (Stockh) 97:619-626

New dimensions in otorhinolaryngology - head and neck surgery, vol. 2.
E. Myers, editor

RESPONSE PATTERN RECOGNITION IN FACIAL EVOKED ELECTROMYOGRAPHY (ELECTRONEUROGRAPHY)

GORDON B. HUGHES, M.D., RICHARD H. NODAR, PH.D., AND MOHAMED A. HAMID, PH.D.

Department of Otolaryngology and Communicative Disorders, The Cleveland Clinic Foundation, 9500 Euclid Avenue, Cleveland, OH 44106 USA

INTRODUCTION

Evoked facial electromyography (electroneurography) is an objective electrophysiologic measurement and recording of a muscle compound action potential, used to determine prognosis for recovery in patients with facial paralysis. When a typical response is identified using ideal stimulus intensity guidelines in normal subjects, test-retest variability is 6.4% (range 2.2-10.2%).[1] Either unimodal or bimodal responses may be observed. In normal subjects, latency-based time measurements are less variable than amplitude-based peak-to-peak measurements; linear peak-to-peak measurements are less variable than geometric curve-area responses.[2] However, in some subjects the response can be distored or unrecognizable due to improper test technique or inherent neuromuscular factors (which are not known at this time). The purpose of this prospective study of 23 normal, adult volunteers was to 1) determine the test technique which most readily yields identifiable responses and 2) to determine with this "ideal" technique whether responses in normal subjects are always easily recognized.

MATERIALS AND METHODS

In 23 normal, healthy subjects, test methodology developed in previous studies[3,4] was applied using ideal stimulus intensity guidelines,[1,2] varying only the polarity (not position) of the bipolar stimulus electrode. That is, the positive electrode (anode) either was placed behind the ear in the mandibulomastoid groove or in front of the ear in direct line with the recording electrode at the lateral nasal ala. Two trials at each polarity were repeated to insure response stability. The compound action potential (CAP) was identified independently by two examiners. When the examiners concurred, the response was considered "definite". When the examiners initially did not agree, the response was considered "probable". A comparison of response patterns was made between both electrode polarities.

RESULTS

When the positive electrode was placed behind the ear (with the cathode/ "stimulating" electrode in front), a negative (downward) stimulus artifact resulted (Figure 1). When the positive electrode was placed in front of the ear, a positive (upward) stimulus artifact resulted (Figure 2). The CAP was more easily identified when the stimulus artifact was negative. Twenty two responses were "definite"; one was "probable". Nineteen responses were unimodal; four were bimodal. The average latency (onset of response) was 3.9 msec (range 2.6-5.0); the average response duration was 1.6 msec (range 1.0-2.2). The average linear peak-to-peak CAP measurement was 480 microvolts (range 280-756).

CONCLUSIONS

The positive electrode should be placed behind the ear in the mandibulo-mastoid groove. Although latency measurements may be more variable in patients with disease, such measurements are helpful in identifying a probable response. Amplitude measurements are still more variable than latency (in normal subjects) but generally do not influence response pattern recognition. Provided proper techniques and ideal stimulus intensities are followed, the CAP is usually easily identified in normal subjects, but not necessarily in all subjects (for reasons that are not clear). These normal subject results must be extrapolated with care to patients with disease.

REFERENCES

1. Hughes GB, Nodar RH, Williams GW (1983): Analysis of test-retest variability in facial electroneurography. Otolaryngol Head-Neck Surg 91:290-293
2. Hughes GB, Nodar RH, Hamid MA, Sismanis A (1984): Response pattern variability in facial electroneurography. Presented at the Fifth International Symposium on the Facial Nerve, Bordeaux, France, September 5
3. Hughes GB, Josey AF, Glasscock ME (1981): Clinical electroneurography: Statistical analysis of controlled measurements in 22 normal subjects. Laryngoscope 91:1834-1846
4. Hughes GB (1982): Electroneurography: Objective prognostic assessment of facial paralysis. Am J Otol 4:73-76

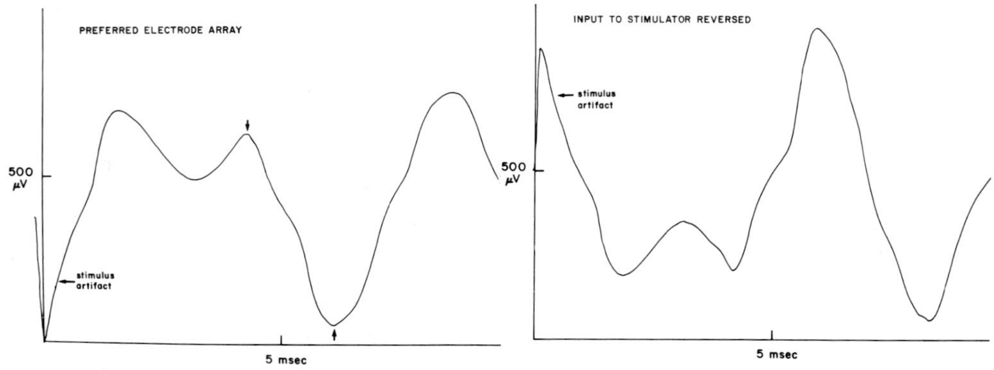

© 1985 Elsevier Science Publishers B.V. (Biomedical Division)
New dimensions in otorhinolaryngclogy - head and neck surgery, vol. 2.
E. Myers, editor

EXPERIENCES IN MOTION SICKNESS PREVENTION

GYÖRGY BODÓ
Department of Otolaryngology, Central Military Hospital, P.O. Box 1. Budapest /Hungary/

In order to prevent motion sickness, we performed two types of experiments. The first set of experiments was aimed to eliminate subjects with high sensitivity to motion sickness.

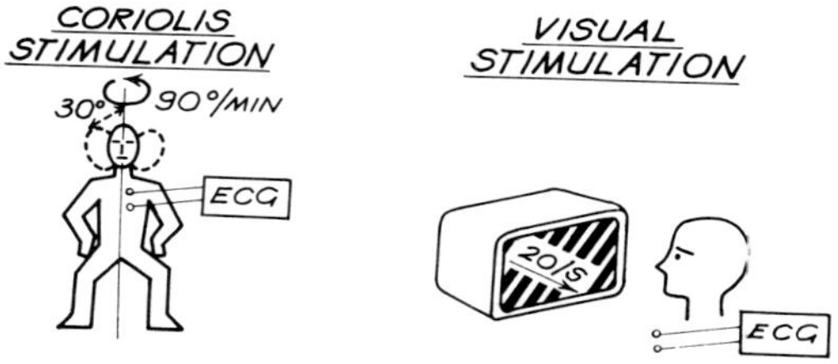

Fig.1. Mass screening selection method.

For screening subjects with a high sensitivity to motion sickness, we applied a method developed in co-operation with LN. Kornilova. We wanted to develop a tolerable method for mass screening and that is why the stimulation was discontinued not by the onset of nausea, but by a change of ± 10/min of the pulse rate. The time from the beginning of the stimulation to the given change in pulse rate was taken the vegetative resistance in minutes.

We have stated that out of 100 healthy young males 53 were sensitive and 10 were resistant to Coriolis stimulation and 17 were sensitive and 37 were resistant to visual stimulation. To both kinds of stimulation 10 subjects were sensitive and 8 were resistant /Thuy/.

The experiments have proved that our method is suitable for mass screening: it is easy to perform, not expensive and relatively quick. About 8% of young males show no changes in pulse rate after 10 minutes, further investigations may be continued in these selected 8% to screen people for special task.

The second set of experiments aimed the pharmacological prevention. In our earlier studies we have concluded that Vinpocetinea vinca minor alcaloid derivate- remarkably decreases the experimental kinetosis. The compound is issued by Chemical Works of Gedeon Richter Ltd. Budapest under the name of Cavinton.

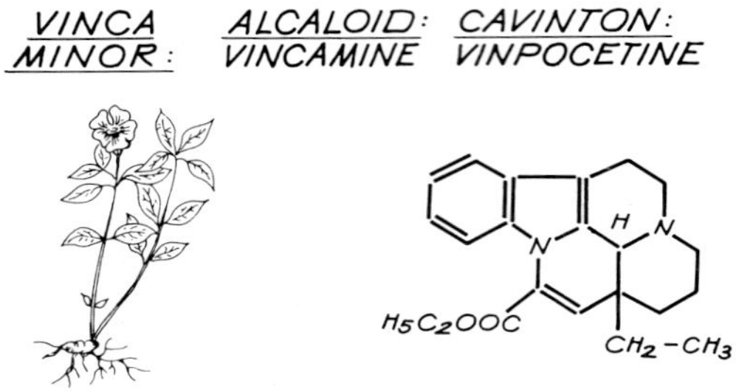

Fig. 2. The chemistry of Cavinton.

It was found that experimental kinetosis induced by Coriolis stimulation in 30 healthy young males was decreased by Cavinton with a moderate improvement of the psychic perfomance. Similar results were obtained by investigators of the Institute of Biomedical Problems in Moscow.

In order to increase this favourable effect, we have administered Cavinton in combination with Scopolamine and Dimenhydrinate, as well as with methyldopa /Dopegyt/ and selegilinum hydrochloricum /Jumex/. But these combinations did not improve the efficacy of Cavinton.

Summing up it can be concluded that Cavinton actually decreases experimental motion sickness. The onset time of the experimental kinetosis could not be really influenced by combination with the above mentioned drugs.

REFERENCES

Bodó G, Hartmann J /1979/ Ther hung 27:2-4

Bodó G, Kotovskaya AR, Galle RR, Gavrilova LN, Gusakova GA, Smirnov VA /1982/ Kosm Biol Aviakosm Med 16: 49-51

Dichgans J, Brandt Th /1973/ Acta Otolaryngol 76: 339-348

Kornilova LN, Shakieva VA, Yakovleva IYA /1982/ Kosm Biol Aviakosm Med 16: 67-70

Matsnev EI, Bodó G, /1984/ Aviat Space Environ Med 55: 281-286

Thuy Tran Le : /1984/ Cand. Thesis, Budapest

New dimensions in otorhinolaryngology - head and neck surgery, vol. 2.
E. Myers, editor

CLINICAL EVALUATION OF THE INFERIOR VESTIBULAR NERVE FUNCTION

HELOISA HELENA CAOVILLA; MAURICIO MALAVASI GANANÇA; PEDRO LUIZ MANGABEIRA ALBERNAZ
Dept. of Otorhinolaryngology, Escola Paulista de Medicina,
Rua Botucatū 834 - 04023 São Paulo - Brazil

INTRODUCTION

Electronystagmography (ENG) has been considered, so far, the best way to detect and analyse eye motion. But the method has limitations, even with the use of two channels, as rotatory and oblique nystagmus can not be recorded.

Pansini and Padovan[1] proposed a three-channel recording technique which they have named vectornystagmography (VENG). On performing a large number of vestibular examinations with VENG in the last nine years, Mangabeira Albernaz et alii[2] could compare its results to those of conventional ENG. They have concluded that with VENG the number of errors in diagnosis was significantly smaller than with one or two-channel ENG tracing.

The main advantage of VENG is the possibility of recording oblique or rotatory nystagmus in addition to horizontal eye movements.Vertical nystagmus can be recorded with a second ENG channel, but oblique or rotatory movements demand VENG. Furthermore, through VENG it is possible to determin from the vectogram the real slow phase eye speed concerning every direction of the nystagmus. Consequently, errors in measuring the intensity of the responses can be avoided.

Our main interest in VENG has been the possibility of studying the oblique nystagmus elicited by vertical canals stimulation . The diagnosis of superior or posterior canals unilateral lesions can only be determined because very often no vestibular compensation occurs for the vertical canals function, even in cases with perfect compensation in the lateral canals, according to Oramas[3] and Mangabeira Albernaz and Ganança[4].

The stimulation of each posterior semicircular canal alone also implies in recording responses involving the inferior vestibular nerve and its central connections. Ganança and Mangabeira Albernaz [5] pointed out that the resulting oblique nystagmus become the first clinical recording of the inferior vestibular nerve, including its CNS pathways.

MATERIAL AND METHODS

The study was performed on 46 patients who presented dizziness of peripheral vestibular origin, confirmed by a thorough otorhinolaryngological and neurological evaluation. A complete otoneurological investigation was carried out including an ear, nose and throat examination, audiological evaluation and vectornystagmographic recordings of spontaneous, gaze and positional nystagmus, eye-tracking and optokinetic tests, torsion swing stimulation and caloric test.

The eye movements were recorded through a Berger Vectornystagmograph VN-106/3 recorder. A detailed description of the method has been given by Mangabeira Albernaz and Ganança[4].

The stimulation of each of the vertical canals has been performed by means of the torsion swing test, placing the patient's head tilted 60° backwards and 45° to either side.

The torsion swing results were assessed by using both the frequency and the slow phase eye speed of perrotatory nystagmus, which was performed in accordance with the criteria established by Mangabeira Albernaz et alii[2].

RESULTS

In this study, we could see that vestibular compsensation in the vertical canals was non-existing or markdely reduced in 43.5 % of 46 cases suffering from labyrinthine patients, even when the lateral canals showed perfect compensation.

Altered responses limited to the posterior canal or inferior vestibular nerve have been seen in 17 (36.9 %) of the cases.

These representative findings suggested that the specific exploration of the vertical canals and inferior vestibular nerve may become an important routine clinical vestibular test in the near future.

In our experience, VENG proved to be a very sensitive test, as to the detection of semicircular canals alterations. In this way, we could verify that the slow phase eye speed seemed to be a much more sensitive parameter than the nystagmus frequency.

The high incidence of vertical canals alterations and also the possibility of inferior vestibular nerve lesions identification leads us to include their sistematic study on the otoneurological evaluation in a mandatory way.

REFERENCES

1. Pansini M, Padovan I (1969) - Three derivations in electronystagmography. Acta oto-laryng (Stockh) 67:303-309
2. Mangabeira Albernaz PL, Ganança MM, Caovilla HH, Ito Y.I., Castro HD (1984) - An Atlas of Vector-nystagmography. Aché, São Paulo.
3. Oramas RH (1972) - Electronistagmografia de los canales verticales. Otolaringológica 10:279-292.
4. Mangabeira Albernaz PL, Ganança MM (1976) - Vertigem. Moderna, São Paulo.
5. Ganança MM, Mangabeira Albernaz PL (1976) - Guia Prático de Labirintologia. Aché, São Paulo.

New dimensions in otorhinolaryngology - head and neck surgery, vol. 2.
E. Myers, editor

CAN THE CHAIR TEST DETERMINE THE SIDE OF VESTIBULAR DYSFUNCTION?

MOHAMED A. HAMID, PH.D., DIC, GORDON B. HUGHES, M.D. AND MARK O'KEEFE, B.A.

Department of Otolaryngology and Communicative Disorders, The Cleveland Clinic Foundation, Cleveland, Ohio, USA

PURPOSE

This preliminary, retrospective review of 90 patients with vestibular dysfunction was designed to test the hypothesis that chair asymmetry could predict the side of vestibular dysfunction.

MATERIALS AND METHODS

Criteria for selecting patients were: 1) clinical evidence of active vestibular dysfunction, 2) significant unilateral caloric canal paresis and 3) abnormal asymmetry on Sinusoidal Harmonic Acceleration[SHA].

All patients underwent complete neuro-otologic examination and vestibular testing. Caloric test was performed using $\pm 7^{o}C$ irrigations. Short format Sinusoidal Harmonic Acceleration[SHA]was performed using frequency range .01-.16 Hz[1]. Caloric canal paresis [%CP] was regarded as abnormal if greater than 30%. SHA responses were digitally analyzed to compute phase[latency], asymmetry and gain as a function of frequency. Values outside tolerance limits [mean $\pm$ 2.02SD] were considered abnormal[2]. Patients were divided into two categories: category (A) included patients with abnormal chair latency [Fig. 1A] and category (B) included patients with normal chair latency [Fig. 1B]. Latency was regarded abnormal if the slope of the regression line between phase and frequency was greater than 2.02 SD.

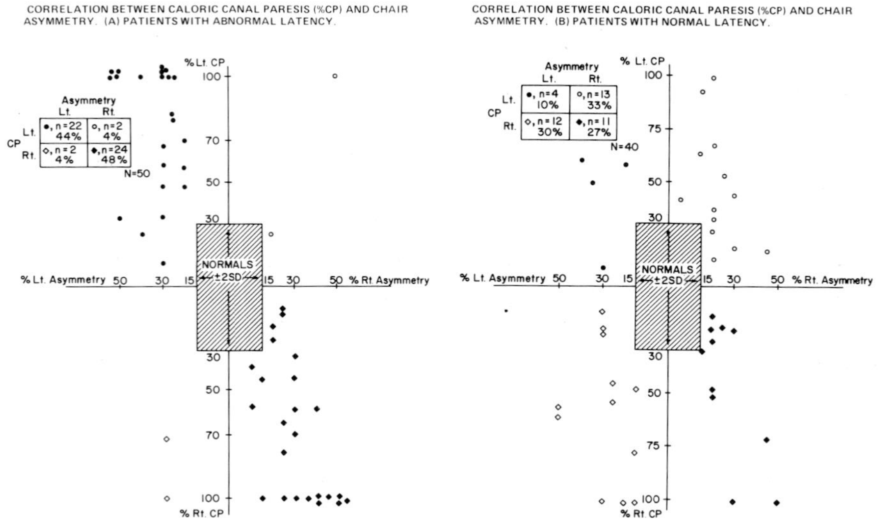

Figure 1: Scatter diagrams of patient results.

RESULTS AND DISCUSSION

Figure 1 shows scatter diagrams of percentage canal paresis [ordinate] and percentage asymmetry [abscissa] for each patient's category. Figiure 1A [patients with abnormal latency] shows that 92% of patients had chair asymmetry and canal paresis on the same side [i.e. Rt. asymmetry and Rt. CP, and vice versa]. Figure 1B [patients with normal latency] shows that only 37% had asymmetry towards the decreased caloric side. Statistical analysis confirmed high association between chair asymmetry and side of canal paresis when latency was abnormal [P=.Ø5].

CONCLUSION

Results of this study indicate that chair asymmetry can predict the side of vestibular lesion in 92% of patients when latency is abnormal. In patients with normal latency, chair asymmetry merely reflects vestibular shift and does not correlate with the side of lesion.

BIBLIOGRAPHY

1) Hamid, M.A: [1983] Reducing the Simple Harmonic Acceleration Test Time. Adv. Oto-rhino-laryng., 3Ø:165-17Ø [Karger-Basel].

2) Remington, R.D. and Schork, M.A: [1985] Statistics with Applications to the Biological and Health Sciences. Prentice-Hall, New Jersey.

© 1985 Elsevier Science Publishers B.V. (Biomedical Division)
New dimensions in otorhinolaryngology – head and neck surgery, vol. 2.
E. Myers, editor

Investigations into the precision of Barany's theory of caloric labyrinthine reaction

by Heinz Joachim Scholtz and Uwe Sievert

In spite of many new techniques the caloric test is a method of utmost importance for investigating the lateral semicircular canal. The elucidation of the underlying physical priniples goes back to Barany and is supported by many physiological and clinical investigations. But there are peculiarities of this reaction which cannot be explained by the concept of Barany:

1. The appearance of a caloric nystagmus at a pessimum position which we have recently proved again by extensive investigations in 114 healthy test persons or in gravity-free conditions found during the investigations on board the space lab 1.
2. The stronger reaction of a caloric stimulation at a normal position with face up than in the reverse body position with face down.

In performing the caloric test at different positions of the head according to Jongkees, the so-called superior area in which a cold stimulation produces a nystagmus to the opposite side covers about 200°. The so-called inferior area in which a cold irrigation produces a nystagmus to the stimulated side covers more than 140°. There are two indifferent areas between them with differing reversing points of the nystagmus for cold and warm stimulation respectively.

In our investigations with 10 healthy persons aged between 19 and 39 years we tried to answer the question how the caloric reaction proceeds in detail at the two optimum positions of the superior or inferior area. The tests were carried out on 2 days. On the first day irrigation was made with water at 44°C, on the second day with water at 30°C. Alternatingly, the calorisation began in the first test person with face up in the following sequence: left ear, right ear, change of position, left ear, right ear. The opposite position with face down was chosen for the next test person. The nystagmus registered by electro-oculography was analysed according to total duration, number of beats, amplitude and total frequency as well as according to maximal slow phase velocity.

Results: All test persons noticed the feeling of mobility to be essentially less in the inferior area. For all nystagmus parameters determined the ratio of stimulating response in the inferior area to that in the superior area was calculated from each stimulated ear (tab. 1).

		total dur.	total beats	total ampl.	total frequ.	max. spv
44°C	$\bar{x}$	0,74	0,57	0,44	0,76	0,56
(n=19)	s	0,19	0,23	0,22	0,22	0,21
30°C	$\bar{x}$	0,79	0,63	0,48	0,78	0,68
(n=20)	s	0,24	0,35	0,31	0,25	0,19

Tab. 1.Ratio of response in the inferior area to that in the superior one

With equal responses in both areas the ratio number would be equal to 1. In our tests, however, a lesser response generally exists in the inferior area. In this respect, the differences are statistically significant for the parameters maximal slow phase velocity and total frequency. But there is no significant difference between the findings obtained for warm irrigation and those for cold irrigation.

Discussion: The weaker nystagmus parameters in the inferior area can be explained as follows: Stimulating the hair cells in the lateral semicircular canal is not only elicited by an endolymph flow on the basis of a calorically induced gradient of density in the gravitational field of the earth. Rather a change in the volume of perilymph and endolymph caused by caloric conditions is first expected to appear at calorisation in a limited area below the ampulla. The differing responses in both areas can be explained by the equal or opposite effect of these components. In the superior area both components will, in each case, lead to an intensification of stimulation and vice versa. We are fully aware of the fact that further experiments are required for ensuring our hypothesis.

Address: Prof.Dr. H.J. Scholtz, ENT-Clinic, Wilhelm-Pieck-University of Rostock, GDR 25 Rostock, Doberaner-Str. 137

New dimensions in otorhinolaryngology - head and neck surgery, vol. 2.
E. Myers, editor

NON-VESTIBULAR CONTAMINATION OF ROTATORY TESTING FOR VESTIBULAR DIAGNOSIS

DAG HYDÉN, BIRGITTA LARSBY AND LARS ÖDKVIST
Department of Otolaryngology, University Hospital, S-581 85 Linköping (Sweden)

INTRODUCTION

In order to adequately measure compensatory eye movements of vestibular origin, it is necessary to minimize the influence from non-vestibular mechanisms. This study was carried out to assess the characteristics of different non-vestibular contamination and find the most adequate way of vestibulo-ocular reflex testing.

MATERIAL AND METHODS

Fifteen normal subjects, 7 patients with bilateral vestibular loss and 34 patients with unilateral vestibular loss were investigated in a broad frequency-band rotatory test. Eye movements were recorded by EOG. Head movements were recorded by an angular rate sensor attached to a biteboard. Gain(slow phase eye velocity/head velocity) was calculated. Measurements were performed in light and darkness during 40 sec trials with different fixation tasks.

RESULTS

Results show that non-vestibular mechanisms(predictive motor programs and visual tracking reflexes) control the eye movement response at lower oscillatory frequencies provided a sinusoidal stimulation is used in light. With increasing frequencies the non-vestibular influence is successively reduced and at 2.5 - 3 Hz valuable vestibular information can be sampled(fig. 1). If a randomized test pattern is used the non-vestibular influence from prediction is eliminated allowing more adequate vestibular results at lower frequencies. In darkness subjects can modulate their compensatory eye movements in a purposeful way up to 2 Hz during sinusoidal stimulation. This predictive capability is not at hand if random oscillation is used. These results are in accordance with our earlier findings in normal subjects and patients(1-4).

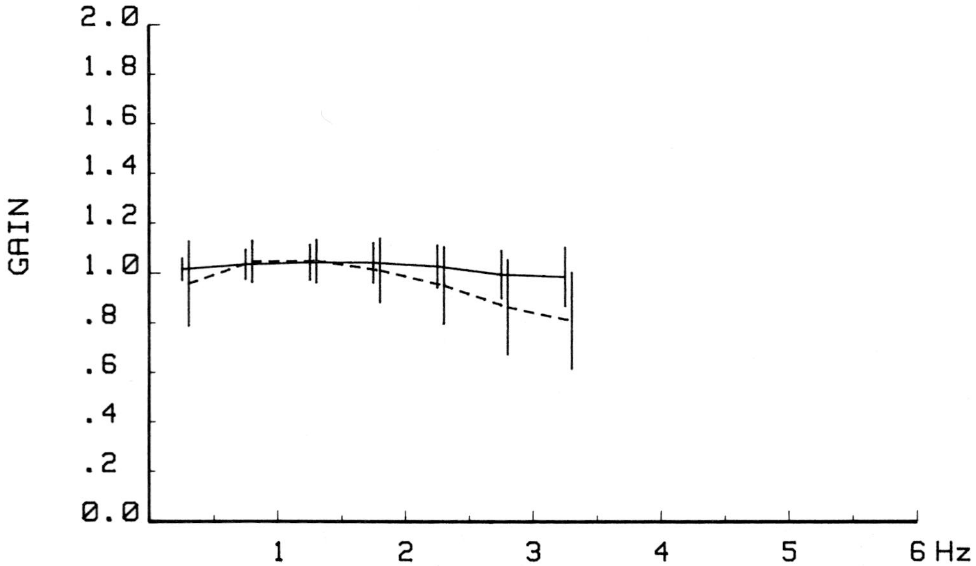

Fig. 1. Mean gain(eye velocity/head velocity) ± 1 SD as a function of frequency during fixation of a stationary target in 34 patients with a unilateral acoustic neuroma(-----). The mean values ± 1 SD in 15 normal subjects are also indicated(——).

CONCLUSION

Adequate vestibulo-ocular testing can only be done in a rotatory test if a high-frequency sinusoidal stimulation(2.5-3 Hz) is used or if a random test pattern is used. This holds true for measurements both in light and darkness.

REFERENCES

1. Hydén D, Istl Y, Schwarz D (1982) Human visuo-vestibular interaction as a basis for quantitative clinical diagnostics. Acta Otolaryngol 94:487-493
2. Hydén D, Larsby B, Schwarz D, Ödkvist LM (1983) Quantification of slow compensatory eye movements in patients with bilateral vestibular loss. Acta Otolaryngol 96:199-206
3. Istl YE, Hydén D, Schwarz DWF (1983) Quantification of localization of vestibular loss in unilaterally labyrinthectomized patients using a precise rotatory test. Acta Otolaryngol 96:437-445
4. Larsby B, Hydén D, Ödkvist LM (1984) Gain and phase characteristics of compensatory eye movements in light and darkness. A study with a broad frequency-band rotatory test. Acta Otolaryngol 97:223-232

New dimensions in otorhinolaryngology - head and neck surgery, vol. 2.
E. Myers, editor

THE FAST PHASE EYE-SPEED OF POST CALORIC NYSTAGMUS IN NORMALS: A VECTORNYSTAGMOGRAPHIC STUDY

YASUKO IMASATO ITO, MAURICIO MALAVASI GANANÇA, PEDRO LUIZ MANGABEIRA ALBERNAZ.
Dept. of Otorhinolaringology, Escola Paulista de Medicina, Rua Botucatu, 740 - 3º andar, 04023, São Paulo, Brazil

INTRODUCTION

The advantages of using vectornystagmography (VNG) over the use of electronystagmography (ENG) has been pointed out [1].

Through VNG it is possible to record nystagmus in any direction (horizontal, vertical, obliquous and horizonto-rotatory), and it also enables us to determine, via the vectorgram, the real angular velocity of the slow and fast phases, even when the nystagmus is not quite horizontal.

Our studies showed us the value of the real slow phase eye-speed as one of the major parameters in the evaluation of the vestibular system. However, we shouldn't neglect the fast phase eye-speed diagnostic value in several vestibular problems.

Vectornystagmographic studies of the fast phase have previously been done with the spontaneous [2], optokinetic [3] and perrotatory nystagmus [4]. In this study the fast phase eye-speed was evaluated in order to establish the normal critical limits concerning the post caloric maximum values.

MATERIAL AND METHODS

A group of 38 apparently normal cases, whose ages varied between 20 and 40 years, was submitted to vectornystagmography. The fast phase eye-speed was accurately measured from the VNG three chanels [1].

RESULTS

The findings obtained from the 38 patients were the following:

1) A wide variability of the absolute values, in degrees per second, ranging from 13.0 to 619.0^{o}/s, the mean value was 88.8^{o}/s, with a standard deviation of 65.1^{o}/s and superior and inferior conficence limits (95%) of 216.4^{o}/s and zero, respectively;
2) Concerning the nystagmus directional preponderance, the extreme value was 56.0%, with the mean value of 2.0%, the standard deviation of 20.0% and the superior confidence limit (95%) of 41.2%;
3) In relation to the labyrinthine preponderance, the extreme value was 86.0%, with the mean value of 3.0%, the standard deviation of 23.0% and the superior confidence limit (95%) of 48.1%.

CONCLUSIONS

1) The normal absolute values of the real maximum fast phase eye-speed of post caloric nystagmus ranged from zero to 216.4°/s.
2) The normal relative values of both nystagmus directional and labyrinthine preponderance were 41.2% and 48.1%, respectively.
3) The determination of these normal limits may identify the abnormal quantitative deviations on vestibular syndromes, when the critical values are overexceeded.

REFERENCES

1) Mangabeira Albernaz PL, Ganança MM, Caovilla HH, Ito YI, Castro HD (1984) Atlas de Vecto-electronistagmografia, Achê, São Paulo.
2) Bertollucci PHF, Ganança MM, Lima JGC, Caovilla HH, Mangabeira Albernaz PL (1983) Da direção e da velocidade angular real da componente rápida do nistagmo espontâneo, Acta AWHO 2: 22-34.
3) Mainardi MT, Caovilla HH, Ganança MM, Mangabeira Albernaz PL (1985) Da componente rápida do nistagmo optocinético vertical à vecto-electronistagmografia. Acta AWHO 4: 34-43.
4) Munhoz MSL, Caovilla HH, Ganança MM, Mangabeira Albernaz PL (1984) Da velocidade angular real máxima da componente rápida do nistagmo per-rotatório em indivíduos normais. Acta AWHO 3: 27-36.

New dimensions in otorhinolaryngology - head and neck surgery, vol. 2.
E. Myers, editor

EFFECTS OF VISUAL TARGET ON BODY SWAY

MASATO KIKUKAWA, YOSHIKAZU MIYASHITA and KIICHIRO TAGUCHI
Dept. of Otolaryngology, Shinshu University School of Medicine, Matsumoto, Japan

INTRODUCTION

The body equilibrium can be influenced by vision, especially the modality and mobility of the visual target which we have studied for several years (Taguchi and Yoda, 1976; Kikukawa and Taguchi, 1983). Visual steadiness depends on the size of visual target and the distance between eyes and target. In this study we investigated the effects of the distance between eyes and target on the movements of the body's center of gravity (abbreviated to CG) in normal adults.

MATERIALS AND METHODS

Ten healthy adults, aged 21 to 30, were asked to participate in this study.

The straingauge type stabilometer, a data recorder and a microcomputer were applied to record and analyze the CG movement. The locus length was calculated during 1 minute of standing looking at the target of white cross which was placed at 0.5, 2.5 and 5.0 meter in front of the subject. To remove the effects caused by fatigue, subjects took a rest for 5 minutes between each test run. At the end of the test eyes closing condition was applied.

RESULTS

Fig.1 shows the length of the movement of CG while looking at the target which has different distance between eyes and target in the light room. Though there were indivisual differences in the length of the movement of CG, the changes showed almost the same tendencies. Namely, the length of the movement of CG increased with increase of the distance between eyes and target. T-test showed significant differences between 0.5 m group and 2.5 m group (P 0.05), and between 2.5 m group and 5.0 m group (P 0.05). However, no significant differences were observed between 5.0 m group and the eyes closed group.

Fig.2 shows the area of the movement of CG while looking at the target which has different distance between eyes and target in the light room. As seen in the length of the movement of CG, the area of the movement of CG also increased with increase of distance between eyes and target. T-test showed significant differences between 0.5 m group and 2.5 m group (P 0.01), and between 2.5 m group and 5.0 m group (P 0.05). No significant difference was observed between 5.0 m group and the eyes closed one.

To remove the influence of nearby peripheral visual field such as ceiling and walls a small lamp was used as a target in the dark room. The length and the area of the movement of CG while looking at the small lamp target were calculated. No significant differences were observed among three different groups because of too large individual differences. However, significant differences were obtained between length and area with eyes closed and those with eyes open in the dark room.

DISCUSSION

From this experiment, we have observed the relationship between body sway and the distance between eyes and target, and the results suggest that in the body sway experiment it is necessary to determine the distance between eyes and target. In the dark room, psychological effect for subject, dark adaptation time of retina and problem of individual physical differences seem to complicate the results.

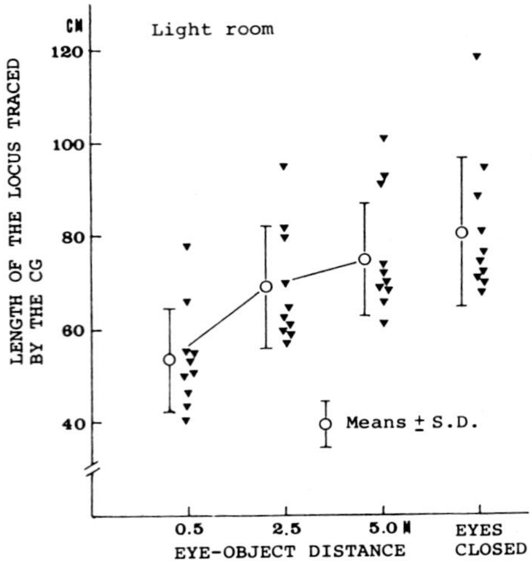

Fig. 1. Length of the locus traced by the CG.

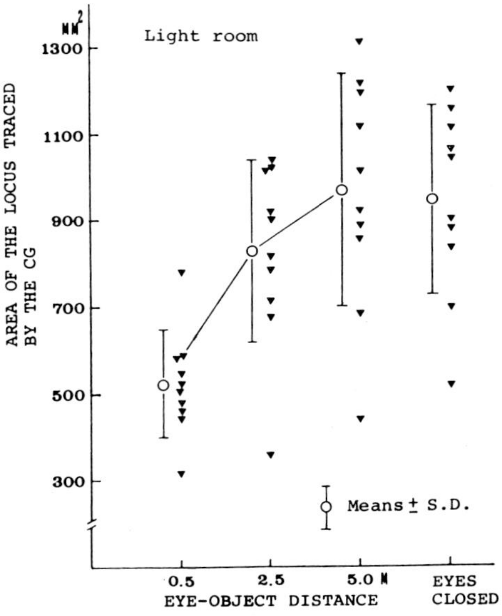

Fig. 2. Area of the locus traced by the CG.

REFERENCES

1. Taguchi K. & Yoda M.(1976). Effects of optokinetic stimulation on the center of gravity. Proceed. Fifth Extraord. Meet. Barany Soci. (Kyoto),pp 347-351
2. Kikukawa M. & Taguchi K.(1983). The movements of the head and the body's center of gravity while eye tracking. Agressologie 24:75-76

© 1985 Elsevier Science Publishers B.V. (Biomedical Division)
New dimensions in otorhinolaryngology - head and neck surgery, vol. 2.
E. Myers, editor

QUANTITATIVE MEASUREMENT OF VISUAL VESTIBULO-OCULAR INTERACTION USING SINUSOIDAL ROTATION IN PATIENTS WITH VERTIGO

HIDETO KOBAYASHI, KANEMASA MIZUKOSHI, YUKIO WATANABE, and NAOKI OHASHI

Department of Otolaryngology, Toyama Medical and Pharmaceutical University, 2630 Sugitani, Toyama City 930-01 JAPAN

INTRODUCTION

In order to investigate interaction of the visual and vestibular systems in patients with vertigo, we measured the vestibulo-ocular reflex (VOR) gain and the visual vestibulo-ocular reflex (VVOR) gain in patients with peripheral vestibular disorders and central nervous system disorders.

METHODS

Test Subjects

Thirteen normal subjects, one hundred and thirty three peripheral vestibular disorders, and eighty four central nervous system disorders were measured. Of 133 peripheral vestibular disorders, 49 had definite Meniere's disease, 46 had sudden deafness, and 38 had benign paroxysmal positional vertigo (BPPV). The 84 patients with central nervous system disorders were divided into three categories as follows: 23 cases of cerebellar lesions, 33 cases of brain stem lesions, and 28 cases of combined cerebellar and brain stem lesions.

Test Procedures

The test subjects were rotated sinusoidally in the center of the optokinetic drum. The chair was rotated for a period of 10 seconds (i,e, 0.1 Hz) with an amplitude of 120° (peak velocity: $75.4^{\circ}/s$). The interval between stripes on the OK drum was thirty degrees. During this test battery, the VOR and VVOR gains in the maximum slow phase velocities were measured first with eyes closed (VOR test) and then with eyes open in the illuminated OK drum (VVOR test).

Analysis Technique

Eye movements were recorded by means of ENG and the data were analyzed by a PDP 11/34 computer system.

RESULTS AND COMMENTS

Normal Limits of the VOR and VVOR Tests

Normal limits of the VOR and VVOR tests were calculated for the nystagmus responses in the 13 normal subjects. From these normal values of the VOR and VVOR gains and those ratios, the normal limits of DP% were also calculated for clinical use, as we have already reported.

Patients with Peripheral Vestibular Disorders

In comparing the VOR and VVOR gains in the patients with the three different diseases, we observed a VOR-DP with normal VVOR gain more frequently in patients with Meniere's disease (24 cases out of 49) and sudden deafness (16 cases out of 46) than in those with BPPV. In patients with sudden deafness, VOR-DP with normal VVOR gain was more frequently observed in those with vertigo than in those without vertigo. However, VVOR responses in peripheral patients were usually normal, in spite of the frequent presence of spontaneous nystagmus. As reported by Baloh et al., visual and vestibular reflexes interact in such a way that the visual optokinetic response almost completely dominates the nystagmic response during the VVOR tests. In each category of abnormal VOR/VVOR gains patients, spontaneous nystagmus was revealed at a constant rate of about 20 - 25 %. But abnormal caloric responses (i.e. CP and DP) were frequently seen in the VOR-DP patients.

Central Nervous System Disorders

Of the 84 patients with central nervous system disorders, decreased VOR gain and VVOR gain were more frequently observed in patients with brain stem lesions (15 cases out of 33) and in combined cerebellar and brain stem lesion patients (10 cases out of 28). The rate of decrease paralleled the decline of the patients' state. However, in the cerebellar lesion patients, abnormal VOR with normal VVOR gains were more frequently seen (8 cases out of 23). In the patients of CNS disorders, decreased VOR and VVOR gains were associated with diminution of OKN, but not always associated with abnormal visual fixation of caloric nystagmus. So there might have been some difference between VVOR and visual fixation of caloric nystagmus.

CONCLUSION

In comparing our VOR and VVOR observations with other otoneurological findings, we have concluded that although the VOR and VVOR test battery cannot replace other otoneurological examinations, it can provide additional vital information for evaluation of vertigo. This is especially useful in the evaluation of vestibular compensation.

REFERENCES

1. Baloh RW et al.(1982) In: Honrubia V, Brazier MAB (eds) Nystagmus and Vertigo. Academic Press, New York, pp 231-240
2. Mizukoshi K et al.(1984) Acta Otolaryngol(Stock), Suppl. 406: 178-181
3. Watanabe Y et al.(1983) Adv Oto-Rhino-Laryngol 30, 187-192

© 1985 Elsevier Science Publishers B.V. (Biomedical Division)
New dimensions in otorhinolaryngology - head and neck surgery, vol. 2.
E. Myers, editor

CHANGE IN VESTIBULAR-OCULOMOTOR FUNCTION DUE TO TRANSDERMALLY APPLIED SCOPOLAMINE

BIRGITTA LARSBY, JAN THELL, DAG HYDÉN AND LARS ÖDKVIST
Department of Otolaryngology, University Hospital, S-581 85 Linköping(Sweden)

INTRODUCTION

Scopolamine has been known for a long time to be a very effective drug against motion sickness(1). Oral and intramuscular administration have however been associated with undesirable side effects such as drowsiness, blurred vision and dry mouth. With Scopoderm®, scopolamine is delivered at a constant rate through the intact skin. This delivering system eliminates high blood concentrations of scopolamine and thereby most side effects are reduced giving a therapeutically effective level during 72 hours. The aim of this study was to investigate the effect of Scopoderm® on normal vestibular-oculomotor function and then use the data to make suggestions about where and how scopolamine might excert its antimotion sickness action.

MATERIALS AND METHODS

Fifteen healthy volunteers with a mean age of 38 years participated in this study. The study was designed as a randomized double blind cross-over test. The transdermal therapeutic system is programmed to deliver 5 ug scopolamine base if placed behind the ear. One patch Scopoderm® or placebo was applied to the test subject at least 12 hours before testing. Vestibulo-oculomotor tests included saccade test, a calcric test, a broad frequency rotatory test in light and darkness, a test of the ability to visually suppress the vestibulo-ocular reflex(VOR) during rotatory stimulation and a broad frequency smooth pursuit test. The rotatory test, the visual suppression test and the smooth pursuit test were carried out both with predictable sinusoidal stimulation and with unpredictable pseudorandomized stimulation. Eye movements provoked by the different stimulations were recorded by EOG. For more information about the test procedures see Larsby et al.(2). For statistical analyses of differences between Scopoderm® and placebo a t-test for paired samples was used. Differences between samples were considered statistically significant when $p<0.05$.

RESULTS

In the saccade test, the caloric test and the rotatory test in light and darkness no effect due to Scopoderm® was observed. In the visual suppression test a statistically significant gain increase during scopolamine treatment was observed in the lower frequency area of stimulation. Gain is defined as eye velocity divided by head velocity. The gain increase was only seen when a predictable sinusoidal frequency stimulation was used. The ability to make smooth following movements was also significantly reduced due to scopolamine. The reduction in gain was seen during sinusoidal frequency sweep stimulation in the frequency range from 0.5 - 1 Hz.

DISCUSSION

Motion sickness is often explained as conflicting information between sensory receptors. During a conflicting visual-vestibular stimulation at the visual suppression test in this study a significant difference was noticed for scopolamine as compared to placebo. It is suggested for example by Robinson(3) that visual suppression shares common neuronal pathways with the smooth pursuit system. This is also underlined by the fact that most patients showing an impaired visual suppression also exhibit a deteriorated smooth pursuit. It is thus not surprising that scopolamine also effects the smooth pursuit function in this study.

The results from this study indicate that scopolamine does not so much block the afferent input as it modulates integrative functions at the level of the vestibular nuclei or/and the cerebellum.

REFERENCES

1. Brand JJ, Perry WLH (1966) Drugs used in motion sickness. Pharmacol Rev 18:895
2. Larsby B, Hydén D, Ödkvist LM (1984) Gain and Phase Characteristics of Compensatory Eye Movements in Light and Darkness. Acta Otolaryngol (Stockh) 97:223
3. Robinson DA (1982) In: Lennerstrand, Zee, Keller (eds) Functional Basis of Ocular Motolity Disorders. Pergamon Press, Oxford pp 5-13

© 1985 Elsevier Science Publishers B.V. (Biomedical Division)
New dimensions in otorhinolaryngology - head and neck surgery, vol. 2.
E. Myers, editor

OPTOKINETIC NYSTAGMUS IN PATIENTS WITH CEREBRAL LESIONS

M.YANAGIDA, T.TOKITA, K.AMANO, K.MIZUTA
Dept. of Otolaryngology, Gifu University School of Medicine, Gifu, Japan

This report presents the characteristics of optokinetic nystagmus (OKN) in patients with cerebral lesions as found by the relation between OKN and target movement.

MATERIALS AND METHOD

The study was conducted in 4 patients with occipital lobe lesion, 4 with frontal lobe lesion, 6 with parietal lobe lesion.

An Ohm-type rotating cylinder was rotated with an angular acceleration of $2°/s^2$ for 90 sec. OKN, induced by optokinetic stimulus, and signals of stripes moving in front of the subject were sampled at 100 Hz for 90 sec and fed to a PDP-12 computer through an A-D converter. Stripe movements were calculated from the stripe signals using Lagrange's square interpolation formula. The nystagmus waves and stripe movements were displayed in superimposition on a cathode ray tube.

RESULTS

OKN of patients with occipital lobe lesion: OKN abnormalities in 4 cases were as follows. Abnormalities were found in both rotational directions, especially more clearly in rotation towards the impaired side. When the cylinder was rotated towards the impaired side, saccadic and delayed pursuit movements, and defect of catching movement were observed. When the cylinder was rotated towards the normal side, unstable fixation was found and pursuit movement didn't match the stripe movement. Typical OKN is shown in Fig. 1. The oblique line stands for the stripe movement and the cogwheel wave represents the nystagmus. (Fig. 1)
OKN of patients with frontal lobe lesion: OKN abnormalities in 4 cases were as follows. Abnormalities were observed in both rotational directions, especially more clearly in the rotation towards the impaired side. Delayed pursuit movement, abnormal amplitude and high frequent nystagmus were observed. Typical OKN is shown in Fig. 2. (Fig. 2)
OKN of patients with parietal lobe lesion: OKN abnormalities in 6 cases were as follows. Abnormalities were observed clearly in the rotation towards the impaired side and less clearly in the rotation towards the normal side. When the cylinder was rotated towards the impaired side, irregular pursuit, square wave jerk, staircase pattern, and delayed initiation of catching movement were observed. When the cylinder was rotated towards the normal side, delayed pursuit movement and catching error were observed. Typical OKN is shown in Fig. 3. (Fig. 3)

Fig. 1. Occipital lobe lesion
Right-thalamic hemorrhage
35 y.o. Male

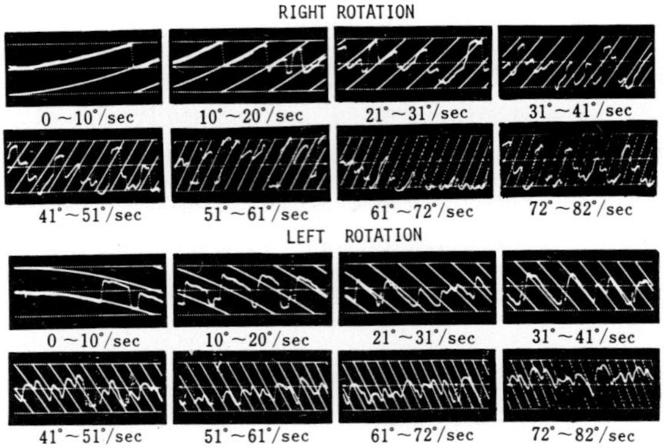

Fig. 2. Frontal lobe lesion
Right-head injery
44 y.o. Male

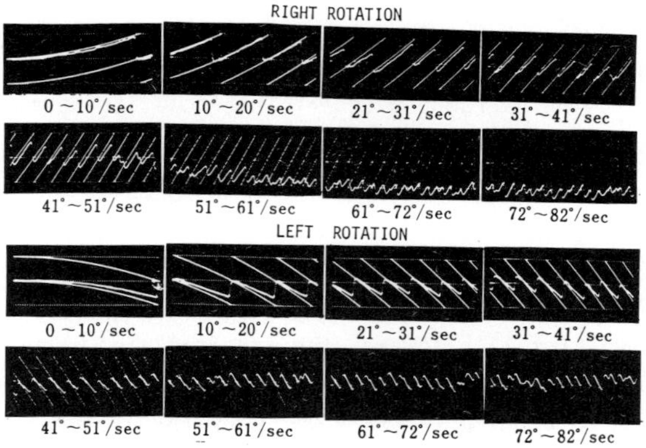

Fig. 3. Parietal lobe lesion
Left-meningioma
57 y.o. Female

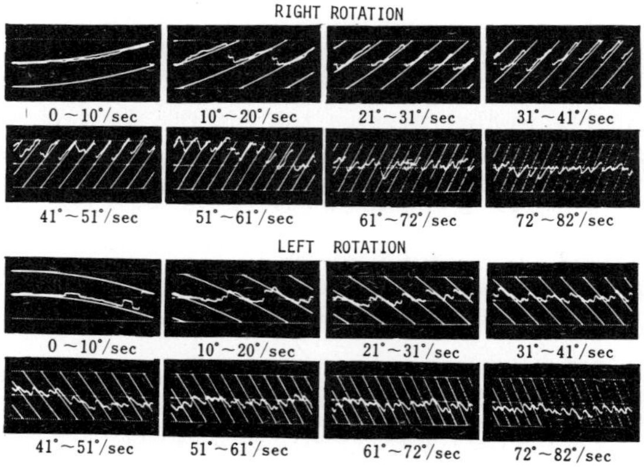

New dimensions in otorhinolaryngology - head and neck surgery, vol. 2.
E. Myers, editor

HAEMOSTATIC STUDY IN PATIENTS WITH VERTIGO AND THE EFFECT OF ANTI-PLATELET DRUG

YUTAKA NODA[1], MASAHARU URA[1], MARIKO NAKAMURA[2], TADAYOSHI KOSUGI[2]
Departments of Otorhinolaryngology[1] and Physiology[2], School of Medicine, University of the Ryukyus, Okinawa, Japan

INTRODUCTION

It has been reported that insufficiency of the cerebral circulation is important in the pathogenesis of some cases of vertigo[1]. On the other hand, it has been shown that platelet function plays an important role in relation to the cerebral circulation[2], while the coagulation-fibrinolysis system is of course significantly involved in the circulation. In the present study, therefore, haemostatic study was procedured in the patients with vertigo and the effect of an antiplatelet drug (Dilazep dihydrochloride) in improving the objective findings and subjective symptoms was assessed.

MATERIALS AND METHODS

Sixteen patients with vertigo (4 males and 12 females) were studied. Blood sample were taken with sodium citrate as anticoagulant (blood:sodium citrate=9:1 by volume) for estimating the levels of fibrinogen, antiplasmin activity and antithrombin activity and for measuring the platelet aggregating activity, and with aprotinin as antiplasminic agent for fibrin-degradation product (FDP) measurement. Furthermore, serum was employed for estimating the levels of α_2-macroglobulin, α_1-antitrypsin, plasminogen and CI-inactivator. Dilazep dihydrochloride was administered as an antiplatelet drug (300 mg/day) and the above parameters were determined before and after the administration. In order to assess the effect of the antiplatelet drug on the patients with vertigo, functional examinations of equilibrium (righting reflex, gait test, stepping test, pointing test, vertical writing test, spontaneous nystagmus, provoked nystagmus, caloric test and eye tracking test) were undertaken before and after 1-2 weeks of Dilazep administration. After the administration of Dilazep, the decreased frequency and intensity of vertigo, disappearance of nausea and tinnitus were examined as to the improvement of subjective symptoms. As for the objective finding, the improvement of some results of functional examination were judged, and especially disappearance of abnormal nystagmus such as spontaneous nystagmus and improvement of the stepping test was determined.

RESULTS

Coagulation-fibrinolysis system and platelet function. The difference in fibrinogen content, plasminogen content and FDP level between the healthy adults and patients with vertigo before and after the administration of Dilazep was thus not significant (data not shown). The difference in α_2-macroglobulin content, α_1-antitrypsin content and CI-inactivator content between the healthy adults and patients with vertigo before and after the administration of Dilazep was not significant (data not shown). Furthermore, as shown in Fig. 1 the difference in antiplasmin activity and antithrombin activity between the healthy adults and patients with vertigo before and after the administration was significant ($p < 0.001$) based on the t-test. In addition, the difference in antithrombin activity between the healthy adults and patients with vertigo before and after the administration was significant.

As shown in Fig. 2, the difference in ADP-and collagen-induced platelet aggregations between the healthy adults and patients with vertigo before and after the administration of Dilazep was significant ($p < 0.001$).

Effect of antiplatelet drug on the vertigo

Following the administration of Dilazep to the patients with vertigo, improvement of the subjective symptoms and objective findings was noted in 68.8 % of all patients with vertigo studied in this paper.

DISCUSSION

It has been reported by Bomholt (1980) that in patients with Meniere's disease, hypofibrinolysis occurred in the circulating blood based on the results of determinations of the fibrinolytic system[3]. Furthermore, Bomholt's findings indicated that the changeable clinical symptoms of Meniere's disease depend on recurrent thrombus formation and stasis in the circulating blood of inner ear. From the present study, it is suggested that in patients with vertigo a decreased antiplasmin activity, decreased antithrombin activity and enhanced platelet aggregation may tend to lead to thrombus formation on the occurrence of circulatory insufficiency in the inner ear. Our results also indicate that administration of an antiplatelet drug[4),5)] can be useful for improving the circulatory insufficiency in the inner ear.

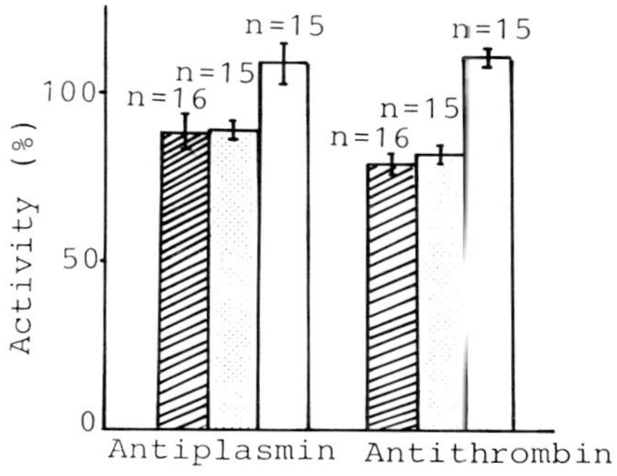

Fig. 1. Antiplasmin activity (left) and antithrombin activity (right) in patients with vertigo before and after administration of Dilazep. Shaded columns, before administration of Dilazep in vertigo; stippled columns, after administration of Dilazep in vertigo: open columns, healthy adults: all data show means ± standard error. The values of n indicate the numbers of patients with vertigo and healthy adults, respectively.

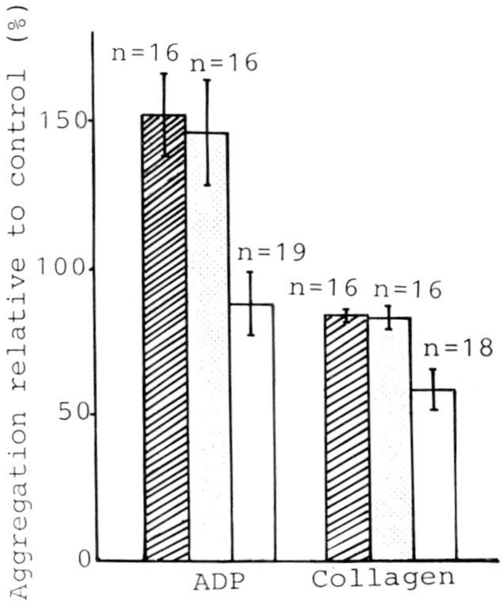

Fig. 2. ADP-induced platelet aggregation (left) and collagen -induced platelet aggregation (right) in patients with vertigo before and after administration of Dilazep. Shading and other details as in Fig. 1.

REFERENCES

1. Harada Y (1978) Statistical observations of vertigo. Otologia (Fukuoka) 24:778-780

2. Yasuda A, Satoh S, Oshima N (1982) Effect of Dilazep dihydrochloride on microvascular blood flow. J Jap Coll Angiol 22(6): 387-391

3. Bomholt A (1980) Hypofibrinolysis in Meniere's disease -Preliminary report- Arch Otorhinolaryngol 226:101-105

4. Sumiyoshi A, et al. (1981) The inhibitory effect of Dilazep on in vivo accumulation of platelets onto damaged aorta in rabbit. I. Quantitative radioisotopic analysis. Thromb Res 23:381-386

5. Suzuki E, et al. (1981) Effect of Comelian (Dilazep) to cerebral arteriosclerosis. -Effect to platelet aggregation and adhesion- The Clinical Report 15(2):384-392

New dimensions in otorhinolaryngology – head and neck surgery, vol. 2.
E. Myers, editor

QUANTIFICATION OF SMOOTH PURSUIT PATTERNS (BETWEEN SMOOTH ,SACCADIC AND ATAXIC PATTERNS)

NAOKI OHASHI,YUKIO WATANABE,HIDETO KOBAYASHI AND KANEMASA MIZUKOSHI

Department of Otolaryngology, Faculty of Medicine, Toyama Medical and Pharmaceutical University, 2630 Sugitani Toyama City, 930-01 Japan

INTRODUCTION

Even after computers began to be used for the measurement of smooth pursuit, however, no trial to compare quantitatively among smooth patterns, saccadic patterns and ataxic patterns had been made up to the present. In the present paper, 23 pathological patients whose routine eye tracking tests were diagnosed as saccadic pattern and 7 pathological patients whose routine eye tracking tests were diagnosed as ataxic patterns underwent the authors' new smooth pursuit examination in the horizontal direction. Comparison of five parameters (amplitude gain, retinal error velocity, maximum velocity, maximum acceleration and phase lag) among three subjects' groups (23 saccadic (pathological) patients, 7 ataxic (pathological) patients and 10 smooth (normal) subjects) was performed. In addition to this, the relationship between amplitude gain and retinal error velocity (REV) was also investigated.

MATERIAL AND METHODS

Prior to this new smooth pursuit examination, routine eye tracking tests with 0.3 Hz sinusoidal wave of 10 degrees amplitude were performed. Eye movements obtained by the routine eye tracking tests were diagnosed as "smooth patterns", "saccadic patterns" or "ataxic patterns" on the ENG recording paper by the authors' visualization in every subject. 10 healthy volunteers whose routine eye tracking tests were diagnosed as "smooth patterns" were collected as the normal subjects. A new target wave (the continuously changing sinusoidal wave) was developed by the authors using a microcomputer (CBM 8032)[1]. The target wave consisted of 20 sinusoidal waves from 0.1 to 2.0 Hz with 10 degrees amplitude in the horizontal direction. The eye movements were recorded into a data-recorder at first and afterwards converted in an off-line method to digital data with a 12 bit A/D converter with the same microcomputer(CBM8032). Five parameters (amplitude gain, retinal error velocity, maximum velocity, maximum acceleration and phase lag) were obtained and the relationship between amplitude gain and retinal error velocity was investigated.

RESULTS

There were no recogrizable differences between saccadic patterns and ataxic patterns in amplitude gain, retinal error velocity, maximum velocity and maximum acceleration. Phase lag was, however, recognized markedly in 30 pathological patients, more markedly in 7 ataxic patterns than in 23 saccadic patterns. The relationship between amplitude gain and the retinal error velocity of saccadic patterns and ataxic patterns were almost all included within the normal ranges.

DISCUSSION

It is well known that in tracking sinusoidal target movements, human subjects exhibit predictive behavior that dramatically improves the quality of tracking.[2]. The studies by Stark et al.[3],Gauthern G.M.[4] et al. Lisberger[2] elucidated that the phase relationship between the target waves and the eye movements played a great role in prediction of smooth pursuit. In the present experiment, phase advance was observed from 0.1 to 2.0 Hz in 10 normal subjects, which reflected the normal predictive function of smooth pursuit with this target wave. Phase lag was, however, recognized markedly in 30 pathological patients, more markedly in 7 ataxic patterns than in 23 saccadic patterns. This led to the conclusions that these 30 pathological patients had an impaired predictive function of smooth pursuit and the predictive function was particularly damaged in pathological patients whose smooth pursuits were ataxic.

CONCLUSIONS

(1)Phase relationship between target movements and eye movements was the most prominent factor for distinguishing smooth pursuit pattern differences.

(2)There was no clear relationship between the affected sites and the pattern differences.

(3)Pathological patients whose smooth pursuits were ataxic had a more impaired predictive control of smooth pursuit.

REFERENCES

1:Ohashi,N.;Watanabe,Y.;Kobayashi,H. ; and Mizukoshi,K.: Quantitative measurement of smooth pursuit using a continuously changing sinusoidal wave in normal subjects. ORL 47:49-56(1985)

2:Lisberger,S.G.;Evinger,C.;Johanson ,G.W. and Fuchs,A.F: Relation between eye acceleration and retinal image velocity during fovealsmooth pursuit in man and monkey. Journal of Neurophysiology 46: 229-249(1981)

3:Stark,L and Vossius,G.: Predictive control of eye tracking movements IRE TRANSACTIONS ON HUMAN FACTORS IN ELECTRONICS September:52-57(1962)

4:Gauthier,G.M. and Hofferer,J.m.: Eye tracking of self-moved targets in the absence of vision. Exp.Brain Res.26:121-139(1976)

© 1985 Elsevier Science Publishers B.V. (Biomedical Division)
New dimensions in otorhinolaryngology - head and neck surgery, vol. 2.
E. Myers, editor

DIAZEPAM IN THE TREATMENT AND PREVENTION OF MOTION SICKNESS

JAI H. RYU, PH.D. AND ROBERT I. KOHUT, M.D.
Section on Otolaryngology, Department of Surgery,
Bowman Gray School of Medicine, Wake Forest University,
Winston-Salem, North Carolina 27103

INTRODUCTION

A large number of anti-motion sickness drugs are currently available, and while the effects of these drugs have been studied by various investigators in clinics and laboratories[1], there is still controversy over their site of action, mechanism, and relative effectiveness. Diazepam, a derivative of benzodiazepine, has an extremely widespread usage in medicine. The purpose of this paper is to describe the effects of diazepam on the vestibular system.

MATERIALS AND METHODS

Twenty-four adult cats were used in this study. They were anesthetized with an intraperitoneal injection of 35 mg/kg pentobarbital sodium. The surgical details, the placement of microelectrodes in the vestibular nuclei, the recording systems, the methods of data processing and drug administration have been described elsewhere.[2,3] The neural resting discharge rate and the neural response to stimulation of thirteen semicircular canal neurons and eleven otolithic neurons were recorded and analyzed. A dose level of 0.4 mg/kg of diazepam was used, as this has been determined to be the physiological dose for CNS study in the cat.[4] For control studies one ml of Ringer's solution (the volume of fluid used for the drug experiment) was injected five minutes prior to the drug injection. Histologic evaluations of the brain stems of the animals were performed to verify electrode site at time of recording. These techniques were previously described.[2]

RESULTS

The control study showed that no effect was produced by the injection of Ringer's solution on either resting discharge rate or on the neural response to vestibular stimulation.

Resting Discharge Rate: At six minutes post-injection of diazepam, the average resting discharge rate of semicircular canal neurons was depressed more than 60% (Fig. 1). This activity returned to the initial level about one hour post-injection. The average resting discharge rate of otolithic neurons was depressed also after injection of 0.4 mg/kg diazepam (Fig. 1). The level of decline was more prolonged in the otolithic neurons than semicircular canal neurons. The average time for otolithic neurons to recover normal resting discharge rate was more than 130 minutes. In some cases, the resting discharge rate of otolithic neurons was depressed to the point of effacing resting activity for more than 20 minutes.

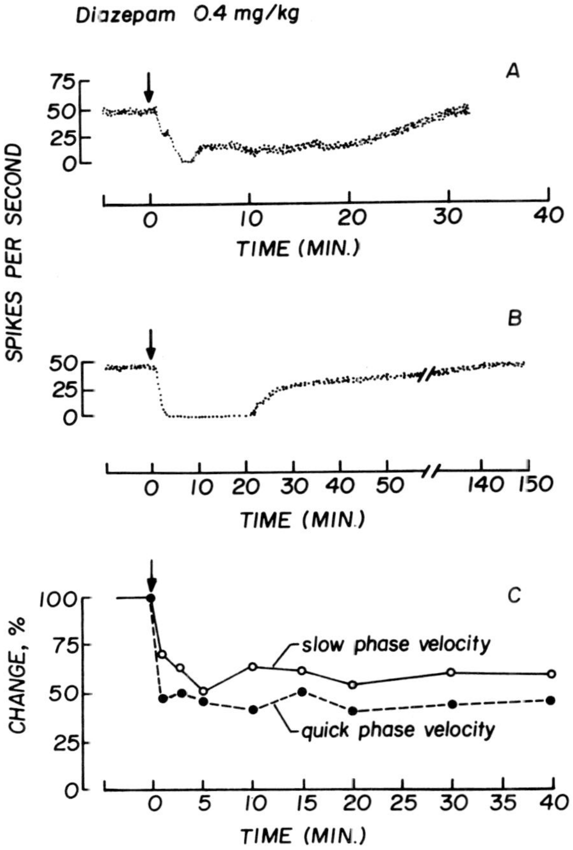

Fig. 1 Change in the frequency histogram of the resting activity of the vestibular neuron over time. Arrows indicate time of diazepam (0.4 mg/kg) injection. The resting activity changes are statistically significant for both (A) the semicircular canal neuron, and (B) otolithic neuron, and (C) percent changes of slow and quick phase velocity of nystagmus.

Neural Response: At 30 minute post-injection of diazepam, the neural response to vestibular stimulation had declined to 42% of the pre-injection level for semicircular canal neurons and to 44.7% for otolithic neurons. Examination of brain stem sections revealed that the data was obtained from neurons well within the vestibular nuclei.

DISCUSSION

It has been reported that diazepam has a certain selective affect upon mesencephalic reticular neurons, controlling sensory input without inducing somnolence or sleep.[5,6] The effect of diazepam on post-labyrinthectomy nystagmus[7] indicated that all parameters of nystagmus were depressed immediately after injection of diazepam. Furthermore, fast component velocity was more strongly affected by the drug than other parameters.

A reasonable speculation, based on these experimental data and other studies, concerning the effect of diazepam, is that it is mediated through a blocking of reticular activating neurons in the vestibulo-reticulo-oculomotor system.

CONCLUSION

Since diazepam suppresses both semicircular canal and otolithic neurons in the vestibular nuclei, it suggests that diazepam should be an effective drug in the prevention and treatment of motion sickness and may provide relief from motion intolerance characteristic of various vestibular disease.

REFERENCES

1. Wood CD: Use of drugs in the prevention of motion sickness. In Fourth Symposium on the Role of the Vestibular Organs in Space Exploration. NASA SP-187:101-107, 1968.
2. Ryu JH, McCabe BF: Neural activity in the vestibular nuclei of the cat. Annals of ORL, 82:1-29, Suppl. 9, 1973.
3. Sekitani T, McCabe BF, Ryu JH: Drug effects on the medial vestibular nucleus. Arch Otolaryng, 93:581-589, 1971.
4. Barnes CD, Eltherington LG: Drug Dosage in Laboratory Animals. A Handbook. Berkeley, Calif., University of California Press, 1964.
5. Przybyla AC, Wang SC: Locus of central depressant action of diazepam. J Pharmacol Exp Ther, 163:439-477, 1968.
6. Hernandez-Peon R, Rojas-Ramirez JA, et al: An experimental study of anticonvulsive and relaxant action of Valium. Int J Neuropharmacol, 3:405-412, 1964.
7. McCabe BF, Sekitani T, Ryu JH: Drug effects on postlabyrinthectomy nystagmus. Arch Otolaryng, 98: 310-313, 1973.

New dimensions in otorhinolaryngology - head and neck surgery, vol. 2.
E. Myers, editor

POSITIONAL VERTIGO - TREATMENT WITH EPHEDRINE NASAL DOUCHE

K.U.SHAH

Paper read at XIII World Congress of Otolaryngology,MIAMI,U.S.A

INTRODUCTION

Positional Vertigo includes all cases of Vertigo and /or unsteadiness with normal auditory and vestibular tests. Most Otologists consider search for the primary cause to be futile and no Otologist is satisfied with the treatment of Vertigo.

The results of Ephedrine Nasal Douche in 46 fully investigated cases are presented, 34 cases(approx.74%) had infective foci.

TABLE 1

Total Cases.	46		
Cure	32	(70%)	91% benefitted by this simple treatment in a short time.
Relief with mild recurrence.	10	(21%)	
No change.	4	(9%)	

TABLE 2

Controlled series	13 cases.	
	Normal Saline	Ephedrine Douche
Cure	0	10(76.90%)
Partial Relief	1 (7.70%)	1(7.70%)
No change	12 (92.30%)	2(15.40%)

EVOLUTION OF EPHEDRINE NASAL DOUCHE

Ephedrine Nasal Douche was thought of for sinus headache in 50's and for Positional Vertigo since 1976 with good results. Ephedrine Hydrochloride was the obvious choice for its decongestant effect.

PROCEDURE

The procedure is simple and without any complication but effective in 2-3 weeks time. The patient bends head forwards and downwards. While he holds the breath,1% Ephedrine solution in normal saline is pushed in the nasal cavities with higginsons Rubber syringe. Ephedrine solution lines the nasal mucosa and mucosa of Eusta Tube opening and drains out immediately. Within 2 weeks we are able to say if this treatment is going to work.

Prof.Emeritus, Grant Medical College,
Hon.E.N.T Surgeon, Jaslok Hospital - Bombay 400 026(INDIA)

DISCUSSION

Barany(1921) first described postural nystagmus later known as Positional Vertigo and thought it due to otolith disease.

Wright(1938)nited the presence of infective foci in nose and throat and suspected eustachian tube pathology.

Hallpike (1952) agreed with Barany that the utricle is the seat of pathology. He also agreed with Wright that upper respiratory infection or acute febrile illness was associated with Positional Vertigo in a large number of cases.

Lindsay(1960) produced Positional Vertigo by section of utricular nerve or nerve to lateral canal.

Tumarkin(1966) called it middle ear malfunction because of good results with grommet insertion.

The Otologists in the past have recorded the following in Positional Vertigo.

1, Utricle as the seat of pathology.
2. Association of upper respiratory infection.
3. Eustachian Tube Dysfunction.
4. Middle ear Malfunction

Anatomically stapes is in very close proximity of utricle.

CONCLUSION

We are entitled to doubt every accepted pattern of thought for if existing ideas are not called in question, research is at an end. A new theory is put forward - a theory that is not proved any more than the other interpretations are.

The only hypothesis which will explain the many isolated observations in the literature is as stated earlier, that Positional Vertigo is a disease of utricle and is due to Eusta Tube Dysfunction with some pathological change at oval window.

The whole thing sounds ridiculous and yet we know it works. The results can be achieved by those who try it.

REFERENCES

1. SHAH K.U (1961: Treatment of Sinus headache with Ephedrine Nasal Wash:IND.J.of Medi.Science 874-879.
2. SHAH K.U;SHAH ANAND(1981):Labyrinthene Vertigo. Treatment with Ephedrine Nasal Douche.J.Asso.of Physi of India. 819-823.
3. BARANY R.(1921);DIAGNOSE VON KARANKHEITSER CHEINUNGE IN BEREICHE DES OTOLITHENAPPARATES ACTA. OTOLARNGO 434-437

4. WRIGHT AJ91938) Aural Vertigo.J.Laryngo and otiology 97-112

5. HALLPIKE C.S. : DIX M.R(1952):The Pathology,Symptoms-Etiology and diagnosis of certain common disorders of the vestibular system. J.Laryngo and Otology:987-1016.

6. LINDSAY JR:FERNANDES C(1960): Positional Nystagmus in Man and Animals. J.Nerve.Ment.Dis.488-495.

7. TUMARKIN A (1966):Thoughts on the treatment of Labyrintho-pathy. Ann-oto-Rhino Laryngo:1041-1053.

New dimensions in otorhinolaryngology – head and neck surgery, vol. 2.
E. Myers, editor

CLINICAL SIGNIFICANCE OF CHANGE IN ANGULATION OF SHOULDERS WHILE STEPPING

KIICHIRO TAGUCHI, KIYOSHI WADA AND MASATO KIKUKAWA
Department of Otolaryngology, Shinshu University School of Medicine, 3-1-1 Asahi, Matsumoto (Japan)

INTRODUCTION

Equilibrium disturbance is one of the most spectacular symptoms in peripheral vestibular disorders. Stepping in the same position with eyes closed or blindholded with a band shows dynamic equilibrium or an ability to maintain the balanced posture while moving. This study deals with the change of shoulder angulation and its variance in normal persons and subjects with several vestibular disorders in order to evaluate ataxia.

MATERIAL AND METHODS

Subjects

Subjects with peripheral vestibular disorders were 20 patients with Ménière's disease, 10 with vestibular neuronitis, 20 with sudden deafness accompanied by vestibular insufficiency and 10 with other peripheral vestibular disorders. Control subjects were 20 healthy adults without any history of vertigo.

Apparatus

The bilateral shoulder angulation with respect to the center of gravity was recorded using a polarized light goniometer (1) and a data recorder. The recorded data on the magnetic tape was fed into a computer to calculate the real value of change in shoulder angulation at the stepping speeds of 0.8 to 2.0 steps/sec.

RESULTS

In the preliminary study the control subjects showed the most stable results at the stepping speed of 1.2 steps/sec. No statistically significant differences were obtained between the changes of angulation with eyes open and those with eyes closed in both shoulders ($p<0.001$).

Figure 1 shows the real values of changes in shoulder angulation during stepping movements in normal subjects and the patients with peripheral vestibular disorders. The patients with peripheral vestibular disorders showed characteristic results in which the

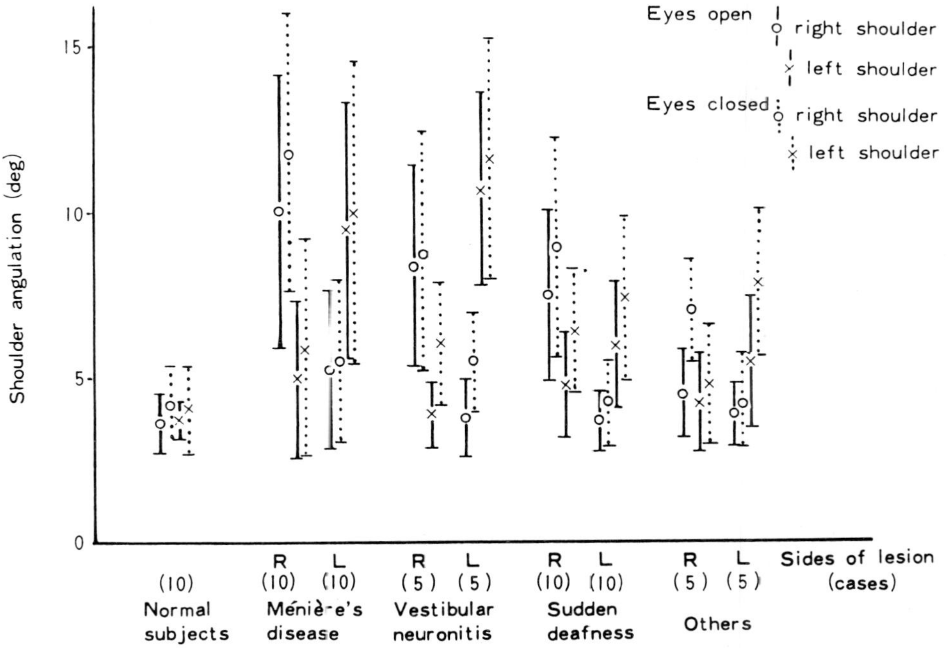

Fig. 1. Shoulder angulation while stepping at the speed of 1.2 steps/sec

shoulder of the same side with affected ear presented larger values and wider distribution as compared with those of the intact side. The patients with Ménière's disease and sudden deafness revealed remarkable changes depending on the stage of the disease.

DISCUSSION AND CONCLUSION

Stepping movement can disclose latent equilibrium disorders, which may be a prodromal symptom of severe vestibular lesions. Fukuda stated the significance of stepping deviation in labyrinthine lesion (2). Our findings corroborated the mechanism of the stepping deviation in the patients with vestibular disorders.

REFERENCES

1. Grieve DW (1969) The assessment of gait. Physiotherapy 56:452-460
2. Fukuda T (1959) The stepping test. Two phases of the labyrinthine reflex. Acta Otolaryngol 50:95-108

New dimensions in otorhinolaryngology - head and neck surgery, vol. 2.
E. Myers, editor

IMMUNOHISTOCHEMICAL STUDY OF COCHLEAR CELLS USING MONOCLONAL KERATIN ANTIBODY AE1

SHAN-RONG SHI AND STEVEN K. JUHN
Dept. of Otolaryngology, University of Minnesota Medical School, Minneapolis, Minnesota, 55455, USA

INTRODUCTION

An identification of various components of the cochlear tissue is important in understanding the function of the cochlea. Immunohistochemical identification and localization of several substances have been reported in the past. However, the localization of keratin in the cochlear tissues using avidin-biotin-peroxidase complex method with monoclonal antibody has has not been reported. It has been reported that keratin antibody AE1 is a reliable marker for simple epithelia, particularly columnar and cuboidal epithelium.

MATERIALS AND METHODS

Temporal bones from chinchillas and guinea pigs were removed under anesthesia and fixed in 3% paraformaldehyde and 0.1% glutaraldehyde in 0.1M phosphate buffer solution (PBS) at pH 7.2-7.4. They were dehydrated and embedded in Epon or in JB-4. After microdissection, all blocks were cut at 2μ with glass knives using LKB ultramicrotome. In order to stain with monoclonal keratin antibody, Epon from the sections on the slide was removed with sodium ethotide and absolute ethanol (1:5) for 5 minutes. After etching procedure, the specimen were incubated with methanolic hydrogen peroxide for 30 minutes to block endogenous peroxidase activity. Trypsinization (25 mg trypsin in 150 ml of 0.134% calcium chloride, pH adjusted to 7.8) for Epon-embedded sections and 0.1% trypsin for 1 hour for JB-4 embedded slides was applied. Mouse monoclonal keratin antibody AE1 was used with avidin-biotin-peroxidase complex (ABC) kits for antibody staining [1]. Keratin localization was determined by a 3-10 minute incubation of the sections with freshly prepared solution containing 10 mg of 3-amino-9-ethylcarbazole (AEC) and 2.5 ml of N.N. dimethyl-formamide in 50 ml of 0.1M acetate buffer (pH 4.9) to which 1 drop of 30% hydrogen peroxide was added. The incubation of tissue sections in the substrate was terminated prior to the development of nonspecific background staining. For every immunohistochemical staining procedure, phosphate buffer (0.1M) instead of monoclonal keratin antibody AE1 was used as a negative control and the auricle skin taken from the same animal as positive control group.

RESULTS

Strongly positive staining with AE1 was observed in the following cells: reticular laminae of both outer and inner hair cells; Hensen's cells; spiral prominence cells (SPC); external sulcus cells (ESC); and a few marginal cells located on the upper end of the stria vascularis (SV) adjacent to Reissner's membrane. Weakly positive staining cells were: marginal cells of SV; Reissner's membrane; Boettcher's cells. Epon-embedded sections showed positively staining interdental cells of the spiral limbus, part of Claudius cells and inner sulcus cells.

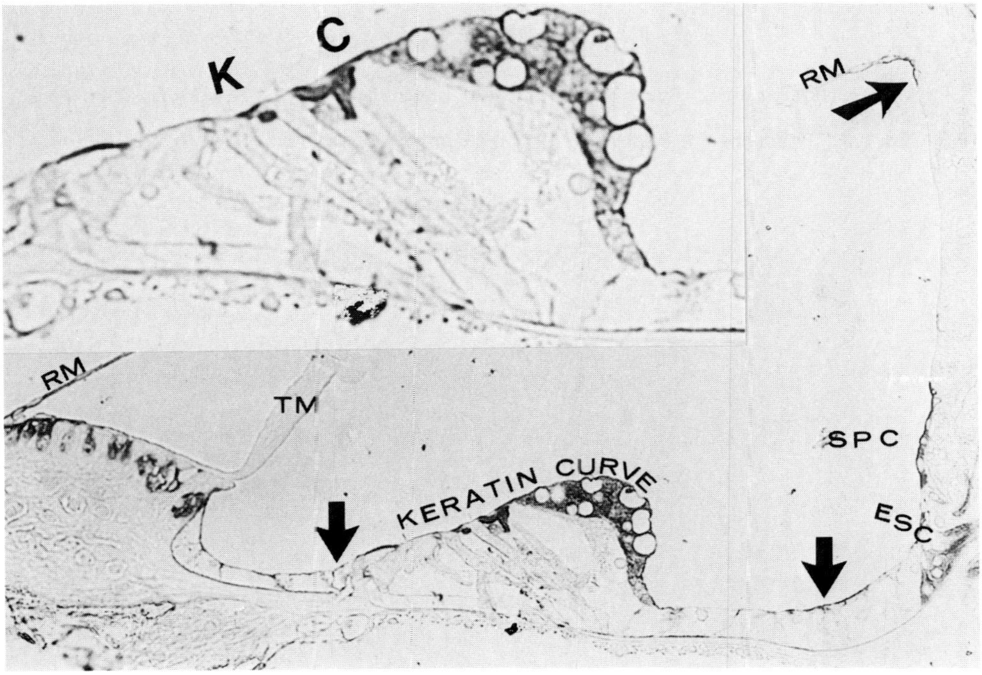

Fig. 1. Keratin localization in the cochlea of guinea pig. Insert: higher magnification. No counterstain.

COMMENTS

The preliminary data of the present study provide the possibility of reliable identification of keratin localization in the cochlear tissues using monoclonal keratin antibody AE1 with Avidin-Biotin-Peroxidase complex method. Flock et al. [2] have previously reported the keratin localization in the reticular lamina. The possible functions of "keratin curve" composed of reticular laminae and Hensen's cells (Fig. 1) might serve as barrier between endolymph and cortilymph. Among the cochlear mechanics, "keratin curve" may play an important role in maintaining the stiffness of the hair cell system. This may play a role in protecting the hair cells from acoustic trauma. Although the significance of AE1 positive cells in the various parts of the cochlear tissues needs to be further defined, the application of this immunohistochemical staining method using monoclonal keratin antibody AE1 with ABC might provide valuable tool to examine the composition of inner ear tissues under physiological and pathological conditions.

ACKNOWLEDGEMENTS

The authors thank Drs. Harold F. Schuknecht, Max L. Goodman, Michael M. Paparella, Arndt J. Duvall, Chen-en Lu, T-T Sun for their advice and assistance.

REFERENCES

1. Shi SR, Goodman ML, Bhan AK, Pilch BZ, Chen LB, Sun T-T (1984) Am J Pathol 117:53.
2. Flock A, Bretscher A, Weber K (1982) Hearing Res 6:75.

© 1985 Elsevier Science Publishers B.V. (Biomedical Division)
New dimensions in otorhinolaryngology - head and neck surgery, vol. 2.
E. Myers, editor

STUDIES OF THE DEVELOPMENT OF THE OTIC CAPSULE IN RATS

KAZUYA SHIMADA

Department of Otorhinolaryngology, Tokyo Jikei University School of Medicine, 3-25-8 Nishi-shinbashi, Minato Tokyo Japan

The otic capsule is known to be the cartilage bone that takes unique developmental course and the physiological characters. We have observed developmental courses and ossification process of the otic capsule in the embryo of young rats. The main purpose of this experiment is to clarify the mitotic activity of the cartilage model and the relationship between ossification process and the development of membranous labyrynth. Development of superior semicircular canal of the otic capsule is discussed in this presentation.

MATERIAL AND METHODS

The animals used in this experiment were the rats ranging in age from Day 18 prenatal to Day 5 postnatal. The mitotic activity was observed by colchicine technique. The animals were injected intraperitoneally with 1 μg of colchicine/g of body weight at 11.00 am and the otic capsules were collected at 2.00 pm. Sections were cut serially at 4 μm and stained with hematoxylin and eosin, Masson's trychrome and alcian blue. The rats in the control group were decapitated at 11.00 am and sections were made in the same manner as that for the treated group. Cell counts were under oil immersion utilizing an ocular net micrometer.

RESULTS

The number of cells in arrested metaphase were encountered at various areas. Mitotic activity at the anterior area was higher than that at other areas in the anterior half of the superior semicircular canal. Mitotic cells at the anterior area were observed to be 2% of the total cells encountered. Mitotic activity was gradually decreasing towards the posterior. The difference between the anterior area and other areas was statistically significant at the 1% level. Mitotic activity was the lowest at the anterior area and no great difference in activity was observed at other areas in the posterior half of the superior semicircular canal. The difference of activity between that at the anterior area and other areas was statistically significant at the 1% level.

The otic capsule on Day 18 prenatal is composed of mature cartilage and membranous labyrinth which appears as a thickened pseudostratified layer. The epithelium of membranous labyrinth loses its stratification with aging and becomes a simple columnar epithelium. Hypertrophic cartilage cells are observed at the ampulla of the superior semicircular canal in the newborn. Mitotic activity weakened throughout the otic capsule, it was observed at the foot plate of the stapes and membranous labyrinth. Hypertrophy of the cartilage cells which began at the ampulla gradually proceed to the curvature. Ossification process at the ampulla of the superior semicircular canal in 5-day-old rats. Ossification was observed at the otic capsule adjacent to crista ampullaris. It seems that ossification at early stage protect crista ampullaris. Ossification center was analyzed by electron probe X-ray microanalysis. The elements analyzed were sulphur of acid mucopolysaccharides, calcium of hydroxy apatite and magnesium. There is a peak of sulphur at the stage prior to ossification. Calcium and magnesium was increasing in the ossification center and the sulphur was on the decrease.

DISCUSSION

Mitotic cycle divides into mitotic stage including prophase, metaphase, anaphase and telophase and interphase. Colchicine has been used for study to solve mitotic rate, mitotic duration and turn-over time by arresting mitosis. It has been shown that arrested metaphase has become pycnotic or been disintegrated and disappeared. The development of the membranous labyrinth derived, precedes that of the osseus labyrinth derived from the mesoderm. We have already demonstrated that there is regional differences in concentration of acid mucopolysaccharides in a developing otic capsule.

These results lead us to the following conclusions. It is available for explanation that three dimensional figure of the otic capsule has three axises of co-ordinate, X, Y, and λ. Axis Y indicates width, X indicates length and λ indicates ^{35}S activity derived from sulphur. λ max is observed at the posterior tip of otic capsule where is push vector, λ min is observed at the anterior tip which is extension vector. ^{35}S activity of acid mucopolysaccarides is inversely proportional to arresting metaphase of cartilage cells. These facts coincided with concept of the second low of thermodynamics.

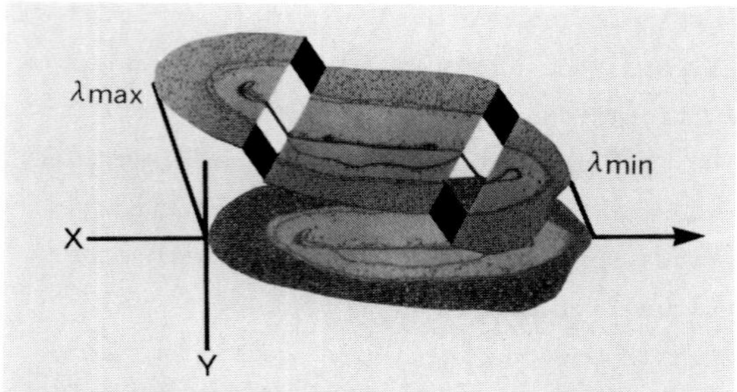

CONCENTRATIVE GRADIENT OF ACIDE MUCOPOLYSACCHARIDE

REFERENCES

1. Shimada K (1972) Studies on the metabolism of chondroitin sulfate in developmental otic capsule. Ear Research Japan. Vol.3. pp48-49

2. Yamazaki Y, Shimada K (1973) Study on the metabolism of acid mucopoly-sacchalides in otic capsule. Ear Research Japan Vol.4 pp 5-6

3. Shimada K (1976) Observations on the otic capsule by automicroprobe. Ear Reseach Japan. Vol. 7 pp9-11

4. Shimada K, Yamazaki Y (1976) Studies on the ossification of the otic capsule. Ear Reseach Japan Vol. 7 pp12-14

5. Shimada K, Takiguchi K, Honda Y (1980) Studies on the development of the otic capsule using colchicine technique. Ear Reseach Japan Vol.11 pp 1-3

6. Shimada K (1984) Studies of the development of the otic capsule and membanous labylinth in the rats. Ear Reseach Japan. Vol. 15 pp87-90.

7. Chiba M (1966) Estimation of mitotic rate and mitotic duration in the internal enamel epithelium of the rat maxillary incisor using a colchicine technique Archs Oral Biol Vol. 11 pp803-814.

New dimensions in otorhinolaryngology - head and neck surgery, vol. 2.
E. Myers, editor

SURGICAL ANATOMY OF THE GUINEA PIG MIDDLE EAR

DENNIS S. THAKOR and TERRENCE W. FRANK

Department of Otolaryngology, University of Wisconsin School of Medicine, Madison, WI 53792 (USA)

INTRODUCTION

The guinea pig is frequently used for otologic experimentation, often because its inner ear is readily accessible. We review the anatomy of the middle ear, and evaluate five surgical approaches.

MATERIAL AND METHODS

Anatomical dissections were performed on guinea pig ears and temporal bones. Large tympanic bullae contain the middle and inner ear structures. The tympanic membrane is held in place by its fibrous annulus. The malleus handle is flared inferiorly; superiorly, the malleus is hinged to a thin scutum. The malleus head is fused to the body of the incus. The incudostapedial joint partially overhangs the round window. The stapes sits in a narrow recess above the round window and below the facial nerve. The facial nerve follows a course similar to that through the human middle ear, but exits the skull through a foramen just posterior to the external auditory canal. The chorda tympani comes off the facial nerve posterior to the incus, passes between the malleus and incus, and exits the middle ear anteriorly.

RESULTS

Five surgical approaches are evaluated, with emphasis on the round window exposure which each offers. The strong and weak points of each approach are noted.

The anterior approach is made difficult by the proximity to the mandible and facial and jugular veins. It offers good exposure to the anterior middle ear space, but the tympanic membrane, tensor tympani, ossicles, and cochlea obstruct the round window.

The inferior approach offers good exposure of the hypotympanum and apical turn of the cochlea, but the tympanic membrane, malleus, and cochlea block the round window.

The superior approach widely exposes the epitympanum. The head of the malleus, body of the incus, tensor tympani, part of the vestibular labyrinth, and anterior middle ear space can be seen well. The round window is obstructed by the chorda tympani, vestibular labyrinth, facial nerve, incus, and stapes.

The posterior approach must avoid the facial nerve. The posterior middle ear and cochlea are accessible. It is possible to manipulate the round window from this approach, although the round window is somewhat tangential to the axis of view.

The trans-canal approach is quick and nearly bloodless. By peeling the posterior-superior tympanic membrane from the scutum and posterior handle of the malleus, it is possible to expose the round window and incudo-stapedial joint. The round window is nearly perpendicular to the axis of view, and it is easy to rupture it or pipette material onto or through it. The small myringotomy heals rapidly, usually within one week.

CONCLUSIONS

The guinea pig is a convenient model for otologic experimentation. Several approaches to various parts of the middle ear are available. We prefer the trans-canal approach for round window manipulation.

REFERENCES

1. Asarch, Richard, et al (1975) Ann Otol 84: 250-255
2. Rogers, Kenneth A., Snow, James B. (1968) Ann Oto Rhino Laryngo 77(1): 66-71

New dimensions in otorhinolaryngology - head and neck surgery, vol. 2.
E. Myers, editor

PROPRANOLOL'S EFFECT ON AUDITORY-NERVE RESPONSES IS DUE TO ITS LOCAL ANESTHETIC PROPERTIES

RICHARD P. WIKHOLM and MICHAEL L. WIEDERHOLD

Division of Otorhinolaryngology, University of Texas Health Science Center, San Antonio, TX, USA 78284

INTRODUCTION

Propranolol has recently been shown to lower metabolic activity in all areas of the brain directly associated with hearing (1). In one study of tinnitus patients in which 20% were taking propranolol it was shown that their tinnitus was reduced when the medication was discontinued (2). When administered systemically or locally in cochlear perilymph, propranolol reduces auditory nerve (N1) and brainstem responses to acoustic stimuli but has minimal effects on the cochlear microphonic (CM) response (M. L. Wiederhold, unpublished results). Propranolol has both beta-adrenergic blocking properties as well as local anesthetic (membrane stabilizing) properties. This study was undertaken to investigate the site and mechanism of propranolol's observed auditory effects.

MATERIALS AND METHODS

Using mongrel cats deeply anesthetized with diallyl-barbituric acid anesthesia, the cat's pinnas were removed and a hollow earbar sound delivery system was placed in the cartilagenous external auditory canal. The bulla was opened widely on one side allowing an easy approach to the round window from the dorsolateral aspect. A hole was cauterized in the round window membrane and a silastic tipped infusion needle was placed into the scala tympani of the basal turn of the cochlea. Several agents similar in structure but with varying pharmacologic activities were dissolved in artificial perilymph and infused into the basal turn of the cat cochlea at a rate of 8 ul/minute. High frequency filtered clicks were applied thru the hollow ear bar and dose response relations obtained. Responses were recorded using the infusion needle in the scala tympani as a recording electrode. Averaging of responses was performed with a PDP 11/44 computer. Dose response relations were obtained for d-propranolol, l-propranolol, timolol, nadalol and dimethisoquine for their effects on N1 and CM response. At each dose an intensity function was obtained by measuring responses at 10 dB intervals over a 70 dB range.

RESULTS AND DISCUSSION

Propranolol was found to reduce the amplitude of the N1 auditory nerve response to high frequency filtered clicks in a dose dependent manner evident from 3 to 300 uM. A 50% reduction in N1 amplitude was achieved at approximately 20 uM, the ED 50. Timolol was found to have similar effects on N1 amplitude with an ED 50 of 100 uM. Neither drug had more than a 10 to 20% effect on CM amplitude at the highest doses. As a beta blocker timolol should be equally effective at concentrations 5 to 10 times lower than those required for propranolol. Recent reports indicate a small local anesthetic effect of timolol. When the separate isomeres of propranolol were compared, their dose response curves were found to be nearly identical, both having ED 50's of 20 uM. As a beta blocker, the l-isomer should have similar effects at concentrations 1000 fold lower than those required for the d-isomer, whereas the local anesthetic properties of the two isomeres is the same. Dimethisoquine is a local anesthetic structurally similar to propranolol but lacking beta blocking properties. This agent was also found to reduce N1 amplitude with a dose response curve virtually identical to that for propranolol. Nadalol is a beta blocker which has no local anesthetic effects. Nadalol was found to have no dose dependent effects in concentrations up to 1 mM.

The results lead us to conclude that the effects of propranolol on auditory nerve responses are due to its local anesthetic properties and not its beta blocking effects. The results also suggest rational for use of nadalol in patients on beta blockers with auditory complaints.

ACKNOWLEDGEMENTS

This work was supported by a Deafness Research Foundation grant awarded to M.W.

REFERENCES

1. Savaki, H.E., Kadebaro, M. Jehle, J., Sokoloff, L.: Alpha- and Beta-Adrenoreceptor Blockers have Opposite Effects on Energy Metabolism of the Central Auditory System Nature 276: 521-523, 1978.

2. Mostyn, R.H.L.: Tinnitus and Propranolol. Brit. Med. J. 2:766, 1969.

© 1985 Elsevier Science Publishers B.V. (Biomedical Division)
New dimensions in otorhinolaryngology - head and neck surgery, vol. 2.
E. Myers, editor

MOTILITY OF ISOLATED MAMMALIAN OUTER HAIR CELLS

HANS P.ZENNER
Dept. of Otolaryngology, University of Wuerzburg, D-8700 Wuerzburg

Motile responses of cochlear hair cells CHCs open new perspectives for the understanding of cochlear hearing mechanisms and hearing disorders located in HCs.

Isolated mammalian cochlear hair cells

Many experimental procedures that require a homogeneous cell population cannot be applied to mammalian inner ear research. Biochemical, virological and immunological approaches to hair cells are frequently prevented because experimental material is contaminated by non-hair cells. In the present study we describe a method for the study of living isolated mammalian outer hair cells (OHCs) which has overcome some of the complexities in dealing with the heterogenous organ of Corti.

Recently electrophysiological giga seal whole cell recordings of single OHC prepared by this approach revealed negative cell potentials ranging from -32 mV to -67 mV (1).

In vivo the apical part of mammalian hair cells is exposed to the unique K^+ rich environment of the endolymphatic space. The fluctuating hearing loss of Ménière's disease is thought to be accompanied by endolymphatic hydrops and by a leakage of membranes lining the endolymphatic space, leading to K^+ intoxication of hair cells (2,3,4). It has also been postulated that damage of hair cells can occur by entry into the Nuel space of K^+ rich endolymph through holes in the reticular lamina resulting from certain types of noise trauma (5).

K^+-induced HC contractions

Elucidation of HC motility has come from two lines of experiments. One follows from, that exposure of the lateral and basal membrane parts of living OHCs to increasing bath K^+concentrations resulted in a sustained reversible depolarization of the cell (1). Here, we report that by depolarization of the cell membrane in the presence of 25-125 mM K^+/Cl^- a sustained contraction of OHC was induced (6). This was followed by relaxation in the presence of artificial perilymph containing 5.4 mM K^+/Cl^-. By alternating these procedures OHCs were made to undergo as many as five cycles of contraction and relaxation. External

Ca^{2+} was not required for the initial contraction but was essential for relaxation. Following repeated contraction/relaxation cycles the cytoplasm of individual OHCs exhibited a filamentous network.

ATP-induced HC contractions

The second originates in the observation of permeabilized OHC, that contracted in the presence of ATP and Ca^{2+}. This contraction was inhibited by cytochalasin B, indicating the presence of an actin-dependent motile mechanism. Studies, using fluorescent labelled phalloidin allowed monitoring of an actin-polymerizing process during ATP-induced contraction of OHCs (7).

REFERENCES

1. Gitter A, Zenner HP, Frömter A (1984): Patch clamp studies on mammalian in ear hair cells. Worksh.noise analysis,Leuven (Belgium),abstr.

2. Dohlmann GF (1976) : On the mechanism of the Ménière' attack.Arch. Oto-rhinolaryngol. 212: 301-307

3. Jahnke K (1977) :Zur Pathogenese der akuten Symptome des Morbus Ménière. Laryngol.Rhinol.Otol. 56:402-406

4. Schuknecht HF (1976): Pathophysiology of endolymphatic hydrops. Arch. Otorhinolaryngol. 212: 253-262

5. Bohne BA (1976): In:Henderson D, HAmernick RP, Dosanjhand DS, Mills JH,Eds.) Raven Press, New York: 41-68

6. Zenner HP, Zimmermann U, Schmitt U (1985): Reversible contraction of isolated mammalian cochlear hair cells. Hearing Research, in press

7. Zenner HP, Drenckhahn, in preparation

ACKNOWLEDGEMENT

This research was supported by DFG grant Ze 149/2-2

© 1985 Elsevier Science Publishers B.V. (Biomedical Division)
New dimensions in otorhinolaryngology - head and neck surgery, vol. 2.
E. Myers, editor

GROWTH OF FRONTAL SINUS WITH AGE
- AN X-RAY TOMOGRAPHIC STUDY -

YUJI ARASHI, TAKIO MABUCHI AND MASAMI TSUTSUMI

Department of Otorhinolaryngology, Kyorin University, School of Medicine, 6-20-2 Shinkawa, Mitaka City, Tokyo (Japan)

In order to determine growth of frontal sinus with age, the frontal sinus was measured using X-ray tomography in a total of 1,942 Japanese cases without paranasal sinusal diseases (984 males and 958 females) aging from 4 to 59 years. The data obtained were treated statistically with following results.

1) The frontal sinus was found to be present in 84% at the age of 10 years and 96% at 19 years for male cases and in 74% and 96%, respectively, for female cases. Thus, it appears that the frontal sinus is present in a high percentage of subjects even under 10 years of age and that at least until 19 years of age presence or absence of the frontal sinus in determined. When comparisons are made between the left side and the right side, the frontal sinus was detected with higher incidences in the left side for both sexes.

2) The width of frontal sinus shows growth-degree much greater than that seen in the frontal bone from about 6 to 8 years of age for both sexes. The growth almost completes until 16 to 18 years for males and 12 to 14 years for females. For male cases four growth patterns were seen in both left and right sides. On the other hand, the growth in the left side showed four patterns, whereas no pattern was observed in the right side.

3) The growth in the height of frontal sinus started and completed at about the same periods as observed for the growth in the width of frontal sinus. However, some difference was seen in growth with age. For males the growth in the right side proceeded at a constant rate, but in the left side three patterns were found. On the other hand, for females there were three patterns in the right side and four patterns in the left side.

4) The global growth rate of frontal sinus (maximal width of frontal sinus + maximal height of frontal sinus/maximal width of orbita x 100) was examined as one of the index for growth of the frontal sinus. It was found that growth-degree much greater than that observed for the frontal bone starts from about 6 to 8 years for both males and females. Four patterns were seen in growth in the left side for both males and females, while in the right side for females no pattern was noted in growth. The growth almost completed until 18 to 19 years for males and until 12 to 14 years for females.

5) Marginal morphology tended to be more complexed with age for both males and females. In addition, there was a tendency that the greater the frontal

sinus is the more complexed became the marginal morphology.

6) For both sexes, high positive correlation was seen in growth between the width and the height of frontal sinus and also in growth of height of frontal sinus between left and right. Thus, it is considered that the frontal sinus shows growth in both width and height harmoniously.

7) In the growth of frontal sinus difference was seen between the right side and the left side, with superiority in growth in the left side. It was postulated that this difference may be explained by the fact that difference in aeration in the nasal cavity between the left and right sides originated from deviations of nasal septum is involved in pneumatization of frontal sinus.

New dimensions in otorhinolaryngology - head and neck surgery, vol. 2.
E. Myers, editor

THE ULTRASTRUCTURE OF THE HUMAN ANTRAL MUCOSA IN CHRONIC SINUSITIS. A FREEZE-FRACTURE STUDY

RUDOLF AUST, ANDERS KÖLING & HELGE RASK-ANDERSEN

Department of Oto-rhino-laryngology, University Hospital, S-751 85 Uppsala (Sweden)

INTRODUCTION

Recently, we reported on the freeze-fracture ultrastructure of the normal paranasal sinus mucosa (1). The aim of the present study was to analyse the epithelial ultrastructure of the mucosa in chronic sinusitis using the freeze-fracture technique.

MATERIAL AND METHODS

From five patients with a history of chronic sinusitis and typical radiological findings undergoing radical surgical operation, pieces of mucous membrane were collected. The preparation procedure for obtaining freeze-fracture replicas has been described in detail previously (1).

OBSERVATIONS

Generally, the mucous membrane was thickened. Areas of squamous metaplasia were seen together with loss of cilia. Most interest was directed towards remaining ciliated epithelium and in particular its apical region.

In the apical part of the epithelial cells typical tight junctions appeared either as belt-like meshworks of branching and anastomosing thin ridges on the E-face or as corresponding furrows on the P-face (Fig.). The junctional belts were not seldom disrupted and the number of strands was frequently reduced as compared to normal antral epithelium.

In the neck region of the cilia intramembranous particles could be seen. They were organized into 5-7 strands and they surrounded the base lying in parallel.

DISCUSSION

Morphological changes in the mucous membrane at chronic sinuitis has been reported from studies using light microscopy (2) and thin-section transmission electron microscopy as well as scanning electron microscopy (For review: 3). The general morphological findings in our study were in concordance with these earlier reports.

The tight junction, or zonula occludence, was first described by Farquhar and Palade (4) as the most luminal element of the junctional complex which links cells of various forms of epithelia. Claude and Goodenough (5)correlated leakiness with the freeze-fracture morphology of the tight junctions. These studies provided a direct structure-function correlation at the molecular level between the number and arrangement of sealing elements of a given zonula occludens.

In the present study we found in epithelium from mucous membranes in patients suffering from chronic maxillary sinuitis both a reduced number of junctional strands and discontinous areas in the band-like arrangement of tight junctions. Theoretically, this could imply increased "leakiness" in this epithelium under inflammatory conditions. Further physiological investigations seem, however, motivated before definite conclusions can be drawn.

The morphology of ciliary necklaces in the present material showed no major changes as compared to normal antral mucosa (1).

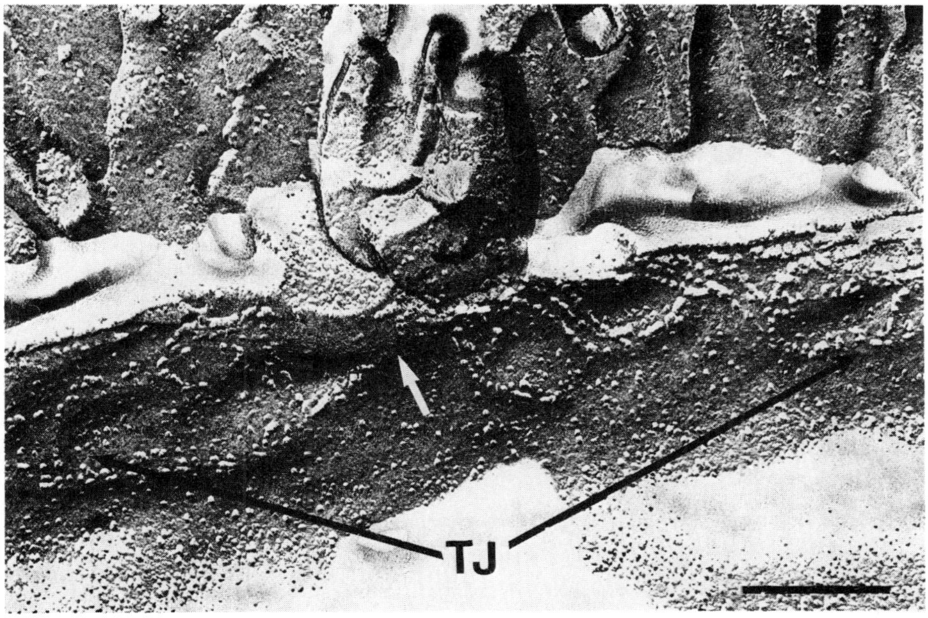

Fig. Photomicrograph of a freeze-fracture replica from mucosa in chronic sinuitis. TJ = tight junction. White arrow indicates discontinuous area of the junction. Scale bar 0.2 um.

REFERENCES

1. Köling A, Aust R, Rask-Andersen H, Hoffstedt M (1985) Rhinology 23:11-17
2. Bauer E (1960) Mschr Ohrenheilk 94:43-52
3. Sanchez-Fernandez JM, Rivera-Pomar JM, Macias JA (1983) Revue de Laryngologie 104:45-53
4. Farquhar MG, Palade GE (1963) J Cell Biol 17:375-412
5. Claude P, Goodenough DA (1973) J Cell Biol 58:390-400

New dimensions in otorhinolaryngology - head and neck surgery, vol. 2.
E. Myers, editor

THE SAFETY OF FRONTAL SINUS FAT OBLITERATION WHEN SINUS WALLS ARE MISSING

PAUL J. DONALD, AND MALCOLM ETTIN, University of California, Davis

INTRODUCTION

In the management of severe frontal sinus fractures, a frequent therapeutic dilemma is posed when significant portions of the sinus walls are missing, Often during cleansing of the wound, the debridement removes significant portions of either the anterior or posterior wall; and some form of surgical restoration of the sinus is required. Removal of the remaining anterior wall of the frontal sinus, and collapse of the forehead skin against the posterior wall or frontal lobe dura is safe, but leaves the frontal lobes relatively unprotected, as well as an unsightly cosmetic deformity. The excision of the sinus lining and fat obliteration of the sinus is advocated by some,[1,2,3] but in our hands has been frequently followed by the later formation of a mucopyocele. To test the safety of the fat obliteration operation in frontal sinuses with missing walls, the following experiment was designed.

MATERIALS AND METHODS

Nine cats were anesthetized with pentabarbitol and, under sterile technique, had an osteoplastic flap of the frontal sinus performed. Meticulous excision of the frontal sinus mucosa was done. All of the sinus wall was removed in eight sinuses; four the anterior and four the posterior wall. One-half of one wall was excised in ten sinuses; six the anterior and four the posterior.

All animals were sacrificed at three months, and the sinuses fixed in celloidin. The tissues were cut at 20 μ thickness, stained with hematoxylin and eosin, and examined under light microscopy.

RESULTS

The table displays the results of the experiment. Either epithelialization, infection, or both were found in 50% of the sinuses. These complications were independent of either the amount or location of wall excised. This reinforces our contention that fat obliteration in frontal sinuses with significant portions of the anterior or posterior walls missing is unsafe. The proposed pathophysiological mechanism presumed here is that of fat absorption and subsequent mucosal ingrowth. Fat requires a rich vascular bed on which to survive.[4,5] This is normally supplied by the drilling down of the inner bony table while ridding the frontal sinus cavity of all its mucosa.[6] When a significant surface of the fat graft is exposed to the impoverished blood supply of dura or subcutaneous tissue or, worse still, the absence of vascularity of a dural graft or bony free fragment, then fat absorption takes place. The graft retracts, usually away from the frontonasal duct, allowing the ingrowth of ductal epithelium into the residual sinus cavity. This new mucosa behaves in a characteristically pathologic way, often resulting in mucocoele formation and infection.[7,8,9]

TABLE: CAT FRONTAL SINUSES, THREE MONTHS FOLLOWING PARTIAL SINUS WALL EXCISION AND FAT OBLITERATION.

A) Right Sinus

Cat No.	Wall - % Removed	Infection	Epithelialization	Fat Obliteration
1	anterior - 100	X	X	
2	anterior - 50			X
3	anterior - 50		X	X
4	anterior - 50	X	X	
5	posterior - 100			X
6	posterior - 100			X
7	posterior - 50	X	X	
8	posterior - 50	X	X	
9	anterior - 100	X		

B) Left Sinus

Cat No.	Wall - % Removed	Infection	Epithelialization	Fat Obliteration
1	anterior - 100	X	X	
2	anterior - 50			X
3	anterior - 50			X
4	anterior - 50	X		
5	posterior - 100			X
6	posterior - 100			X
7	posterior - 50	X	X	
8	posterior - 50		X	
9	anterior - 100			X

REFERENCES

1. Lyons D, Rybak L, Maisel R, et al (1980) Treatment of frontal sinus fractures. Presentation at meeting of the AAO.

2. Olson NR (1982) Frontal sinus ablation. Letter to the editor. Arch Otolaryngol 108:749

3. Duval AJ, Montgomery WW (1981) Management of frontal sinus fractures (functional/obliterative). Presentation at meeting of the AAFPRS.

4. Peer LA (1977) Transplantation of fat. In: Plastic & Reconstructive Surgery. Converse JM, McCarthy JG (eds) W.B. Saunders, Philadelphia, pp 251-261.

5. Williams BH, Crepeau RK (1979) Free dermal fat flaps to the face. Annals Plastic Surg 3:1-12

6. Montgomery WW (1969) The fate of adipose implants in the bony cavity. Laryngoscope 74:816-827

7. Donald PJ (1979) The tenacity of the frontal sinus mucosa. Otolaryngol Head Neck Surg 87:557-566

8. Lotta JS, Schall RJ (1934) The histology of the epithelium of the paranasal sinuses under various conditions. Ann Otol Rhinol Laryngol 43:945-971

9. Schenck NL (1975) Frontal sinus disease: III Experimental and clinical factors in failure of the frontal osteoplastic operation. Laryngoscope 85:76-92

New dimensions in otorhinolaryngology - head and neck surgery, vol. 2.
E. Myers, editor

ASPECTS OF PROTEASE TREATMENT OF CHRONIC INFLAMMATION II. ROLE AND FATE OF ADMINISTERED PROTEASE

S. FUJISAKI*, T. NAKAMURA, S. KUROKAWA, M. MITANI, J. YOSHIDA and M. NAKAMURA
*Fujisaki Institute, 2-56 Bingo-cho, #2 Nomura Bldg., Higashi-ku, Osaka 541, (JAPAN)

INTRODUCTION

About twenty years have passed since we first used oral administration of pronase on human chronic paranasal sinusitis. This therapy was put into practical use only after it had borne the brunt of critism based on the accepted knowlege that chronic paranasal sinusitis nearly always defies drug therapy and that enzyme molecules are too large to be absorbed from the intestinal walls. We gave pronase, an excellent proteolytic enzyme produced from *Streptomyces griseus*, to experimental animals, and engaged in biochemical studies of effects of protease administration.

MATERIAL AND METHODS

Pronase was radio-labeled with iodine-125, and α_2-macroglobulin, a protease inhibitor in serum was carbon-14[1,2]. Male Sprague-Dawley SPF rats and rabbits weighing about 200g and 1.5kg, respectively, were used in all experiments. Sephacryl S-300 was obtained from Pharmacia Fine Chemicals. All other materials were either reagent grade or the purest commercial source available.

RESULTS AND DISCUSSION

Formation of complex of pronase with α_2-macroglobulin. When pronase is incubated with serum *in vitro*, one of 65K apparent mol. wt. produce components of 75K mol. wt. which complexed with α_2-macroglobulin. This complex was also obtained with plasma after intravenously injection.

Absorption of pronase from intestinal tract. Labeled pronase was administered into rat duodenum, and the appearence of radioactivity in the blood was followed as a measure of intestinal absorption. The intestinal absorption continued for about 60 min after administration of the labeled pronase, and more than 3% of the total radioactivity administered was generally detected in the blood. We can't practically detect the free form of pronase in the blood stream.

Proteolytic activity of the complex. The complex of pronase with α_2-macro=globulin in serum retains both elastase-like activity toward succinyl-alanyl-alanyl-alanyl-para nitro aniline and trypsin-like activity toward benzoyl arginine para nitro aniline such as chemically synthetic substrates, but inhibits its activity toward casein as protein substrate.

Fate of the complex in blood stream. If we intravenously administered the complex of pronase with α_2-macroglobulin that formed previously, the complex with α_2-macroglobulin disappeared from the blood within 15 min, whereas that with α_1-proteinase inhibitor remained circulating for a much longer period of time. It was found that liver, kidney, lung and granuloma were accumulated the labeled pronase - α_2-macroglobulin complex. These observation suggested that pronase administered was incorporated into lymphocytes, macrophages, phagocytes and fibroblasts, which present an α_2-macroglobulin receptor.

Fate of the complex in inflammatory tissues. We introduced inflammation to the skin of rat according to Hans and Selye method. When the radioactivity appearing in the exudates from granuloma pouch were measured after administra= tion of the labeled pronase, it was increased to 1% of the total radioactivity administered was detected in the exudates. It was found that pronase was accumulated in the exudates to higher extent than serum albumin which was used as a control, and that both pronase and α_2-macroglobulin were converted to small fragments in the exudates.

Role of α_2-macroglobulin - protease complex on inflammation. These results suggested that protease administered was absorbed on duodenum, transported to blood, formed a complex with α_2-macroglobulin, masked proteolytic activity toward proteins, disappeared from blood stream, incorporated to different cells which were possessed of receptor for complex, degraded to small fragments, released from cells. We present a brief discussion of the structural and func= tional aspects of α_2-macroglobulin[3]. Recently the primary structure of the tetrameric plasma glycoprotein human α_2-macroglobulin has been determined[4]. The comparison of sequences and structure from α_2-macroglobulin with human complement components C3, C4 and C5 indicates that these are evolutionary related closely. Unique internal thiolester site also found in the complement components C3 and C4. Amino-terminal end of the alpha chains were released C3a, anaphylatoxin fragment, and C5a, chemotactic factor, respectively. We guessed that α_2-macroglobulin may be present these fragments of inflammatory effector. It is likely that inflammatory proteases and administered protease and serum inhibitors play certain important roles in the process of inflammation.

REFERENCES

1. Hunter WH, Greengard FC (1962) Nature 194:495
2. Martin DD, Ravel JM (1978) Anal. Biochem. 49:593
3. James K (1980) Trends Biochem. Sci. 5:43
4. Lars SJ, Stepanik TM, Kristensen T, Wierbicki DM, Jones CM, Lonblad PB, Magnusson S, Petersen TE (1984) J.Biol.Chem. 259:8318-8327

© 1985 Elsevier Science Publishers B.V. (Biomedical Division)
New dimensions in otorhinolaryngology - head and neck surgery, vol. 2.
E. Myers, editor

CLINICAL SIGNIFICANCE OF EOG (ELECTRO-OLFACTOGRAM) FOR THE OBJECTIVE OLFACTORY EXAMINATION

MICHIHIRO KAMIDE, MITSURU FURUKAWA, RYOZO UMEDA
Depertment of Otorhinolaryngology, School of Medicine, Kanazawa University, 13-1 Takaramachi, Kanazawa, Ishikawa, Japan

INTRODUCTION

The potential that is produced by an odorous stimulation to the olfactory epithelium has been called the EOG (Electro-olfactogram)[1]. The technique of the EOG might be a useful method for olfactory studies. We introduce the recent fundamental and clinical studies using the EOG.

EOG IN RABBITS

The nasal bone was removed and the olfactory region was exposed, so that we placed the electrode on the first endoturbinate where the olfactory epithelium exsisted anatomically[2], and stimulated with the odorous substances. We obtained the slow negative potential that is the EOG (Fig. 1). After nasal irrigation with 5% zinc sulfate solution, the olfactory epithelium was histopathologically degenerated[2], and the EOG disappeared (Fig. 2). But after irrigation with distilled water, the olfactory epithelium was not degenerated and we obtained the normal EOG. Therefore, it was presumed that the EOG originated in the olfactory epithelium.

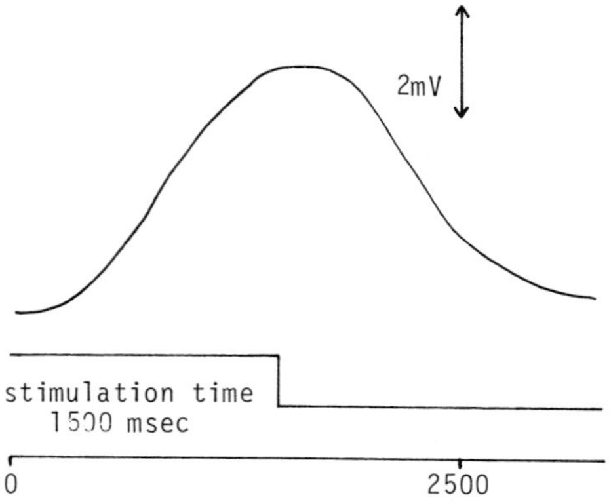

Fig. 1. Typical EOG in persons with normal sense of smell. Latency is 100 -200 msec, peak latency is 1600-1800 msec and amplitude is 2-6 mV.

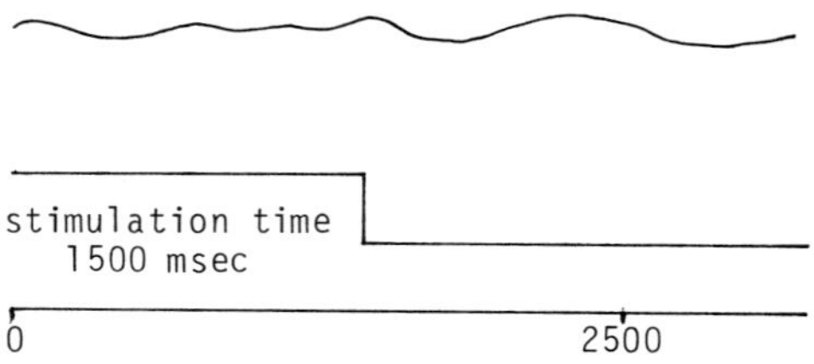

Fig. 2. EOG after nasal irrigation with 5% zinc sulfate solution. Olfactory epithelium is histopathologically degenerated.

CLINICAL APPLICATION OF THE EOG

The electrode and the odorous stimulation tube were connected with Olympus selfoscope SES 1711D, so that we could set them on the olfactory portion. When the persons with normal sense of smell were stimulated with Scatol, the slow negative potentials simillar to those in rabbits were obtained. But, when the same persons were stimulated with no odorous substance, we could not obtaine the EOG. In persons with normal sense of smell, the EOG evoked by the odorous substance was obtained in about 68%. In persons with peripheral dysosmia, the EOG was obtained in about 26%, and in anosmia the EOG was not obtained. In persons with central dysosmia, the EOG was obtained in about 69%, as same as in persons with normal sense of smell, and in spite of the anosmia, the EOG was obtained.

A CASE REPORT

The patient was a forty two years old female whose chief complaints were headache and unilateral hyposmia from two months ago. There was no remarkable finding in her nasal cavity and roentogenography of olfactory clefts and paranasal sinuses. The standard olfactory acuity test and the intravenous olfaction test widely used in Japan[3] revealed only right side severe hyposmia, but the typical slow negative potential was recorded in each sides. As the EOG originated from the olfactory epithelium under the fundamental examination of rabbits, we considered that hyposmia in this case was due to central disorder. As RI angiography, CT scan and right carotid angiography showed a typical frontal fossa tumor, total removal of tumor was performed by neurosurgeon. Histological examination revealed a typical meningioma with psammoma body and micronecrosis.

CONCLUSION

The EOG could be applied one of the useful objective examination of differential diagnosis in olfactory disturbance.

REFERENCES

1. Kamide M (1980) J Juzen Med Soc 89:1-23
2. Otosson D (1971) Handbook of Sensory Physiology, Springer Verlag., 4:95-131
3. Zusho H (1983) Rhinology 21:281-285

New dimensions in otorhinolaryngology – head and neck surgery, vol. 2.
E. Myers, editor

AMIDOLYTIC AND FIBRINOLYTIC ACTIVITY OF TISSUE PLASMINOGEN ACTIVATOR FROM PARANASAL MUCOUS MEMBRANE IN CHRONIC SINUSITIS

TADAYOSHI KOSUGI[1)], MASAHARU URA[2)], YUTAKA NODA[2)]
Departments of Physiology[1)] and Otorhinolaryngology[2)], School of Medicine, University of the Ryukyus, Okinawa, Japan

INTRODUCTION

In the otorhinolaryngological field, large amounts of tissue plasminogen activator (t-PA) have been reported to exist in the nasal and paranasal mucous membrane[1),2),3),4)].

Furthermore, it has been suggested that t-PA in paranasal mucous membrane with chronic sinusitis and antrochoanal polyp played an important role to enlarge and proliferate the mucous membrane[5)]. On the other hand, from the recent studies on thrombolytic therapy, it has been known that t-PA from melanoma cell was more useful to lyse the thrombus than urokinase. The present paper deals with t-PA from the paranasal mucous membrane of patients with chronic sinusitis, and attempts to clarify some of biochemical properties of t-PA, compared with those of urokinase, which may play an important role in lysing the thrombus.

MATERIALS AND METHODS

At first, acetone powder was prepared from paranasal mucous membrane in chronic sinusitis[6)]. 50 ml of 2 M KCl was added to 1.0 g of acetone powder, and the suspended solution was stirred at 4°C for overnight. After centrifugation at 10,000 g for 20 minutes, the resultant supernatant was used as the crude extract in the subsequent experiment. Zn-imminodiacetate-sepharose was equilibrated with 20 mM phosphate buffer (pH 8.0) containing 2 M KCl and 0.02 % Tween 80. The crude extract was applied to this Zn-imminodiacetate-sepharose and was washed with 20 mM phosphate buffer (pH 8.0) containing 0.02 % Tween 80. The elution was carried out using 20 mM phosphate buffer (pH 8.0) containing 0.02 % Tween 80 and 50 mM EDTA. The active fraction eluated from Zn-imminodiacetate-sepharose was collected and the collected eluates was then applied to lysine-sepharose. The lysine-sepharose was equilibrated with 20 mM phosphate buffer (pH 8.0) containing 0.02 % Tween 80 and was washed with the above buffer and the same buffer containing 0.15 M NaCl.

The elution was carried out using the same buffer containing 1 M KSCN. The amidolytic activity was estimated using synthetic substrate, S-2288. The fibrinolytic activity was determined by means of fibrin plate. Fibrinogen was purchased from Miles Laboratory.

RESULTS

1) Lysine-sepharose affinity chromatography of t-PA from paranasal mucous membrane

The starting buffer for elution was 20 mM phosphate-buffer containing 0.02 % Tween 80-0.15 M NaCl, and at the time when the eluted volume reached 30 ml, the column was eluated with the starting buffer containing 1 M KSCN. As shown in Figure 1, the active fraction of amidolytic activity was eluted from tube No. 35 to tube No. 40, and the active fraction of fibrinolytic activity was eluted from tube No. 40 to tube No. 60. These active fraction was collected and on the subsequent experiment, the collected fraction was used as a preparation of t-PA from paranasal mucous membrane.

2) Binding to fibrin of UK and t-PA from paranasal mucous membrane

As shown in Figure 2, the binding to fibrin of t-PA from paranasal mucous membrane was stronger than that of UK. Furthermore, the binding to human fibrin of t-PA and UK was stronger than that to bovine fibrin.

DISCUSSION

It has been clarified that t-PA from paranasal mucous membrane has the high affinity to human fibrin. Furthermore, the fibrinolytic activity of UK was easy to inactivate by human plasma but it of t-PA from paranasal mucous membrane was resistant to inactivate. On the above-mentioned character of t-PA from paranasal mucous membrane, it was suggested that t-PA from paranasal mucous membrane was more effective and useful to thrombolyse than UK.

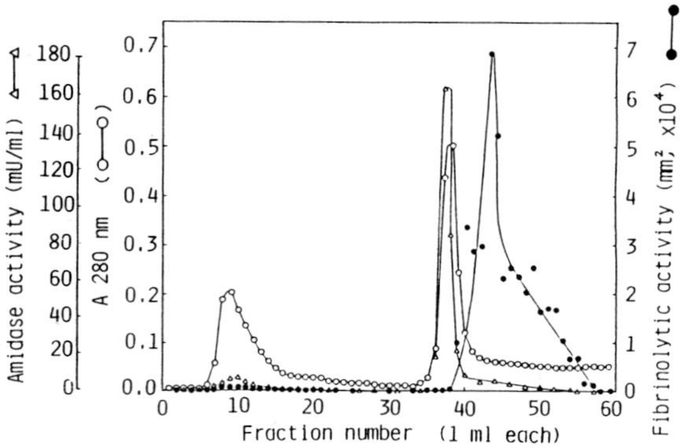

Fig. 1. Lysine-sepharose affinity chromatography. Amidase activity was determined using S-2288, and fibrinolytic activity was determined by means of fibrin plate.

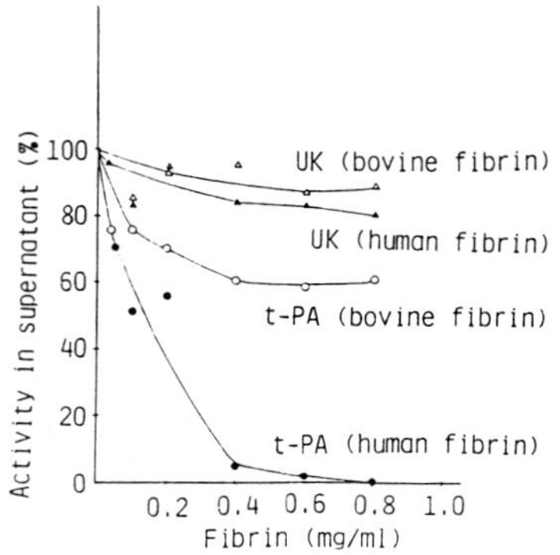

Fig. 2. Binding to fibrin of UK and t-PA from paranasal mucous membrane. After UK or t-PA was incubated with various concentration of fibrinogen and thrombin, the fibrinolytic activity of supernatant of this mixture was measured. Decreased activity in supernatant indicates strong affinity to fibrin.

REFERENCES

1. Sasaki Y, Okamoto S, Ohwada K, Nishibata T. (1959) Some observations on a remarkable fibrinolytic activity in the extract of nasal tissues and related tissue. Keio J Med 8: 235-246

2. Sasaki Y (1968) The electrophoretic analysis of the nasal fibrinolytic enzyme. Acta Otolaryngol 65:346-358

3. Kosugi T, Takagi I, Matsuo O, Mihara H, Morimitsu T, Hirano K, Hamaya, M. (1981) Characteristics of tissue plasminogen activator from paranasal mucous membrane in chronic sinusitis -Tissue plasminogen activator with low molecular weight- Rhinology, Suppl. 2:105-130

4. Kosugi T, et al. (1981) Differences in physicochemical properties between tissue plasminogen activator from human paranasal mucous membrane and pig heart. Auris Nasus Larynx 8:77-80

5. Kosugi T, et al. (1982) Differentiation of proactivator from tissue plasminogen activator with low molecular weight in the paranasal mucous membrane. Auris Nasus Larynx 9:99-104

6. Kosugi T, et al. (1982) Characteristics of tissue plasminogen activator from paranasal mucous membrane in chronic sinusitis. Ann Oto Rhin Laryng 91(1):101-105

© 1985 Elsevier Science Publishers B.V. (Biomedical Division)
New dimensions in otorhinolaryngology - head and neck surgery, vol. 2.
E. Myers, editor

ELECTRONMICROSCOPIC HISTOCHEMISTRY OF THE SEROUS SECRETORY GRANULES IN THE HUMAN NASAL AND SALIVARY GLANDS

M MACHINO, M TACHIBANA, M HIRAYAMA*, H HAMA and O MIZUKOSHI

Department of Otolaryngology, Kyoto Prefectural University of Medicine, Kyoto, Japan 606 *Department of Otorhinolaryngology, Matsushita Hospital, Moriguchi, Osaka, Japan 570

INTRODUCTION

Electron microscopy has demonstrated that the matrix within the serous secretory granule is mainly composed of two substructures; the electron opaque central core and the electron lucent rim surrounding the central core. We made an attempt to trace the morphological relationship between substances in the matrix and the two substructures. Using electron microscopic histochemistry, amylase, lysozyme and glycoconjugates were studied in the serous secretory granule of the human nasal and salivary glandular cells.

MATERIALS AND METHODS

Tissues of the inferior turbinate, parotid and submaxillary glands were obtained surgically from patients. Tissues were fixed in 1% glutaraldehyde, dehydrated in ethanol, and embedded in Epon 812. Thin sections were mounted on uncoated nickel or copper grids. (a) Immunogold staining by protein A-gold (pAg) technique. Sections on some nickel grids were incubated in the diluted (1:400) goat antiserum to human amylase and in pAg solution (a particle, 5 or 15 nm). Sections on the other nickel grids were incubated in the diluted (1:2000) goat antiserum to human lysozyme and in pAg (15 nm). (b) Simultaneous staining of both enzymes by double labelling technique[1]. Antigenic sites of amylase were labelled with small gold particles (5 nm) and ones of lysozyme with large gold particles (15 nm). Staining with lectin-gold complex. Sections on the copper grids were incubated in wheat germ agglutinin (WGA)-gold solution.

RESULTS AND DISCUSSICNS

Amylase localised cver the rim and lysozyme over the central core (Fig. 1). WGA binding sites localised over the rim (Fig. 2). Controls for the specificity of the reactions were satisfactory.

Amylase tended to disperse in the rim with rich glycoconjugates. Lysozyme tended to localise in the central core. Functional significance of the distributional dissociation of both enzymes in a serous secretory granule is unkown[2].

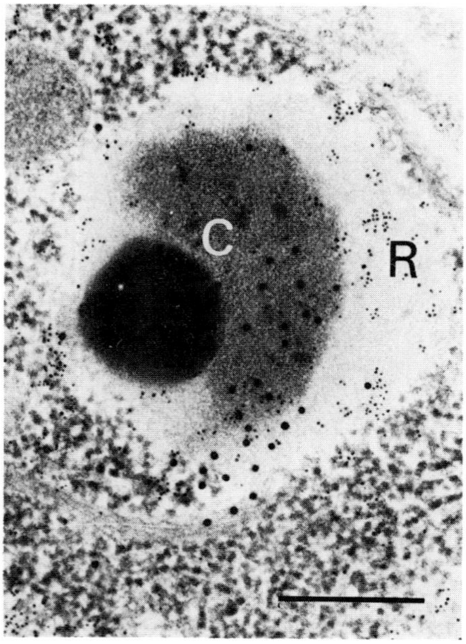

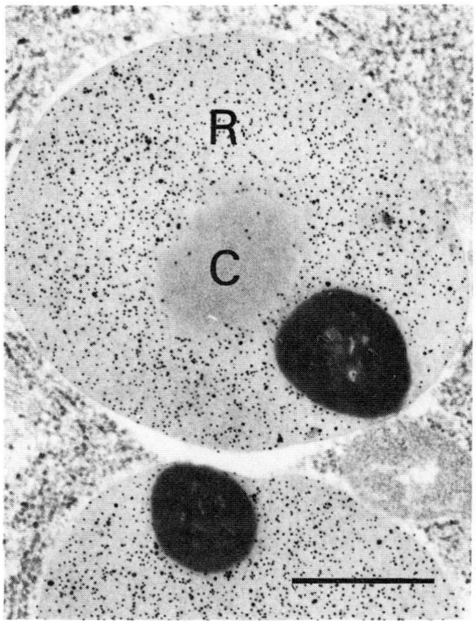

Fig. 1. Simultaneous localisation of amylase and lysozyme. Amylase (as revealed by the small gold particles) localised over the rim and lysozyme (as revealed by the large gold particles) over the central core. Fig. 2. Staining with WGA-gold complex. Rim was stained heavily. Counterstained with uranyl acetate and lead citrate. C: central core, R: rim. Scale bar = 0.5 nm.

REFERENCES

1. Bendayan M, Stephens H (1984) In: Polak JM, Varndell IM (eds) Immunolabelling for Electron Microscopy. Elsevier, Amsterdam, pp 143-154

2. Varndell IM, Polak JM (1984) In: Polak JM. Varndell IM (eds) Immunolabelling for Electron Microscopy. Elsevier, Amsterdam, pp 155-177

New dimensions in otorhinolaryngology – head and neck surgery, vol. 2.
E. Myers, editor

PRELIMINARY OBSERVATIONS ON MEDIATORS IN RHINOVIRUS-INDUCED COLDS

ROBERT NACLERIO, JACK GWALTNEY, OWEN HENDLEY, CLAUS BAUMGARTEN, ANN KAGEY-SOBOTKA, DENISE BARTENFELDER, PAT BEASLEY, LAWRENCE LICHTENSTEIN, DAVID PROUD
Departments of Otolaryngology and Medicine, Johns Hopkins University, Baltimore, Maryland, and University of Virginia, Charlottesville, Virginia

INTRODUCTION

Rhinovirus infections cause 1/3 of all upper respiratory tract infections and are the major cause for absence from work and school. Thus, it is surprising that relatively few investigations into the pathophysiology of this disease have been done. To further our understanding of the pathophysiology of rhinovirus infections, we inoculated volunteers with live virus, assessed their symptoms, and collected their nasal secretions for the measurement of inflammatory mediators. The aim of these investigations is to identify one or more mediators which are responsible for inducing the symptoms of the infections.

MATERIAL AND METHODS

Study Design. Thirteen healthy volunteers, students attending the University of Virginia, with negative serum titers of neutralizing antibody to the type of rhinovirus used for inoculation were recruited.

We collected secretions by nasal lavage with normal saline as previously described (1). The lavages began prior to inoculation with either type 39 rhinovirus (n=9) or placebo (n=4) and continued every 4 hours for the next 5 days. During the experiment, subjects were placed in isolation. Symptom diaries were obtained before each nasal lavage. The symptoms of nasal congestion, sneezing, rhinorrhea, headache, cough, and malaise, were assessed individually on a scale of 0 to 4.

Mediator Assays. The nasal lavages were centrifuged and then frozen until they were assayed. The assays for histamine, albumin, TAME-esterase activity, and kinins are all standard, previously described techniques (1,2).

RESULTS

During the study, 7 subjects became ill (feeling of having had a cold plus a total symptom score of >15) and infected (increase in the serum titer of neutralizing antibody and/or a positive nose or throat culture for rhinovirus). Two subjects inoculated with the virus became infected but did not develop symptoms. The 4 placebo inoculations did not cause symptoms or infection. Results for the parameters measured are listed in Table 1. The subjects are divided into 2 groups, ill and non-ill, based on the presence or absence of symptoms.

TABLE I

AVERAGE DAILY RESULTS (mean ± SD)

DAY	1	2	3	4	5
ILL					
Symptoms	.3±.3[d]	3.9±2.2[c]	3.6±2[b]	2.5±1.0[b]	1.6±.9[b]
Kinins (ng/ml)	.09±.01[d]	1.6±1.3[a]	2.7±1.7[b]	1.8±.9[b]	1.2±.8[d]
TAME ($CPMx10^{-3}$)	2.5±1.2[d]	8.0±5.3[a]	8.1±3.4[b]	4.9±2.9[d]	4.0±2.8[d]
Albumin (µg/ml)	15.1± 8[d]	206±224[d]	335±253[a]	165±113[a]	106±113[a]
Histamine (ng/ml)	1.4±.8[d]	1.3±.9[d]	1.2±.4[d]	1.1±.2[d]	1.2±.1[d]
NON-ILL					
Symptoms	.4±.4	.7±.9	.6±7	.5±.6	.2±4
Kinins (ng/ml)	.07±.03	.12±.09	.2±.19	.2±.2	.8±1.4
TAME ($CPMx10^{-3}$)	1.8±.5	2.1±1.2	2.5±1.1	2.4±1.1	2.7±.6
Albumin (µg/ml)	26±25	29±15	33±11	44±15	38±32
Histamine (ng/ml)	2.0±2.0	2.9±3.1	2.8±3.4	3.0±4.0	1.9±2.1

a = $p < .05$, b = $p < 0.01$, c = $p < .001$, d = NS

DISCUSSION

We have demonstrated a temporal association between the occurrence of symptoms induced by rhinovirus infection and increases in the levels of kinins, albumin, and TAME-esterase activity but not in the level of histamine. Kinins are potent inflammatory peptides with the ability to induce all the symptoms of rhinovirus-induced colds. However, documenting their presence during the symptoms does not prove that kinins are responsible for them. The increase in TAME-esterase activity probably represents activity induced by glandular and plasma kallikrein, enzymes capable of generating kinins. Since albumin is not produced in the nose, the increases found suggest that there is an increase in nasal vascular permeability, which probably contributes to the increase in nasal secretions. Histamine, which comes only from mast cells or basophils, did not change during the course of the experiments. Therefore, we conclude that these cells are not involved in the pathophysiology of rhinovirus-induced colds. In total, these results show that this method of study has great potential for adding to our knowledge about the pathophysiology of this illness. Once the mediators causing the symptoms of rhinovirus colds are defined, there is a potential for defining new therapeutic agents.

REFERENCES

1. Naclerio RM, Meier HL, Kagey-Sobotka A, Adkinson NF Jr, Meyers DA, Norman PS, Lichtenstein, LM (1983) Am Rev Respir Dis 128:597-602.

2. Proud D, Togias A, Naclerio RM, Crush SA, Norman PS, Lichtenstein LM (1983) J Clin Invest 72:1678-1685.

© 1985 Elsevier Science Publishers B.V. (Biomedical Division)
New dimensions in otorhinolaryngology - head and neck surgery, vol. 2.
E. Myers, editor

QUANTITATIVE ANALYSIS OF SIALIC ACID AND L-FUCOSE IN PATIENTS WITH CHRONIC SINUSITIS OR NASAL ALLERGY

KAZUAKI OGAWA, KAZUNORI ITOH, AKIHIRO UCHIZONO, MASARU OHYAMA
Department of Otolaryngology, Faculty of Medicine, Kagoshima University, Kagoshima Japan

Quantitative analysis of sialic acid and L-fucose in the serum, tissue extract and nasal secretion of patients with chronic sinusitis or nasal allergy was performed to clarify the pathogenesis of these diseases. Sialic acid was measured by the thiobarbituric acid method of Aminoff and L-fucose by the cysteine sulfate method of Winzler.

1) There was no significant difference in serum sialic acid concentration among normal volunteers (n=15), patients with nasal allergy (n=21) and those with chronic sinusitis (n=11) (see fig.1). The concentration of serum fucose was significantly higher in patients with nasal allergy (20.7±8.4mg/dl) or chronic sinusitis (38.1±20.6mg/dl) than in the normal volunteers (9.8±4.8mg/dl) (see fig.1). Moreover, there was a significant correlation between the serum fucose level and the X-ray findings of the sinuses or rhinoscopic finding of nasal polyps in the patients with chronic sinusitis (see fig.2).

2) The concentration of sialic and was higher in the maxillary mucosa of patients with chronic sinustitis (0.99±0.29mg/ml, n=9) and nasal polyp (0.99±0.74mg/ml, n=9) than in the inferior turbinates of those with nasal allergy (0.38±0.22mg/ml, n=4). In contrast, the concentration of fucose was higher in the inferior turbinates of patients with nasal allergy (1.41±0.43mg/ml, n=4) than in those with maxillary mucosa of chronic sinusitis (0.69±0.34mg/ml, n=9) or nasal polyp (0.48±0.14mg/ml, n=7) (see fig.3).

3) Concentrations of both sialic acid and fucose were significantly higher in nasal secretions (1.51±0.66mg/ml, n=26, 1.41±0.61mg/ml, n=20) and retention fluid in the maxillary antrum (0.99±0.29mg/ml, n=9, 0.54±0.28mg/ml, n=4) of patients with chronic sinusitis that in those with nasal secretions due to nasal allery (0.42±0.33mg/ml, n=11, 0.24±0.12mg/ml, n=11) (see fig.4).

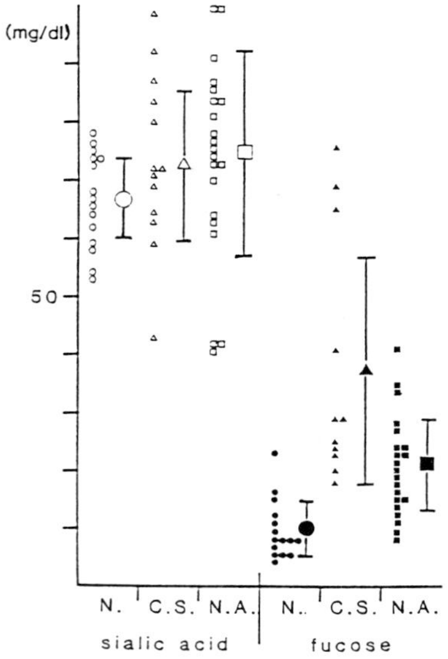

Fig.1 Quantity of serum sialic acid and fucose in normal volunteers and patients with chronic sinusitis or nasal allergy

N. normal volunteer
C.S. chronic sinusitis
N.A. nasal allergy
○ 67.0 ± 7.9 mg/dl (n = 15)
△ 73.9 ± 15.4 mg/dl (n = 11)
□ 74.6 ± 18.4 mg/dl (n = 21)
● 9.8 ± 4.8 mg/dl (n = 15)
▲ 38.1 ± 20.6 mg/dl (n = 11)
■ 20.7 ± 8.4 mg/dl (n = 21)
▲ > ● (P < 0.005)
■ > ● (P < 0.005)
▲ > ■ (P < 0.005)

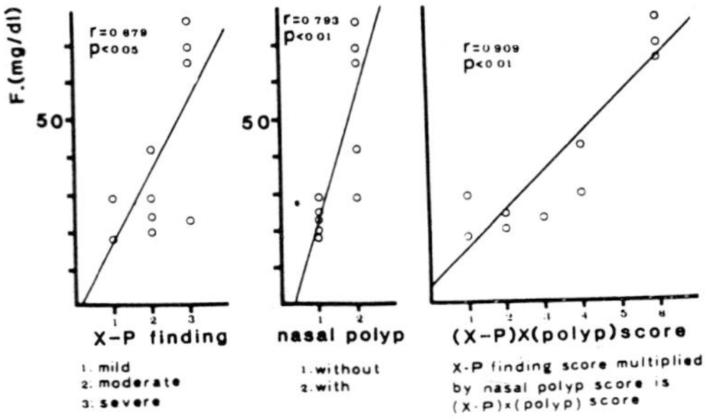

Fig.2 Correlation between serum fucose and some clinical findings of chronic sinusitis

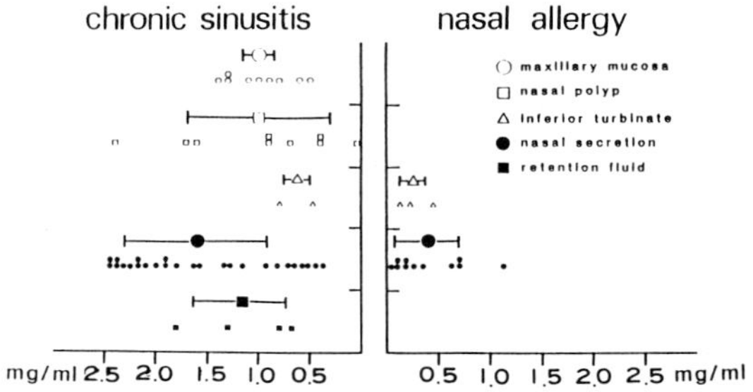

Fig.3 Quantitative analysis of sialic acid of tissue extracts, nasal secretions and retention fluids in the patients with chronic sinusitis or nasal allergy

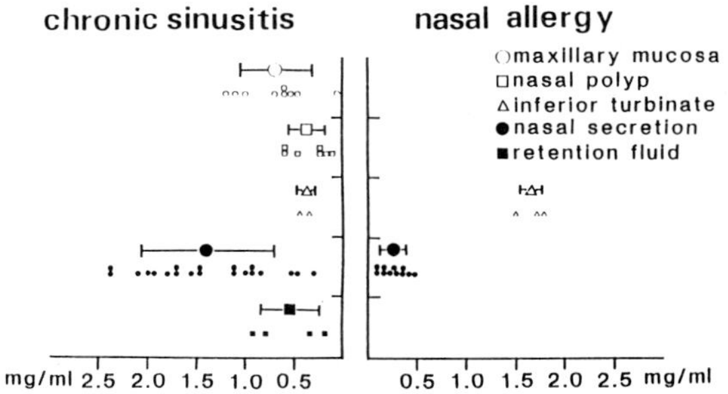

Fig.4 Quantitative analysis of L-fucose of tissue extracts, nasal secretions and retention fluids in the patients with chronic sinusitis or nasal allergy

© 1985 Elsevier Science Publishers B.V. (Biomedical Division)
New dimensions in otorhinolaryngology - head and neck surgery, vol. 2.
E. Myers, editor

COMPARATIVE HISTOCHEMICAL STUDY OF GLYCOCONJUGATES OF NASAL AND PARANASAL MUCOSA IN MAMMALIAN

KAZUYO TANAKA , KOZO FUKAMI , MASARU OHYAMA
Department of Otolaryngology, Faculty of Medicine,
Kagoshima university, Kagoshima, Japan

INTRODUCTION

Glicoconjugates are divided broadly into glycoprotein, preteoglycan and glycolipid. In recent years a special attention to glycoprotein and proteoglycan of them have been focused in a sphere of histochemistry.

In this study, the glycoconjugates of nasal and paranasal mucosa in some mammalian were studied histochemically from the point of view of their function and character among the different species.

MATERIAL AND METHODS

Nasal and paranasal mucosa were used in tow normal rabbits, three normal cats, six normal monkeys, five rabbits with experimentally induced sinusitis and 20 patients with chronic sinusitis.

After AB-PAS method, HID-AB method and HE staining, light microscopic observations were performed, and for observation by erectron microscope, PA-TCH-SP method was used.

RESULTS

In nasal and paranasal mucosa, goblet cells contain large amounts of sulfomucin independent of species. It may play a functional role in point of mucosal defence and lubication during the mucociliary transport.

In the glandular cells of human nasal mucosa, it was found mainly sulfomucin, in the mucous cells of upper area and sialomucin in those of deeper area. While, in paranasal mucosa, there were few secretory cells and they have a little amount of glycoconjugates.

The secretory cells of cat nasal mucosa contained much more sulfomucin as compared with the others.

It was of interest that there was a characteristic feature in the glandular cells of rabbit, showing nasal mucosa contained mainly sulfomucin and paranasal mucosa contained only neutral glycoprotein.

In the rabbit with the experimental sinusitis, their mucosa were stained as well as that of normal rabbit.

REFERENCES

1. Spicer SS (1980) Am J Anat 158: 93-109
2. Taete LG (1981) Am J Anat 162: 243-263
3. Spicer SS (1979) J Histochem Cytochem 27:1182-1184
4. Ohyama M (1984) Pathobiochemistry of chronic sinusitis, Shibundo, Kagoshima, pp 132-135
5. Spicer SS (1981) J Histochem Cytochem 29:994-1002
6. Fukami K (1986) Pract Otol KYOTO 79 (in press)

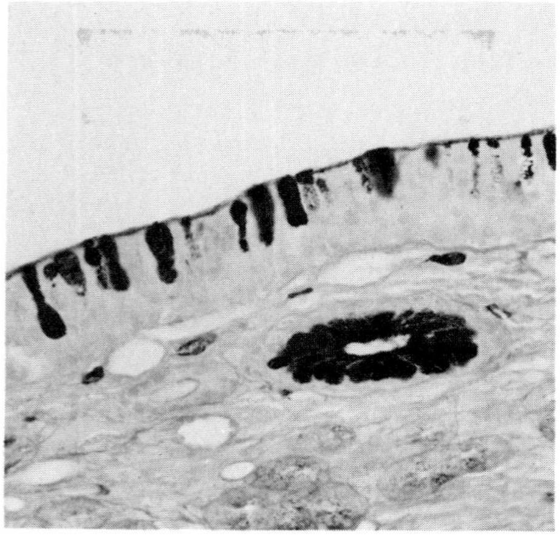

Fig.1 monkey nasal mucosa stained with HID-AB

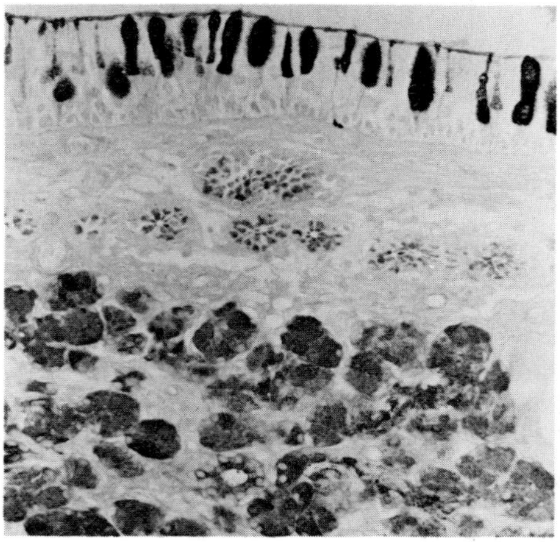

Fig.2 monkey nasal mucosa stained with AB-PAS

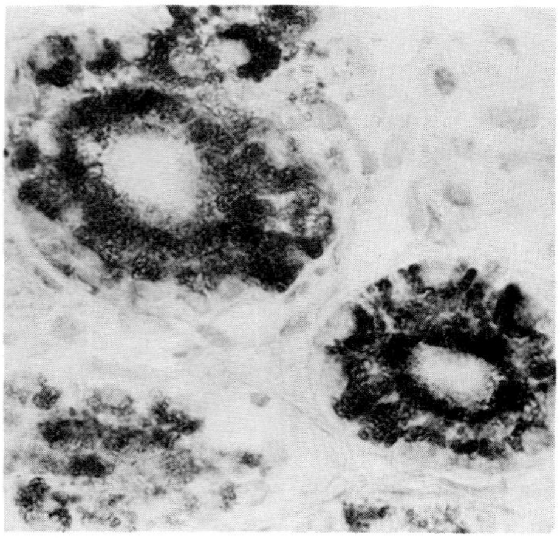

Fig.3 monkey paranasal mucosa stained with HID-AB

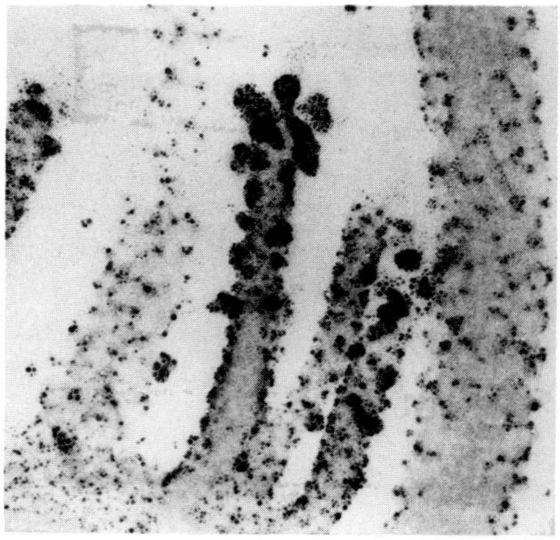

Fig.4 monkey nasal mucosa stained with PA-TCH-SP

New dimensions in otorhinolaryngology - head and neck surgery, vol. 2.
E. Myers, editor

IMMUNOHISTOCHEMICAL AND BIOCHEMICAL STUDY OF COMPLEMENT IN NASAL AND PARANASAL DISEASES

AKIHIRO UCHIZONO, YUTAKA HANAMURE, SHIGERU FURUTA AND MASARU OHYAMA
Department of Otolaryngology, Faculty of Medicine, Kagoshima University, 1208-1 Usuki-cho, Kagoshima, Japan

INTRODUCTION

It has been pointed out that there are important roles of the complement system in the mucosal pathology of the nasal and paranasal cavity. This paper is concerned with immunochemical and immunohistochemical studies of the complement in these subjects.

MATERIALS AND METHODS

Distribution of C3 and C5

The distribution of C3 and C5 in the mucous membrane of the nose were studied with PAP method. Inferior turbinates and nasal polyps of the patients with chronic sinusitis and inferior turbinates of the patients with nasal allergy were used.

Concentration of C3, C4 and C5

Complement proteins C3, C4 and C5 in nasal discharges, extracts of tissue and sera of the patients with the nasal and paranasal diseases were measured using the single radial immunodiffusion method.

RESULTS

Immunohistochemical studies

C3 was diffusely noted in capillaries and lamina propria of the nasal mucous membrane and nasal polyp. On the other hand, no specific distribution of C5 was seen in this study.

Immunochemical studies

Figure 1 shows the complement proteins in sera. In both patients with chronic sinusitis and nasal allergy, C3, C4 and C5 concentration showed in normal range. But in comparing both chronic sinusitis and nasal allergy, the latter seemed to show the tendency of low concentration.

Figure 2 shows the results of the nasal secretions and tissue extracts. All of C3, C4 and C5 in the nasal secretions of the patients with chronic sinusitis had about one forth to one sixth that of the normal serum level. On the other hand, in those of patients with nasal allergy, no component was detected. Futhermore, in those of of patients with acute rhinitis,only C5 was detected to have a normal serum level. In the extracts of the maxillary mucosa,C3 and C4 were detected to be relatively less than in the nasal secretions. Conversely,C5 was detected to be relatively more than in the nasal discharges.

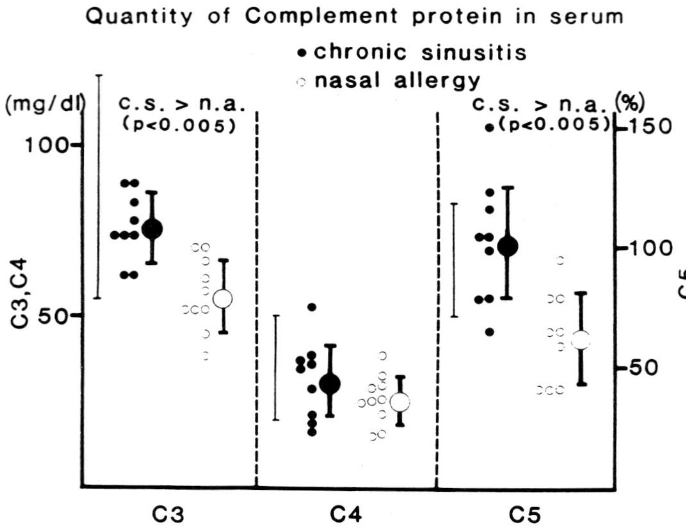

Fig. 1. Complement proteins in sera

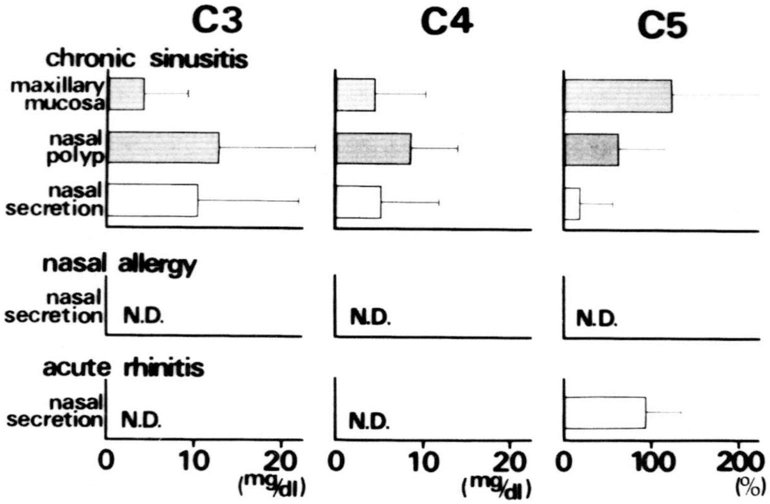

Fig.2. Complement proteins in nasal discharges and tissue extracts

New dimensions in otorhinolaryngology - head and neck surgery, vol. 2.
E. Myers, editor

ABSORBANCE SPECTROPHOTOMETRIC ANALYSIS FOR THE MUCOUS MEMBRANE IN NASAL AND PARANASAL SINUS DISEASES

HIROMI YANO, SHIGERU FURUTA, SUMIJI YASHIKAWA AND MASARU OHYAMA
Department of Otolaryngology, Faculty of Medicine, Kagoshima University, 1208-1 Usuki-cho, Kagoshima, Japan

INTRODUÇTION

By converting the reflectance spectra with a computer, absorbance spectra of various mucosal pathologies in the nose were analized, and tried mesurement of the blood flow volume of the nasal mucosa using hydrogen decomposition in order to compare with the results of spectral analysis.

MATERIAL AND METHODS

Fig. 1 shows the Blockdiagram of our reflectance spectrophotometer system. After hitting by the natural light on the subject through fibers, the reflectance light was accumulated coxially and absorbance spectral curve was extracted through photometer mediating computer. To compare each curves, we defined the spectral strength (A1 and A2, as shown in Fig. 2, which absorbance spectral shape in normal volunteer indicates in the curve.).

RESULTS

Fig. 3 shows time cource mesurement of absorbance spectra in the inferior turbinate mucosa before and after laryngectomy in the patients with laryngeal cancer. Fig. 4 shows various degrees of spectral changes of the inferior turbinates mucosa in 20 cases who received laryngectomy during follow up period. Fig. 5 is representation cases of absorbance spectra from the nasal mucosa with allergic rhinitis. In these cases, mean values of A1 and A2 were 13.35 and 15.53 respectively, in spite of the average value of 14.58 and 15.48 in normal volunteers. Table. 1 shows the relationship between strength of absorbance spectra and blood flow volume. As compared to normal group, in the group with allergy, blood flow volume was slightly less and strength of absorbance spectra was lower. In the group with chronic nasosinusitis, the result was more distinctly.
The color tone of the mucous membrane of the superior respiratory tract including nasal one, which had been grasped only subjectively, came able to be expressed as figures and recorded.

Therefore, we believe that this method may be effective for clinical practice.

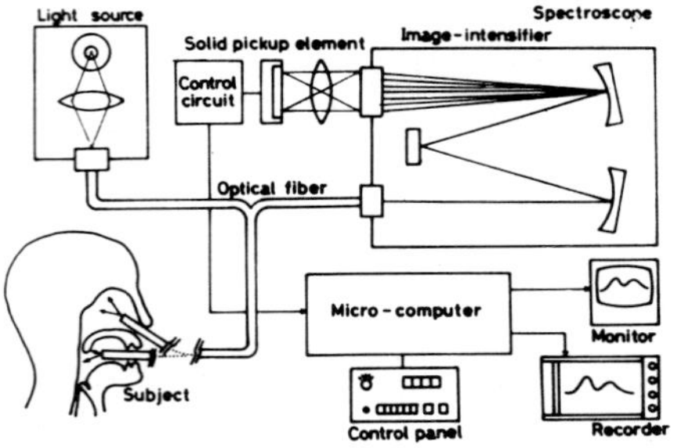

Fig. 1

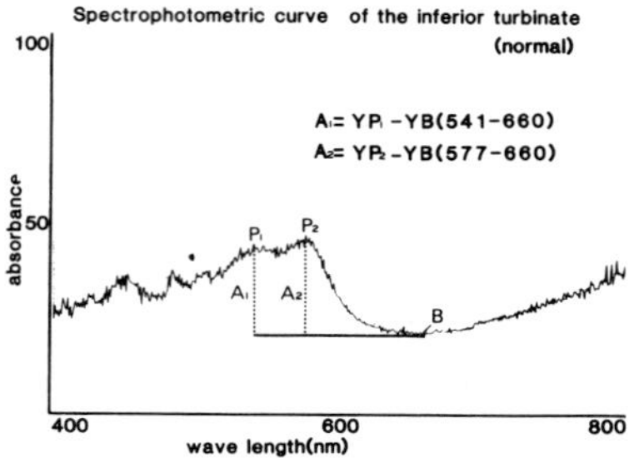

Fig. 2

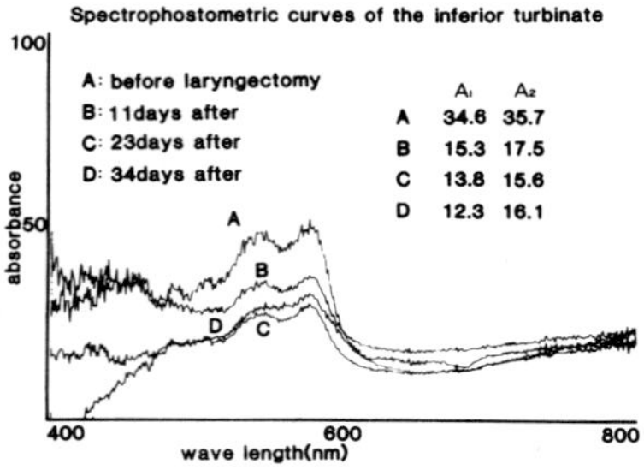

Fig. 3

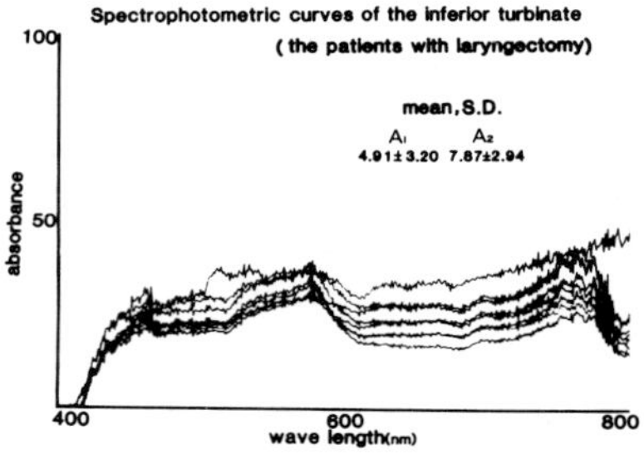

Fig. 4

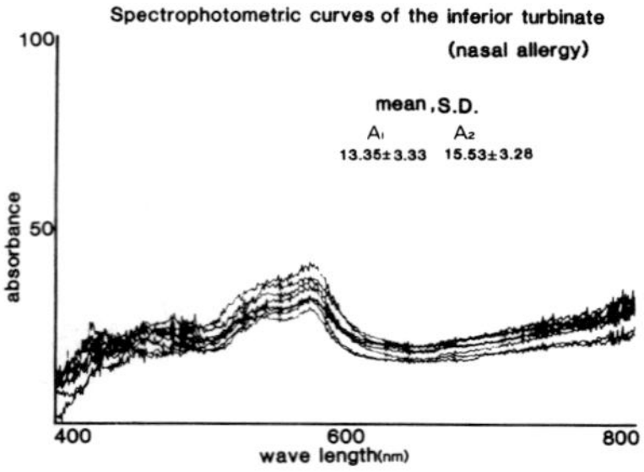

Fig. 5

ABSORBANCE INDEX AND BLOOD FLOW

		NORMAL	SINUSITIS CHR.	NASAL ALLERGY
ABSORBANCE INDEX	A_1	22.3	19.3	13.35
	A_2	24.9	21.9	15.53
BLOOD FLOW (ml/min/100g)		144.1	126.3	98.7

Fig. 6

REFERENCE

1 . MASARU OHYAMA . et al. : Reflectance spectrophotometric studies on mucosal pathology of the upper airway. Laryngoscope, 92 : 1168-1172 , 1982 .

New dimensions in otorhinolaryngology - head and neck surgery, vol. 2.
E. Myers, editor

MORPHOLOGICAL BASES OF ECHOLOCATION IN THE BAT: RHINOLOPHUS FERRUMEQUINUM

J. SLOCKER, L. CABEZUDO, J. ANTOLI-CANDELA, F. ANTOLI-CANDELA
Departamento de Otorrinolaringología, Centro Ramón y Cajal, Madrid, España

INTRODUCTION

The larynx of the bat emits pulses of high frequency sounds. The echoes of these sounds are received by the ear, coded and delivered to the CNS to be analyzed. This information allows them to get oriented in space and hunt their prey in complete darkness. The bat's high frequency emitter and receptor organs have been studied to establish the morphological bases of Echolocation.

MATERIAL AND METHODS

The larynges and both ears of seven specimens of Rhinolophus ferrumequinum (RF), were processed with the Schuknecht's histological technique. Serial 20 µm thick sections were obtained in the three perpendicular planes. Every third section was stained in hematoxylin-eosin for a quantitative study under the light microscope.

RESULTS

The larynx of the RF is a tubular formation situated in a high position on the animal's neck. Its upper orifice opens into the rhinopharynx by means of a chimney like structure which is formed by the epiglotic cartilage and the ary-epiglotic ligaments. The epiglotis appears in contact with the soft palate, so there is no direct comunication between nasal and oral cavities. From the latter, two pharyngeal alimentary ducts emerge, ending posteriorly in the esophagus.

The cartilaginous skeleton of the RF is basically similar to that found in other mammals. However, it presents many osteocartilaginous expansions which serve for the anchoring of a large muscular system. The posterior cricoarytenoid and cricothyroid muscles wrap around the larynx and are so developed that they hide the other intrinsic muscles. The thyroid and cricoid cartilages show many areas of ossification. In contrast, the arytenoids have a fully cartilaginous consistence. Their apical tips fuse in the middle line forming an arch covered by a common perichomdrium. They also have an unusual anterosuperior placement of the interarytenoid muscle.

In the laryngeal lumen the vocal membranes have a laminar structure and run parallel to the vocal muscle from the vocal apophysis of the arytenoids to the thyroid angle. At the level of their insertion, on their posterior end, they widen markedly acquireing a ligamentous apperance hardened by cartilage. They project towards the middle line and are covered by a flat epithelial lining.

In the middle ear cavity, as in other bats (1), the ossicular chain is firmly attached to its walls. The tensor tympany muscle has an enormeous size but it has few muscular fibers. Its tendinous portion occupies more than 50% of the volume. The Os Quartum (2) is also found in the stapedial muscle.

In the cochlea: The cochlear duct has an average of 12,61 mm of length and its examination reveals a great development os the anchoring system of the basilar membrane, spiral limbus, spiral ligament and both osseous spiral laminas (Fig. 1).

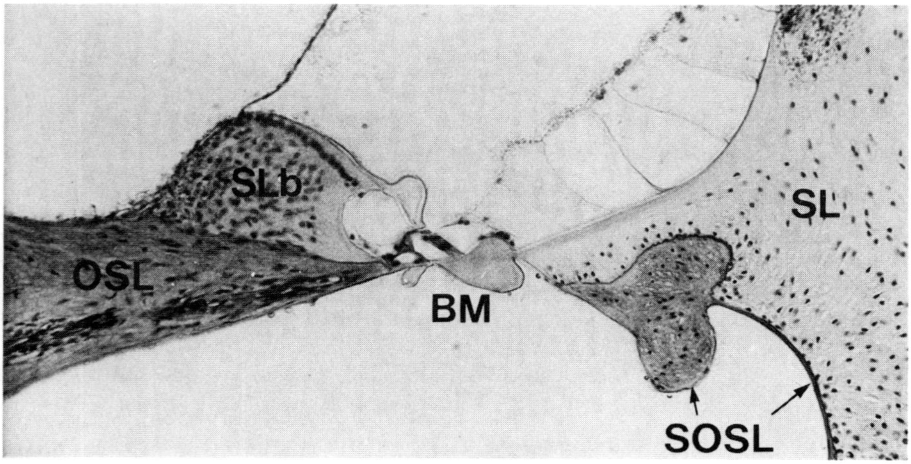

Fig. 1. A section of the Cochlear Duct showing: The Osseous Spiral Lamina (OSL), the Secundary Osseous Spiral Lamina (SOSL), the Spiral Limbus (SLb), the Spiral Ligament (SL) and the Basilar Membrane (BM). Notice the great lanceolate shaped enlargment of SOSL, and the thickening of BM at this level.

The secundary osseous spiral lamina is present even at the level of the apex, showing a considerable broadening of a lanceolate shape along the basal turn. The basilar membrane has two pronounced thickenings in the areas of the "pars tecta" and "pars pectinata", its narrowest point being halway along the cochlear lenght (Fig. 2).

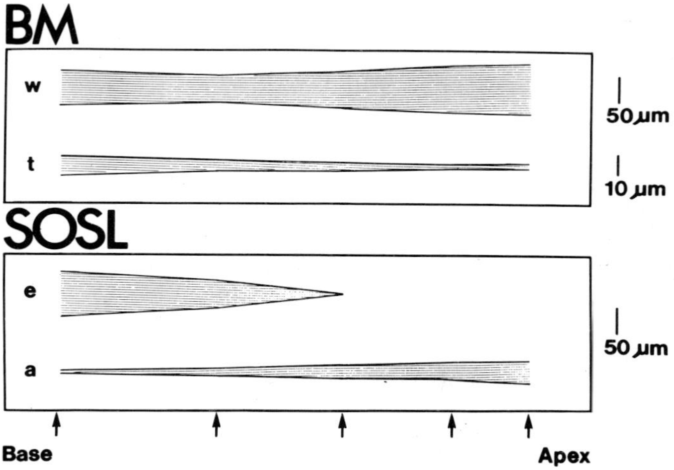

Fig. 2. Schematic representation of the Basilar Membrane (BM) and the Secundary Osseous Spiral Lamina (SOSL). w) represents the width, t) the thickness, e) the width of the enlargement of SOSL and a) the thickness of its attachment to the endostal surface of the Cochlear Capsule. Arrows indicate the localization of the measured points along the Cochlear Duct.

CONCLUSIONS

The above described structure of the emitter and receptor organs of the RF could account for Echolocation. As in other bats (3, 4), the laminar structure of the vocal membranes are subjected to the powerful tensile action of extremly developed muscles. These are anchored on a partialy ossified cartilaginous skeleton with little mobility. The closure of the glottis needed for the increase of the subglottic preassure (3) can't be achieved by the thin vocal membranes, but by its posterior "ligamentous" broadening. In the ear, the characteristics of the ossicular chain facilitate the transmission of ultrasounds (1), and so do the long basal turn of the cochlea. The particular disposition of the osseous spiral lamina and the thickening of the basilar membrane in this area (5), might make the region sensitive to a shorter range of high frequencies than in other bats.

REFERENCES

1. Henson, O.W. (1970). Biology of Bats II, 181-262.
2. Klaauw, C.J. van der. (1923). Z. Anat. EntwGesch, 69: 32-83.
3. Griffiths, T.A. (1983). Mammalia, 47: 377-394.
4. Griffin, D.R. (1952). Fed. Proc., 11:59.
5. Bruns, V. (1980). Anat. Embriol., 161: 29-50.

© 1985 Elsevier Science Publishers B.V. (Biomedical Division)
New dimensions in otorhinolaryngology - head and neck surgery, vol. 2.
E. Myers, editor

COMPARATIVE ANALYSIS OF TISSUE ALTERATIONS FOUND IN THE TONSIL BEDS OF DOGS OPERATED THROUGH CONVENTIONAL SURGERY OR USING CO2 LASER

MARCO ELISABETSKY, LUIZ CARLOS DA COSTA GAYOTTO, JOÃO BATISTA FERREIRA, ELISARIO PEREIRA NETO
Faculdade de Medicina da Universidade de São Paulo - Brasil

INTRODUCTION

LASER (Light Amplification by Stimulated Emission of Radiation) has been used for several purposes, being nowadays a noteworthy resource for biological research and a promising therapeutic instrument in Medical Science. The first Laser system was developed by Maiman in 1960 using ruby cristal. Other forms of Laser such as Argonium, Neodimium, Helium, Neonium, CO_2, etc, were subsequently developed.

In Otholaryngology pulsatile Lasers were tried by different authors between 1965 and 1967. A CO_2 continuous form of Laser has been developed, its energy being totally absorbed by the biological tissues; consequently it became feasible the making of incisions and even the removal or vaporization of tissues. Strong and Jako initiated in 1971 the use in human larynx this type of continuous CO_2 Laser.

In medical literature the hemostatic effect of Laser is widely described, but its result on healing is scarcely described, frequently contraditory, reason why this paper is presented.

MATERIAL AND METHODS

Twelve dogs weighing between 25 and 35 Kgs. were used for this experiment, divided into three groups A, B and C with 4 dogs each. Those of group A were submited to bi-lateral tonsilectomy using CO_2 Laser; the ones of group B were operated using conventional technique and those of group C were operated on the left side using CO_2 Laser and on the right side by conventional technique. The animals sacrifice was performed, half of each group in the 9th day and the other half on the 16th day.

The tonsil beds were ressected and submitted to macroscopic examination by the pathologists, and the microscopic examination was done using standardized cuts of 4μ thickness.

The following variables were investigated: fibrin, edema, vascular neo-formation, vase-dilation, volume of the endotelial cells, inflammatory cells, comprising neutrophils, eosinophils, lymphocytes, plasmocytes, besides the mesenchimal cells, including histiocytes cells and fibroblasts.

Macroscopically what was noticed in the tonsil beds of the dogs sacrificed in the 9th and 16th days, was the following: in those operated by the conventional technique, the aspect was of shallow bottom, and early signs of cicatrization: in those operated by Laser we noticed that the tonsil beds became deep and wide wounds, with irregular and dark bottoms and delayed cicatrization.

Microscopically it was noticed that on the 9th day the exsudative phenomena were more intense in the dogs operated with Laser: statistically significative differences were noticed between both techniques regarding the quantification of edema, fibrin, and specially that of neutrophiles with high significance ($p < 0{,}001$).

Regarding the evolution of the inflammatory phenomena of the 9th and 16th days, it was noticed a reduction of the vaso-exsudative reaction in both groups, as well as lower degree of inflammatory infiltrate.

CONCLUSIONS

The healing process of dogs tonsil beds operated with Laser is delayed when compared with conventional technique. The conventional technique yields a faster maturation of the granulation tissue, an early healing and a faster reepitelization.

REFERENCES

1. Mester E (1976) Clinical results of wound healing stimulation with Laser and experimental studies of the action mechanism. In: Kaplan I., ed - Proceedings of the 1st. International Symposium on Laser Surgery. Jerusalem, Jerusalem Academic Press, p. 190-213.
2. Strong MS, Jako GJ (1972) Laser surgery in the larynx. Early clinical experience with continuous CO2 Laser. Ann Otol 81: 791-798.
3. Verscheren RJ, Oldhoff J The carbon dioxide Laser. A new surgical tool. Archivum Chirurgicum Neerlandicum vol 27 nº 3 199-207, (1975).

© 1985 Elsevier Science Publishers B.V. (Biomedical Division)
New dimensions in otorhinolaryngology - head and neck surgery, vol. 2.
E. Myers, editor

A NEW TECHNIQUE FOR TOTAL SEPTAL RECONSTRUCTION IN CHILDREN

SLOBODAN B. JUGO, and IVO F. PADOVAN
Depts. of Otolaryngology, Muhlenberg Community Hospital, Greenville, Kentucky, USA, and University of Zagreb, YUGOSLAVIA

INTRODUCTION

Severe postraumatic deformities of the ventrocaudal and ventrocranial septum in children continue to present serious challenge to the modern rhinosurgeon. Conservative septoplastic techniques through Cottle's approach have produced an untolerably high rate of recurrences of insufficient restoration of the function of the nose (1-2). Decortication (external) rhinoplasty has been pioneered by Rethi (3), and Sercer (4), and fully developed by Padovan (5). The first report of external rhinoplasty in children was published in 1960. Hage (6) used this technique for excision of a nasal glioma in two children and found no alteration of the growth of the nose due to temporary elevation of the nasal skin. Encouraged by this report the authors developed a method for a total septal reconstruction through decortication approach.

SURGICAL TECHNIQUE

A circumferential incision along the caudal border of the lower lateral cartilage is made on both sides and connected with a V-shaped transcolumellar incision. By careful sharp dissection, the skin is elevated over the lower lateral cartilages. The nose is further skeletonized up to the nasal bones. The lower lateral cartilages are retracted with two skin hooks and the loose connective tissue in between is cut with scissors. The septal tip is identified, and elevation of the mucoperichondrium is started with a Cottle's knife. At first, elevation is directed cranially and posteriorly. The septal cartilage is then separated from the upper lateral cartilages but the K-area is not violated. Only after this maneuver, is elevation of the mucoperichondrium carried out inferiorly and caudally. The fibers of the septopremaxillary ligament are approached and dissected in a retrograde fashion. After sufficient elevation of the mucoperichondrium is achieved, the septal cartilage is incised approximatelly 5 mm ventrocaudally to the K-area. The cut is extended posteriorly and inferiorly leaving a rim of about 2-3 mm of cartilage in contact with the perpendicular plate of the ethmoid bone. The septal cartilage is dislocated from the vomerian groove and removed. It is very important to excise the entire septal cartilage in a single piece so that a sufficiently large straight part will be obtained for subsequent grafting. The cartilage is carefully examined and an imprint of the ventrocaudal part is drawn with a marker on the drape sheet. This imprint is then translated to the straight part of the cartilage so that grafted cartilage will be a perfect replica of the ventrocaudal septum. The cartilage implant is carefully positioned in the ventrôcaudal septal space and sutured with several 4-o dexon sutures to the upper lateral cartilages and to the fibers of the septopremaxillary ligament. The remainder of the cartilage is straightened by crushing and is positioned in the posterior part of the septal sac. The nasal skin is replaced and the incisions are meticulously closed with 5-o nylon and 4-o dexon.

RESULTS and CONCLUSSION

There were twenty four children (5-12 y old) operated using the external approach in the period between July 1978 and April 1985. The results of total septal reconstruction in all operated children were very satisfactory and none of the children required reoperation. The reimplanted cartilage has shown remarkable survival capacity providing solid support for the nasal tip and dorsum in all patients. Also, the grafted cartilage appeared to continue to grow maintaining the normal development of the nose. The authors conclude that external rhinoplasty approach is useful in correcting severe septal deformities in children

REFERENCES

1. Pirsig W. (1984) Laryngol. Rhinol. Otol. 63: 17o-18o.
2. Schultz-Coulon H.J. (1983) HNO 31:6-9.
3. Rethi A.C. (1934) Rev. Chir. Plast. 2: 85-1o6.
4. Sercer A. (1957) Rev. Laryngol. Otol. Rhinol. 3-4:161-168
5. Padovan I. (1966) Symp. Orl. Iug. 3-4:354-36o.
6. Hage J. (1960) Brit. J. Plast. Surg. 12:327-339.

© 1985 Elsevier Science Publishers B.V. (Biomedical Division)
New dimensions in otorhinolaryngology – head and neck surgery, vol. 2.
E. Myers, editor

CORRECTION OF NASAL SEPTAL PERFORATION THROUGH EXTERNAL RHINOPLASTY APPROACH

WALAE H. ABOUSHELEB AND HASSAN M. MOUSTAFA
E.N.T. DEPARTMENT, TANTA UNIVERSITY. EGYPT

INTRODUCTION

Nasal septal perforation is considered one of the difficult problems to solve. Septal trauma is the commonest aetiological factor in producing nasoseptal perforation. Many procedures had been done to correct septal perforation. Cottle (1958) closes septal perforations of 2 or 3 cm. in diameter, Gollom (1968) used the reverse flap technique to close nasoseptal perforation.

External rhinoplasty approach has been recently used to close nasoseptal perforation. Goodman and Stralzow (1978, 1982) are the pioneers to correct nasoseptal perforation through external rhinoplasty approach.

PATIENTS AND PROCEDURE

Twelve patients with antrior caudal septal perforation were operated upon through external rhinoplasty approach.

10 cases were due to repeated electric csutery to treat nasal bleeding and 2 cases were due to tomplicated S.M.R.

PROCEDURE

All patients were done under general anaethesia an inverted mid columellar incision with bilateral rim extension of the lower lateral cartilage. Dissection and raising of the skin from the dorsal nasoseptal structure. Careful elevation of the mucoperichonderium flaps on both sides of the cartilagenous septum with refreshing the edges of the perforation. Two vertical or transeverse release incisions parallel to the long axis of the septal perforation. Fixation of autogenous septal cartilage or bone graft with intact perichondrium or periostium to close the perforation. Suture of the edges of the perforation by 5 zero chromic catgut and through and through sutures of the graft to assure its fixation.

RESULTS

Septal perforation was closed in 8 cases. Two cases in which the perforation was narrowed to about tow thirds of its original diameter. Failure of closure in two cases.

DISCUSSION

The reverse flap technique used by Gollom (1968) depends mainly on the vascular supply of the constructed flaps. Failure of this method is expected in large septal perforations which needs a large flap to close. Goodman and Stralzow (1978, 1982) used the external rhinoplasty approach to close septal perforation. The main advantages of this exposure that it does not interfere or compromise the airway passage or causing any deformity. The vascular supply of the bilateral pedicled flap is not interfered.

The result of our work coincide with the opinion of Goodman and Stralzow. We found the exposure is free enough to enable proper dissection, flap construction and fixation of the required graft. The survival rate of the graft with intact perichondrium or periostium was very good. Packing of the nose for 5 days under cover of local and systemic antibiotics is quite sufficient for fixation of the graft in position. We found that there is no need for sialastic sheeting of the nasal cavity.

REFERENCES

- Joseph Gollom: "Perforation of the nasal septum, the reverse flap technique. Arch. Otolaryng VoL. 88; Nov. 1968.
- Cottle, M.H. : Nasal Atrophy, Atrophic Rhinitis, Ozena, Medical and surgical treatment : Repair of Septal Perdorations, International College of Surgeons, 29 : 472-483, April 1958.
- Stralzow, V. and Goodman, W.S. : Nasoseptal perforation, closure by external septo-rhinoplasty, Journal of Otolaryng. Vol. 7, Nov. 1, 1978.
- Goodman, W.S. and Stralzow, : "Surgical closure of nasoseptal perforation. Laryngoscope, 1982 Feb., Vol. 92 (2) P. 121-4.

© 1985 Elsevier Science Publishers B.V. (Biomedical Division)
New dimensions in otorhinolaryngology - head and neck surgery, vol. 2.
E. Myers, editor

PREDICTING SUCCESS OF SURGICAL TREATMENT IN OBSTRUCTIVE SLEEP APNEA

VINOD K. ANAND, M.D., Division of Otolaryngology; MILTON KRAMER, M.D., LARRY SCHOEN, Ph.D., Division of Somnology, University of Mississippi Medical Center, 2500 North State Street, Jackson, Mississippi USA

Several reports have emerged in the recent literature regarding the effectiveness of Palatopharyngoplasty for the treatment of Obstructive Sleep Apnea. However, there remains a need to establish criterion for identifying patient subgroups that would benefit most from such surgical therapy. Another major area of controversy is the definition of success. The results of different therapeutic modalities are difficult to compare, because success continues to be measured by varying yardsticks such as improvements in snoring, excessive daytime sleepiness, etc. The preoperative standards of polysomnographic monitoring are not being rigidly applied in determining postoperative improvements in a significant number of cases.

The following report deals with our experience of surgical treatment of Obstructive Sleep Apnea in 30 patients at the University of Mississippi Medical Center from 1982 until 1935. All 30 patients underwent postoperative polysomnography three to six weeks following surgery. A retrospective analysis was performed to define factors which were associated with poor surgical outcome.

On the basis of postoperative polysomnography, surgical response was categorized into three main groups. Patients with a 90% or greater improvement in Apnea Index were classified as responders, and 57% of our patients belong to this group. Another 23% were classified as moderate responders on the basis of Apnea Index improvement between 50 - 89% over the preoperative levels. The nonresponders had a less than 50% improvement in Apnea Index, and they constituted 20% of the group. All but one nonresponder reported improvement in snoring and excessive daytime sleepiness. A review of the preoperative clinical analysis revealed that patients classified as responders had a significantly higher incidence of tonsillar enlargement. Our subjective clinical impression showed a greater incidence of hypopharyngeal mucosal redundancy and epiglottic floppiness in the nonresponder group. There were no statistically significant differences in the pre- and postsurgical weights among the responders and nonresponders.

Computed tomographic measurements were obtained in the awake stage in all 30 patients preoperatively. These measurements were obtained from the narrowest areas and revealed considerable reductions from the normals. Also, there was considerable variation within the group. The hypopharyngeal dimensions in the nonresponder group were reduced in contrast to those classified as responders.

Based on cephalometric observations, patients were excluded from undergoing Palatopharyngoplasty. Somnocinefluoroscopy provided information about the nature of obstruction, but because of our limited application, a valid conclusion as to its predictive reliability could not be made.

One or more of the following procedures were performed in one stage based on the preoperative assessment. Palatopharyngoplasty was done in all 30 patients; 21 patients required tonsillectomy. Septoplasty and turbinectomy were done in 15 patients each, and three patients required nasal polypectomy. The improved rates of surgical success may be explained due to simultaneous correction of perceived nasal deformities. A careful analysis of Apnea Indices disclosed that the response to surgical intervention occurred in the severest group, and the response was proportional to the preoperative Apnea Index. Six patients were considered nonresponders, and we closely analyzed reasons for failure. Three patients who had moderately severe Obstructive Sleep Apnea also had marked hypopharyngeal narrowing both clinically and on computed tomography and somnocinefluoroscopy. One patient had choanal narrowing such that a fiberoptic scope could not be passed. This patient also had asthma and nasal allergies. Another patient had nasopharyngeal stenosis from a previous adenotonsillectomy. The requirement for barbiturates for controlling seizures in one patient may have been responsible for poor surgical outcome. Thus, a retrospective analysis disclosed apparent causes of failure in five out of six patients.

CONCLUSIONS

1. Palatopharyngoplasty in conjunction with corrective surgery of nasal passages is effective in treatment of Obstructive Sleep Apnea. In our series, Apnea Index was reduced by more than 90% in 57% of patients; in 80% of patients, an improvement of greater than 50% reduction in Apnea Index was achieved.
2. The severity of apnea preoperatively correlated with the degree of postsurgical reduction in Apnea Index.
3. Most predictable surgical results were observed in patients having tonsillar enlargement associated with oropharyngeal airway compromise.
4. Redundancy of hypopharyngeal mucosa, epiglottic floppiness, severely reduced hypopharyngeal airway on CT scan and choanal narrowing indicate probable surgical failure with Palatopharyngoplasty.
5. No correlation was observed between preoperative body weights, postsurgical weight loss and improvements in Apnea Indices with surgery.
6. Retrospective analysis disclosed apparent causes of failure in five out of six nonresponders.

ACKNOWLEDGEMENTS

The authors wish to acknowledge the editorial assistance in preparation of this manuscript by Ms. Denise Fletcher.

© 1985 Elsevier Science Publishers B.V. (Biomedical Division)
New dimensions in otorhinolaryngology - head and neck surgery, vol. 2.
E. Myers, editor

SURGICAL MANAGEMENT OF EAR LOBE KELOIDS SECONDARY TO EAR PIERCING USING A NEWER COMPRESSION DEVICE

HERBERT L. BAKER, M.D., Chief, Otolaryngology Section, Veterans Administration Medical Center, Portland, Oregon, USA and REGINALD BAUGH, M.D., Department of Otolaryngology, University of Michigan, Ann Arbor, Michigan, USA

Ear lobe keloids may become more common since the recent fad of male ear piercing. The author's preferrred treatment of this problem consists of subtotal surgical or CO_2 laser removal of keloids in combination with intralesional steroid injection and placement of a compression device where pressure can be regulated at the site of the excised lesion. The description and diagram of this new compression device will be described. A five year personal experience at the University of Michigan Medical Center, the Oregon Health Sciences University as well as recent experience at Emanuel Hospital will be reviewed. Since the use of the new Baker keloid ear clamp there has been no recurrence or post-op complications with six months to one year followup in our early experience. Our findings are consistent with the literature which suggests that constant light pressure is an effective means of preventing post-excisional recurrence of keloid lesions. We used this method as the initial treatment and preserve radiation therapy and other modes of treatment for possible recurrent lesions.

INTRODUCTION

Factors associated with increased probability of developing a keloid are: a) trauma, b) tension, c) race, d) location, e) age, and f) genetic predisposition.

In review of the literature the most common modalities that have been suggested are surgical excision in combination with: 1) radiation therapy, 2) steroid therapy, or 3) pressure.

MATERIALS & METHODS

In the author's personal experience since 1978 at University of Michigan Medical Center, the most reliable method of teatment of keloids had been a combination of subtotal excision and intralesional steroid injection with Kenalog 20 to 30 mg per cc and pressure. Until recently the pressure was difficult to maintain on the ear lobule when using ski band or taping technique. Since the development of this ear clamp we have evaluated ten patients in an ongoing prospective study to determine the effectiveness of this clamp device in combination with subtotal excision and intralesional steroid treatment.

Several authors have reportedly used pressure devices such as the Snyder button compression[1], and the Brent spring pressure device with varied success[2]. Several complications have been reported with these devices which include trauma and infection when placing sutures through the ear lobe and pressure sores using the spring pressure device due to inability to regulate pressure. In contrast, we advocate the Baker ear lobe clamp where the amount of pressure can be regulated as illustrated in Figure 1.

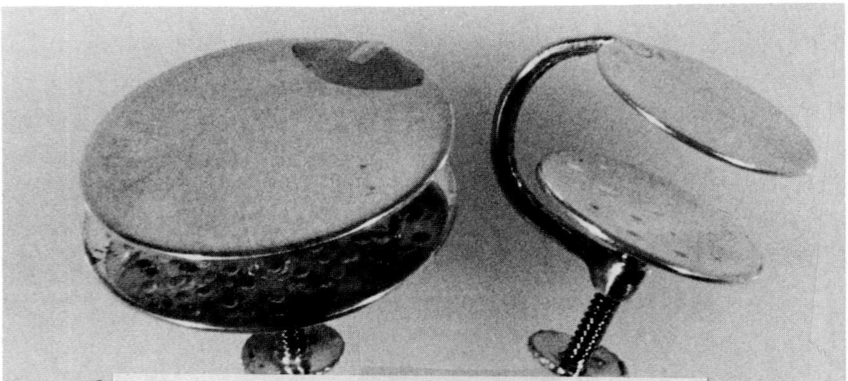

Figure 1. The Baker adjustable keloid ear clamp

In conclusion, we feel that this is the most conservative and effective means of currently treating ear lobule keloids. Use of subtotal excision of the keloid with scalpel, and intraoperative steroid injections with postoperative pressure using the Baker ear lobe clamp device is the best initial treatment. The use of routine radiation therapy for benign lesions should be questioned because of cost effectiveness and potential future risk to the patient. This seems to be an excellent initial non-invasive, safe, simple approach which would allow greater advantage to the patient. Also will avoid possible complications of hypo- or hyperpigmentation and skin atrophy with long term steroid use. Patient compliance will be improved by avoiding multiple injections that could traumatize the area further and cause recurrence of keloids as well as eliminate the possible risks of complications from radiation therapy in the future.

REFERENCES

1. Snyder GS (1974) British J Plastic Surgery 27:186-187

2. Brent B (1978) Ann Plast Surg 1:579-581

© 1985 Elsevier Science Publishers B.V. (Biomedical Division)
New dimensions in otorhinolaryngology - head and neck surgery, vol. 2.
E. Myers, editor

FACIAL RECONSTRUCTION WITH IMPLANTS OF POROUS POLYETHYLENE

ALEXANDER BERGHAUS, M.D.

ENT-Department, Klinikum Steglitz, Free University of Berlin, Hindenburgdamm 30, D-1000 Berlin 45 (West Germany)

Porous polyethylene is a sintered synthetic with a pore size of approximately 150 µ. The material can easily be formed with the scalpel or thermoplastically and is sterilized with ethylene oxide gas. In the ear, nose and throat field it has so far only become known for its use in the replacement of auditory ossicles.

Experimental animal studies have shown that there is ingrowth into the pores of both connective tissue and bone.

Since, moreover, the danger of infection appears to be relatively low, we have used porous polyethylene for the correction of various defects in the head and neck area.

For the correction of forehead defects, a profile plate of porous polyethylene is formed thermoplastically on a plaster model (Fig. 1).

After an arcuate incision behind the hairline, the defect cavity is filled with a multiply perforated block of porous polyethylene, which can easily be shaped to the required size with the scalpel. Final profiling is done by putting on the prepared profile plate and fixing it with fibrin glue. This type of operation has so far been performed in four patients. In one patient, the defect cavity was filled with iliac crest bone. The roentgenogram before and 2 years after the correction shows the expected ossification of the defect area in this case. But also in cases where filling was accomplished with the perforated synthetic plate, the roentgenogram later shows an obliteration with bone or dense connective tissue. The results were satisfactory in all cases. This material even permits correction of large defects where the skin has grown directly onto the dura.

The maximal postoperative observation period is about three years. There were no complications in any of the cases. The cosmetic result is lasting; resorption has so far not been observed.

The favorable properties of porous polyethylene have induced us to also use it as a frame for reconstruction of the external ear. We use a light implant without edges or points, as shown in Fig. 2. If necessary, it can be reduced in size intraoperatively and used for partial ear reconstructions. For a microtia operation, the implant is covered with the temporalis fascia, the so-called "fan-flap" according to FOX and EDGERTON. This reduces the risk of postoperative complications. We have implanted such frames five times. None of the implants for correction of microtia have had to be removed. The synthetic frame was particularly suitable in a case of abscess-forming pericondritis of the external ear. The nearly totally destroyed auricular cartilage was replaced by a polyethylene frame after the acute inflammation had been brought under control. Three years later, the relief is satisfactory; the retroauricular fold is normally formed.

If the results obtained continue to be favorable, porous polyethylene could obviate the removal of autogenous bone or cartilage for reconstructive surgery in the head and neck region.

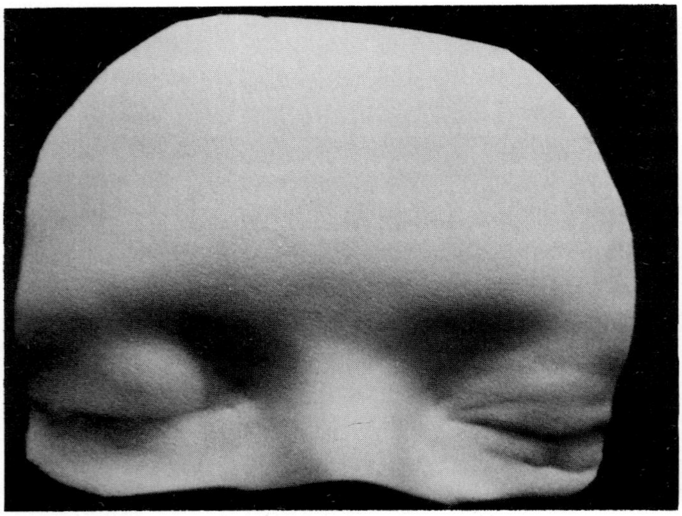

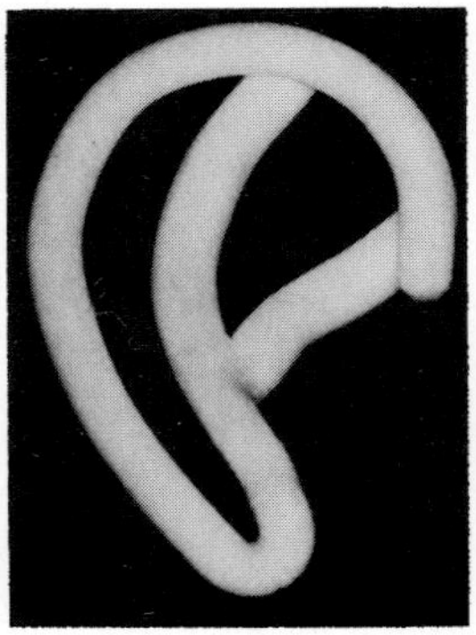

Fig. 1 (left). Profile plate of porous polyethylene cut to the desired shape intraoperatively.

Fig. 2 (right). Framework of PHDPE for auricular reconstruction.

REFERENCES

Berghaus A (1985) Porous polyethylene in reconstructive head and neck surgery. Arch Otolaryngol 111:154-160

New dimensions in otorhinolaryngology - head and neck surgery, vol. 2.
E. Myers, editor

SERIAL EXCISION IN MANAGEMENT OF FACIAL SCARS AND KELOIDS

HEMENDRA N. BHATNAGAR

10 School Street, Waterville, Maine 04901 U.S.A.

Excision of large facial hypertrophic scars and keloids even when combined with skin grafting may not produce quite aesthetic results. Serial excision combined with advancement flaps offers an excellent alternative. The lesion is serially excised over a period of time. The surrounding skin is advanced from all around in such a fashion that the reconstructed lines fall at natural creases or folds. Sometimes it is not possible to do so and one has to compromise in order to achieve the objective.

Keloids are generally managed by excision, intralesional steroids and radiation. Excision of large areas requires free skin grafts or a combination of various flaps. No one modality is best suited for all lesions alike.

Children present special problems in rehabilitation because of constantly changing growth patterns in an active and exposed area such as the face. The scars and keloids rapidly proliferate in such tissues which are subject to stress and tension during the growth period. Rehabilitation may take several years. Results are, however, gratifying with serial excision in combination with advancement flaps.

CASE REPORT

A seven year old white boy presented with extensive delayed hypertrophic scars and keloids of the face as a result of gasoloine burns an year earlier. The lesions involved both sides of face, chin and the neck with some contractures. The tissue was massive , firm pink and at places as thick as 3 cm. Some of these showed deep pits filled with sebaceous material.

Initial treatment consisted of intralesional steroids with Dermojet for about four months. On an average 15 ml of steroid was injected at three week interval. This reduced the bulk of the massive tissue which became rather soft and flat. Adrenal function was monitored and tests were normal.

The next stages consisted of repeated combinations of segmental and serial excisions with advancement facial and cervical flaps and steroid injections from time to time for a period of about three years. He was followed for five years without evidence of hypertrophic scars and keloids.

Figures 1 thru 12, reproduced with kind permission of the publisher (1), illustrate the various stages and results.

REFERENCES

1. Bhatnagar,HN (1984) In:Ward PH, Berman WE (eds) Plastic and Reconstructive Surgery of Head and Neck. Proceedings of the Fourth International Symposium. The CV Mosby Company, St. Louis pp 483-487

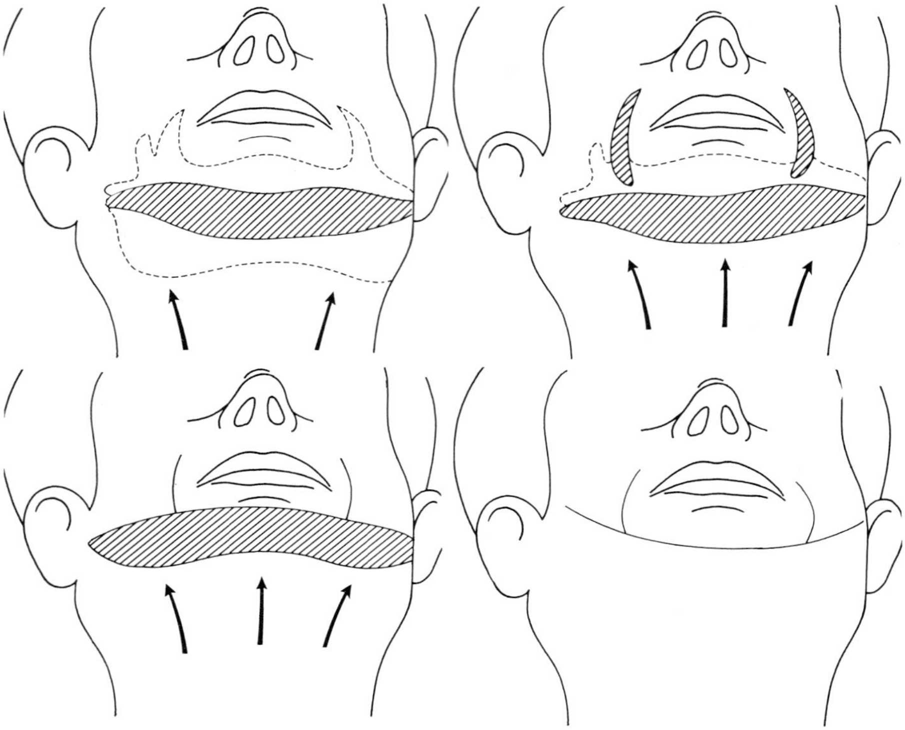

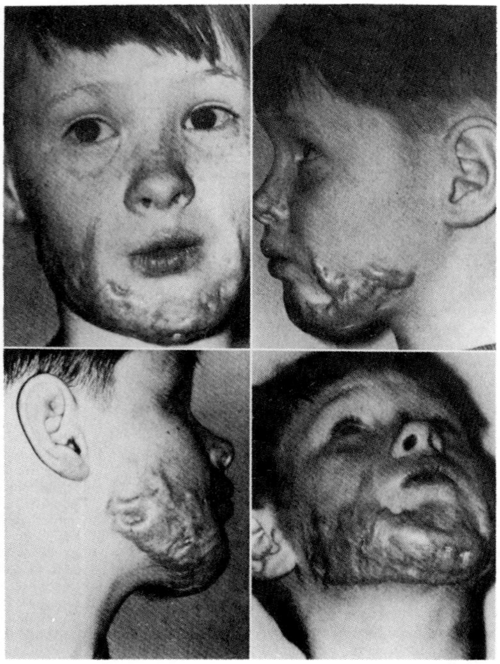

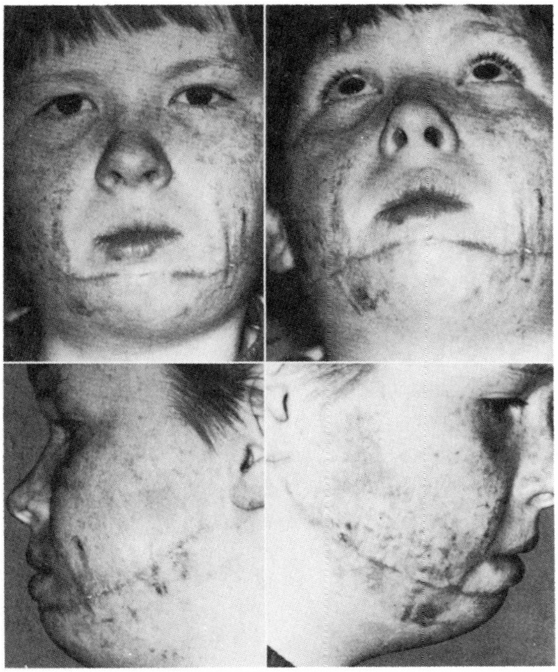

New dimensions in otorhinolaryngology – head and neck surgery, vol. 2.
E. Myers, editor

PAROTID GLAND SURGERY: A TWENTY-FIVE YEAR EXPERIENCE AT BAYLOR COLLEGE OF MEDICINE

BOBBY R. ALFORD, M.D., CHARLES D. KATZ, M.D., JAMES H. ATKINS, JR., M.D.

Department of Otorhinolaryngology and Communicative Sciences, Baylor College of Medicine, One Baylor Plaza, Houston, Texas 77030 (U.S.A.)

INTRODUCTION

An attempt to compare the experience with parotid gland surgery at Baylor College of Medicine to other large series[1-6] revealed inconsistencies in the literature which made interpretation difficult. Some studies refer solely to neoplasms of parotid origin while others include neoplasms of supporting tissue, inflammatory masses, and other "pseudotumors." The inclusion of previously treated and recurrent lesions is variable. The term "primary" refers to "parotid origin" in some articles and to "non-recurrent" in others. We present our findings in 1349 patients and the classification structure which simplified comparison between studies.

MATERIALS AND METHODS

Parotid gland surgery at three private hospitals, one county hospital, and the Veterans Administration Medical Center from 1960-1984 was retrospectively evaluated. Previously treated and recurrent lesions were included. Parotidectomies performed during extended neck dissections for unrelated malignancies were excluded. The original histopathologic diagnoses were accepted without re-examination of the surgical specimens. Follow-up was obtained by contacting the surgeon or personally reviewing the chart.

RESULTS AND DISCUSSION

1349 patients underwent parotid surgery in the 25 year period. No mass was present in 132 patients (74 trauma, 45 abscesses, 3 fistulas, and 10 cutaneous malignancies). The classification of the 1217 patients with masses is shown in Table 1.

TABLE 1

CLASSIFICATION OF PAROTID MASSES

Neoplasms of Parotid Origin
Neoplasms of Extra-Parotid Origin
Inflammatory Diseases
Non-Neoplastic, Non-Inflammatory Lesions

Neoplasms of parotid origin accounted for 57.3% (698 cases) of parotid masses. This is consistent with reports which include all pathology groups in Table 1[7], but is much lower than reports which exclude neoplasms of extra-parotid origin and/or inflammation. In accordance with other studies, 14.2% of these neoplasms were malignant and 85.8% benign. The histopathologic distribution, patient characteristics, and physical findings of malignant and benign neoplasms of parotid origin were similar to those of other series.

14.6% of parotid masses were neoplasms of extra-parotid origin. The malignant types included metastatic and invasive squamous cell carcinoma, melanoma, lymphoma, and basal cell carcinoma and accounted for 65.7% of this class. Hemangiomas, lymphangiomas, lipomas, pilomatrixomas, and schwannomas comprised the remaining 34.3%.

Chronic sialadenitis, granulomatous disorders, and lymphadenitis accounted for 18.8% of parotid masses. The frequency with which these inflammatory disorders simulate parotid neoplasms is overlooked in studies which limit themselves to neoplastic diseases.

Non-neoplastic, non-inflammatory lesions include cysts, lymphoid hyperplasia (without an inflammatory component), and ectopic salivary gland tissue. They made up 8.9% of parotid masses. 30 masses (2.5%) had no pathologic diagnosis.

CONCLUSION

Our classification system and avoidance of the term "primary" facilitated comparison between our experience and previous studies. The distribution and characteristics of neoplasms of parotid origin was similar to other reports. There were a significant number of parotid masses with extra-glandular or inflammatory origins.

ACKNOWLEDGEMENTS

We would like to express our gratitude to S. Donald Greenberg, M.D. (Department of Pathology, Baylor College of Medicine) for his assistance.

REFERENCES

1. Eneroth CM (1970) Acta Otolaryngol Suppl 263:174
2. Woods JE, Chong GC, Beahrs OH (1975) Am J Surg 130:460
3. Sharkey FE (1977) Am J Clin Pathol 67:272
4. Spiro RH, Huvos AG, Strong EW (1975) Am J Surg 130:452
5. Beahrs OH, Woolner LB, Carveth SW, and Devine KD (1960) Arch Surg 80:890
6. Foote FW and Frazell EL (1953) Cancer 6:1065
7. Gallia LJ, Johnson JT (1981) The Laryngoscope 91:512

New dimensions in otorhinolaryngology - head and neck surgery, vol. 2.
E. Myers, editor

THE ROLE OF RADIOTHERAPY IN TREATMENT OF MALIGNANT TUMORS OF THE TRACHEA*

M. E. BARAKA

Assistant Professor & Consultant E.N.T. Surgeon, Department of Otolaryngology, King Faisal University, Dammam, Saudi Arabia

SUMMARY

The clinical presentation and pathological findings in 37 patients with a malignant tumor of the trachea are reviewed. Treatment with radical radiotherapy resulted in a 5-year survival rate in excess of 40%.

MATERIAL & METHODS

Between the years 1971-81, 37 cases were treated at the Christie Hospital and Holt Radium Institute, Manchester, England.

Survival curves were calculated using the life table method and survival between different groups was compared using the Logrant test of statistical significance.

SYMPTOMATOLOGY

TABLE
Symptoms in the 37 patients.

Symptom	Cough	Stridor	Dyspnea	Hemoptysis	Wt. loss	Dysphagia	Hoarseness	Neck nodes
No. Patients	24	20	19	14	11	8	8	5

DIAGNOSIS

All cases were diagnosed by direct examination. Soft tissue views of the neck and tomography were found to be very helpful in diagnosing and delineating the extent of the growth.

PATHOLOGY

Twenty-eight cases were squamous cell carcinomas. One tumor was an anaplastic tumor of thymic origin.

TREATMENT

Treatment is by external beam therapy using mega voltage x rays. The volume irradiated is based on clinical and radiological findings. When radical treatment is attempted the technique used varies according to the site of the primary lesion. Cervical lesions are treated by means of a parallel opposed pair of fields, delivering a dose of 5250 cGy in 16 exposures over 21 days. Intrathoracic lesions are treated by a 3-field technique, delivering 5250 cGy in 15 exposures over 21 days.

Twenty patients had palliative treatment and 16 patients were given radical treatment. One patient was treated by sternotomy and partial resection of the tumor.

RESULTS

Of the 16 cases who had radical treatment 6 are alive. Of the 20 patients who had palliative radiotherapy 1 is alive.

The overall 5-year survival rate for all patients was 20% (Graph 1). The 5-year survival rate following radical radiotherapy was 40% (Graph 2).

CONCLUSIONS

Prospects of prolonged cure are very small in malignant tracheal tumors, so that a less mutilating form of treatment should be adopted. Radical radiotherapy resulted in a 5-year survival of over 40%.

*Article first appeared in the Annals of the Royal College of Surgeons of England, January 1984, vol 66, pp 27-29.

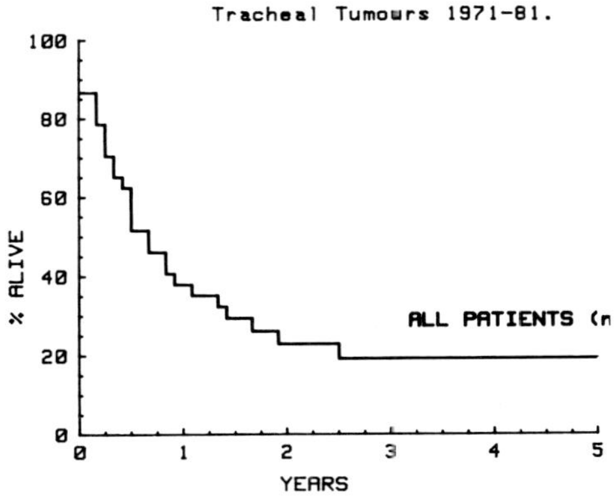

Graph 1. Five-year survival curve for all patients.

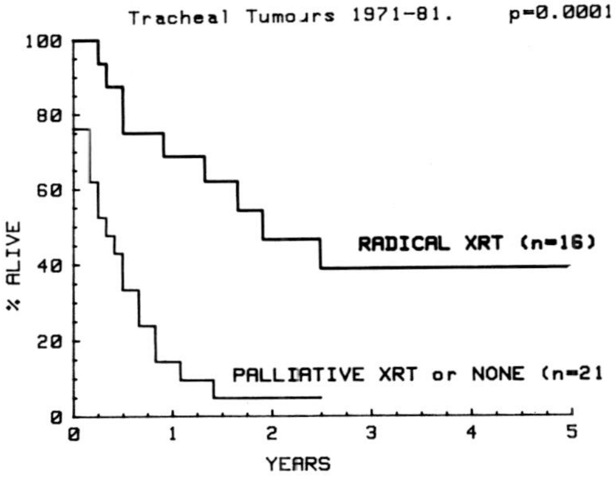

Graph 2. Survival curves of patients treated with palliative & radical radiotherapy.

New dimensions in otorhinolaryngology - head and neck surgery, vol. 2.
E. Myers, editor

SURGICAL SALVAGE AFTER HIGH-DOSE IRRADIATION FAILURE IN PATIENTS WITH HEAD AND NECK CANCER

GREG A. CARL, M.D., JAMES A. DUNCAVAGE, M.D., ROBERT J. TOOHILL, M.D., AND THOMAS W. GROSSMAN, M.D.

Department of Otolaryngology, Medical College of Wisconsin, Milwaukee, Wisconsin, U.S.A., and the Surgical Service of the Veterans Administration Medical Center, Milwaukee, Wisconsin, U.S.A.

Surgical salvage of patients with persistent or recurrent cancer of the head and neck can be attempted following high-dose irradiation for tumors that 1) normally respond well to that modality, 2) were not resected initially due to patient refusal, and 3) were considered unresectable prior to the institution of irradiation.

Forty-six patients were salvaged with 53 surgical procedures over the past seven years. The range of radiation dosage given as the first course of treatment was 5220 to 9000 rads, with the median being 7000 rads. The time interval between the completion of irradiation and surgical salvage for persistent or recurrent disease ranged from one month to seven years, with a median of six months.

Surgical extent was rated on a scale of I to IV. I included local excision to radical neck dissection. II included excision involving transgression of pharynx or larynx. III involved excision requiring regional flaps for closure. IV included excision whose extent required multi-stage reconstruction using multiple regional flaps with or without gastric pull-up.

Complications by surgical extent are as follow:

TABLE I

COMPLICATIONS BY SURGICAL EXTENT

Surgical Extent	# Patients	# Procedures	Incidence of Complications	% Surgical Death
I	8	12	0	0
II	30	31	38%	3%
III	3	5	80%	0
IV	5	5	100%	40%

Outcome by surgical extent is as follows:

TABLE II

OUTCOME BY SURGICAL EXTENT

Surgical Extent	Alive, NED	Alive, w/ ca	Died, w/ ca	Died, Other Causes	Lost to Follow-up
I	0	1	3	4	0
II	13	1	9	5*	2
III	3	0	0	0	0
IV	0	0	3	2**	0

*One surgical death
**Both surgical deaths

Outcome by specific site is as follows:

TABLE III

OUTCOME BY SITE

	Larynx	Pharynx	Oral Cavity	Sinus	Salivary Gland	Neck, Unknown P°
Alive, NED	13	3	0	0	0	0
Alive, w/ ca	0	1	1	0	0	0
Died, w/ca	3	5	3	1	1	2
Died, Other Causes	2	3	3	0	0	0
Surgical Death	1	2	0	0	0	0
Lost to Follow-up	1	1	0	0	0	0
Total	20	15	7	1	1	2

It was concluded that although surgical salvage after high-dose irradiation can be attempted, a higher incidence of wound complications should be expected. Best results at this institution were obtained with those patients suffering from laryngeal lesions. Special care in surgical technique including perioperative antibiotics, cold-knife scalpel incisions only, care in flap retraction, and avoidance of the use of electrocautery is advocated.

New dimensions in otorhinolaryngology – head and neck surgery, vol. 2.
E. Myers, editor

PARALLEL HISTOLOGIC MARGINS FOR HEAD AND NECK CANCER

TERENCE M. DAVIDSON, PARVIZ HAGHIGHI, ROBERT W. ASTARITA
University of California, San Diego; VAH, San Diego, California USA

Microscopically controlled margins are the standard of care for aggressive malignant epidermoid and basal cell skin cancers. The same concept has been used for 122 consecutive patients with epidermoid carcinoma in the upper aerodigestive tract. The local control rate has been 94%, an impressive figure for these aggressive neoplasms with a known disturbingly high local recurrence rate.

Beginning in July of 1979 and extending through the end of April 1985, 122 new patients with biopsy-proven epidermoid carcinoma have been fully evaluated and all the surgical candidates included. All these patients had a primary neoplasm and had surgery as the initial treatment modality.

In all cases the primary tumor was resected first. A 1 cm margin of normal tissue, both mucosal and soft tissue, was included about the clinically evident tumor.[1,2] Parallel histologic sections similar to those initially recommended by Mohs were cut, mapped and histologically examined. Where tumor inflammation or surface dysplastic changes were identified, additional directed excisions (called Levels I, II, III, etc.) were cut, mapped and examined until all traceable tumor was resected.

The majority of patients had advanced tumors (mean T = T3).

The most interesting observations are evidenced in Table 1. Sixty-eight percent of the patients required a Level II or higher excision. This means that a 1 cm margin of normal tissue around these neoplasms left microscopic disease in the patient. This disease was submucosal and too small to be clinically evident.

TABLE 1
PARALLEL SECTION LEVELS

	ORAL CAVITY	OROPHARYNX	LARYNX	HYPOPHARYNX	NOSE & PARANASAL SINUSES	TOTAL	%	
I	16	4	13	6		39	32%	
II	20	22	12	6	2	62	51%	68%
III or more	6	5	5	4	1	21	17%	
TOTAL	42	31	30	16	3	122	100%	

Figure 1 is a typical example of microscopic spread. Directed excision removed the histologic abnormalities. The high local control rate implies that this is an effective means of eradicating the primary tumor.

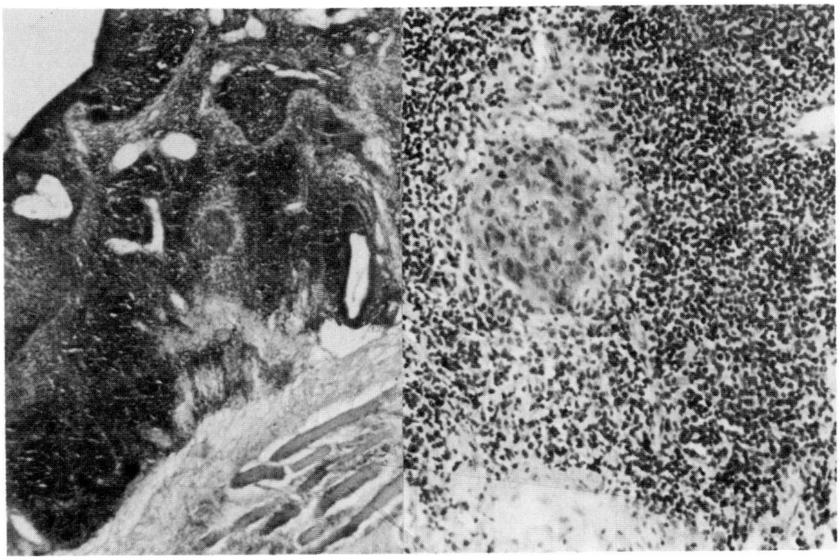

Figure 1. (a) Low power magnification. Note cord of tumor in the submucosa. (b) High power magnification of tumor cord. Note surrounding inflammation.

Seventy-nine patients were tabluated two years following surgery. This includes no patients lost to follow-up (Table 2). Thirty-nine percent died within 2 years of surgery. None had local disease at the time of death. Forty-eight patients (62%) lived 2 years; 45 (95%) had no local recurrence.

TABLE 2

SUMMARY AND STATISTICS OF 79 PATIENTS	No.	Percent
Total Patients, Median T = T3	79	100%
Lost to follow-up	0	0%
Died before 2 years without evidence of local disease at time of death	31	39%
Local recurrence	3	4%
No local disease (2 years or more)	45	57%
Patients alive 2 years	48	100%
Local recurrence	3	6%
No local disease	45	94%

The local control rate for patients with a two-year follow-up is 94%, an experience very similar to the cure rates with cutaneous chemosurgery. These local control rates are exceptionally good for advanced neoplasms.

REFERENCES

1. Davidson TM, Nahum AM, Astarita RW (1981) Otolaryngol Head & Neck Surg 89:224

2. Davidson TM, Nahum AM, Haghighi P, Astarita RW, Saltzstein SL, Seagren S (1984) Arch Otolaryngol 110:193

© 1985 Elsevier Science Publishers B.V. (Biomedical Division)
New dimensions in otorhinolaryngology - head and neck surgery, vol. 2.
E. Myers, editor

CERVICAL METASTASIS FROM THE URINARY BLADDER: A RARE DIAGNOSIS

D. EDELSTEIN MD, W. LAWSON MD DDS, M. TANNENBAUM MD PhD

Dept. of Otolaryngology, Manhattan Eye, Ear and Throat Hospital
Depts. of Otolaryngology and Pathology, Mount Sinai School of Medicine
New York, New York, U.S.A.

INTRODUCTION

The patient with a cervical mass from an occult primary tumor presents one of the most difficult diagnostic problems in head and neck surgery. This paper reviews the case of a 65 year old patient with a neck mass originating from a previously undiagnosed transitional cell bladder carcinoma. It represents the first documented case of bladder carcinoma metastases involving the external carotid artery and encasing the hypoglossal nerve. A review of the literature demonstrates that bladder carcinoma metastases to the soft tissues of the head and neck in the absence of widespread or bony disease are very rare.

CASE REPORT

The case presented is that of a 65 year old white male who, when first seen in October 1983, complained of a firm, right neck mass which had been increasing in size over the previous 9 months. One month prior to admission, the patient had noted occasional hoarseness with progressive dysphagia, although he had not experienced any weight loss, hemoptysis, hematuria or other systemic symptoms. Physical examination revealed a 6X3 centimeter, rock-hard, fixed, right upper neck mass. C.T. scanning and angiography confirmed the presence of a large, enhancing mass adjacent to the upper, right carotid artery. Negative results were obtained from a battery of diagnostic tests, including panendoscopy with multiple biopsies, a barium swallow, thyroid and bone scans, an intravenous pyelogram, and C.T. scanning of the chest and abdomen. During routine urinalysis, however, the patient exhibited microhematuria with abnormal cells. Cystoscopy revealed a transitional cell carcinoma on the lateral bladder wall. An extended right radical neck dissection was performed, which demonstrated the involvement of the external carotid artery and the hypoglossal nerve. Pathologic study confirmed the source of the neck mass to be transitional cell carcinoma from the urinary bladder. The patient died 12 months later of diffuse disease.

DISCUSSION

Bladder tumors tend to reveal distant metastases late. In clinical studies only 4-17% of patients showed metastases, but post-mortem studies indicate that this figure may be as high as 70%.[1] Most metastases are to regional nodes followed by the lungs, bone, liver, adrenal gland and the intestine.[2] Transitional cell carcinoma rarely metastasizes to the neck or to the soft tissues of the head. Although there are multiple reports of metastases to the brain and skull, there are few reports of metastases involving the eye, skin, tongue, mandible and neck. Indeed, a literature review reveals just 14 reports of bladder metastases to the neck of which only three are well documented.[3,4,5,6,7,8]

In reviewing 18 major series of cervical metastases of unknown primary sources conducted during the last 26 years, in only 2 of the 1,457 cases, or less than 0.1% of all cases, was bladder carcinoma determined to be the primary site of origin. The percentage of determinate cases ranged from 14 to 42%.[3,8] Even with the advent of C.T. scanning in recent years, the percentage of primary lesions found has not improved. This highlights the possibility that more bladder sources may exist but remain undetected. It is important to note in this respect that roughly one third of all determinate cases of cervical metastases involve infraclavicular sources. While the most common infraclavicular sites are the lung and abdomen, other genitourinary sites (i.e. kidney) are well documented.

The case presented is an unusual cervical metastasis from the urinary bladder. As demonstrated by this patient, bladder tumors are often clinically silent, highly vascular and present with distant metastases. The significance of this case lies not only in its rarity, but in the fact that its occurence may be more frequent.

REFERENCES

1. Fetter TR, Bogaev JG, McCuskey B, Seres JL (1959) J of Urol 81:746-748
2. Babaian RJ, Johnson DE, Llamas L, Ayala AG (1980) Urology 16:142-144
3. Comess MS, Beahrs OH, Dockerty MB (1957) Surg Gynec Obstet 104:607-617
4. Edwab RR, Roberts MJ, Sole MS, Mahoney WD, Rappapart SC (1981) J of Oral Surg 39:972-974
5. Flocks RH and Boatman DL (1973) Laryngoscope 83:1527-1539
6. Greenfield H (1941) Radiology 37:181-185
7. Hendrick JW (1967) In: Conley J (ed) Proceedings of the International Workshop on Cancer of the Head and Neck. Butterworth, New York, pp41-55
8. Nordstrom DG, Tewfik HH, Latourette HB (1979) Int J Radiation Oncology Biol. Phys 5:73-76

© 1985 Elsevier Science Publishers B.V. (Biomedical Division)
New dimensions in otorhinolaryngology - head and neck surgery, vol. 2.
E. Myers, editor

APPRAISAL OF FINE NEEDLE ASPIRATION BIOPSY OF CERVICAL METASTASES

UCG ENGZELL
ENT Unit, Department of Surgery, University of Hong Kong, Hong Kong

Reliable morphological diagnosis is crucial in the correct management of patients with neck metastases. Fine-needle aspiration biopsy (FNA) offers a time-saving, simple, safe and economical method of achieving such diagnosis.

Conventional open biopsy of cervical metastases has been shown to significantly increase the rate of complications of wound necrosis, regional recurrence and distant metastases[1] and thus should be avoided whenever possible.

After more than 15 years of clinical experience with FNA in Scandinavia, Africa, and Asia the following advantages of this method are stressed in comparison with open biopsy of cervical metastases:

	Aspiration Biopsy	Open Biopsy
Safety	+	-
Convenience	+	-
Simplicity	+	-
Versatility	+	-
Reliability	+	+
Specificity	+	+
Low cost	+	-
Time-saving	+	-

Safety

The safety of FNA has been documented in the literature. We[2] made a 5 year followup study of 656 patients with neck metastases and 459 patients with prostatic carcinoma and a 10 year followup study of 124 patients with pleomorphic adenoma of salivary glands without finding any evidence of needle track recurrence. Experimental studies[2] with FNA carried cut on Vx2 carcinoma metastases in rabbits have shown that there is leakage of tumour cells at the puncture site of the metastases. If such tumour spillage occurs in clinical work it is probably small enough to be clinically insignificant. By cannulating the efferent vein and lymph vessel we could analyse the draining blood and lymph. There was no evidence of tumour spread caused by FNA.

Convenience

FNA of neck tumours causes little or no discomfort to the patient. The technique is easy to learn and the equipment is simple and non-expensive.

Reliability

FNA is as reliable as open biopsy of neck metastases. The accuracy is well over 90%[3]. The number of false negative results have been less than 7% in several series reported in the literature. It should be emphasised that even if repeated FNA shows negative results malignancy cannot be completely ruled out in clinically suspected cases.

Specificity

There are two aspects of the specificity of FNA. The risk of getting false positive cytology results is minimal. However, branchial and dermoid cysts may yield squamous epithelial cells which can be undistinguishable from well differentiated squamous carcinoma cells and cause erroneous cytological diagnosis[3]. The other aspect is the possibility by cytology to specify the type of malignancy and the probable site of the primary in cases of cervical metastases from occult primaries. In this aspect there are so far limitations in comparison with conventional histology. With acquired microscopic experience and possibly with electron microscopy and cytometry such limitations should be overcome.

Low cost

The low cost of FNA as compared to excision biopsy was stressed by Frable and Frable[4] in 1982. They estimated the patient costs to be $75.- for FNA and $2310.- for excision biopsy of a neck mass. Zajicek[5] in 1974 calculated that the Karolinska University Hospital made savings of $2mil. yearly by using FNA.

Conclusion

The application of FNA to diagnose cervical metastases is not a new concept and it is surprising that it has not, until recently, been more widely accepted and practised. The benefit of the method has long been underestimated and confidence in FNA will rapidly accompany increased experience with its use.

REFERENCES

1. McGuirt WF, McCabe BF (1978) Laryngoscope 88:594
2. Engzell U et al (1971) Acta Radiol 10:385
3. Engzell U et al (1971) Acta Otolaryng 72:138
4. Frable MAS, Frable JF (1982) Laryngoscope 92:1414
5. Zajicek J (1974) Personal Communication

New dimensions in otorhinolaryngology – head and neck surgery, vol. 2.
E. Myers, editor

SCINTISCANNING OF LOW GRADE MALIGNANCIES OF THE PAROTID GLAND

SHIGENORI HARAGUCHI (1), YASUSHI MURAKAMI (2), TAKESHI MARUYAMA (2), HIDEKI TATENO (2), AKIKO FUJIMURA (2), YASUKO URAO (2)

(1) Dept. of Otolaryngology, Saiseikai YOKOHAMA South Hospital, Kanagawa, Japan
(2) Dept. of Otolaryngology, School of Medicine, Keio University, Tokyo, Japan

INTRODUCTION

$^{99m}TcO_4^-$ and ^{67}Ga-citrate scintigraphies have recently applied to parotid gland tumors for differential diagnosis from inflmmatory lesion, certification of adenolymphoma, and preoperative estimation of malignancy grade. The reliability and diagnostic criteria of these supplimental methods have not established over the world. However, our previous report (1) in Japan pointed out diagnostic advantage of RI scintigraphy, especially in malignancy grade diagnosis. Except adenolymphoma and oxyphilic cell adenoma, parotid neoplasm indicated high rate of focal defective image in $^{99m}TcO_4^-$ scintigraphy, which is easily discriminated from other causes of parotid swelling. In ^{67}Ga-citrate scintigram, highly malignant tumors showed high rate of focal hot image in accordance with the tumor site, whereas benign neoplasms seldom showed hot scan. Only hypercellular typed pleomorphic adenoma and purulental fluid in the tumor had the inclination of false positive. Low grade malignant tumors such as mucoepidermoid tumors and acinic cell tumors did not show the same appearence as neither benign or high grade malignant tumors. In this report, the results of RI scintigraphy are compared among subgroups of the low grade malignant neoplasms.

MATERIALS AND METHODS

13 mucoepidermoid tumors (METs) and three acinic celltumors (ACTs) we experienced during 1975-1984 were examined by RI scintigraphy ($^{99m}TcO_4^-$ and/or ^{67}Ga-citrate). The METs were subdivided as well (6 cases), moderately (one case), and poorly differentiated types (6 cases) according to Healey's classification (2).

Scintigraphic findings were classified as symmetrcal, focal defect, focal hot, diffuse increased uptake, and diffuse decreased uptake image both in $^{99m}TcO_4^-$ and ^{67}Ga-citrate scan.

RESULTS

A. $^{99m}TcO_4^-$ scintigraphy

TABLE 1
TC SCAN IN PAROTID LOW GRADE MALIGNANCIES

	focal defect	symmetrical
well diff. MET	1	5
mod.diff. MET	1	
poorly diff. MET	4	
ACT	3	
total	9	5

MET: mucoepidermoid tumor
ACT: acinic cell timor

None of the tumors were represented as focal hot, diffuse increased uptake, or diffuse decreased uptake. Well differentiated METs had an inclination to show symmetrical (or normal) images (5/6). A single moderately differentiated and all of the poorly differentiated METs and ACTs were imaged as focal defects (table 1).

B. ^{67}Ga-citrate scintigraphy

TABLE 2
GA SCAN IN PAROTID LOW GRADE MALIGNANCIES

	focal defect	focal hot	diffuse increased	symmetrical
well diff. MET	1		2	
mod. diff. MET		1		
poorly diff. MET		4		2
ACT		1	1	1
total	1	6	3	3

None of the well differentiated METs showed focal hot image. While, four of six cases of poorly differentiated METs showed focal hot images. Totally almost a half cases were imaged as focal hot, that means less positive rates than highly malignant parotid tumors (75 % in our 16 cases).

DISCUSSION

IN $^{99m}TcO_4^-$ scan, intraparotid neoplasms are generally represented as focal defect images with some exceptions such as adenolymphoma, oxyphilic cell adenoma, and a part of mucous producing papillary adenocarcinoma. Such exceptinal tumors show remarkable Tc accumulation. In ^{67}Ga-citrate scan, high malignant neoplsns show hot images corresponding to the location of the tumor, while benign tumors seldom accumulate Ga activity.

The results of well differentiated mucoepidermoid tumors in $^{99m}TcO_4^-$ give rise to a hyposthesis that they have potentiality to accumulate ^{99m}Tc to the same extent of normal salivry gland. Such an inclination was not seen in poorly differentiated mucoepidermoid tumors.

^{67}Ga-citrate scan often showed focal hot image in pooly differentiated tumors like the other highly malignant tumors. While, well differntiated tumors did not seem to have strong activity to accumulate ^{67}Ga.

REFERENCES

(1) Haraguchi, S.: Diagnostic evaluation of RI scintigraphy in parotid gland tumors. J. Lpn. Otol. Soc. 88:518-532, 1985

(2) Healey, W. V., Perzin, K. H., and Smith, L.: Mucoepidermoid carcinoma of salivary gland origin. Cancer 26:368-388, 1970

© 1985 Elsevier Science Publishers B.V. (Biomedical Division)
New dimensions in otorhinolaryngology - head and neck surgery, vol. 2.
E. Myers, editor

ENTERAL NUTRITION IN HEAD AND NECK CANCER SURGERY

HILL JH, LYGIZOS NA, DEUTSCH EC, CORRIGAN R, LAKE I, APPLEBAUM EL

Department of Otolaryngology-Head and Neck Surgery, University of Illinois College of Medicine at Chicago, 1855 W. Taylor St., Suite 2.42, Chicago, Illinois 60612, USA

INTRODUCTION

Suboptimal nutrition is associated with head and neck cancer. There is a direct correspondence between deviation from nutritive norms pretreatment and treatment-associated complications[1,2,3] The value of short-term presurgical nutritional rehabilitation in preventing or reducing the severity of surgical complications has not been proven.[4]

MATERIAL AND METHODS

Thirty-four patients for this prospective study were randomized into either the experimental or the control group if they had operable squamous cell cancer and satisfied criteria of a fair or poor nutritional status and/or a prognostic nutritional index (PNI) greater than or equal to 21%. The nutritional status was determined by the Blackburn scheme.[5] Delayed hypersensitivity (DH) was determined with the multitest CMI.[6] An anergic patient was given a zero score. Other patients were given scores of two or one as indicated by the standard table developed for the CMI. The PNI is a formula based on variables statistically determined as the most predictive of surgical outcome.[7]

The experimental group of seventeen patients received high nitrogen enteral supplementation on the average of 2700 Kcal per day for 14 days prior to surgery. The supplement had a total calorie/protein ratio of 150:1. These patients were reevaluated nutritionally the day before surgery, and they underwent surgery on or about the fourteenth day after initial contact. The control group received no presurgical nutritional supplementation beyond their customary diet and underwent surgery as soon as possible after initial contact. Tumors were reevaluated every three days during the supplementation period. In the postoperative period, all thirty-four patients received enteral feeding at or above presurgical calorie and protein levels at least until the time of hospital discharge.

RESULTS

The average number of days between initial contact and surgery was 13 in the control group (with a range of 3-22) and 20 in the experimental group (with a range of 14-26).

As a result of the two-week supplementation, average body weight increased by 2.1%, the creatinine/height index increased by 3.22% (CV=3.00%), the total lymphocyte count increased by 9.32% (CV=2.50%), and the number of positive delayed hypersensitivity responses increased by 13%. No primary tumor increased significantly in size during the period of supplementation. The lymph node classification however, changed in two patients, and in one of these patients resectability may have been reduced.

Fifteen of 34 or 44% developed postsurgical complications. Most significant were death (2), incision separation (3), pharyngocutaneous fistula (3), and pneumonitis (3). There were approximately the same number of minor complications in each group (Table I). However, six of 17 or 35% of control patients died or experienced major morbidity compared to 2 of 17 or 12% of experimental patients. This represents a 23% difference in complication rate between the two groups and a 66% proportional reduction in complication rate for the experimental group.

TABLE I - ADVERSE POSTOPERATIVE EVENTS: SUMMARY

COMPLICATION	CONTROL	EXPERIMENTAL
MINOR	4	6
MAJOR	4	2
MORTALITIES	2	0
	6 (35%)	2 (12%)

Whether this difference in mortality and complication rate can be attributed to the nutritional supplementation alone can be answered by comparing predisposing factors between the uncomplicated and complicated cases. The experimental and control groups were well matched for these factors. In the complicated subgroup both deaths occurred in patients who had undergone prior therapy, and there were more patients requiring surgery for oropharyngeal tumors with fewer patients requiring total laryngectomy. The complicated group underwent procedures on the average one and one-half hours longer than the control group, and there were fewer good nutritional status people in the complicated group.

DISCUSSION

Multiple factors predisposing to postsurgical complications and mortality have been suggested.[8] Of these factors, only the nutritional status is potentially remediable prior to surgery. From this pilot study we suggest that significant improvement in nutritional status can be obtained from a short period before surgery of intensive nutritional supplementation, that this improvement can be obtained without significantly altering resectability, and that presurgical nutritional supplementation combined with standard postoperative nutritional support will reduce the postsurgical complication rate in head and neck cancer surgery.

ACKNOWLEDGEMENTS

A gift from Ross Laboratories, Columbus, Ohio 43216 supported this pilot project. We gratefully acknowledge the efforts of Ms. Linda Collins in preparing this manuscript.

REFERENCES - AVAILABLE UPON REQUEST

New dimensions in otorhinolaryngology – head and neck surgery, vol. 2.
E. Myers, editor

PHONATRY FISTULOPLASTY IN LARYNGECTOMY

DRES.J.ALGABA.,A.ZULUETA.,J.J.CAMACHO.,J.C.VEA

NUESTRA SEÑORA DE ARANZAZU HOSPITAL, SAN SEBASTIAN, SPAIN

INTRODUCTION

In the last four years we have been doing phonatory phistuloplasties in old laryngectomy patients,mostly the Blom-Singer(2) technique,but there are some other patients to whom the cricoides was kept at the time of the laryngectomy,and therefore it is impossible to make the Blom-Singer technique.For These cases we use a personal technique as a modification to the Amatsu(1)technique.

TECHNIQUE

It is simple and consists on a tracheoesophagus fistula.Therefore all the upper part of the trachea is isolated.The former part of cricoides and the firts tracheal ring is removed,afterwards the mucopericondrio precricoideo is saved and the cricoideo seal is removed.

The fistula is made in the mucopericondrio,and its consistence makes it possible to remain there,and prevents feeding from

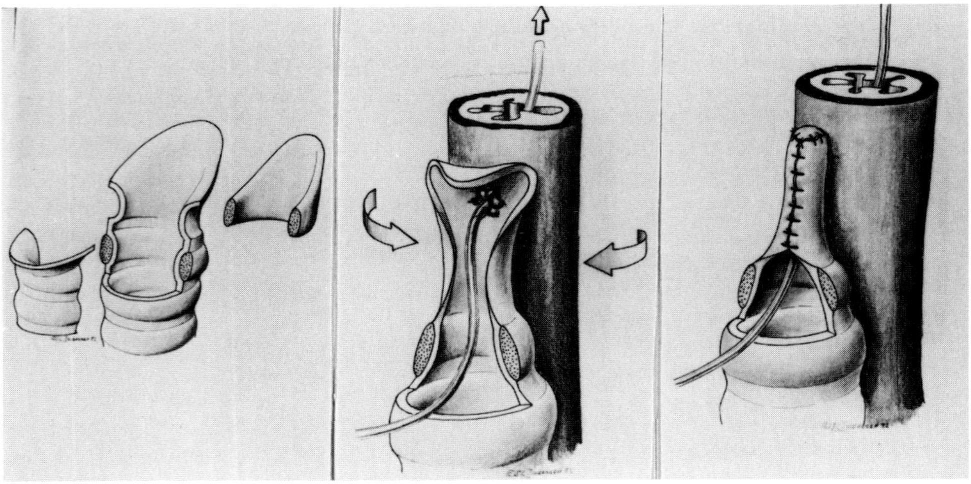

Different stages of the operation

passing to the trachea.An upright cut is made of aproximately 1cm. and another similar cut in the oesophagus making suture from its sides to the mucopericoncrio precricoideo.

A catheter is put through the fistula and suture is made in the middle line of the sides parts of the mucopericondrio,creating, thus,the tunnel.Tissue is replaced and sutured to the sides of future tracheostome.A feeding-tube is put in,which will be removed after 8-10 days.At the 12th day,the catheter of the fistula is removed and replaced by a silk string.

RESULTS

Up to the moment,we have used this technique with 19 patients, and we think that the results must be evaluated from three different points of view.1st=Voice quality,2nd=Correct feeding,3rd=Fistula maintenance.

1st= All patients have a strong,rithmic and fluid voice,not having needed any phoniatric instruction.

2nd=Feeding is correct and only six cases there was some saliva and we put a Blom-Singer prothesis.

3rd=In two patients there was an inclination to the closing of the fistula,therefore we also put a prothesis.All the other patients speak and eat without any kind of prothesis.

COMMENTS

This is a simple technique with a normal postoperative,and with great phonatory and swallowing advantages,mostly because the fistula is upright,and is only opened by the tracheal air pressure.

It is also possible to place a speaking prothesis to these patients so that there is no need to cover the tracheostome with the finger.

REFERENCES

1. Amatsu M.(1978) A new one-stage surgical technique for postlaryngectomy speech.Arch.Otol.Rhino-Laryngol.220/1-2,149-152.

2. Blom E.C.,Singer M.Z.(1980) Una técnica endoscopica para el restablecimiento de la voz después de una laringectomía.Presentado en la reunión anual de la Asociación laringologica Americana.Palm Beach.Florida.15 de Abril.

New dimensions in otorhinolaryngology - head and neck surgery, vol. 2.
E. Myers, editor

VERRUCOUS CARCINOMA OF THE LARYNX

AVELLANEDA, R., ALVAREZ-BUYLLA, M., AVELLANEDA, R.M., TRASERRA, J.
Servicio de Otorrinolaringología, Hospital Clínico y Provincial, Barcelona, Spain

The Verrucous Carcinoma of the larynx, also known as Verrucous Acantosis or Malignant Verrucous Keratosis, is not common but creates great diagnostic problems, both pathologically and clinically.

PATHOLOGY

This has to do with a type of epidermoid carcinoma which is difficult to diagnose due to similarity to benign papilloma. The characteristic difference is that, in the cavity of some well-defined papillae, there hardly exists a conjunctive-vascular axis. This is constituted by well-differentiated and structured epidermoid cells, with no cellular abnormalities, but wich in depth separates trabeculae that penetrate the subjacent tissues with keratosic ballon formations, necrosis zones and reaction to foreign bodies. The tumor is surrounded by an inflamatory reaction. A layer of keratin appears to coat its surface.

As it evolves, it invades the neighbouring tissue, erodes and destroys the cartilages until it errupts on the skin's surface.

At present two types seen identificable. In one, the papillae are very near one another; in the other, much farther apart, viral inclusions are noted in its structure. There would be a differenciation between an irritative etiology (tobacco) and a viral one (infectious). however, in the Clinic, they are treated in the same mannes.

MATERIAL AND METHODS

23 cases of Verrucous Carcinoma of the larynx are studied, found from 1.146 larynx cancers treated between 1973 and 1983. They have all been operated on and studied sistematically in a series of cuts from the surgical specimens.

DISCUSSION AND RESULTS

All the patients studied were cronic smokers of more than 20 cigarettes a day. Age varied between 38 and 72, with an average of 55 years old, which coincides with the statistics presented by Leroux-Robert and Batsakis.

SYMPTOMATOLOGY, EXPLORATION AND LOCALIZATION

Dysphonia is the most common sympton. We found it the first manifestation in 21 cases (91.3%). The other two remaining cases began with dyspnea together with a subglotic localization.

It looks like a tumor having a greyish-white exofittic papillomatous aspect with finger-like formations that grow at the expense of any zone of the larynx but with clear predominance in the glottic region.

In our cases we find the following implantations: Supraglottic: 4 (17.3%), Glottic: 13 (56.5%), Subglottic: 2 (8.6%), TRANSGLOTTIC: 4 (17.3%)

DIAGNOSIS

In general the major problem is that a rapidly growing tumor, relapsed on removal, does not agree with the repeatedly negative biopsy results.In our cases the result was positive for 34.8% (8 patients) on the first biopsy, 30.4% on the second biopsy, while in only three cases was it necessary to perform 3 biopsies and in two patients the positive result was not registered until the fourth.

The biopsy must be made very deep, bypassing the basal in order to find the invasion and trabecular infiltration and the inflammatory substratum.

EVOLUTION

Treated correctly the Verrucous Carcinoma has a good prognosis. The problem is that derived from difficulty in diagnosing which leads on occasion, to a progressive growth on the surface towards the larynx airway, giving an obstructive situation (4 emergency tracheotomies in our cases) and deeply infiltrating neighbouring tissues until it moves outwardly toward the skin, usually through the anterior comissure.

The lymphatic nodes are never affected by neoplasy. It's relatively common that in depth inflamation and the perichondrial phenomena bring on inflamatory nodes whose differential character consists of painful throbbing.

TREATMENT

Treatment is exclusively surgical. Complete extirpation is always the solution. Radiotherapy is definitely ruled out here, as much for its radioresistence as the risk of anaplasic degeneration and perichondrial phenomena.

New dimensions in otorhinolaryngology - head and neck surgery, vol. 2.
E. Myers, editor

ENIGMA OF POST-RADIATION OEDEMA AND RESIDUAL OR RECURRENT CARCINOMA OF THE LARYNX AND LARYNGOPHARYNX

Sudhir Bahadur and S.K. Kacker
Department of Otolaryngology,
All India Institute of Medical Sciences,
New Delhi - 110 029

Persistence of significant laryngeal oedema following radiotherapy presents the surgeon with a diagnostic dilemma. Though the oedema may represent a prolonged response to irradiation, the possibility of residual carcinoma must be considered. Several authors have commented upon it and have suggested frequent biopsies to prove the presence of residual of recurrent neoplasm[1,2]. However, difficulty of obtaining a positive biopsy in a post-irradiated case is well known, and repeated negative biopsies do not exclude the presence of a residual tumour.

Material and Methods

The present paper studies 63 histopathologically proven cases of carcinoma of the larynx and laryngopharynx which had received full curative radiotherapy earlier. These cases underwent salvage radical surgery on clinical suspicion of residual/recurrent tumour, manifested by persistence of significant laryngeal oedema and/or fixation of the larynx. No positive biopsies were obtained following radiotherapy. Besides, 10 cases of carcinoma of the larynx have been included in which a planned regime of preoperative radiotherapy (5,500 rads) following by radical surgery was carried out.

Ages of the patients varied from 18 years to 75 years. However, the maximum number of patients (51 of 73 patients) belonged to the age group between 41-60 years. There were 64 males and 9 females.

OBSERVATIONS

Site and stage of the disease at initial presentation is described in the table. There were 49 cases with lesions in the endolarynx, whereas the remaining 24 cases had laryngopharyngeal lesions.

Sixty patients (80%) had either stage III or IV disease. Twenty two patients (30.0%) had lymph node metastasis in the neck and in these a radical neck dissection alongwith excision of the primary lesion was carried out.

(Site and stage of the disease).

Site	No. of cases	Stage			
		I	II	III	IV
Supraglottic	9	-	3	2	4
Glottic	31	2	7	16	6
Transglottic	7	-	-	3	4
Subglottic	2	-	-	-	2
Pyriform fossa	20	-	1	9	10
Postcricoid	4	-	-	1	3
Total No. of Cases	73	2	11	31	29

In all cases, the resected specimens were examined histopathologically. Fifty eight of 63 cases (92%) which had received full curative radiotherapy showed presence of a residual tumour in their operative specimens. Five cases (8%) showed no evidence of residual cancer. Of 10 cases undergoing a planned protocol of preoperative radiotherapy and surgery, 9 (90%) showed evidence of tumour in the resected specimens. Thus, 67 of 73 cases in the present series exhibited evidence of residual/recurrent lesions.

Histological study of our larynges suggested that persistence of oedema with or without fixation of the larynx after radiation is strongly indicative of a residual/recurrent tumour, and that biopsy may be unwarranted. Repeated negative biopsies do not exclude the presence of a tumour and in fact only delay the subsequent treatment with total laryngectomy. To await a positive biopsy very often means waiting too long and the patient forfeits his chance of cure by surgery.

It had been our practice in earlier years to obtain a positive biopsy before proceeding for the radical surgery, in radiation failed cases. The biopsies were mostly inconclusive and it would often be difficult to convince the patients for the urgent need of surgery. Finally, when they did agree for surgery because of increase in severity of the symptoms, the lesion would be much larger than was orginally seen and was associated with poor prognosis. A planned combined regime of preoperative radiotherapy and surgery is recommended for advanced lesions.

References

1. Ward, P.H., Calcaterra, T.C., Kagan, A.R. (1975) Laryngoscope, 85, 522-529
2. Lederman, M. (1970): The Journal of Laryngology and Otology, 84:867.

© 1985 Elsevier Science Publishers B.V. (Biomedical Division)
New dimensions in otorhinolaryngology - head and neck surgery, vol. 2.
E. Myers, editor

ETIOLOGY AND MANAGEMENT OF PHARYNGEAL FISTULAE FOLLOWING LARYNGECTOMY

Sudhir Bahadur and S.K. Kacker
Department of Otolaryngology
All India Institute of Medical Sciences,
New Delhi - 110 029

The occurrence of a pharyngocutaneous fistula following laryngectomy often mars healing of the wound, increases morbidity and prolongs the hospitalization of the patient. Preoperative radiotherapy is known to be an important contributory factor to formation of the pharyngeal fistula[1,2] The present paper attempts to assess the role of various factors in the etiology of pharyngocutaneous fistulae and discusses the management of these cases.

Material and Methods:

This study consists of 156 patients of carcinoma of the larynx and laryngopharynx which underwent radical surgery. Mean age of the patients was 52 years. There were 139 males and 17 females patients.

One hundred and fourteen (73%) cases had endolaryngeal lesions, while the remaining 42 (27%) were laryngopharyngeal lesions.

A majority of the patients had advanced disease when first seen. Eighty two percent cases presented with stage III and IV lesions, whereas only 28 cases (18%) had stage I and II disease. Neck node involvement occurred in 56 cases (35%). All cases with palpable nodalmetastasis underwent radical neck dissection.

Results

Incidence of pharyngeal fistulae and mode of therapy

Mode of Therapy	No. of cases	Fistulae	Spontaneous healing	Required repair	Residual lesion
Primary surgery (14 patients received post-operative RT)	76	15(20%)	14	-	1
Radiation failed salvage surgery (6,500 rads)	69	45(64%)	25	18	2
Planned pre-operative Radiotherapy surgery (5,500 rads)	11	4(36%)	-	4	-
TOTAL :	156	65(41%)	29(61%)	22(37%)	3(2%

We feel that preoperative radiotherapy is the single most important factor in causing a high incidence of pharyngeal fistulae following laryngectomy. Dose of radiotherapy and the interval between the latter and subsequent radical surgery are thus important (table). Cases receiving full curative radiotherapy and undergoing salvage surgery (interval between radiotherapy and surgery being greater than six weeks) were maximally associated with formation of pharyngocutaneous fistulae. Stage of the disease and additional surgery in the form of radical neck dissection does not seem to influence formation of a fistula.

Post operative sepsis has been blamed to be an important factor in causation of fistulae. Commonest organisms found for the infection were gram negative bacilli.

However, postoperative infection was also mostly seen in heavily irradiated patients.

Proper and meticulous care of the local tissues help in early healing. However, type of skin incisions and the type of suture material used for pharyngeal reconstruction do not seem to influence the incidence of pharyngeal fistulae.

We have found suction drainage to be very useful in ensuring good healing. The corrugated rubber drains used in earlier years were associated with high incidence of fistulae.

Once the fistula has occurred initial problem is management of the infected wound. An important surgical dressing is application of a free skin graft over the raw surface.

Of 64 fistulae (41%) observed in this series, in 39 (61%) cases the fistulae healed spontaneously within 6-8 weeks. Only 22 fistulae (37%) required surgical repair. Type II and III fistulae were treated by bringing tissues from elsewhere, such as utilising the deltopectoral and/or the pectoralis major myocutaneous flaps. In type I fistulae local tissues were used for repair.

References

1. Meyers, E. (1972): Archives of Otolaryngology 95:10
2. Briant, TDR (1975) Laryngoscope 85:829.

New dimensions in otorhinolaryngology – head and neck surgery, vol. 2.
E. Myers, editor

SPEECH RESULTS OF BRANDENBURG'S NEOGLOTTIC PROCEDURE

JAMES H. BRANDENBURG, DIANE M. BLESS, BARRY SALINSKY

Division of Otolaryngology, Department of Surgery, University of Wisconsin-Madison, University of Wisconsin Hospital and Clinics, 600 Highland Avenue, Madison, WI 53792, USA

INTRODUCTION

The purpose of this preliminary study was to report on quantitative measures of speech results in a group of patients undergoing total laryngectomy and the Brandenburg Neoglottic procedure. More specifically, this study attempted to quantify the vocal characteristics of patients using neoglottic speech in order to compare the frequency, intensity, rate of speaking, and acceptability of neoglottic speech with normative data reported in the literature for esophageal, T-E prostheses,and normal speakers.

MATERIAL AND METHODS

Surgical Procedure

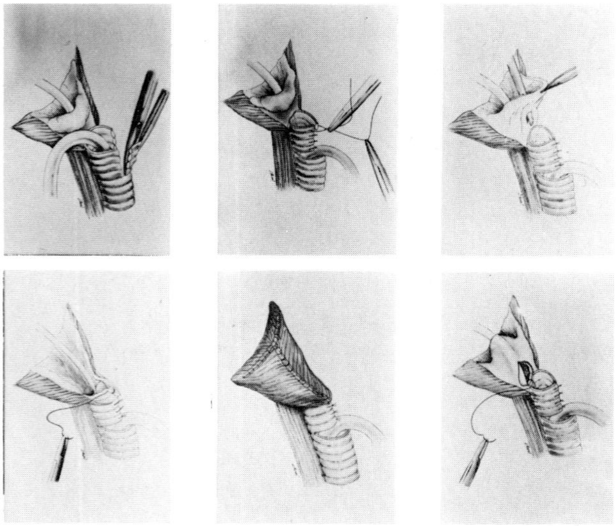

Following removal of the larynx, including the hyoid bone and cricoid cartilage, the neoglottis is constructed from the upper four tracheal rings and upper esophagus. An anterior segment approximately 1 cm in width is removed. The walls are then reapproximated anteriorly in such a fashion as to create a triangular-shaped tube which becomes the neoglottis. The newly created tube is partially dissected away from the esophagus and mobilized. A suture is secured transversely through the newly created tube about 1 cm below the superior end of the neoglottic tube. This produces a tuck in the posterior wall of the neoglottis forming an hourglass configuration of the lumen. The final steps involve connecting the neoglottis to the upper esophagus. The lower margin of the pharyngeostoma is reflected on itself and sutured to the anterior and anterolateral portion of the upper margin of the neoglottis. This forms a flap of mucous membrane overhanging the opening of the tube creating a "neoepiglottis" when serves to prevent aspiration.

Subjects and Speech Sampled

Fifteen laryngectomies who had undergone the neoglottis reconstructive procedure following the total laryngectomy performed by the same surgeon at the University of Wisconsin Hospital and Clinics, Madison, Wisconsin served as subjects. Speech samples were recorded during a variety of tasks including sustained vowel production, conversational speech and reading. The speech samples were analyzed for mean and range of frequency, mean and range of intensity, syllable and word rate, and level of acceptability.

RESULTS AND DISCUSSION

Quantitative analyses of speech following Brandenburg's neoglottic reconstruction are encouraging. Preliminary results indicate that vocal parameters of frequency (mean 79 Hz, range 55-114 Hz), intensity (mean 68, range 18 dB), maximum phonation time (27 seconds) and rate (5.49 syllables/second, 130 words/per/min) are superior to those reported for good esophageal speakers and compare favorably to those reported for speakers with prosthetic T-E shunts. In addition, the speech of neoglottic speakers is judged to be generally acceptable, even by naive judges, and generally preferable to good esophageal speakers. Finally, although it was beyond the scope of this paper to describe the source of vibration in these speakers, evidence is presented from videostroboscopic images that demonstrates the esophageal opening into the oro-pharynx clearly makes some contribution .

ACKNOWLEDGMENTS

We gratefully acknowledge the efforts of Maria Cavicchio and Stanley Ewanowski in recording some these subjects.

New dimensions in otorhinolaryngology - head and neck surgery, vol. 2.
E. Myers, editor

CHONDRONECROSIS OF THE LARYNX

FRANCIS L. MCNELIS, M.D., F.A.C.S.

Department of Otolaryngology, Rhode Island Hospital,
Providence, Rhode Island, (U.S.A.)

Chondritis or chondronecrosis of the larynx and especially of the cricoid cartilage is an infrequent occurrence with modern improved techniques for radiotherapeutic irradication of primary squamous cell carcinoma. Perichondritis in the form of laryngeal and especially arytenoid edema is more often seen, but the diagnosis seldom made as it is felt unwise to biopsy intact tissue at this stage. Careful follow-up to rule out a possible recurrence must be made.

The author has observed three cases in the past three years of clinical chondronecrosis of the larynx each following radiation therapy:

1. LL Seventy-five-year-old male given 6500 rads with currative intent for T3 NO MO supraglottic squamous cell carcinoma in 1974. He was symptom free until 1983 when he experienced progressive symptoms of dysphagia, weight loss and stridor requiring first a tracheostomy and then followed by gastrostomy. An ulceration was found in the post cricoid area measuring 1x1 cm and exhibiting bare cartilage. When he failed to respond to conservative management a laryngectomy was carried out. Histology of the post cricoid ulceration showed carcinoma in situ with microinvasion. Margins of the resection were clear of disease.

2. FD Seventy-two-year-old female who had out of state x-ray therapy of an unknown amount to the left tonsillar area in 1951 for malignancy. She was a pack a day cigarette smoker and enjoyed one martini a day. In 1982 she developed a carcinoma at the base of the epiglottis extending into the supralaryngeal area, but not involving the true cords. A supraglottic laryngectomy was carried out, but

poor healing was experienced and the patient developed chondronecrosis at the margins of resection. This required subsequent laryngectomy with prompt healing and no tumor in the remaining specimen.

3. AK Fifty-eight-year-old male with metastatic node in the right neck and no primary lesion found. He was treated with split dosage x-ray of 6800 rads in combination with Cis Platinum. This was followed by chemotherapy with multiple agents on a monthly basis. He initially did well, but after six months developed increasing soreness of throat, burning and dysphagia. He was admitted in acute stridor and required tracheostomy. At that time laryngoscopy was performed and the marked edema of the arytenoids was found to be the cause of his stridor. Further passage of the scope into the post cricoid area showed an area of bare cartilage 1 cm in diameter and consistent with chondronecrosis of the cricoid cartilage. Biopsy showed no evidence of tumor. He also was treated with gastrostomy and after ten months of keeping the area at rest it was found to heal and both the tracheostomy and gastrostomy was discontinued.

The common finding in these three cases was the prior use of x-ray therapy many years before in cases one and two and the combination with chemotherapy in case number three. Healing may occur by placing the diseased area at rest by tracheostomy and gastrostomy as in case three. However, when improvement does not occur as in case one recurrent disease must be suspected. Case number two probably should not have been treated by conservation surgery because of the previous irradiation therapy administered thirty-one years before. However, the patient would not at first accept total laryngectomy.

These three cases are felt to be a valuable contribution to the mode of occurrence and management of a relatively uncommon disease (clinical laryngeal chondronecrosis) in modern laryngology.

New dimensions in otorhinolaryngology - head and neck surgery, vol. 2.
E. Myers, editor

VOCAL CORD AUGMENTATION: CHARACTERISTICS OF COLLAGEN VS. TEFLON IN THE CANINE LARYNX

ROBERT J. FEDER, M.D., STEPHEN A. GELLER, M.D., ROBERT KASSEL, M.D., RICHARD MERTENS, M.D., ALFRED S. LAVORATO, PhD, CCC

ROBERT J. FEDER, M.D., ATTENDING DIV. OTOLARYNGOLOGY, STEPHEN GELLER, M.D., CHIEF, DEPT. OF PATHOLOGY: ROBERT KASSEL, M.D., RESIDENT DEPT. OF SURGERY; RICHARD MERTENS, M.D., FELLOW DEPT. OF PATHOLOGY: CEDARS-SINAI MEDICAL CENTER, LOS ANGELES, CA.

CEDARS-SINAI MEDICAL TOWERS, 8635 WEST THIRD STREET, SUITE 465W
LOS ANGELES, CA. 90048

INTRODUCTION

Bruning[1] introduced hard paraffin for vocal cord augmentation in 1911. Complications and the formation of pariffinomas led to its abandonment thereafter. Teflon* was introduced by Arnold[2] in 1962 and remains the bioimplant of choice. Gelfoam[R**] was introduced by Schramm[3] et al as an interim implant for vocal cord augmentation of the unilaterally paralyzed vocal cord and may be injected to allow patients to determine vocal quality before injection of a permanent material such as Teflon. It is absorbed in tissue anywhere within 6 to 10 weeks. Ford[4] reported on the use of collagen (ZydermII[R***]), in which he cited a canine experiment to fill surgically created defects. Since that study, both Ford and the senior author, Feder[5], have injected human subjects for unilateral vocal cord paralysis, surgically created scarring and defects. The senior author felt that collagen appeared to disperse differently than did teflon and display slightly different characteristics during the injection. To compare the characteristics of collagen and teflon, the canine larynx was chosen to study these observations.

MATERIALS AND METHODS

Each of five dogs were injected into the most lateral portion of the vocal cord through the ventricle directly adjacent to the mid-membranous cord. The left cord of each animal was injected utilizing a protype piston gun with approximately 0.2cc of collagen. A similar quantity of teflon was injected into the right cord of each experimental animal with a Bruning syringe. Teflon was injected through a #19 needle and the collagen delivered through a #27 needle. Dogs 1 & 2 received 4 mg. of dexamethasone IV during surgery and an equal dose the following day. The dogs were sacrificed at varying intervals; dog #1 after 48 hours; dog #2 after 14 days; dogs 3, 4 and 5 within one hour of injection. Excised larynges were fixed in 10% neutral buffered formalin for periods ranging from 5 to 32 days prior to further dissection. The specimens were then bisected in the midplane, exposing both vocal cords. Vertical sections of the true vocal cords were taken parallel to the free edge of the cord and lateral to the bulk of the injected bolus of teflon or collagen, such that the majority of each vocal cord was excised in a single tissue block. Following dehydration in graded alcohols, xylenes and

---

* TEFLON-THE MENTOR O AND O INC.; HINGHAM, MA.
** GELFOAM - UPJOHN CO.; KALAMAZOO, MICHIGAN
*** ZYDERM II-COLLAGEN CORP.; PALO ALTO, CA.

subsequent embedding in paraffin, 5 micron thick sections were cut from the lateral surface of each block after leveling into the injection site. Sections were stained with Hematoxylin and Eosin and Masson's trichrome stain, using standard histologic methods and were then examined by light microscopy.

RESULTS

Dog #1, sacrificed after 48 hours, exhibited early capsule formation around a campact bolus of teflon. A significant number of multinucleated giant cells and a marked inflammatory response was noted. The collagen formed a loose bolus with mild inflammatory reaction primarily of mononuclear cells, a few segmented cells but no giant cells. Dog #2 was sacrificed after 14 days. The teflon in the right cord exhibited many multinucleated giant cells and a thick fibrous capsule. The collagen in the left cord was found to be in a loose bolus. There was no capsule and no evidence of reaction. No side effects or airway compromise was encountered in either dogs 1 or 2. Dogs 3, 4 and 5 were sacrificed immediately following injection. During sectioning, the teflon was lost in a single bolus. The collagen persisted after sectioning and stained readily.

CONCLUSIONS

Comparative studies appear to reveal that collagen is somewhat more easily injected and appears to extrude less readily through the entry needle than does teflon. This may be a function of viscosity and needle size, with teflon requiring a 19 gauge needle and collagen a 27 gauge for injection. The larger needle hole may be allowing for greater extrusion. Collagen appears to form a less compact bolus. No capsule is formed around the collagen even after 14 days. Teflon exhibits an early capsule after 48 hours. No conclusions could be made regarding dispersion in muscle since the lateral ventricle region of the vocal cord in the dog is poor in muscle fibers. This study would lead us to conclude that an additional group of animals should be injected in a region of greater muscle mass. A second study is to begin shortly which will include injection of collagen and teflon directly into the vocalis medially so as to place the implant in a region that contains a greater number of muscle fibers and allows for additional observations on dispersion. Collagen is absorbed although at a slower rate then gelfoam.

Supported by
The Henry J. Rubin, M.D. Research Fund, Cedars-Sinai Medical Center
Collagen Corporation, Palo Alto, Ca.

BIBLIOGRAPHY

1. Brunings W. Uber eine Behandlungsmethode der Rekerrenskahmung Verhandl Ver. Deutsch. Laryng. 18;93 (525) 151 (533) 1911
2. Arnold GE. Vocal Rehabilitation of Paralytic Dysphonia. IV Technique of Intracordal Injection, Arch. Otolaryng. 76; 358-368, 1962
3. Schramm VL May M Lavorato AS. Gelfoam Paste Injection for Vocal Cord Paralysis: Temporary Rehabilitation of Glottic Incompetence. Laryngoscope 88;1978: 1268-1273
4. Ford CN Martin DW Warner TF. Injectable Collagen in Laryngeal Rehabilitation. Laryngoscope. 94;1984: 513-518
5. Feder RJ. Lavorato AS. Collagen Augmentation for Early Unilateral Vocal Cord Paralysis and Asthenia Laryngis: A Preliminary Report. Presented So. Cal. Chap. ACS 1/85 Submitted for Publication

© 1985 Elsevier Science Publishers B.V. (Biomedical Division)
New dimensions in otorhinolaryngology – head and neck surgery, vol. 2.
E. Myers, editor

NEO-LARYNX (A NEW OPERATION)

P. GHOSH. P.O. BOX 1492, BOROKO, PAPUA NEW GUINEA

INTRODUCTION

After experimenting on dog [I], 'Neo-Larynx' was constructed on humans, offering alaryngeal speech[2]. Development of neoglottic stenosis, after initial phonation, was a problem. To obviate this a few modifications were reported [3, 4]. A new operation has been devised, as follows, for preventing stenosis.

OPERATIVE PROCEDURE

After a low tracheostomy, a total laryngectomy is performed. The trachea is separated from the oesophagus for 2.5 cm. A full-thickness tongue-shaped flap is raised from the posterior tracheal wall, based superiorly, which would be the neo-epiglottis (Fig Ia, FL, NE). Its base is 5 mm below the upper margin of trachea. An ancoring stitch is applied to the neo-epiglottis (Fig-Ib, AT (NE). A slant transverse incision is made through the anterior oesophageal wall at the level of the base of the neo-epiglottis (TC, Fig-Ib). Anchoring stitches are applied near the ends of TC (Fig-Ib, AT (O). An inferiorly based mucosal flap, raised from the posterolateral tracheal wall, is passed over the inferior margin of TC and stitched with 3-0 chromic catgut. The neo-epiglottis is passed into the lumen of oesophagus through the TC which would form the neo-glottis (Fig-Ia &b and INSET, NG). This is done by tractions on AT (NE) & AT (O), (Fig-Ib). Trachea and oesophagus are stitched together with 3-0 chr.catgut (Fig-Ia, CS). A rectangular plastic sheet is passed through the neo-glottis and kept for three weeks. The upper end of trachea is closed with 3-0 chr. catgut (Fig-Ia,Cst). Finally, the pharynx and the skin wound are closed as usual. Postoperative managements are as after total laryngectomy. A fenestrated tracheostomy tube is inserted after removal of the plastic sheet after three weeks and the patient is asked to phonate after closing the tube with a finger and he readily does so.

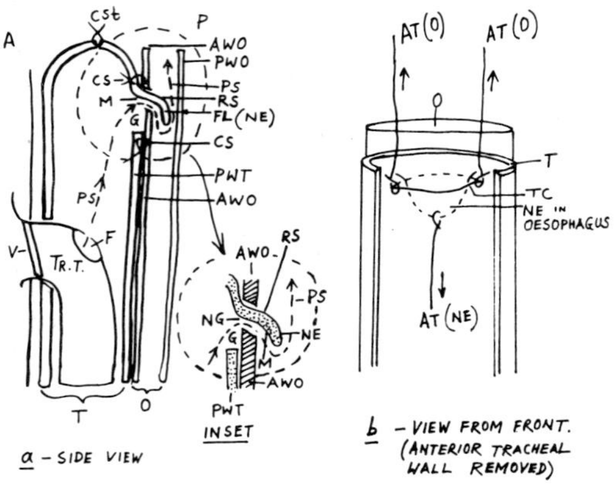

FIG-1

FIG- A-ANTERIOR, P-POSTERIOR, CSt-CATGUT STITCH IN TRACHEA, AWO -ANTERIOR WALL OF OESOPHAGUS, PWO-POSTERIOR WALL OF OESOPHAGUS, CS-CATGUT STITCHES, PS-PHONETIC STREAM, RS-RAW EXTERNAL SURFACE OF NEOEPIGLOTTIS, FL-TRACHEAL FLAP, NE-NEOEPIGLOTTIS, M-MUCOSAL SURFACE OF NEOEPIGLOTTIS, NG-NEOGLOTTIS, G-GAP IN POSTERIOR TRACHEAL WALL FILLED UP BY AWO, PWT-POSTERIOR WALL OF TRACHEA, F-FENESTRA IN TRACHEOSTOMY TUBE, TR.T.-TRACHEOSTOMY TUBE, V-SPEAKING VALVE, T-TRACHEA, O-OESOPHAGUS, INSET-NEOGLOTTIS REGION, AT(O)-ANCHORING SILK IN OESOPHAGEAL WALL, AT(NE)-ANCHORING THREAD FROM NEOEPIGLOTTIS, ↑↓ -DIRECTIONS OF TRACTION ON THREADS, TC-TRANSVERSE CUT.

OBSERVATIONS AND DISCUSSION

The lips of the neo-glottis are mucosa-lined and this minimises the occurrence of stenosis. Aspiration into the trachea is prevented by the neo-epiglottis and the sphincteric action of the muscles around the neoglottis [4]. The patient develop-es 'tracheo-oesophageal' speech (cf.-conventional pharyngo-oesophageal one) immediately after removal of the plastic sheet and no strenuous training and practice are necessary. Skiagraphs (Fig-2A & B) show interrupted air shadows in oesophagus and pharynx at rest (R) and continuous phonetic stream (PS) during phonation (P) respectively. This speech is more physiological than the conventional one since the pressure of the phonetic stream, produced by natural bellows, is higher than that produced in the alimentary canal and is pleasantly continuous (cf. interrupted pharyngo-oesophageal one) and the patient does not get exhausted during phonation. The operation can be performed even after radical neck dissection without compromising the principles of cancer surgery.

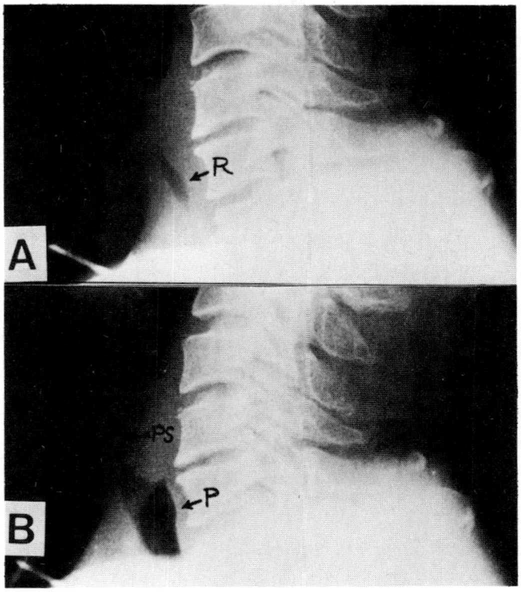

REFERENCES

1. Ghosh, P. (1976): Vertical Tracheo-oesophagoplasty, Indian. J. Otolaryngology, 28:164.
2. Ghosh, P. (1977): Transverse Tracheo-oesophagoplasty, The J. Laryngology and Oto., 9I:I077.
3. Ghosh, P. (1980): Phonosurgery, Bihar Journal of Otolaryngology (India), I:29.
4. Ghosh, P. (I980): Modification of Transverse Tracheo-oesophagoplasty, India J. Otolaryngology, 36:I03

© 1985 Elsevier Science Publishers B.V. (Biomedical Division)
New dimensions in otorhinolaryngology - head and neck surgery, vol. 2.
E. Myers, editor

SYSTEMIC COMPLICATIONS OF ACUTE EPIGLOTTITIS

CARLOS GONZALEZ, M.D.; J. CARLTON GARTNER, M.D.; MARGARETHA L. CASSELBRANT, M.D., PH.D.; MARGARET A. KENNA, M.D.

Departments of Otolaryngology and Pediatrics, University of Pittsburgh School of Medicine and Children's Hospital of Pittsburgh, Pittsburgh, PA

INTRODUCTION

Acute epiglottitis is one of the most dramatic and potentially fatal diseases of childhood. The clinical course is usually fulminant, progressing to complete airway obstruction within hours. *Haemophilus influenzae* type B is recovered from over 90% of blood cultures when performed prior to antibiotic therapy. Despite the high incidence of *H. influenzae* type B bacteremia associated with acute epiglottitis, few patients suffer associated septic complications. Branefors-Helander[1] reported four cases of meningitis in 15 children with epiglottitis. Molteni[2] reviewed 72 patients with acute epiglottitis and noted a 25% incidence of pneumonia as well as cervical adenitis. They encountered no cases of meningitis associated with acute epiglottitis. In contrast, Davis et al.[3] at Children's Hospital of Pittsburgh noted only five cases of pneumonia and three cases of cervical adenitis in 100 consecutive cases of acute epiglottitis. They noted no cases of acute epiglottitis associated with meningitis or severe septicemia. Our recent experience with a two-year-old child with acute epiglottitis complicated by septic shock prompted this report.

CASE REPORT

A.H. is a two-year-old white boy who was doing well until approximately two days prior to admission when he developed signs and symptoms of upper respiratory infection. On December 19, 1984, the patient's breathing difficulty increased and was accompanied by inspiratory stridor. The child suddenly had an acute respiratory arrest and required intubation. The child was then transferred to Children's Hospital of Pittsburgh. Direct laryngoscopy, at that time, established the diagnosis of acute epiglottitis. Blood cultures and epiglottic swab cultures grew *H. influenzae* type B. During the first week of hospitalization, our patient went into septic shock and respiratory failure, cardiovascular collapse and dessiminated intravascular coagulation. Treatment included cefatoxime and ampicillin and ventilator support as well as vasopressors. In addition, the child required a tracheotomy for prolonged intubation, amputation for (L) foot gangrene, jejunal resection for ischemic bowel disease and peritoneal and hemodialysis for renal failure.

The child was decannulated and discharged after a four month hospital stay. The child has no neurological sequelae and is doing well.

DISCUSSION

Complications of acute epiglottitis have been reported to vary between 1%-37%.[4] These complications should be divided into noninfectious and infectious in origin (Table I). Noninfectious complications are secondary to regional disease and acute upper airway obstruction. They include respiratory arrest, cardiac arrest, anoxic encephalopathy and pulmonary edema. These complications of acute epiglottitis are well recognized and have been preventable with prompt airway control. The infections complications of acute epiglottitis are secondary to the bacteremic episode and, as such, are true systemic complications. These include meningitis, pneumonia, cervical adenitis and septic shock. Use of appropriate high dose intravenous antibiotic therapy should reduce the incidence of these complications. In conclusion, this case stresses that acute epiglottitis is a systemic disease with regional manifestations. Although prompt airway management has been paramount in reducing the noninfectious complications of acute epiglottitis, expedient high dose antibiotic therapy is also important to avert the infectious complications of this disease.

TABLE I

COMPLICATIONS OF EPIGLOTTITIS

Pathophysiology	Systemic Bacteremia	Regional Airway Obstruction
	Pneumonia	Respiratory Arrest
	Meningitis	Cardiac Arrest
	Cervical Adenitis	Anoxic Encephalopathy
	Septic Shock	Pulmonary Edema

REFERENCES

1. Branefors-Helander, P. and Jeppssor, P.: Acute Epiglottitis. Scand. J. Infect. Dis., 7:103-111, 1975.
2. Molteni, R.: Epiglottitis: Incidence of Extraepiglottic Infection. Pediatrics, 58:526-531, 1976.
3. Davis, H., et al.: Acute Upper Airway Obstruction: Croup and Epiglottitis. Ped. Cl. N.A., 28(4):859-880, 1981.
4. Baugh, R. and Baker, S.R.: Epiglottitis in Children: Review of 24 Cases. Otolaryngol. Head & Neck Surg., 90:157-162, 1982.

© 1985 Elsevier Science Publishers B.V. (Biomedical Division)
New dimensions in otorhinolaryngology – head and neck surgery, vol. 2.
E. Myers, editor

PHARYNGEAL CONSTRICTOR MYOTOMY AND SPEECH REHABILITATION OF THE LARYNGECTOMY PATIENT

JULIAN HENLEY, M.D., F.A.C.S., CHARLES R. SOULIERE, JR., M.D.
Yale New Haven Hospital and St. Raphaels Hospital

INTRODUCTION

Twenty percent of patients fail to develop or maintain TE speech after laryngectomy (4,5). Previous studies by us (3) and Singer (6) suggested the possibility of airflow induced pharyngospasm as the basis of TE speech failures. We report five patients with documented pharyngospasm who developed TE speech only after secondary middle and inferior constrictor myotomy.

MATERIAL AND METHODS

Five laryngectomy patients had failed to develop speech despite trials with three different laryngeal prostheses (Singer-Blom, Panje, Henley-Cohn). All had patent TE fisulae and documented correct placement of the prosthesis. Video cervical fluoroesophago-scopy, and temporary pharyngeal plexus nerve blockade demonstrated airflow induced pharyngospasm. All patients underwent constrictor myotomy with successful acquisition of TE speech postoperatively.

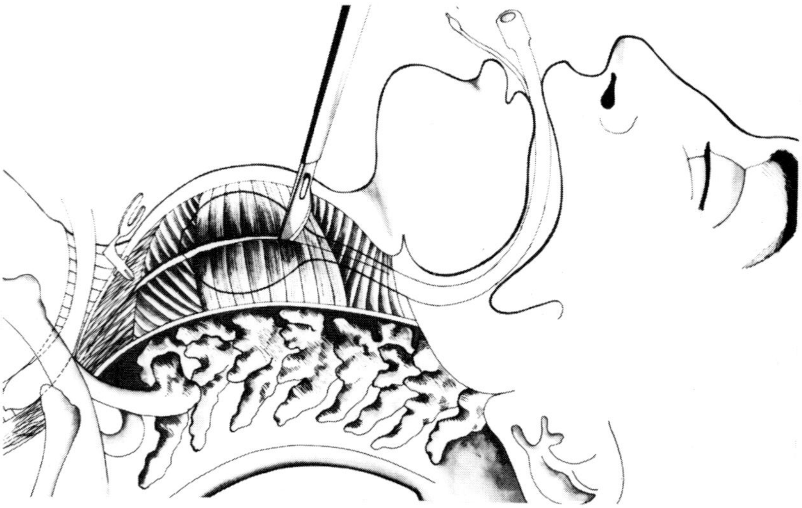

RESULTS AND DISCUSSION

The TE insertion procedure described previously by the senior author is performed on outpatient basis under local anesthesia with little morbidity (3). However, a subpopulation of patients fail to develop effective speech, despite adequate time and intensive training. In evaluating these patients several of questions need to be addressed.

1. Is speech device dependent? - Previous studies of a group of patients each being fitted with three devices in sequence (Singer-Blom, Panje, Henley-Cohn) clearly demonstrated that there are distinct differences in speech loudness, fluency, and effort that are related to device choice (3). Our biased experience has been with the Storz Henley-Cohn device which has shown itself over the past several years to have low air resistance (Table 1), low extrusion rate, low maintenance, and longevity without removal.

2. Does the patient have pharyngeal constrictor spasm blocking the outflow of air from the pharynx? - A video cervical esophagoscopy can be used to document pharyngospasm. A temporary Xylocaine block of the pharyngeal plexus is performed, and if TE speech is acquired, we proceed to inferior and middle constrictor myotomy.

We have found it to be crucial to incise both the inferior and middle constrictors (Fig. 2). We have had no significant complications despite previous neck disection or radiotherapy, and all previous TE speech failures have attained excellent prosthetic speech after constrictor myotomy.

CONCLUSIONS

1. A number of patients remain unable to speak with TE

prosthesis despite optimal device choice.

2. Such patients should be evaluated for pharyngeal spasm.

3. Surgical constrictor myotomy is very effective.

4. Surgical myotomy may make TE fistula devices obsolete. Patients previously unable to learn esophageal speech may become excellent unaided esophageal speakers.

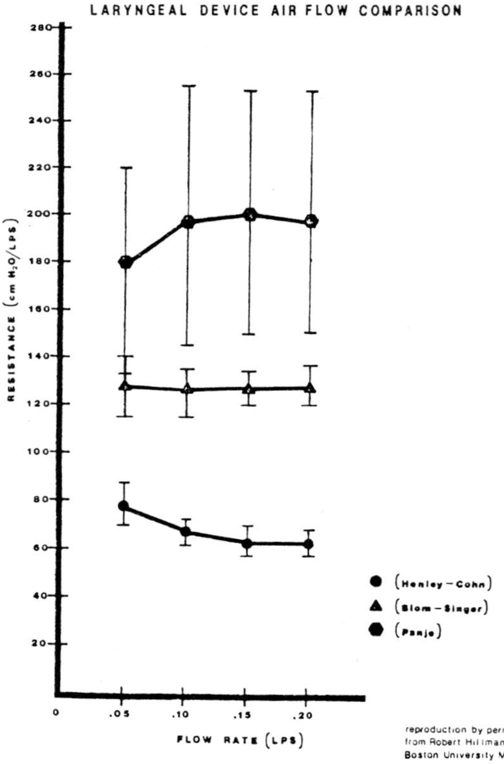

reproduction by permission
from Robert Hillman, et al.
Boston University Medical School

REFERENCES

1. Singer MI, Blom ED (198Ø) Ann Otol 89:529
2. Panje WR (1981) Ann Otol 9Ø:116
3. Henley-Cohn JL, Hausfeld JN, Jakubczak GJ (1984) Laryngoscope 94:43
4. Wetmore SJ, Johns ME, Baker SR (1981) Arch Otol 1Ø7:674
5. Singer MI, Blom ED, Hamaker RC (1981) Ann Otol 9Ø:498
6. Singer MI, Blom ED (1981) Arch Otol 1Ø7:674
7. Kirchner JA, Scatliff JH, Dey FL, Shedd DP (1963) Laryngoscope 73:18
8. Winans CS, Reichbach SJ, Walddrgo WF (1974) Arch Otol 99:1Ø
9. Henley-Cohn, JL (1981) Laryngoscope 91:1957

New dimensions in otorhinolaryngology - head and neck surgery, vol. 2.
E. Myers, editor

LARYNGEAL DYNAMICS IN DYSARTHRIC SPEECH

HAJIME HIROSE, SEIJI NIIMI AND MASAYUKI SAWASHIMA
Research Institute of Logopedics and phoniatrics, Faculty of Medicine, University of Tokyo, 7-3-1 Hongo Tokyo (Japan)

INTRODUCTION

This paper will present the preliminary results of an analysis of laryngeal maneuvers during speech production in selected cases of different types of dysarthria. For analyzing this laryngeal articulatory behavior, the techniques of photoglottography and electromyography were used.

SUBJECTS AND METHOD

Recordings were made in 2 cases of parkinsonism and 3 cases of amyotrophic lateral sclerosis (ALS). As a control, a normal speaker also served as a subject. The subjects were required to repeat the Japanese monosyllables as quickly and regularly as possible. In addition, selected Japanese words were uttered with a frame sentence.

A fiberscope was inserted through a nostril of each subject. The fiberscope was attached to a video-camera and, while the glottal maneuvers were displayed on a monitor screen, the illuminating light modulated by the glottal gestures was sensed by a photo-transister attached to the anterior neck on the trachea. The signals were recorded on a PCM data-recorder. Meaningful words embedded in a carrier phrase were also recorded.

Separate from the glottographic recordings, electromyographic signals were recorded from the thyroarytenoid muscle during sustained phonation and respiration.

RESULTS AND COMMENTS

In normal subject, the glottis opened and closed regularly for the rhythmical repetition of the monosyllable which consisted of a voiceless consonant and vowel.

In ALS subjects, the pattern of the repetitive gestures of the glottis quickly became irregular, and the glottal opening also became smaller. The repetition gestures were often preceded by an interval of glottal opening with an abrupt air intake and followed by a choking gesture associated with an outbreak of coughing. The choking gesture seemed to be the result of tight reflex closure of the glottis corresponding to increasing spasticity.

It was noted that parkinsonian subjects tended to automatically repeat the same articulatory gesture, or to "stutter", during speech. It was also noted that there was limitation of vocal fold movements in parkinsonian subjects. EMG examination on one of our parkinsonian patients revealed that the number of NMU discharges for phonation, or for the concomittant vocal fold adduction, was not reduced, and there were no pathological discharge patterns such as polyphasic or highamplitude voltages. On the other hand, persistent firing was seen even during the period of inspiration in which thyroarytenoid activity was suppressed in normal cases. These findings would seem to indicate that there is no evidence of neurogenic paralysis in this case, but that there is a loss of the reciprocal suppression of the thyroarytenoid during inspiration.

Hypokinetic patterns in parkinsonism in terms of a reduction in the range of movements can be related to a deterioration in the reciprocal adjustment of the antagonistic muscles. The limitation of the vocal fold movement in these cases must be one example of this type of pathology. The EMG patterns of persistent discharge in the thyroarytenoid even during inspiration must be taken as a physiological evidence of parkinsonian rigidity as described by Leanderson and his colleagues (1).

Although EMG signals were not recorded from the functionally antagonistic muscle, the posterior cricoarytenoid in this case, it seems probable that the apparent limitation of vocal fold mobility is due to a rigidity of the laryngeal muscles in parkinsonism. In other words, the apparent limitation of vocal fold movement should not simply be taken as a paralysis of the vocal folds.

REFERENCE

1. Leanderson R. Meyerson BA and Persson A (1972): Lip muscle function in Parkinsonian dysarthria. Acta ololaryngol 74: 354-357.

New dimensions in otorhinolaryngology – head and neck surgery, vol. 2.
E. Myers, editor

ACUTE LARYNGEAL TRAUMA

Edward E. Jacobs, M.D., William W. Montgomery, M.D., William G. Lavelle, M.D.; Harvard Medical School, Boston, MA, USA

This report summarizes the principals of surgical treatment of acute laryngeal trauma with particular focus on the use of the Montgomery® Laryngeal Stent to prevent subsequent stenosis and laryngeal dysfunction. The current method of management is derived from the authors' experience over the last 20 years involving 179 cases of laryngeal trauma at the Massachusetts Eye and Ear Infirmary.

The vast majority of severe laryngeal injuries are due to external blunt trauma related to motor vehicle accidents and sports mishaps. Optimal management entails prompt support of vital functions, comprehensive evaluation of injury severity and early definitive surgical intervention to restore anatomical and functional integrity.

Methods

Severe laryngeal injuries manifested by gross clinical abnormalities including mucosal lacerations, exposed and displaced cartilages and vocal cord paralysis usually require open surgical repair. In most cases the recommended surgical strategy includes: (1) vertical midline laryngofissure, (2) reduction of displaced cartilages, (3) removal of devitalized tissue, (4) closure of mucosal lacerations and (5) support with a Montgomery® Laryngeal Stent.*

**Available from: Boston Medical Products, Inc. 100 Charles River Plaza, Boston, MA USA 02114*

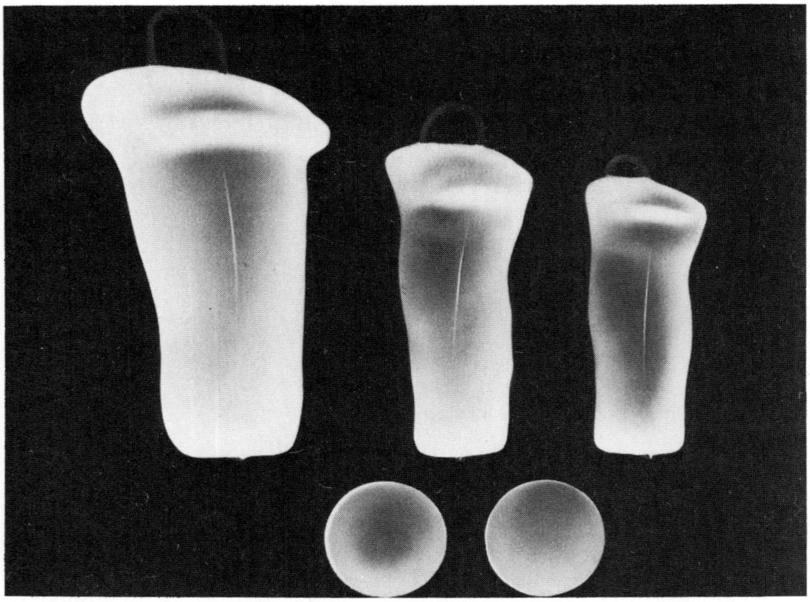

The Montgomery® Laryngeal Stent is designed specifically to prevent larygneal stenosis and is therefore used in conjuction with reconstructive procedures involving both acute and chronic laryngeal injuries. The advantages of the Montgomery® Laryngeal Stent include (1) non-reactive soft silicone construction to decrease granulation and cicatrix, (2) preformed contour to maintain the proper relations of the vocal cords, supraglottic and subglottic structures, (3) three sizes specific for male, female and child, (4) superior ligature loop to aid in endoscopic removal 3 - 6 weeks after insertion.

Summary

Severe laryngeal trauma requires open surgical repair to prevent subsequent laryngeal stenosis and dysfunction. The Montgomery® Laryngeal Stent has been used successfully for over 20 years in the management of severe acute laryngeal trauma.

© 1985 Elsevier Science Publishers B V. (Biomedical Division)
New dimensions in otorhinolaryngology - head and neck surgery, vol. 2.
E. Myers, editor

JITTER CHARACTERISTIC OF VOICE PRODUCTION AFTER AMATSU TRACHEOESOPHAGEAL SHUNT OPERATION

MINORU KINISHI, MUTSUO AMATSU

Department of Otolaryngology, Kobe University School of Medicine
Kusunoki-cho, Chuo-ku, Kobe, Japan

INTRODUCTION

During the past nine years, we have been performing the tracheoesophageal (TE) shunt operation for the purpose of voice restoration following total laryngectomy.[1] The basic idea of this technique is to divert the pulmonary air through the TE shunt into the esophagus where the vibration occurs and sound is produced.

This study was designed to explore the pitch perturbation during vowel phonation obtained through the TE shunt.

SUBJECTS AND METHODS

SUBJECTS

Ten laryngeal speakers, twenty TE speakers, and five esophageal speakers were subjected to various measurements. The laryngeal speakers had no history of voice or speech disorders. Periods of speech for the TE and the esophageal speakers ranged 2 months to 7 years, and 2 years to 14 years respectively.

METHODS

Audiotape recording were made of each subject producing a series of sustained vowel. The computer program provided duration for each cycle with a resolution of 0.05 msec. Period-by-period measurement was used to obtain seven acoustic measures: (1) mean period, (2) standard deviation of period, (3) mean fundamental frequency, (4) mean jitter, (5) average perturbation, (6) jitter ratio, and (7) relative average perturbation. Mean jitter was calculated by measuring the difference between each consecutive pair of vocal period, and obtaining the average of the differences. Average perturbation was the average of the absolute differences between three point moving and vocal period. Jitter ratio and relative average perturbation measures were used to facilitate comparisons of variation in absolute value with varying mean fundamental frequencies.

RESULTS

The results obtained were summerized in Table I.

DISCUSSION

The fundamental frequency perturbation measures indicate that both alaryngeal groups had greater jitter values and perturbation values than the laryngeal group. In the alaryngeal groups, the TE speakers had lower values of jitter ratio and relative average perturbation compared to the esophageal speakers.

When the two alaryngeal groups regulate fundamental frequency, the biomechanical and neuromuscular events not only differ from these of laryngeal speakers, but differ from each other.

The vibratory source is the same in both alaryngeal speakers, while air supply mechanism is different. In the TE speech, driving the pulmonary air through the TE shunt into esophagus results in more stable air supply than air inhalation of the conventional esophageal speech. Stable air-flow in TE speech results in more stable pitch perturbation than the esophageal speech.

CONCLUSION

AMATSU TE speech surpasses the conventional esophageal speech in the pitch perturbation measurements, because pulmonary air reserve supplies the stable air-flow to regulate the stability of the fundamental frequency.

TABLE I Means of mean period, standard deviation of period, mean Fo, mean jitter, average perturbation, jitter ratio, and relative average perturbation for laryngeal, TE, and esophageal speakers.

Variable	Laryngeal	TE	Esophageal
Mean Period (msec)	7.2	14.7	14.6
Standard Deviation of Period (msec)	0.09	0.50	1.22
Mean Fo (Hz)	149	83	73
Mean Jitter (msec)	0.07	0.47	0.82
Average Perturbation (msec)	0.04	0.29	0.45
Jitter Ratio	10	30	58
Relative Average Perturbation(10^{-3})	6	18	38

REFERENCE

1. Amatsu M (1980) A one stage surgical technique for postlaryngectomy voice rehabilitation. Laryngoscope 90:1378-1386

© 1985 Elsevier Science Publishers B.V. (Biomedical Division)
New dimensions in otorhinolaryngology – head and neck surgery, vol. 2.
E. Myers, editor

HIGH FREQUENCY JET VENTILATION: A USEFUL TECHNIQUE FOR ENDOSCOPY AND SURGERY OF THE AIRWAY

GREG RENNER MD, GREG LOVE MD, HERBERT FERRARI MD

Departments of Otolaryngology and Anesthesiology, University of Missouri School of Medicine, Columbia Missouri (United States)

INTRODUCTION

High Frequency Jet Ventilation (HFJV) is a method of mechanical ventilation which is uniquely different from more conventional techniques and can offer clear advantages for endoscopic surgery of the airway. Ventilatory rates are typically 100-150/min with tidal volumes of only 3-5ml/kg. Ventilatory gas is delivered under high pressure (55psi) to a special ventilator which is set to regulate the rate, flow pattern and driving pressure of gas to the patient. The system must overcome the resistance of a narrow canula to the airway. Klain recommends that the expiratory airway be at least 10 times larger than the ventilating canula.

Adequate ventilary exchange has been shown using the jet ventilator with conventional respiratory rates. The primary reason for the use of high frequency rates is to protect the airway from aspiration. Using a canine model, Klain showed reverse movement of laryngeally aspirated fluid with rates greater than 100/min, provided expiration is no more than 50% of the cycle.

MATERIAL AND METHODS

In 1982 a protocol was set up for selected patients undergoing airway endoscopy at the University of Missouri-Columbia. Patients were premedicated with a narcotic and anticholinergic agent. Anesthetic induction was performed using pentothal intravenously. This was continued using intravenous fentanyl and inhalation of nitrous oxide 60% - oxygen 40%. Additional pentothal was given as needed. Succinylcholine was given intravenously immediately prior to canulation and continued through the case by drip infusion. Blood pressure, EKG and heart sounds were monitored continously and arterial blood gases taken every 5 minutes.

Once the patient was anesthetized a 14 gauge, 2 inch catheter was inserted through the cricothyroid membrane. The jet ventilator (IDC-VS 600) was connected to the patient's catheter via tubing and locking connector. Ventilating rate was initially set at 150/min for patients without a history of pulmonary disease and at 100-150/min for those with a history of obstructive or restrictive pulmonary disease and at 40% for those with mild to moderate chronic obstructive pulmonary disease. Driving pressure was set at 0.35psi/kg body weight.

RESULTS

Twenty-four adult male patients were administered HFJV and successfully underwent endoscopic diagnostic and operative procedures. Serial arterial blood gas evaluation was shown acceptable throughout the procedures with good oxygenation at an FiO_2 of 0.4. Serial evaluation showed a pH range of 7.30-7.39 with a median of 7.36, pCO_2 34-55mmHg with a median of 46mmHg and pO_2 112-165mmHg with a median of 147mmHg. Blood pressure and pulse were kept within 20% of preoperative levels.

There have been no deaths or serious morbidity incurred in this patient sample. One patient who had a history of chronic obstructive pulmonary disease with bullous emphysema experienced an episode of airway expiratory obstruction during endoscopic examination of the pyriform sinuses. Upon awakening the patient was asymptomatic but a postoperative chest x-ray revealed a unilateral pneumothorax of less than 10%, which resolved without intervention by the fifth postoperative day.

DISCUSSION

Though low volumes are given with each burst, a collective volume can accumulate quite rapidly because of the rapid rate. The greatest danger in using HFJV is the chance for pneumothorax. This potentially hazardous complication should be extremely unlikely in the absence of prolonged expiratory obstruction. Both the anesthesiologist and the surgeon must be constantly on vigil to insure a constant adequate airway for expiration. Expiratory sounds are clearly audible in the unobstructed airway. If at any time expiratory flow is occluded, the jet ventilator should be immediately shut off until the airway is again secured.

A lesser disadvantage with HFJV is a tendency for hemorrhage from procedures done on the larynx to be blown upward towards the face of the endoscopist, requiring a need for protective facial shielding.

It is our opinion that HFJV is a very useful technique for selected cases of diagnostic and operative endoscopic procedures when unobstructed access to the airway is important. We have begun expanding our capabilities with HFJV by using other methods of laryngeal intubation. It is likely that HFJV will continue to develop an expanding role in ventilatory support for airway endoscopic surgery.

References

1. Klain M, Smith RB (1977) Crit Care Med 5:280-287

2. Marquez J, Fine J, Klain M, et al (1982) Anesth 57:A464

3. Sjostrand U (1977) Acta Anaesth Scand: Suppl 64

4. Jonzon A, Oberg PA, Sedin G, Sjostrand U (1970) Acta Physiol Scand 80:21A

© 1985 Elsevier Science Publishers B.V. (Biomedical Division)
New dimensions in otorhinolaryngology - head and neck surgery, vol. 2.
E. Myers, editor

ENDOSCOPIC LASER ARYTENOIDECTOMY

ROMEO Y. LIM, MD, FACS

Chief of Surgery, The Eye and Ear Clinic of Charleston, WV; Clinical Associate Professor of Otolaryngology, West Virginia Medical Center, Charleston Division, P.O. Box 3107, Charleston, WV 25331 (U.S.A.)

INTRODUCTION

Bilateral abductor paralysis of the vocal cords from varying causes results in either a severe obstruction or in a marginal compromise of the laryngeal airway.[1] Thornell's[2] endoscopic arytenoidectomy offers the most direct and simplest method of lateral mobilization of the vocal cord, since this does not require an external incision and it provides immediate assessment of the airway.[3] This procedure, however, using conventional forceps and blades has drawbacks such as bleeding, technical difficulty and unnecessary scarring. The carbon dioxide laser for laryngeal surgery as introduced by Strong and Jako[4] in 1972, has enhanced the effectiveness and predictable results of the Thornell procedure; in terms of excellent hemostasis, improved visualization, ease of manipulation and minimal cicatrization.

MATERIALS AND METHODS

From 1977 to the present, a total of 22 patients underwent an endoscopic laser arytenoidectomy at the Eye and Ear Clinic of Charleston, WV using the Coherent 450 carbon dioxide laser, coupled with a Zeiss operating microscope, for bilateral abductor vocal cord paralysis. The youngest patient was 15 years old; the oldest 91 years old. There were 16 women and 6 men. The causes of the bilateral abductor vocal cord paralysis were: 10 from thyroidectomy, 5 neurologic, 2 neck trauma, 1 post radiation, and 4 from prolonged endotracheal tube arytenoid subluxation. Twelve patients had a previous tracheostomy while the other 10, with marginal airway, did not have a tracheostomy. Mirror or fiberoptic laryngoscopy revealed a midline fixation of the vocal cords (postintubation arytenoid subluxation) or a 1.0 mm. - 1.5 mm. glottic opening. Patients without the tracheostomy manifested labored stridorous breathing and exertional dyspnea. The symptom duration varied from 3 months to 2 years.

General endotracheal anesthesia, using an aluminum wrapped #6 silicone tube, was used in 19 patients. Intravenous diazepam (Valium), coupled with dyclonine hydrochloride (Dyclone) topical anesthesia and superior laryngeal nerve block with lidocaine hydrochloride (Xylocaine) 1%, was used in one patient. Exposure of the arytenoid was accomplished by anterior displacment of the endotracheal tube with the Jako laryngoscope. Commonly, a power setting of 18-20 watts and 0.2-0.5 second duration was used. The arytenoid mucosa was first laser incised down to the cartilage. The cartilage was then grasped with a microlaryngeal cup forcep, and with traction, this was laser separated and excised from its mucosal attachment. The vocal process was included with the resection. Redundant arytenoid mucosa, prominent overlapping ventricular bands and hyperplastic vocal cord mucosa were also laser trimmed.

Steroids were administered neither intraoperatively nor postoperatively. Humidification was however, provided postoperatively. Patients with a previous tracheostomy were decannulated 3 days postsurgically. Patients without a tracheostomy were discharged the day after surgery. There was no postoperative bleeding, pain or edema except in a 72-year old patient who required an immediate postoperative tracheostomy for a severe laryngeal edema and was subsquently decannulated 3 days later. All patients had an improved laryngeal airway (absence of stridor and exertional dyspnea) and all had an intelligible phonation. Healing was complete in 3 weeks. The postoperative glottic opening was approximately 4-5 mm. Postoperative speech counseling was provided as a supportive measure. Absence of scarring and laryngeal airway compromise was evident in all patients after a follow-up period of 1-8 years.

DISCUSSION

The eight-year experience with the carbon dioxide laser has shown that the laser is a very useful tool for endoscopic arytenoidectomy. Despite the variable redundancy and thickness of the arytenoid mucosa, the cartilage could easily be excised from its mucosa with absence of bleeding in a short time. The laryngoscope, suction, cup forceps and laser are the only instruments needed for endoscopic arytenoidectomy.

The laser's added capability to trim redundant arytenoid mucosa, prominent obstructing ventricular bands and hyperplastic vocal cord mucosa without causing bleeding or edema ensures the restoration of an adequate laryngeal airway in a one-step procedure.

REFERENCES

1. Newman, MH, and Work, WP: Arytenoidectomy revisited. Laryngoscope 1976;86: 840-849
2. Thornell, WC: Intralaryngeal approach for arytenoidectomy in bilateral abductor paralysis of the vocal cords, a preliminary report. Arch Otolaryngol 1948;47:505-508
3. McFarland GE: Arytenoidectomy. Paper presented at the Annual Meeting of the American Laryngological, Rhinological and Otological Society, Iowa City, May 5, 1977
4. Strong, MS, Jako GJ: Laser surgery in the larynx. Early clinical experience with continuous CO_2 laser. Ann Otol Rhinol Laryngol 1972;81:791-798

© 1985 Elsevier Science Publishers B.V. (Biomedical Division)
New dimensions in otorhinolaryngology - head and neck surgery, vol. 2.
E. Myers, editor

THE SOLUTION IN FUNCTIONAL REHABILITATION AFTER DESTRUCTION OF THE LARYNX: THE TRACHEOSTOMA CLOSED

RODOLPHE MEYER, Centre de Chirurgie plastique, Avenue Marc-Dufour 4,Lausanne (Switzerland) and ENT Unit, Centre Hospitalier Universitaire Vaudois, Lausanne (Director: Prof.M.Savary)

INTRODUCTION

Apart from all voice problems the final goal after subtotal laryngectomy is reconstruction of an airway without a tracheostoma. Until now this was possible only in cases of partial laryngectomies. In five of such cases, MAJER of Vienna succeeded, in 1958, in performing a cricohyoidopexy leaving the cricoid cartilage, the epiglottis, and the hyoid bone intact. The cricoid ring had been fixed to the hyoid. The epiglottis and the base of the tongue prevented the passage of saliva and alimentary fluid into the lower airway. Up to now, MAJER (1) had no more opportunity to develop his promising procedure. PIQUET (2) (1980) took over and used the same conservative cricohyoidoepiglottopexy, leaving the epiglottis intact as MAJER did. In addition, he preserved one arytenoïd cartilage as suggested by LABAYLE. PIQUET's experience has shown that a closed airway is possible only in cases where the cricoid can be left intact.

FRITZ (3) (1974) tried to solve this difficult problem by mobilizing the tracheal stump more anteriorly towards the chin. This allowed a maximal anteropexy by suturing the anterior circumference to the floor of the mouth between the two digastric muscles. The posterior wall of the trachea formed a vertical line passing through the hyoïd bone. Unfortunately, the author did not succeed to close the airway by covering the gutter between the two stomas because of the collapsing of the transverse horizontal sublingual tract of the new air passage. In a second case the patient died before the multistage procedure was completed.

We went a step further with this procedure. We had the opportunity to treat two selected cases. In order to build a closed rigid bayonet-shaped pharyngo-laryngo-tracheal airway, a multistage procedure is necessary. Due to the complexity of this operation such a venture is possible only in young well motivated patients willing to undergo any surgical attempt to get rid of the tracheostoma. In two young women we succeeded to reconstruct a bayonet-shaped laryngo-tracheal segment permitting free respiration and deglutition without aspiration and with acceptable restoration of voice.

CASES AND METHODS

Case 1: Following irradiation for thyroid carcinoma, a young female patient sustained subtotal destruction of the cartilaginous framework of the larynx and of the superior part of the trachea. This resulted in laryngeal atresia, laryngo-hypopharyngeal fistula, and necrosis of the hypopharynx and prevertebral ligament.

In the first intervention, a left pectoralis major myocutaneous flap was used to repair the fistula that was at the level of the destroyed cricoid and to reconstruct the stenosed pharyngo-esophageal segment. The hypopharynx had to be enlarged from the right side using a right pectoralis major myocutaneous flap.(Fig. 1 in a second intervention, as we have done in 38 other cases.(4)

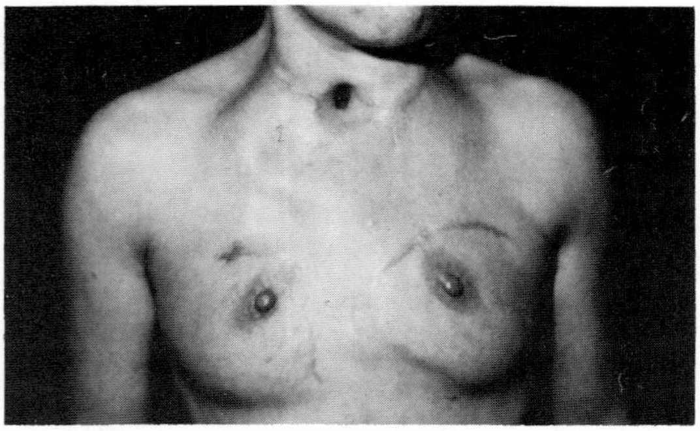

Fig. 1.) Pat. after pharyngoesophageal reconstruction.

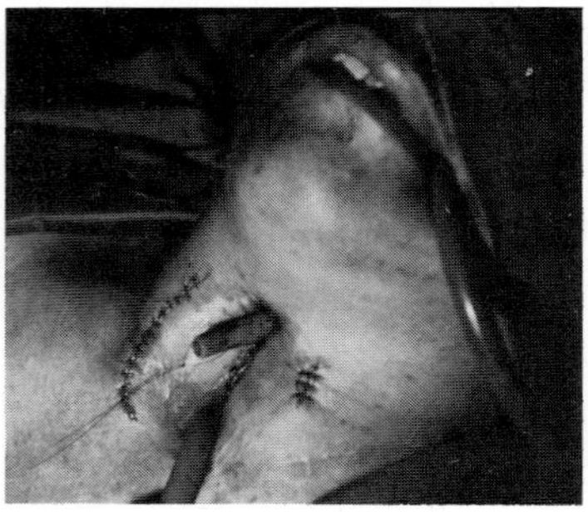

Fig. 2.) Montgomery stent in laryngostomy.

The next three operations were performed in order to reestablish the obstructed laryngo-tracheal airway. The larynx was opened above the rudimentary cords creating an external communication 5 cm above the tracheostomy. The laryngostomy was maintained at an adequate caliber by a Montgomery stent.(Fig.2) To reconstruct a rigid closed passage between the two stomata, the two lateral walls were first reconstructed by reinforcing the skin with costal cartilage. This formed a gutter. Next, the anterior wall was created by a folded regional flap equally reinforced by cartilage from the ear. A Portex tube acted as a luminal splint in the new bayonet-shaped air tract for four months before the tracheostoma was closed with another composite flap. With a skin expander and prostheses the breasts could be remodeled. (Fig.3).

Finally the patient could breathe well, swallow without aspiration, and speak understandably with a closed airway (Fig.4).

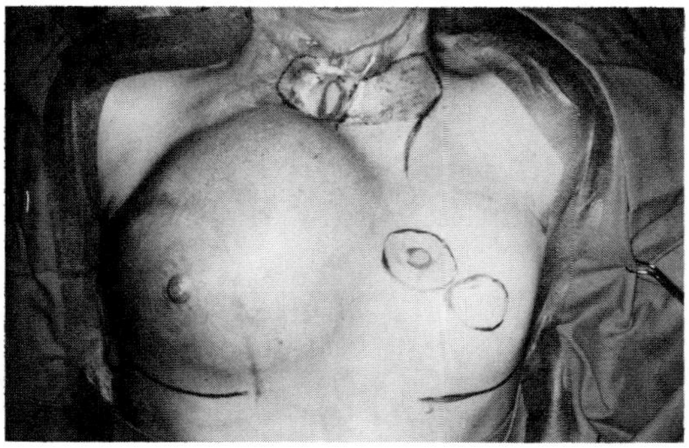

Fig. 3.) Stome before closure

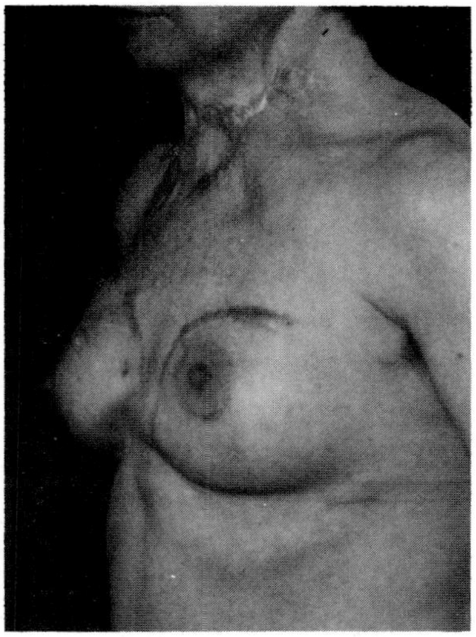

Fig. 4.) Result with closed airway.

Case 2: 8 years ago we had a similar case of laryngo-tracheal reconstruction that was first published in 1976 (5) and reported again in the book "Reconstructive Surgery of the Trachea" (MEYER-FLEMMING 1982) (6). The patient was a 40 year old female with subtotal destruction of the larynx and the upper segment of the trachea after irradiation for struma maligna. After five operations in three years a good functional result was obtained. For this purpose a local flap, a delto-pectoral flap, and other local flaps reinforced with cartilage were used.

According to our two-stage method for reconstruction in tracheal stenoses, (7 and 8) the superior part of the new laryngo-tracheal air tract was built in the first and second operation with a trap door flap. Rib cartilage grafts were inserted into subcutaneous pockets on either side of the lower part forming a gutter where only posterior wall was present. During the third intervention a submental flap was used for lining and a right delto-pectoral flap for the external coverage. A crescent shaped rib cartilage was interposed replacing the virtually absent hyoid and thyroid cartilages. With three more flaps, we closed the lower open part of the cervical trachea. After this repair the patient could breathe and swallow properly and phonate adequately.

In both cases the X-rays showed that the air passage was bayonet-shaped.(Fig. 5 and 6).

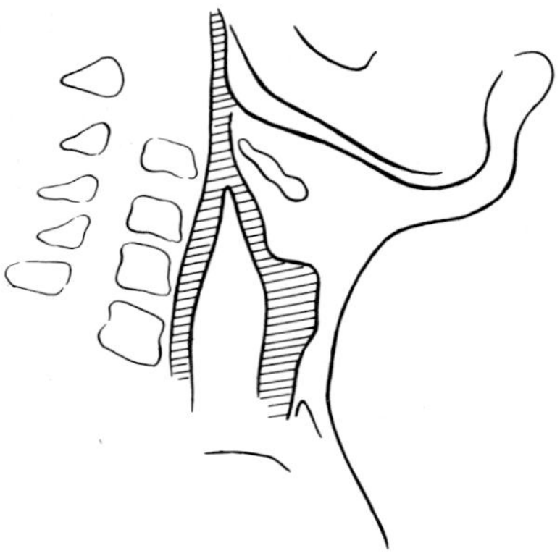

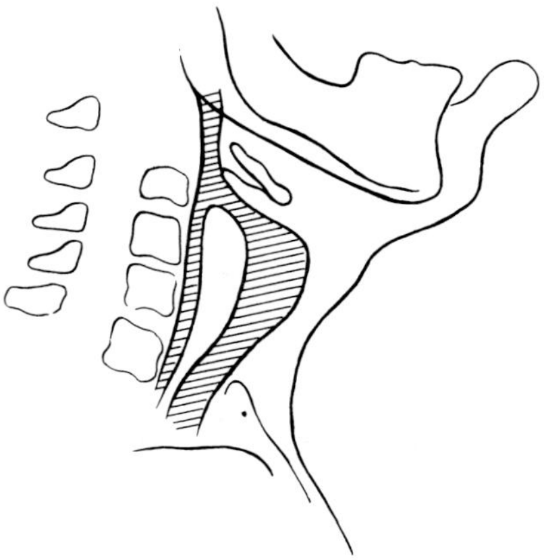

Fig.5.) Case 1 New airway in Xeroradiography Fig6.) Case 2 Same bayonet shape of airway

SUMMARY

We report two cases where after a subtotal destruction of the larynx, it was possible to rebuild the airway (bayonet-shaped) allowing free respiration and undisturbed deglutition. Both cases concerned young females having undergone tracheotomy and radiotherapy for thyroid carcinoma. The structures of the laryngeal vestibule, glottis, and subglottis were nonexistent and the airpassages closed.We believe that this successful method of laryngo-tracheal reconstruction may also be applied in cases after laryngectomy where only a part of the epiglottis and aryepiglottic folds are present.

REFERENCES

1. Majer EM, Rieder W, Ueber eine Modifikation der Laryngektomie unter Erhaltung der Luftwege. Arch.Ohren-Nasen-Kehlkopfheilkd. 1958, 173, 442.
2. Piquet JJ, Desaulty A, Hoffman Y et Decroix G, Indications et résultats de la laryngectomie sus-glottique dans les cancers du vestibule laryngée. Rev.Laryng. 93,289, 1972.
3. Labayle J., La chirurgie partielle du larynx, état actuel de la question. Rev. Laryngol.Otol.Rhinol., 1970, 91, 495, 510.
4. Fritz K., Versuche in der Wiederherstellenden Kehlkopfchirurgie. Wien.Klin. Wnhr. 86 421-423 1974
5. Meyer R, Brupbacher JP and Brown WL, Pharyngo-esophageal reconstruction by myocutaneous flaps. Chir.plast. 6, 249, 1982.
6. Meyer R, Kesselring UK, Hertig P and Poget M, Subtotal reconstruction of the larynx and the cervical trachea. Chir.Plast.3, 253, 1976
7. Meyer R. with collaboration of Flemming I, Reconstructive surgery of the trachea. Thieme Verlag - Stuttgart, Thieme Stratton Inc., New York 1982.
8. Meyer R., New concepts in laryngotracheal reconstruction.Trans.Amer.Acad. Ophtal.Otolaryng. 76: 758-765,1972.

© 1985 Elsevier Science Publishers B.V. (Biomedical Division)
New dimensions in otorhinolaryngology – head and neck surgery, vol. 2.
E. Myers, editor

REVISED SILICONE TRACHEAL T-TUBE (SAFE-T-TUBE)

WILLIAM W. MONTGOMERY, M.D.
Professor of Otolaryngology, Harvard Medical School, Boston, MA, United States of America

INTRODUCTION

The silicone tracheal T-Tube has been modified to prevent accidental displacement of the extraluminal portion of the T-Tube into the trachea. During 21 years usage of the tracheal T-Tube this complication has been rare, but on the other hand, significant, for it has been fatal. Ridges and grooves have been constructed on the extraluminal portion of the Montgomery® Safe-T-Tube so that a ring can be attached to prevent posterior displacement. Drainage grooves have also been added along the long axis to aid in the drainage of secretions and to differentiate it from the silicone tracheal cannula on which there is only one longitudinal groove.

DESCRIPTION

The Silicone Tracheal T-Tube has now been widely used for 21 years with considerable success: (1) to support the repaired or reconstructed cervical trachea and subglottic space, (2) for support following injury to the trachea, (3) with segmental resection of the cervical trachea and end-to-end anastomosis, (4) to support the intrathoracic tracheal stenosis, and (5) as a substitute for the cervical or thoracic trachea which cannot be repaired.

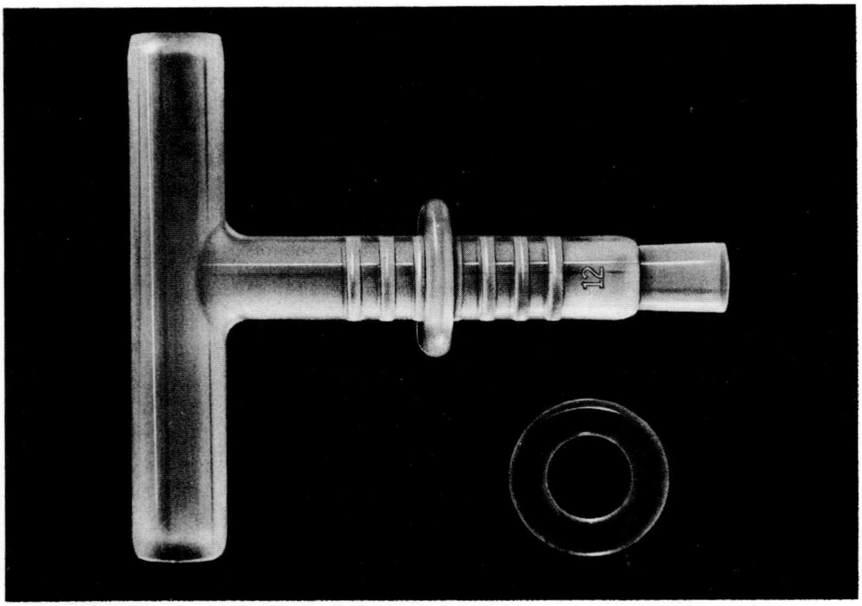

The Safe-T-Tube was designed in order to prevent the accidental displacement of the T-Tube in a posterior direction. This complication has been fatal. The addition of ridges and grooves to the extraluminal portion of the Montgomery® Safe-T-Tube allow for a ring washer to be applied thus preventing posterior displacement of the tube into the trachea. The ridges and grooves are not present on the innermost portion of the extraluminal limb of the Safe-T-Tube (arrow) so that this portion can still be bent superiorly and inferiorly to facilitate suctioning and also allow for easy insertion of the Safe-T-Tube by the surgeon. Ridges are absent on the superior and inferior aspect of the extraluminal portion of the Safe-T-Tube. These grooves allow for drainage during the immediate postoperative period and distinguish the Safe-T-Tube from the silicone tracheal cannula which has only one groove (on its inferior aspect).

LASER SURGERY IN TRACHEAL OBSTRUCTION

J.J.M. VAN OVERBEEK., E.TH. EDENS, P.E. HOEKSEMA, ENT-department, University Hospital Groningen, P.O. Box 30.001, 9700 RB Groningen (The Netherlands)

It is a striking phenomenon that no or hardly any edema is to be seen after laser treatment of laryngeal and tracheal diseases. This effect, as well as minimal bleeding and rapid healing, are important advantages of the laser in the treatment of obstructing lesions in this region.

In our clinic we use the CO_2 laser (Sharplan) as well as the Nd-YAG laser (Medilas), sometimes employing both systems in the same patient. With the CO_2 laser tissue can be vaporized and cut while the Nd-YAG laser gives more a coagulation effect.

The CO_2 laser beam is guided in the trachea by an adapter with micromanipulator on an operation microscope through a especially designed micro-tracheal scope (Fig. 1). In this technique injection ventilation is used. In cases of more distal trachea obstruction CO_2 laser energy is brought in by a rigid bronchoscope on the Sharplan coupler with joystick manipulator.

The Nd-YAG laser beam is used with the aid of an Olympus flexible bronchoscope or a special rigid Wolf device.We have succesfully treated a variety of traumatic and surgical stenoses and malignant lesions.

Instruments, techniques and several cases are demonstrated by slides.

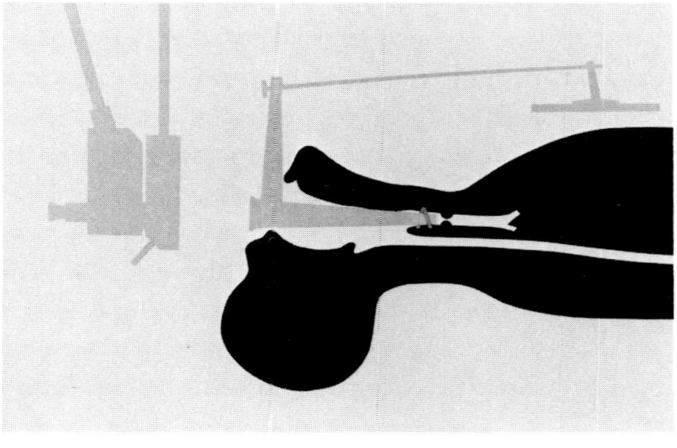

Fig. 1. Diagram showing microtracheal scope in position.

New dimensions in otorhinolaryngology - head and neck surgery, vol. 2.
E. Myers, editor

OSSICULAR ARTHROPLASTY

G. DONALD ALBERS, M.D.

Department of Otolaryngology, Blodgett Memorial Medical Center, Grand Rapids, Michigan, U.S.A.

Greater recognition should be given to the smallest joint in the human body. Frequently involved in lack of continuity, the incudo-stapedial articulation may be disrupted by congenital defects, middle ear disease, neoplasms, iatrogenic factors, and other forms of trauma, particularly skull fractures.

Hough[1] has been a major contributor to our knowledge of traumatic ossicular defects. Gaps between the incus and stapes occurred in over 82% of skull fractures in his series. Nager[2] classified congenital ossicular defects showing partial absence of the lenticular process of the incus and fusion with the malleus.

Middle ear diseases; such as, cholesteatoma, polyps, and granulations, may result in an incus stapes gap. Eustachian tube dysfunction may produce an atelectatic middle ear and a poorer prognosis for surgical repair.

Austin[3] reviewed ossicular reconstruction operations and stressed the importance of controlling the original disease before proceeding with a tympanoplasty. He concluded that it is imperative to avoid artificial prostheses and restore an energy coupler within the tympanic membrane. An ossicular lever system must also be maintained to enhance sound transmission.

Janzen[4] advocated an ossiculoplasty using a hemi-incus interposition of autogenous bone grafts. The incus was fabricated with an L-shaped prosthesis, and a deep socket was drilled for a tight fit with the capitulum of the stapes. He used histoacryl glue to maintain a good position against the malleus handle near the center of the tympanic membrane.

Ossicular continuity should be restored whenever possible. An arthroplasty of the incudo-stapedial joint may restore more natural hearing and maintain protection against acoustic trauma. After using the usual assortment of synthetic prosthesis and various cartilage, bone, and stainless steel devices; we have found that a homogenous incus works the best. This can be fabricated to form a bony sleeve for the long process of the patient's incus and a right angled socket for the capitulum of the stapes. A diamond burr 0.5 to 1.0 millimeter in size can be used with saline irrigation to prevent burning of the bone. The gap between the long process of the incus and the stirrup should be less than 0.09 or 3/32 of an inch. Careful fitting of the prosthesis demands gentle contact with the stapes to prevent subluxation and inner ear damage. The fabricated unit must not be too large as it should not rest on the facial canal or touch the promontory.

Operative technique includes microsurgical measuring tools and drills. A dependable incus holder can be used for microscopic drilling. A new micromanipulator may have some advantages when connected to a microdrill. An angled measuring device can measure degrees of incus gaps and predict accurate diameter and length of the prosthesis from 1/32 to 6/32 of an inch. Tapering of the bony sleeve matches the shape of the abnormal long process of the incus. Glue may help to stabilize this connection.

Analysis of 16 documented cases of ossicular arthroplasties during the past six years show that out of ten cases with attic defects or perforations, seven had otorrhea while three had cholesteatomas. Fusion of a displaced incus was present in each of two severe skull fractures. Eustachian tube narrowing was present in eight instances. Incus gaps were classified as +1 if less than 0.03 (5 cases), +2 if 0.06 (10 cases), and +3 if 0.09 (1 case).

Preoperative audiograms showed an average air of 49 decibels with an average bone of 19 decibels and an air bone gap of 30.5. Postoperative average air was 28.6 decibels for one month, 33.4 for one year, and 38.7 for two years. Closure of the air bone gap to 10dB or less at one year postop was 33% whereas closure to 20dB was 53%. Less improvement in hearing was seen in patients who had cholesteatomas, tympanosclerosis, and narrow eustachian tubes.

Preformed prosthesis would be preferred if they would be tolerated by the host and not slip. A hollow gold tube with a right angled socket and burnished inside has been cast and will be evaluated.

SUMMARY

Incus-stapes gaps should be considered in moderate to severe, conductive hearing losses; particularly if tympanograms show considerable compliance.

Causes of ossicular discontinuity are: congenital, traumatic, middle ear disease, neoplastic, and iatrogenic.

An ossicular arthroplasty may help to restore more physiologic motion and improved hearing when eustachian tube function is adequate and middle ear disease has been eliminated.

REFERENCES

1. Hough, J. V. D.: Incudostapedial Joint Separation. Laryngoscope., 69: 644-664, 1959.
2. Nager, G. T.: Aural Atresia: Anatomy and Surgery. Postgrad. Med., 29: 529, 1961.
3. Austin, D. F.: Ossicular Reconstruction. Arch. Otolaryngol., 94: 525-535, 1971.
4. Janzen, V. D.: Ossiculoplasty Using A Hemi-Incus Interposition. J. Otolaryngol., 13:4: 211-212, 1984.

New dimensions in otorhinolaryngology - head and neck surgery, vol. 2.
E. Myers, editor

MIDDLE EAR SILICONE SHEETING IN TYPE I TYMPANOPLASTIES

CIRÍACO CRISTÓVÃO TAVARES ATHERINO
Serviço ORL, Hospital de Ipanema, INAMPS, Rio de Janeiro, Brasil.

We analysed 2 series of 18 successful type I tympanoplasties, the first one with a circular 0.005 inches Silicone film over the promontory and the other without. The technique used in all cases was the same, with a posterior tympano-meatal flap and a medial temporalis fascia graft. The lesions were limited to the tympanum and Middle Ear mucosa. The Silicone film was used whenever there was degenerated mucosa, which was removed, or with a flat tympanic cavity to prevent adhesions. The follow-up ranged from 4 to 20 months.

The audiological results were similar in both series (air-bone gap closed within 10 dB in 0.5, 1 and 2 KHz, and good discrimination scores). In the 1st series the preoperative air-bone gaps had been greater than those of the 2nd series; this could be explainede by the disease degree presented in the 1st group. Also in the 1st group (with Silicone) we noted tympanosclerotic plaques in the tympanum in 4 cases (22.22%) while in the 2nd group this did not occur. The plaques had no relationship to the original defect, but they were always located marginally, in low movement tympanic areas.

Tympanosclerosis would not be a disease but an unusual healing process closely related to the tissue mechanisms of damage and repair[1,2]. There is an increase of the collagen deposits together with an hyaline degeneration of the fibrous layer (lamina propria) that can occur in all Middle Ear surfaces[3]. Schiff et al[3,4] suggested that tympanosclerosis would have an immunologic component that would occur in the Middle Ear after a mucosa injury; and a genetic component too, thus explaining its low incidence in children,which have a high index of Middle Ear inflammation. This also could be the reason for the high tympanosclerosis rate among Esquimo children and American indians.

There are many kinds of inflammatory reaction involved in the tympanic healing in tympanoplasty. All of them have in common the production of ground substance which, if infiltrated by the proper cells, can produce collagen. This almost disappear as a part of the normal repair process in the majority of the surgical observations. The temporalis fascia itself is replaced by fibrocytic infiltration and collagen deposition[5]. The enzyme collagenase controls the collagen production. The relative concentration of collagenase and its inhibitor decides the place and the extent of collagen resorption. Collagenase is synthesized under control of specific stimuli (hormones, lymphokines, prostaglandins, etc). Thus, inflammation can activate it[3]. The activation degree seems to obey to an individual immunologic code. As well as it seems to occur a deficiency of collagen degradation in the origin of tympanosclerosis, the contrary would explain those cases in which the tympanoplasty fails without an apparent cause, perhaps due to an exaggeration of the destructive phase of the healing process, beyond the extent of connective tissue production[6].

The excellence of the Silicone when used in the Middle Ear is only slightly dulled by the fact that ciliar function is impaired even by the contact with the most inert substance[7]. However, there is some variability among the results reported by several authors regarding the inflammatory reaction degree it causes[8,9].

But why only 4 patients developed the lesion ? One of them had his 2 ears operated, one with Silicone sheeting and the other without; tympanosclerosis only developed in the ear with the Silicone sheet.

It seems that the introduction of a new irritative factor (Silicone) along with immunologic and genetic patterns[3,4] would be important to the development of the lesion in the reported cases.

The 0.005 inches Silicone film is a good implant for chronic otitis media surgery. It didn't interfere with the sound conduction mechanism and the same is true regarding the tympanosclerotic plaques noted. However, the real origin of these observations remains obscure and more work is needed to clear it up.

REFERENCES

1. Gibb AG (1983) J Laryngol Otol 97(sup.8):63.
2. Birchall JP, Pearman K, Dawes JDK (1982) J Laryngol Otol 96:797.
3. Schiff M et al (1980) Ann Otol 89(sup.70):1.
4. Schiff M (1983) Ann Otol 92:635.
5. Perkins R (1975) Ann Otol 84:518.
6. Abramson M et al (1984) Otolaryngol Clinics North Amer 17:353.
7. McKelvie P (1976) In: Hinchcliffe R, Harrison D(eds) Scientific Foundations of Otolaryngology. Year Book Medical Publishers, Chicago, pp.762-766.
8. Falbe-Hansen J, Tos M (1975) Ann Otol 84:315.
9. Kitchens GG, Gross CW (1976) Arch Otolaryngol 102:547.

© 1985 Elsevier Science Publishers B.V. (Biomedical Division)
New dimensions in otorhinolaryngology – head and neck surgery, vol. 2.
E. Myers, editor

THE USE OF PRE-SCULPTED HOMOLOGOUS CARTILAGE TRANSPLANTS IN OSSICULAR REPLACEMENT

RICHARD A. CHOLE

Department of Otolaryngology, University of California, Davis, School of Medicine, 4301 X St., #208, Sacramento, California 95817 U.S.A.

INTRODUCTION

Ossicular reconstruction with self-stabilizing replacement prostheses has proven to be an effective way of reconstituting the ossicular chain. Alloplastic materials used for these prostheses, however, may extrude through the tympanic membrane due to the foreign body reaction that they often induce. The use of a similarly shaped strut fashioned from homologous cartilage was proposed as an alternative to alloplastic materials.[1] In this clinical investigation, 102 pre-sculpted homologous cartilage struts were implanted for the purposes of reconstruction of the ossicular chain.

MATERIAL AND METHODS

One hundred two patients between the ages of 5 and 73 underwent ossicular reconstruction with 70% alcohol stored, pre-sculpted ossicular replacement struts (Lions Eye & Tissue Bank, UCDMC, Sacramento, CA 95817). The cartilage struts were fashioned from costo-chondral cartilage obtained from cadaver donors from four to twenty years of age. They were fashioned into 'blanks' with 8mm stems and stored in 70% ethyl alcohol. At the time of surgery, the blank was rehydrated in saline for 30 minutes. The blank was then sculpted to serve as a partial ossicular replacement strut (Fig. 1) or a total ossicular replacement strut (Fig. 2).

These procedures were sometimes done in one stage with mastoidectomy and sometimes staged after the ear had stabilized. Procedures were performed by faculty and residents at the University of California, Davis Medical Center.

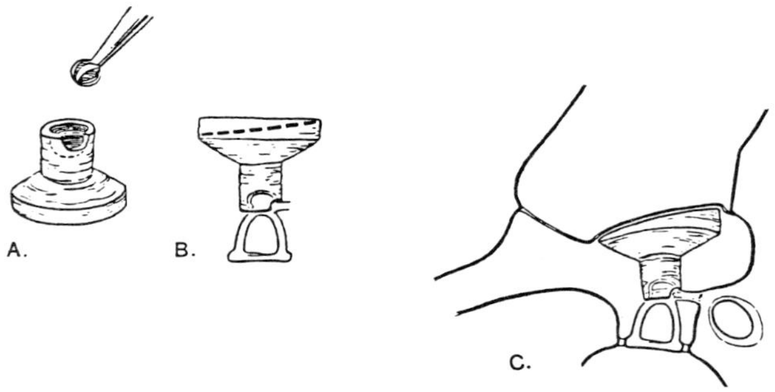

Fig. 1. The pre-sculpted cartilage blank is trimmed to the proper length and a socket for the capitulum with a notch for the stapedial tendon created (A & B). The head of the strut may be trimmed (B & C) to conform to the angle of the tympanic membrane.

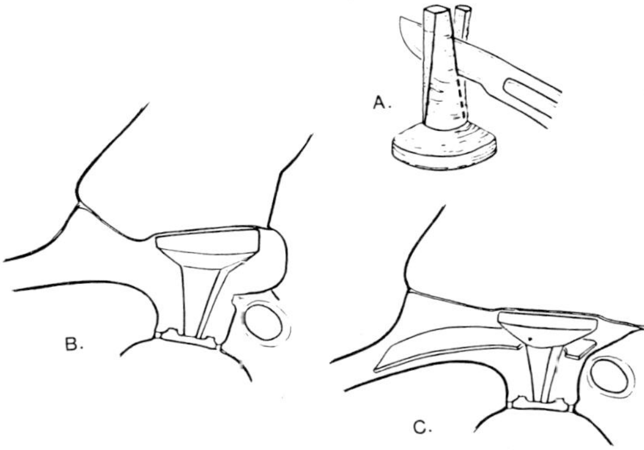

Fig. 2. For total ossicular replacement, the cartilage blank is trimmed by thinning the stem after proper length is determined. (A) This type of strut can be used when the canal wall is intact (B) or in an open procedure (C). In (C) a silastic sheet is shown which often helps to prevent middle ear adhesions.

RESULTS

Of the 102 transplants in this study, no extrusions occurred in the follow-up period of 4 to 84 months. Three of the 102 implants have partially resorbed due to recurrent cholesteatoma (2) or infection (1). Some patients experienced bouts of otitis without deterioration of hearing. In patients available for long-term hearing assessment (n = 51), hearing was stable (see Table 1).

TABLE 1

HEARING RESULTS N=102					HEARING STABILITY N=51	
	Mean A-B Gap	S.D.	A-B Gap	% of Patients		% of Post-Op Hearing
PORP	16.9	11.1	0-10dB	25.5	At One Yr.	98.2
TORP	17.8	9.6	0-20dB	64.7	At Three Yrs.	96.0
	P=NS		0-30dB	88.2		
			0-40dB	97.1		

The cases were analyzed to compare the effects of various factors on hearing. The Student t-test for independent variables was used in statistical analysis. Surprisingly, the presence of mucosal inflammation, concurrent or past mastoidectomy or myringoplasty had no significant effect on the hearing result (p = ns).

Total or partial ossicular replacement with pre-sculpted homologous cartilage is an effective, reliable alternative for ossicular reconstruction. The complications of exposure can be avoided and long-term hearing stability attained with this method.

REFERENCE

1. Chole RA (1982) Arch Otolaryngol 108:560-562

New dimensions in otorhinolaryngology - head and neck surgery, vol. 2.
E. Myers, editor

THE SUBSTITUTION OF THE EAR-DRUM WITH CORNEA TRANSPLANT

M.CORRADI, D.VOROSMARTHY
ENT Department of the Railway Hospital Budapest, Hungary

Several materials have been used for grafting tympanic membrane perforations. Most widely used is the temporal fascia, wich has proved to be quite successful in the majority of cases, especially in those of smaller size.

For the closure of tympanic membrane perforations cornea has been used at our department since 1976, becouse its histological construction and physical properties are similar to the ear-drum. Cadaver cornea, not older than 24 hours were obtained. The removal of the cornea can be carried out in its whole or lamellated. It is kept for 30 minutes in Penicillin-Streptomycin solution, than rinsed with BSS. After such simple treatment the cornea is ready for transplantation, but in case of need, it can be stored for a few day in a wet chamber at low temperature in refrigerator.

At the beginning we prefered using cornea in full thickness, but the thickness of the transplantatum was found to be of little significance, becouse it is becoming thinner with time. The cornea-disc should be placed between the epithelium and stratum proprium of the marginal region of the perforated tympanic membrane. Due to the physical properties of the cornea, that is to say to its high desnity and tensil strength, there is no need to assure holding the graft in situ by placing Gelfoam into the middle ear. The external ear-canal is closed with Gelfoam and gauze plag for 5 to 6 days postoperation.

On days 10 to 14 as a rule, the transplantatum showes a mild superfitial inflammatory reaction, manifested by moderat sweating, returning to normal within a few days without any special medication.

In the first and secund month after operation at the edges of transplantated disc intensiv vascularisation is seen. It is more intensiv, than by fascia graft.

The grafte cornea remands oedematic and opalescent throughout some two or three month. This is followed by gradual thinning and the graft becomes fo be bright and sometimes transparent. At this point the transit of the transplantatum to the tympanic membrane cannot be distinguished any longer. In other cases the grafte disc is thinner than its surroundings, translucid and showing clear demarcation from the ear-drum.

Secundary perforations developed in 9% of the patients. These were usuelly situated at the anterior-inferior part of the tympanic membrane, largely occuring after myringoplasties, when the anterior edge of the membrane was extremely narrow. In order to prevent this, a flange was prepared by drill, thus widening the surface available for the holding of the graft.

Should secundary perforation be developed, the cornea-graft must be totally removed and replaced by a new one.

By tympanometric examination during the first potoperativ year the novomembrane appears to be more stiff and more tense, than normal.

Since 1976 we have performed kerato-myringoplasty in a total of 250 cases. Of these in 227 patients, that is in 91% of cases, the operation resulted in primary and permanent recovery.

As the next slide showes, good results were obtained also in functional terms.

Improvment in hearing		n	%
air-bone gap closed		107	43,1
Improvement between 250-2000 Hz	by30 dB	62	24,8
	by20 dB	38	15,3
	by10 dB	13	5,8
No change		24	9,5
Declined		6	1,5
TOTAL		250	100

It is belived, that from the experience we obtained during 250 kerato-myringoplasties, it can be concluded, that the cornea appears to be highly suitable for the grafting of tympanic membrane.

New dimensions in otorhinolaryngology – head and neck surgery, vol. 2.
E. Myers, editor

DOUBLE FLAP TYMPANOPLASTY

LUIZ F. P. DEMOURA,MD
Mount Clemens, Michigan

This paper consists of a study of over 1000 cases of tympanoplasty and mastoidectomy that were performed by the author from July 1972 to May 1985. The patients were followed up from over six months to over one year.

The patient is brought to the operating room and put in a supine position. He is intubated, and the head is turned to the side opposite that of the ear that is to be operated on. The hair around the ear is shaved about three fingers, and polymyxin (Neosporin) ointment is used to keep the hair away from the operating field. The aptient is prepared and draped in the usual fashion for ear surgery. The retroauricaularea and canal are infiltrated with lidocaine (Xylocaine) 1% with epinephrine 1:100,000. the incision is made in the retroauricular area. A large piece of fascia from the temporal muscle is removed to close the perforation and is kept outside to dry. A "T" incision is made with a Bovie all the way to the periosteum, and the periosteum is elevated from the mastoid all the way to the external auditroy canal, which is entered. After the bleeding has been controlled, the self-retainer retractor is applied, and the skin of the canal is ellevated all the way to the annulus. The annulus is also elevated away from the bone, and the middle ear is entered. The skin of the canal is cut with scissors all the way to the annulus and, from the annulus, all the way to the perforation. The perforation edges are removed to make a bed for the graft. The superior flap is then developed all the way to the malleus head, and the inferior flap is developed all the way to the round window level. After this is done, mastoidectomy is performed using high-speed drills in the beginningand diamond drills at the end. The lateral canal, short process of the incus, and the head of the malleus are identified. If there is difficulty in removing the lesion, the facial recess is opened. The connection between the tympanic membrane and the oval window is made by use ofthe bones of the ear, when possible, to replace homografts or plastic prostheses. After this is accomplished, a Silastic sheet is put into the middl ear from the eustachian tube to the oval window, and the fascia is put beneath the remainder of the tympanic membrane resting on the ear canal,with the superior and inferior flaps in their original positions, to hold the flaps against the bone.

The annulus is also put irto original position. The ear canal is then packed with Vaseline guaze and polymyxin and neomycin (Cortisporin). The retroauriolar area is closed using 3-0 chromic catgut for the muscle and 5-0 nylon for the skin. The ear is examined through the microscope and Vaseline guaze with Cortispoirn is put on the canal. A large, bulky dressing is applied.

The patient stays in the hospital for one more day and is followed up with office visits. In seven days from the date of surgery, the sutures are removed. Three weeks after surgery, the packing is removed. An audiogram is done six weeks from date of surgery and again after three months, six months, and one year; thereafter, it is done yearly.

The results that have been achieved in over 1000 of the operations in this clinic are as follows: (!) the infection is gone in 90%, (2) the hearing has improved in 70%, (3) 10% require second surgical procedures and (4) part of the hearing is lost and the infeciton remains in less that 1%.

The analysis of results and pictures of the surgical procedure are presented.

© 1985 Elsevier Science Publishers B.V. (Biomedical Division)
New dimensions in otorhinolaryngology – head and neck surgery, vol. 2.
E. Myers, editor

TECHNIQUES FOR THE RECONSTRUCTION OF RADICAL CAVITIES

ROBERTO FILIPO, MAURIZIO BARBARA, ELIO DE SETA

Audiology Department, ENT Clinic, 'La Sapienza' University
Viale del Polclinico, 00185 Rome (Italy)

INTRODUCTION

The surgical rehabilitation of radical cavities is motivated due to various problems linked to the symptoms (otalgia, otorrhea, debris), to the development of new microsurgical techniques and also due to newly developed expectations on the part of the radicalized patient who requires social integration. The key to middle ear rehabilitation is the reconstruction of the posterior canal wall and the obliteration of the anterior and posterior epitympanum. The obliteration of the epitympanum is important in order to prevent the formation of retraction pockets.

MATERIALS AND METHODS

Our technique is based on the fundamental principles of full-thickness obliteration of the pre-existing cavity and of the reconstruction of the bony wall leaving the remaining posterior cavity empty.

Regarding the outcome of radical surgery, it is important to carry out a accurate evaluation of residual epitympanic structures; in fact, in some cases we may find these structures removed uniquely adjacent to the antrum. In this case a simple reconstruction of the posterior canal wall is sufficient to cover the bony defect. The canal wall curvature must however leave adequate space for the reconstruction by TORPs and PORPs, often impossible when preformed walls are used as those in Ceravital.

We cannot use posterior canal walls in Ceravital when the destruction of the epitympanum is almost total, so we revert to the use of a more malleable material (cartilage) or to a full-thickness obliteration procedure.

Generally speaking, in reconstructive techniques it must be stressed that obliteration of the epitympanum should be performed with the full-thickness method in order to avoid the possible formation of retraction pockets. In our experience with rehabilitation of radical cavities (42 cases) we used three different techniques:

- Posterior canal wall reconstruction with Ceravital;
- Full-thickness obliteration of the mastoid cavity with costal cartilage + bone patè + Tissucol;
- Full-thickness obliteration of the mastoid cavity with spongy bone tissue taken from the tibia and stabilized with fibrin glue.

New dimensions in otorhinolaryngology - head and neck surgery, vol. 2.
E. Myers, editor

CLOSURE OF NON-MARGINAL TYMPANIC PERFORATIONS USING VENTILATING TUBES

GEORGE N. GEORGOPOULOS
Athens, Greece

Small but permanent tympanic membrane perforations, resulting from an otitis media or a half-successful tympanoplasty, often persist because of inadequate function of the eustachian tube.

Using polyethylene tubes of different sizes (from 1.4 to 2.4 mm in diameter) as well as a combination of ventilating tube and silastic patch of 7 mm diameter (——(‾—+), placed over or through a non-marginal perforation, we succeeded in closing about 50% of perforations 5 mm or less in diameter.

Our technique

After tympanometric evidence that the eustachian tube is not obstructed, we place a tube of adequate gauge, as an office procedure, in combination with medical measures aiming to restore the tubal function. Before placing the tube, the edges of perforation are rubbed gently with a cotton ball soaked with Lindocain 10% solution. A month later we check the patient again and if extrusion of the tube has left a smaller perforation we re-insert a smaller gauge tube and wait until the new extrusion of the tube, with or without closure of the perforation. If the tubal function is restored within normal, the perforation usually closes.

On the contrary, if the perforation persists, that means that the middle ear spaces need supplementary ventilation besides the eustachian tube. In this case the perforation can be fitted with a permanent-type ventilating tube.

© 1985 Elsevier Science Publishers B.V. (Biomedical Division)
New dimensions in otorhinolaryngology - head and neck surgery, vol. 2.
E. Myers, editor

EAR CARTILAGE PALISADE TYMPANO-EPITYMPANUM-,ANTRUM-AND MASTOID-PLASTIES WITH HYPOTENSION - 10.000 CASES

Joachim HEERMANN, KRUPP HOSPITAL, D 43 ESSEN, WEST GERMANY

Fascia temporalis tympanoplasties are spontaneously covered with local epithelium preserving the selfcleaning process in the ear canal (Heermann, H. 1960, Storrs 1961). While the primary results are excellent, we noticed poor long term results in 2,300 cases. - In 1962 we advised to use the ear cartilage (Goodhill 1967) for reconstruction of the drum (Jansen 1963). Autogenous cartilage is used from the auricle (larger pieces and consequent enlargement of the auditory canal) and from the tragus (Heermann, J. 1962). Multiple parallel pieces of cartilage achieve the normal shape of the drum and the auditory canal. The ANULUS-STAPES-PLATE (1962) in type III tympanoplasty collects the movement of one radius of the new drum, as the handle of the malleus does under normal conditions. This reconstruction is more stable and easier to perform than any other prothesis or incus interposition. No bony fixation is possible with the cartilage. The TUNNEL-PLASTY (1964-67) reconstructs the tympano-metal niche and the entrance of the tube. The EPITYMPANUM-ANTRUM-PLASTY (1962-67) allows ventilation of the antrum via a tunnel of parallel pieces of cartilage fixed by selftension replacing the bony canal wall. In absence of the stapes a COLUMELLA-TUNNEL-PLASTY (1970) is used or a prothesis with sector resection or a type IV palisade plasty. MASTOIDPLASTY (1962-67) is performed with parallel wedges of cartilage and perichondrium, as we see no advantage in ventilating a drilled out mastoid cavity because of wide spread cholesteatoma. In cases with extreme pneumatisation the mastoid tip is removed as well. An expanding postoperative cholesteatoma will press the cartilage grafts into the external auditory canal, whereas after osteoplasty of the auditory canal wall the patient runs to an uncertain percentage the same risk as before the operation. "Second look" operations are of uncertain value, because

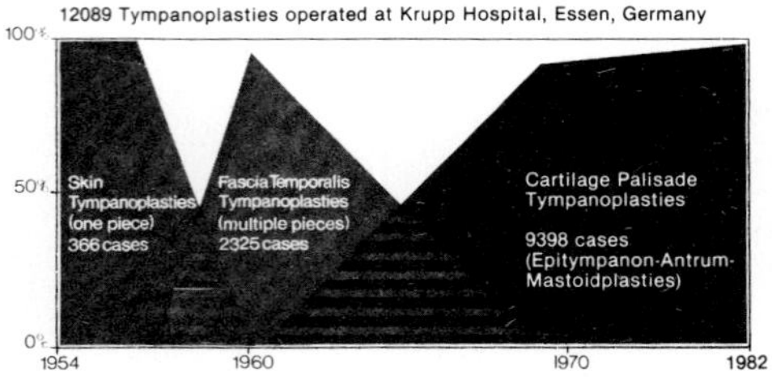

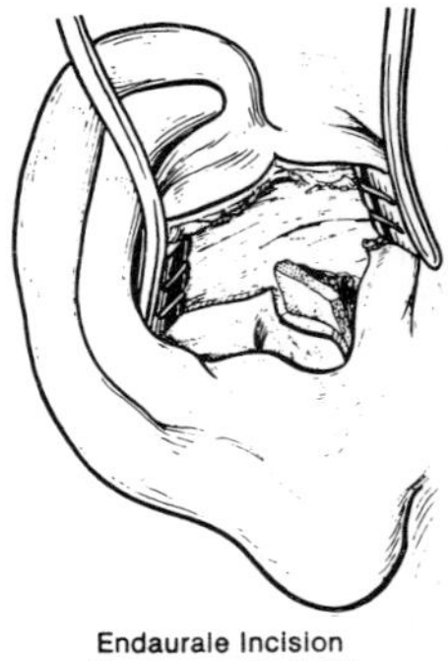

Endaurale Incision
(Heermann, H. 1930)
Tragusknorpelentnahme
(Heermann, J. 1962)

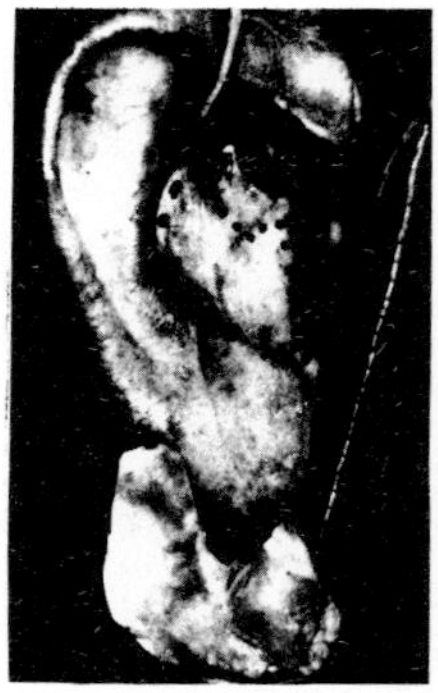

Ohrmuschelknorpelentnahme
von retroaurikulär

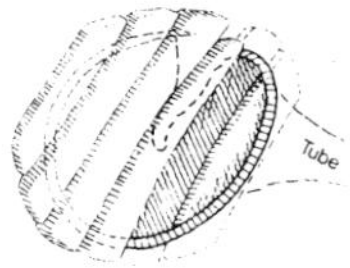

Palisaden-Plastik I

we noticed very small cholesteatomas in 25-years-old plasties. HYPOTENSION is important to achieve good results: Flunitrazepam, Chlorpromazine, Isoflurane, Nitroglycerine. The SEMI-SITTING-FOWLER-POSITION of the patient has 3 advantages: 1) lowest blood pressure in the operating field

2) liquids run out of the operating field without suction

3) microscope focused by head motions of the surgeon.

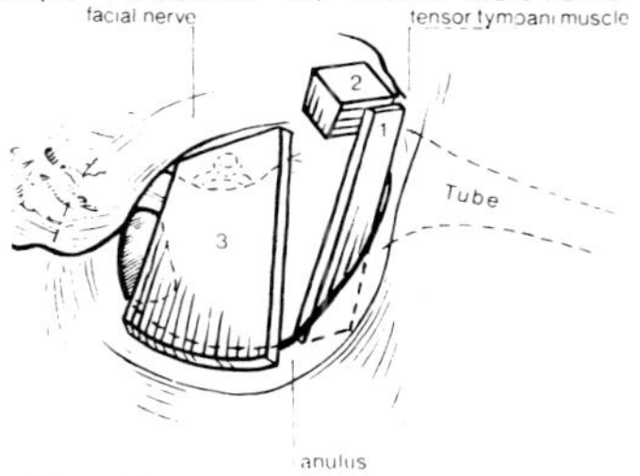

Tunnelplastik am Tubeneingang und Plastik III

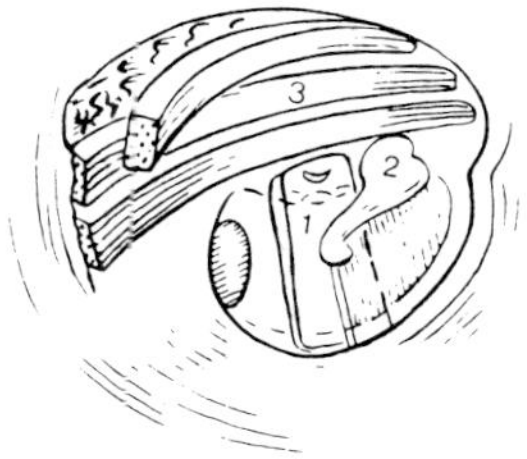

Palisader-Epitympanum-Antrumplastik

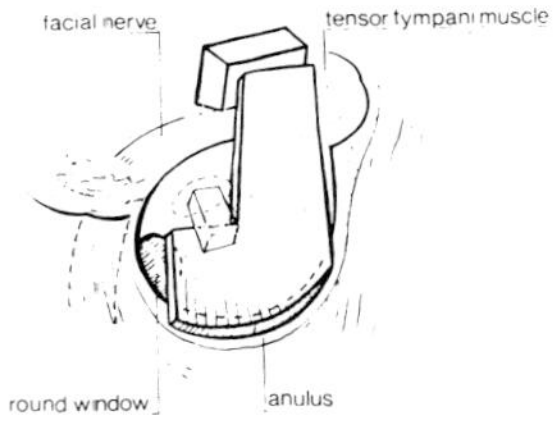

Columellaplastik

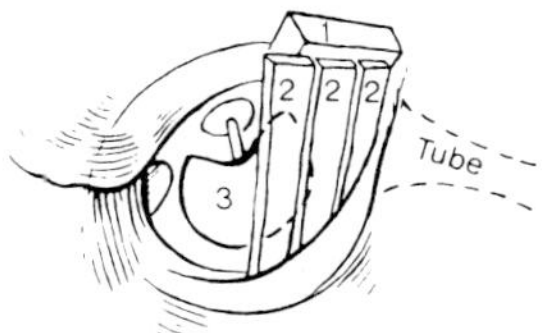

Palisaden-Prothesenplastik

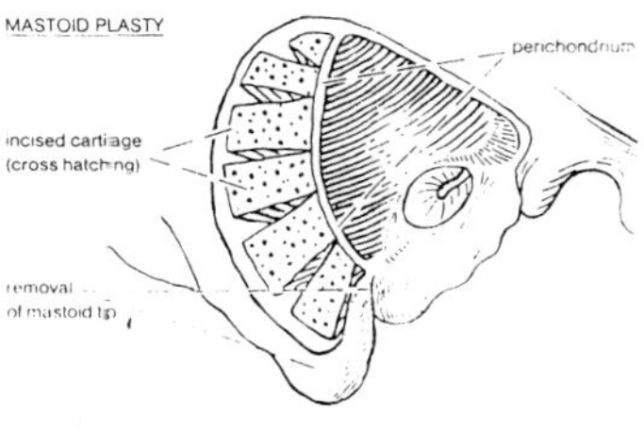

REFERENCES

Ely, E. T.: Haut-Transplantation bei chronischer Eiterung des Mittelohres. Z. Ohrenheilk. **10,** 146 (1881)

Goodhill, V.: Tragal perichondrium and cartilage in Tympanoplasty. Arch. Otolaryng. **85,** 480 (1967)

Heermann, H.: Trommelfellplastik mit Fasciengewebe vom Musculus temporalis nach Begradigung der vorderen Gehörgangswand (Filmvortr. Aachen 1960). HNO **9,** 136 (1961)

Heermann, J.: Erfahrungen mit frei transplantiertem Faszien-Bindegewebe des Musculus temporalis bei Tympanoplastiken und Verkleinerung der Radikalhöhle. Knorpelbrücke vom Stapes zum unteren Trommelfellrand. Z. Laryng. Rhinol. **41,** 141 (1962)

Heermann, J.: Trichterförmige Faszienplastik des Trommelfelles aus mehreren Stücken mit Knorpelbrücke zum Stapes nach Radikaloperationen des Ohres und das Gehör bei dickerem Trommelfell. Arch. Ohr.-, Nas.-, Kehlk.-Heilk. **180,** 556 (1962)

Heermann, J.: Sieben Jahre Faszien-Knorpel-Dachschindel-Tympanoplastik und Antrum-Mastoidplastik. Z. Laryng. Rhinol. **46,** 370 (1967)

Heermann, J.: Fascia and cartilage palisade tympanoplasty. Arch. Otolaryng. **91,** 228 (1970)

Heermann, J.: Entwicklung von der Haut- zur Faszien- und zur Knorpeltympanoplastik (Epitympano-Antrum-Mastoidplastik). Laryng. Rhinol. **56,** 277 (1977)

Heermann, J.: Cartilage palisade tympano-epitympano-antrum-mastoidplasties. XI World Congress on Otorhinol., Buenos Aires, 1977

Heermann, J.: Auricular cartilage palisade tympano-, epitympano-, antrum- and mastoid-plasties. Clin. Otolaryngol. **3,** 443 (1978)

Jansen, C.: Stapesersatz durch Knorpel. Acta Oto-Laryng. (Stockh.) **54,** 262 (1962)

Jansen, C.: Cartilage tympanoplasty. Laryngoscope **13,** 1288 (1963)

Leopold, G.: Virchows Arch. path. Anat. **84,** 283 (1881). Zit. n.: Denecke u. Meyer: Nasenplastik. Berlin, Göttingen, Heidelberg: Springer 1964

Plester, D.: Vortr. Politzer Soc. Clin. Otolaryngol. **3** (1978)

Shea, J. Jr.: Plastipore total ossicular replacement prosthesis. Laryngoscope **86,** 239 (1976)

Strauss, P.: Vergleich von Amboßinterposition und Kunststoffcolumella bei der Tympanoplastik. Laryng. Rhinol. **58,** 15 (1979)

Utech, H.: Bessere Endhörergebnisse bei der Tympanoplastik durch Veränderung der Operationstechnik. Z. Laryng. Rhinol. **39,** 367 (1960)

Wiegand, H.: Knorpelpalisaden und doppelschichtiges Transplantat als Trommelfellersatz. HNO **26,** 233 (1978)

Wullstein, H.: Collegium Oto-Rhino-Laryngologicum, London 1954 (pers. Mitt.)

New dimensions in otorhinolaryngology - head and neck surgery, vol. 2.
E. Myers, editor

INCUS INTERPOSITION

PROFESSOR M. JALISI
E.N.T. Department, Jinnah Postgraduate Medical Centre,Karachi, (Pakistan)

Incus Interposition or Incus Transposition is a fairly new technique. It is a form of OSSICOPLASTY. In this operation, we TRANSPOSE or INTERPOSE the REMODELED or SCULPTURED Long or Short INCUS GRAFT to RE-ESTABLISH the DE-ESTABLISHED or broken down SOUND CONDUCTING middle ear OSSICULAR CHAIN. So far we have done and followed up 112 cases during the last two years. The present is a report on them.

INDICATIONS

The main indication responsible for the great majority of cases is the NECROSIS OF THE LONG PROCESS OF INCUS, usually because of C.S.O.M., sometime because of inadvertant crimping during Stapedectomy, and rarely after middle ear trauma causing fracture of the process. The next important indication is DISLOCATION OF THE INCUS, either due to callous use of aditus seeker in simple mastoidectomy or due to middle ear trauma causing subluxation of the incudo-stapedial joint. A good third indication is FIXED MALLEUS SYNDROME either congenital or postinflammatory. Recently we have had experience of doing the operation in TYMPANO-SCLEROSIS with more than satisfactory results.

CONTRAINDICATIONS

Just as in other Plastic reconstructive procedures INFECTION remains the chief hazard. In the presence of active infection in the middle ear, no graft will take, whether it be fascia or bone. Similarly a NON-FUNCTIONING BLOCKED EUSTACHEAN TUBEobviates the operation. In fact the commonest of all complications accounting for almost 50% of the failures namely LATERALIZATION OF THE GRAFT results from an obstructed auditory tube.

In addition one must remember that no matter what we do with middle ear transformer, functional gain will just not occur in presence of any appreciable degree of SENSORI-NEURAL LOSS or NERVE DEAFNESS.

MATERIALS

Both AUTOGRAFT or HOMOGRA_FT INCUS can be used. For AUTOGRAFTS, our Practice is to sculpture the bone, rinse it thoroughly in normal saline, treat it with 70% alcohol for 20 minutes, and then rinse it again in normal saline before using. For HOMOGRAFTS, the assicle should be removed within 12 hours of the death of an otherwise healthy individual. It is then preserved either in 70% alcohol or 1:5000 solution of cialit at low temperature.

METHODS

1. Remodeling or Sculpturing. For horizontal interposition the ossicle is first cut to size and then drilled through the centre. The average diameter of the hole is 0.65 mm to 0.8 mm. This is just enough to allow the head of the stapes Protrude.

In more popular vartical placement, 5.76 mm to 6.5 mm long grafts are sculptured to fit between the handle of malleus and the Foot Plate of stapes and 3-4.5 mm short grafts are modeled to bridge between the handle of malleus and the head of stapes. In either case, the lateral end of the graft is drilled a saddle indentation measuring 2mm x 1.75 mm. The medial end of the graft is kept flat if it has to go on the foot plate or burred a cup 0.65 mm - 0.8mm in diameter to accomodate the stapecial head.

2. Positioning. One can interpose the ossicle horizontally as well as vertically. We prefer the later position. It is easier, allows good visibility during operation, and in confirmity with the normal anatomy.

3. Stabilization. The factors which help in stabilizing the graft are tensor tympani which is inserted in the malleus neck, malleal through saddle indentation at the lateral end of the graft, and chorda tympani. In addition, one may use a drop of glue to obtain fixation.

CASES

In the 112 cases under study the indications were as follows:

1.	NECROSIS OF THE LONG PROCESS	94
2.	DISLOCATION/SUBLUXATION OF THE INCUS/INCUDO-STAPEDIAL JOINT	10
3.	FIXED MALLEUS SYNDROME	6
4.	TYMPANO SCLEROSIS	2

We used AUTOGRAFT INCUS in 96 cases and HOMOGRAFT INCUS in 16 cases.

Initially, we did 7 HORIZONTAL interpositions. Since, we are transposing in the VERTICAL manner.

RESULTS

The follow up results of the operation are as under:

Postop. A/B gap		Number	%
0 - 10	db	14	12.5
10- 20	db	30	26.8
20-30	db	28	25.0
Over 30	db	40	35.7

If 30 db is regarded as threshold(upper limit), the success rate is 64.3% which is quite satisfactory.

Of 40 failures, 12 have been revised. The findings are as below:

1. Lateralization--------------- 7
2. Displacement----------------- 3
3. Fixity----------------------- 2

ADVICE

To improve results in Incus Transposition as well as in other Ossiculoplastic/Tympanoplastic Procedures, we suggest the following:

1. AVOID ALL CONTRAINDICATIONS
2. STAGING
3. SYSTEMETIC EPITYMPANECTOMY
4. PROPER MEASUREMENTS
5. GOOD SCULPTURING
6. ADEQUATE STABILIZATION
7. TRANSMASTOID DRAINAGE
8. RECONSTRUCTION OF MEDICAL ATTAC WALL
9. USE OF THICK SIALASTIC SHEETING.

1. Tympanoplasty, J.V.D. Hough
   Otolaryngology I, Alan Gibb, et. al., 1982
2. Middle ear transformer reconstruction-
   Manfield F.W. Smith
   Otolaryngology I, Alan Gibb, et. al., 1982
3. Preoperative evaluation of tympanoplasties,
   Pedro L. Mangabeira - Albernas,
   Ear Clinic International, Vol. 2,
   Paparella, et. al., 1982.
4. Causes of failures & complications in tympanoplasty,
   R.J. Bellucci.
   Ear Clinic International, Vol.2,
   Paparella, et. al., 1982.
5. General review of surgical methods in the treatment
   of C.O.M.,
   Sergio Prado Angirre, Ear Clinic International,
   Vol. 2, Paparella, et. al., 1982
6. Total reconstruction of Ossicular Chain,
   Ugo P. Fisch,
   Ear Clinic International, Vol.3,
   Paparella, et. al., 1983.
7. Prefabricated Allograft Ossiculo-Plasty,
   Victor Goodhill,
   Ear Clinic International, Vol.3,
   Paparella, et. al., 1983
8. Tympanosclerosis, Alan Gibb,
   Proceeding of 6th British Academic Conference in
   ORL, Bristol, July, 1983.

New dimensions in otorhinolaryngology - head and neck surgery, vol. 2.
E. Myers, editor

STATISTICAL ANALYSIS OF RESULTS IN VARIOUS TYPES OF OSSICULOPLASTIES

S.K. KACKER

Professor & Head, Department of Otolaryngology, All-India Institute of Medical Sciences, Ansari Nagar, New Delhi-110 029, India.

INTRODUCTION

The discharging ears due to chronic suppurative otitis media are the most common cause of hearing loss in India (ICMR, 1983).

These days it is possible to get a dry ear with adequate air containing middle ear in nine out of ten cases where such a surgery is attempted. However, the results in making the hearing normal in cases with the involvement of ossicles is not yet possible with certainty.

MATERIALS AND METHODS

This is a retrospective study carried out on patients operated in the Department of Otorhinolaryngology of the All-India Institute of Medical Sciences, from 1971-1984. A total of 164 cases of primary teflon piston stapedectomy followed up for 5 years or more and 190 cases of ossiculoplasties followed up for 1 year or more have been analysed. In all the cases a healed air containing middle ear with intact tympanic membrane was a pre-requisite for ossiculoplasty. This included myringoplasty cases and also cases with tympanomastoidectomy with repair of diseased tympanic membrane. The ossiculoplasty was usually done 6-8 months after the first operation, if the middle ear healed and tympanic membrane was intact but conductive deafness persisted. In any cases having recurrent ear discharge or with residual or recurrent perforation, ossiculoplasty was not done.

OBSERVATIONS

The summary of various results seen in different types of damages of ossicles is shown in Table No.1.

TABLE I : SHOWING RESULTS OF OSSICULAR REPAIR

S.No.	Type of damage	No.of cases	AC/BC closed to within 15 dB	Failures
1.	Long process incus necrosis	12	10 (83%)	2 (17%)
2.	Total incus necrosis	60	40 (67%)	20 (33%)
3.	Stapes fixation(Otospongiosis)	164	142 (85%)	22 (15%)
4.	Incus stapes damage (inflammatory) Revision Surgery	23	18 (78%)	5 (22%)
5.	Incus stapes damage failed stapes surgery Revision Surgery	37	24 (65%)	13 (35%)
6.	All ossicles damage except footplate	26	12 (44%)	14 (56%)

Statistical Analysis: 3 Vs 1, 3 Vs 4, 2 Vs 4 and 4 Vs 5 = are not statistically significant.

6 Vs 4 ($P < 0.05$) just significant.

3 Vs 2 and 3 Vs 5 ($P < 0.01$) significant.

3 Vs 6 ($P < 0.001$) highly significant.

DISCUSSION

The observations reported in this study have clearly shown that results obtained by stapedectomy techniques in Otospongiosis, are better and more lasting than those seen in ossiculoplasty done for correcting the sequlae of chronic suppurative otitis media. The causes of defective sound transmission after surgery are lack of contact, loose contact, fixation to the promontary or other walls of the middle ear, lack of aeration of middle ear, defective vibration of repaired tympanic membrane, fibrous fixation of ossicles or loss of contact after initial adequate placement. Antigenic rejection of ossicle has been blamed for late failures.

Our results have failed to give conclusive proof that our attempts to upgrade the tympanoplasty from type III to type II or type IV to type III has given consistently better and lasting results in such cases. A guarded prognosis of such operations for long term hearing gain should be offered to the patients.

CONCLUSIONS

1. Results of surgical repair of isolated stapes fixation are best of all the techniques of ossiculoplasty.
2. Difference in results of repair of total incus necrosis Vs. partial incus necrosis are statistically significant. Repair of necrosis of long process of incus gives better results ($P < 0.01$).
3. Difference in results are statistically significant in repair of stapes fixation only Vs. repair for stapes fixation and incus necrosis as done after failed stapedectomy ($P < 0.01$).
4. Difference in results are highly statistically significant in repair of stapes fixation and repair of total ossicular loss ($P < 0.001$).
5. Difference in results are just significant statistically in repair of malleus-incus defect Vs. repair of total ossicular loss in inflammatory conditions ($P < 0.05$).

REFERENCES

Indian Council of Medical Research Report (ICMR): Prevalence and etiology of hearing impairment, 1983.

© 1985 Elsevier Science Publishers B.V. (Biomedical Division)
New dimensions in otorhinolaryngology - head and neck surgery, vol. 2.
E. Myers, editor

"WIDEFIELD" MASTOIDOTYMPANOPLASTY

K. J. LEE, M.D., F.A.C.S. and KENNETH E. LEE
Ear Research and Educational Center, Hospital of Saint Raphael, New Haven, CT

Using the "widefield" mastoidotympanoplasty, 97% of 500 patients achieved a safe, dry ear with at least a 24 month post-operative follow-up. Ninety-seven per cent of the grafts remained intact. Out of the 227 cases with cholesteatoma found at the time of surgery, 94.3% had no recurrent cholesteatoma. Ninety-five per cent of those with a Type I Tympanoplasty have closure of the air bone gap to within 10 db; 88% of the Type III to within 25 db, and 72% of the Type IV to within 30 db.

The technique is a refinement of that described in our 1971 publication.[1] The principle of the technique is to perform the mastoid-tympanoplasty through a "wide-field" approach with the "canal wall down":[2]

a. A post-auricular incision is used.

b. A pedical posterior canal skin flap based laterally at the concha supplies a base for quick epithelization of the mastoid cavity (Korner flap). (Figure 1)

c. A wide meatoplasty is made by removing a sufficiently large crescent-shaped piece of conchal cartilage.

d. A wide canalplasty is achieved by removing any anterior osseous bulge and any other bony buttresses.

e. The "canal wall down" technique is used taking down the posterior bony canal completely; exposing the epitympanic space, zygomatic root cells, sino-dural angle, perilabyrinthine cells, facial recess, sinus tympani, mastoid tip cells, protympanum and hypotympanum for thorough removal of disease.

f. Temporalis fascia is used for tympanoplasty; "sculptured," "fitted" ossicular reconstruction or homograft ossicles are used to restore hearing. For the purpose of this study, the incus interposition reconstruction is classified as a "Type III Tympanoplasty."

g. After thorough removal of disease, an inferiorly based muscle pedical graft is used to reduce the cavity size, particularly in the region of the mastoid tip. Care must be taken not to bury any squamous epithelium or any cholesteatoma. (Figure 2)

h. The temporalis fascia graft was packed in the customary rosette fashion using strips of Owen's silk and gelfoam.

i. A smooth telfa roll is used to pack the extenal auditory canal; minimum granulation tissue was encountered postoperatively and the packing was removed with little or no discomfort.

In this series of 500 cases, no iatrogenic facial nerve or semicircular canal injury was encountered. We encountered eight cases of either the middle fossa or posterior fossa dura that were exposed by disease; none of the 8 cases had any untoward postoperative results. One case of CSF leak was encountered after the removal of an extensive cholesteatoma. The leak was successfully corrected with a fascia graft coupled with a musculoplasty flap. Six cases of horizontal semicircular canal fistula were found at the time of the surgery secondary to cholesteatoma invasion. The cholesteatoma was meticulously removed and the fistula in each instance repaired successfully with a fascia graft. One posterior semicircular canal was similarly treated. No total sensori-neural deafness was encountered in any of the cases. Five Type III Tympanoplasty patients suffered sensorineural hearing loss ranging from 5 db to 25 db with an average of 14 db. Four of the 72 Type IV cases had sensorineural hearing loss ranging from 5db to 30 db, averaging 15 db. None of the Type I patients suffered sensorineural loss.

We had one case of post-operative perichondritis which was successfully treated with "through and through" penrose drain and Keflex antibiotic therapy. None of the cases resulted in a displeasing auricular appearance.

It is important to note that it is practically impossible to eliminate completely the mastoid cavity. However, the combination of a wide meatoplasty, canalplasty, and the use of muscle pedical graft helps to equalize the size of the "opening" to the size of the "cavity." The use of the Korner flap accelerates epithelization of the cavity. Thus, the mastoid cavity becomes self-cleansing and free of debris and drainage. This leads to a high success rate of achieving a safe, dry ear; with minimum rate of cholesteatoma recurrence and with reasonably good post-operative hearing.

REFERENCES

1. Lee, K. J. and Schuknecht, H.F. (1971) Laryngoscope 81:529-543
2. Lee, K. J. and Lee, Kenneth E. (1985) Laryngoscope 95:107-110

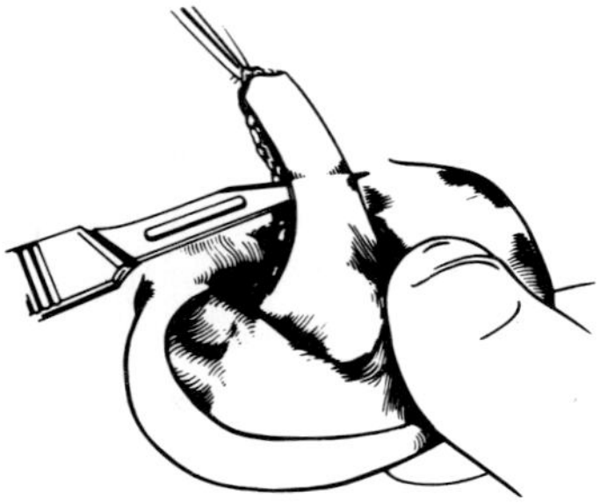

Fig.1. Korner flap

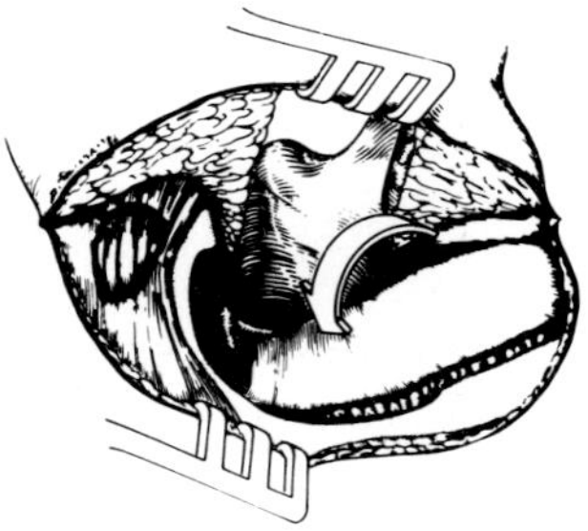

Fig.2. Musculoplasty flap

© 1985 Elsevier Science Publishers B.V. (Biomedical Division)
New dimensions in otorhinolaryngology - head and neck surgery, vol. 2.
E. Myers, editor

MIRINGOPLASTY:100 CASES OF EXPERIENCE AND RESULTS

A.MORELLO,G.MORELLO,G.CASTRO
Centro Medico Delfos.Av.Hospital Militar 151.Barcelona.Spain

INTRODUCTION

The tympanic membrane is a principal element in the transfer of sound stimuli from the environement to the ossicular structures of the middle ear.

There are many causes of tympanic membrane perforations and these are categorized in three goups:A)Traumatic.B)Tumor.C)Postotitic consecuence of a general or local,either acute or chronic disease;this last category being the most frecuent.

We denominate Miringoplasty in the surgical act as being based on the singular reconstruction of the tympanic membrane perforation.

MATERIAL AND METHODS

In this presentation we deal with 100 cases between the age or 14 and 65 affected by tympanic perforation in dry ears,on whom we have surgically intervined using a temporalis fascia autograft(House 1961,Garcia-Ibanez 1974 and other autors).Previously we had used the perichondrium autograft(Castro 1978).We shall classify these cases by referring to the perforation's type and location,without using any other distinctions.

The following cases have been excluded from this study:A)When the tympanic perforation is located anteriorly and we are not able to see in totality its anterior edge.B)In which there has been reintervention.C)When the tympanic remains are totally sclerosed and there is a sclerotic blockage in the ossicular chain or its remains.

The classification is as follows:Anterior perforations 11;Posterior perforations 25;Central perforations 38;and Total perforations 26.

SURGICAL PROCEDURE

The intervention is usually performed using a base sedation followed by local anesthesia.A supra-auricular point is infiltrated in order to extract temporalis fascia grafting,plus four conventional points in the E.A.C.We use the transmeatic approach,realized by means of an ear speculum.

After eliminating the epithelium at the perforation's edges and scraping them raw,the surgical incision is made in the E.A.C.at 8 or 10 mm.from the tympanic annulus.If we compare the tympanic frame to the face of a clock,the incision is made from 12 o'clock to 6 o'clock if the perforation is posterior or continuing to the superior edge of the perforation in its most anterior part in the other cases.In continuation we separate,raise and fold over the tympanomeatal flap,revealing the malleus handle and the perforation's antero-superior edge.We place the grafting on 2 or 3 tyni fibrin sponges or cover the grafting internally with a layer of fibrin thus facilitating its placement under the malleus handle and the tympanic remains.If the handle is extremely oblique,we section its point.;this done and having checked the coverage of the perforation,the middle ear is filled with sponges to avoid the neotympano's collapse,and the flap is returned to its place.Sponge and gauze in the E.A.C.

RESULTS

We shall evaluate the results as Reconstructive and Functional.In reference to Reconstructive the results are as follows:

A)Total closure of the perforation ----92----92%

B)Persistence of the perforation ---- 8----8%

In respect to Functional results,we have obtain:auditive improvement in 89% of the cases;an auditive level equal to the preoperative in 8%;and an auditive decrease in 3% of the cases.Auditive gain is measured in dB,referred to the shortening of the gap in conversational frequencies and to the total number:A)1 to 10 dB---40%.B)11 to 20 dB---43%.C)21 to 30 dB---6%.

CONCLUSIONS

We feel the use of this surgical technique is interesting due to:1)The procedure's lack of agresiveness.2)The brief duration in surgery.3)Low cost intervention.4)Anatomo-functional restitution of the tympano-ossicular system(in case of integral chain),since the malleus handle remains placed between the grafting and the flap,helping to avoid the neotympano's lateral movement and gain a physiological transmission of sound.5)In cases of interrupted chain with mobil stapes.audition can be improved by supporting the grafting on the stapes.6)The formation of Cholesteatoma balls is avoided.7)Short postoperative recuperation time.8)The results obtained.

This surgical procedure,as much on the Reconstructive level as Functional, permits us to positively evaluate the use of said method and its validity in surgery at the present time.

REFERENCES

1. House,W.Sheehy,J.Miringoplasty.Arch.Otolaryngol 73:407.1961.

2. Garcia-Ibanez,E.Comunicacion Curso Diseccion Hueso Temporal.1974.

3. Castro,G.Sanlley,J.Miringoplastia Simple.Anal O.R.L. Iber-Am Vol V:451-458.1978.

New dimensions in otorhinolaryngology – head and neck surgery, vol. 2.
E. Myers, editor

¿ CAN CHRONIC EXPOSURE TO " CIVILIZED NOISE " HAVE AN EFFECT ON HEARING ?

MARCOS V. GOYCOOLEA, MD MS PhD
HORTENSIA G. GOYCOOLEA, Audiologist
CORINA R. FARFAN, Audiologist
LEONARDO G. RODRIGUEZ, MD
GUMARO C. MARTINEZ, MD

From the Chilean Military Hospital and Audia, Santtiago Chile.

INTRODUCTION :

There are many questions about the effect that living in modern civilization might have on hearing, and doubts as to how much influence can chronic exposure to " civilized noise" have on aging and hearing.

There have been interesting studies on the subject, particulary in isolated communities (1,2). However, it has been extremely difficult from an epidemiological standpoint to control all the variables and ultimately compare individuals with all factors being equal except exposure to noise.

In an effort to clarify some of these questions we selected a unique population such as the natives who live in Easter Island, " the most isolated inhabited place in the world ", also called " the island of the great silence " (3,4). This is a genetically homogeneous population (875 natives), recently censed, in which every individual has a complete medical record, is educated and has no language barriers. Moreover, many natives have lived in " modern civilization " for years and have returned to the island. We have been able to compare groups of individuals who have all factors in common except having nor being exposed to life in "civilized societies".

MATERIAL AND METHODS :

Ninety natives, aged 45 years and older were evaluated. They represent 59,6 o/o of the natives population over 45 years old (5). They were divided in groups :

Those who I Had always lived in the island (54)
II Had lived in the Continent from 3 to 5 years (19)
III Had lived in the Continent over 5 years (17)

All subjects underwent a complet ENT examination by a Board Certified Otolaryngologist. Before they were examined a questionnaire was completed that included questions as to years spent in the island and in civilization. Natives were tested in a quiet room (not a sound proof chamber). Testing was done by two fully trained audiologists and included pure tones and discrimination in all of them.

PURE TONE AUDIOMETRY

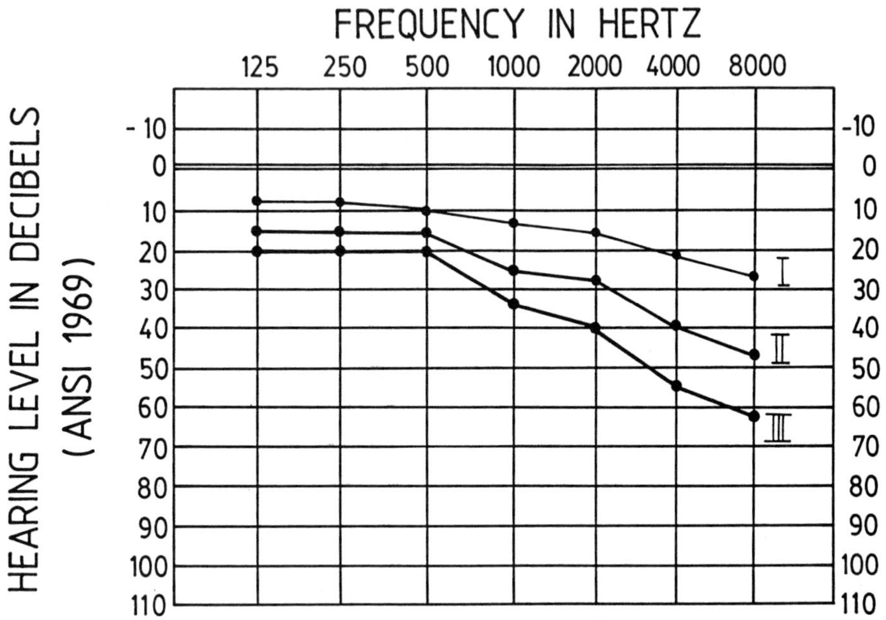

AVERAGE AUDIOGRAMAS

I ALWAYS LIVED LIVED IN THE ISLAND.

II LIVED IN THE CONTINENT 3 TO 5 YEARS.

III LIVED IN THE CONTINENT OVER 5 YEARS.

AVERAGE DISCRIMINATION SCORES

	RIGHT EAR	LEFT EAR
GROUP I	96%	96%
GROUP II	91%	89%
GROUP III	90%	85%

For clinical examination we used a complete set up for otoscopy, tuning forks testing (512 and 1024 Hertz), Rhinoscopy, pharyngeal, nasopharyngeal and laryngeal examination.

Audiological testing was done by using a Qualitone model NB audiometer (ANSI 69) and a Beltone portable audiometer model 12 - D (ISO-64), equiped with TDH - 39 earphones. For reporting purposes ISO - 64 was converted to ANSI 69

R E S U L T S :

RESULTS ARE SUMMARIZED IN TABLE I :

D I S C U S S I O N :

By comparing average hearing levels of the different groups according to years spent living in " civilized societies ", it is clear that people over 45 years old who have not left the island have better hearing than those who have lived 3 to 5 years in " MODERN CIVILIZATION ... In turn, those living 3 to 5 years in " CIVILIZED SOCIETIES " have better hearing than those living 6 years or more. It should be mentioned that we studied a representative group of (59.6 o/o of the total population over 45 years old) a genetically homogeneous population of natives, with no genetic sensorineural deafness, descendants of persons (3,4), practically all family related, with regular birth certificates, no language barriers, with complete medical records and recently censed. Based on these observations we can conclude that members of an isolated population living in a low ambient noise have better hearing, than members of the same group who have lived in " CIVILIZED SOCIETIES ", and that the degree of hearing loss acquired in modern civilization seems to be directly proportional to the number of years spent in it.

REFERENCES :

1.- *ROSEN S et al (1962) Presbycusis study of a relatively noise free population in the Sudan Ann Otol 71 : 727 - 743.*

2.- *HINCHCLIFFE R (1964) Hearing levels of elderly in Jamaica Ann Otol 73 : 1012 - 1019.*

3.- *HEYERDHAL T (1958) Aku - Aku. Rand MacNally and Co.*

4.- *FISHER R (1980) In : Mysteries of the Ancient World. Publications Division, National Geographic Society. Washington DC pp 192 - 214.*

5.- *NATIONAL CENSUS (1984) Chilean National Institute of Statistics.*

New dimensions in otorhinolaryngology - head and neck surgery, vol. 2.
E. Myers, editor

DIAGNOSTIC AND TREATMENT MANAGEMENT OF MALIGNANT EXTERNAL OTITIS (MEO)

DIAMANTE V., HAEDO G., ORFILA D. AND FAERMAN I.

Otorhinolaryngology and Endocrinology Service, Spanish Hospital, 2975 Belgrano Ave. 1209, Buenos Aires, Argentina

INTRODUCTION

This disease was clinically described by Chadler in 1968 as an external otitis caused by Pseudomonas aeruginosa in diabetic and elderly patients, and having a generally poor prognosis.

Physiopathology

Temporal bones from diabetic patients are known to present a thick layer of collagen, poorly vascularized, extending from the cartilagenous surface towards the dermis and which expands along the periosteum of the skull base, from the meatus.

Pseudomonas aeruginosa

Reaches these soft infratemporal tissues and attacks the bone, causing the well - known complications.

MATERIAL AND METHODS

Diagnosis

Typical clinical signs and symptoms include purulent otorrhea, severe earache and characteristic granulations in the external auditory canal, specially in elderly diabetic patients.

Basic complementary studies consist of laboratory tests to confirm diabetes, secretion cultures to recognize the presence of Pseudomonas aeruginosa and biopsy histology to rule out alternative pathologies. Besides X-rays and CT scanning, accessory studies include scintigraphy with Tc 99 to reveal early bone invasion and with Ga 64 to follow the inflamatory process.

Classification

Clinically, two main forms may be discerned: 1-early or localized MEO; and 2-late or widespread MEO, with or without complications.

Clinical Progress

The course of the disease depends on the early confirmation of diagnosis, on the clinical form and on the treatment administered. Complications include: facial palsy, IX,X,XI and XII nerve cranial paralysis. Sigmoid sinus thromboflebitis, meningitis, and endocranial infection. Besides, there are general complications arising from prolonged hospitalization.

Treatment

Once diagnosed, the patient is hospitalized and therapy started from three angles: 1-local treatment, 2-systemic antibiotic administration and 3-diabetic and clinical monitoring. Local treatment consists in daily examinations of the external ear by means of boric acid and drops of lemon juice, removal of bone detritus and cryctherapic applications to clear away granulations.

Antibiotics are given by endovenous route, associating a beta-lactamic drug with an aminoglucoside. On occasion 3rd. generation cephalosporins have been employed. In case of poor response to antibiotics or recurrent disease, hyperbaric treatment is given.

Surgery

Surgery is only necessary for the removal of bone detritus.

Curative criteria

Normal otoscopy, lack of pain, and normal erythrosedimentation are positive indications which should be confirmed by Ga scintigraphy.

Material

Ten patients were studied by our method. Average age was 69 years. Sex ratio was 9 males: 1 female. Clinical forms were: 4 cases of early MEO, 2 of late and 4 of late with complications.

RESULTS

All 20 patients made satisfactory recovery. However, in one there was definitive facial palsy, in another facial paresia and in a third spinal nerve paralysis. Mortality was nil.

DISCUSSION

The authors believe MEO is an essentially curable disease. The infection was found to spread through soft tissue at the skull base, rather than temporal bone pneumatization. There fore there is no advantage in removin mastoid bone while leaving infectious foci untouched. Lastly, extreme care should be taken in simple routine examination in elderly and/or diabetic patients.

REFERENCES

1. Simonic. Parisier. Nuclear scanning in necrotizing progressive Malignant external otitis. Laryngoscope 92: September 1982.
2. Joseph Nadol. Histopathology of pseudomonas osteomyelitis of the temporal bone, starting as malignal external otitis. American Jurnel of Otolaryngology. Vol. 1 Number 5. November 1980.
3. Mader. Malignant external otitis. Cure with adjunctive hyperbaric oxygentherapy. Arch. Otolaryng. Jan. 1982.
4. Czernobilsky. Ostfeld. Malignant external otitis early histopathologic changes and pathogenic mechanism. Laryngoscope juin 1981, 965 - 970.
5. David Neal G. and George Gates. Invasive pseudomonas osteitis of the temporal bone. American Journal of Otology (Vol. 4 Number 4. April 1983).

© 1985 Elsevier Science Publishers B.V. (Biomedical Division)
New dimensions in otorhinolaryngology - head and neck surgery, vol. 2.
E. Myers, editor

SURGICAL TREATMENT OF GLOMUS TUMORS-TECHNIQUES AND RESULTS

Michael J. Holliday, Nathan E. Nachlas, David W. Kennedy, George T. Nager

Depts. of Otolaryngology-Head and Neck Surgery, The Johns Hopkins University School of Medicine, Baltimore, Maryland, U.S.A.

INTRODUCTION

Surgical treatment of glomus tumors, particularly of glomus jugulare tumors has changed considerably during the past 10-15 years. Classifications of inoperability have been modified because of new approaches and instrumentation development. As a result, cure and complication rates with surgery have improved, paralleling development of neuro-otology as a subspeciality. This stimulated us to review our institutional experience with these neoplasms over the past 25 years. Forty-four cases have been identified. We have seen definite trends to change in therapy and expect to see long term results reflective of present data on cure rates.

MATERIAL AND METHODS

Our cases were derived from review of diagnosis indexing of the Surgical Pathology Dept. at The Johns Hopkins Hospital as well as from operative notes of the authors. Forty-three of the 44 cases identified were diagnosed and treated at The Johns Hopkins Hospital. One case was treated at an affiliated hospital. No search was performed at affiliated hospitals per se and therefore reflects the experience of the major institution only. The medical records including pathology, operative, radiology and audiology reports as well as outpatient notes were reviewed on all patients which it was available.

RESULTS

Between 1960 and 1985, 44 cases were identified. 39 of these cases were treated from 1970 to present date. All had biopsy proven diagnosis. 26 (59%) were glomus jugulare, 14 (39%) were glomus tympanicum, 3 (7%) glomus vagale and 1 (2%) glomus caroticum. Because of similarity in course and in treatment, the glomus caroticum case will be included in the glomus jugulare group elsewhere in this report. There has been a steady increase in cases with each decade. 25 cases or 57% were treated between 1980-85. Treatment has been by surgery alone in 23 cases, combined surgery and radiation in 19 cases and radiation alone following biopsy in 2 cases.

In the past 5 years, 17 of 25 patients (68%) were treated by surgery alone compared with 6 of 19 (32%) the prior 20 years. The first surgical procedure of an extended type such as infratemporal fossa approach or combined 2 stage neurosurgical neuro-otologic was performed in 1979. Since that time these procedures have outnumbered other forms of surgical therapy so that 13 of 25 otolaryngology procedures for glomus tumor between 1980 and present were extended procedures. There have been no surgical deaths. Followup has varied from 1 month to 25 years in 40 patients. In 4 patients followup was not available. None of 8 tympanicum, 11 jugulare and 3 vagale tumors treated with surgery alone have evidence of any tumor persistence to date. Three of 4 tympanicum and 3 of 13 jugulare tumors treated by combined surgery and radiation had evidence of tumor persistence at last followup. One jugulare tumor treated by radiation alone was free of disease. Both pre and postoperative audiometry was available in 29 of the 41 tumors excluding vagale tumors. Of those treated by surgery alone 9 were unchanged, 3 were improved and 4 had worse hearing postoperatively. Those patients with combined treatment had 6 unchanged and 5 worse postoperatively with none improved and 3 of the 6 unchanged having anacusis ears preoperatively. The one patient with radiation alone had improved hearing post radiation.

DISCUSSION

Recognition of extension of glomus jugulare tumors along the jugular bulb as well as the internal carotid artery has led to more aggressive surgical treatment in recent years. Removal of the jugular bulb when invasion is present and skeletonization and/or facial nerve rerouting or grafting should increase surgical cure rate. Better diagnostic procedures including digital subtraction angiography and high resolution CT scanning has increased diagnostic acumen as well as treatment planning ability. It is possible that some tumors previously felt to be extensive tympanicum tumors in the past might more likely be classified as jugulare tumors today. Preoperative embolization has cut down on required blood replacement. Two stage planned neurosurgical neuro-otologic procedures for tumors with intracranial extension through creation of false dural barriers have changed previously inoperable tumors into surgically resectable lesions. There has been a trend to increased attempts at hearing preservation and canal preservation or reconstruction whenever possible. Facial nerve rerouting allows exposure but is avoided when possible to prevent risk of nerve degeneration and undesirable synkinetic activity. Access to the internal carotid artery may be gained through the infratemporal fossa approach as well as an extended facial recess approach combined with extended posterior hypotympanotomy. All of the options have been utilized in selected cases. Radiotherapy remains a useful adjunct if tumor removal is incomplete or in poor surgical risks or the very elderly.

New dimensions in otorhinolaryngology – head and neck surgery, vol. 2.
E. Myers, editor

CLASSIFICATION OF INNER EAR ANOMALIES BY HIGH RESOLUTION CT-SCANNING OF THE TEMPORAL BONE

MICHIO ISONO, M.D., KIYOTAKA MURATA, M.D. AND FUMIHIKO OHTA, M.D.
Department of Otolaryngology, Kinki University School of Medicine, Osaka Japan

INTRODUCTION

Visualization of the architectural features of the labyrinthine capsule is rather difficult by ordinary radiological techniques including even tomography (Valvassori [1], Frey [2], Phelps [3]), while detailed classification of anomalies can be achieved by histological examination of the inner ear. High resolution CT-scanning of the temporal bone was carried out in our clinic in order to classify inner ear anomalies into more detailed groups than previously. Radiological classification of malformations of the inner ear may lend significant assistance to facilitating diagnoses of hearing and maldevelopment.

MATERIALS AND METHODS

High resolution CT-scanning revealed anomalies of the labyrinthine capsule in 50 ears in our clinic from Nov, 1980 to the end of 1984. They consisted of 23 ears with total deafness, 11 with profound deafness, 8 with high tone loss, 2 with a flat type audiogram of moderate hearing loss, 4 with fluctuant hearing and 2 with normal hearing or contour. Tomography was sliced at intervals of 1.5 mm and each was scanned, using a General Electric CT/T 8800 or Siemens Somatom DR-3, for 10 slices parallel to the plane which contained the orbitomeatal line and the vestibules on both sides. Ten slices consisted of 7 above the plane, 2 below it and one on the same plane. The window level was fitted to +100 and the window width of 2000 or 4000 HFU was used.

RESULTS

Following are the maldevelopment of the inner ear identified by high resolution CT-scanning of the temporal bone.

1) Agenesis of the whole labyrinthine capsule in 1 ear.
2) Maldevelopment of the cochlea.
    a. Agenesis in 5 ears.
    b. Slight protrusion of the cochlear growth in 3 ears.
    c. Poor cochlear turning in 16 ears.
3) Maldevelopment of the semicircular canal.
    a. Agenesis of all the semicircular canals (s.c.) in 5 ears.

b. Anterior s.c. without posterior and lateral s.c. in 8 ears.
c. Anterior s.c. without hypoplasia of posterior s.c. and aplasia of lateral s.c. in 4 ears.
d. Anterior and posterior s.c. with hypoplasia of lateral s.c. in 3 ears.

4) Maldevelopment of the vestibule.
   a. Enlargement in 25 ears.
   b. Deformation in 11 ears.
   c. Smallness in 4 ears.
5) Deformation of the internal acoustic meatus.
   a. Enlargement in 15 ears.
   b. Normal in 19 ears.
   c. Narrowing in 16 ears.

COMMENTS

Accumulation of high resolution CT-scannings of the temporal bone may provide detailed classification of inner ear anomalies, which contributes significantly to otological diagnoses. It may allow delineation of the pathological background for unilateral total deafness, idiopathic progressive sensorineural hearing loss and fluctuant hearing of children with a hearing aid. The last-mentioned hearing impairment may result from recurrent acute acoustic trauma in an immature ear. The detailed classification of inner ear anomalies may also help vastly for dismissing risks of misdiagnosis by polytomography and for obtaining measurable or variable diagnosis of maldevelopment.

REFERENCES

1. Valvassori G E, Naunton R F and Lindsay J R (1969) Inner ear anomalies: Clinical and histopathological considerations. Ann Otol 78:929-938
2. Frey K W (1965) Die Tomographie der Labyrinthmissbildungen. Fortschr Roentgenstr 102:1-13
3. Phelps P D (1974) Congenital lesions of the inner ear, demonstrated by tomography. Arch Otolaryngol 100:11-18

© 1985 Elsevier Science Publishers B.V. (Biomedical Division)
New dimensions in otorhinolaryngology - head and neck surgery, vol. 2.
E. Myers, editor

OTOLOGIC INVOLVEMENT IN HISTIOCYTOSIS X

D.W. KENNEDY, G.T. NAGER, A. SHIKHANI, W. ZINKHAM

Departments of Otolaryngology-Head & Neck Surgery and Pediatrics, The Johns Hopkins University, School of Medicine, Baltimore, Maryland, U.S.A.

INTRODUCTION

Histiocytosis is an uncommon disease with protean manifestations. Because of the wide variety of clinical presentation in the head and neck area, the otolaryngologist must be aware of the disorder, its forms of presentation, the possible courses of the disease, and its therapy.

Lichtenstein[1] recommended that eosinophilic granuloma, Hand-Schuller-Christian disease and Letterer Siwe disease should be grouped together under one term "Histiocytosis X", denoting their common origin from the histiocyte, but unknown etiology. This classification is still debated[2], but close clinical and pathological relationships between the different manifestations of Histiocytosis X remain. The prognosis in Histiocytosis is difficult to predict[3], but is related to the number of sites of involvement and to the presence of organ dysfunction arising from the disease. Treatment may consist of surgery, readiotherapy, chemotherapy or observation and careful follow up.

Previous reports[4,5] have indicated significant differences in the incidence of otologic involvement. A study was undertaken to further evaluate the presentation, manifestations and clinical course of otologic involvement in this disorder.

MATERIAL AND METHODS

Fifty five cases of Histiocytosis X evaluated at The Johns Hopkins Hospital between 1945 and 1984 were reviewed for the study. The age at onset of disease in the cases reviewed varied between birth and fifty five years of age. Males outnumbered females in the study by 32 to 23. Thirteen patients had unifocal eosinophilic granuloma (24%). Soft tissue involvement was present in twenty-eight patients (51%) and involvement in the head and neck area was present in thirty-five (63%). Cases with otologic involvement were evaluated in detail.

RESULTS

Of the fifty-five patients in the series, fifteen (27.3%) had evidence of otologic involvement. The mean age at onset in patients with otologic disease was younger (2.9 years) than for the group as a whole (8.5 years). By far the most common presentations were recurrent otitis (9 patients) and skin or scalp lesions (9 patients). Other presentations, including bony lesions, diabetes insipidus, fever, hepatosplenomegally and generalized lymphadenopathy were present with less frequency. Only two patients in the group had unifocal disease, and the incidence of soft tissue involvement (73%) was considerably higher than for the group as a whole.

The most frequent otologic manifestation was chronic otitis occurring in thirteen patients (87%). Lytic temporal bone defects were also present in eight patients (53%). Isolated lytic lesions of the temporal bone were present in two cases. The vast majority of the patients had bilateral involvement (87%). In several of the patients the external auditory canal was noted to be a sensitive indicator of overall disease activity.

DISCUSSION

Although an uncommon disorder, Histiocytosis frequently presents with manifestations in the head and neck area. The study suggests that patients with otologic involvement are likely to present earlier and have a greater likelihood of soft tissue involvement. This implies more aggressive disease, and a more guarded prognosis than for the disorder as a whole.

The otologist has an important role both in the diagnosis and in the long term follow up of Histiocytosis X. As isolated temporal bone involvement is uncommon, complete evaluation of these cases is mandatory, and surgery is rarely indicated as the primary therapeutic modality. In patients with otologic involvement, the external auditory canal may provide a sensitive indicator of disease activity during treatment and follow up.

REFERENCES

1. Lichtenstein L(1953) Histiocytosis X: Integration of Eosinophilic Granuloma of Bone, "Letterer-Siwe Disease" and "Schuller-Christian Disease", As Related Manifestations of a Single Nosological Entity. Arch Path 56:84-102

2. Cline MJ, Golde DW (1973) A Review and Reevaluation of the Histiocytic Disorders. AM J Med 55:49-60

3. Zinkham WH(1976) Multifocal Eosinophilic Granuloma: Natural History, Etiology and Management. Am J Med 60:457-463

4. Tos M (1966) A survey of Hand-Schuller-Christian's Disease in Otolaryngology. Acta Otolaryngol 62:218-228

5. McCaffrey T, McDonald T (1979) Histiocytosis X of the Ear and Temporal Bone: Review of 22 cases. Laryngoscope 89:1735-1742

New dimensions in otorhinolaryngology – head and neck surgery, vol. 2.
E. Myers, editor

POSITIONAL NYSTAGMUS IN NORMAL SUBJECTS - ELECTRONYSTAGMOGRAPHIC STUDY

LAVINSKY, LUIZ - Faculdade de Medicina - Universidade Federal do Rio Grande do Sul - Rua 24 de Outubro 1086 - Porto Alegre - 90.000 - RS (Brazil)

INTRODUCTION

The meaning of the positional nystagmus is stil a controverted subject, whereas neither its origin localization, nor its patological aspects - including the normality limits - are until this moment clearly defined.

The present study presents the investigations developed with o homogenius group, which selection followed rather rigid criteria, so that both from the clinical and the otorhinolaryngologic points of view it would offer the proper conditions of a normal group of study.

The objective of this study is to colaborate in the characterization of the normality patterns and of the topodiagnostic value of the positional test.

MATERIALS AND METHODS

The study was performed in volunteers from the Brazilian Air Force, who were at the 5th Regional Air Comand, Rio Grande do Sul, Brazil. All were males, ages varying between 19 and 20.

All subjects submitted to an exaustive clinical selection and otorhinolaryngologic, audiologic and otoneurologic evaluation, and 50 volunteers considered normal were left.

The group of normal subjects was submitted to a positional test, though electronystragmography, woth two register channels - vertical and horizontal - with open eyes and, afterwards, closed.

RESULTS AND CONCLUSIONS

1 - The occurency of positional nystagmus is significantly ($p<0.05$) common in normal subjects.

2 - The positional nystagmus, in the positional test woth closed eyes, in significantly greater ($p<0.05$) than when performed with open eyes.

3 - During the positional test in normal subjects, there was no vertigo or vegetative symptomatology.

4 - The number of cases of normal individuals with positional test wihout the positional nystagmus in significantly greater ($p<0.05$) with open eyes than when the positional test is performed with eyes closed.

5 - The maximum values of the different parameters to establish the normality criteria of the positional test (95% safety margin) are the following:

EYES NYSTAGMUS	OPEN		CLOSED	
	HORIZONTAL	VERTICAL	HORIZONTAL	VERTICAL
§ VACL - Maximum (^{o}/s)	4	5	13	20
§ VACL - Average-Maximum (^{o}/s)	3	4	7	12
§ Frequency in 10 s	3	3	6	9
§ Total number of positions with nystagmus	8	6	8	8

6 - The number of positive positions with eyes closed, both of horizontal and vertical nystagmus, do not seem to be useful to the definition of normality, whereas nystagmatic responses appear in all positions in normal subjects (95% confidence limit).

7 - In normal subjects, especially when the horizontal nystagmus with closed eyes are studied, the presence of positional nystagmus of alternating direction (45,75%) and alternating in the same position (12,5%) is frequent.

8 - In normal subjects the vertical positional nystagmus generally have a fixed position both with eyes open (95%) and with eyes closed (89,35%).

9 - The Vertical positional nystagmus with fixed ascendent direction happens in 97,56% of the cases, when the patients has the eyes closed, and in 84,62% when the eyes are open.

10 - The direction of the positional nystagmus, when the individual is lying on his/her side, has a significantly greater incidence ($p<0.05$) in the direction opposite the ear of the side on which the individual in lying.

11 - The incidence of nystagmatic response in normal subjects does not vary with the different positions of the positional test.

12 - There was no evidence of a significant correlation ($p>0.05$) between the intensity scales of the caloric test and the intensity scales of the positional test in normal subjects.

REFERENCES

1. BARBER, R.W. & WRIGHT, Grace. Positional nystagmus in normal. *Advances in Oto-Rhino-Laryngology,* Basel, 19:276-85, 1973.
2. CAWTHORNE, Terence. Positional vertigo. *Annals of Otology, Rhinology and Laryngology.* St. Louis, Mo., 63:481, 1954.
3. DIX, M.R. Positional nystagmus of central type and its neural mechanism. *Acta Oto-Laringol.,* GBR, 95:56-(585-8), 1983.
4. FERNANDEZ, Cesar; ALZATE, Rene; LINDSAY, John R. Experimental observations on postural nystagmus in the cat. *Annals of Otology, Rhinology and Laryngology,* St. Louis, Mo., 68:816-29, 1959.
5. JONGKEES, L.B.W. & PHILIPSZOON, A.J. The posture test. *Acta Oto-Laryngology* Suppl., Stockholm, 139:17-43, 1964.

New dimensions in otorhinolaryngology – head and neck surgery, vol. 2.
E. Myers, editor

STUDY OF THE LABYRINTHINE FUNCTION AND PSYCHOMOTRICITY IN THE SEVERELY DEAF

LAVINSKY, LUIZ - Faculdade de Medicina - Universidade Federal do Rio Grande do Sul- Rua 24 de Outubro 1086 - Porto Alegre - 90.000 - RS (Brazil)

INTRODUCTION

The hypothesis which generated this investigation is based in the fact that the patients who present severe otopathy would very often suffer from severe hearing losses, and would have the possibility of having alterations in the labyrinthine function without clearly definible symptomatology, due to the age of onset of the process.

This situation, when associated to proprioceptive, cerebellar, visual disturbances, as well as to disturbance in the development of the cerebral hemisphere dominance (laterality), would cause disturbances in posture, balance, and in the development of motor ability. These would then cause psychomotor disturbances which would then affect the learning process. There would be serious consequences over the development of language, reading and writing abilities and over the intelectual aspects.

The objective of this study is to investiqate a group of severe deafs and their labyrinthine function broadly, as well as their pscychomotricity, viewing the establishment of a relation between them.

MATERIALS AND METHODS

The investigation was carried out in 50 children, from 4 to 14 years old, from the Educational Center for Hearing Deficients, in Porto Alegre, Brasil. All children were severe deafs (65 db or more in both ears), without labyrinthine symptomatology in the present or in the past, and without clinical or neurological problems added to the hearing loss.

The investigation was broad and included a clinical and otorhinolaryngologic evaluation (more particulary the otologic and otoneurologic), labyrinthine evaluation through electronystagmography, studying the spontaneous and positional nystagmus, with open and closed eyes, the semi-spontaneous, optokinetic and perrotatory nystagmus, as well as the pendular eyetracking. It followed the methodology referred to by MM Ganança[1] and L Lavinsky[2]. To decide on normality and its topodiagnostic classification, the methods referred to by MM Ganança[1] were used.

The psychomotor examination evaluated the elementar motricity with the study of the manual dynamics coordination, the general dynamics coordination and visual motor coordination of pre-school children and the body perception through the study of balance. The Ozeretski-Guilmain tests were used, according to Pierre Vayer's[5] systematization. The visual motor coordination of school children followed Bender's test, according to E. Kopitz. The laterality study followed the observations n. 2,3 and 9 of the "Harris Tests of Lateral Dominance", also systematized by Pierre Vayer.

Trough these tests the developmental age was studied as to each potenciality in study. We considered the chronological age as ideal (100%), and established the psychomotor performance percentual, as well as the average of all psychomotor performance percentuals, of all tests - average psychomotor performance.

RESULTS AND CONCLUSIONS

Through a broader evaluation of the labyrinthine function than the one found in the literature, plus the quantitative analysis od the average psychomotor retardation and of each test separatedly, it was possible to reach the following statements about the labyrinthine function ot the severe deaf and its probable repercussion over the motor performance; That there is a high incidence of abnormal electronystagmopgraphyc findings, independent from the probable topographic diagnosis (peripheral, central of mixed) in all tests performed; that there was retardation of the psychomotor profile, in different proportions, in all members of the group studied, and high incidence of alterations in the development of the cerebral predominance (laterality); that there was no significant difference in the psychomotor performance degree in terms of the chronological age of the studied hanficapped; that in spite of the several correlations of the results, the cases is which the labyrinthine tests were normal did not show a significantly different psychomotor perfcrmance when compared to those who had the labyrinthine tests abnormal; that there is no relation of proportion between the directional preponderance ot the torsion swing stimulation test and the percentage of average psychomotor performance.

REFERENCES

1. GANANÇA, M.M. A eletronistagmografia no diagnóstico otoneurológico. In: LOPES Filho, O. *Temas de Otorrinolaringologia*. São Paulo, Manole, 1978. v.3. p. 161-80.
2. LAVINSKY, L. *Do nistagmo posicional em normais; estudo eletronistagmográfico*. Rio de Janeiro, 1979. Dissertação (Mestrado Otorrinolaringologia). Centro de Ciências Médicas e Biológicas da Pontifícia Universidade Católica do Rio de Janeiro.
3. QUIROS, J.B. & SCHARGER, O.L. *Neuropsychological fundamentals in learning disabilities*. San Rafael, Academic Theraphy Publications, 1977.
4. RAPIN, I. Hypoactive labyrinths and motor development. *Clin. Pediatr.*, Philadelphia, 13:922-37, 1974.
5. VAYER, P. *El niño frente al mundo*. Barcelona, Editorial Didático-Médica, 1973. p. 70-96.

New dimensions in otorhinolaryngology – head and neck surgery, vol. 2.
E. Myers, editor

ACUTE AIR-WAY OBSTRUCTION IN THE PAEDIATRIC AGE-GROUP

S. MAHINDRA, G. SAHOO, M.A. MEHAR AND R.K. BHAGAT
Otolaryngology Deptt., Lady Hardinge Medical College, N.Delhi. INDIA

INTRODUCTION

Acute air-way obstruction of rapid onset, often endangering life is commonly encountered in infants and young children in our country. Most cases present as acute respiratory emergencies. Unless the patency of the air-way is not immediately restored, the condition may prove rapidly fatal. Hence our interest in the subject.

METHOD AND MATERIAL

The present study is based on 1091 cases of upper air-way obstruction, selected at random, who attended the Lady Hardinge Medical College and the associated hospitals from Sept. 1971 to Aug. 1983. Their age-group ranged between 2 days to 7 years. Direct laryngoscopy was done as a routine in all cases, after recording brief history, systemic and local examination and the management decided on the basis of D/L findings. Laryngeal swab, X-ray chest etc. were done as indicated. 471 of these cases presented as acute respiratory emergencies and were hospitalized.

OBSERVATIONS AND COMMENTS

Routine direct laryngoscopy in our study consisting of 1091 cases of acute air-way obstruction in the paediatric age-group revealed acute infection ? viral in 83% cases, since of the 34% laryngeal swabs, 77% were reported negative. Of the positive cases, the commonest organism was Staph. pyogenes. Ps. pyocyaneus and E. coli were however isolated in few cases. 25% cases of this group presented signs of lower respiratory infection, X-ray chest revealing opacities in 9.8% cases of acute laryngo-tracheo-bronchitis.

Viral neuritis caused bilateral abductor palsy in 5% cases in our series. Two cases had associated 9th nerve palsy as well.

Allergy was the underlying factor in 40% cases in our series. 70% of these cases presented signs of superadded infection.

Congenital anomalies in the form of laryngomalacia, infantile epiglottis and web formation were seen in 18% cases. We had 8 cases of multiple papilloma of the larynx.

Intensive antibiotics were used in all cases of acute infection in our series. Initially Pencillin, Streptomycin and Sulphadiazine formed the usual therapy. Later Erythromycin was used routinally. unless the sensitivity report indicated Tetracycline, Chloromycetin, Gentamycin or Kanamycin. Ampicillin was the drug of choice during the seventies, but lately because of poor response to this drug Erythromycin has replaced it with excellent results. Corticoids, including intra-venous dexona have been freely used both in cases of severe infection as well as in those of allergy. Symptomatic treatment such as antiallergic drugs, expectorants, O_2 inhalations, decongestants, nasal drops, mucolytic agents and steam-tents was used as indicated.

Tracheostomy was done in 23.7% cases. Intubation as pre-tracheostomy procedure was used in emergency cases only for lack of intensive care facilities. Emphysema, wound infection and maggot formation in 2 cases were some of the complications of tracheostomy in our series. We had two cases of difficult decanulation who required prolonged nasotracheal intubation. There was no morbidity in our series and the overall mortality was 2.8%.

Maximum cases were seen during Mar./Apr. and Aug./Sept. 95% cases in our series were below 3 years of age, the youngest a 2 days old baby. 63.5% cases were males inspite of the male sex being more precious in our country. The condition is of rapid onset as 89% cases presented within 48 hours. Hoarse voice, dyspnoea, fever, noisy respiration and croupy-cough formed the usual clinical picture in our study.

SUMMARY

- Acute infection? viral was responsible in 83% of our cases.
  25% of these were of acute laryngo-tracheo-bronchitis.
  Viral Neuritis accounted for another 5%.
- Allergy was the underlying factor in 40% cases. 70% of these presented signs of superadded infection.
- Congenital anomalies in the presence of mild infection resulted in "Out of Proportion" air-way obstruction in 18% of cases.
- Tracheostomy for relief of air-way obstruction was done in 23.7% cases.
- An overall mortality of 2.8% was noted in our series.

ACKNOWLEDGEMENT

We are grateful to the Principal, Lady Hardinge Medical College for her kind permission to publish this study.

New dimensions in otorhinolaryngology - head and neck surgery, vol. 2.
E. Myers, editor

QUANTITATIVE AND QUALITATIVE DIAGNOSES OF CHILDREN WITH VOICE DISORDERS

MF PEDERSEN (1), S MØLLER (2), K ERIKSEN (3) & U SØNDERGAARD (4)
Copenhagen Singing School, the Health Service, Copenhagen School Systems, Sjælør Boulevard 135, DK-2500 Valby, Denmark

In a clinical setting it seems necessary to use both quantitative and qualitative methods for the evaluation of voice disorders. Such an attempt has earlier been made in adults (1). In this study 110 school children were submitted by 35 logopeds to the phoniatric laboratory at the Copenhagen Singing School. The qualitative diagnosis was carried out traditionally with laryngological anamnesis and objective examination. The quantitative methods were stroboscopy, fundamental frequency measured with electroglottographic registration of 2000 cycles during reading of a standard text, phonetograms and phonation time. This method has been used in normal children in earlier studies (2, 3, 4).

Table I shows the diagnoses together with results of practicable stroboscopies. Other diagnoses found were 3 cases with chronic allergic voice disorder, 5 with mutational problems, 4 with dysodia and 1 had left recurrent nerve paralysis. 55% were between 8-10 years old, 33 were girls.

The heaviest voice disorder was fibrous nodules and here all but 1 had insufficient glottis closure; only 3 were girls. The age was 9.9 years with SD 2 years, which was much narrower than for the other diseases. Of course the reason could be psychological maladaption to male puberty, but a purely biological reason could be increasing sensitivity to strain of the tissue in the age 8-10 years due to the completion of the cover layers of the vocal chords at the same time as the endocrinological development accelerates. Also allergy at the beginning of puberty could not be excluded. The means of the variables, fundamental frequency, the lowest and highest frequency in the phonetogram and their location on the ordinate (in dB) together with intensity ranges at 262 and 523 Hz are shown in Table II together with the results of the analysis by linear regression with age as the independent variable, taking into account both the development by age and the different ages in the normal and pathological material. No slopes and levels showed significant differences between the disorders (II-VI).

Phonetograms by microprocessing seem relevant in a clinical situation, possibly together with Fo/noise before and after treatment.

REFERENCES

1. Pedersen MF, Eriksen K, Heramb S (1980) Proc XVIII Congr Int Ass Logoped Phoniatr Wash, pp. 621-626

2. Pedersen MF, Kitzing P, Krabbe S, Heramb S (1982) Acta Otolaryngol Suppl 386: 189-192

3. Pedersen MF, Munk E, Bennett P, Møller S (1984) Proc X Int Congr Phon Sci Utrecht, pp 604-608

4. Pedersen MF, Møller S, Krabbe S, Munk E, Bennett P, Kitzing P (1984) Acta Otolaryngol Suppl 412: 46-49 and 138

TABLE I

DIAGNOSES OF VOICE DISORDERS

Stroboscopy	Functional dysphonia	Nodules		Laryngitis		Others	Total	%
		oedematous	fibrous	chronic	acute recid.			
Closure insufficient	11	9	20	4	0	3	34	37
Movements								
irregular	23	28	20	12	2	6	74	82
tense	19	27	20	12	2	6	79	88
loose	3	1	0	2	0	0		
Diagnosis total (%)	41	31	19	14.5	1.8	14.3		

TABLE II.

QUANTITATIVE ANALYSIS. Results of analysis of linear repression by age

Means		Total	Normals I	Voice disorders II-VI	Common slope/level I-VI	
Average Fo	(Hz)	244	299	260	-	
Fmin	(Hz)	168	141	197	-	
	(dB)	60	61	58	+	(+)
Fmax	(Hz)	921	1130	710	+	(-)
	(dB)	85	88	82	+	(+)
Intensity						
range 262 Hz	(dB)	22.4	26.6	17.4	+	(-)
range 523 Hz	(dB)	18.6	23.3	11.3	-	
Tone range						
singing	(semi	29	36	22	-	
reading	tones)	4.25	4.29	4.21	+	(+)

-: Significant differences ($P < 0.05$) in slopes.

+: Non-significant differences in slopes.

(-): Significant differences in levels ($P < 0.05$) comparable when common slopes.

(+): Non-significant differences in levels comparable when common slopes.

New dimensions in otorhinolaryngology – head and neck surgery, vol. 2.
E. Myers, editor

LASER APPLICATION IN OTOLARYNGOLOGY

WANG QI

Department of otolaryngology, Wuhan Medical College, Second Hospital, People's Republec of China

Laser, a main CO2 device, has been used for the treatment of ENT disease, including chronic hypertrophic rhinitis,epistaxis,surperficial localized angioma, nevus and warts with good results, Laser therapy in tonsillitis and malignant tumor has also proved to be satisfactory.

Different laser devices, including CO2 laser,Ar, Helium-Neon, Nd-YAG,etc. have been used in this study. The main purpose is to select a specific dosage for a particular lesion as mentioned above. For example, in the treatment of chronic hypertrophic rhinitis, using a 40-watt CO2 laser, nasal ventilation was improved a few minute after treatment in 95.24% of our cases. After 1 to 3 doses of treatment, the hypertrophied lower nasal concha was markedly reduced in size and the mucous membranes locked fairly smooth. The brief method is described as follows. After surface anesthesia, the CO2 laser focusing tube is placed near the hypertrophic portion of the lower nasal concha, and applies dispersing intermittent irradiation to the local lesion.

An alternate method using a 10 to 15-watt CO2 laser can be applied for the treatment of nevi and warts in the ear and nose, and the face and neck as well. If the applied power is excessive, a sunken scar will appear after treatment. In contrast, appropriate dosage does not damage the normal skin. Generally only one treatment is necessary, leaving no scar or only a superficial with occasional depigmentation or pigmentation. Localized telangiectasia and children's telangioma were also treated using this method with good results. The lesion could be completely disposed of by vaporization. A 15-watt CO2 laser device was used for tonsillectomy, no bleeding was seen in the incision wound and little postoperative pain was ensued for 156 patients receiving this treatment. The operative techni was a modified procedure of tonsillectomy using guillotine. A cotton swab was use to separate the blade and the enlarged tonsil, the exposed padicle can thus be resected by the laser. A 20-watt CO_2 laser may also be used in many surgical procedures, such as megarhinophyma excision, accessory auricle excision, separa-

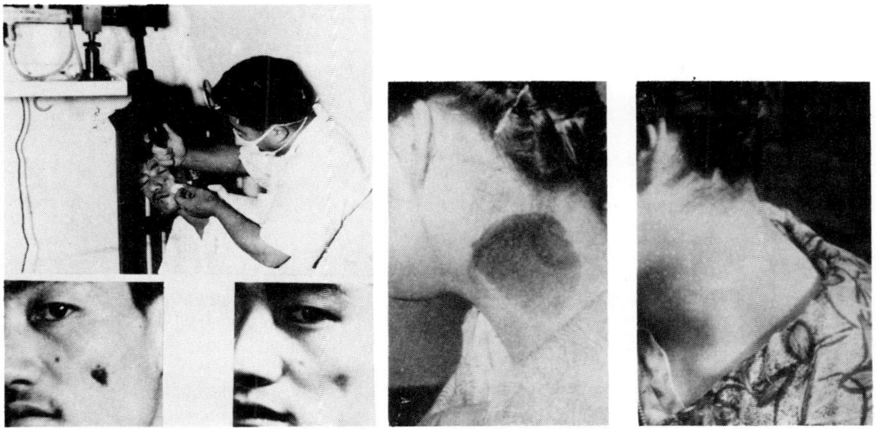

Figure. The melanin nevus. Left patient treated with a high powered laser post operatively showed indurated scar. Right patient treated with appropriate laser power showed little scarring at the operative site.

tion of nasal space adhesion, and superficial tumor excision.

Either surgical resection or vaporization or both can be used effectively for the treatment of certain neoplasma once the lesion are exposes sufficiently. These neoplasma include laryngeal carcinoma, skin carcinoma, and some intracranial tumors. In the case of maxillary sinus carcinoma, cryotherapy followed laser treatment has been shown to be effective. some cases have been followed up for 3-5 years with no signs of recurrence.

Using high energy-beam scanning method, relatively large-surfaced tumors can be treated, the rate of lightsport scanning is adjusted according to the depth of pathologic changes. Treatment is continued until the lesions disappear. Ar laser and CO_2 laser has been used for the treatment of angioma, large vacularis nevus and melanoma.

REFERENCE

Wang Qi (1979): Laser in Otolaryngology. Chinese Medical Journal, 92 (12) 857-861.

New dimensions in otorhinolaryngology – head and neck surgery, vol. 2.
E. Myers, editor

"Severe Trauma of the Trachea, Pharynx and Larynx"

De la Rosa, Juan Francisco, M. D.*; Cardona, Raul M. D.**; Gonzalez, Fernando, M.D.***; Galvez, Carlos M.D.****; MacDonald Rodolfo, M.D.*****

Introduction

The purpose of this work is to describe tracheal, pharyngeal and laryngeal trauma and the different therapeutic approaches. We know that neck trauma should be treated as fast as possible, for the structures in this area are of vital importance and early and careful treatment can be the difference between life and death.

It is essential that repair of the damaged structure be made having in mind the anatomy of the area,for good function will depend on this point. All problems should be resolved primarily for later complications that result from a bad anatomical repair, pose problems that are more difficult to solve due to sequelae that will prevent the patient from adapting again to society.

In this paper we are presenting our experiences and suggestions in management and treatment as well as the importance of pre- and post-operatory assessment of injuries that, if not treated adequeately, will leave sequelae that can limit swallowing, phonation and/or ventilation.

Material and Methods

From October 1981 to May 1985 63,312 patients with multiple traumas were hospitalized in the Surgery Department of the Roosevelt Hospital in Guatemala, C. A. 60 patients with neck injuries required surgical examination and 12 had severe tracheal, pharyngeal and laryngeal trauma, and patients were treated as a whole in the

* Chief of the O.R.L. Section
** Chief of Residents
*** Third Year Resident
**** Chief of Residents
***** Head of Section
Surgery Department of the Roosevelt Hospital
Guatemala, Central America

Section of Otorhinolaryngology.

Results

Age and Sex. Ages ranged between 10 and 60 years of age, average 30 years. The most affected decades were the third and fourth decades of life. There were 34 patients -- 11 males, 1 female, 8 farmers, 2 army officers, 1 house wife, 1 salesman, and 10 were referred to other hospital centers.

Trauma mechanisms

As shown on Table 1, 9 were stab wounds, 2 gun shot wounds and 1 closed trauma, resulting from a car accident. In gun shot wounds, bullets were of a 45 caliber; in knife injuries, one case was suicide attempt and the other eight, homicide attempts.

Table No. 1

Injuries	Cases
Knife	9
Gun shot	2
Car accident	1
Total	12

Evolution time. In 4 cases, patients received medical care in the first 24 hours after trauma. In 5 cases, 24 to 48 hours after, and in 3 cases, more than 72 hours had elapsed. In this last group a patient was referred to us 5 days after he was injured.

Types of Injury. As shown on Table 2, there were four cases with total pharyngeal, laryngeal section that were treated with lavage and debridement, anatomical repair of the structures and distal tracheostomy. In one of the cases, a gastrostomy tube was placed to feed the patient and three other patients were fed by means of a nasogastric tube. A pen rose was placed for wound drainage and was removed on the 5th day of the post operatory period. There was complete tracheal section and one of the patients underwent distal tracheostomy and was sent afterwards to our institution where resection and end-to end anastomosis of the trachea was practiced, together with distal tracheostomy. Another case was total traumatic section of the trachea. The patient was intubated, end-to-end anastomosis was practiced and nasotracheal intubation was left for 48 hours. The patient who suffered partial tracheal resection was treated with resection and end-to-end anastomosis with distal tracheostomy. In two cases the pharynx was perforated and the right primitive carotid artery was injured. Treatment involved primary closure of the pahrynx and in one the primitive carotid artery was ligated successfully and without neurologic sequelae. In another case, primary closure of the pharynx and end-to-end anastomosis were performed. The patients course was not satisfactory and there was brain involvement that will be discussed later. In other two cases, there was tracheolaryngeal injury. Anatomic repair was the surgical approach, leaving a tracheostomy tube in one and a nasotracheal tube in another.

Table No. 2

Injury	Cases
Partial tracheal section	1
Total tracheal section	3
Total pharyngeal laryngeal section	4
Pharynx perforation and injury primitive carotid artery	2
Section of the trachea and the larynx	2
Total	12

Associated injuries. In four cases there was section of the upper laryngeal nerve. One case of section of the right recurrent nerve. Two cases of injury of the primitive carotid artery.

Morbi-mortality rates

There were no infections of the surgical wound; in one of the cases there was crico-tracheal stenosis that required a tracheo-fistula and the placement of a teflon mold that was removed 6 weeks after with successful results. Another case developed paralysis of the right vocal chord secondary to section of the recurrent. The patient was on speech therapy with an 80% recovery. Another patient developed brain edema with endocraneal hypertension and another had bronchoaspiration when being fed with a nasogastric tube.

Two patients died. One because of bronchoaspiration on the 6th day after surgery. The other after intracraneal hypertension. Autopsy studies showed hemorrhagic brain infarct.

Conclusions

a) As in every surgery, in-depth knowledge of the anatomical area is basic for adequate and funciontal repair of these structures.

b) When sections are above the vocal chords and there is no lesion of the great vessels, patients breathe through the wound.

c) Meticulous lavage and debridement are basic for this type of lesions.

d) In all cases of severe tracheal-pharyngeal-laryngeal trauma and adequate air way must be provided by distal tracheostomy or naso-tracheal tube.

e) Nasogastric tube or gastrostomy will be necessary to feed the patient.

Recommendations

We recommend the primary closure of anatomical lesions regardless of the evolution time, in order to prevent sequelae in swallowing, phonation and respiration.

New dimensions in otorhinolaryngology - head and neck surgery, vol. 2.
E. Myers, editor

COMPLICATIONS OF CO_2 LASER SURGERY IN LARYNGOLOGY: 1992 CASES

Dr. Jean Abitbol, Chief of ENT Department
Hopital de Passy 75016
Paris, FRANCE

In the field of laryngology, particularly phonosurgery, the CO_2 laser appears to be the instrument of choice in my hands. In the past seven years, I have performed laser surgery in 1992 cases.

COMPLICATIONS DURING SURGERY

1: HEMORRAGE. It appears only when the arterioles exceed 1mm in dia- diameter, particularly the arteries from the anterior commissure and the posterior commissure. We coagulate arytenoid artery if it is necessary by electrocoagulation prior to laser surgery.

2: REFLECTS FROM ANY SHINY SURFACE. Instruments should preferably be black and ebonized to avoid reflection.

3 CASES: 2 cases of reflected laser beam from shiny suction tube to free edge of opposite normal cord, one on the anterior commissure artery. All healed well.

Abrasions of vocal cords by aluminum protecting the tube in three cases. We avoid this complication now, eliminate extubation coughing, by using a green gauze steeped in xylocaine fixed under the glottis. With such a gauze, we protect trachea, the crico thyroid membrane and also the cuff of the E.T. tube.

Pachydemia of one vocal cord: 5 cases. Post-operative dysplasia has increased. We observed inflamation for 5 weeks then the epithelium thickened to pachydermia.

By dynamic vocal exploration, we noticed the vocal cords to be edematous, erythematous decreased wave motion, vocal pitch control was poor.

3: PARALYZED VOCAL CORD. We observed 2 cases. I did a cordectomy for carcinoma T1 in these 2 patients. In coagulating the arytenoid arteries, the final branches of the recurrent nerve were destroyed also. The cord stayed paralyzed after 3 years following.

4: OTHER COMPLICATIONS ABOUT MUCOSA. We noticed 4 types of complications:

a: Persistant oedema in 5 cases which needed cortisone therapy. The voice did not come back entirely even after speech therapy.

b: Vascular corditis are more a reaction of the muscle that appears just after surgery and disappears after 8 months of voice therapy.

c: Infections and laryngitis are very rare.

COMPLICATIONS INVOLVING TYPE OF LESIONS OPERATED. In my experience, as conventional techniques, we observed recurrences:

30% for web lesions, 38% for granuloma.

Papillomas need at least three operations in 1½ years.

Exceptionally we noticed recurrences for nodules: cases we observed were patients who did not want to have any speech therapy. So the same effects lead to the same lesions.

Sulcus Glottidis: Vaporizing the sulcus creates a sticking space between the vocal ligament and mucosa. After surgery, very little waves could be seen in strobofiberscopy. On 11 cases, we noticed 9 failures. Actually, laser seems to be contraindicated for the sulcus.

HOW TO PREVENT SUCH COMPLICATIONS

1: Power of the laser beam must be very well known, 10w. seems the best level.

2: Time of shooting is very important too; continuous firing is dangerous, section is too deep, thermal effect is too high. The best way seems to shoot with length of 1/10 second and with very fast impulse. By that technique, you avoid thermic effects and bleeding.

3: Angle of shooting is the third fundamental element of good results. 90^{0} angle avoid to have a big spot on the vocal cord, the energy is not absorbed by the under mucosa. If not, the more tangential we are, the more thermic effect we will observe.

4: Other parameters are important also such as a very precise beam with a good focus, an unreflective tool, a green gauze steeped in xylocaine fixed under the lower edge of the glottis, and a very deep anesthesia.

CONCLUSIONS

After having observed my and other patients, laser is a very interesting tool in most lesions described which need phonosurgery. Sulcus seems very difficult by such techniques. Anyway, in future, taking care about the balance between thermal effect and vaporized effect remains fundamental. With conventional techniques, we never see mucosa thermic effects. In some precise indications we think that the two ways are very helpful in phonosurgery.

New dimensions in otorhinolaryngology – head and neck surgery, vol. 2.
E. Myers, editor

NEW TRACHEOSTOMA FLAP VALVE FOR SURGICAL SPEECH RECONSTRUCTION

WARYAM SINGH

Department of Otorhinolaryngology, Bangour General Hospital, Broxburn, West Lothian, Scotland (U.K.)

INTRODUCTION

The newer surgical fistula procedures provide a very effective way of producing a good intelligible speech. In all these procedures manual occlusion of tracheostoma is required for speech production. Finger occlusion of stoma for speech production is embarrassing in that it draws attention to stoma. It is unhygienic and at times inconvenient. Patient is inhibited to speak with finger occlusion, if hands are dirty or both hands are busy driving or busy eating or dancing or sporting activity.

The new tracheostoma flap valve eliminates the use of finger to close stoma for speech.

MATERIAL AND METHODS

The tracheostoma flap valve consists of a Plastic PVC valve button with a metallic valve body. The inner end of the button is variable in size to suit the patient's tracheostoma. The external end of the button is constant in size. It has a groove which snap fits with the rib on the valve body. The valve body has a flap (0.035cm thick) hinged on the front of its floor and a screw to adjust the sensitivity of the flap. The flap valve fits snugly into the valve button. The composite system is air tight and self retaining. (Fig. 1). Air flow back pressure at the stoma is no problem as the valve is not dependent on any adhesives to hold it.

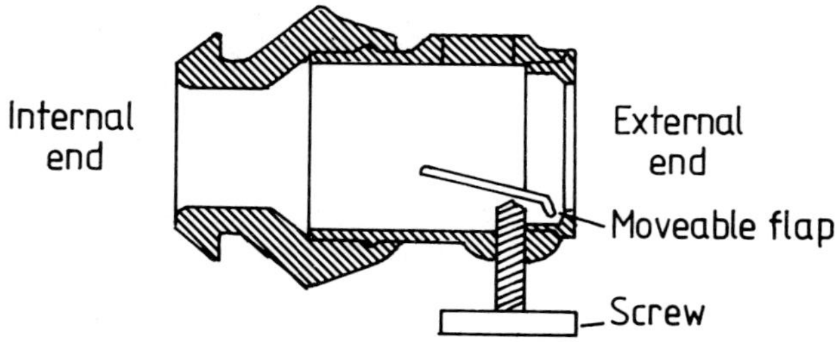

Fig. 1 Section showing component part of valve.

During normal quiet breathing, and routine physical activity the flap valve remains open where it has been set by the screw manually. (Fig. 2). When the patient desires to speak with exhaled air, the flap valve closes. (Fig. 3.) but automatically re-opens when one stops speaking. During coughing and strenuous physical exertion the valve can be temporarily removed.

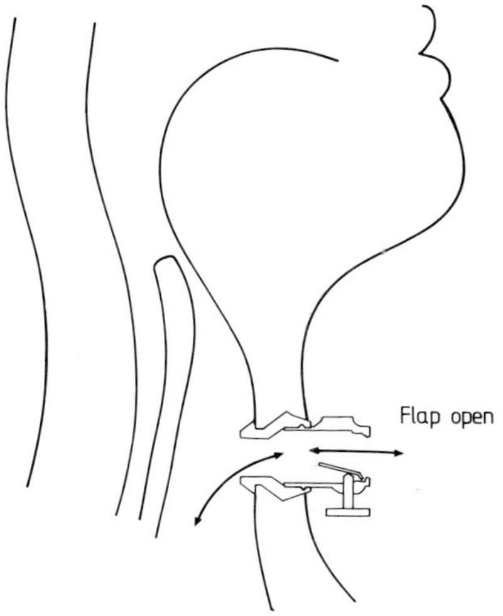

Fig. 2. Open position of the valve (during breathing)

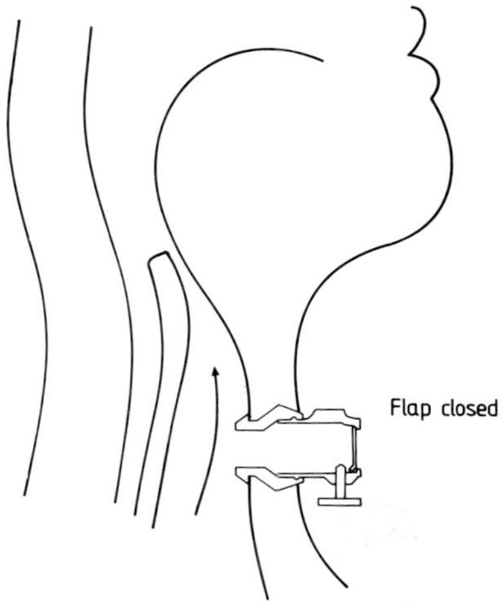

Fig. 3. Closed position of the valve (during speech)

VOCAL EFFICIENCY EVALUATION

The tracheostoma flap valve has been used by 9 patients (8 patients with near total laryngectomy with myomucosal shunt and 1 with tracheo-oesophageal fistula) for over a period of one year. All the 9 patients took a few seconds to a minute to insert the valve and speak immediately without prior training. The patients report that their speech seems clearer and more natural than by using finger occlusion. Psychologically it was a great morale booster as they could work as well as talk at the same time. The vocal efficiency measurements are very encouraging: the quality of speech is the same both with finger occlusion and with the tracheostoma flap valve.

New dimensions in otorhinolaryngology - head and neck surgery, vol. 2.
E. Myers, editor

VOICE PROSTHESES: SURGERY, EVALUATION AND RESULTS

HANS-P.ZENNER, I.F.HERRMANN and H.PFRANG

Depts. of Otolaryngology and Psychology, University of Wuerzburg,
D-8700 Wuerzburg, W.-Germany

INTRODUCTION

130 patients have undergone prosthetic voice restoration using primary or secondary tracheo-pharyngeal-(TP)-shunt techniques (1,2). Objective analysis of the success or failure has been assessed according to two major criteria: (i) the ability to swallow without aspiration; (ii) the production of vocal sounds that allowed for speech rehabilitation with less than 10% intelligibility loss as measured by to the PLT-test according to ZENNER (3,4)**. Furthermore, the role of radiotherapy has been evaluated to determine its effect on each of these two criteria.

The secondary TP-puncture

In 53 patients we performed an outpatient endoscopic procedure using a large esophagoscope (5). Speech intelligibility and intelligibility loss were determined according to (3,4) using the PLT-test (PLTT) (Fig.1). 60 % of the patients developed speech with an intelligibility loss of less than 10%, whereas only 10% of the controls - the esophageal speakers - belonged to this group.

Glottoplasty - the primary technique (8)

To increase overall intelligibility we developed a procedure that (i) decreases airflow resistance (1,2,6),(ii) creates a voice shunt during wide field laryngectomy (1,2,6),(iii) make use of a low pressure valved prosthesis* and (iv) reproducibly creates a uniform tracheostoma (1,2,6).

77 patients underwent the primary shunt procedure,(i) 54 individuals without and (ii) 23 including dorsal myotomy. In the series of 54 patients without myotomy 33 laryngectomees (61%) achieved fluent voice, the PLTT (3,4) revealing an intelligibility loss of less than 10 %. This is similar to the secondary technique (60 %) and superior to the esophageal speech (10%). In contrast (ii) following additional intraoperative dorsal myotomy 19 patients (82%) produced excellent speech as judged by the PLTT indicating an intelligibility loss of

* Fa.Koss, Geisenheim, W.-Germany
** available upon request (english version in preparation)

less than 10%. Thus, 10% of esophageal speakers, 60% of prosthetic speakers without myotomy and 80% of patients with voice prostheses and pharyngeal myotomy mastered to use a telephone at a 90%-100% intelligibility level (Fig. 1a).

REFERENCES

1. Herrmann IF, Kley W (1981): The glottoplasty. Proc.World Congr.ORL (L.Surjan,Ed.) Budapest
2. Zenner HP, Herrmann IF (1984): A new versatile technique for primary and secondary surgical voice restoration following laryngectomy. In: Plast. Reconstr.Surg.(P.Ward and W.Bergmann,Eds.)Mosby Press,pp.1102-1106
3. Zenner HP, Pfrang H (1985): Ein Sprachverständlichkeitstest für Laryngektomierte. Laryngol.Rhinol.Otol.,in press
4. Zenner HP (1985): The Post-Laryngectomy-Telephone-Test.In:Voice restoration following laryngectomy (IF Herrmann and M Singer,Eds) Springer,in press
5. Zenner HP :The tracheo-pharyngeal puncture (s.Ref.4)
6. Herrmann IF (s.Ref.4)
7. Herrmann IF ,Zenner HP (1982): Pharynxrekonstruktion mit Stimmrehabilitation Arch.Otorhinolaryngol. 235:703
8. Herrmann,I.F.,J.Buchwald and H.P.Zenner:Die Glottoplastik-Eine neue Methode zur chirurgischen Stimmrehabilitation. HNO 1984,23:294-301

FIGURE 1

INTELLIGIBILITY EXAMPLES OF PATIENTS WITH DIFFERENT ALARYNGEAL SPEECH MODES

Intelligibility loss (IL) was determined using the PLT-Test (Post-Laryngectomy-Telephone-Test) according to (3,4).

(a) Primary TE-shunt, low pressure valve prosthesis (ESKA-Herrmann) and myotomy

(b) Esophageal Speech (c) Control:normal speaker

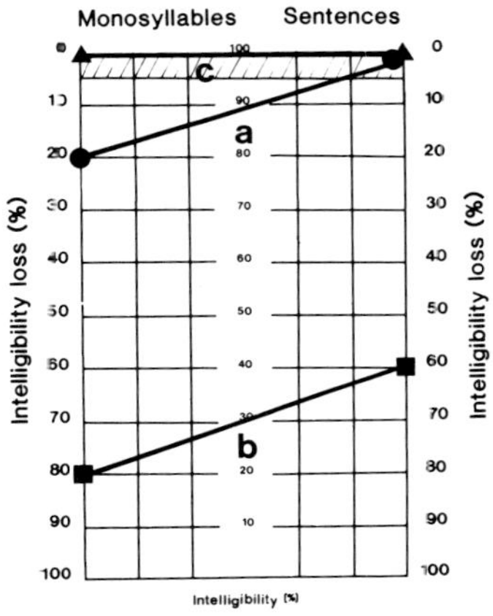

New dimensions in otorhinolaryngology – head and neck surgery, vol. 2.
E. Myers, editor

MUCORMYCOSIS WITH RHINO-ORBITAL AND CEREBRAL INVOLVEMENT

O.L.MENDONÇA CRUZ, E.S.HARON, E.GENTA, L.J.PAIVA.
Hospital das Clínicas da Universidade de São Paulo. Rua Eneas de Carvalho Aguiar 255 - 6º andar - 05403 - São Paulo - Brasil

INTRODUCTION

Mucormycosis is the designation of a group of infections caused by fungi belonging to the order Mucorales. These fungi are widespread in nature and are frequently found in upper respiratory tract of normal persons, presenting minimal pathogenicity (Lehrer R.I. et al, 1980). These infections usually occur in immunocompromised patients, Diabetes Mellitus being the most commonly recognized underlying disease associated with Mucormycosis.

Among the clinical forms reported, the rhino-orbital involvement shows typical clinical manifestations which allow early diagnosis and treatment improving the survival rate even in cases with cerebral complications.

CASE REPORTS

Case 1: A 29-year-old white woman admitted to the Hospital das Clínicas da Universidade de São Paulo with ketoacidosis, right purulent nasal discharge, necrosis of the homolateral hemi-palate, right facial paralysis, proptosis and unilateral lost of vision.CT showed clouding of maxillary, ethmoid and sphenoid sinuses and a posterior fossa abcess (Fig. 1). Biopsy specimens taken at surgical debridment confirmed the presence of Mucormycosis. Therapy with Amphotericin B was initiated. Nine months later, the patients was discharged with good general conditions and complete resolution of the cerebral abcess (Fig. 2).

Case 2: This fifth-five-year-old woman has a four year history of Diabetes Mellitus and was admitted at the Emergency Room with ketoacidosis and a sudden onset of right palpebral swelling, ptosis, proptosis and unilateral loss of vision. CT disclosed clouding of all paranasal sinuses on the right side and a right frontal lobe abcess. Two surgical debridments were performed associated with Amphotericin B and general supportive measures. Although the cerebral abcess showed only partial regression with the treatment, the patient was discharged six months later in good clinical and neurological conditions.

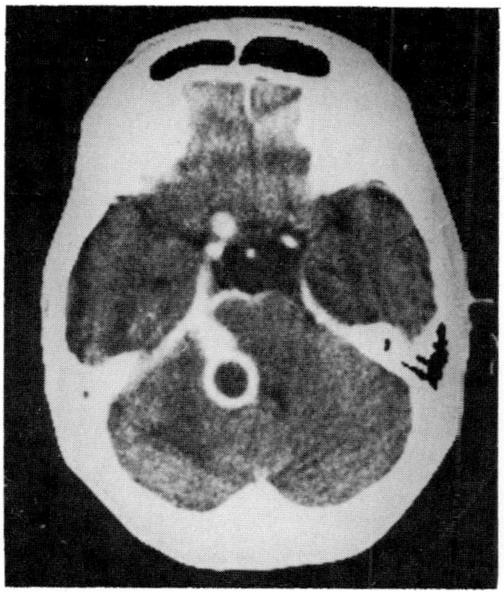

Fig.1 Posterior fossa abcess

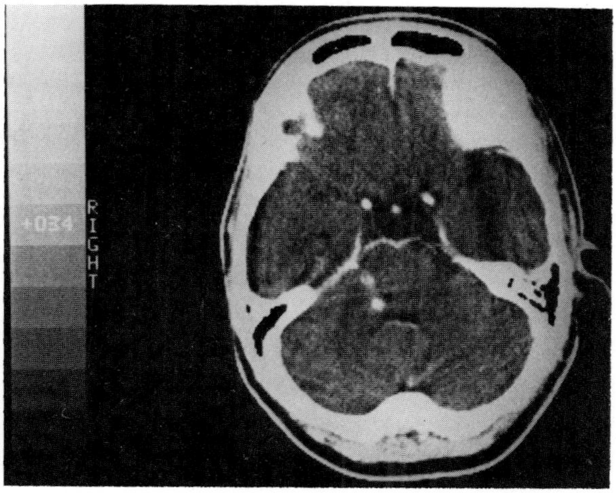

Fig.2 Resolution of the abcess

COMMENTS

The most common features of nasal, sinus cavities and orbital Mucormycosis are unilateral necrotic aspects of mucous nasal membrane with encompasses the inferior turbinate, ptosis and proptosis.

The invasion of the CNS by zygomycetes occurs either by direct extension from lesions in the nose, paranasal sinuses or orbit, or by hematogenous progression usually by direct invasion of vessel walls or secondary to infected emboli (Salaki JS et al, 1984).

The cases presented confirm the efficacy of repeated local debridment of necrotic tissues associated with high doses of Amphotericin B and supportive therapy especially enteral hyperalimentation. These procedures were sufficent in our cases to control the cerebral involvement avoiding neurosurgical approach, which is sometimes extremely difficult as showed by case nº 1.

REFERENCES

1. Blitzer A, Lawson W, Meiers BR, Biller HF (1980):Patient survival factors in paranasal sinus mucormycosis. The Laryngoscope 90:635-648.
2. Lehrer RI, Howard DH, Sypherd PS, Edwards JE, Segal GP, Winston DJ(1980):Mucormycosis. Annals of Internal Medicine 93(Part 1):93-108.
3. Salaki JS, Louria DB, Chmel H (1984): Fungal and yeast infections of the central nervous system. Medicine 63 (Nº 2):108-132.

© 1985 Elsevier Science Publishers B.V. (Biomedical Division)
New dimensions in otorhinolaryngology – head and neck surgery, vol. 2.
E. Myers, editor

THE EXTERNAL FRONTO-ETHMOIDAL APPROACH

André PECH, Michel ZANARET, Jean-Marc THOMASSIN, Jean-Michel TRIGLIA, Maurice CANNONI

Clinique O.R.L. - C.H.U. TIMONE 13385 - MARSEILLE (FRANCE)

The exeresis of certain benign tumors of the fronto-ethmoidal sinus, together with surgical treatment of serious frontal sinusitis with complications, seems to call for an external fronto-ethmoidal approach, simultaneously and clearly exposing the frontal sinus, the ethmoidal sinus and the nasal fossae. A fronto-nasal bone flap cut in one piece from the anterior wall of the area, is the only solution affording wide access.

THE TECHNIQUE : The principe entailed here hinges on the removal of an osseous bone flap cut in one piece from the anterior wall of the frontal sinus, the bone itself, the rising ascending branch of the maxilla and the internal orbital ridge through a para-lateronasal approach.

The detachment : - Of the cutaneous periosteal layer : the flap is folded back. The levator palpebrae and check ligament, the lacrimal sac and the lacrimal ducts are reclinated sub-periosteally. The canthus insertion point in the bone is noted. - Of the muco-periosteal layer : detached below the osseous hood of the bone itself. - Cutting out the bone flap : This is done using a jigsaw leaving a clean and narrow kerf (see diagram).

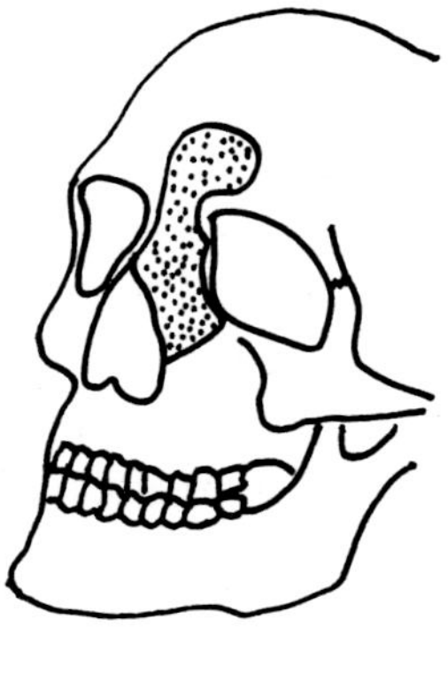

The fronto-nasal bone flap

- The sinus stage : Once the bone flap has been removed, the frontal sinus and the naso-frontal canal are immediatly visible and the nasal fossae are clearly exposed. An ethmoidectomy can be carried out without difficulty -either anterior or total- and the sphenoidal sinus can be opened wide. - The closure : a large caliber Portex drain is positioned in the fronto-nasal opening. The bone flap is put back in place by osteosynthesis. A canthopexis is then carriec out accross the bone flap. The lacrimal ducts return spontaneously to their anatomic position.

CASE STUDIES

. Benign tumors (10 cases) : 5 fronto-ethmoidal osteomae, 4 fronto-ethmoidal mucoceles and 1 inverted papilloma. Exeresis of tumors was always total. No recurrences have been recorded to date.

. Serious frontal sinusitis (11 cases) : No patient required further surgery afterwards. The preoperational fistulae did not reappear. 2 cases presented an inflammatory periorbital tumefaction regressive under medical treatment. As regards functional after-effects, we have observed neither canthal dysmorphia nor lacrimation. The aesthetic sequelae are acceptable in all cases ; scarring is minimal in elderly patients.

INDICATIONS FOR THIS TECHNIQUE

In tumoral pathology : All lesions of the frontal sinus extending beyond the anterior ethmoid should be treated externally and by this fronto-ethmoidal osteoplastic approach which offers great safety in the exeresis. This applies for osteomae and mucoceles of the fronto-ethmoidal system with inverted papillomata which require wide access.

In infectious pathology : It is indicated, in general, for iatrogenic sinusitis where there has already been surgical treatment via an external approach and which are, in most cases, accompanied by prints of fistulized sinusitis on the skin ; rarely, in cases of serious sinusitis coupled with ocular or endocranial symptomes ; exceptionally, for certain sinusitis which resist both medical treatment and surgical treatment of the drainage and endo-nasal ethmoidectomy type.
In cases of serious frontal sinusitis, we consider preferable to reaerate the sinus than to sclude it. The operations favored at the moment are more or less distant offshoots of LYNCH's fronto-ethmoidectomy, via a passage of discarded bone. We consider that the fronto-ethmoidal approach by bone flap is preferable. It retains the principle of LYNCH's fronto-ethmoidectomy, whilst adding to it the advantages of an osteo-plastic bone flap. Through the use of a scanner, we were able to visualize the difficulties of this reaeration. This lec us to maintain the drainage by the Portex drain for 6 months. To promote reaeration, it further requires eradication of only those mucous lesions considered irreversible and preservation of healthy mucous zones, creation of a vast opening towards the nasal fossae through systematic ablation of the middle concha so as to arrive at a real nasalization of the frontal sinus, closure if need be of an osseous defect at the level of the anterior wall of the bone flap using autogenous material.

REFERENCE : Pech A., Freche Ch.,Cannoni M., Rouvier P. et Coll.
Etat actuel de la Chirurgie des Sinus Masson Editeur (Paris) 1982

© 1985 Elsevier Science Publishers B.V. (Biomedical Division)
New dimensions in otorhinolaryngology - head and neck surgery, vol. 2.
E. Myers, editor

CENTRO FACIAL APPROACH FOR THE SURGICAL TREATMENT OF JUVENILE ANGIOFIBROMA

J.R.ARRIETA(1) J.CORVERA(2) M.A. GARCIA(3) A. CHI(4)

Otorrinolaringology Department from General Hospital Dr. Manuel Gea González. Secretaría de Salubridad y Asistencia. Calzada de Tlalpan 4800 C.P.14000 México D.F.

INTRODUCTION

Traditionally Juvenile Angiofibroma has been surgically approach through the palate and in some cases combined with lateral rhinotomy. In our experience with these approaches the visualization of the tumor is very poor, and the tumor is excised through palpation and generally there is tearring of the tumor, with the risk of reimcidence and of a greater bleeding.

In choosing the surgical approach we have to take into account that the rate of reimcidence of these tumors is up to 50%.[1] The difficult for a satisfactory surgical approach of the nasopharyux is testified by the 55 different surgical approaches described in the literature.[2]

The Juvenile Angiofibroma according to it's location, surgeon's preference and experience can be approched through the palate with a vertical insition in the midline, in the form of a S or U insition, through Caldwell Luc with or without the Denker modification; through the gingivolabial region in the maxillar tuberosity; through lateral rhinotomy, external ethmoidectomy, transmandibular and through the pharynx in the suprahyoid region.[3]

We prefer to use the centro-facial approach because of the following advantages: easy access; adequate sight and direct extirpation of the base of implantation; in case to be needed the insition can be extended to the maxillary sinus and to the pterigomaxillary fosae; there is an easy surgical reparation; no need of tracheostomy, patient can be feeded early, and patient hospital stay is shortered.

MATERIAL

The centro-facial aprroach was used in three male patients of 15, 18 and 19 years old, with clinical diagnosis of Juvenile Angiofibroma, confirmed with computed Axial Tomography and with histopathological studies. The quantity of blood loosen in the three patients were: 300, 500 and 500 mls. There were no complications. The esthetic result of the scars was good. The Surgery approach was done at the General Hospital Dr. Manuel Gea González, in May, June and July, 1984.

TECHNIQUE

All patients were with general anesthesia with orotracheal intubation and controlled hypotension, local infiltration with 2% Xylocaine and adrenaline 1:60,000. Insition in the midline of the nasal dorsum, dividing the columnella in two, if the tumor was confined to the rhinopharynx the insition is directed towards the nasal groove (Fig.1) medial osteotomy with 8 mms. chicel, transverse osteotomy, with Striker drill, lateral osteotomy with 2 mms. chicel, extirpation of the tumor including the perostium, tumor was extracted through the mouth, the rhinopharynx is occluded with Gelfoam and gauze, which was previously inpregnated with antibiotic. The surgical wound is sutured in two planes; if the tumor is invading the maxillary sinus and the pterigomasillar fosae the insition can be prolong to the midline of the superior lip and to the gingivovestibular region.(Fig.2) a Caldwell Luc Procedure is done with Denker modification, excition of the tumor and insition sutured in the conventional planes.

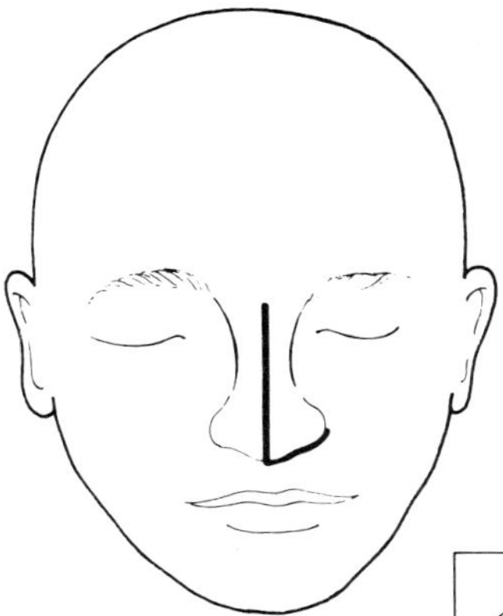

FIG. 1

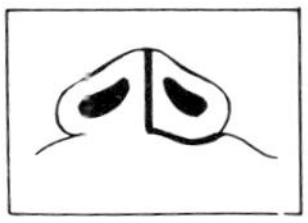

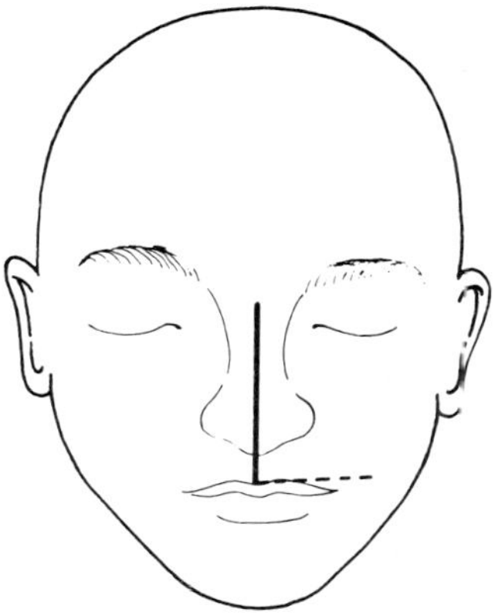

FIG. 2

COMMENT AND CONCLUSIONS

In our experience the transpalate approach for the surgical treatement of the Juvenile Angiofibroma does not provide a good visualization of the tumor, the tumor is excised exclusively through palpation and generally there is tearring of the tumor, with the risk of reimcidence and of a greater bleeding.

That is why, we decided to practice the Centro Facial approach with it's variety of extension to the nasal alae and gingivolabial region in combination with gingivovestibular insition.

Through the Centro Facial approach the visualization of the base of implantation is excellent, allowing a precise exsition and in case of invation to the maxillary antrum or to the pterigomaxillar fosae, the gingivovestibular extension allows also and adequate vision.

The only possible disadvantage of this technique is the scar in the face; although it has not been a negative influence in our patients, it could be for others, but the advantages are clear, and we believe this is an excellent approach for the exsition of the Juvenile Angiofibroma.

REFERENCES

1. Paparella-Shumrick (1982), Otorrinolaringology, Head and Neck, 2nd ed. Ed. Panamerican Medical, pp 2083-2084
2. Waldman SR, Howard LL (1981), Surgical experience with nasopharyngeal angiofibromas, Arch Otolaryngol, 107:677-682
3. Hall L, Wilkins S (1968), Nasopharyngeal Fibroma, The American Journal of Surgery, 116:530-537

© 1985 Elsevier Science Publishers B.V. (Biomedical Division)
New dimensions in otorhinolaryngology - head and neck surgery, vol. 2.
E. Myers, editor

INVERTED FOLLICULAR KERATOSIS OF THE NASAL VESTIBULE

JACQUELYNNE P. COREY, M.D., AND GORDON G. KEYES, D.D.S.
Depts. of Otolaryngology and Oral Pathology, West Virginia University, Morgantown, WV 26506 (United States)

Inverted follicular keratosis is a benign lesion usually occurring on the face in white males in their 60's. Clinically it is often diagnosed as a cutaneous horn, wart, basal cell, papilloma, or seborrheic keratosis.[1] We report here a case of inverted follicular keratosis occurring in the nasal vestibule. All previously reported cases have been on the skin. (Fig. 1)

A 57 year old white female presented with a one month history of a sensitive "growth" in the right nasal vestibule which bled easily. Examination of the head and neck was remarkable only for a 0.5 cm. sessile papillomatous lesion in the right nasal vestibule. The lesion was excisionally biopsied under local anesthesia, and the initial pathologic diagnosis was squamous cell carcinoma. Radiation therapy and/or radical surgical excision was planned. Upon reviewing the pathology slides for presentation to the Tumor Board, a revised diagnosis, confirmed by consulting pathologists, of inverted follicular keratosis was made. Ten months of follow-up have revealed no recurrences.

Previously Reported Sites of Inverted Follicular Keratosis

FIG 1

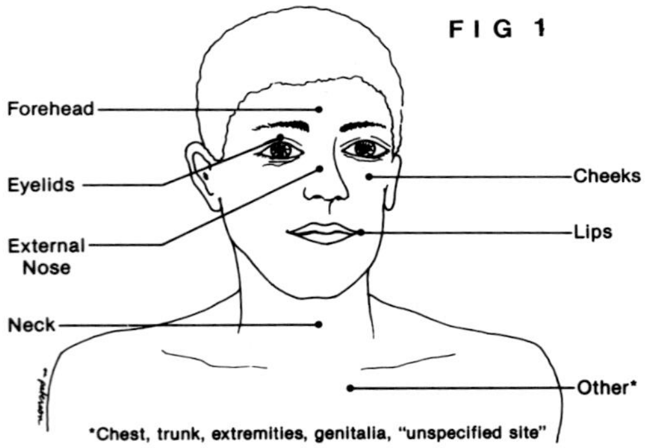

Sections of the submitted specimen show a well-defined, discrete lesion that is both exophytic and endophytic. The surface is papillary and covered with epidermis that has a distinct central keratin plug. Proliferating beneath the surface of the lesions are two types of epithelial cells. Centrally, there are cells that are typically squamoid in nature which are surrounded by more basaloid cells. (Fig. 2) This arrangement is seen throughout the specimen. In addition, numerous squamous eddies can be seen. (Fig,3)

Inverted follicular keratosis occurs primarily on the face in middle-aged

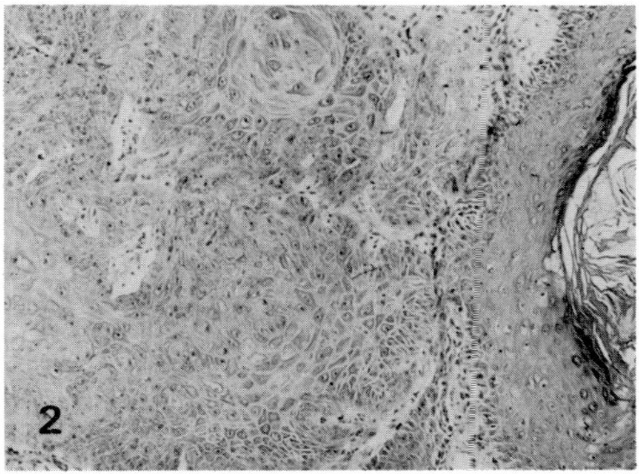

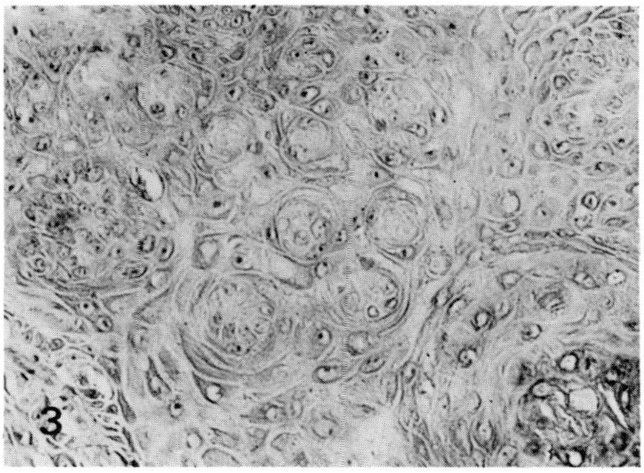

to elderly males. Most lesions are single, present for several months, and asymptomatic except for mild bleeding, itching, or "scabbing". They usually appear pink to grey, soft, and raised 5 mm. from the surface, ranging in size from 3-10 mm.[2] The histologic distinctiveness of the inverted follicular keratosis is controversial. Some authors feel it is a distinct pathologic entity.[3] Others are of the belief that this tumor is a variant of such conditions as seborrheic keratosis[4] and verruca vulgares[5]. The presence of squamous eddies is distinctive in this lesion but not specific[6]. Coupled with other histologic features, the squamous eddies allow the recognition of a small group of cutaneous hyperplastic processes that are benign and should not be confused with squamous cell carcinoma. The lack of significant cytologic atypia, the well-defined epithelial connective tissue interface, and the discrete, localized nature of inverted follicular keratosis help make the separation. The presence of squamous eddies is helpful as well. The separation of inverted follicular keratosis and related lesions from squamous cell carcinoma is the significant consideration here.

1. Azzopardi, A.G., and Laurini, R.; J. Clin. Path. 23, 465-471, 1975.
2. Mehregan, A.; Arch. Derm. 89, 117-123, 1964.
3. Mehregan, A.; Am. J. Dermatopath. 5:467, 1983.
4. Lever, A.; Am. J. Dermatopath., 5:575, 1983.
5. Uanoff, M.; Am. J. Dermatopath, 5:475, 1983.
6. Speilvogel, R., et. al.; Am. J. Dermatopath, 5:427, 1983.

© 1985 Elsevier Science Publishers B.V. (Biomedical Division)
New dimensions in otorhinolaryngology - head and neck surgery, vol. 2.
E. Myers, editor

JUVENILE NASOPHARYNGEAL ANGIOFIBROMA (JNA) IN SYRIA

M. A. HAJJAR, M. D.
DAMASCUS UNIVERSITY, DAMASCUS, SYRIA

INTRODUCTION

Juvenile nasopharyngeal angiofibroma (JNA) is a rare benign tumors which occurs in adolescent males. The incidence rate of JNA is 1/6000 - 1/16000 of all E.N.T. diseases. Although JNA is histologically benign, it has locally invasive features producing soft tissue and bone destruction into the pterygo maxillary space, the nose, the sinuses, and even, on rare occasions, the intracranial area.

Surgical extripation is the treatment of choice. If untreated, it is often produce life threatening expistaxis and extensions into neighbouring structures.

CLINICAL MATERIAL

30 patients with JNA have been treated surgically at Damascus University hospital (Al-Mouassat) in Syria from 1972 - 1984.

The incidence rate of JNA in Syria of all E.N.T. diseases is 1/1000 - 1/2000, which is higher than what reported in the literature.

All the 30 patients treated here were males, and most of them adolescents (median age 15 years, range 10 - 22 years). Patients typically presented with severe recurrent expistaxis and/or nasal obstruction, less commonly with facial deformity. Symptoms had persisted 4 to 24 months (average 14 months). 20 of these have been followed from 5 to 10 years, the rest for from 6 months to 2 years.

INVESTIGATION

The history and physical examination usually indicate the dominant side of involuement. Radiological investigation included plain films, angiograms, and, recently computed axial tomography CT SCAN. Although, angiography supports the diagnosis of JNA, however, CT SCAN delineated the sphenoid and pterygo maxillary space extension very clearly. Accurate localization of the tumor is important in the choice of the surgical approach.

TREATMENT AND RESULTS

All 30 patients with JNA operated on primarily by the author. 29 patients underwent surgical excison through the transpalatal approach, and in one patient a combined transpalatal buccal approach for lateral, maxillary and sphenoid sinuses, and pterygo maxillary space extensions which produced signs of facial asymmetry. Only five patients treated early in the series had external carotid artery ligation.

The blood loss during surgery range 500cc - 2500cc with an average blood loss 1500cc. The sizes of tumors excised range 5 X 3 X 2 CM^3 - 4 X 15 X 18CM^3 with an average size 3 X 8 X 10 CM^3.

I have never utilized biopsy as a pre-operative diagnostic method in any of these cases. Only one patient developed moderate hemorrhage post operatively upon removal the nasopharyngeal pack. He required only placing the pack again in the nasopharynx to control the bleeding.

Of all 30 of patients of JNA treated surgically, only one recurrence occured after six months of surgery. This required secondary surgery and have remained free of tumor for three years.

The palatal incision healed nicely in all cases without functional deficiency in any of these patients.

DISCUSSION

The incidence rate of JNA in Syria appears higher than what is reported in the literature. Since almost all patients with JNA in Syria are treated at Damascus University Hospital (Al-Mouassat).

The transpalatal approach gives an excellent and direct exposure of the naso-pharynx, and provides removal of the entire tumor, and also, controls excessive bleeding.

There were, neither significant morbidity, nor intraoperative death among these series. The recurrence rate considerably low, only one patient out of 30 patients. Radiotherapy never been used in treating these benign tumors or to reduce hemorrhage during surgery.

SUMMARY

30 patients of JNA treated surgically by the author in the past 12 years utilizing the transpalatal approach. There were no morbidity or intraoperative death. There was only one recurrent case underwent secondary surgery with no further recurrence after three years of follow-up.

New dimensions in otorhinolaryngology - head and neck surgery, vol. 2.
E. Myers, editor

EXTENSIVE NASOPHARYNGEAL ANGIOFIBROMA WITH INTRACRANIAL INVOLVEMENT

M. H. KHERADPIR
University of Tehran, Tehran, Iran

Angiofibroma is relatively rare, locally slow expansive, histologically benign tumor found exclusively in males, usually starting at the time of permanent dentition eruption. From 1965 to 1984 a hundred cases were diagnosed and managed by differentmedical and surgical techniques. All patients have been males, and have been between the ages of ten and twenty, whose duration of disease was between one to six years. The purpose of this report is twofold:

First, is a long term follow-up of our patients, resulting in the best way for diagnosis, by taking a complete history of patient's age, sex, symptoms, physical findings, extent and appearence of the tumor. Consistent characteristics are seen on radiography **(plate 1)**,ct and ct scan **(plate 2)**. Final confirmation of this tumor should be made by angiography **(plate 3)**. Subtraction technique is very important for post operative arteriography to rule out persistant tumors. We have concluded, surgery is exclusive treatment of choice. Even though radiation demonstrated a marked decrease in the mass and vascularity, serious short and long term complications are reasons for its avoidance, and irradiation is reserved for palliation, or those legions deemed surgically unapproachable. **(Plate 4)**

Angiofibroma can extend to mid, ant cranial fossa by erroding greater wing, body of sphenoid or vault of nose and ethmoid cells. It extends to the orbit through sup, inf orbital fissures, ethmoid cells and maxillary sinuses; produces orbital cellulitis, proptosis, papilledema, visual acuity decreasse and headache. Once this tumor occupies ant, mid cranial fossa usually seperates from the duramatter easily, but when the tumor penetrates into the brain **(because delayed diagnosis and different modality of treatment)** needs some kind of neurosurgery, and mortality rate is high.

Plate 1

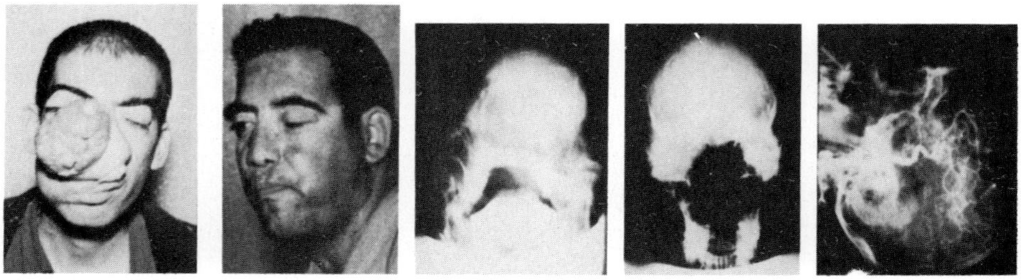

pre operation post op(5 yrs) pre and post radiology pre op arteriograph

SURGICAL TECHNIQUE

Accurate removal with minimal complication is the goal. Several approaches have been used in the past to gain access to the neoplasm. These include any or all of the following: piecemal removal, Caldwell-Luc, transpalatal, lateral rhinotomy, cerical, and sublabialretomaxxillary. Surgicall procedure selected should be determined by location, extension, surgeon experience and existing facility. In our recent series all tumors were removed by extended sublabial retromaxillary approach, with the aid of midline incission on the external nose. Sublabial incission extends from the pyriform aperture on opposite side of the tumor to the maxillary tuberosity and a little further onto molarbone. After preparing the muco-periostal flap, insert a long ribbon gauze between the posterolateral wall of maxilla and periostum, while gradually pushing it inside, til it contacts the sphenopalatan fossa and press hard on internal maxillary artery, and bringing it to complete obstruction.By removing ant, lat, and post wall of maxillary sinuses, and sometimes ascending process of maxilla and nasal bone, wegain access to the tumor.**(in this huge kind of angiofibroma usually these bones are eroded by the tumor itself.)**

With the aid of the index finger we follow the periphery of the tumor and take it out from all sinuses and cavity that it occupied. Once the tumor has been completely exposed and mobolized, knife and rongercan be used to incise through the nasal mucosa and periosteum of the post phyrangeal wall, just inf to the rim of the tumor. The tumor is then removed and the cavity is washed by warm water and examined thorougly for any residual tumor or dural dehiscence, and at this time we put fixation suture or clips on the internal maxillary artery or any bleeding vessels on the base of the skull or in the orbit. The brain, optic nerve, covernous sinus, or any combination of three can be vulnerable to damage with removal of some type of angiofibroma.

Plate 2

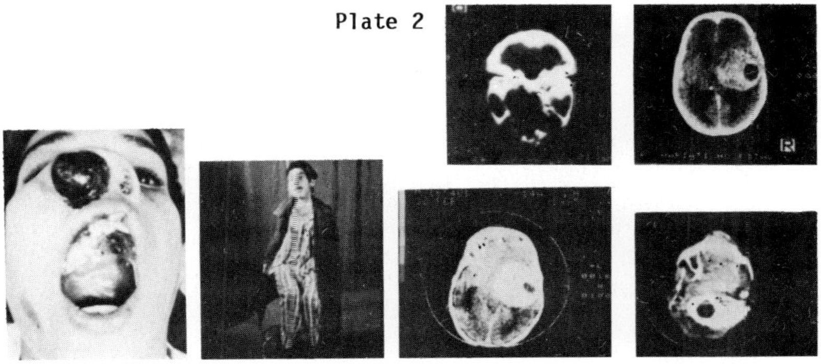

pre operation post operation pre and post operation ct scans

Second, to suggest a new theory about etiology and patogenesis: vascular granulation tissue **(nidus vascularis)** which penetrates normally into developing facial and skull base bone and replace them to fully developed cells and sinuses, behave in an uncontrolled manner like a neoplasm by the effect of some foreign agent, which may be trauma at time of puberty. **(Nearly all our patients had experienced trauma.)** That is why a supposedly benign tumor should grow to the base of the skull rather than into the path of least resistance, as would be expected. **(Performing its natural function as nature forces it to do.) Another interesting point is that more of morphological characteristics during puberty are retained in the skull of adulescent female than that of adulescent male.**

Plate 3

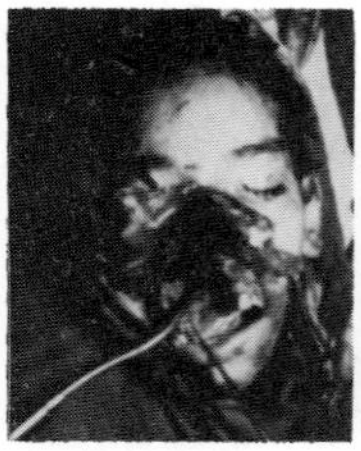

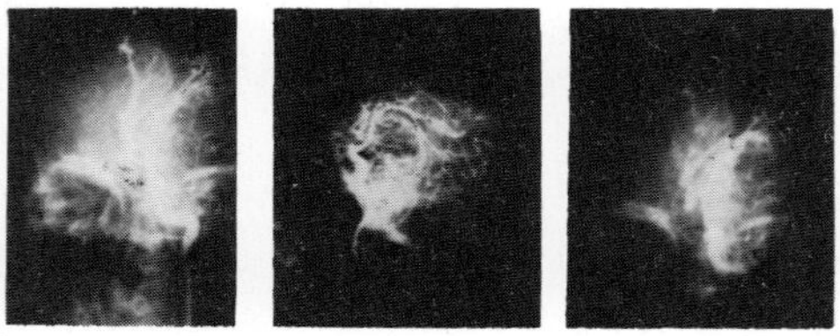

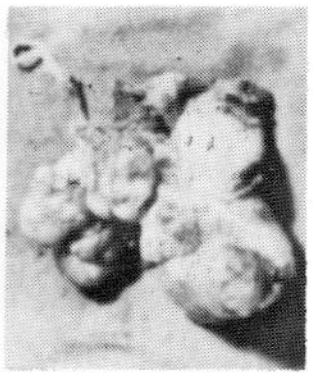

patient in plate 2 during operation

angiograms of patient

its mass

Plate 4

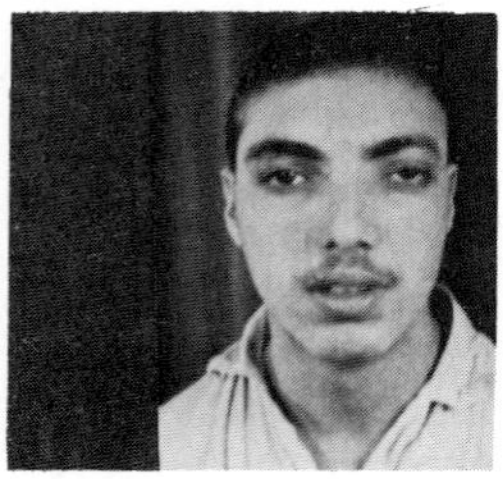

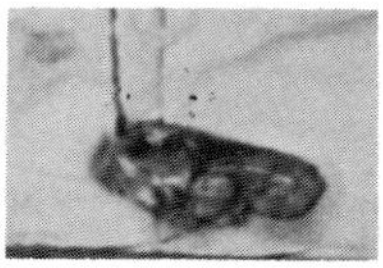

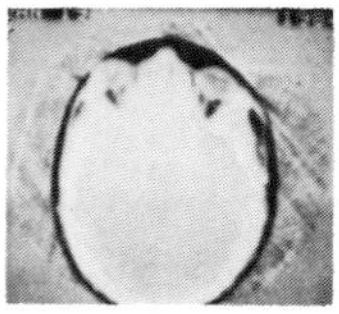

patient w/marked proptosis irradiated

marked decrease in the mass after irradiation

ct scan

© 1985 Elsevier Science Publishers B.V. (Biomedical Division)
New dimensions in otorhinolaryngology – head and neck surgery, vol. 2.
E. Myers, editor

NASOPHARYNGEAL ANGIOFIBROMA
RECENT ADVANCES IN TOPODIAGNOSIS AND TREATMENT

JOSE ANTONIO PINTO and ALEXANDRE FELIPPU NETO
Dept. of Otolaringology, Hospital Ibirapuera
Av. Rubem Berta, 3350 - São Paulo, Brasil

INTRODUCTION

Angiofibroma is considered the most common benign tumor the nasopharynx.

This rare neoplasm (0,5% of all neoplasms of the head and neck), highly vascular, grows pressing the surrounding structures, displacing and destroying the bones without infiltration.

At the present time there remains controversies concerning the etiology, site of origin, diagnostic procedures and treatment of this tumor[1,2,3,4,5]

MATERIAL AND METHODS

Correlations among the physical examination, radiology (CT) and surgical findings in 32 patients treated from 1975 to 1984 at Hospital Ibirapuera, São Paulo, Brasil, lead us to the following considerations:

1 - The most frequent site of origin of the angiofibromas is in the posterolateral wall of the nasal cavity and not in the nasopharynx[5]. More specifcly the point of origin is around the sphenopalatine foramem and the posterior end of the middle turbinate.

From this site it spreads to nasal cavity, nasopharynx, sphenoid, ethmoid and maxillary sinuses, pterygomaxillary fossa and middle and anterior cranial fossa.

2 - Computed tomography (CT) is the ideal method of evaluation of the nasopharyngeal angiofibroma, particularly to delineate the location, the extension and intracranial invasion. It is used as the decisive curative criterion and to detect the recurrences of the disease.

Angiography has been recommended only in large tumors with intracranial invasion.

3 - Surgical resection is the treatment of choice and sublabial incision with transantral-retromaxillary approach under magnification is prefered. No external incisions are required. Previous ligation of internal maxillary artery is an unvaryng procedure.

This technique was used in our last 17 patients.
In 3 cases with intracranial invasion the tumors were removed by this approach without necessity of combined intracranial and extracranial excision (IEE). The IEE may be used when the neoplasm receive vascular supply from the internal carotid artery or there are gross intracranial involvement.
Intraoperative bleeding was minimal and the necessity of blood transfusions decreased.
Presurgical embolization and tracheotomy were not required.
Estrogens were administrated prior to surgery to decrease the vascularity of the tumors.

RESULTS
An accurate knowledgment of the site and extension of the tumour allows the use of a conservative surgical technique to remove the nasopharyngeal angiofibromas with minimal risk and morbidity. Seventeen patients in the last seven years were submitted to an extended sublabial and transantral-retromaxillary approach. Only one patient required a second operation and sixteen are free of disease.

CONCLUSION
It is emphasized the anatomical source of the angiofibromas, the better pre and post-operative evaluation through CT scanning and the good results with the surgical resection through the sublabial transantral retromaxillary approach.

REFERENCES

1 - Conley J, Healey WV, Blaugraund SM, et al (1968): Nasopharyngeal angiofibroma in the juvenile. Surg Gynecol Obstet 126:825-837.
2 - Neel HB, et al (1973): Juvenile Angiofibroma: Review of 120 cases.
The American Journal of Surgery 126:547-556.
3 - Ward PH, Thompson R , Calcaterra T, et al: (1974) Juvenile angiofibroma: A more rational therapeutic approach based upon clinical and experimental evidence. Laryngoscope 84:2181-2194.
4 - Briant TDR, Fitzpatrick PJ, Berman JM (1978): Nasopharyngeal angiofibroma: A 20-year study. Laryngoscope 88:1247-1251.
5 - Chandler JR, et al (1984): Nasopharyngeal angiofibromas: Staging and management. Ann Otol Rhinol Laryngol 93:322-329.

New dimensions in otorhinolaryngology - head and neck surgery, vol. 2.
E. Myers, editor

ASTHMA AND NASAL POLYPS

GUY A. SETTIPANE, M.D., DONALD E. KLEIN, M.D. AND MARY D. LEKAS, M.D.
(Brown University) 95 Pitman Street, Providence, RI 02906, U.S.A.

Nasal polyps have been an enigma as far back as man can remember. Hippocrates developed surgical methods for nasal polypectomy. Nasal polyps are frequently associated with asthma, especially in the triad of asthma, nasal polyps, and aspirin intolerance. For several years, the medical literature has had anecdotal reports that surgical, nasal polypectomy may cause or aggravate asthma. We decided to look at this question using modern day technology and strict clinical criteria.

The mechanism as to how stimuli in the nasal-sino area can affect asthma is through the Rhini-Sino-Bronchial Reflex.[1] Stimulation of this H_1-receptors, irritant receptors, or the cholinergic receptors can cause this reflex mechanism. This is why one must not neglect treatment of the sinuses when treating asthma.

We recently reviewed 167 patients with verified nasal polyps and a history of one or more polypectomy. In addition, 40% of those that had one polypectomy required another polypectomy because of recurrances. Our data suggests that patients with positive allergy skin tests (pollen, animal dander, or molds) have a progressively higher rate of repeated polypectomies.

Our data also reveals that IgE mediated disease is not the cause of polyps, but when present may contribute to episodes of exacerbation. Seventy-one percent of cases with nasal polyps are associated with asthma, especially the intrinsic or non allergic type of asthma. The triad of asthma, aspirin intolerance and nasal polyps is associated with intrinsic or non allergic asthma.[2,3]

In our division[4] 10 patients with nasal polyps and no history of asthma or abnormal pulmonary function tests were studied. Methacholine challenge tests done before and about 5 months after polypectomy were similar. In a report by Miles-Lawrence et al,[5] similar data were obtained. They studied 16 patients and performed methacholine challenge tests 1 month prior to polypectomy and up to 1 year following polypectomy. They found essentially no change in methacholine sensitivity. It appears that polypectomy does not increase the risk of developing asthma or making asthma worse.

In order to correlate these results to clinical conditions, we compared a pulmonary function test (PFT) in 8 patients before and an average of 3 months after polypectomy and found PFT essentially unchanged. In six steroid-dependent asthmatics, the steroid dose for control of asthma before and up to 6 months following polypectomy also was essentially unchanged. When patients had both asthma and nasal polyps (119), the onset of asthma occurred first 61% of the time, followed by the development of nasal polyps 10 years later. Therefore, nasal polyps usually occur after the onset of asthma and does not cause it.

In summary, nasal polyposis is a highly recurrent disease despite polypectomy. Nasal polyps are frequently associated with intrinsic (non allergic) asthma, and are not caused by an IgE mechanism. However, coexisting allergies can aggravate polyps. Pulmonary function test and steroid dose requirement were essentially the same before and after polypectomy. Polypectomy does not cause or aggravate asthma.

REFERENCES

1. Rhinitis (1st ed) GA Settipane, M.D. (ed) NER Allergy Proceedings, Providence, RI (USA) 1984
2. Settipane GA, Chafee FH, Nasal Polyps in asthma and rhinitis: a review of 6,037 patients. J Allergy Clin Immunol 59:17-21, 1977
3. Settipane GA, Chafee FH, Klein DE. A critical evaluation of aspirin challenge in patients with nasal polyps. J Allergy Clin Immunol 69:Part 2, 148, 1982
4. Downing E, Braman S, Settipane GA. Bronchial reactivity in patients with nasal polyposis and the effects of polypectomy. J Allergy Clin Immunol 69: Part 2, 102, 1982 (abst)
5. Miles-Lawrence R, Kaplan M, Chang K. Methacholine sensitivity in nasal polyposis and the effects of polypectomy. J Allergy Clin Immunol 69:Part 2, 102, 1982 (abst)

New dimensions in otorhinolaryngology - head and neck surgery, vol. 2.
E. Myers, editor

MICROSURGICAL SPHENOETHMOIDECTOMY

HERBERT SILVERSTEIN, M.D., ALAN B. McDANIEL, M.D.
Ear Research Foundation, 1921 Floyd Street, Sarasota, FL 33579

INTRODUCTION

Polypoid rhinosinusitis is a relatively common problem, occurring in 4% of the adult population and in 7% of adult asthmatics. Multiple etiologic factors include inhalent allergies, chronic bacterial sinusitis, and metabolic abnormalities, including the "aspirin triad" (nasal polyps, asthma, and aspirin sensitivity), and cystic fibrosis.

METHOD

Standard surgical treatment for this condition is either snare polypectomy or intra-nasal ethmoidectomy with monocular vision and only one hand free to operate. The usual result is incomplete removal and frequent recurrence. In July, 1975, we began performing microsurgical sphenoethmoidectomy. An operating microscope with a 300mm lens, straight eye-pieces, and a Sony video camera are used. The surgeon is seated and a self-retaining retractor exposes the nasal cavity (a modified Leyla retractor and modified set-screw speculum). An Essar suction irrigator is held in one hand and standard instruments are used in the other hand. Polyps are removed from the nasal cavity and the middle turbinate is resected. A complete ethmoidectomy is performed, followed by a complete sphenoidectomy. Finally, the inferior turbinates are cauterized. Hemostasis is achieved using bipolar cautery and where necessary, Surgicel (R) and Avitene (R). Advantages of this procedure include operating from a seated position with both hands free, enjoying magnified, binocular vision. The scrub nurse observes via the monitor and can anticipate the surgeon's needs. Suction irrigation constantly keeps the field clear and a sphenoidectomy is easily permitted. This results in thorough removal of disease and minimized recurrence.

PATIENTS

Thirty-one patients have undergone microsurgical sphenoethmoidectomy from July, 1975, to October, 1984. Fourteen (45%) had previously had surgery for polyps. Twenty-eight patients had bilateral disease. Twenty-nine had allergic polyps and three were aspirin sensitive. In nineteen patients, allergic desensitization immuno-therapy was used after operation. The average follow-up time was 2.1 years and 32% had greater than 3 years follow-up.

RESULTS

Twenty-eight (90%) are free of disease. Three patients have had recurrence at one, four and seven years; none received effective desensitization therapy. Complications after revision operations were hemmorhage (2) and streptococcal meningitis (1). Primary procedures were complicated by delayed epistaxis (1) and transient diplopia (1). Four patients have had recurring purulent sinusitis, one severely.

DISCUSSION

The advantages of this technique allow more vigorous and effective completion of sphenoethmoidectomy. Allergic desensitization immuno-therapy may aid in reducing recurrences. Surgical complications will be reduced through the use of the microscope but will be higher among patients with multiple previous sinus operations. Since our initial report, Dixon has added a second series to the literature, in which he supports our conclusions (2). As in 1979 (1), we feel that extensive microsurgery with postoperative immunotherapy will result in a longer or more permanent cure of polypoid sinusitis. We will continue to use this approach in the treatment of this complex disease.

REFERENCES

1. Silverstein H (1980): In: Johnson F and Spencer J Jr. (eds) Allergy, Immunology and Medical Treatment. Year Book Medical Publishers, Chicago, Illinois, pp 95-99

2. Dixon HS (1983): Microscopic Sinus Surgery, Transnasal Ethmoidectomy and Sphenoidectomy. Laryngoscope 93:440-444

© 1985 Elsevier Science Publishers B.V. (Biomedical Division)
New dimensions in otorhinolaryngology - head and neck surgery, vol. 2.
E. Myers, editor

ECTOPIC MENINGIOMA OF THE NOSE AND PARANASAL SINUSES

CIRÍACO CRISTÓVÃO T. ATHERINO, ROSEMARY GARCIA, LEOPOLDO J. LOPES
Serviços ORL and Anatomia Patológica, Hospital de Ipanema, INAMPS, Rio de Janeiro, Brasil.

Primary and secondary meningiomas occurring outside the CNS are uncommon. To the best of our knowledge there are 21 cases of nasal and paranasal meningiomas related.

CASE REPORT

On August 18th, 1983, a 76-year-old white man reported a 16-year history of progressive chronic nasal obstruction, epistaxis and frequent frontal headaches. Four years ago he was interned in another Hospital due to his first episode of epistaxis, and a wide surgical approach was performed there on October 24th, 1979, whereupon the extraction of a large, hard, well encapsulated tumor was carried out. The tumor was implanted in the higher portion of the left nasal fossa. The patient was discharged one week later, free of symptomatology, thus remaining for 1 year, after which time he again began to feel a progressive nasal obstruction along with a fetid greenish discharge, epistaxis and intense frontal headaches. The E.N.T. examination revealed a hard, reddish tumoral tissue, painless to palpation, occupying both nasal fossae and producing septal deviation to the right. The plain X-Rays and tomograms showed the extension of the involvement but proved to be insufficient for a therapeutical elaboration. A CT study was then made and showed a mass in the left nasal cavity extending to the right nasal fossa, to the maxillary sinuses, mainly to the left, and to the ethmoidal cells and nasopharynx to the left. The cerebral parenchima was isodense with no evidence of expansive lesion or vascular alteration. The ophthalmological and neurological examinations showed no alterations.

As the endocranium had not been involved we decided upon a surgical sublabial approach according to Kretschmann[1,2]. Due to its size the tumor was removed in fragments showing implantation at the level of the left nasal fossa roof and no adhesions to the occupied sinuses. The histological chart suggested the diagnosis of a meningothelial meningioma. The patient was discharged one week later and is still assymptomatic.

DISCUSSION

The extracranial meningiomas may be divided in 4 groups [3,4]: (1) primary extracranial meningiomas extending directly out of the skull; (2) extracranial meningiomas arising from arachnoidal cell rests of cranial nerve sheathes; (3) meningiomas having no demonstrable connection with foramina or cranial nerves; (4) metastasis of intracranial meningiomas. The case described would belong in the third group.

Concerning the symptomatology, there are no singular characteristics which may enable the differentiation from other neoplasias in this area[5]. The patients may present nasal obstruction, headaches, epistaxis, anosmia or hyposmia, exophthalmos or facial deformity [6]. In all cases which have been reported the diagnosis was provided by the histology of the surgical specimen. The plain X-Rays and tomograms are useful mainly for the verification of the extracranial involvement. The CT was permitted a better evaluation of the tumor and its extensions, confirming or denying an intracranial invasion, thus being helpful in the therapeutical planning [6].

The recommended treatment is a surgical exeresis of the lesion and the prognosis following this seems to be good [5,7,8].

REFERENCES

1. Kirschner M (1937) Tratado de Técnica Operatoria General y Especial, tomo III, Editorial Labor S.A., Barcelona, pp.106-108.
2. Anand VK, Conley JJ (1983) Laryngoscope 93:1483-1484.
3. Batsakis JG (1979) Tumors of the Head and Neck, 2nd ed., Williams & Wilkins Co., Baltimores, pp.347-348.
4. Kjeldesberg CR, Minckler J (1972) Cancer 29:153-156.
5. Ho K-L (1980) Cancer 46:1442-1447.
6. Persky MS, Som ML (1978) ORL 86:714-720.
7. Leroux-Robert J, Guiot G, Paquelin F, Prache H (1966) Annales Otolaryngologie (Paris) 83-617-638.
8. Manni JJ (1983) J Laryngol Otol 97:657-660.

© 1985 Elsevier Science Publishers B.V. (Biomedical Division)
New dimensions in otorhinolaryngology - head and neck surgery, vol. 2.
E. Myers, editor

JUVENILE NASOPHARYNGEAL ANGIOFIBROMA (JNA)

MICROSURGICAL APPROACH IN 25 CASES AS UNIQUE TREATMENT

ALEJANDRO E. TERZIAN- CARLOS NACONECY

1st. Catedra de ORL- Hospital de clinicas -Universidad de Buenos Aires-ARGENTINA-
Chairman: Prof. Dr. Juan Carlos Arauz

INTRODUCTION

The JNA is an uncommon. highly vascular, locally invasive, non capsulated tumor, with the highest incidence in male adolescents. It's origin is located predominantly in the posterior nares or nasopharynx, and spreads in order of frequency into the nasal cavity, sphenoidal sinus, pterigomaxillary space, ethmoidal sinus, maxillary sinus, and subtemporalis space. Through the inferior and superior orbital fissuraes, reaches the orbital apex and the middle cranial fossae.

In order to reach the tumoral spreads, many surgical approaches have been advocated, and not infrequentely more than one technique should be combined.

This paper reports our experience with JNA through a sublabial transantral deep microsurgical technique.

MATERIAL AND METHODS

From 1979 to 1984, 25 patients with histologically confirmed JNA were seen in the Clinic's Hospital of Buenos Aires University. All were males aged 7 to 23 years old (media 13). 16 patients were primary cases, whereas 9 secondary with initial treatment elsewhere.

Epistaxis was seen in all patients (100%), others symptcms included: nasal obstruction, 84%- nasal discharge, 72%-facial deformity, 20%- unilateral proptosis 16%- hypoacusia, 12%- headache, 8%- bilateral proptosis, 4% and blurred vision, 4%.

History, physical findings, angiography and CT scan showed to be adequate elements to establish the diagnosis and the extention of the tumor. Lately we believe that angiography can be avoided, as it doesn't modify our surgical strategy. Biopsy should not be mandatory, nevertheless all cases had intraoperatory biopsy.

According to Fisch and Chandler, we agree that is necessary to stage this pathology, for its adequate therapy and case reporting. Keeping in mind the common origin of this tumor, the classification is helpfull to determinate the differents extentions in the surroundings structures with the aid of CT scan's findings. Following Chandler, we had 2 cases in stage I,1 in II, 19 in III,and 3 with intracranial extentions IV.

As in otehr tumoral processes of the anterior base of skull we approach these areas performing a unilateral sublabial incision and a wide antrotomy, removing enterily removing entirely the posterior and internal wall of the maxillary sinus and from there to all the above mentioned areas. Intracranial extensions are no problem thanks to this wide exposure. Under normal anatomic conditions we would not be able to reach easily the above mentioned areas, but the tumor itself modifies anatomy in such a way that these deep structures become widely available to the surgeon just by following the same path of tumoral growth.

As one of the first manouvers is the ligation and section of all branches of the internal maxillary artery, hemorrage becomes a minor problem. The tumor is gently dissected from the adjacents structures, specially elevating the periostium towards the tumor, and withdrawning it through the same incisional approach. If the tumor is completly removed, bleeding ceases immediately.

Packing is not necessary. The nasal and oral airways are free allowing normal breathing and immediate nourishment, as in minor antral surgery.

RESULTS

The treatment plan outlined has result in a tumor cure in 24 of 25 patients. In one patient, part of the tumor was left in place because of the high risk to produce tears in the cavernous sinus duramater. No symptoms were reported in this case after 3 years control.

Follow-up varies from 6 to 72 months. All cases are asymptomatic. Postoperatory control included clinical evaluaction and periodicaly CT scan studies. No recurrences were recorded.

CONCLUSIONS

Thanks to this operative strategy :

1. The postoperative period is smooth and brief as in antrotomy.
2. Let us immediate free airways.
3. Allows immediate normal oral nourishment.
4. Needs minimun nursing and medical care.
5. Shortens hospital stay. No more than 3 or 5 days.
6. Shows no surgical or other complications. No mortality.
7. No recurrences, except one whereas part of the tumor was left in place.
8. No needs of preoperative procedures (hormonotheraphy, radiotherapy, embolizations,criotherapy or arterial ligations).
9. Avoids: previous tracheostomy, external scars, pharyngostome possibility mandibular osteotomies, facial nerve injury, conductive hypoacusia or temporomandibular disfunction.

REPRINTS: Dr. Alejandro Ernesto Terzian
Ecuador 1428- 4°
1425-Buenos Aires-ARGENTINA

New dimensions in otorhinolaryngclogy - head and neck surgery, vol. 2.
E. Myers, editor

INNER EAR LESIONS AND OPTOKINETIC NYSTAGUS

SETSUKO TAKEMORI,* YOJIRO SEKI, and TADASHI AIBA**
*Neurotology, **Neurosurgery, Toranomon Hospital
Toranomon 2-2-2, Minato-ku, Tokyo, Japan

INTRODUCTION

In cases of inner ear or vestibular nerve lesions, optokinetic nystagmus (OKN) shows some different responses between the right and left OKN. The purpose of this study is to clarify how the inner ear or vestibular nerve lesions affect the optokinetic nystagmus.

SUBJECTS

Normal	20 persons	
Pathological cases	27 cases	
Unilateral complete labyrinthectomy		16 cases
Unilateral vestibular neurectomy		3 cases
Bilateral labyrinthine afunctions		8 cases

METHODS

Optokinetic nystagmus was evoked by an electrically rotating OKN drum which had 12 black strips inside. The velocity of the drum rotation was measured by a microcomputer and the constant drum velocity of 30, 45 and 87°/sec for 30 seconds were used.

DC recordings of horizontal and vertical eye movements were performed by using sliver plate electrodes. Eye movements were recorded by electro-oculography (EOG) and they were analyzed by a microcomputer. The slow and quick phase velocity of optokinetic nystagmus were calculated by this computer. The sampling time was 5msec and the high cut filter was 1,000Hz.

The mean values of the slow and quick phase velocity of the optokinetic nystagmus at each velocity for 30 seconds were used for this study, and their standard deviations were also calculated.

The labyrinthectomy was done under the general anesthesia. The post-auricular incision was taken and the mastoidectomy was performed. The three semi-circular canals and the vestibule were opened and the membraneous labyrinth was destroyed. The retromastoid craniectomy was done for the vestibular neurectomy, and the cerebellopontine angle was exposed. After the VIIth and VIIIth nerves had been identified, the VIIIth nerve was cut. The bilateral labyrinthine afunction was caused by streptomycin sulfate injection in 2 cases and by dialysis in 3 cases of chronic renal diseases. The etiology was unknown in 3 cases.

RESULTS and CONCLUSION

The slow and quick phase velocity of optokinetic nystagmus showed a big difference between the right and left optokinetic nystagmus soon after the unilateral labyrinthectomy. The slow and quick phase velocity of optokinetic nystagmus to the direction of the spontaneous nystagmus was larger than those to the other direction. The slow and quick phase velocity of the optokinetic nystagmus to the direction of the spontaneous nystagmus, which was the optokinetic nystagmus to the contralateral side, was within normal limits and those of the optokinetic nystagmus to the ipsilateral side was less than normal.

The difference of the optokinetic nystagmus was larger as the drum velocity became higher. This difference of optokinetic nystagmus between the right and left was still seen even after the spontaneous nystagmus to the contralateral side had disappeared. The difference started to disappear from the lower velocity of optokinetic nystagmus drum. The difference of the optokinetic nystagmus between the right and left at the 30°/sec drum velocity was seen for 10 - 14 days after the unilateral labyrinthectomy. The optokinetic nystagmus at the 87°/sec drum velocity showed the difference between the right and left for 2- 3 months.

The difference between the right and left optokinetic nystagmus in cases of unilateral vestibular neurectomy showed the same results as those after the unilateral complete labyrinthectomy.

In cases of bilateral labyrinthine afunctions, the slow and quick phase velocity of optokinetic nystagmus were within normal limits or reduced.

Thus, the inner ear or vestibular nerve affects the slow and quick phase velocity of optokinetic nystagmus.

© 1985 Elsevier Science Publishers B.V. (Biomedical Division)
New dimensions in otorhinolaryngology - head and neck surgery, vol. 2.
E. Myers, editor

"A NEW METABOLIC APPROACH TO HEADACHE AND DIZZINESS"

WILLIAM R. UPDEGRAFF, M.D., P.C.
202 Hooker Avenue, Poughkeepsie, New York 12603 U. S. A.

INTRODUCTION

The occurrence of impaired glucose/insulin metabolism is vastly underestimated and underdiagnosed in a large group of patients with idiopathic vertigo and headache. This statement is supported by a 15-year comprehensive biochemical and nutritional assessment of 2186 patients. Eight hundred and ninety-seven were diagnosed as having muscle contraction headache or migraine, and the remaining 1289 patients suffered from dizziness. Hyperinsulinism attributed to abnormal glucose/insulin ratios in these patients. That is why Kraft (Table I) 1975 advises combining insulin tolerance testing with glucose tolerance testing. The control of hyperinsulinism is achieved by nutritional management. Approximately ninety-seven percent of 2186 patients with dizziness and/or headache have been relieved of their symptoms by correcting their glucose/insulin ratios.

MATERIAL AND METHODS

Laboratory Orders for Patients with Vertigo and/or Headache

1) Six-hour Glucose Tolerance Test with INSULIN levels, including the 15-minute, 1/2 hour and 3 1/2 hour levels.
2) Fractionated Catecholamines, at 4th hour of Glucose/Insulin Tol. Test.
3) Fasting Cholesterol.
4) Triglycerides.
5) HDL Cholesterol.

TABLE I

KRAFT'S INSULIN TOLERANCE PATTERNS

Pattern I	1/2 or 1 hour Peak Value (Normal)	27%
Pattern II	Normal Peak, Delayed Return (Abnormal Pattern)	27%
Pattern III-A	Second Hour Delay Peak, Abnormal Insulin Pattern	33%
Pattern III-B	Third Hour Delayed Peak, Abnormal Insulin Pattern	8%

DIETARY MANAGEMENT

The calorie and protein requirement for each patient is calculated by the Registered Dietician and individualized nutritional support is then provided. The total percentage of carbohydrate is reduced to between 20 and 27 percent of the total caloric intake to maintain an acceptable insulin response and avoid an excessive production of insulin. We attempt not to have more than 10 to 13 grams of ingested fruit and milk carbohydrate at the same meal feeding. Tests on our patients have shown that the assimilation of these two carbohydrates dovetail each other and cause a surplus of insulin to be produced when taken at the same time. (Updegraff and Koniz, 1978)

The basic working calorie plans are: 1636 calories, 2005 calories and 2365 calories. Each plan is tailored to the individual's caloric energy expenditure by adjusting the fat intake.

The meal pattern is designed with three small meals and three to five snacks depending on the patient's schedule. This frequent feeding pattern helps to normalize insulin levels and maintain optimal circulating glucose levels. After three months, the patient is gradually allowed to eat three meals a day plus a bedtime snack. Then the carbohydrate intake is increased up to 160 grams, depending upon the patient's glucose/insulin tolerance curve.

The expertise of a Registered Dietician plays a key role in patient rehabilitation. Handing out a diet sheet results in poor compliance. Patients are educated in the importance of their diet as related to biochemical need. A therapeutic alliance is formed between the physician, registered dietician, nurse and the patient.

RESULTS

Dietary interviews conducted on our patients revealed irregular and poor dietary habits. Three-day dietary surveys showed a high percentage of naked, empty calories in the form of refined carbohydrates, alcohol, or saturated fats. With few exceptions, the patients reviewed were hyperinsulinemic and had abnormal glucose/insulin ratios. Treating functional hyperinsulinism by regulation of the diet, discontinuance of smoking, and a sustained exercise program resulted in decreased insulin resistance, increased insulin sensitivity and normal glucose/insulin ratios.

DISCUSSION

The usual medical modalities for the treatment of vertigo and headache have not appreciably improved the quality of life for many patients.

Surgery for Meniere's Disease is resorted to far more often than necessary. Our nutritional approach can be made useful in maintaining a successful surgical result while lessening the incidence of regression and failure.

Migraine headaches are frequently found in patients with Meniere's Disease. Abnormal insulin patterns are the earliest expression of impaired carbohydrate and nutrient metabolism. Patients experienced complete relief of headache and dizziness when the therapeutic goal of glucose/insulin homeostasis was achieved.

REFERENCES

1. Kraft, J.R., M.D. (1975) Detection of Diabetes Mellitus in Situ (occult diabetes), Laboratory Medicine. 6:1, 10-22
2. Updegraff, W.R., M.D. (April 1977) Impaired Carbohydrate Metabolism and Idiopathic Meniere's Disease, Ear, Nose and Throat Journal, New York

© 1985 Elsevier Science Publishers B.V. (Biomedical Division)
New dimensions in otorhinolaryngology - head and neck surgery, vol. 2.
E. Myers, editor

SOME ANALYSIS ON STABILOGRAMS WITH LOADING TECHNIQUES

HARUO WAKUTANI, MASARU KISHIMOTO, HIROSHI MACHIZUKA, HIROSHI MORI, TORU INAMORI, TAKEO KUMOI
Hyogo college of medicine, Nishinomiya, Hyogo, Japan

INTRODUCTION

The stabilography seems to be the most proper way to analyse the human body sway. Many studies have been documented[1,2], but yet they are not still fully clear enough for clinical use. So we have studied some new techniques with loadings to evaluate the human body sway.

SUBJECTS AND METHODS

1) A platform which roles with sign wave of 0-0.6 Hz within 2.5 degree was made. On this platform, a force plate was placed and test subjects were standing erect on it. The stabilograms were recorded for 100 seconds with the frequency of 0,0.05,0.075,0.1,0.15, 0.2,0.3,0.4, and 0.5 Hz of rolling. Following three groups were sutdied.

group	cases in 1)	cases in 2)
A. NORMAL GROUP	100	37
B. VESTIBULAR (DISTURBANCE) GROUP	15	10
C. CENTRAL (DISTURBANCE) GROUP	12	27

The stabilograms were analysed by frequency analysis and by cross correlation analysis between the center of gravity and the slant of the platform.

2) On the force plate, subjects were standing erect and they were pushed laterally by their iliac region with a stick in a moment, and the stabilogram was recorded for 10 seconds after this pulse-like stimulation. The stabilograms were avaraged 10 times, and the damping coefficient was calculated.

RESULTS

1) In order to indicate the range of the frequecy of power spectrum involved, we measured highest freequencies of the spectrum as index (upper limit of power:UL).

In vestibular group, there is no obvious differences from normal group. But in central group, the value of ULs are significantly heigher than that of in normal group, especially at 0.05 Hz of the loading (fig.1).

And with the cross correlation analysis, we noticed the phase shift between movements of center of gravity and slant of the platform.

In central group, the preceding of center of gravity is much more obvious than that of nomal and vestibular group (fig 2).

2) In the second type of stimulation, normal subjects once shifted to the direction of stimulus force, and then returned to the neutral position rapidly with following slight

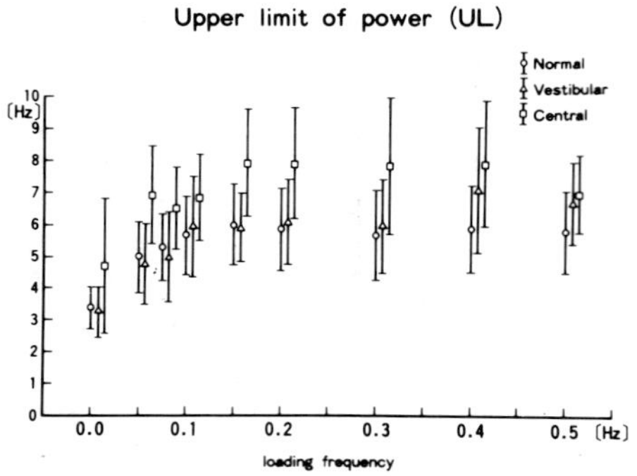

Fig. 1. Average and S.D. of upper limit of power spectrum(UL)

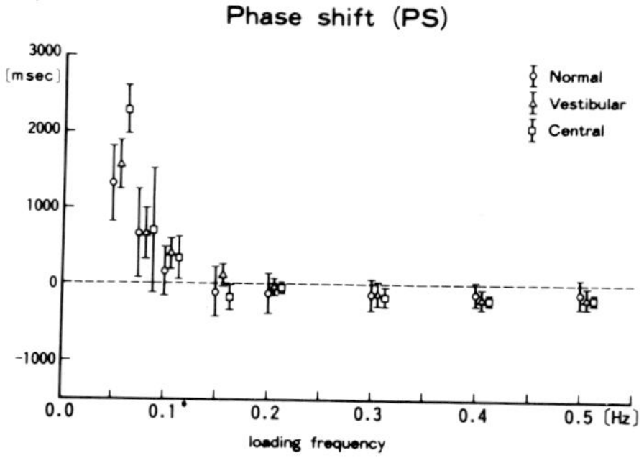

Fig. 2. Average and S.D. of phase shift(PS) (preceding)

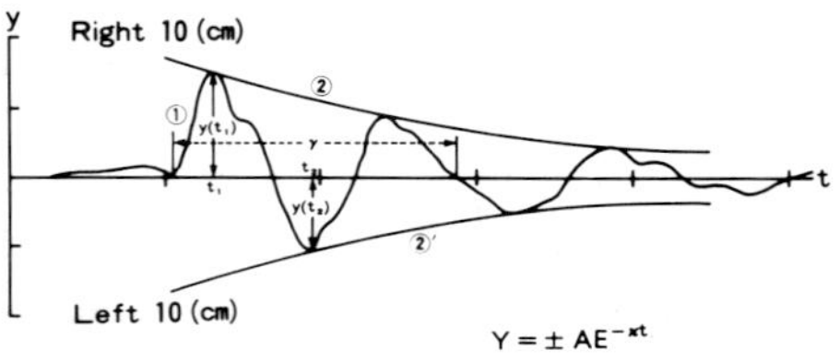

Fig. 3. Oscillation of center of gravity and its damping curve.

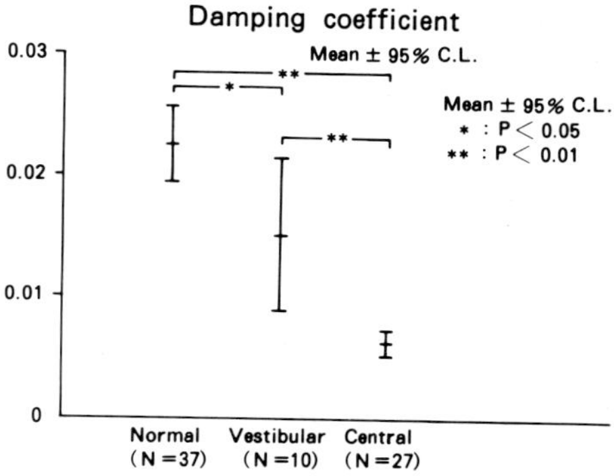

Fig. 4. Average and S.D. of damping coefficients(DC)

oscillations around the neutral position.

In vestibular and central groups, following oscillations of center of gravity continued longer than in normal group. Calcuated damping coefficient (DC) of oscillations are given (fig.3).

Vestibular group has no obvious differences from normal group in this parameter. But in central group, the value of DC is obviously lower than the other two groups (fig.4).

With these three parameters, we are able to distinguish central group from normal and vestibural group.

SUMMARY

We studied stabilography with two types of loadings, and noticed that we can distinguish central group from normal and vestibural group with our new three parameters, i.e. UL,PS, ans DC. These studies suggest that the usefullnese of stabilography with loading for clinical application.

REFERENCES

1.Koles Z.T.,Castelein R.D. (1981) In:The relationship between body sway and foot pressure in normal man. J. Medic. Engin. Technol. Vol.4:228-238

2.Suga H.,Takemori . (1970) In:Measurement of body movement and its clinical appication. J.J. Physiol.20:296-308

© 1985 Elsevier Science Publishers B V. (Biomedical Division)
New dimensions in otorhinolaryngology – head and neck surgery, vol. 2.
E. Myers, editor

LOCALIZATION OF BRAINSTEM LESIONS BY COMBINED USE OF OPTOKINETIC NYSTAGMUS & FIXATION-SUPPRESSION OF CALORIC NYSTAGMUS

JIN WATANABE, ISAO KATO, TADASHI NAKAMURA, KOJI HARADA, TOMOHIKO HASEGAWA, RYOJI KANAYAMA and YOSHIO KOIKE
Department of Otolaryngology, Yamagata University School of Medicine, 990-23 Yamagata, Japan

INTRODUCTION

Both optokinetic nystagmus (OKN) and fixation-suppression of caloric nystagmus have been proposed as useful diagnostic tools for assessment of infratentorial lesions. However, despite all efforts to establish diagnostic values in the brainstem lesions over the years, localizing values of deranged OKN and failure of fixation-suppression (FFS) against a discrete lesion site have not been established as yet. In the present study, slow phase OKN velocities against lesion sites was investigated on 28 patients who showed FFS and also discrete unilateral lesions by CT at different levels of the brainstem. Then, the efficacy of combined use of OKN and fixation-suppression for the localizing lesion site was evaluated from the neurological point of view.

MATERIALS AND METHODS

One hundred eight of 2240 patients from 1979 to 1984 who visited the EOG laboratory showed FFS. Forty-three of 108 patients showed FFS in only one direction with slow phase velocity (Type III)(Kato et al., 1980). Twenty-eight of 43 patients showed a discrete unilateral lesion. Patients with ocular dissociation were discarded, because such eye conditions have valuable diagnostic significance in themselves.

Electrodes (Ag-AgCl) were placed in a conventional way. Horizontal eye movements were recorded with DC-EOG (0-20 Hz; -3dB) and rectified by amplifiers with a time constant of 0.03 sec to obtain slow phase velocity of nystagmus. Caloric stimulus was 50 ml water at temperatures of 30° and 44°C during an irrigation period of 20 sec. During the maximum intensity of slow phase velocity, the patients were requested to fix their gaze upon a light spot 3 m away for 10 sec. Thus, a percent reduction in slow phase velocity was established. OKN stripes (white-4°, black-26°) were rotated in both clockwise and counterclockwise direction at angular acceleration of 1.2°/sec for 100 sec.

RESULTS

Twenty-eight patients are tabulated in Table I according to lesion site at each level of the brainstem.

The relationship between the direction of OKN limitation and FFS against the lesion site is summarized in Table II according to each level of the brainstem.

TABLE 1

Lesion site	Case No
Midbrain	6
Pons	14
Medulla	8
Total	28

Medulla*; Wallenberg's syndrome

TABLE 2

Lesion site	OKN	FFS	Case No
Midbrain	I	I	5
Pons(ventral)	I	B	6
(dorsal)	C	C	2
Medulla*	I	I	4
	C	I	4
SCP	I	C	1
MCP	I	C	6

I; ipsilateral to lesion, C; contralateral to lesion, B; bilateral, SCP; superior cerebellar peduncle, MCP; middle cerebellar peduncle, *Medulla; Wallenberg's syndrome

DISCUSSION AND CONCLUSION

As outlined in Table II, the basic pattern of EOG in brainstem lesions is that OKN velocity and fixation-suppression were impaired toward the lesion site. In lesions in the dorsal tegmentum of the pons, however, EOG patterns against lesion sites were quite opposite, suggesting the oculomotor decussation in the dorsal area of the pons. In patients with lesions in both the superior and the middle cerebellar peduncle, the relationship between the direction of OKN limitation and FFS was dissociate.

Based on this finding, there is a possibility that the inferior cerebellar peduncle may be involved in 4 patients with Wallenberg's syndrome whose direction of OKN limitation and FFS were dissociate. On this matter, however, further investigations must be needed.

It may conclude that these test batteries possibly provide some additional information for neurological test.

© 1985 Elsevier Science Publishers B.V. (Biomedical Division)
New dimensions in otorhinolaryngology - head and neck surgery, vol. 2.
E. Myers, editor

DIFFERENTIAL DIAGNOSIS OF CEREBELLOPONTINE ANGLE NEURINOMAS

HIROYA YAMAGUCHI YUTAKA YOSHIMOTO*
Depertment of E. N. T. Tokyo Senbai Hospital (Japan)
*Depertment of E. N. T. Teikyo Univ. (Japan)

INTRODUCTION

Among the tumors of the cerebellopontine angle (CPA), acoustic tumor is the most frequent. There are many reports related tc the acoustic tumor. Recently, due to the improvement in diagnostic methods, such as C T scan, very small acoustic tumor can now be diagnosed.

Now acoustic tumor of the CPA is a very rare case. If the tumor is not an acoustic tumor, it is difficult to diagnose correctly before the operation.

So we tried to differencial diagnose the tumor of the CPA neurinoma.

MATERIALS AND CASES

We experienced the following cases, which were confirmed by the operations.

Acoustic Neurinoma	74 cases
Neurinoma of IX, X, XI th C.N.	2 cases
Neurinoma of the V th C.N.	5 cases

RESULTS

Neurinomas of the IX, X, XI th C.N. were observed dilation of jugural foramen, and obstructive of internal jugural vein with retrograde-juguranography (1).

The degrees of the hearing loss and the caloric response are not always the same.

With the enlargement of the tumor, the impairments of VII, VIII, XII th C.N. should be occured (2).

There are three types among in the trigeminal neurinoma, so-called root type , ganglion type and combined type (3).

The tumor of the root type grows into posterior cranial fossa and its symptoms are resemble with the acoustic tumor.

But the tumor of ganglion type grows into middle cranial fossa and is hard to diagonse. For this type, especially C T scan is very useful.

Neurinomas of the V th C.N. were diaosed dilation of the oval foramen and obstruction of internal jugural vein.

Hearingloss and canalis paresis are not usual.

With the enlargement of the tumor impairments of the III, IV, VI, VII, VIII, IX, X, XI th C.N. were occurred.

CONCLUSION

The differential diagnostic points of CPA neurinoma are as follows.

	acoustic neurinoma	trigeminal neurinoma	IX,X,XIth C.N. neurinoma
X-Ray film findings	Dilation of internal auditory canal	Dilation of foramen ovale clearcut defect of apex of petrous bone	Dilation of jugural foramen Obstruction of internal jugural vein
Audiogram Caloric Test	both severely impaired	dissociation (+)	dissociation (+)
Development of C.N. disturbance	VII - V VI - IX X - XII	Root type V - III,IV,VI,VII VIII,IX,X,XI Ganglion type V - III,IV,VI	- VII,VIII,XII

REFERENCES

1 Gejrot, T. : With spicial Reference to the Diagnostic Value of Retrograde Juguranography, Acta Otolaryng. 57 : 450-458, 1963

2 HIROYA YAMAGUCHI et al : Intracranial neurinoma of the Jugural Foramen. Equilibrium Research : 37. 46-51, 1978

3 Kundsen, V. , et al. : Neurinoma of the gasserian Ganglion and the trigeminal Root. Acta Neurochirurugica, 26 : 159-164, 1972.

© 1985 Elsevier Science Publishers B.V. (Biomedical Division)
New dimensions in otorhinolaryngolcgy - head and neck surgery, vol. 2.
E. Myers, editor

CLINICAL AND STATISTICAL OBSERVATIONS ON ACOUSTIC TUMORS WITH SUDDEN DEAFNESS

YUTAKA YOSHIMOTO* AND HIROYA YAMAGUCHI**

*Dept. of Otolaryngology, Teikyo University School of Medicine, Kaga 2-11-1, Itabashi-ku,Tokyo (Japan), **Dept. of Otolaryngology, Senbai-Kosha Tokyo Hospital, Tokyo (Japan)

INTRODUCTION

Sudden deafness include not only cases which the so-called sudden deafness of unknown etiology but also ones which arise from several kinds of diseases. Acoustic tumors present rarely sudden deafness as the initial symptom. However, no statistical study have been tried because such cases are relatively rare. In this report, clinical and statistical observations were made on 13 acoustic tumor patients presenting sudden deafness and following results were obtained.

RESULTS

The onset of acoustic tumors presenting sudden deafness was also preceded by symptoms of upper respiratory tract infection in 4 of 13 patients (31%). We are inclined to presume that those patients with acoustic tumor had upper respiratory tract infection only by chance. In 6 of 13 acoustic tumor, its onset was accompanied with rotatory vertigo. Special care should be exercised when examining patients of the acoustic tumor with sudden deafness because those cases may be often confused with the so-called sudden deafness.

Ten patients, or 77%, had an average hearing level of 60 dB or more. There was only one patient who had 30 dB or lower hearing level. According to the audiograms, the gradual high tone loss type was most frequently recognized in these cases.

Some gaze nystagmus was recognized in 9 of 13 cases. Bilateral gaze nystagmus was noted in 5 patients, or 38%, and those patients were suspected of having some brainstem disturbance. The positional nystagmus test revealed positive findings in 11 cases of 13 cases or 88% of these cases.

The caloric nystagmus test indicated that all 13 patients had a diminished response to the test. As many as 8 of 13 patients, or 62%, had no reaction to irrigation of ice-water.

Abnormalities suggestive of brainstem disorder, such as inhibition of optokinetic nystagmus, were elicited by the optokinetic nystagmus test in 9 cases, or 70%. The eye tracking test revealed signs of the brainstem disorder, such as saccadic and ataxic waves were present in 7 of 13 cases.

It was found that 11 of 13 patients (85%) had neurological symptoms of cranial nerves excluding the VII cranial nerve.

Plain X-ray films revealed abnormality of the internal auditory canal in 9 patients, or 70%. Tomograms were abnormal in 10 patients, or 77%. Many of sudden deafness show an abnormality on X-ray examination of the internal auditory canal. 12 of 13 cases, or 92%, had an abnormality on the conventional CT examination. All patients were positive for contrast enhancement. There was only one patient who had a small tumor of 1 cm in diameter. It was only on the metrizamide CT cisternograph that the tumor was visualized in this case.

SUMMARY AND CONCLUSION

Based on the results of the present study, there was a significant difference in the frequency of such abnormalities as gaze nystagmus, canal paresis in the caloric (nystagmus) test, inhibition of optokinetic nystagmus, dilatation of the internal auditory canal and cranial nerve signs. While, there was no significant difference in such symptoms as preceding upper respiratory tract infection and rotatory vertigo at the onset of sudden deafness.

The cases where the patient presenting with sudden deafness should be examined for acoustic tumors include patients; (1) with retrocochlear deafness, (2) with no response at all to treatment, (3) with progressive deafness, (4) with central nystagmus (e.g. bilateral gaze nystagmus), (5) with absent response to caloric stimulation, (6) with a positive finding of internal auditory meatus on the X-ray and (7) with symptoms of cranial nerves except VIII cranial nerve.

© 1985 Elsevier Science Publishers B.V. (Biomedical Division)
New dimensions in otorhinolaryngology - head and neck surgery, vol. 2.
E. Myers, editor

TYMPANIC THERMOMETRY IN CALORIC TESTS

ALBERTO ZUÑIGA, ARISTIDE ZUÑIGA
Centro Diagnóstico Oído - Nariz - Garganta, Providencia 701-B, Santiago, Chile.

INTRODUCTION

Tympanic thermometry describes ear's thermal behavior during caloric stimulation as time function.

MATERIAL AND METHODS

In 25 normal individuals, ages between 18 and 24 years old (13 women and 12 men, in 20°C ± 2.5°C environment), basal tympanic temperature was measured. External ear canal was irrigated with 320 cc of water (± 20 cc) at different temperatures between 25°C and 48°C during 40 seconds.

Temperature control before and during caloric test was made with sensor applied under direct vision on the tympanic membrane's inferior quadrants (T.M.). Temperature was read in a digital electronic thermometer (constant current) for a range of 25°C to 48°C with error ± 0.2°C (1-2).

Temperature was checked, every 10 second, during the water irrigation up to 400 seconds, keeping the sensor fixed at 0 level on T.M., through the otoscope used to perform the irrigation.

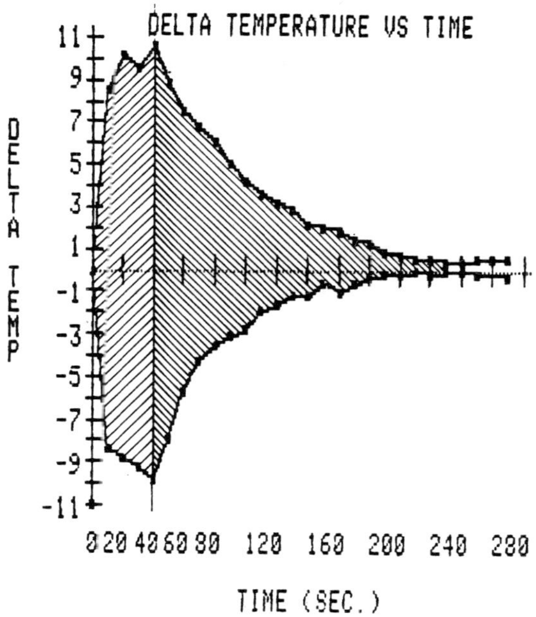

Fig. 1 Experimental thermal stimulatory and recovery periods (hot and cold)

RESULTS

Basal tympanic temperature (BTT) mean average was 37.6°C ± 0.1°C S.D. Caloric test's two fundamental periods are: Stimulatory and Recovery periods.

I. Stimulatory Period. It corresponds to the irrigation time of the external ear canal (Fig. 1).

a) Fast period of heating or colding in the first 10 seconds of the stimulation.

b) Stabilization period. In the following 30 sec. thermal stabilization is attained at pretended level. T.M. thermal equilibrium is in relation to the temperature of the water used in the irrigation and the thermic capacity and resistance characteristics of the surrounding tissues.

II. Recovery Period. Thermal recovery curve behavior is one of exponential function type (Fig. 1) depending on:
1. BTT: Basal tympanic temperature.
2. MTT: Maximal tympanic temperature after 40 seconds of irrigation.
3. RC : Time constant with a theoretical value of 63% of $\triangle t_0^o$ ($\triangle t_0^o$ = MTT − BTT)

Its mathematical equation is represented in figure 2.
Fitness of observed values and predicted values for the recovery curve is shown in figure 3.

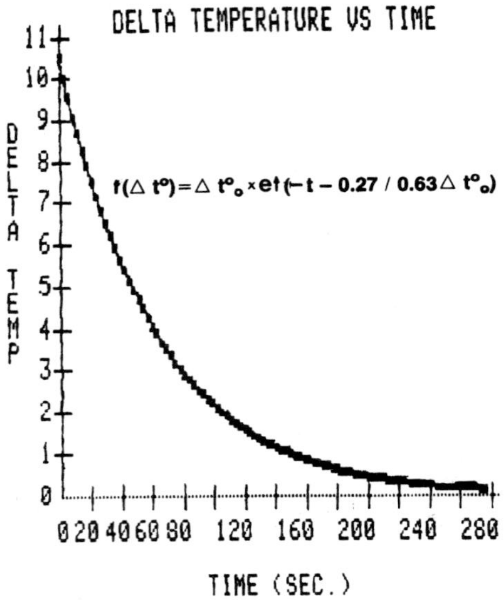

Fig. 2 Thermal recovery curve equation for experimental design

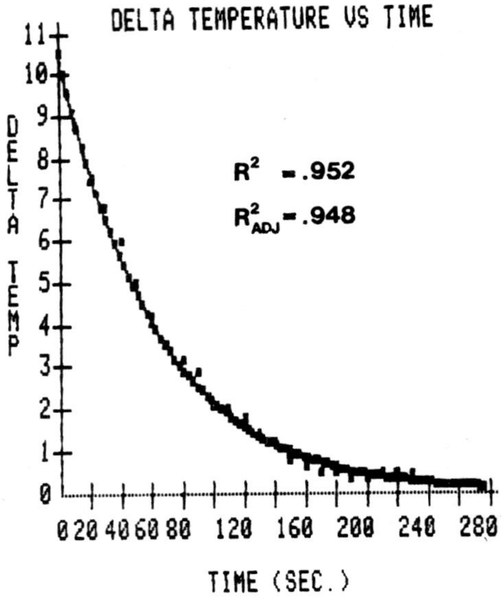

Fig. 3 Fitness of theoretical and experimental values ($\triangle t^o_o$ = 10.5 C°)

COMMENTS
a) We assume constant R.C. values in cold and hot stimulations. Experimental mean average value: 68.5 sec ± 18.95 S.D. and 59.0 sec ± 13.19 S.D. for hot and cold stimulations respectively.
b) Total duration of thermal recovery period is accepted up to 5 R.C. values.
c) Experimental fluctuations of the recovery curve around BTT are observed between 200 sec and 300 sec. Sometimes an over recuperation occurs (colder than BTT with hot stimulus or warmer than BTT with cold stimulus).
d) Temperature recovery curves are symmetrical in comparable cold and hot stimulus.
e) Practical clinical applications involve use of expected referential curves obtained with equation for any given single value of $\triangle t_0^o$.

AKNOWLEDGEMENTS
We wish to thank Professor José Pascual from the Mathematics Institute, Universidad Católica Valparaíso and Rodrigo Zúñiga, Agronomy student University of Chile for their colaboration in the computational and mathematical work-up of this paper.

REFERENCES
1. Zúñiga C., Aristide. Temperatura timpánica. Instrumentación y exploración clínica en el oído normal y patológico Rev. de Otorrinolaring. 34:53-62, 1975.

2. Zúñiga, Alberto y Zúñiga, Aristide. Valoración objetiva del estímulo utilizado en la prueba calórica de Hallpike. Rev. de Otorrinolaring. 35:20-26, 1975.

New dimensions in otorhinolaryngology - head and neck surgery, vol. 2.
E. Myers, editor

SENSORINEURAL HEARING LOSS IN HYPOTHYROIDISM

MK AGARWAL, OP GUPTA

Department of Otolaryngology, Institute of Medical Sciences, Banaras Hindu University, Varanasi, India

INTRODUCTION

The impairment of auditory function is found not only in Pendred's syndrome and cretins but also in adults suffering from acquired hypothyroidism[1]. In the present study, a battery of audiological and vestibular function tests have been performed in 72 cases of confirmed hypothyroidism.

MATERIALS AND METHODS

The severity of hypothyroidism was graded as mild, moderate or severe depending upon serum protein-bound iodine estimation. The incidence of hearing impairment, tinnitus and vertigo was correlated with the severity of the disease. The site of lesion causing sensorineural hearing impairment in 25 cases was pinpointed audiologically. The age of the patients varied from 8 to 49 years with females outnumbering males by a ratio of 2.4:1. Idiopathic hypothyroidism was present in 66 cases (91.6%), cretinism in 3 children (4.2%), while there was one case each of hypothyroidism due to an extrinsic carcinoma of larynx infiltrating the thyroid gland, prolonged treatment of thyrotoxicosis with neomercazole and total thyroidectomy in a case of carcinoma thyroid. The hypothyroidism was confirmed by estimating serum cholesterol level, serum protein-bound iodine level and 24-hour iodine uptake by the thyroid.

RESULTS

The hypothyroidism was graded as mild, moderate and severe according to protein-bound iodine levels at 3.1-3.5 mcg, 2.6-3.0 mcg and 2.0-2.5 mcg, respectively. The appearance of the tympanic membrane as well as the eustachian tube functions were within normal limits in all the cases. The tuning fork tests as well as pure tone audiometry revealed bilateral symmetrical sensorineural hearing impairment in 25 cases (34.7%) which showed linear relationship with the severity of hypothyroidism. The remaining 6 cases had conductive hearing impairment. The pure tone audiometric curve in all the patients having sensorineural hearing impairment was of flat type, the difference in speech frequencies being 10 db or less. Such a curve has been categorized as type III by Schuknecht[2] and it signifies atrophy of stria vascularis. Tinnitus was present only in 7.0% cases who had either moderate or severe grade of hypothyroidism. Giddiness was noted in 21 cases (29.1%). The vestibular tests did not reveal any functional deficit though the feeling of giddiness experienced during the tests was similar to the vertigo complained of by the patients.

The battery of audiological tests done in 25 cases having sensorineural hearing impairment revealed presence of type III curve on puretone audiometry, good or normal speech discrimination score, absence of tone decay, roll-over index below 0.5 and loudness discomfort level in the range of 45-80 db in all these cases thus establishing the site of lesion to be cochlea.

CONCLUSIONS

Our investigations show that the hearing impairment occurs more frequently than vertigo in hypothyroidism while tinnitus is present rarely. The incidence of all these symptoms goes on increasing with the increase in the severity of hypothyroidism. The hearing loss in acquired hypothyroidism is always bilaterally symmetrical, mild to moderate in severity, mainly progressive and sensorineural with cochlea as the site of lesion. There is definite subjective improvement on becoming euthyroid but audiometry does not confirm it. The cretins have usually severe sensorineural hearing impairment. Tinnitus is intermittent and of low buzzing character. The vestibular function tests reveal no abnormality even if the subjective vertigo is present.

REFERENCES

1. Bircher H (1883) Der Endemische Kropf. Basel Quoted by Stephens SDG (1970) J Laryngol Otol 84:317-321
2. Schuknecht HF (1964) Arch Otolaryngol 80:369-382.

New dimensions in otorhinolaryngology - head and neck surgery, vol. 2.
E. Myers, editor

TINNITUS: A CLINICAL STUDY

LUCIO A. CASTAGNO,MD

SYDNEY CASTAGNO,MD,PhD

Department of Otolaryngology,Federal University of Pelotas School of Medicine.
Rua General Osorio,1585. Pelotas,96100,Brazil

INTRODUCTION

Tinnitus is a symptom present in several diseases.The differencial diagnosis may be time consuming and sometimes expensive.This work was designed to investigate clinical characteristics of the tinnitus patient and to estabilish etiological correlations.The final goal would be to instruct the general physician to achieve a useful tinnitus diagnosis with a clinical history.

MATERIAL AND METHODS

One hundred fifty one patients with tinnitus as a chief complaint were studied between January 1983 and January 1984.A complete otolaryngological exam was done in all patients.Tonal audiometry,SISI test,impedance audiometry and tinnitus matching were done in some of them.A clinical characteristics study was conducted in 76 patients with a standard questionaire.All data were fed into a computer and statistical correlations (Chi square analysis) were estabilished.

RESULTS

Tinnitus multiple etiologies were grouped in four major groups: secundary to sensorineural pathology,secundary to hearing conduction disorder,idiopathic,and tinnitus of extra-auditory origin (table I).

TABLE I: Tinnitus etiologies (n= 151)

Group	Disease		Total per group (%)
IDIOPATHIC			63 (41.7%)
EXTRA-AUDITORY	Carotid stenosis........	2	2 (1.4%)
SENSORINEURAL	Presbiacusys............	22	
	Acoustic trauma.........	18	
	Undetermined............	11	
	Meniere's disease.......	5	
	Drugs...................	1	57 (37.7%)
CONDUCTION	SOM-tube dysfunction....	11	
	Otosclerosis............	5	
	AOM.....................	5	
	COM.....................	5	
	Undetermined............	3	29 (19.2%)

Sex distribution was unremarkable.There was a higher incidence of tinnitus in patients over 45 years (63.6%) and just four (2.6%) were under 15.A marked relationship was found among tinnitus in patients under 45 and conduction disorder with patients over 45 and sensorineural disease at a significance level of p=0.0003.

Tinnitus started suddenly in 12(15.8%) patients and insidiously in 64(84.2%).It was present for more than a year in 59(77.6%),for less than a year and more than a month in 13(17.1%),and in just 4(5.3%) patients it was present for less than a month.These features indicate a slow progressive chronic disease for most patients.An important relationship among tinnitus sudden onset and conduction disorder with insidious onset and sensorineural pathology was found (p=0.0222).

Tinnitus was continuous in 61(80.3%) patients and pulsatile in 15(19.7%).A significant (p=0.0118) was found among continuous tinnitus and sensorineural pathology with pulsatile tinnitus and hearing conduction disorder.

DISCUSSION

Etiological site of lesion diagnosis was not possible in 63(41.7%) patients. It was feasible in 88(58.3%).However one must realize that this site of lesion diagnosis might not be the precise site of tinnitus production (Goldstein).

Several clinico-etiological relationships were estabilished (table II),but some overlap exist among these clinical categories.

TABLE II: Tinnitus clinico-etiological relationships

Group	Age	Onset	Type	Etiology
CONDUCTION	<45	Sudden	Pulsatile	SOM-tube dysfunction (38%)
SENSORINEURAL	≥ 45	Insidious	Continuous	Presbiacusys-Acoustic trauma(70%)

REFERENCES

1. Castagno L (1985) J Bras Med,in press.
2. Douek E (1981) Ciba Foundation Symposium 85:4-15.
3. Feldman H (1979) First International Tinnitus Seminar:60-70.
4. Goldstein B, Shulman A (1979) First International Tinnitus Seminar:33-45.
5. Hazell J (1981) Ciba Foundation Symposium 85:35-53.
6. Johson R, Goodwin B (1979) First International Tinnitus Seminar:48-60.
7. Pulec J et al (1978) Ann Otol 87:821-833.
8. Vernon J, Meikle M (1981) Ciba Foundation Symposium 85:239-262.

© 1985 Elsevier Science Publishers B.V. (Biomedical Division)
New dimensions in otorhinolaryngology – head and neck surgery, vol. 2.
E. Myers, editor

COMPARATIVE RESULTS OF TINNITUS. TREATMENT BY MESOTHERAPY AND ELECTROSTIMULATION

HENRI MARTIN - CHRISTOS MARCOPOULOS

Clinique d'Oto-rhino-laryngologie et d'Audiophonologie de l'hopital Edouard Herriot - 69 003 Lyon

The aim of this study is to compare the results obtained in the treatment of tinnitus by the Electrostimulation (50 cases) and the Mesotherapy (100 cases) which is not studied rigorously till now. This study deals with various aetiologies of permanent, fixed invalidating tinnitus which is resistant to all other treatments. An extensive examination of these patients was performed including a medical history, audiometry, tinnitus and blood tests.

MATERIALS AND METHODS

A - Mesotherapy

A simple syringe with a special needle of label 4/mm length and 4/10mm diameter is used to inject Peridil Heparine which is composed of,

- mono ethanolamine nicotinate
- sodium heparinate
- procaine
- sodium mercuro thiolate

The quantity of injection used for each ear is 0,5 ml, it is administered intradermally in the peri-auricular area by multi-injections once weekly for four weeks.

B - Electrostimulation and Electroacoustistimulation

The electrostimulator Tino-top controlled by a microprocessor system was at our disposition. The parameters of the treatment are preprogrammed. The parameters of the treatment are preprogrammed as,

- electrostimulation 7 volts
- acousticstimulation 60 volts
- time-switch 45 min

The intensity of alternating current and acoustic signals are adjusted according to the sensibility of patients. The machine emits simultaneously synchronised acoustics and electric signals. The frequency of the impulses is 5/min with a 2 sec interval between each. The electrical signals are transmitted by subcutaneous electrodes implanted in the middle cervicolateral area.

The treatment requires 6 sessions, once weekly with 45' sec duration each.

RESULT

The four following criterial are obtained

1. Slight amelioration (+) :
   Tinnitus intensity is diminished at least by about a 1/3
2. Fluctuating amelioration (~) :
   The fixed and continious tinnitus becomes unstable in intensity and frequency during the day
3. Satisfying amelioration (++) :
   Tinnitus intensity becomes very feeble
4. Very satisfying amelioration (+++) :
   Total disappearance of tinnitus

The groups 1 and 2 are considered as medium results.

The groups 3 and 4 are considered successful when their favourable results are prolonged for a sufficient time.

TABLE I

COMPARISON OF THE TINNITUS TREATMENTS BY MESOTHERAPY AND ELECTROSTIMULATIONS WITH THE RESULTS OBTAINED IN THE PRESENT STUDY BY THIS TWO METHODS

	Mesotherapy		Electrostimulation	
Total or subtotal amelioration	21 %	46 %	14 %	32 %
Slight amelioration	25 %		18 %	
Failure	54 %		68 %	
Number of patients	100		50	

TABLE II
OURS OBSERVATIONS ACORDING THE AETIOLOGY IS DIVIDED AS FOLLOWING (values in parentheses are % of success)

Factors	Number of patients	
	Mesotherapy	Electrostimulations
Presbyacusis	26 (19 %)	14 (21 %)
Acoustic trauma	33 (27 %)	16 (19 %)
Otosclerosis	5	2
Viral	9	5
Menier's disease	2	1
None found (x)	20	12

It is impossible in certain affections to establish sufficient statistics.

We have only studied here the percentages of success and failure concerning specialy first two affections of Table II.

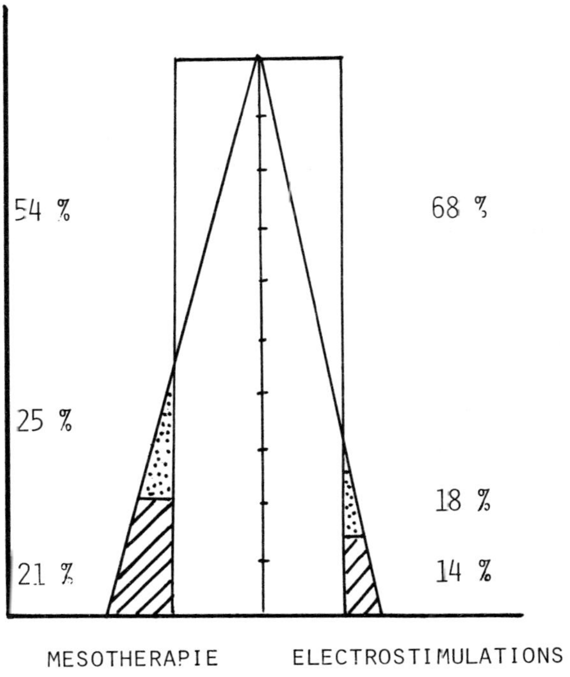

© 1985 Elsevier Science Publishers B.V. (Biomedical Division)
New dimensions in otorhinolaryngology – head and neck surgery, vol. 2.
E. Myers, editor

TEMPORARY RELIEF OF SEVERE TINNITUS BY TRANSCUTANEOUS ELECTROTHERAPY

B. MEYER, MD ; D.MARIDAT, MD ; C. BEYRAND, MD ; F. CHABOLLE, MD .

Laboratoire de Recherches O.R.L. (Pr. C.H. CHOUARD)
C.H.U. PARIS, Saint-Antoine, FRANCE

In cases of total deafness associated with tinnitus we had frequently noticed a decrease of tinnitus during electrical stimulation test and complete suppression by the permanent use of cochlear implant. (1-2)

So, we had tried a transcutaneous electrotherapy in any cases of severe tinnitus whatever had been the audition.

Since 1981 we have reported that about 1/3 of patients experience considerable relief following such a transcutaneous electrotherapy. (3-4)

We felt it would be of interest to review our 566 cases, the more so as reviewing some patients, for other pathologies some months or years later, their results seemed not so good as we thought.

MATERIEL AND METHODS

The stimulation has been standardized by using the "MEDTRONIC'S NEUROMOD BICANAL", wich supplies with square waves, 0.08 ms in duration, a range from 0 to 10 volts, and 2 sorts of frequency : either a square wave at 85Hz, or a salve of 7 impulsions at 3Hz.

Since some months, we have used a simultaneous electrical and acoustical stimulation. The electrical stimulation is a sinusoïd wave at 144 Hz ; the acoustical stimulation is a decreasing sound (250Hz, from 50 to 100dB) during 10 secondes, delivered 6 times a minute.

In both type of therapy, the treatment is half an hour long.

The therapy has been begun after research of an etiology and failure of usual therapeutic attempts.

Before begining a precise information is given to patients concerning the results that may wait. Indeed, during stimulation, they can notice faint or none modification of their tinnitus, that must be considered as a failure. On the contrary a definite improvement with post-effect during some hours to some days will be a succes. At least 4 tests are necessary in order to use the two types of frequency and, so, to juge wether if the test is positive (T+) or negative (T-). When less than 4 tests has been performed, results are said uncertain (T?).

It is very important to advise patient that tinnitus cannot be cured by such an electrical stimulation. As well as can be, he will feel an improvement during some days.

When the tests are positive we propose to continue the therapy either at the hospital or at home by renting or buying a device.

In order to know the results months or years later, we investigated asking the patients if electro stimulation had been a success (R+) or a failure (R-).

RESULTS AND DISCUSSION

Of the 566 patients tested since 6 months at least, 24.9% had a positive test, 40.6% a negative test and 34.5% a uncertain test.

We can admit the pessimist hypothesis of considering all the uncertain test as negative. So, only 24.9% of patients would be really positive.

In the other hand, we could omit this uncertain group and study the 371 patients with complete tests. In this case we have 38% of positive test, this rate corresponding to the results we have already published some years ago.

Concerning the investigation, we have got 224 responses (39.6%) with a positive response in only 15,6% and negative in 84,3% of cases. This discordance of positive results between tests and responses could have been induced by an inequal repartition of responses among the different test groups, and more precisely a majority of responses among the negative test group. But, in fact, there is no significant difference (37.6% ± 8 in T+ ; 39.1% ± 6.4 in T- and 41.5% ± 7 in T?). So the three groups answered the same rate.

The detail of responses in each group shows that in positive test-group there are 37.7% of positive response. In negative test group there are 98.9% of negative response, one patient noticing a spontaneous good result after 5 negative tests which could be a coincidence. At last, in uncertain test-group there are 17,3% of positive responses.

By calculation we can know what would have been this uncertain test-group if the test had been complete and so distribute it in the 2 groups, with a theorical result of 40,8% of positive test wich is statistically similar to the results when we suppress the uncertain test-group.

So, it is the optimist hypothesis which is true.

How explain the discordance between the results confessed by the patient during tests and later by the investigation ?

We have studied several criteria without finding any correlation with the different results. These criteria are sex, age, duration, breakdown, etiology, type of tinnitus, side and intensity noticed on a psychophysical scale. The number of cases in each etiology is too small to allow a significative study.

Eventhough the relation is evident between intensity and presence of breakdown (53% when intensity is >12 and 33% when intensity is <12) we have not found more failures in these cases .

As for the simultaneous electrical and acoustical stimulation, only ten patients have a sufficent delay of study. But we can consider this technic does not bring something more in so far as it is possible to conclude with a so little sample of patients.

One can think that a part of patients has been disappointed not to be really cure eventhough they had been informed about expected results.

Other considered as a failure, the impossibility to continue the therapy. Indeed many patients do not live in Paris and in their country they could not be cured by a specialist. In the other hand, many people living in Paris could not come in hospital for professional reasons (50% of patients are less than 60 years old) or for physical problems (20% are more than 70 years old).

As for renting or buying a device, it was very often refused for economical reasons, social insurance do not yet helping these patients.

At last we can think about the psychotherapic effect of the test, the patient having a repeated contact with the otologist and hoping a great success by this technic.

Whatever is the explanation of this discordance we must wonder what is the true rate of success between 15% and about 1/3 of patients. This uncertainty must lead us to refine the tests, to try to better understand the physiopathology of each case of tinnitus and to look for other sorts of electroherapy such as stimulation by an implanted device in the middle ear. Indeed, we have noticed as other authors (5), the high frequency of success concerning tinnitus by using cochlear implant wich contrasts with the modest results with transcutaneous electrotherapy.

REFERENCES

1) HATTON D.S., ERULKAR S.D., ROSENBERG P.E., (1960) Some preliminary observations on the effect of galvanic current on tinnitus arium. Laryngoscope 70 /123-130.

2) PIALOUX P., CHOUARD C.H., MEYER B., FUGAIN C., (1979). Indications and results of the multichannel cochlear implant. Acta Otolaryngol (Stockh) 87 : 185-189.

3) CHOUARD C.H., MEYER B., MARIDAT D., (1981). Transcutaneous electrotherapy for severe tinnitus. Acta Otolaryngol (Stockh) 91 : 415-422.

4) CHOUARD C.H., MARIDAT D., LACOMBE H., CANDAU P., (1982). Traitement des bourdonnements d'oreille par stimulation électrique percutanée. Ann. Otolaryng. (Paris) 99 : 1-6.

5) THEDINGER B., HOUSE W.F., EDGERTON B.J., (1985) Cochlear implant for tinnitus. Case reports. Ann. Oto Rhinol Laryngol. 94 :10-13.

New dimensions in otorhinolaryngology - head and neck surgery, vol. 2.
E. Myers, editor

SEVERE HYPERSOMNIA AND SLEEP APNEA CAUSED BY FOODS

SORAYA HOOVER, M.D.

Disabling Hypersomnia, snoring with or without sleep apnea, has been treated by C.N.S. Stimulants, surgery of the soft palate and nasal airway with mixed results initially and definite recurrence in the patients who do not change their diet. Seven cases are presented in which this acquired sleep disorder was found to be caused by foods.

Diagnosing the sleep inducing foods was done by:

1. *In vitro estimation of the IGE by the RAST method. This identified the foods that had high IGE which they were eating daily.*
2. *Intradermal provocation with these foods followed - to single out the foods that produced sleep. The intradermal method was chosen so that the patient and the technician injecting the food antigen cannot identify the nature of the food. Not all the foods that have high IGE produce sleep; some produce heachaches, others produce post nasal drip, or any other symptom.*
3. *The patients were started on a simple rotating diet. They were instructed to eat one or two items of food every four to six hours and take note of the effects the foods gave them. They were to avoid complex foods like fruit salads, mixed salads, fried meats and breaded poultry. The neutralizing doses of the food antigens were prepared and food antigen therapy was begun. Six patients had two shots a week; one patient refused the shots so that her food antigen therapy was given in the sublingual way. It was found that therapy helped them to eliminate the foods and decreased their craving for them.*
4. *By the end of the first week, the patients had managed to eliminate the sleep inducing foods completely. As the change started, they became more alert and felt like their old selves as they were prior to the onset of the sleep disorder. In three months they started re-introducing the sleep inducing foods once every two weeks and then slowly once a week. It was found that they were able to do so. However, they would get severe hypersomnia if they indulged again in those foods.*

	Sex	Age	Color	Obesity	Nasal Airway Obstr.	Soft palate size & movs.
1.	M	40	W	present	partial	normal
2.	M	36	W	present	complete	normal
3.	F	29	B	no	intermittent	normal
4.	M	40	B	no	partial	normal
5.	F	52	W	present	partial	normal
6.	F	32	W	no	intermittent	normal
7.	F	61	W	no	intermittent	normal

The Sleep Inducing Foods

Case 1 -	Case 2 -	Case 3 -	Case 4 -	Case 5 -	Case 6 -	Case 7 -
Wheat	Wheat	Rice	Beef	Wheat	Wheat	Milk
eggs	corn	corn	corn	onions	pecans	peanuts
	pork	pork	eggs		bananas	bananas
	fish	cheese	fish			
	potatoes					

Discussion

It was found that food generates an action potential in the buccal mucosa. This was measured by means of micro electrode techniques (11). The action potential was also measured in the same manner to drop with the intradermal prick. Those initiate a nervous stimulus that is carried by the nerve axon to other synthesized nerve cells and the hypthalamus is stimulated. It is assumed that the sleep center in the anterior hypothalamus is the target organ for these allergic reactions. In experimental animals, stimulation of the anterior hypothalamus produces sleep. On the other hand, bilateral distruction of the anterior hypothalamus causes the animal to die from severe exhaustion due to intense wakefulness. Herberg (3) noted the striking similarity between the prodromal stage of migrane and lesions of the anterior hypothalamus, especially regarding hypersomnia, hyperphagia and fluid retention. Also, the hypothalamus area (2,10) was found to allow penetration of food antigens that will produce further stimulation of that area. Serotonin is secreted by the sleep areas while the wakefulness areas in the lateral hypothalamus secrete norepinephrine (14). Measured increase in plasma serotonin and norepinephrine after consumption of eggs in a case of eggs induced bradycardia and severe chest pain. This shows hypothalamic stimulation by the eggs antigen reaction *that was transmitted via the para sympathetic system and phagus nerve to the heart.*

AUTONOMIC CONTROL CENTERS OF THE BRAIN

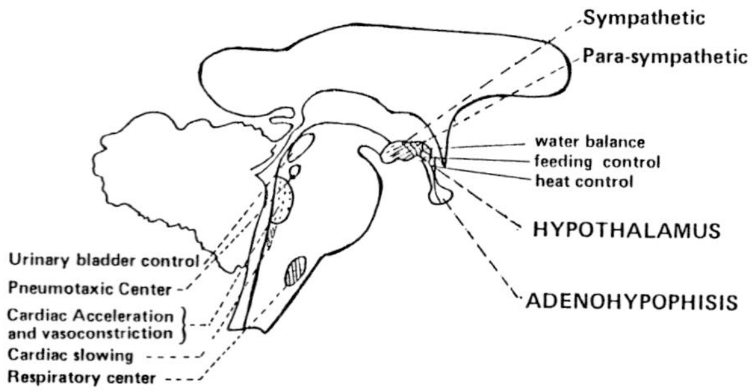

Treatment by eliminating the sleep inducing foods corrects the sleep disorder as well as they hyperphagia and the fluid retention. It is believed that the acquired hypersomnia, snoring and sleep apnea is caused by the engorged congested soft tissue in the pharynx, soft palate, base of the tongue and nasal airway areas. And this is why the uvulo-palatopharyngo-plasty has such a high rate of of recurrence in the patients that do not change their diets. The improved airway is believed to increase the P02 and will stimulate the wakefulness center

in the *<u>lateral</u>* *hypothalamus. Also, by cutting out the soft palate, there is less tissue to be engorged and lax due to the effect of those sleep inducing foods on the hypothalamus. The second patient had severe nasal airway obstruction, large tonsils and an adenoid pad-like shadow on the lateral x-ray film of the neck. He refused any surgery. Eliminating the sleep inducing foods, together with the food antigen therapy, controlled his sleep disorder and he is back working now. E.E.G.'s done on cases 1,2 4 after eating the sleep inducing foods showed a pattern of sleep and when the EEG's were repeated after giving the neutralizing dose of the food antigens by injection, the pattern reverted to normal. This confirms that stimuli from the buccal mucosa and from the injection site in the arm have been transmitted to the cerebral cortex.*

Follow-up of Cases 6 and 7 is four years now and the rest varies between 1 year, 4 months and 3 years. Case one had this disorder for four years and was on Retalin three times a day. He was disabled due to his hypersomnia. He wets and soils when asleep. He has been recovered now for the past two years.

<u>Summary</u>

This presentation involves seven patients with severe hypersomnia and snoring, two of which have sleep apnea. Diagnosing the sleep inducing foods accurately was discussed. Treatment was successful by elimination of these foods together with food antigen therapy either by injection or sublingual. Discussion of the mechanism involved in stimulation of the sleep center in the hypothalamus was presented.

<u>References</u>

1. *Food Allergy in Migrane, J. Monro, J. Brostoff, C. Carni, K. Zikha. The Lancet. July 5, 1980.*
2. *The Entry into the Brain of Large Molecules Derived From Dietary Protein. Hemings W.A. (1967 a & b). The Proceedings of the Royal Society London Series B, 200, 175.*
3. *The Hypothalamus and Aminergic Pathways in Migrane, L.J. Herberg. Modern Topics (Ed. by Pearce, J.) Cap 9 Wm. Heinmann Medical Books Ltd., London.*
4. *Is Migrane Food Allergy, E.J. Wilson, J. Carter, C.M. et al. Lancet 1983, 2 (8355)(865-8).*
5. *Blockade by Antidepressants Selectively Block Nor-epinephrine Uptake. European J. of Pharmacology 104 (1984) 277-286. Richelson & M. Pfenning.*
6. *Clinical Features of Migrane as a Manifestation of Allergic Disease. C.W.M. Wilson, J.G. Kirker, H. Warnes, M. O'Malley. Post Graduate Medical J. Sept. 1980 56, 617-621.*
7. *Is Migrane a Manifestation of Food Allergy? R.N. Podell, Post Graduate Medical Journal 54, 231, Jonson E.S., 1978.*
8. *A Basis for Migrane Therapy - The Autonomic Theory Re-appraised. Post Graduate Medical Journal 54, 231. Jonson E.S., 1978.*

9. *Absence of the Blood Brain Barrier from Certain Areas of the C.N.S., Journal of Pharmacology 132, 133. Wilson C.W.M. & Brodie B.B., 1961.*

10. *The effect of Reserpine on Uptake of Epinephrine in Brain and Certain Areas Outside the Blood Brain Barrier, Wilson C.W.M., Murray, A.W. and Titus, 1962, Journal of Pharmacology 135, 11.*

11. *An Alternative Hypothesis for the Immune Response Based on the Buccal Absorption and Action of Sodium Cromoglycate, Wilson C.W.M. and Sharma S.C. (1979) The Mast Cell, Ed. by Pepys J & Edward A.M., p. 455, Pitman Publishing Co., London.*

12. *Recognition of Food Allergic Patients and Their Allergins by the Rast Technique, Wraith, Merret, Roth, Yman and T.G. Merret. Clinical Allergy, 1979, Vol 9, pages 25-36.*

13. *Clinical Ecology, Dickey L.D., Editory, Springfield, Illinois, 1976.*

14. *Report of a Case of Eggs Induced Bradycardia and Severe Chest Pain, Antonetti C., Hoover S. (to be published).*

© 1985 Elsevier Science Publishers B.V. (Biomedical Division)
New dimensions in otorhinolaryngology - head and neck surgery, vol. 2.
E. Myers, editor

THE ROLE OF HYDROGEN PEROXIDE-INDUCED HISTAMINE RELEASE FROM HUMAN BASOPHILS

HIROSHI OGASAWARA*, TETSUZO FUJITANI, ELLIOT MIDDLETON JR**

* Dept. of Otolaryngology,Hyogo College of Medicine,Mukogawacho,Nishinomiya 663 Japan. ** State University of New York,Buffalo,NY,USA.

INTRODUCTION

During the phagocytosis by polymorphonuclear leukocytes and monocytes, oxygen consumption is increased, active oxygen is generated, and glucose catabolism through the hexose monophosphate pathway is increased. Rat mast cells and human mast cells as well as human leukemic basophils induce parallel release of superoxide anion (O_2^-) and histamine by anti-IgE[1]. Rat mast cells induce release of histamine by xanthine oxidase and hypoxanthine, and hydrogen peroxide (H_2O_2)[2]. We measured histamine release (HR) by human leukocyte suspension enriched in basophils mixed with neutrophil or eosinophil fraction and opsonized zymosan, and studied the effect of H_2O_2 on HR from human basophils.

MATERIAL AND METHODS

The dextran plasma was collected from heparinized venous blood from allergic patients. 1.099, 1.091, 1.078 and 1.071 g/ml Percoll solution and cell suspension were carefully overlaid from bottom to top in a polypropylene tube. The tube was centrifuged at 1600G for 20 min, then we collected from each layer in 2.5X10^6/ml the cell fractions rich in monocytes and lymphocytes, basophils, neutrophils, and eosinophils. Histamine was determined by a fluorometric technique ,O_2^- generation was measured by reduction of 50 uM ferricytochrome C, and H_2O_2 generation was measured by the horseradish peroxidase-scopoletin fluorescence technique. Data are expressed as means±SD. Significance was determined by the paired student t-test.

RESULS

When basophils (Ba 3.1,Mo 3.0,Ly 93.8,Ne 0.1%) were incubated with opsonized zymosan, HR was 3.1±3.1%, and O_2^- and H_2O_2 were not generated. But addition of neutrophils (Ne 98.8,Ly 0.9,Eo 0.3%) into the above suspension resulted in a significant increased of HR to 15.7±1.1% ($P<0.05$), O_2^- generation to 1.629 nmol/min, and H_2O_2 generation to 0.238 nmol/min. Also, addition of eosinophils (Eo 89.0, Ne 9.8, Ly 1.2%) resulted in a significant increased of HR to 14.8±2.0%, O_2^- generation to 2.813 nmol/min, and H_2O_2 generation to 0.306 nmol/min. When a catalase was added to neutrophil-opsonized zymosan mixture, H_2O_2 generation was decreased by 73.8% and HR was decreased by 58.7%. Alpha-tocopherol did not decrease H_2O_2 generation, but HR was decreased by 33.8%. Superoxide disumutase and D-mannitol did not decrease either HR or H_2O_2 generation. When basophils were suspended in cell-free supernatants in which $2.5x10^6$ neutrophils had been treated previously with opsonized zymosan, HR was seen, but catalase inhibited these HR. Therefore, this HR from basophils was caused mainly by H_2O_2 and partly by singlet oxygen.

H_2O_2-induced HR reached a plateau in 20 min. As shown in the figure, the maximum HR was observed in concentration of 20 to 100 uM H_2O_2, but less or higher concentration of H_2O_2 showed low HR. Low concentration of H_2O_2 seemed to augment anti-IgE or Dermatophagoides farinae-mediated HR. But, both HR were inhibited in high concentration of H_2O_2. Forty minutes incubation with 100uM H_2O_2 and anti-IgE reduced HR by 79% compared with anti-IgE alone, and further 40 min incubation inhibited HR completly. By addition of catalase after 40 min incubation, HR was enhanced by 137%. H_2O_2-induced HR was Ca^{++} and glucose dependent, and also inhibited by 2-deoxy-glucose. Theophylline which increased the cyclic-AMP did not have an effect on H_2O_2-induced HR.

DISCUSSION

These studies demonstrate that HR from cell fractions rich in human basophils was produced by incubation with autologous neutrophils or eosinophils and opsonized zymosan. This HR was caused mainly by H_2O_2, and not by complement or another substance. 100 uM H_2O_2 was not cytolytic, and H_2O_2-induced HR was Ca^{++} and energy dependent and cyclic-AMP independent, like A23187 or strontium-induced HR. Previous study of the effect of 3 flavonoids (quercetin,taxifolin,apigenin) on anti-IgE-stimulated HR and H_2O_2 generation, suggested that H_2O_2 was not required for HR but was another aspect of basophi activation. The present results suggest that low concentration of H_2O_2 potentiates the release process, however, a high concentration of H_2O_2 protects the release process. On the other hand, extracellular H_2O_2 was soon reduced by neutrophils or eosinophils in the same manner. H_2O_2 plays a significant role on HR from basophils in vivo in patients allergic or nonallergic diseases.

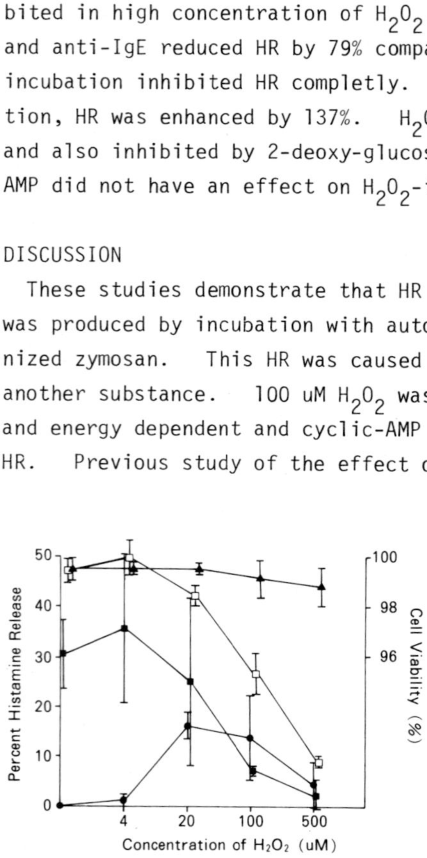

The effect of H_2O_2 on HR.
The data present as the mean+SD of 2 experiments with triplicate samples. H_2O_2 alone(●—●), H_2O_2+anti-IgE(■—■), H_2O_2+D.farinae (□—□), cell viability(▲—▲).

REFERENCES

1. Henderson WR,Kaliner M, J Clin Invest 61: 187,1978.
2. Ohmori H etc,Biochem Pharmacol 29:741, 1980.

New dimensions in otorhinolaryngology - head and neck surgery, vol. 2.
E. Myers, editor

CLINICAL EFFECT OF NEW ANTI-ALLERGIC DRUG, TRANILAST, IN NASAL ALLERGY

SATOSHI OGINO, ICHIRO OKAWACHI, TAMOTSU HARADA, MORIHIRO IRIFUNE AND TORU MATSUNAGA
Department of Otolaryngology, Osaka University Medical School, Osaka (Japan)

INTRODUCTION

Recently, the patients suffering from nasal allergy has been markedly increasing in Japan. Several kinds of therapies are available for the treatment of this disease, and drug therapy can occupy an important position. In the drug therapy, besides anti-histamines and corticosteroids, drugs which inhibit the release of chemical mediators from mast cells have recently been researched, developed and used. DSCG(disodium cromoglycate) is a typical drug in this category. In this study, we have used Tranilast, a new anti-allergic drug originated in Japan. This compound has the same mechanism as DSCG, but can be given orally unlike DSCG. We have studied clinical effects of Tranilast on nasal allergy.

DRUG

Tranilast is a compound of a cinnamic acid derivative extracted from leaves of nandin or Nandina Domestica, and antranilic acid. Its chemical name is N-(3,4-dimethoxycinnamoyl) antranilic acid and in Japan its pharmaceutical preparaions are called Rizaben.

SUBJECTS AND METHODS

The subjects were those suffering from nasal allergy who visited our Allergy Clinic and the other 9 participating institutions from July 1983 through Februaly 1984. Patients were diagnosed from allergic skin test, RAST, nasal provocation test and eosinophils in nasal discharge. One capsule containing 100mg of Tranilast was given to adults three times daily, and to children a daily dosage of 5mg/kg was divided into 3 times. All patients were treated for 4 weeks or longer.

RESULTS AND DISCUSSION

The subjects were 104 cases in total; 63 males and 41 females. The improvement rates after 4 weeks of administration were 78.6%

for sneezing, 76.2% for nasal discharge, and 63.2% for nasal obstruction.

When the overall efficacy was compared by the length of administration period, the rate of effectiveness tended to become higher as the administration period was prolonged.

The time of appearance of efficacy was studied, and in 22 cases (21.2%) the efficacy became apparent within 1 week and in 58 cases (55.8%) within 2 weeks, showing in more than a half of the patients the efficasy was manifested within 2 weeks. Generally speaking, the onset of efficacy of this drug seems rather slow.

The effect were studied according to the background factors. Though in many factors there was no significant difference in efficacy, significant differences in effectiveness were detected with age, age of onset and IgE values. Regarding age, younger patients showed higher effectiveness. A similar tendency was seen with the age of onset. Those who had the age of onset at 5 years old or younger showed the highest effectiveness rate. When the subjects were divided into two groups at a serum IgE values of 400IU/ml, a group having 400IU/ml or higher showed better effects than the other group of lower than 400IU/ml.

In one patients an adverse effect of slight abdominal pain was noted, but the medication could be continued.

In the studies on the action of Tranilast, it has been reported to inhibit homologous passive cutaneous anaphylaxis and rat experimental asthma in a dose-dependent manner, and also inhibit rabbit Arthus reaction.[1,2] However, the drug does not inhibit spontaneous histamine release or affect histamine release induced by Compound 48/80. Additionally Tranilast does not show any direct anti-histaminic effects. Clinically Tranilast was found to be effective on asthma in a well-controlled double blind trial.[3]

As mentioned above, although the onset of effects of Tranilast was rather slow, the drug was found to be safe and effective on nasal allergy. And especially in children and those whose onset of the disease was in childhood excellent effects were obtained.

REFERENCES

1. Koda A, et al (1976) J Allergy Clin Immunol 57:396-407
2. Azuma H, et al (1976) Br J Pharmac 58:483-488
3. Yamamura Y, et al (1979) Igaku No Ayumi 108:252-273

New dimensions in otorhinolaryngology - head and neck surgery, vol. 2.
E. Myers, editor

THE RUNNING NOSE. ITS TREATMENT

ROGER ROOS
2 Rue du Vieux Marché aux Vins STRASBOURG 67000 (FRANCE)

The Running Nose is a very common discomfort and one of the most frequent causes for Ear Nose and Throat consultation. Many patients suffer from what they call a year around cold. Very often the patient himself or herself will make a very precise differential diagnosis eliminating first a vasomotor rhinitis because the airway is not obstructed, an acute infection because these are no signs of infection and finally an allergy such as hay fever which occurs between May and September because the chronic running nose runs all year round and more so in winter and the flow is waterlike wetting the handkerchief.

The case history of most patients is one of many years of discomfort. Some patients have been suffering from this aperiodic rhinitis for 10 or 20 years or more. Usually all sorts of treatments have already been tried to no effect.

The lack of success in treating this rhinitis often leads the patient to an allergologist. Desensitization however almost always fails even though skin tests are positive.

It is this case history which made me try another approach.

DIAGNOSIS

The main symptom of aperiodic rhinitis is a running nose. This flow is aperiodic. It has no season and is a chronic all year round symptom appearing even when there is a low pollen concentration and no hay fever in winter.

Skin tests permitted to conclude that patients afflicted with aperiodic rhinitis practically always have positive tests to microbes.

The skin test. This test is done by a sub cutaneous injection of 0,1 milliliter of C. C. B. vaccine.

The C. C. B. vaccine is a product of the Institut Pasteur in France and is composed of bacteria killed by heat and put in an isotonic solution of sodium chloride (Nacl).

For 1 ml of C. C. B. vaccine :

Streptococcus groups A D G K .... 2 500 million
(hemolyticus and viridans)
Neisseria Catarrhalis and Flava .... 750 million
Pneumococcus .... 750 million.

The test usually has a late reaction and can be read after 12 hours. Usually the test is strongly positive with a little oedema and a large red halo. The patient must be warned about this.

TREATMENT

We desensitize our patients using the Proetz technique.

In 20 cc of a physiological saline solution we put 0,2 ml of C. C. B. vaccine. At the next sitting we put 0,4 ml of C. C. B. in 20 cc of saline. Then at the next sitting we put 0,8 ml of C. C. B. and at the next sitting 1,6 ml of C. C. B. At the last sitting 2 ml are used diluted in 20 cc of physiological saline solution. A laps of three or four days is left between two sittings.

RESULTS AND FOLLOW UP

After the third sitting the patient usually notices the first results and the nose becomes normal after the fifth and last sitting. In other words the nose no longer drips and runs.

Just like in other desensitizations the results are not durable if the patient is not followed up. We favor a perennial type of desensitization seeing the patient three times a year for a recall of the desensitization. We do this once in September, once in January and once in April. For the recall we use 1 ml of C. C. B. vaccine in 20 cc of saline. Usually we follow the patient for four or five years and then stop the desensitization.

CONCLUSION

Our results with this technique over the past fifteen years have been excellent. In case of a recurrence after having stopped the desensitization for a few years one can always start all over again with the same good results. I have also used this technique in cases of chronic atrophic rhinitis with fairly good results.

© 1985 Elsevier Science Publishers B.V. (Biomedical Division)
New dimensions in otorhinolaryngology - head and neck surgery, vol. 2.
E. Myers, editor

GASTRIC MUCOSAL PATTERN IN ALLERGIC RHINITIS

DR. S. SELVANARAYANAN

INTRODUCTION

Allergic rhinitis is common in women amounting to 60% of the cases examined. We observed that some of the patient with nasal Allergy were also found to have received antacids and antichlinergic treatment for their "Gas" problem.

Patients of nasal allergy complained the symptoms being worse in the early morning hours when the acid content of the stomach is high, compared with the rest of the day even though they live in the same antigenic surroundings throughout the day.

This observation initiated us to take up this study as to correlate allergy-acid relationship. Thus we have taken up 80 cases of allergic rhinitis and studied the fractional test meal.

MATERIAL AND METHODS

Cases with the history of sneezing, rhinorrhea and nasal stuffiness and itching sensation in the nasal cavity were chosen in the age group of 15 to 50 years. Amongst these 48 were females. 32 were males and 20 control subjects. Patients who were on corticosteroids or Antihistamines or analgesics or oral contraceptives or oral Antihypertensive drugs were excluded.

PROCEDURE

Ryle's tube is passed in the morning hours on empty stomach and the resting contents are aspirated and analysed. One print of the barley gruel is administued and time noted. Samples of gastric contents are aspirated every 15 minutes for 2½ hours and analysed. Titration was done with IN NAOH using Topher's indicator for free acid and phenolpthalein indicator for total acid, and plotted against the graph.

INFERENCE

In our series 36 cases had shown free acidity in the resting juice varying between 20-40 units and total acidity exceeding beyond 30 units. Following gruel free acidity exceeded 60 units and total acidity 80 units.

DISCUSSION

In allergic states the antigen antibody reaction results in the release of histamine which is responsible for all the symptoms locally in the nose. The same substance viz., the released histamine may activate the gastric mucosa thereby increasing the free acid content of the stomach.

The frequency of aspirin tolerance in the asthmatic group is an undebtable fact and the rate of asprin sensitivity in patients with rhinitis alone was found to be 0.7%.

It is observed Ulcero-genic drugs like asprin and indomethocin make the individual more susceptible for allergic rhinitis, possibly, by activation of the complement pathway, and through mediator mechanism i.e., degrannulation of the mast cells and thus liberation of histamine. It is not that the nasal mucosa is already sensitised for the drug but the nasal mucosa is the target tissue for the change in P.H. of the stomach that is conveyed to the nasal tissue by humoral mechanism. This fact may explain why food allergy is always accompanied by inhalant allergy.

Flemstrona and coworkers 1976 suggest that asprin may contribute to sensitization and allergic reactions to potentially antigenic food materials by facilitating their easy absorption from the stomach. The high incidence of sensitivity to foodstuffs in asprin sensitive individual would be one argument in support of this suggestion.

CONCLUSION

In allergic rhinitis which results from antigen antibody reaction, the histamine released from the nasal tissue, induces the parietal cells of the stomach and thus the acidity. Even though, the direct estimation of the nasal histamine content and the severity of the antigen and antibody reaction could not be done, we can estimate indirectly by measuring the free acidity of the gastric juice. Thus, it was proposed to take up a comparative study to correlate the nasal allergy with free acidity of the stomach.

REFERENCES

1. M.H. LESSOR - Immunological and Clinical Aspects of Allergy 42-43, 54.
2. FREDERIC SPEER - Food Allergy 8-9 (1983)
3. M.H. LESSOR - Clinical reactions to food 111, 136-137, 140, 143.
4. Aspects of Allergy & Applied Immunology R. VISWANATHAN & R.K. SANYAL 91-105-113.
5. Text Book of Biochemistry - A.V.S.S. RAMARAO 170-177
6. Asprin and the Salicilates - K.D. RAINSFORD - 102 - 236-237
7. Biogenesis and Physicology of Histamine - GEORGE KAHLSON AND ELSA ROSENGREN 95-162.

© 1985 Elsevier Science Publishers B.V. (Biomedical Division)
New dimensions in otorhinolaryngology – head and neck surgery, vol. 2.
E. Myers, editor

ASPIRIN SENSITIVITY, BRONCHIAL ASTHMA AND NASAL POLYPS. MEDICAL AND SURGICAL ASPECTS FOR THE OTOLARYNGOLOGIST

ISAAC SHUBICH, M.D.

Chairman, Dept. Of Otolaryngology. Children's Hospital.
Mexico City, Mexico

INTRODUCTION

Sensitivity to A.S.A as well as cross sensitivity to non steroid anti- inflamatory drugs (NSAID) has been documented together with bronchial asthma, as part of the clinical problem on this patients, since 1919 by Cooke [1].

Samter, Beers and others, observed the frequent presentation of rhinosinusitis and nasal polyps, completing the classical triad. Patients that refered idiosincrasy to dyes and other chemical compounds, such as tartrazine, parabens, antioxidants, sodium benzoate & others, were also described [2].

Due to the relative frequency and importance of this problem, which the practicing Otolaryngologist faces, this paper was selected in order to contribute for it's proper management.

MATERIAL AND METHODS

Between 1979 and 1984, a total of 18 patients were studied and followed for a minimum of 6 months, up to 5 years.

The age range was of 18 to 69 years when first seen. The mean age was 44 years old, corresponding to 10 female and 8 male patients. The study included a complete history & physical examination, routine laboratory tests, immunological and allergy workup (Immunoglobulins, skin test to inhalant antigens, RAST and nasal cytology), pulmonary function tests in most of the patients, Chest and paranasal sinus X rays, and on 4 patients, a challenge test to tartrazine (azo- yellow), was done. Medical and surgical aspects of the management, as well as other measures, such as pulmonary rehabilitation, were recorded.

TABLE 1.
CLINICAL DISTRIBUTION N: 18

No. Of Patients: F/M	* A.S.A Sens.	Bronchial spasm	Polyps & Rhinosinusitis
Female/Male	9/8	9/8	8/7
Age range	(22-60)	(18-69)	(18-69)
Mean age	39	44	44
N.S.A.I.D cross-sen.	8/7	Dye reactions	1/4

* Female/male (only one female without A.S.A sensitivity, but positive to N.S.A.I. D.

TABLE 2.

DIAGNOSIS: Positive findings.

	Sinus X Rays	Chest X Rays	Atopy Immunol	Pumonary funct.
Female pts. N: 10	9 pts.	3 pts.	3 pts.	4 pts.
Male pts. N: 8	7 pts.	3 pts.	3 pts.	2 pts.

TABLE 3.

MEDICAL THERAPY.

N: 18

	No. Of pts. treated
Bronchodilators	17
Steroids (inhaled)	16
Antihistamines	16
Steroids (oral or IM)	13
Antibiotics	11
Acetominophen	9
Antichlinergic (local or syst.)	9
Cromolyn (inhaled)	6
Sympathostimulants	6
Ketothiphen	4
Other drugs (not related)	15

TABLE 4.

SURGICAL THERAPY/ OTHER MEASURES.

N:18

	No. Of pts. treated
Caldwell- Luc/ethmoid surgery	6
Intranasal polypectomy	12
Septoplasty	7
Vidian neurectomy	2
Inhalant immunotherapy	6
Physical (pulmonary) rehab.	16
A.S.A desensitization program	4

RESULTS

The overall result with medical, surgical & other neasures recorded was the following:

4 patients seen from 6 months up to 4 years, had a good result: no recurrence of asthma attacks, nasal cavity free of polyps and minimal or no rhinitis. Preventive measures consisting in avoidance of all drugs & chemicals involved, has been satisfactory. One patient continues with antigen immunotherapy, and another has an aspirin desensitization program.

10 patients obtained a moderate result (6 months to 5 years of follow- up). Several signs & symptoms have reappeared, although non - severe.

Four patients have been without clinical improvement, in spite of therapy, and continue with constant care.

COMMENTS

Potential mechanisms of hypersensitivity to A.S.A and all other drugs - chemical compounds mentioned before, have been documented[3]. Prostaglandin biosynthesis inhibition at the cyclo-oxygenase pathway seems the possible explanation, with a shift to the leukotriene production & resulting tissue reaction after this.

Onset is frequent at about 18- 20 years of age; atopy has been found on 20 % of cases, nasal polyps in 60- 80 %, ocular symptoms and bronchial asthma, each up to 80 % and skin manifestations, such as urticaria or edema in 10 %. Preventive measures mainly with those drugs & chemical substances involved are important, since even a fatal overcome is a possibility. Pulmonary function tests, challenge tests and evaluation are done based upon the FEV_1 responses.[4]

REFERENCES

1. Cooke RA (1919) Allergy in drug idiosincasy. JAMA 73: 759.

2. Weber RW et al (1979) Incidence of bronchoconstriction due to aspirin, azo dyes, and preservatives in a population of perennial asthmatics. J. Allergy Clin. Immunol. 64: 32-37.

3. Poole MD, Pillsbury HC (1985) Prostaglandins and other metabolites of arachidonic acid. Arch. Otolaryngol. 111:317

4. Lumry WR, Curd JG and Stevenson DD (1984) Aspirin sensitivity asthma and rhinosinusitis: current concepts and recent advances. Ear, Nose & Throat journal. 63: 66-77.

New dimensions in otorhinolaryngology - head and neck surgery, vol. 2.
E. Myers, editor

SECRETORY OTITIS MEDIA IN CASE OF ATOPIC-ALLERGIC AND NON-ALLERGIC PATIENTS

MAGDOLNA STEPPER
Dept. of Otolaryngology, Makó-Hospital, Makó.Hungary, H-6900

Secretory otitis media /SOM/ as disturbance of Eustachian tube functions /ventillation, clearance, protection/ was at first described by Adam Politzer, an otologist of Hungarian origin in 1867. Its aetiology and correlation to different atopic-allergic and non-allergic diseases has been discussed several times since then.

MATERIAL AND METHODS

SOM occurence and its frequency have been followed by us at the Makó-Hospital,Outpatient Dept. of Allergy and Outpatient Dept. of Otolaryngology from 1979 to 1983

FREQUENCY TABLE

Cases		SOM occurence	Percentage
Atopic-allergic p.:	950	79	8.31%
Non-allergic p.	:72 650	112	0.15%

Comparisons have been made according to age and sex.No difference was found according to sex.In case of allergic patients it occured most frequently in the age group of 0-3 yrs. /10%/, while in case of non-allergic patients in the age group of 15-30 yrs. /0.23%/. SOM occured very frequently together with rhinopathia connected with food allergy and rhinitis allergica in case of atopic-allergic children,while in adults it occured most frequently together with rhinitis allergica and nasal polyposis.In childhood in the case of non-allergic patients it occured together with rhinosinusitis and adenoids while in adults it was most frequently associated with rhinosinusitis,deformity of the nasal septum, virus infection, tumors of nasopharynx.

We could differentiate between our allergic and non-allergic patients concerning the location of SOM /one-folded, Two-folded/, the time of recovery, its recidivism and the quality of middle ear effusion.

The 73.21% of non-allergic patients developed one-folded SOM, while it was only 3.80% in case allergic patients, 96.20% was two-folded. After the treatment of basic diseases, the time of recovery in case of non-allergic patients was one week in 83.04% and in all cases of allergic patients over 3 weeks.The recidivism of SOM in case of non-allergic patients was 7.14% while in case of allergic patients it was 78.48%. The type of middle ear effusion in case of non-allergic patients was serous: 91.08%, sero-mucoid: 8.92%, mucoid was not found in this group, while in case of allergic patients the middle ear effusion was serous: 2.53%, sero-mucoid: 62.03%, mucoid: 35.44%. The middle ear effusion was not tested citologically in each case, so it was not taken into account.

The therapy in case of non-allergic patients was the following: after the treatment of basic diseases we applied myringotomy and daily aspiration of effusion, and in case of necessity insertion of ventillation tube. The treatment of SOM can be the most problematic in case of allergic children, because neither children with food allergy nor children with respiratory allergy show any sign of complaint. Conductive hearing loss about 40 dB. is hardly explorable especially among children with food allergy and the environment doesn't recognise it. In the early childhood delayed speech development occured very often. In these cases myringotomy, aspiration of middle ear effusion and insertion of ventillation tube were applied and food allergy was treated, too. In case of adult allergic patients first the basic diseases and three weeks later the SOM were freed from symptoms but especially in cases of patients with nasal polyps the recidivism was very frequent even after its removal.

RESULTS

Having followed the patients of a 5-year period, the conclusion can be drawn, that there are great differences between atopic-allergic and non-allergic patients concerning the frequency of SOM, its location, time of recovery, recidivism and the quality of middle ear effusion.

Bibliographical data will be given by the author on request.

© 1985 Elsevier Science Publishers B.V. (Biomedical Division)
New dimensions in otorhinolaryngology - head and neck surgery, vol. 2.
E. Myers, editor

QUANTITATIVE NASAL PROVOCATION TEST WITH RHINOGRAPH

NOBUO USUI, AKIO IWATA, MARI UCHIYAMA, and MERI TSUKASA
Laboratory of Otorhinolaryngology Ohashi Hospital, Toho University School of Medicine, Tokyo

MATERIALS AND METHOD

We studied a method for quantitatively evaluating the response of the nasal mucous membrane to provocation using antigen disks whereby the nasal respiratory resistance is measured continuously with a rhinograph.

The test was tried on 62 patients with nasal allergy (33 males and 29 females) aged 9 yr to 66 yr (mean age : 31 yr).

RESULTS

Classification and patterns of the response curve by the nasal provocation test

The response curve in the nasal respiratory resistance provocation test was classified by patterns into six types as follows.

1) Normal type: where the provocation test is negative. 2) Incremental type: where the nasal respiratory resistance increases with the lapse of time. 3) Delayed incremental type: where the nasal respiratory resistance starts to respond after the certain lapse of time. 4) Mountain type: where the nasal respiratory resistance responds for a certain period but gradually returns to the original state. 5) Mountainvalley type: where an element of the incremental type has been superimposed upon the non-specific response, that is, the nasal respiratory resistance increases sharply at the beginning in response to the non-specific stimulation, becomes gradually stable and starts rising again with the increase in the nasal respiratory resistance by provocation itself. 6) Sharp increase-sharp decrease type: where the nasal respiratory resistance is increased sharply by non-specific stimulation and then becomes gradually stable. At one time, this type might have been evaluated to be false positive to the provocation test, but this should correctly evaluated as negative.

Analysis of the response curves by the nasal provocation test

Three parameters can be derived from the graph.

1) Rrs.N: The value of the stable nasal respiratory resistance within the initial one minute of the measurement. 2) ΔRrs.N: This is an inclication in rise when nasal respiratory resistance is increasing in the provocation test, and this can be calculated by $\tan\Theta$. This indicates the intensity of the response of the nasal mucous membrane. 3) Ta: This represents the duration for the beginning rise of nasal respiratory resistance in response to the provocation

test, reflecting the degree of the sensibility of the nasal mucous membrane.

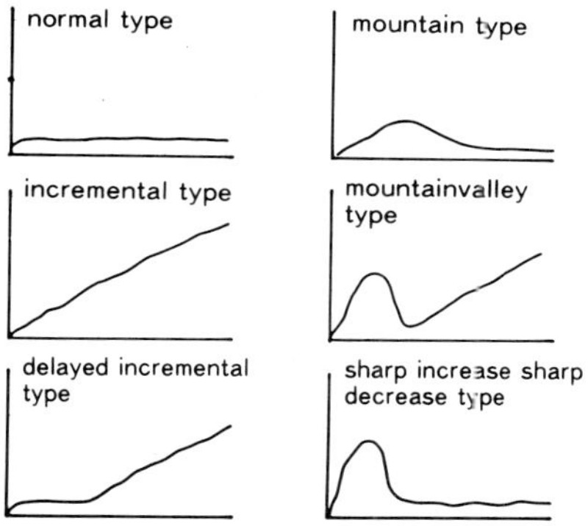

Fig. 1. Classification of the response curves in nasal respiratory resistance provocation test

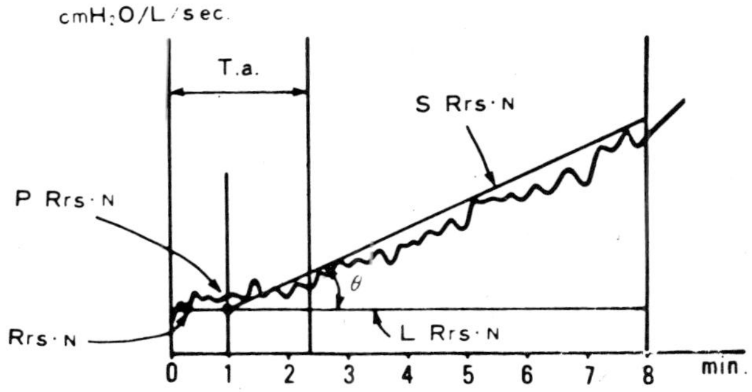

Fig. 2. The method of analysis of the response curve obtained in nasal provocation test

SUMMARY

1) The state of response to nasal provocation was represented by a graph. 2) The response curves in nasal respiratory resistance provocation test were classified into 6 types by their pattern. 3) Irrespective of whether the antigen was house dust or pollens, the pattern of response curve fell under one of the 6 categories. 4) In cases evaluated as false positive in the past while being categorized in the sharp increase-sharp decrease type in the present test, the response to provocation was negative. 5) The response curves in nasal respiratory provocation test were analyzed, and 3 parameters, Rrs.N, ΔRrs.N and Ta were obtained. 6) It was impossible to analyze the sharp increase-sharp decrease type of curves, a part of the mountainvalley type curves and the curves with Rrs.N elevated from the outset.

© 1985 Elsevier Science Publishers B.V. (Biomedical Division)
New dimensions in otorhinolaryngology - head and neck surgery, vol. 2.
E. Myers, editor

INTEGRATING ALLERGY IN OTOLARYNGIC TRAINING

ALAN J. SERRINS, M.D.

Clinical Associate Professor, Director of Allergy and Immunology Training Program, Director of the ENT Allergy Clinic, Department of Otolaryngology, University of Miami School of Medicine, Miami, Florida (USA)

It has been estimated that there are presently as many as 40 million patients in the United States who have significant upper airway allergy. Those physicians who currently include allergy as an active part of their practice number approximately 6000 including less than 2000 otolaryngologists. This would mean that there are approximately 7000 allergy patients for practicing general allergist or ENT allergist, a staggering number that could not be adequately treated by immunotherapy because of the continuous follow up that is required, unless the number of allergists is greatly increased. The otolaryngologist as the regional expert in upper respiratory anatomy, physiology and disease, is the only specialist adequately trained to properly and completely examine these areas. He is the logical physician to initially diagnose and treat these problems. Moreover, the patient or referring physician will select the otolaryngologist to evaluate complaints in the nasal-sinus areas, as well as the head and neck in general. It is up to us to adequately assess and identify these problems and treat them as ENT allergists or to refer them to those who will.

A simple one page screening allergy questionaire filled out by the patient can quickly point toward the potential candidate for further evaluation, including skin testing and immunotherapy.

If the patient has minimal or occasional symptoms, treatment with antihistamines, decongestants or topical steroids once or twice a year is sufficient. It is not sufficient for those patients with persisting or debilitating symptoms. A more detailed allergy questionaire is given to those patients selected for further evaluation in our practice and clinical teaching.

Serial endpoint titration (SET) has been the otolaryngologists primary diagnostic test for inhalant allergy since it was proposed and later published by Herbert J. Rinkel in 1949 and further refined by James Willoughby, et al.

Following the discovery of IgE by the Ishizakas in 1966, rapid development of In Vitro tests that identify specific IgE was developed by Johannson and Wide in 1967. The scoring system and technique were subsequently modified by Richard Fadal and Donald Nalebuff in 1977, which allowed for the initiation of immuno-therapy with a safe starting dose by the use of an In Vitro test (modified RAST) for the first time. Majid Ali and coworkers subsequently developed an enzymatic method of identifying specific IgE using microtitre technology.

Allergy today is increasingly understood in immunologic terms. We are treating a Type I, IgE mediated disease demonstrated by RAST or micro-Elisa. Skin tests also demonstrate IgE mediation, as well as other mediators such as SRSA (Leukotrienes), histamine, ECFA, PAF, NCF, heparin, Bradykinin, serotonin, etc.

Other immunologic methods such as immuncdiffusion and nephelometry can be used to rule out immune dysfunction and deficiency.

As an initial group chosen to evaluate the IP system for the southeastern United States during the past three years, we have accumulated convincingly reliable data from over 40,000 tests to confidently use the IP micro-Elisa as our principal inhalant allergen diagnostic technique, until 2 months ago. We were using this method in our office laboratory, and it was the accepted method for testing allergy patients in our medical school's otolaryngology training program. However, because of recent quality control problems modified (RAST) is now the exclusive In Vitro technique.

The teaching program of the University of Miami School of Medicine requires all otolaryngology residents to spend a minimum of four months in our office as part of their allergy-immunology training, as well as attending the ENT allergy clinic at the Jackson Memorial Hospital Medical Center. Clinical and Laboratory methods are emphasized. The routine workup of patients with suspected inhalant allergy is a thorough history, including a review of a detailed allergy questionaire and physical examination. Sinus x-rays are usually obtained to rule out unidentified or suspected pathology. Careful examination of the nose is followed by a nasal cytogram. Cell collection has been enhanced by using the plastic rhino-probe.

We then obtain a venous blood sample and run a CBC and nephalometric determinations of serum proteins including IgE, IgA, IgM, C3, C4 and alpha 1-antitrypsin to help rule out immune deficiency and immune dysfunction. This also gives us a baseline study prior to starting the patients in our allergy program. The remaining serum is frozen so that we can run them in batches and another aliguot is frozen to run a total IgE and a modified (RAST) specific IgE inhalant screen of ten antigens. If one or more of these assays is a Class II or higher or 2 or more class I's or higher, we then run the complete series of inhalants. I have chosen 3 panels of ten allergens that have clinical significance in the south Florida area. These panels contain a total of thirty allergens which represent a complete battery of tests. We have chosen the conservative approach in this new technique using modified RAST minus two as a starting dose. We presently confirm this with a single 4 mm intradermal wheal as a vial test. If this is below 12 mm in diameter at the end of 10 minutes, this becomes the actual starting dose. If it is greater than 12 mm we go 1 dilution weaker or until a wheal is found smaller than 12 mm and this becomes the starting dose. We then have the patient come in for weekly injections of 0.10, 0.20, 0.30, 0.40 and 0.50 ml. The next strongest dilutions are then made up with progression of the build up through the #2 dilution. Thus far, we have had no systemic reactions and minimal problems from local reactions from the modified RAST. The number of inhalants treated by this approach averages 10-15 allergens, far less than 30-35 by the serial endpoint titration. This method has earned the enthusiastic support and confidence of the technical and medical staff.

From the otolaryngology resident's standpoint, switching over to the IP micro-Elisa tests for inhalants and now the modified RAST has allowed for a greater number of patients to be tested and followed in our ENT allergy clinic.

In conclusion, an inhalant allergy workup for immediate Type I hypersensitivity to house dust mite, molds, pollens and animal danders has been replaced by modified RAST at this time. These techniques are now standard and are incorporated into the teaching program in the allergy immunology section of the Department of Otolaryngology - Head and Neck Surgery of the University of Miami School of Medicine. A private clinical faculty office, laboratory outpatient clinic and didactic instruction round out the teaching and learning experince that is required to complete the residency program.

It is the intent of those who are responsible for teaching in the Department to provide the resident staff with exposure and experience in these new laboratory methods so that they will be increasingly knowledgeable and competent in this dynamic and changing field.

Otolaryngology which has pioneered in so many aspects of medicine holds great promise for an undeniable and expanding role in allergy diagnosis and treatment.

© 1985 Elsevier Science Publishers B.V. (Biomedical Division)
New dimensions in otorhinolaryngology - head and neck surgery, vol. 2.
E. Myers, editor

VASO-MOTOR ASSESSMENT BY CUTANEOUS TESTING IN VASO-MOTOR RHINITIS

M. WAYOFF*, D.A. MONERET VAUTRIN, P. GAZEL

* E.N.T. Department, University of Medicine (54000 NANCY - FRANCE)

In many patients, allergic or not, the clinical symptomatology is modulated by personal autonomic reactions. It seems interesting to assess the general vaso-motor behaviour for each patient. We used a four substances battery for cutaneous vasomotor testing :

* Papaverine relaxes directly the smooth muscles of blood vessels.
* Acecholine leads to vaso-dilatation via a parasympathetic effect.
* Histamine is a vaso-dilatating mediator both directly and indirectly.
* 48/80 coumpound, codeine are histamino-releasing agents.

METHODOLOGY

Intracutaneous injections of these substances are located on back's skin. Different data are noticed : dilutions for which pseudo-whealing appear. Or little value for stronger dilutions such reactions are significant for 1.I00 to 1.I0 000 titrations.

I. Papaverine investigate the basal vascular tone. The lack of reaction indicated a general hypersympathicotony, especially if the tests with the three other substances are negative or weak.

2. Acecholine is injected with a scale on increasing concentrations : 0.02 mgr, 0.2 mgr, 2 mgr. Normaly, the I.I0 test is the only to give a wheal less than or equal to 25 mm. In some cases, an important reaction was seen with the first or second concentration, this increased reactivity being in favour of a cholinergic mechanism for the vasomotor rhinitis.

3. Histamine reactivity was studied with a series of increasing concentrations : 0.I0, 0.I, 1 and I0 µg. In the normal 20 to 40 years subject (most often the case for V.M.R. patients), the reaction threshold seemed to be about 1 µg..

4. 48/80 is used to study the patients histamine releasing potential. We used doses of I0, 1, 0.I and 0.0I µg. The criteria used were the same as with histamine. We separated thus those patients who presented an increased suceptibility to histamine whilst having a normal histamine releasing potential.

The vasomotor tests are very sensitive, and can be modified by small doses of neuroleptic, anti-histamine or anti-cholinergic drugs. These tests are also perfectly reproducible in the same patient several months later. They are always carried out in parallel to allergic skin tests. The reactions to various allergens is better interpreted when the patient's vasomotor behaviour is known. For many patients, this assessment is completed by an isoprenaline perfusion test, calcemia, magnesemia, electromyographic study. The goal of this investigation is to demonstrate clinical and biological features of neural and cellular non-specific hyper-excitability.

RESULTS

This methodology was developed in a prospective study of 405 patients (222 men and I83 women).

Allergic rhinitis 48 %, Vaso-motor rhinitis 35 %, Mixed forms I7 %.

History, clinical symptomatology, rhinoscopy, X.rays do not drive towards a precise etio-pathology. Autonomic system dysbalance play a major part in the expressivity of clinical picture and his correction enhances always other treatments, in atopic as well as in pseudoallergic patients.

We think that the vaso-motor assessment by cutaneous tests is a very prac-tictal sight for "in vivo" pathological processes evaluation and consequently for treatment decision making.

Thus, in the vaso-motor rhinitis group, we found 62 to 68 %, with non-specific hyperexcitability, 56 %; with histamine hypersensibility; 46 % Mg++ globular deficiency.

CLINICAL AND DIAGNOSIS APPLICATION

In 60 %, a predominant vaso-motor disturbance seems to be obvious. We can separate 3 main types of vaso-motor rhinitis :

I. Histamine rhinitis (30 to 45 %), which is clinically similar to the allergic rhinitis.

2. Sympathetic (hyperreactivity) or angiospastic rhinitis (20 to 25 %) : sneezing fits are frequent, RAYNAUD'S phenomenon often present. Skin reactions to papaverine are either weak or absent, making it impossible to interpret the reactions to the other test drugs. The isoprenaline test is positive. Non specific hypersensitivity is frequent.

3. Cholinergic rhinitis (IO %) : It is very badly tolerated by the patient.

REFERENCES

I. Van Cauwenberge P, Grote JJ (I984) Nasal hypernasality. Scientific Soc for Med Information, Gent Belgium

2. Wayoff M, Moneret-Vautrin DA and Al (I980) Diagnostic étiopathogénique des rhinites vaso-motrices. Acta ORL belg 34:II9-I30

New dimensions in otorhinolaryngology - head and neck surgery, vol. 2.
E. Myers, editor

ULTRASTRUCTURE OF THE MUSCLE SPINDLE IN THE ARYTENOID MUSCLE OF HUMAN LARYNX

M.HIRAYAMA (1)*, M.MACHINO (2)**, M.TACHIBANA (3)**, AND O.MIZUKOSHI (4)**
Dept. of Otorhinolaryngology,
* Matsushita Hospital,Osaka, 570
** Kyoto Prefectural University of Medicine, Kyoto, Japan

INTRODUCTION

Muscle spindles are skeletal muscle proprioceptors that are highly sensitive to the length and tension of the muscle fibers among which they lie.
Mammalian muscle spirdles generally contain at least two kinds of intrafusal fibers : nuclear bag fibers.and nuclear chain fibers. However, the intrinsic muscles of the human larynx have not been studied in such detail.
The pattern of innervation of the intrafusal fibers by fusimctor axon is of interest when exploring how control is effected. Here are presented the two types of intrafusal fibers that we found having nerve endings in the arytenoid muscle.

MATERIALS AND METHODS.

A muscle of the human larynx, the arytenoid muscle, was obtained after a laryngectomy. This muscle was fixed in 2% glutaraldehyde and post fixed in 1% Osmium tetroxide.

The specimen was embbeded in Epon 812 and serially sectioned 20μm thick using a steel knife. Sections including one muscle spindle, which was the only one we foud, were selected and cemented onto support blocks befcre being cut again in transverse or longitudinal section.
The motor and sensory nerve supply to the intrafusal fibers were then explored under light and electron-microscopes.

RESULTS

This muscle spindle had a diameter of about 70μm, and eight intrafusal fibers at its equatorial region.

Two nuclear bag fibers and six nuclear chain fibers were present.

Nuclear bag fibers lacked myofilaments at their central area in the equatorial region.

The myofibrils of the two nucler bag fibers were poorly separated by a sparse sarcoplasmic reticulum.

The sensory nerve fibers of these fibers had the annulospiral or varicose endings that contain many mitochondria and lie deep in the muscle fibers in the equatorial region. One of the two nuclear bag fibers we inspected had a motor nerve endings with a small sole area, poorly developed postsynaptic foldings at the outside of the equatoiral region.

These myofibrils of the six nuclear chain fibers were relatively, well delineated by a sarcoplamic reticulum,and the mitochondria were more numerous and larger than those of the nuclear bag fibers.

The motor nerver endings had a sole area of moderate size and poorly developed postsynaptic foldings.
There were also small, simple motor nerve endings with no postsynaptic foldings.

SUMMARY

The diamter of the muscle spindle was about 70μm. There were eight intrafusal fibers, of two types, nuclear bag and nuclear chain fibers.

The sensory nerve endings of the nuclear bag fibers were annulospiral or varicose. Nuclear chain fibers had two kinds of motor nerve endings, of different size and complexity.

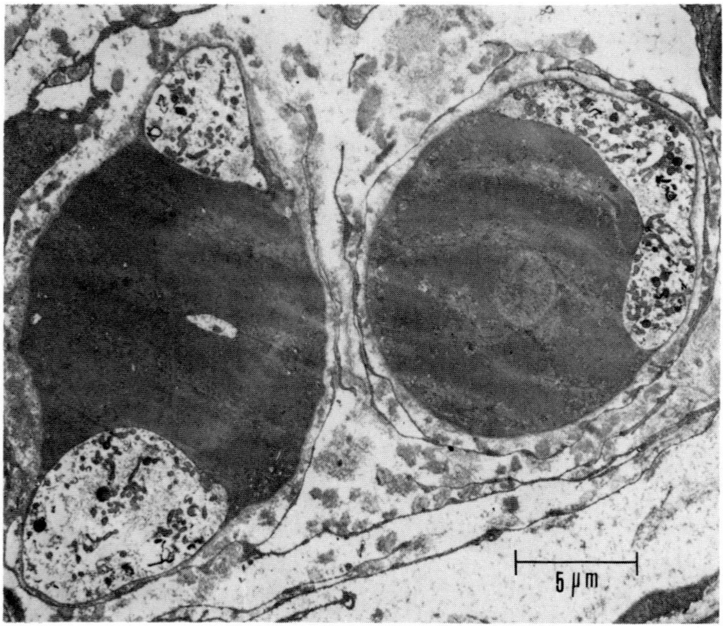

Sensory nerve endings of two nuclear bag fibers.

REFERENCES

1. Baken, R.J. (1971) J. speech and Hearing Research. 14, 513~518,
2. Banks, R.W. (1981) J. Anat., 133, 4, 571~591,
3. Grim, M. (1967) Folia Morphologica, XV 2, 124~131,
4. Kucera, J. (1984) Cell Tissue Res. 236, 383~391,
5. Kattou, Y, H.Okamura (1983) J. Oto,Japan, 86, 6, 661~665
6. Lucas Keene, M.F. (1961) J. Anat, 95, 25~29

© 1985 Elsevier Science Publishers B.V. (Biomedical Division)
New dimensions in otorhinolaryngology - head and neck surgery, vol. 2.
E. Myers, editor

MORPHOLOGICAL STUDY OF MUSCLE SPINDLES IN INTRINSIC LARYNGEAL MUSCLES OF HUMAN LARYNX

YOICHI KATTO M.D., HIROSHI OKAMURA M.D. AND NAOAKI YANAGIHARA M.D.

Dept. of Otolaryngology,Yawatahama Municipal Hospital,Ehime,JAPAN and
Dept, of Otolaryngology,University of Ehime School of Medicine,Ehime,JAPAN

INTRODUCTION

There has been little information available to the morphology of muscle spindles in the human intrinsic laryngeal muscles. Obviously more detailed information of muscle spindles is necessary for understanding the function of muscles in phonation,swallowing and respiration. In the present study,we examine the distribution of muscle spindles in the human laryngeal muscles by histological serial sections,and also describe their fine structual features evidenced by using a transmission electron microscopy.

MATERIAL AND METHODS

The intrinsic laryngeal muscles were obtaind from patients of laryngeal cancer at operation. The muscles were fixed with 4% glutaraldehyde and were cut into a few segments. The specimens were embedded in JB-4 EMBEDDING KIT and serially sectioned transversely and then were staind with Lee's Methylen-blue-basic fucsin solution. Some of the specimens were also embedded in Epoxy-resin and prepared for an electron microscopic examination.

RESULTS

Muscle spindles were found in all the intrinsic laryngeal muscles except the lateral cricoarytenoid,which was not examined yet. Their number and size varied in different muscles,as summarized in Table 1. The largest spindle found in the posterior cricoarytenoid was about 1800 micron in length,containing 6 intrafusal fibers,whereas the smallest one in the cricothyroid was shorter than 700 micron in length,containing only one or three intrafusal fibers.

A muscle spindle encountered in the interarytenoid was also examined with an electron microscope. The muscle spindle contained two large and two small intrafusal fibers which resembled ordinaly extrafusal fibers in myofibral organization. (Figure 1). The sensory endings innervating the intrafusal fibers were devoid of Schwann cell investment and often penetrated the sarcoplasm to terminate within the fiber. Unlike muscle spindles observed in other skeletal muscles,the muscle spindle in the interarytenoid was characterized by abundant collagenous fibrils investing the intrafusal fibers. Moreover,a number of capillaries were present in the capsule.

TABLE 1

MORPHOLOGICAL CARACTERISTICS OF MUSCLE SPINDLES IN INTRINSIC LARYNGEAL MUSCLES

MUSCLE	No.spindles	LENGTH mean in	WIDTH micron	No.intrafusals
Interarytenoid	7	-	78.4	1 - 5
Post.Cricoarytenoid	4	1435	78.5	1 - 6
Cricothyroid	3	713	46.7	1 - 3
Thyroarytenoid	2	925	45.0	1 - 4

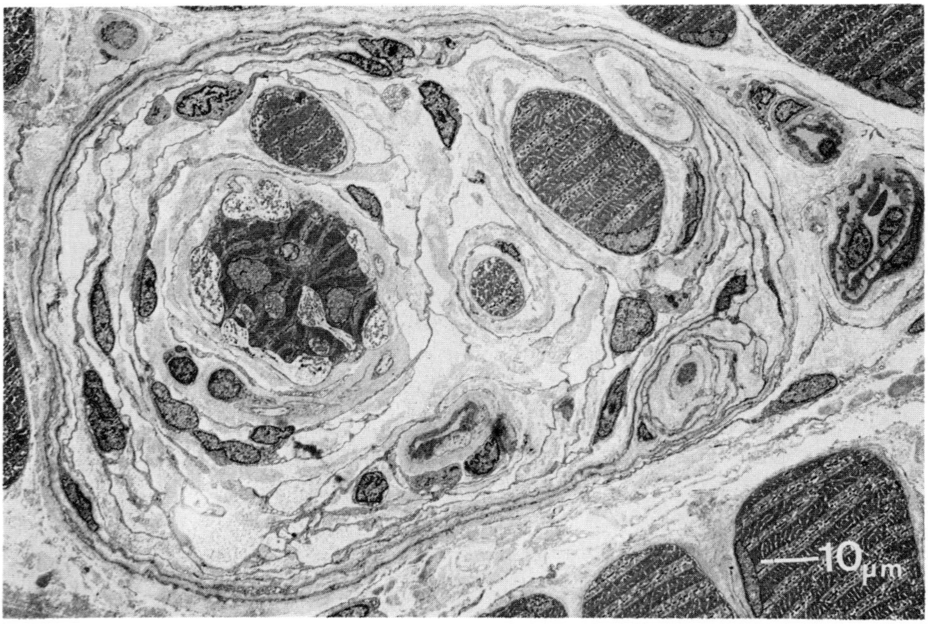

Fig.1 Transverse section through the capsular region of a spindle in the interarytenoid muscle(an electron microscopic view).

REFERENCES

1.Baken RJ (1971) Neuromuscular spindle in intrinsic muscle of human larynx J Speech Hear Res 14: 513-518

2.Barker D (1974) Morphology of muscle receptor In: Handbook of Sensory physiology. III. Pt.2,Muscle Receptors (edited by Hunt CC),p.1-190, Berlin: Springer-Verlag.

New dimensions in otorhinolaryngology - head and neck surgery, vol. 2.
E. Myers, editor

TRANSPLANT OF LARYNGEAL CARTILAGINOUS STRUCTURE IN DOGS EXPERIMENTAL STUDY.

Dr. Alvarez Vicent and Mingorance Lopez

INTRODUCTION

After the laryngeal functional technique of endolaryngeal draining (1), in the cases of tumorous infiltration the problem of the cartilage is posed , and the possibility of replacing same in order to initiate new functional surgical techniques.

The study was based on the fact that cartilaginous tissue, because of its special characteristics, is the tissue which can most easily be transplanted; in addition, the larynx does not need autonomous mobility in its cartilage, since the nearby tissues make up for this perfectly well. The easy with which autologous implants are made in human larynxes led us, in an experimental way, to carry out transplants with homologous laryngeal cartilage in dogs. The parameters studied were tolerance, functional results and a histopathological study of the parts.

MATERIAL AND METHODS

The study was carried out on 20 dogs of a similar size, and which were not related by blood. Perochondrium-removed cartilage is transplanted, with exhaustive conservation of receptor muscles and endolaryngeal mucous membrane. Two dogs are operated on at the same time, and the cartilage from one is transplanted into the other, and viceversa; this begins with hemithyroids and continues until the transplant of thyroids and epiglottis is complete, maintaining the cricoid cartilage. The procedure is performed in five rounds of four dogs each. In each round, the amount of transplanted tissue is increased.

The cartilaginous sutures are made with fine dexon and the muscular sutures with cagut. Tracheotomy cannula sutured to the skin until possible decannulation. Antibiotherapy and azathioprine. Introvenous feeding the first six days and after six months, the dogs were slaughtered in order to make the histological study.

RESULTS

Rejection: Elimination of the epiglottis in the first 15 days in those 4 dogs in which the epiglottis was transplanted independently of the rest of the thyroids.

Clinical functional results: Death of one dog during anaesthesia. Emergence of food during the first six days. Two pneumonias by inhalation which were taken care of with antibiotherapy. Decannulation between the 7th and the 15th days. There were no dyspneic problems, feeding was normal after 20 days and the dogs barking and growling were acceptable. All survived and were slaughtered after 6 months for study of their larynx.

Histological results: The parts have been examined by means of seried sections, enclosed in parafin and dyed with hematoxiline-eosin. Sections have been made at all levels, (the greatest number in the thyroid cartilage), using nitric acid to decalcify.

The sections show an integral epithelium. In the striated-type muscles no alterations are detected. The mucous glands are found preserved. No inflammatory infiltrations nor granulmatosic reaction is found at any level.

Diverse particular features are noted in the cross section of the thyroid cartilage. The rear half of the thyroid cartilage appears artefacted (change in tissue structure), and is detached from the connecting cartilage which integrates the corresponding perichondrium. In some cases, this portion has a solution of continuity with the preceding part, whereas in other cases there is perfect continuity and changes of bone metaplasia are even observed at the level where both parts join. In no case is there necrosis or cellular degeneration, The cartilaginous matrix is normal in appearance and the chondrocitary nucleii show no atypical features or variations.

CONCLUSION

No rejection and very acceptable functional results.

REFERENCES

1. ALVAREZ VICENT. Laryngectimie fontionelle selon la technique de levidement sous-perichondral du larynx. Ann. Otolaryng.: Paris, 1975. T.92. pp. 61-72.

New dimensions in otorhinolaryngology - head and neck surgery, vol. 2.
E. Myers, editor

AFFERENT PROJECTIONS TO THE NUCLEUS AMBIGUUS IN THE BRAIN STEM OF THE CAT

TAKAO MITSUMASU*, YOSHIKAZU YOSHIDA*, MINORU HIRANO*, TAKESHI KANASEKI**
*Department of Otolaryngology, School of Medicine, Kurume University, Kurume,
**Department of Anatomy, Faculty of Medicine, Kyushu University, Fukuoka (Japan)

INTRODUCTION

Several investigations can be found in the literature regarding the descending projections to the nucleus ambiguus(AMB). However, there are some obscure points about these projections. Then, we conducted a series of investigations aimed at establishing a comprehensive concept of the afferent projections to AMB using anterograde and retrograde axonal transport of WGA - HRP.

MATERIAL AND METHODS

71 cats were used in this investigation.

The present study divided into 2 stages.

The 1st stage

WGA - HRP was injected into AMB. Then retrogradely labeled cell bodies and anterogradely labeled axon terminals were evaluated in the brain stem.

The 2nd stage

WGA - HRP was injected into the sites labeled cell bodies were seen in the 1st stage individually.

RESULTS

The 1st stage

In the midbrain, labeled cell bodies were found in the lateral and ventrolateral part of the periaqueductal gray (PAG) bilaterally with ipsilateral predominance.

In the pons, labeled cell bodies were seen in the ipsilateral nucleus parabrachialis (nPB).

In the medulla oblongata, labeled cell bodies were recognized in the bilateral nucleus tractus solitarii (nTS) except the rostral part of the nucleus with ipsilateral predominance. Furthermore, labeled cell bodies and labeled axon terminals were found in the contralateral AMB and reticular formation around AMB.

The 2nd stage

After WGA - HRP injection into PAG, labeled axon terminals were seen in the bilateral AMB only caudal part of the nucleus.

Following WGA - HRP injection into nPB, labeled axon terminals were found in AMB ipsilaterally.

After WGA - HRP injection into nTS, neumerous labeled terminals were seen in AMB bilaterally with ipsilateral predominance.

CONCLUSION

AMB received projections from the PAG, the ipsilateral nPB, the middle and caudal part of the bilateral nTS, the contralateral AMB and the contralateral reticular formation around AMB.

REFERENCES

1. Jürgens U, Rratt R (1979) Role of the periaqueductral gray in vocal expression of emotion. Brain Res 167:367-378

2. Westlund KN, Coulter JD (1980) Descending projections of the locus coeruleous and subcoeruleus, medial parabrachial nuclei in monkey. Axonal transport study and dopamine-β- hydroxyrase immuniocytochemistry. Brain Res Review 2:235-264

3. Takeuchi Y et al. Parabrachial nucleus neurons projecting to the lower brain stem and the spinal cord. A study in the cat by the Fink-Heimer and the horseradish peroxidase methods. Exp Neurol 70:403-413

© 1985 Elsevier Science Publishers B.V. (Biomedical Division)
New dimensions in otorhinolaryngology - head and neck surgery, vol. 2.
E. Myers, editor

CENTRAL LOCATION OF EFFERENT NEURONS SUPPLYING THE LARYNGEAL AND THE VAGAL NERVES — AN HRP STUDY IN MONKEYS —

Y YOSHIDA, T MIYAZAKI, T MITSUMASU, M HIRANO AND *T KANASEKI
Dept. of Otorhinolaryngology and Head and Neck Surgery, Kurume University, School of Medicine, Kurume, and *Dept. of Anatomy, Faculty of Medicine, Kyushu University, Fukuoka, Japan

INTRODUCTION

The topographic representation of the laryngeal motoneurons has been determined in several kinds of animals. There was, however, only one study with primates, which was reported by Furstenberg et al.[1] The purpose of the present study was to demonstrate the topographic representation of the laryngeal motoneurons of monkeys.

MATERIAL AND METHOD

Thirty-two monkeys (macaca fuscata) weighing 2-4.5 kg were used. Investigation was performed on the cricothyroid muscle (CT) in 6, the abductor muscle (Abd) in 5, the adductor muscle (Add) in 9, the recurrent laryngeal nerve (RLN) in 6 and the vagal nerve in 6 monkeys. Details of the procedures of horseradish peroxidase (HRP) injection, histochemical reaction and examining specimens were described elsewhere.[2]

RESULTS

Following injection of HRP into CT, Abd, Add and RLN, labeled neurons were found ipsilaterally mainly in the nucleus ambiguus (AMB) including the retrofacial nucleus (RF). CT cell column extended from the level caudal to the facial nucleus to the level caudal to the middle of the inferior olivary nucleus (IO). CT neurons were scattered around the outer area of the compact cell group of AMB. Abd neurons distributed from the level of the most caudal part of the CT cell column to the level rostral to the caudal end of IO. They were slightly scattered in the medial part of AMB. Also a few labeled cells were situated in the reticular formation. Add cell column extended from the level immediately caudal to the rostral end of Abd cell column to the level of the caudal end of IO. Add neurons were aggregated in the lateral part of AMB and were sparse in the middle part of the nucleus. RLN neurons were found between the level rostral to the middle of IO and that of the caudal end of IO. They showed a compact form in the lateral part of AMB and were scattered in the dorsomedial part of the nucleus. Vagal neurons investigated at the level of the nodose ganglion were found throughout AMB (including RF) and the retroambigual nucleus, and were also seen in the dorsal motor nucleus ipsilaterally. The neurons in the former two nuclei were distributed from the caudal part of the facial nucleus to C_2 whereas the neurons in the latter nucleus were found between the level of the rostral part of IO and C_2. The RF and AMB neurons were slightly compact while the dorsal motor nucleus of the vagus neurons were tightly packed. The retroambigual neurons were sparse.

DISCUSSION

The rostrocaudal pattern of distribution of motoneurons for CT, Abd, Add and RLN was similar to the results of our previous study of cats.[3] According to Furstenberg et al., in the rostrocaudal distribution of laryngeal motoneurons of a monkey, CT neurons was located the most rostral while Add neurons was situated the most caudal. Abd neurons were found between CT neurons and Add neurons.[1] In the present study, the Abd neurons were located more caudally, than those in the report by Furstenberg et al..[1] The arrangement of CT, Abd and Add motoneurons in transverse plane was different compared with that of cats.[3] These arrangement of the laryngeal motoneurons indicates different pattern between animal species.

REFERENCES

1. Furstenberg AC, Magielski JE (1955) A motor pattern in the nucleus ambiguus. its clinical significance, Ann Otol Rhinol Laryngol 64: 788-793.
2. Yoshida Y, Mitsumasu T, Miyazaki T, Hirano M, Kanaseki T (1984) Distribution of motoneurons in the brain stem of monkeys innervating the larynx. Brain Res Bull 13: 413-419.
3. Yoshida Y, Miyazaki T, Hirano M, Shin T, Kanaseki T (1982) Arrangement of motoneurons innervating the intrinsic laryngeal muscles of cats as demonstrated by horseradish peroxidase. Acta Otolaryngol 94: 329-334.

© 1985 Elsevier Science Publishers B.V. (Biomedical Division)
New dimensions in otorhinolaryngology - head and neck surgery, vol. 2.
E. Myers, editor

DNA CLASSIFICATION OF HUMAN PITUITARY TUMOURS

MATTI ANNIKO[1], BERNHARD TRIBUKAIT[2] and JAN WERSÄLL[3]

1- Department of Otolaryngology - Head & Neck Surgery, University of Umeå, Umeå, Sweden
2- Department of Medical Radiobiology, Karolinska Institute, Stockholm, Sweden
3- Department of Otolaryngology, Karolinska Hospital, Stockholm, Sweden

INTRODUCTION

The nuclear DNA content of a cell can be studied quantitatively by means of flow-cytofluorometry or single cell analysis or qualitatively by analyzing individual chromosomes in individual mitotic dispersed cells. The relationship between nuclear DNA content and its expression of biological properties and/or clinical parameters varies considerably between the different types of human tumours (1-2). Earlier studies on human pituitary tumours have been focused on ploidy levels with regard to clinical parameters (3-4) whereas the present material, the so far largest one, is directed towards analyses of the cell cycle, in particular the proliferation rate.

PATIENT MATERIAL AND METHODS

The present study is based on 80 patients with pituitary tumours. All patients underwent prior to surgery a complete endocrinological, ophthalmological and roentgenological investigation (3). The tumours are subdivided according to their endocrinological type: GH secreting -31 tumours, concomitant secretion of GH and PRL -15 tumours, prolactinomas -12 tumours, TSH-secreting -2 tumours, ACTH-secreting -7 tumours, and non-secreting -13 tumours.

The technique for flow-cytofluorometry has been described earlier (4). Pieces from all pituitary tumours were taken for morphological analysis at the light microscopic level (epon-embedded, 1 μm thick sections stained with toluidine blue).

RESULTS

Light microscopy showed a benign type of morphology in all pituitary tumours.

In the total material 39 tumours (49%) were diploid and 41 tumours (51%) were aneuploid. In acromegaly with a concomitant secretion of GH and PRL and in prolactinomas aneuploidy occurred in 67%. Tumours secreting GH only and ACTH-secreting tumours revealed aneuploidy in approximately 45% but in non-secreting tumours aneuploidy occurred only in 31%. Seven cases with two cell lines were identified, all occurring in tumours causing acromegaly. Seventy-three tumours had only one cell line. The total number of cell lines was thus 37.

The aneuploid cell lines (totally 45) were grouped accordingly: hypodiploid (1.5c - <2c) - 5/45, 2.2c - 3c - 27/45 and >3c - 13/45 cell lines. There was no tumour with a nuclear DNA content above 4c. Polyploidization did not occur. Aneuploidy alone or levels of aneuploidy did not correlate with age or sex of the patients.

The proliferation rate of the tumours was determined according to the S-phase: low (below 5% of the total cell population), moderate (5-10%) and high (>10%). For technical reasons determination of cell phase was successful in only 69 tumours. The percentage of S-phase cells can be low (<5%) in also aneuploid tumours (5/36 cell lines; 13%). In diploid tumours the corresponding rate was 8/33 (24%). This difference became even more obvious when comparing the two sexes. In females, 28% of the diploid tumours had a proliferation rate below 5% whereas only 4% of the aneuploid tumours. In males, a low proliferation rate occurred in 19% of the diploid and 27% of the aneuploid tumours. A high proliferation rate (>10% S-phase cells) was determined in 6% (males) and 16% (females) of the diploid tumours and 26% (males) and 35% (females) of the aneuploid tumours.

There is no obvious tendency for an increased proliferation rate with increasing age. Most pituitary tumours in the present material were found in patients between 30 and 70 years of age. In the age group 30-39 years a high proliferation rate occurred in 1/7 of diploid and 3/6 of aneuploid tumours. During the next decade (40-49 years) the corresponding rates were 1/7 respectively 3/12; during 50-59 years of age at 1/9 respectively 4/8, and, during 60-69 years of age the incidence was 0/3 respectively 3/6. Likewisely this difference in proliferation rate between diploid and aneuploid pituitary tumours merely reflects the incidence of aneuploid tumours and is not directly correlated with patient age.

The comparison of the proliferation rate in individual endocrinological types of tumours shows a difference ($p>0.05$) between diploid and aneuploid tumours only in those with secretion of GH only. In the total material the S-phase in diploid tumours averaged $6.93 \pm 2.85\%$ and in aneuploid tumours $8.91 \pm 4.11\%$ being significantly different ($p<0.05$).

CONCLUSIONS

1. The flow-cytofluorometric technique is suitable for the assessment of both ploidy level and proliferation rate in solid human pituitary tumours.

2. Pituitary tumours can be subdivided according to their nuclear DNA content and proliferation rate.

3. A high incidence of aneuploidy indicating a nuclear malignant transformation occurs but varies considerably with regard to endocrinological type of tumour.

4. Pituitary tumours have a homogenous nuclear DNA content independent of site of biopsy for DNA analysis.

5. The majority of pituitary tumours has only one cell line. So far at most two cell lines have been identified, all in tumours causing acromegaly.

6. A significantly higher proliferation rate ($p<0.05$) occurs in aneuploid tumours as compared with diploid ones.

ACKNOWLEDGEMENTS

This study was supported by the Ragnar and Torsten Söderberg Foundation (M.A.) and the Cancer Society in Stockholm (B.T.).

REFERENCES

1. Sandberg AA (1980) On chromosomes in human cancer and leukemia. Elsevier, New York
2. Tribukait B, Hammarberg C, Rubio C (1983) Acta Pathol Microbiol Scand [A] 91:89-95
3. Anniko M, Holm L-E, Tribukait B, Werner S, Wersäll J (1981) Acta Otolaryngol (Stockh) Suppl 379:21-28
4. Anniko M, Tribukait B (1985) DNA pattern of human pituitary tumours. Am J Otolaryngol In press

New dimensions in otorhinolaryngology - head and neck surgery, vol. 2.
E. Myers, editor

UNUSUAL CAUSES OF SLEEP APNEA SYNDROME

ISRAEL BRAMA, SHLOMO TAICHER, ISAAC GAY

Department of ENT and Dentistry, Hadassah University Hospital, Kiryat Hadassah, Jerusalem, Israel

INTRODUCTION

Sleep apnea is a potentially lethal condition that is more prevalent than commonly suspected. A broad spectrum of causes leading to obstructive sleep apnea has been described including adenoid and tonsil hypertrophy, mandibular malformations, nasal obstruction, macroglossia, acromegaly, Down's syndrome, myxedema, craniofacial abnormalities and obesity. Two unusual cases of upper airway obstruction causing severe sleep apnea are described: one case was obstructed by the *anterior* part of the tongue and the other by the uvula. In both cases uvulopalatopharyngoplasty operation (uppp) is contraindicated.

PATIENTS

Two patients with severe sleep apnea were examined in our clinic. The first was a young soldier with normal body weight who complained of excessive daytime sleepiness, he woke several times each night with sensation of choking and a complaint of headache and tiredness after awaking in the morning, he felt depressed and anxious and noted a deterioration in his ability to concentrate. His physical examination was completely normal. Polysomnography revealed 302 obstruction apneas during a six hours sleep period with an average length of 30 seconds. One major symptom was missing in the history and the examination, the snoring phenomenon. The patient and his friends did not observe unusual snoring and neither did we. On observation of the patient during sleep, we noted that the obstruction was caused by the *anterior* part of the tongue which folds backwards behind the uvula causing obstruction of the naso-oro-pharynx. After awaking the patient, we asked him to turn the anterior part of the tongue backwards behind the uvula and he did it easily (Fig. 1). In this case uppp operation is contraindicated because after the operation the obstruction caused by the anterior part of the tongue falling backwards will remain the same. We offered the patient to suture the anterior part of the tongue to the mandibula, but he refused and disappeared.

Patient 2

The second patient aged 20 years had a normal weight, he complained of a choking sensation every night causing him to jump up several times during the night. There was a history of drowsiness and falling asleep during quiet situations such as reading or listening to a lecture. There was no complaint of snoring. An ENT examination disclosed an extremely enlarged uvula touching the suppraglottic area; when lying on the side the uvula protruded through the teeth outside the mouth. There was no doubt that the uvula was falling at the glottic entrance causing airway obstruction at night. Amputation of the uvula was carried out and all the symptoms disappeared.

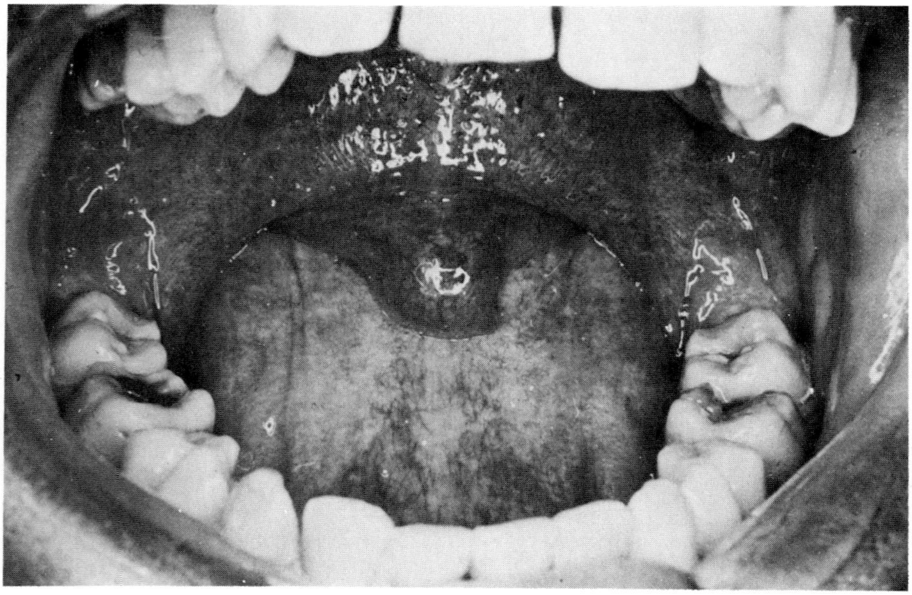

Fig. 1. The tongue behind the uvula.

DISCUSSION

uppp operation is designed to enlarge the potential airspace in the naso-oro-pharynx by removal of redundant tissue from the pharyngopalatial arch. But this new operation is successful only in 50% of the cases as reviewed by Simmons et al.[1] Some of the failures may be due to unusual causes such as case 1. in which the normal weight of patients and absence of snoring lead us to look for the unusual source of the obstruction. The snoring is caused by partial obstruction of the airway, but in complete obstruction as in infants with bilateral choanal atresia or as in our case there is no snoring phenomenon.

REFERENCES

1. Simmons FB, Guileminault, C, Miles LE (1984) The palatopharyngoplasty operation for snoring and sleep apnea: An interim report. Otolaryngol Head & Neck Surg 92: 375-380.

© 1985 Elsevier Science Publishers B.V. (Biomedical Division)
New dimensions in otorhinolaryngology – head and neck surgery, vol. 2.
E. Myers, editor

LITERATURE SEARCHING BY MICROCOMPUTER

KEITH CLARK and J. GAIL NEELY

Department of Otorhinolaryngology, P.O. Box 26307, South Pavilion, University of Oklahoma Health Sciences Center, Oklahoma City, Oklahoma 73126, USA

INTRODUCTION

Computers are directly effecting all of our lives. A wide variety of tasks including wordprocessing, spreadsheet analysis, graphics, and math intensive operations are certainly within the capability of the personal computer. Most medical software deals specifically with the business aspects of a physician's practice. Literature searching is a task that is nicely accomplished by the microcomputer and can improve patient care by selecting pertinent journal articles for the physician. We have implemented computer-generated literature searching in our department to determine if high quality searches could be easily and effectively obtained by the residents and faculty themselves.

MATERIALS AND METHODS

An IBM-PC microcomputer with a Hayes Smartmodem 1200 Baud internal telephone communications modem was used to access the Medline database of the National Library of Medicine. A subscription to this database was purchased from the BRS/Saunders Colleague online retrieval service. The members of our department are only casually acquainted with microcomputers, and each needed an introduction to the computer and literature searching. This was accomplished by computerized self teaching tutorials that came with the computer and the BRS/Saunders Users' Manual.

RESULTS

The required hardware can be purchased in today's market for under $4,000.00. This includes an IBM-PC with monitor and memory, one floppy disk drive, one hard disk drive (optional), and a dot-matrix printer. Memory requirements vary according to the software being used. Only the software that comes with a modem and the operating system software is needed. Wordprocessing and database management software can be used to manipulate the information received during a literature search.

BRS/Saunders charges a $50.00 initial fee to subscribe to their online service and a monthly minimum of $15.00. In our hands the cost per search varied widely depending on the topic being searched. Well defined topics with specific key words were more easily completed and less expensive since multiple searches were not needed. In general the average search yielding 30 articles (with full abstracts) costs under $5.00 based on an hourly rate after 6:00 P.M. of $20.00. Hourly rates during business hours are more expensive.

Since the microcomputer is communicating with another powerful computer by telephone, the process of searching is done by software residing on the remote computer. This software is designed specifically for literature searching. No computer language needs to be learned,the process is reduced to selecting options from menus. By moving through the menus, one selects a time period to search. A keyword or keywords are given to search for and relevant articles are selected. Specific information may be specified such as; language, reviews only, and certain journals or authors only. The information about these articles may then be listed and saved on paper or diskette.

Listing options vary from title, author, and source to 15 different pieces of information including the author's full abstract. BRS/Saunders Colleague service even offers certain journals and textbooks online (may read book or articles on the computer screen). These full text services may also be searched in a similar manner.

There are advantages to performing a search personally. Feedback is immediate and further searching can be done on the basis of a preliminary search. Often key words are not correct for the first search, but just reading the information from one article can reveal useful information for a second very successful search. Furthermore, a more complete search is produced by a searcher who knows the subject material.

DISCUSSION

Computerized literature searching is not new. Medical libraries have provided this service for years. Libraries usually use the simplest of terminals that do not have data storage hardware (disk drives). With a disk drive the search can be saved permanently.

Hardware requirements are minimal. Almost any computer available today can be used, and machines that will suffice can be purchased for under $1,000.

Wordprocessing software is designed to edit textual information. Each literature search is simply a body of text that most wordprocessing software packages can work with. We have edited unwanted article information from searches and even edited a search to the point of being ready to use as a bibliography in a scientific publication.

Database management software allows one to import the information to a structured format. Once organized into the database, the user can then ask a variety of questions about the literature search data. An alphabetized list of journal articles by journal source is routinely produced for our library to use to obtain reprints. As the amount of search material stored on our hard disk grows, we will be able to search through our own library of literature data for specific articles. The possibilities are limited only by the user's database management skills and imagination.

CONCLUSION

Residents and faculty can perform sophisticated computer literature searches without previous computer experience or knowledge. Learning the skill of searching by microcomputer required little time and effort. The information received can be stored for future viewing or listing and may be manipulated by wordprocessing and database software. While the individual physicians must spend their own time to produce a search, the searches are very comprehensive and relevant.

© 1985 Elsevier Science Publishers B.V. (Biomedical Division)
New dimensions in otorhinolaryngology - head and neck surgery, vol. 2.
E. Myers, editor

A MULTIDISCIPLINARY APPROACH TO THE TEMPOROMANDIBULAR JOINT

Claude C. Cody III, M.D., Baylor College of Medicine; James L. McClendon, D.D.S., Clinical Professor, Health Science Center, Houston, Texas

The temporomandibular joint (TMJ) syndrome is beginning to assume increasing attention with dentists, oral surgeons, otolaryngologists, family practitioners and even neurologists. In my practice alone, I see patients several times a month with pain traceable to the jawbone area. Referred pain to the TMJ must then be examined very carefully to determine its exact source of pathological abnormality. This is not always easy. Here, consultations would be very helpful.

Dr. James Costen, an otolaryngologist in 1934, first called attention to patients with severe ear pain with normal-appearing ear canals and drums but with a bite disorder resulting in referred pain to the ear on the ipsilateral ear and occasionally on the contralateral ear. Since Costen's time, there has been more attention paid to the muscles, fascia and tendons in and about the joint, neck, jaw muscles and ligaments with their fascia. Physical medicine and physiotherapy have shown their value in solving some cases of TMJ along with facial, neck and upper body muscles. (MPD) Myofacial Pain Dysfunction. The excellent trigger point manual by Drs. Travell and Simons reviews all the complexes of the TMJ-MPD syndromes. It helps to show the value of consultation to all the involved disciplines in getting the correct diagnosis.

As dental errors become less of primary concern, the dentist has greater motivation to expand his or her understanding and knowledge in a field of temporomandibular apparatus. There are literally millions of people suffering from these problems who currently have nowhere to go. The dentists of the future will use basic dental skills plus increased knowledge to help people, while working more closely with medical colleagues. We are beginning to realize that such a minute thing as high fillings will have a disastrous effect on the entire body. No longer can dentists afford to look upon themselves as being a complete end in themselves with their treatment having little or no effect on the rest of the human structure. One must emphasize the team approach on each patient although the individual patient may be effectively treated by a single modality.

The majority of patients with TMJ disease presents something that they think originates in structures of the ear, nose and throat. It is therefore important for anyone treating TMJ patients to have a thorough understanding of the anatomical relationship between the ear and the TMJ, to be familiar with the many causes of the obscure symptoms--tinnitus and vertigo--and to be aware of the elements and techniques of a good ear, nose and throat examination.

Symptoms of TMJ disorder that are common to the ear, nose and throat problems are tinnitus, vertigo, impaired hearing, fullness in the ear, and pain. It should be pointed out that these are symptoms, not pathological entities, and as such are subjective rather than objective. These symptoms occur in a variety of conditions--central nervous system disorders, pathological coordinations with the external, middle and inner ear, head and neck tumor problems, sinus disease, dental problems and metabolic abnormalities of various allergies and yes, emotional problems, with the exception of impaired hearing which can be evaluated by audiometry. The symptoms cannot ordinarily be measured or tested objectively. Thus, one must rely on a careful history and physical examination and, when indicated, special tests, x-rays and other procedures that help a diagnosis.

The otolaryngologist sees patients complaining of ear pain, sometimes severe. This may be accompanied by tinnitus, such as buzzing, hissing, ringing, pounding and a variety of other sounds. The vertigo frequently complained of, when a patient says it is "dizziness," is not a true objective vertigo. This is more like light-headedness or syncope and ataxia. Some patients with TMJ syndrome may actually experience true vertigo when more than pain is a chief complaint. Patients may complain of hearing loss which cannot be proven by audiometry. A full sensation of the ears with or without subjective loss of hearing may indicate eustachian tube dysfunction, middle ear pathology, and that could mean more otological causes. Thus a full work-up of all of the disciplines is mandatory to get an overall diagnosis of the proper cause.

The most common cause of pain dysfunction in the temporomandibular joint is not bony abnormality but rather muscle spasm. This is divided into three groups: 1) macrotrauma, 2) microtrauma, and 3) stress situations. Macrotrauma includes excessive mandibular opening, as in laughing, yawning, biting, whiplash followed by the momentary inability to close the jaw and as one closes it, a horrendous click occurs. The first symptom is severe pain in the joint area and marked restriction of the opening. Treatment is soft diet, heat, analgesics, muscle relaxants, anti-inflammatories, and a dental occlusion bite plate. Microtraumas are more common and are caused by occlusion discrepancies. They are also caused by clicking and grinding of the teeth (bruxism). The treatment involves treating the damaging habits and after the pain is gone, correction of the occlusal abnormalities. Tension and stress is a significant cause of the TMJ pain dysfunction.

The future holds more hope for the large number of people afflicted with this most severe and perplexing problem.

Second Edition-Diseases of the Temporomandibular Apparatus-A MultiDisciplinary Approach, 1982.

Travell, Janet G.; Simons, David G.: Myofacial Pain and Dysfunction. The Trigger Point Manual: Williams and Williams, 1983.

© 1985 Elsevier Science Publishers B.V. (Biomedical Division)
New dimensions in otorhinolaryngology - head and neck surgery, vol. 2.
E. Myers, editor

SONOGRAPHY OF BRANCHIOGENIC CYSTS - A DIAGNOSTIC FREQUENCY-RELATED APPEARENCE

MATTHAEUS CH. GRASL*, PAUL C. HAJEK**
*First Department of Otorhinolaryngology, **Department of Radiology
University of Vienna School of Medicine, Vienna Austria
A-1097 Vienna, Lazarettgasse 14

INTRODUCTION

The branchiogenic cyst is one of the most frequent cystic mass of the neck. Manifestation is preponderantly in the second and third decade. There exists obscurity about the origin of those cysts (1). The diagnosis basis on history, palpation and in the last years also on sonography. Up to now the branchiogenic cysts supposed to be cystic, echo-free (2). During our research about the value of ultrasound in masses of the neck we noticed, that some cysts figured semisolid to solid (3).

We assume that the reason of the different statements could be on the one hand the content of the cysts and on the other hand the frequency of the used transducers. Therefore we set the reflexibility of the content to dependence on the frequency-related resolution of different transducers.

PATIENTS AND METHODS

23 patients with surgical and histological proven branchiogenic cysts were evaluated sonographically preoperative with a Real-Time-Sector-Scanner (Firm Diasonics). Transducers with the frequency of 3,0 Mega Hertz, 5,0 Mega Hertz and 7,5 Mega Hertz were used in each patient. The content of some of the cysts was analyzed by macro- and microscopy and also by chemistry.

RESULTS

I. Sonography

In all patients there was seen a round up to oval, exactly limited mass, surrounded with a thin smooth echo-dense wall, maximum five millimeters. The diameter of the smallest cyst was 2:1 cm, that of the largest one 7:6 cm. The cysts figured by using the transducer with: 3,0 Mega Hertz always as echo-free - cystic, 5,0 Mega Hertz hypoechoic - semisolid and 7,5 Mega Hertz definite echo-dense - solid.

2. Macro- and microscopy

Inside the analyzed cysts there was a yellowish, viscous, inodorous, homogeneous liquid. The microscopic examination perceived 0,I to 0,2 mm large rhomboedic formations, typical of cholesterol crystals. They were found partly in shape of conglomerations with a size of 0,5 mm and larger. Besides these crystals there was a insignificant quantity of fats, perished cells and sporadic macrophages.

3. Chemistry

The liquid of the cysts consisted of 80 % (w/v) cholesterol on the average (+,- I5 %), fats, traces of albumen and neglectigable amounts of triglycerides, phosphorics and calcium.

DISCUSSION

The sonographically distinction between cervical soft tissues takes as basis their different pattern of echos (2). Because of the high axial resolution of the transducers with the frequency of 5,0 Mega Hertz (about 0,7 mm) and 7,5 Mega Hertz (0,4 - 0,5 mm) the conglomerations of the cholesterol crystals could be demonstrated partly, respectively complete (4). The transducer with 3,5 Mega Hertz and therefore lower axial resolution (I,0 mm) showed the content of the cysts echo-free.

Consequently could be proved that the reflexibilities caused of the cholesterol crystal conglomerations are figured in dependence on the frequency of the used transducers: eighter not, partly or complete.

We consider this fact as typical of branchiogenic cysts and therefore as a distinctive mark to other structures of the neck as: thyreoid gland, lymph nodes, salivary glands, muscles, vessels and cystic masses of another origin.

REFERENCES

I. Stoll W (I980) Laryng Rhinol 59: 585-595
2. Mann EJ (I984) Ultraschall im Kopf-Hals-Bereich. Springer Verlag
3. Hajek PC, Grasl MCH et al. (I985) Assessment of Cervical Lymph Node Pathology by Ultrasound: A Clinical Study. Radiology, in press
4. Glancy JJ (I980) J Clin Ultrasound 8: 27-29

New dimensions in otorhinolaryngology - head and neck surgery, vol. 2.
E. Myers, editor

HUMAN PLEOMORPHIC ADENOMAS TRANSPLANTED TO NUDE MICE

CLAUS BARFOED, NIELS GRÆM, POUL BRETLAU, JØRGEN RYGAARD
ENT-department, Gentofte University Hospital, DK-2900 Hellerup, Denmark, and Pathological-Anatomical Institute, Kommunehospitalet, Copenhagen, Denmark

INTRODUCTION

With this two-species model it is possible to distinguish between murin and human cells by staining with DNA-specific fluorochrome in such a way that the original stromal components can be determined. Labelling with ^{3}H-thymidin has shown that both human epithelial and human mesenchymal cells proliferate.

MATERIAL AND METHODS

The transplantation followed the principles described by Rygaard (1). From 13 pleomorphic adenomas, tumor tissue samples were transplanted to 4-5 mice. The growth of the transplanted tissue was observed weekly until wasting of the animals 52-214 days after transplantation (Table I).

Seven mice, representing 7 different pleomorphic adenomas were selected for autoradiography with ^{3}H-thymidine. An intraperitoneal injection of ^{3}H-thymidine (100 μCI) was given once a day for 5 days. Details have been described in a previous publication (2).

Grafted tissue from 6 mice from second passage, representing 6 pleomorphic adenomas, was selected for heterochromatin studies using a recently described technique (3). Tissue fragments, 8 mm^3 in size, were incubated with trypsin for 18 h, resuspended in fetal calf serum, centrifugated and the resultant cell suspensions were fixed in glacial acetic acid and methanol, dropped on slides, dried and stained with DNA-specific fluorochrome D287-179, dried and mounted with glycerol/0.2 M Na_2HPO_4, and, finally, examined at x1000 in a microscope equipped for examination of fluorescein-isothiocyanate fluorescence. In each slide, 1000 nuclei were counted and analyzed for occurrence of brightly stained heterochromatin regions. For control, 4 types of non-grafted tissue were examined with the same technique. These were: (a) human pleomorphic adenomas; (b) nude mouse umbilical cord; (c) nude mouse costal cartilage, and (d) nude mouse epidermis.

RESULTS

Macroscopic examination (see Table I)

Microscopic examination

All 13 pleomorphic adenomas were represented. In all cases the transplanted tissue showed the characteristic histological picture of pleomorphic adenomas, and the overall histological picture showed no change from the donor tumor to the transplanted tissue.

Autoradiography

The slides prepared for autoradiography were examined by conventional light microscopy. In all cases but one there were labelled cells and both mesenchymal and epithelial cells were labelled. There were from 29 to 217 (mean 59) labelled cells per 1000 cells in the whole tumor, from 15 to 40 (mean 27) in the mesenchymal cells, and from 9 to 87 (mean 31) in the epithelial cells. The difference between the number of labelled mesenchymal and epithelial cells was not significant (Wilcoxon test, p 0.05).

Heterochromatin pattern

There were no fluorescent chromocenters in the slides with test samples of human pleomorphic adenoma, whereas all the cells in the murine samples, cartilage, umbilical cord, and epithelium showed fluorescent chromocenters. In each of the 6 tumors selected for this procedure there were from 30 to 60 (mean 45) murine cells per 1000 human cells in the specimens.

DISCUSSION

Our results show that the nude mouse model is useful for the study of the human pleomorphic adenoma, and we conclude that the proliferation in the tumor takes place in both the mesenchymal and epithelial areas.

TABLE I

Macroscopic results in 64 nude mice hosting human pleomorphic adenomas

Gross examination	Number of mice
Obvious growth of transplanted tumor	39
Tissue survival	8
Waste of mice	9
No take of transplanted tissue	8

REFERENCES

1. Rygaard J (1973) Thymus and self. Immunobiology of the mouse mutant nude. FADL, Copenhagen & J. Wiley, London

2. Barfoed C, Græm N, Bretlau P, Rygaard J (1984) Growth and differentiation of human pleomorphic adenomas in nude mice. Acta Otolaryngol (Stockh), Suppl. 412: 10-12

3. Græm J, Dabelsteen E, Tommerup N (1984) Blood group substances, T_6 antigen and heterochromatin pattern as species markers in the nude mouse-human skin model. Expl Cell Biol 52: 251-259.

New dimensions in otorhinolaryngology - head and neck surgery, vol. 2.
E. Myers, editor

COMPARATIVE HISTOCHEMICAL STUDY OF THE GLYCOCONJUGATES IN THE HUMAN RESPIRATORY MUCOSA

KOZO FUKAMI, MASARU OHYAMA & YUTAKA HANAMURE
Department of Otolaryngology, Faculty of Medicine, Kagoshima University, Kagoshima, Japan

INTRODUCTION

In recent years,particular interest has been focused on the glycoconjugates that are related to membrane functions and play an important role in defence mechanism of mucociliary system. The present study concerns the glycoconjugates in normal respiratory mucosa and pathologic subjects which were studied histochemically to lead to a clearer understanding of their physiologic roles.

MATERIALS AND METHODS

PAS staining, HID-AB methods and horse-raddish peroxidase conjugated lectins (UEA-I, PNA, WGA, DBA, RCA, SBA) were used to stain on three normal nasal mucosa collected from volunteers, 15 ones of the patients with chronic sinusitis, five allergic nasal mucosa, five normal laryngeal and tracheal mucosa collected from the patients with laryngeal cancer and 13 vorcal cord polyps taken by micro-laryngo-surgery.

RESULTS

The larger amounts of sulfo-mucin were observed in laryngeal mucosa than it in nasal mucosa. However, sialomucin were shown much more dominant in nasal mucosa compared with it in laryngeal mucosa. Some sugar residues staind by RCA, PNA ans SBA were detected in several different grades in goblet cells lining epithelium and mucous cells of sub-mucosal gland, while serous cells were unreactive. UEA-I, a specific to fucosyl residue, were observed in all mucous cells and serous cells in nasal gland, whereas only some mucous cells in laryngeal mucosa. As regards to pathological nasal mucosa, the glycoconjugates, while similar in their staining pattern, were different in their amount and reactive intensity depending on their pathological state.
The vorcal cord polyps could be classified into three types according to their staining features with lectin.
These data indicate that expression of membranous glycoprotein in

epithelia differs according to the maturation of the cell from the basal cell to the more mature keratinocyte, and suggest also that lectins may be used beneficially as one of markers in various stages of normal and abnormal differentiation.

REFERENCES
1. Ohyama M (1984) Pathobiochemistry of chronic sinusitis, Shibundo, Kagoshima, pp 14-27
2. Fukami K (1985) J Otolaryngol Jpn 88:449-454
3. Fukami K (1986) Pract Otol KYOTO 79:(in press)
4. Fukami K ; J Jpn Bronchoesophagol Soc (in press)

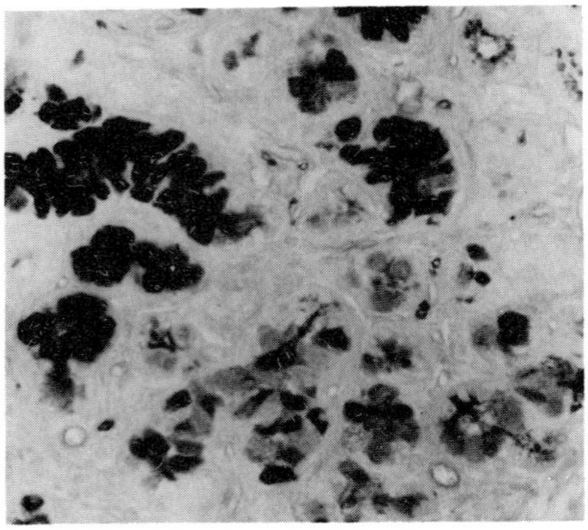

Fig.1 nasal mucosa of sinusitis stained with HID-AB

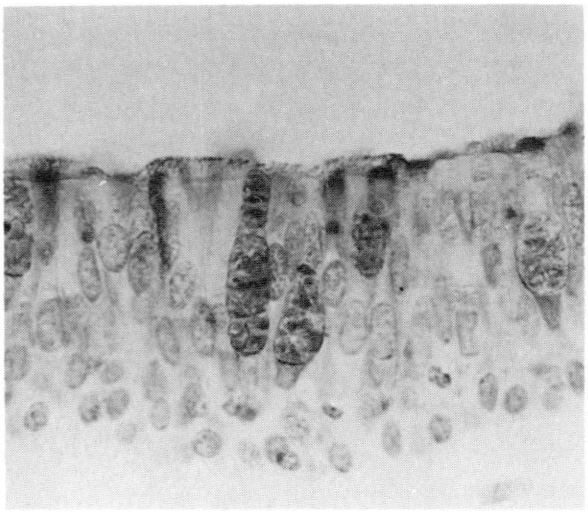

Fig.2 normal nasal mucosa stained with UEA-I

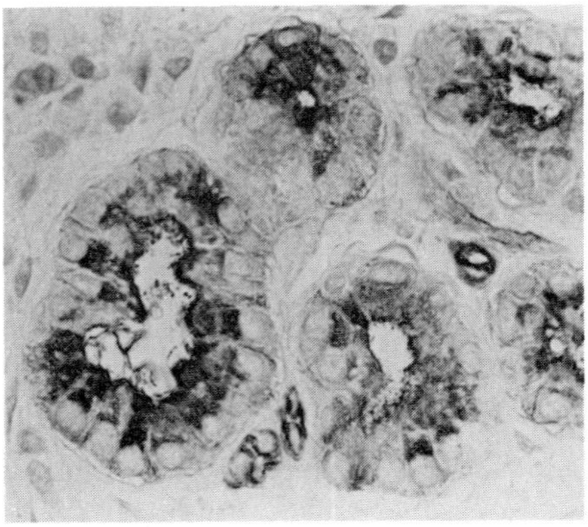

Fig.3 nasal mucosa of sinusitis stained with UEA-I

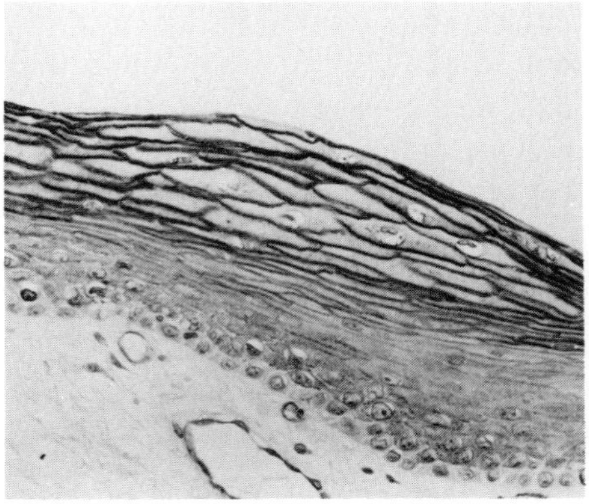

Fig.4 vorcal cord polyp stained with UEA-I

New dimensions in otorhinolaryngclogy - head and neck surgery, vol. 2.
E. Myers, editor

ELECTRON MICROSCOPIC INVESTIGATIONS IN BRONCHIAL SECRETION OF INFANTS AND CHILDREN FOR DETECTING VIRAL INFECTIONS

L. IMREI, P. SOTONYI, T. MARIALIGETI

Apathy Istvan Children's Hospital, Dept. of Pediatric ENT and Bronchology, Budapest, Bethesda u. 3. 1146, and Children's Sanatorium, Dept. of Pediatric Bronchology, Budapest, E otvos u. 2. 1121 (Hungary)

Several methods have been introduced in the latter years in order to prove morphologically the human virus infections. The results verified that electron microscopic morphological methods are quick and they guarantee, among certain and suitable circumstances during 30 minutes, precise and good diagnosis. Our comparative examinations have proved as well that these results can be matched with immunologic and with serologic methods very easily. They are specified, too, in certain circumstances diagnostically.

M. McLean has presented in his book, published in 1984[1], an excellent summarised report about the EM-ic virus detecting methods and about their usefulness in the clinical diagnostical work

We could draw the conclusion from the experiences of our earlier proceedings, which were made from nasal secretion and from biopsy material in infants and children suffering of bronchial asthma in early age, that TEM, SEM, EMC investigations can give important and specific information in connection with the pathomechanism and the diagnosis of viral infection.

The purpose of our present investigations were to clarify whether we could find or not diagnostic-value information if we examine infants' and children's bronchial secretion with EM-negative staining method compared these results with clinical and laboratory data.

MATERIAL AND METHOD

We elaborated bronchial secretions in infants and children who suffered of bronchial asthma in early age. The patients' age was between 6 months and 7 years. They were mostly one and two years old. 23 girls and 15 boys were examined. The bronchological examinations, the suction of bronchial secretion were carried out in summer, June and July, 1984.

During the above mentioned period virus epidemy did not

exist. We did not observe any symptoms of viral infections among our patients. From the 38 patients 6 examinations were not appreciable. We could estimate bronchial secretion in 32 patients only. We could find viruses in the bronchial secretion of 18 patients with Electron Microscopic Negative Staining.

The viruses were as follows: Adeno-, RES, Influenza, Herpeto viridae.

The bacteriological examination results of the pharyngeal secretion were negative. Bronchological deformities - ring anomalies and stenosis could have been observed in 6 cases among the 18 virus positive ones.

Electron Microscopic Negative Staining and bacteriological examination results were negative in 14 cases. We could not find bronchus deformities among these negative cases but we detected bacteriums in the pharyngeal secretions in 5 cases as are Pyocianeus, Pneumococcus, Neisseria.

CONCLUSION

We can summarise our examination results as follows: we could detect viruses in more than 50% of our cases with EM-ic Negative Staining from bronchial secretation in infants and children, who were treated owing to bronchial asthma in early age. On the other hand, we did not detect Bact. from bronchial secretions in the virus positive patients.

REFERENCE

1. McLean Donald M. (1984) Same-day Diagnosis of Human Virus Infections, CRC Press, Boca Raton, Florida

© 1985 Elsevier Science Publishers B.V. (Biomedical Division)
New dimensions in otorhinolaryngology - head and neck surgery, vol. 2.
E. Myers, editor

PENETRATION OF CIPROFLOXACIN INTO NASAL SECRETIONS

GIEBEL W, ULLMANN U, DALHOFF A, KOEPPE P
University E.N.T.-Clinic, Silcherstraße 5, D-7400 Tübingen, GFR

INTRODUCTION

Ciprofloxacin pharmacokinetics are characterized by a high volume distribution indicating an efficient diffusion of the drug into the extravascular space (6,7). Following oral administration the absorption is rapid but the elimination is slow with a half-live time ranging from three to five hours (1,2,4,6).
Nasal secretions are easy to obtain at a free selectable time course without heavy noxes to the volunteers.
The present study was performed to evaluate multiple dose pharmacokinetics and penetration activities of ciprofloxacin.

MATERIAL AND METHODS

Twenty healthy volunteers of both sexes participated in this study. All participants had given their written informed consent and were in good health.
Individual doses of 500 mg ciprofloxacin were administered orally twice daily. Pharmacokinetic profiles were monitored on days 1 and 8 respectively. Blood was taken just before swallowing the tablet and at the following intervals thereafter:

0.5, 1. 1.5, 2, 3, 4, 6, 8 and 12 h.
Nasal secretions were sampled
0.5 1.5, 3, 6 and 12 h.
after administration.

Nasal secretions were collected by placing two pads of dry cotton wool in the nasal cavity 10 min before the various points of time mentioned above and were left there for 20 min.
After removal the pads were eluted in 0.3 ml buffered physiological saline (3).
Ciprofloxacin concentrations were determined microbiologically.
Pharmacokinetic parameters were calculated according to well established known equations. (5)

RESULTS

Ciprofloxacin is rapidly absorbed from the gastrointestinal tract as the data for serum concentrations show (table 1). The elimination from serum is slow with a half live of approximately 4 h.

The diffusion of ciprofloxacin into the extravascular space is almost as rapid as is absorption from the gastrointestinal tract. In nasal secretions ciprofloxacin concentrations peaked approximately 15 to 30 min later than in serum. The maximum of the concentration following the first administration was in nasal secretions 1.4 mg/L and in serum 1.8 mg/L. Following repeated drug administration ciprofloxacin concentration peaked in nasal secretions at 1.9 mg/L and in serum at 2.6 mg/L.

Table 1

Pharmacokinetic constants of ciprofloxacin in serum and nasal secretion

		serum		nasal secretions	
		day 1	day 8	day 1	day 8
C_{max}	(mg/l)	1.8 ± 0.48	2.6 ± 1.21	1.4 ± 0.81	1.9 ±
T_{max}	(min)	79.2 ± 3.3	67.9 ± 35.6	93.0 ± 28	99.0 ±
K_a	(h^{-1})	2.5 ± 0.9	4.8 ± 3.1	2.58 ± 2.1	1.75 ±
$t_{1/2}$	(h)	0.72 ± 0.23	0.37 ± 0.20	-	-
$t_{1/2}$	(h)	4.01 ± 0.86	4.12 ± 0.62	2.12 ± 0.58	2.65 ±
f		-	0.73 ± 0.39	-	0.90 ±

DISCUSSION

Our results are in agreement with previously data for single oral administration of 500 mg ciprofloxacin (1,2,4,6). Similar concentrations as were found here for nasal secretions (1.4 mg/L) were obtained by the skin blister technique (2). So the effective diffusion of ciprofloxacin into the extravascular space was confirmed.

Multiple dose kinetics in the extravascular space were not studied up to now. Although ciprofloxacin levels in nasal secretions increased upon multiple doses and tended to decrease more slowly no relevant accumulation of ciprofloxacin in the intra- und extravascular space was noted.

REFERENCES

1. Brumfitt W, Franklin I, Grady D, Hamilton-Miller J M T, Iliffe A (1984): Changes in the pharmacokinetics of ciprofloxacin and fecal flora during administration of a 7-day course to human volunteers. Antimicrobial Agents and Chemotherapy 26:757-761

2. Crump B, Wise R, Dent J (1983): Pharmacokinetics and tissue penetration of ciprofloxacin. Antimicrobial Agents and Chemotherapy 24:784-786

3. Giebel W, Schönleber K H, Breuninger H, Ullmann U (1979): Quantitative Bestimmung von Protein, Albumin und Antibiotika im Nasensekret gesunder Probanden. Arch Otorhinolaryng 225:149-159

4. Höffken G, Lode H, Prinzing C, Borner K, Koeppe P (1985): Pharmacokinetics of ciprofloxacin after oral and parenteral administration. Antimicrobial Agents and Chemotherapy 27: 375-379

5. Ritschel W A: Handbook of basic pharmacokinetics. (2nd ed.) Drug Intelligence Publications, Hamilton, Il

6. Wingender W, Graefe K H, Gau W, Förster D, Beermann D, Schacht R (1984): Pharmacokinetics of ciprofloxacin after oral and intravenous administration in healthy volunteers. European Journal of Clinical Microbiology 3:355-359

7. Wise R, Lockley R M, Webberly M, Dent J (1984): Pharmacokinetics of intravenously administered ciprofloxacin. Antimicrobial Agents and Chemotherapy 26:208-210

© 1985 Elsevier Science Publishers B.V. (Biomedical Division)
New dimensions in otorhinolaryngology - head and neck surgery, vol. 2.
E. Myers, editor

MEASUREMENT OF VERTEBRAL BLOOD FLOW DURING STELLATE GANGLION BLOCKS WITH ULTRASONIC DOPPLER METHOD

M.SANO, M.TSUDA, K.GOTO AND T.MATSUNAGA
Depts. of Otolaryngology, Osaka University Medical School,
Fukushima-ku, Osaka, Japan

INTRODUCTION

Stellate ganglion blocks induce the increase of blood flow by ceasing the action of the cervical sympathetic nervous system. There have been many publications on the clinical effects by stellate ganglion blocks, but the changes in vertebral blood flow have not been measured during these operations. Before we have investigated the vertebral blood flow in vertigenous patients with ultrasonic Doppler method. With this method, we measured the change of blood flow in the vertebral artery and the common carotid artery in 10 sudden deafness patients during stellate ganglion block.

METHOD

For a testing device, we used the pencil type transcucer(diameter 5 mm), an ultrasonic flow-meter which has audio and analog outlets, an electrocardiograph(Sanei Sokki Co.) for a triggen mode, a medical computer(ATAC-201, Nihon Koden Co.) and X-Y recorder. The projected ultrasonic wave was 5 MHz.

To measure the blood flow velocity of the common carotid and vertebral arteries, the subject was placed in a supine position at rest in a quiet room. After palpation of the common carotid pulse, the ultrasonic transducer was attached to the skin surface on the area below the bifurcating portion of the common carotid artery. To measure the blood flow velocity of the vertebral artery, the examiner applied transducer to the skin between the 1st and 2nd transversal processus of the cervical vertebra below and behind the mastoid processus. We used blood flow index for measuring blood flow rate. This index does not indicate the real blood flow but is proportional to the blood flow in the case of large blood vessel.

RESULT

Fig.1. shows the average change in the common carotid blood flow after stellate ganglion blocks in 10 sudden deafness patients. The vertical axis indicates blood flow index. The blood flow on the blocked side a little increased(P<0.10), but on the unblocked side was not changed.

Fig.2. shows the average change in vertebral blood flow after stellate ganglion blocks. The vertebral blood flow on the blocked side was greately increased(P<0.05), but on the unblocked side was not changed so much.

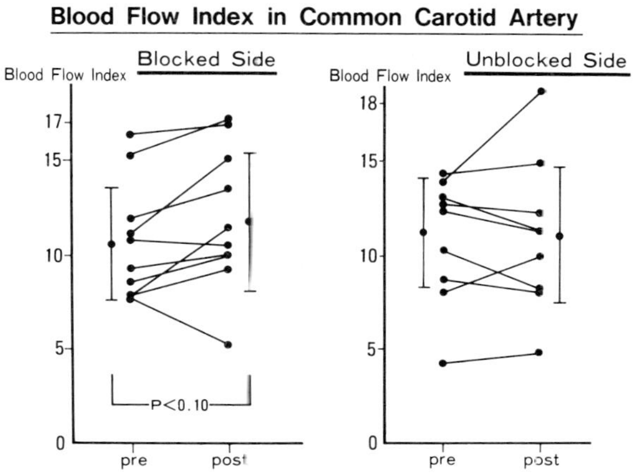

Fig.1. The common carotid blood flow index creased on blocked side.

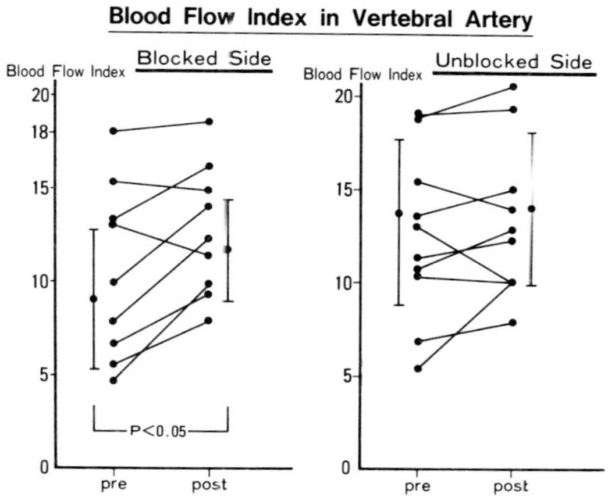

Fig.2. The vertebral blood flow index increased on blocked side.

New dimensions in otorhinolaryngology - head and neck surgery, vol. 2.
E. Myers, editor

DIGITAL SUBTRACTION ANGIOGRAPHY IN PATIENTS WITH CENTRAL VERTIGO

TORU INAMORI, YOSHIO UMETANI, YUKIO TAKAYASU, HARUO WAKUTANI, TAKEO KUMOI
Takarazuka municipal hospital, Hyogo College of Medicine, Hyogo, Japan

INTRODUCTION

Digital subtraction angiography (DSA) is a recently developed non-invasive intravenous angiography which has become possible through real time digital subtraction of X-ray transmission data from an image intensifier and television system. The output signals of the image intensifier-television camera system are digitized by an analog-digital converter. The digital information, 512X512 pixels and 9 bits deep, is fed into the image processing assembly after logarithmic amplification, where 2-8 frames are added and subtracted from mask images for the final digital images. Intravenous digital subtraction angiography was performed in 21 patients.

SUBJECTS

On the patients

1. With intractable dizzy spells of central origin resistant to treatment.
2. With some signs of CNS disturbance.
3. With no significant findings on CT scans.
4. With oneself's request for further study of DSA test.

Performed in 21 patients

Male 9

Female 12

Age 29yrs - 78 yrs (means 50.2 yrs)

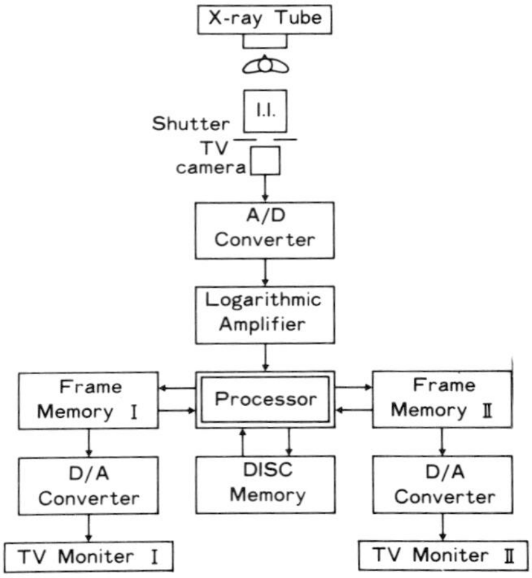

fig.1 Block diagram of DSA

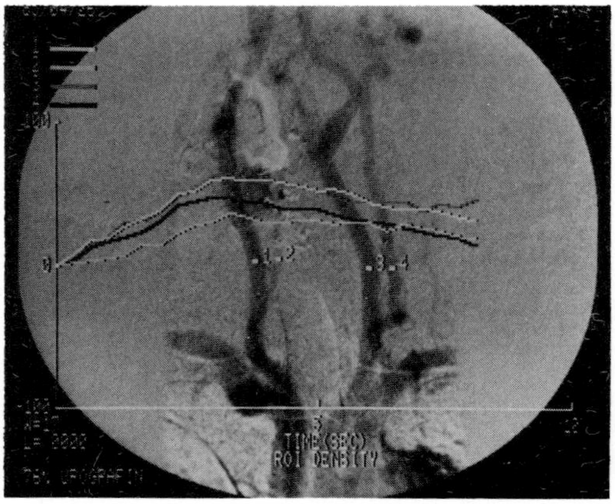

fig.2 DSA photogram in patients with MPPV, showed Rt vertebral aretery stenosis.

RESULTS

		CASES	PERCENTAGE
NORMAL		7	33.3
ABNORMAL		14	66.7
grade	unilateral vertebral obstruction	4	19.0
	stenosis	6	28.6
	reduced flow	2	9.5
	bilateral vertebral stenosis	2	9.5
location	all vertebral region	7	33.3
	partial vertebral (extracranial)	5	23.8
	(intracranial)	2	9.5
bending	neither meander,bending nor kinking	7	33.3
	slightly meander,bending and kinking	5	23.8
	severe meander, bending, and kinking	2	9.5

1. Patients showing the stenosis at almost all are of the vertebral artery are elderly people.
2. Patients who have right vertebral artery stenosis tend to complain clockwise rotatory vertigo and on the contrary patients who have left vertebral artery stenosis tend to complain counter clockwise rotatory vertigo.
3. 3 cases in 4 complete obstruction cases complain vertigo of several hours duration.
4. 4 cases in 5 cases (80%) who have sensorineural hearing loss, showed the same side vertebral artery stenosis predominantly.
5. Both 2 cases with malignant type of paroxysmal positional vertigo revealed vertebral artery stenosis owing to the cervical osteophyte.
6. Both 2 cases presenting Bruns type Nystagmus were recognized to be the vertebral artery stenosis in the palalytic nystagmus side.

DISCUSSION

The advantage of DSA is high contrast resolution which makes it possible to perform intravenous angiography. Since DSA is less invasive, it can be used for screening or repeated examinations. Because a catheter is not inserted into the aretery, DSA has the advantage that the examination is performed in a relatively physiologic condition. Because of real-time observation of the images, there is no need to wait for development of the film as in conventional angiography.

CONCLUSION

DSA's findings were abnormal in 14 of 21 patients (66.7%). DSA is, therefore, considered to be an important aid in the diagnosis of vertigo of the central type.

New dimensions in otorhinolaryngology - head and neck surgery, vol. 2.
E. Myers, editor

ULTRASTRUCTURAL CHANGES WITH CARBON DIOXIDE AND NEODYMIUM YAG LASER CUTANEOUS TISSUE INTERACTION

RONALD ALLEN KIRSCHNER, A.S. Kirschner, Bernard C. McDonnell, J. Bishop, D. DeBias, C. Greene, F. Munson, R. Giuliano

The Institute For Applied Laser Surgery

Suite IL-17, Two Bala Plaza, Bala Cynwyd, Pa. 19004, U.S.A.

The CO2 laser has been utilized for a variety of cutaneous applications for quite some time. The microscopic and ultrastructural changes have been studied and reported at length.

The F.D.A. has recently approved a clinical trial in which the Nd:YAG laser will be employed for the treatment of a number of cutaneous lesions. It behooved us to study the effects of this modality on a laboratory model. The Cooper Lasersonics model 8000 and the Xanar Articulator were utilized in this study.

The Nd:YAG laser is characterized by a wavelength of 1060 nm. The coefficient of absorption of cutaneous tissue is relatively low. To compare, the coefficient with CO2 is 911, and with Nd:YAG it is 231.

The model used for the study was the Mountain White Rabbit. For the active parts of the study, the rabbits were anesthetized using Nembutal delivered through a venocath in small titred amounts. We found that this was the safest way to maintain the animals in a comfortable and humane fashion. Samples were obtained immediately after exposure at varying power settings and exposure durations. The early samples were removed with a power driven cutaneous punch. We found that there was less tissue distortion for the SEM if the samples were removed with a strip technique, which was subsequently used.

At moderate power density applications, we noted an immediate slight blistering effect. SEM examinations of this material demonstrated coagulated liquid which appeared as a small mass lying beneath a zone of necrotic material. There was actually an increase in the tissue volume due to the formation of coagulum. In contrast, the CO2 treated area demonstrates immediate tissue shrinkage due to vapor which is lost as the cellular fluid turns into steam. The CO2 laser incisions presented with a great deal of necrotic material initially. After an eighteen day period, they still exhibited a marked amount of scar tissue. The Nd:YAG exposed tissue demonstrated a great deall less necrotic material initially, and at the eighteen day point the overall healing quality was much better than that of the CO2 exposed specimens when a similar number of joules were applied.

A complete review of our data suggests that the Nd:YAG laser may prove to be an excellent tool for cutaneous plastic surgery.

© 1985 Elsevier Science Publishers B.V. (Biomedical Division)
New dimensions in otorhinolaryngology - head and neck surgery, vol. 2.
E. Myers, editor

ENZYME HISTOCHEMICAL, IMMUNOPATHOLOGICAL AND ULTRASTRUCTURAL STUDIES OF THE LYMPHOID COMPONENT OF PAROTID ADENOLYMPHOMA

TAKESHI MARUYAMA M.D., YASUSHI MURAKAMI M.D. AND SHIGENORI HARAGUCHI M.D.
Dept. of Otolaryngology, School of Medicine, Keio University, Tokyo (Japan)
ATUO MIKATA M.D.
Dept. of Pathology, School of Medicine, Keio University, Tokyo (Japan)

INTRODUCTION

Adenolymphoma of the parotid gland is composed of two histologic components, epithelial and lymphoid.

The purpose of this study was to clarify the origin of the epithelial component of this tumor.

Two theories have long been disputed as the histogenesis of this tumor. One is that the epithelial component originates from the striated duct in the parotid gland and that heavy lymphocytic infiltrations are generated around it due to an unknown cause. The other is that ductal inclusions in the lymph nodes in or around the parotid gland develop into a tumor.

Thus, there is no definite opinion as yet. With regard to these considerations, immunopathological and histochemical studies were undertaken in an attempt to elucidate the origin of the neoplasm.

MATERIALS AND METHODS

Accordingly, in order to supplement the existing results of morphological observations, we tried several test methods to investigate the characteristics of the lymphatic tissues.

All materials used were obtained from 28 patients aged between 42 and 82 years at Keio University Hospital, during the period from 1974 to 1984.

First, in order to clarify the presence of the structures of the lymph node in the tumor lymphatic tissues. HE-stained sections from all cases were examined. Second, surveys of E and EAC rosette formation were undertaken. Third, surface immunoglobulins of the tumor lymphocytes were detected by fluorescein antibody techniques. Fourth, enzyme histochemical studies of the frozen sections and the rosette-forming lymphocytes were carried out in 16 cases. The enzymes analyzed in these studies were: acid phosphatase by the method of Barca, β-glucuronidase by that of Hayashi, α-naphthyl acetate esterase by that of Yam and α-naphthyl butylate esterase by that of Li for the frozen sections and the rosette-forming lymphocytes. Alkaline phosphatase was analyzed by the method of Burston, adenosine triphosphatase by that of Wacstein, 5'-nucleotidase by that of Wacstein and nucleotide diphosphatase by that of Wacstein for the frozen sections. Fifth, PAP techniques were performed in 16 cases as an immunopathological study. Paraffin-embedded tissues were cut into sections 3 μm in thickness and processed for immunopathological staining; IgG, IgA, IgM, κ light chains and λ light chains all being determined. Electron microscopic studies were also done using the usual method in 16 cases.

RESULTS

A light microscopic survey of the HE-stained sections revealed that the lymph node structures, i.e., the lymphatic sinus, the marginal sinus and the trabecula, were found in eight cases (32.3%). Surface immunoglobulins of the lymphocytes were expressed polyclonally, and the T- to B-cell ratio calculated by rosette formation indicated that B cells predominated.

Tests of cell suspension revealed that enzyme activities of T and B cells of the tumor lymphocytes, which were calculated by E and EAC rosette formation, were the same as those of the normal lymph node. Histochemistry of the frozen sections of the tumor tissues showed that the localizations of the activities of the eight enzymes in the tumor lymphatic tissues were the same as those in normal lymph nodes.

Immunopathological studies by PAP method revealed that the distribution of the immunoglobulin-containing cells was almost the same as in normal lymph nodes, and the presence of positive cells in the area just below the epithelium was found to be characteristic of tumor lymphatic tissues.

Finally, the electron microscopic studies showed that tumor lymphocytes had completely the same characteristics as those of the normal lymph node.

CONCLUSION

Based on these results, we concluded that the lymphatic tissues of parotid adenolymphoma are identical with those of the normal lymph node. It was also assumed that the lymphatic tissue of this tumor was composed of the preexisting lymph node.

It was also assumed that the presence of the many immunoglobulin-containing cells in the area just below the epithelial component may indicate an autoimmune reaction between the epithelial component and the lymphatic tissues.

New dimensions in otorhinolaryngology - head and neck surgery, vol. 2.
E. Myers, editor

THE EPITHELIUM OF THE HUMAN WHARTON'S DUCT IN OBSTRUCTIVE SIALADENITIS. A TEM AND SEM STUDY

P PUXEDDU (1), F TESTA-RIVA (2), R SOLINAS (3), G AGUS (4) AND A RIVA (5)

Institutes of Otolaryngology and Anatomy, University of Cagliari,
I 09100, Cagliari, ITALY

INTRODUCTION

In a previous paper on the ultrastructure of normal submandibular main excretory duct (MED) of man we described (1) sporadic ciliated cells interspersed among goblet and principal cells. On the other hand some authors (2, 3) observed numerous ciliated cells in the epithelial lining of the human submandibular ducts in cases of obstructive sialadenitis. No attention, however, was paid to the submandibular MED epithelium in pathology. We considered, therefore, interesting to study the submandibular MED (also known as Wharton's duct) in 4 cases of sialolithiasis in which the obstruction was upstream with respect to the portion of the duct observed.

MATERIAL AND METHODS

Specimens of the submandibular gland were obtained from 3 females and 1 male patients aged 33-50 years at the time of operation from the removal of the entire gland because of obstructive sialadenitis. Tissues were then fixed and processed for TEM and SEM according to the schedule indicated in our previous paper (1).

RESULTS

In all the cases studied, we noticed a considerable increase of goblet and ciliated cells if compared with the normal duct. Cilia (Fig.1) were present in the apex of principal cells and were either uniformly distributed or placed in tufts between the microvilli. In TEM images of ciliogenesis of the acentriolar pathway were frequently observed. The anomalies of cilia most commonly encountered were the atypical microtubule patterns and compound cilia, that is multiple axonemes enclosed within a single cell membrane.

From our results, we consider ciliated cells as principal cells altered by inflammatory desease. In fact, the ciliation in tissues normally devoid of cilia has been described in many pathological states. It is noteworthy that the abnormalities observed by us in the Wharton's duct cilia are very similar to those described in the respiratory epithelium in a variety of pathological states (4).

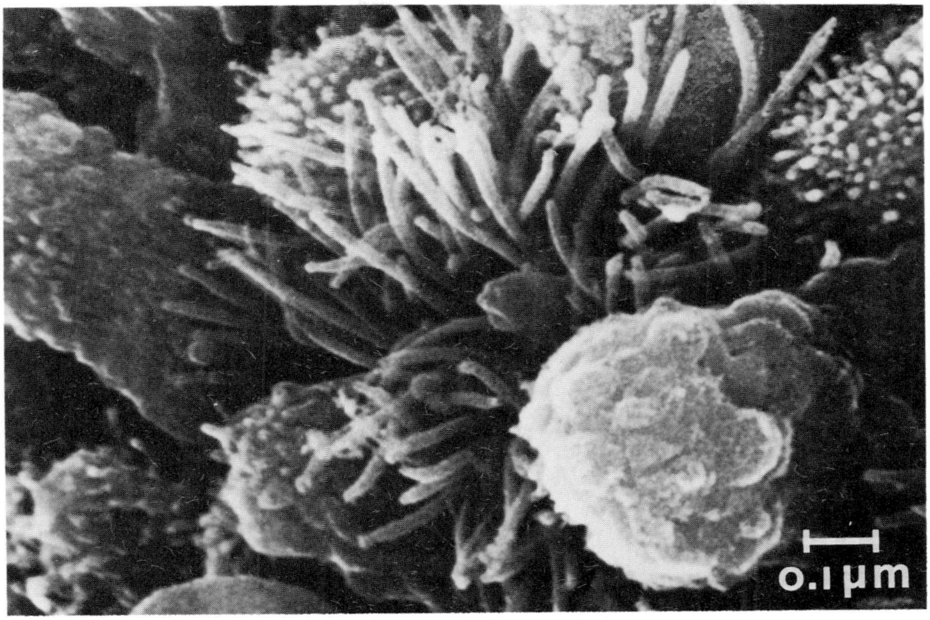

Fig. 1. SEM. Note the presence of several cilia on the apices of principal cells. The cell in the bottom right is a goblet cell.

ACKNOWLEDGEMENTS

This work has been financed by a grant from the Consiglio Nazionale delle Ricerche.

REFERENCES

1. Testa-Riva F, Puxeddu P, Riva A, Diaz G (1981) Am J Anat 160: 381-393

2. Vortel V, Sazama L (1977) Cek Patol 13: 134-137

3. Davies KJ, Garrett JR (1981) J Micr 123: RP1-RP2

4. Herzon FS (1981) Ann Otol Rhinol Laryngol 90 (83): 1-12

New dimensions in otorhinolaryngology – head and neck surgery, vol. 2.
E. Myers, editor

MICROASPIRATION OF GASTRO-ESOPHAGEAL REFLUX IN CHRONIC BRONCHITIS AND ASTHMA

N SANDBERG, I MÅNSSON, U BENGTSSON, S CARLSSON AND M RUTH

Depts. of Otolaryngology, Allergy and Nuclear Medicine, University of Gothenburg, Gothenburg and Central Hospital, Uddevalla, Sweden

INTRODUCTION

Different pulmonary complications are wellknown to occur in patients with gastro-esophageal reflux both in children and adults. Pulmonary fibrosis, recurrent pneumonia, bronchial asthma and chronic bronchitis have been reported in adults (for ref. see Nelson[1], Sandberg[2]).

Gastro-esophageal reflux (GER) during the night could possibly explain the special rhytm which some asthmatics - so-called morning dippers - have with their lowest peak flow rates in the early hours. Small aspirations of gastric content from GER may be the causative factor in air-way complications such as asthma and chronic bronchitis. A modified scintimetric method for objective documentation of small aspirations[3] was applied in asthmatics and in patients with chronic bronchitis combined with GER to elucidate this problem.

METHODS

Tests of GER. 24-hour pH monitoring of the distal esophagus was performed according to DeMeester et al[4] and modified for recording in ambulant patients. The number and duration of reflux episodes during day and night were registered with a computer.

Aspiration of reflux. A non-resorbable radiopharmaceutical (200 MBq ^{99m}Tc - sulfur colloid in 70 ml of water) was deposited intragastrically via a naso-gastric tube at bedtime. In the morning the count rate over the lungs was recorded by a scintillation camera. Broncho-pulmonary aspiration was diagnosed if the count rate was significantly over background in a computerized program. Further technical details are given by Månsson and Carlsson[3].

RESULTS

The relation between the patient´s history (heartburn and/or regurgitation) and result of 24-hour pH monitoring showed in 43 asthmatics that no reflux symptoms were noted in 7 patients with normal pH-test and in 4 with pathologic refluxes. 13 patients had symptoms of reflux but normal pH-tests and 19 had symptoms and pathologic refluxes at the pH-test.
Pathologic refluxes were thus found in 23 patients (53%) and 11 of them had

nocturnal refluxes and reflux symptoms were noted in 32 of the total number of patients.

Scintimetric recordings. Scintimetry has so far been performed in a control group of 9 non-smokers and in 19 patients with respiratory disease combined with GER disease. Nobody in the control group showed aspiration. 9 out of 19 patients had nocturnal asthma and aspiration was demonstrated in 3. 8 patients had chronic bronchitis and in 2 aspiration was found. 2 patients had other respiratory disease and no aspiration was found.

Treatment. The respiratory disease was successfully treated with antireflux procedure in 4 out of 5 patients in whom aspiration was found: One was operated upon and 3 patients got conservative treatment including H_2-blockers.

SUMMARY AND CONCLUSIONS

1. Pathologic reflux was found in patients with asthma or chronic bronchitis.
2. Scintimetry with a new developed technique was found to be a method to detect microaspiration.
3. Antireflux procedures was an effective treatment of the respiratory disease in some patients with aspiration.

REFERENCES

1. Nelson HS (1984) J Allergy Clin Immunol 73:547-556
2. Sandberg N (ed) Function and Disease of the Oesophagus. Scand J Gastroenterol suppl 106 (1984)
3. Månsson I, Carlsson S (1984) Proc 4th World Congr for Bronchology pp 72-73
4. DeMeester T R, Wang C I, Wernly J A, Pellegrini C A, Little A G, Klementschitsch P, Bermudez G, Johnson L F, Skinner D B (1980) J Thorac Cardiovasc Surg 79:656-665

© 1985 Elsevier Science Publishers B.V. (Biomedical Division)
New dimensions in otorhinolaryngology - head and neck surgery, vol. 2.
E. Myers, editor

MURINE SUBRENAL CAPSULE ASSAY FOR SQUAMOUS CELL CARCINOMA OF THE HEAD AND NECK

CHARLES M. STIERNBERG, MD, WM. H. ROTZLER, MD, K. VALYI-NAGY, MD,
JAMES A. HOKANSON, PhD, PRICE HALE, BS, BYRON J. BAILEY, MD
Departments of Otolaryngology and PMCH, University of Texas Medical Branch,
Galveston, Texas 77550, U.S.A.

INTRODUCTION

The murine subrenal capsule (SRC) assay is an in vivo method for rapidly determining the responsiveness of human tumor xenografts to chemotherapeutic agents. The assay allows in situ measurement of small changes in the size of tumor xenografts transplanted beneath the renal capsule of mice.[1] The purposes of this study were to demonstrate growth and rate of growth of squamous cell carcinoma of the head and neck in the SRC assay and to determine the feasibility of using the assay for testing sensitivity of this malignancy to therapeutic agents.

METHODS AND MATERIALS

One hundred and twenty-seven mice were used to perform seven assays, one for a tumor-growth curve and six for testing tumor sensitivity to indomethacin (20 mcg/ml in drinking water) and cisplatin (2 mg/kg/day). Using an operating microscope with ocular micrometer, one-millimeter (16 ocular microunits) fragments of squamous cell carcinoma were implanted beneath the renal capsule of normal immunocompetent mice. Base-line and post-treatment measurements were made of the xenografts, and tumor responsiveness determined by comparing the mean change in tumor sizes of test and control groups. An assay was evaluable if positive growth occurred in the control group and histologic exam confirmed carcinoma in xenografts. The growth curve was calculated by determining the mean change in tumor size in five mice per day on days 3 through 7.

RESULTS

Figure 1 shows the tumor-growth curve for a squamous cell carcinoma. There was significant ($P<0.05$) growth every day except for day 5, and the growth rate declined on day 7. Table I summarizes results of six assays. Carcinoma was confirmed histologically in all assays, and all were evaluable by our criteria. A significant ($P<0.05$) decrease in tumor growth was shown in four of six assays for indomethacin-treated mice and in three of four assays for cisplatin-treated mice.

SUMMARY

Observations in this pilot study lead to the conclusions that squamous cell carcinoma of the head and neck can be grown in the murine SRC assay and significant growth occurs as early as three or four days, as demonstrated by the tumor-growth curve. Collaboration with a pathologist is necessary to assure viable tumor is used and xenografts need to be similar in size (one millimeter). The assay allows cytotoxic therapeutic agents such as cisplatin to be evaluated, but clinical correlations will require comparison with response rates observed in patients. Similar to a study by Stratton et al who used sodium ibuprofen, our results with indomethacin showed that it may retard growth of squamous cell carcinoma.[2] However, considering the mechanism of action of prostaglandin synthetase inhibitors, firm conclusions cannot be stated since the SRC assay is completed within a time frame before the host can produce a significant cellular-immune response.

FIGURE 1 TUMOR-GROWTH CURVE

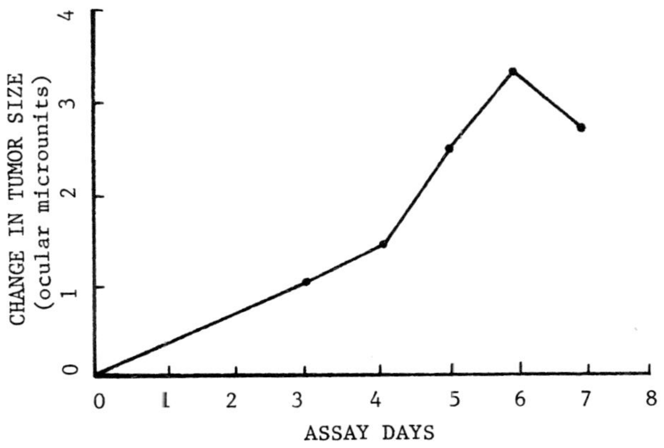

TABLE I COMPARISON OF MEANS FOR CHANGE IN TUMOR SIZES

Assay #	Control Group	Indomethacin Group	Significance Level	Cisplatin	Significance Level
1 (18)*	3.57(7)	0.04(5)	P<0.13	-2.50(6)	P<0.01
2 (18)	2.75(6)	-1.00(6)	0.04	1.67(6)	0.45
3 (12)	5.00(7)	-0.20(5)	0.01	--	--
4 (20)	3.00(6)	0.36(7)	0.01	-1.93(7)	0.01
5 (15)	2.63(8)	0.00(7)	0.16	--	--
6 (19)	4.36(7)	-3.00(6)	0.01	-3.08(6)	0.01

* Number of mice in each assay and group appears in parentheses.

REFERENCES

1. Bogden AE, Kelton DE, Cobb WR, et al (1978): A rapid screening method for testing chemotherapeutic agents against human tumor xenografts. In: Houchens D, Ovejera A (eds) Proceedings of the Symposium on the Use of Athymic (nude) Mice in Cancer Research. New York, Gustav Fiser, pp 231-250.

2. Stratton JA, Braly PS, DiSaia PJ (1984): Response of human adenocarcinoma to chemotherapy: As sole agents and in combination with sodium ibuprofen. Gynecol Oncol 18:145-149.

New dimensions in otorhinolaryngology - head and neck surgery, vol. 2.
E. Myers, editor

A STUDY FOR CHLAMYDIA PSITTACI ISOLATION TECHNIQUE

SUSUMU MUKAI, MD, CHIKAKO MUKAI, MD, ISSEI SUZUKI.
MUKAI Medical Clinic and Microbiological Laboratory,
Yamatominami 2-8-9, 242 Kanagawa, JAPAN

INTRODUCTION

There are much more diseases infected by c.psittci than ever thought.[1-5) For the correct diagnosis for these isolations of the organism are inevitable. To isolate chlamydiae, tissue culture is now the method of choice. The techniques are established for the c.trachomatis. But what extent the isolation techniques for chlamydia trachomatis is useful for those of chlamydia psittaci? We tried to isolate c.psittaci by use with the isolation techniques for c.trachomatis. We also tried to develope a simple technique to isolate c.psittaci that can be used for routine clinical laboratory.

MATERIAL AND METHOD

Material. DEAE-dextran was used to change cell surface membrane charge and cycloheximide for cell metabolism supressor.
C.psittaci meningopneumonitis(MP) are employed to the isolation. Monolayered L cells were used for culture with 2% FCS Eagle's MEM as sustention medium.
Method. Condition A) 30min before the inoculation of MP, L cells were treated with DEAE. B) No treatment was done to the L cells.
Situation After 1hr of MP inoculation with L cells, there was no movement detected. These were incubated with 1) sustention medium and with 2) $2.3X10^{-8}$g/ml of cycloheximide added sustention medium. With inoculation of MP cells, the vials were centrifugalized at 400g for 1hr. After these they were incubated with 3) sustention medium and with 4) $2.3X10^{-8}$g/ml of cycloheximide adde sustention medium. Condition C-1) Both MP and sustention medium and C-2) both MP and $2.3X10^{-8}$g/ml of cycloheximide added sustention medium, L cells were incubated.
Total of condition-situation combinations were as follows;
A-1, A-2, A-3, A-4, B-1, B-2, B-3, B-4, C-1 and C-2.

After 37°C 48hrs incubation of these conditions, infected cells were counted under microscope with Machiavello stain and infected rates were also counted for each combinations' controls.

RESULT (Table-1)

	A1	A2	A3	A4	B1	B2	B3	B4	C1	C2
ICC	7	13	1500	1800	120	240	2340	1390	170	350
IR	0.04	0.52	7.9	72	0.63	9.6	12.3	55.6	o.89	14

(ICC; Infected Cells Count, IR; Infected Rates)

DEAE did not increase L cells affinities for MP. Cycloheximide increased L cells infected rate and the growth of intracytoplasmic inclusions of MP but they did not increase infected cell count. Cultures with Eagl's MEM only increased infected cell count and number of L cells.

DISCUSSION

After the isolation of chlamydiae to detect them is relatively difficult. With cycloheximide added medium chlamydiae are easier detectable than with non added medium, but isolations with Eagl's MEM only augment their infected cells number. So the most effective c,psittaci isolation method is B-3, that is, no treatment before the inoculation of the cells, inoculation with centrifugal force and culture with Eagle's medium added FCS only.

REFERENCES

1. Mukai S, Mukai C, Suzuki I (1981) 82 cases of cervical lymphadenitis caused by ornithosis. XII World Congress of Otorhinolaryngology, Budapest.
2. Mukai S, Mukai C, Asaoka K, Suzuki I (1983) Chlamydial infection with main symptoms of upper cervical lymphadenitis. Jap J Otol 86: 441-45 .
3. Mukai S, Mukai C, Asaoka K, Suzuki I (1985) Chlamydial infection of head and neck. Ear Nose and Throat J 64: 173-179.
4. Mukai S, Mukai C, Asaoka K, Suzuki I (1985) Chlamydia infection with main symptoms of upper cervical lymphadenitis(UCLA)--Isolation of chlamydiae-- Jap J Otol: in print
5. Mukai Susumu (1985) Upper-deep cervical lymphadenitis by chlamydia infection. JOHNS 1:129-132.

New dimensions in otorhinolaryngology - head and neck surgery, vol. 2.
E. Myers, editor

SPECTRUM OF KAPOSI'S SARCOMA OF THE HYPOPHARYNX IN AIDS: ITS DIAGNOSIS, EVALUATION AND MANAGEMENT

C. DANIEL SOOY, M.D., CARL O.M. HO, SUSAN D. WALL*, M.D.

University of California School of Medicine, departments of Otolaryngology-Head and Neck Surgery and Radiology*, San Francisco

The incidence of acquired immunodeficiency syndrome (AIDS) is increasing at a near epidemic rate, with the number of cases doubling every six months. Since its initial description in 1981, 9760 cases of AIDS have been reported to the U.S.A. Centers for Disease Control (as of April 22, 1985).

Characteristic of the acquired immunodeficiency syndrome is a severe depression of the immune system, primarily in the T-cell arm, with a reduction in the helper to suppressor cell ratio. The depressed immunity predisposes the patient to opportunistic infections. Pneumocystis carinii pneumonia is the most frequent life threatening infection. The dermatologic malignancy, Kaposi's sarcoma (KS), is the most common neoplasm.

Recent evidence has implicated a retrovirus as the etiologic agent of AIDS. Three independent laboratories have isolated a new retrovirus from AIDS or ARC patients and reported it as the etiologic agent with Human T-lymphotrophic retrovirus-III (HTLV-III) the most cited retrovirus.

Otolaryngologic and head and neck manifestations of the acquired immunodeficiency syndrome are seen in 41% of AIDS patients.[1] The manifestations include cutaneous lesions of Kaposi's sarcoma with oro and hypopharyngeal lesions seen in 35% of these patients with KS; oral, pharyngeal, laryngeal and esophageal candidal lesions; chronic cough and shortness of breath due to infection with pneumocystis carinii or mycobacterium avium-intracellulare; rapidly enlarging neck masses due to Burkitt's lymphoma; labial or oral lesions of herpes simplex. Some patients also have serous otitis, acute mastoiditis, sensorineural hearing loss, parotid mass, sinusitis, or squamous cell carcinoma. Cervical lymphadenopathy is almost a universal finding.

A single case of obstruction of the hypopharynx due to Kaposi's sarcoma has been reported.[2] Our report is a retrospective review of a series of six patients who represent the spectrum of presentation, complications, evaluation and treatment of Kaposi's sarcoma of the hypopharynx and supraglottic larynx. In these six patients, the violaceous lesions of Kaposi's sarcoma range from a small sessile or pedunculated solitary mass to multiple massive lesions causing airway obstruction.

The median duration from the diagnosis of AIDS to hypopharyngeal complaints in the five symptomatic patients was one month. All of these patients complained of dysphagia while odynophagia, dysphonia, and airway obstruction were each seen in one patient. The severity of symptons correlated well with the extent of the patient's disease although this tumor is commonly asymptomatic.

The treatment of the hypopharyngeal Kaposi's sarcoma lesions was by surgery or radiation therapy in addition to the chemo or immunotherapeutic agents the patients were receiving. These agents included interferon, interlukin 2, vinblastine and vincristine. Single or isolated lesions were excised with the CO_2 laser or by electrocautery. In those patients with multiple diffuse sarcomatous lesions, radiation therapy was our treatment of choice.

Radiation therapy was relatively well tolerated when a total of 2000-3000 R were fractioned over 2 to 4 weeks. A control rate of 95% and an approximate 20% complication rate was obtained.

TABLE I. SUMMARY OF SIX PATIENTS WITH KS OF THE HYPOPHARYNX.

Pt #	Sx	Duration	Lesion	Dx Exams
1	0	-	Mild disease on post. wall with extension to nasopharynx	Ba swallow Biopsy
2	Dyspha	3 mo	1x1cm polypoid post. pharyngeal wall mass	Ba swallow Biopsy
3	Dyspha	21 mo	Disease in left hypo-pharynx; base of tongue	Ba swallow
4	Dyspha	1 mo	Diffuse lesions in oro and hypopharynx	Ba swallow Biopsy
5	Dyspha Dyspho	1 mo 1 mo	Pedunculated lesions on right AE fold, 1.5x2cm, and left epiglottis	CT scan Biopsy
6	Dyspha Airway obst.	1 mo 12 hr	Extensive and diffuse encompassing all visible naso, oro & hypopharynx; entire trachea	CT scan Biopsy

REFERENCES

1. Marcusen DC, Sooy CD (1985) Laryngoscope 95:401
2. Patow CA, Stark TW, et al (1984) Otol Head Neck Surg 92:713

New dimensions in otorhinolaryngology – head and neck surgery, vol. 2.
E. Myers, editor

TOTAL CIRCULAR PHARYNGO-LARYNGECTOMY - THE RADIAL FOREARM FLAP (CHINESE FLAP) IN RECONSTRUCTION OF THE ALIMENTARY CANAL

Michel ZANARET, Guy MAGALON, Jean-Marc THOMASSIN, Régis LEGRE, Maurice CANNONI, André PECH

Clinique O.R.L. - C.H.U. TIMONE 13385 MARSEILLE (FRANCE)
Service de Chirurgie Plastique - C.H.U. TIMONE 13385 MARSEILLE (FRANCE)

The reconstruction of the digestive tube by cervical methods, after total circular pharyngo-laryngectomy continues to pose a number of problems. Musculo-cutaneous flaps, because of their tubulization difficulties and the thickness of the cutaneous layer are, however, an uncertain means of closing total circular pharyngo-laryngectomy. Free visceral plasties give first intention repairs with rapid return of eating but, because of its inherant abdominal stage it, sometimes, leads to fatal complications. The free ante-brachial plasty with a radial pedicle still known as the "Chinese flap" seems to be a satisfactory alternative.

SURGICAL TECHNIQUE

The flap has a roughly rectangular shape centered on the radial artery. Its elngth, suited to the size of the reconstruction work, averages 10 cms. The width is 10 cms in the upper part and 8 cms in the lower. The flap is raised by cutaneous aponeurotic dissection, passing systematically below the radial bundle, in the valley between the flexor carpi radialis and the brachioradialis. Before beginning the vascular dissection stage, the flap is then tubulized on the anterior side of the forearm. The longitudinal suture is carried out on two levels ; the deep cutaneous layer is closed with separate everted stitches knotted in the lumen, whereas the superficial aponeurotic layer is closed with a continuous edge-to-edge suture. The vascular dissection stage is then begun : on the lower part, the superficial veins are bound, as is the entire radial pedicle, on the upper part, the radial artery is dissected up ti its source, thus producing an artery of 2-3 mm in diameter and some 2 to 3 cms long. The deep radial veins are dissected so as to obtain a sufficiently long venous pedicle and the anastomosis between the deep and the superficial system. Dissection of the surface veins of the elbow crease gives a second veinous pedicle of a larger caliber and greater in length that we select in preference.

The operation is carried out concomitantly :
- The cervical stage entails a classic exeresis : total circular pharyngo-laryngectomy with traditionnal curage of one side and functional of the oter. The cutaneous flap is taken to the cervical region. The vascular micro-anastomosis at the neck are carried out after having sutured the posterior layer of the digestive anatomosis so as to stabilize the flap. We prefer to use the facial artery

because of its suitable caliber and of the fact that its length allows adaptation to the positioning of the flap. The end-to-end arterial suture is sewn, using a microscope, with individual stitches of 9/0 thread. The choice of venous anastomosis depends on the venous return. In order to obtain the best possible drainage we connect the vein with the strongest flow directly onto the jugular vein termino laterally. As a safety precaution, we also carry out a second termino-lateral venous suture onto a branch of the Faraboeuf venous trunk. The donor site is filled with a split thickness skin graft. Once the micro-surgical stage is over, we proceed with the anterior side of the digestive sutures after having inserted a gastric probe - we use no temporary gastrostomy.

Between December 1983 and Marc 1985, we performed 9 reconstructions of the alimentary canal using the above described technique. 5 of the patients had been irradiated previously and the other 4 cases had already undergone initial surgery. There were no post-operative mortalities. One patient presented a total necrosis of the flap, this specific case had mild diabetes which decompensated after the operation. We are able to close his pharyngostome by a musculo-cutaneous flap. None of the other patients showed signs of fistulae and deglutition therefore resumed between the 14th and the 21st day. Alimentation posed no particular problem. 4 of the patients who had undergone initial surgery were irradiated in normal doses without post-radiation stenosis developing.

The chinese flap thus seems to us a promising method in the reconstruction on the alimentary canal following total circular pharyngo-laryngectomy, and should thus be weighed against musculo-cutaneous flaps and free visceral plastic surgery. In this comparison, its advantages are clear : Good vascularization leads to great reliability, the thinness of the skin permits troublefree tubulization and a satisfactory suture at the cesophageal junction and, finally, it circumvents the need for an abdominal operation and its inherant dangers.

There are, notwithstanding, some minor inconveniences : the resultant scarring of the forearm. The sacrifice of the radial artery seems however to present no inconvenience ; the fact that a digestive segment is replaced by skin : this open the door to a potential stenosis, especially after radiotherapy. We have, for the moment, had no complications of this kind.

REFERENCES

1. Pech A., Cannoni M., Zanaret M. et Coll. - Pharyngo-laryngectomie totale circulaire. Méthode de reconstruction par un lambeau cutané libre d'avant-bras. Ann. Oto-Laryng. (Paris) 1984, 101 : 535-540

2. Yang Guofan et Ol. - Forearm free skin flap transplantation. National Med. J. China 1981, 61 : 139

3. Zanaret M., Legré R., Kevorkian B. - Pharyngo-laryngectomies totales circulaires. Méthodes de reconstruction de la filière digestive par un lambeau antibrachial à pédicule radial. J. Fr. O.R.L. 1984, 33, 6 : 286-290

New dimensions in otorhinolaryngology - head and neck surgery, vol. 2.
E. Myers, editor

ADJUVANT STRATEGY FOR TREATMENT OF INCURABLE OROPHARYNGEAL MALIGNOMAS

L. Osterwald, D. Gefeller, K. Dahlem and V. Bendel
ENT-clinic of the city of Hannover and Hannover Medical School, Radiotherapy Dept., Hannover, Federal Republic of Germany

Poor results of traditional therapeutic procedures and hopelessness of patients with primarily non-operable tumors or recurrent disease stimulated us to seek for auxiliary strategies:

1.) utilization of cis-platinum (DDP) in low doses as 'radio-sensitizer'
2.) application of extract of mistletoe (Viscum Album Quercus)
3.) Urging the patient to avoid drinking alcoholic beverages and refrain from smoking.

Radiation therapy was given in two series, adding up to 40 Gy and 16 - 26 Gy respectively. Cis-platinum was administered in 20 mg/m² dosage regimen, twice during the first week of treatment, to be repeated the following fourth week as long as the radiation program continued.

During each chemotherapy unit DDP was only given on days exempt from high-voltage treatment, followed by radiation and each unit completed by the second dispensing of the presumed radio-sensitizer.

Patients not treated otherwise before (n=17) showed complete remission in 1/3 and a one-year-survival rate of 70 % (according to the 'life-table method' of CUTTLER and EDERER). However, only half of the cases with recurrent tumor showed partial remission.

Extract of mistletoe was used in more than 20 patients who either had undergone conventional therapy or suffered from intractable progression of the tumor. No scientific analysis of the results achieved can be presented, but despite absence of true cures periods of individual well-being could be increased and further progression of the disease delayed.

Avoiding alcoholic drinks as well as smoking proved to be a major problem in nearly all of our patients and often compliance was poor. In successful individuals particularly amelioration of local growth of the disease could be noted.

© 1985 Elsevier Science Publishers B.V. (Biomedical Division)
New dimensions in otorhinolaryngology - head and neck surgery, vol. 2.
E. Myers, editor

CARCINOMATOUS CHANGES IN PHARYNGEAL DIVERTICULA°

M. E. BARAKA* & S. A. A. SADEK**

*Assistant Prof, Dept of Otolaryngology, King Faisal Univ, Dammam, Saudi Arabia
**Consultant ENT Surgeon, Khor-Fakan Hospital, U.A.E.

INTRODUCTION

In the 10-year period between 1972 and 1982, 70 cases of pharyngeal diverticula were treated by either general surgeons, ENT surgeons or thoracic surgeons at Wythenshawe Hospital, Manchester, England. These cases are now reviewed.

METHODS OF TREATMENT

TABLE

Methods of treatment adopted for all patients.

Method of treatment	Ext. excision & crico-pharyng. myotomy	Dohlman's op.	Dilatation only	Inversion	None	Crico-pharyng. myotomy only	Deep x-ray therapy
No. of pts.	47	9	6	4	3	1	2

HISTOLOGY

Of the 47 patients who underwent external excision of the pouch, in 35 there was a histological record of the excised diverticulum; 32 were reported to be simple pouches and three showed malignant changes.

BRIEF NOTES ON THE THREE CASES WITH MALIGNANT CHANGES

<u>First Case--J.S., aged 76</u>

Presented with a longstanding history of dysphagia, regurgitation of food, cough and weight loss. Radiological investigation confirmed the presence of a pharyngeal pouch. He had total excision of the pouch and cricopharyngeal myotomy.

Histology showed carcinoma in situ. No evidence of invasive tumor.

<u>Second Case--S.F., aged 75</u>

Presented with a two-year history of dysphagia for solids and regurgitation of food eaten hours before. Radiological examination confirmed the presence of a pharyngeal pouch. Esophagoscopy showed the pouch to be full of food particles and there was an annular mass which bled easily on touch. Histology showed squamous carcinoma in situ. No definite evidence of invasive carcinoma in the specimen but very little subepithelial tissue included.

Third Case--A.R., aged 85

This patient had a longstanding history of dysphagia. She was diagnosed clinically and confirmed radiologically to have a pharyngeal diverticulum. Esophagoscopy showed an ulcerating mass on the wall of the pouch. Histology showed a well differentiated squamous cell carcinoma of pharyngeal diverticulum.

DISCUSSION

Frank malignant changes in pharyngeal pouches are rare, having been reported in only a small number of cases (Liberson and Riese, 1960; Carlock and Richter, 1961), and in situ carcinoma has been demonstrated in the literature in fewer instances (Bullock and Synder, 1952).

In this 10-year review of 70 cases of pharyngeal pouch treated at Wythenshawe Hospital, it was found that the percentage with malignant changes was 4.3%. In these malignant cases, the diagnosis was made by endoscopy and/or external approach. In this series the three cases with malignant changes did not show the typical radiological appearances suggestive of carcinoma in a pharyngeal diverticulum.

We therefore conclude that it is mandatory that any patient with a pharyngeal diverticulum should be endoscoped to detect any possible malignancy. Also every excised diverticulum must be sent for histological scrutiny to avoid missing an occult carcinoma or carcinoma in situ.

REFERENCES

1. Bullock WK, Synder EN (1952) Carcinoma in situ occurring in a pharyngeal diverticulum. Cancer, 5:737-739
2. Carlock JH, Richter R (1961) Carcinoma in a pharyngoesophageal diverticulum. Annals of Surgery, 154:259-262
3. Dunhill T (1950) Pharyngeal diverticulum. Brit J Surg, 37:404-415
4. Liberson M, Riese RT (1960) Carcinoma in a large pharyngoesophageal Diverticulum. Gastroenterology, 38:817-820
5. Lindskog GE (1954) Diverticulum of the esophagus. Yale J of Biol and Med, 26: 285-294

°Article first appeared in the Journal of Laryngology & Otology, March 1985, vol. 99, pp. 297-299.

New dimensions in otorhinolaryngology - head and neck surgery, vol. 2.
E. Myers, editor

THE SIGNIFICANCE OF PALPABLE ADENOPATHY IN SQUAMOUS CELL CARCINOMA OF THE PYRIFORM SINUS: A RETROSPECTIVE STUDY OF 41 CASES

MICHAEL BRONIATOWSKI, M.D.

Department of Otolaryngology, Case Western Reserve University School of Medicine, 2074 Abington Road, Cleveland,Ohio 44106 USA

INTRODUCTION

Like all classifications, the TNM system represents a compromise, as there is no better way to precisely evaluate and record size, site of origin and distant spread of malignancies. The benefits gained through its allowing for information exchange and treatment planning may be additionally offset by staging, that creates even more variables. Because the majority of this series comprised advanced node and non node bearing patients in roughly equal numbers, this study was done to verify the accuracy of the staging system in such instances.

MATERIAL AND METHODS

For a period of ten years starting in January 1973, 41 patients with squamous cell carcinoma of the pyriform sinus seen at Case Western Reserve University Hospitals with enough data to be evaluable, were retrospectively staged according to the American Joint Committee of Cancer 1980; among the 39 patients devoid of distant metastasis (M0), 22 initially presented with palpable neck adenopathy (N+), while 17 did not (N0).

TABLE

OVERALL/N0M0 PATIENT DISTRIBUTION BY STAGE

Stage	I	II	III	IV
Number of Patients	1/1	1/1	9/6	30/9
Percent	2.4/6	2.4/6	22/35	73.2/53

Most cases were classified stage IV, while almost all who were N0 belonged in stages III and IV (88%). Survival by the actuarial method using standard error evaluation was therefore computed irrespectively of treatment for these categories in addition to the overall population. Minimum follow up of survivors was 5 years except for 2 patients lost after 1 and 2 years.

RESULTS

Overall survival (Fig. 1) was 27% at 3 years (s=0.08) and 16% at 5 years (s=0.06) and in stage IV patients (Fig. 2), it was 28% at 3 years (s=0.07) and 7% at 5 years (s=0.05). This contrasts with N0 patients (Fig. 3) where 74% survived 3 years (s=0.11) and 61%, 5 years (s=0.03). Thirteen stage IV N+ patients died after a mean of 11.2 months (close to those two M+, 12 and 7 months) and 11 had N2 or N3 lesions. For the 9 T4N0M0 patients who also died, mean survival was 20.5 months, while it was 67 months in the T3N0M0 group.

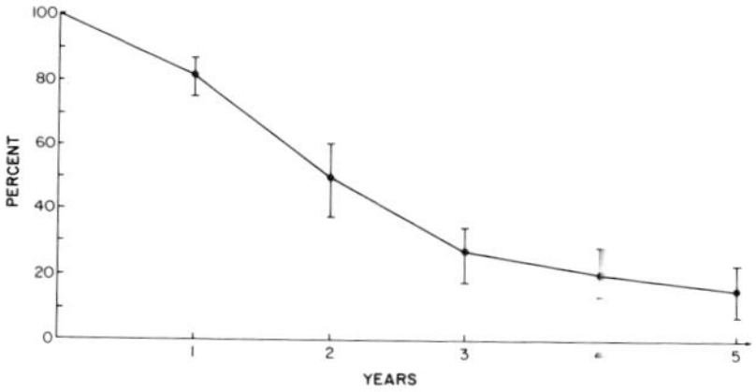

Fig. 1 Overall Survival

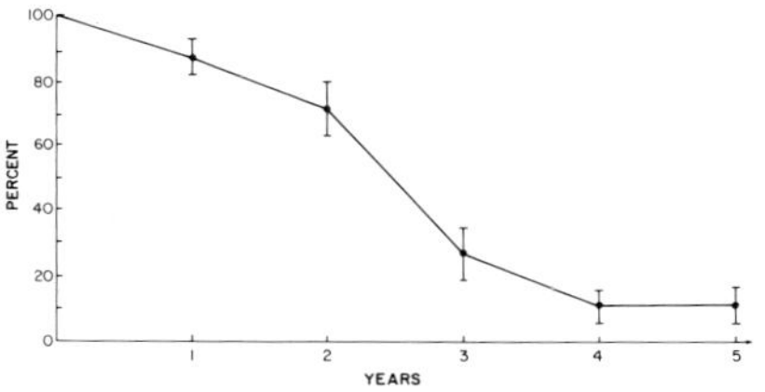

Fig. 2 Stage IV Survival

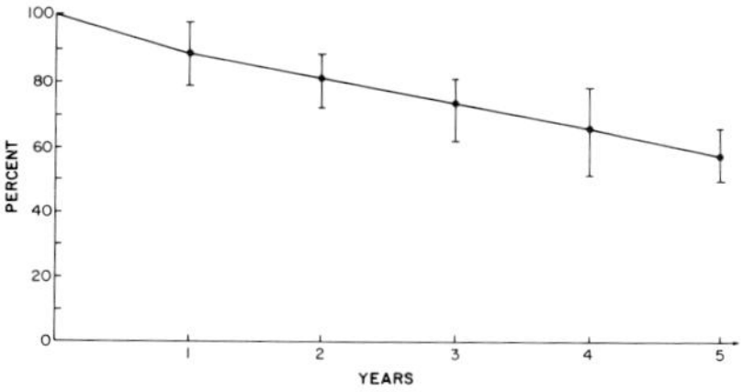

Fig. 3 N0 Patients Survival

DISCUSSION

The overall poor survival of squamous cell carcinoma of the pyriform sinus is verified in this series, where it appears related to a high rate of advanced disease at discovery. While all N+ patients qualify in stages III and IV by definition, 15/17 of those who were N0 did so as well because of high size primaries. A relationship between tumor size and clinical neck disease has not been fully verified here. Hence, higher survival rates from a negative nodal perspective have some value, although clearly, studies on higher numbers are necessary. The better outcome observed in all N0 patients with special attention to those in stage IV, is similar in their laryngeal counterparts where T4N0M0 lesions have been downgraded from stage IV to stageIII.

REFERENCE

Harrison DFN (1979): Intrinsic weakness of the TNM system for classification of laryngeal cancer. ORL 41:241-251.

© 1985 Elsevier Science Publishers B.V. (Biomedical Division)
New dimensions in otorhinolaryngology – head and neck surgery, vol. 2.
E. Myers, editor

PHONATORY FUNCTION OF THE PARTIALLY ABLATED LARYNX

TOMOYUKI HAJI, M.D., STANLEY M. BLAUGRUND, M.D., and WILBUR J. GOULD, M.D.

Vocal Dynamics Lab and ENT Dept., Lenox Hill Hospital
100 East 77 Street, New York, NY 10021, United States

INTRODUCTION

Much has been written about glottic reconstruction after partial laryngectomy. Yet, there exists only little information concerning actual factors responsible for voice production in these patients. This study was undertaken to obtain information on the phonatory characteristics of the partially ablated larynx.

SUBJECTS AND METHODS

Twenty patients were examined[1]. Ten had vertical hemilaryngectomy with arytenoidectomy (H. w A.). All patients underwent glottic reconstruction using the arytenoid replacement procedure with mucosal flap. Six patients had vertical hemilaryngectomy without arytenoidectomy (H. w/o A.) with several reconstructive procedures. Four patients underwent the anterior commissure technique (A.C.T.).

The Olympus ENF fiberscope Type-P was used for visual examination. The Pentax strobe light source Model LS-V was also used to examine detailed vibratory movement. Video recordings were made in each patient. Mean air flow rate (MFR) and maximal phonation time (MPT) were measured in order to examine aerodynamic phonatory function. Fundamental frequency (Fo) and voice range were determined by sound spectrographic analysis. Voice quality was evaluated perceptually by two otolaryngologists and three speech pathologists.

RESULTS

Visual findings. In the H. w A. group, sphincterization of glottic and supraglottic components was noted during voicing. The remaining arytenoid demonstrated remarkable ability to move anteriorly and medially.

Marked hypertrophy of glottic and supraglottic remnants was also noted. Vibratory movement was seen mostly at the supraglottic level.

In the H. w/o A. and A.C.T. groups, less sphincterization was noted. False vocal folds adducted to compensate glottic gap in many cases. Compensatory movement by the contralateral arytenoids was not significant and voicing had more glottic component. In two patients with severe atrophy of both true and false vocal folds, both arytenoids were remarkably hypertrophic and moved anteriorly to strike the epiglottis.

Aerodynamic tests. High MFR was usually associated with noticable glottic or pseudoglottic gap. MPT was roughly related to MFR. When MFR was high, MPT was usually short.

Fo and frequency range. In cases where there was more supraglottic structure involved in voicing the Fo tended to be lower, and where the arytenoids had been saved at surgery, frequency range was found to be wider.

Voice quality. Supraglottic voicing was perceived as being rougher and glottic voicing as more breathy. Rough voice was attributable to excessive secretions and irregular vibrations within the area of voicing. Breathy voice was caused by large glottic or pseudoglottic gap and small amplitude vibration. Marked sphincterization with small amplitude vibration seemed to cause strained voices.

CONCLUSION

Videolaryngofiberscopy in combination with aerodynamic, acoustic and perceptual voice analyses provided us integrated understanding of voicing mechanism of the partially ablated larynx. Further evaluation will establish a data base which will help to improve reconstruction technique and enhance methods of voice rehabilitation.

REFERENCES

1. Blaugrund SM, Gould WJ, Haji T, Meltzer J, Bloch C, Baer T, (1984) Ann. Otol. 93:311-317

New dimensions in otorhinolaryngology – head and neck surgery, vol. 2.
E. Myers, editor

APPLICATION OF CO_2 LASER TO THE CARCINOMA OF THE LARYNX

TETSUZO INOUYE, M.D., Professor and Chairman

Department of Otolaryngology, National Defense Medical College, Tokorozawa, Saitama (Japan)

INTRODUCTION

CO_2 LASER has been widely used for the treatment of benign and malignant tumors in the head and neck area. The LASER provides excellent hemorrhage control by sealing the capillaries. The simultaneous use of CO_2 LASER and Nd-YAG LASER gives even better hemorrhage control. The LASER method of treatment also results in the minimal dissemination of cancer cells improving long term outcome.

MATERIALS AND CASES

We have treated 27 patients with carcinoma of the larynx with 48 operations in 17 months. Resectability of lymph nodes by a radical neck dissection is the indication for use of the LASER (Table1).

TABLE 1

	Tis	T1a	T1b	T2	T3		N0	N1	N2		M0
cases	1	2	8	5	1		24	3	1		27

LOCATION OF TUMORS

One of the difficulties with the use of LASER irradiation to laryngeal lesions is the problem of exposure. Lesions located at the anterior commissure are difficult to expose so that the LASER beam can be directed perpendicularly to get optimal irradiation (Table 2).

TABLE 2

Rt. cord 11, Lt. cord 10, Rt. ventricular band 1, Anterior commissure 8, Posterior commissure 4, Arytenoid area 2, Subglottic space 2, Supraglottic space 5.

We usually use LASER power of 10 to 30 watts, continuous wave, superpulse (Pulse width x repetitive rate), defocused beams to irradiate the lesions. One of the advantages of this superpulse is that it creates the least amount of residual carbon while destroying the tissue. Currently, we are using an instrument which produces both CO_2 and Nd-YAG LASER simultaneously.

PATHOLOGY FACTORS

Of the 27 patients treated by the LASER method, 20 had well differentiated squamous cell carcinomas, 3 had poorly differentiated squamous cell carcinomas, 3 had spindle cell carcinomas and 1 had a muco-epidemoid carcinoma.

RESULTS AND CONCLUSION

Survival rate as of April 1985 is 24/27 (89%) and all of the living patients are tumor free histologically. LASER (CO_2 and Nd-YAG) is an excellent method for the treatment of head and neck tumors. For any one patient, LASER surgery may be repeated for a total of three operations, at which time total laryngectomy should be considered.

REFERENCES

1. Holinger, L.: Treatment of severe subglottic stenosis without tracheotomy, Ann.Otol.Rhinol.Laryngol., 91:407-412, 1982.
2. Dedo, H. et al: Laryngeal papilloma: Results of treatment with the CO_2 LASER and podophyllum, Ann.Otol.Rhinol.Laryngol., 91:425-430, 1982.
3. Healy, G. et al.: Complications of CO_2 laser surgery of the aerodigestive tract: Experience of 4416 cases, Otolaryngology Head and Neck surgery, 92(1):13-18, 1984.
4. Inouye, T. et al.: Application of CO_2 and Nd-YAG LASER to Head and Neck Tumors, The Journal of Japan Society for LASER Medicine 5(3):305-308, 1985.

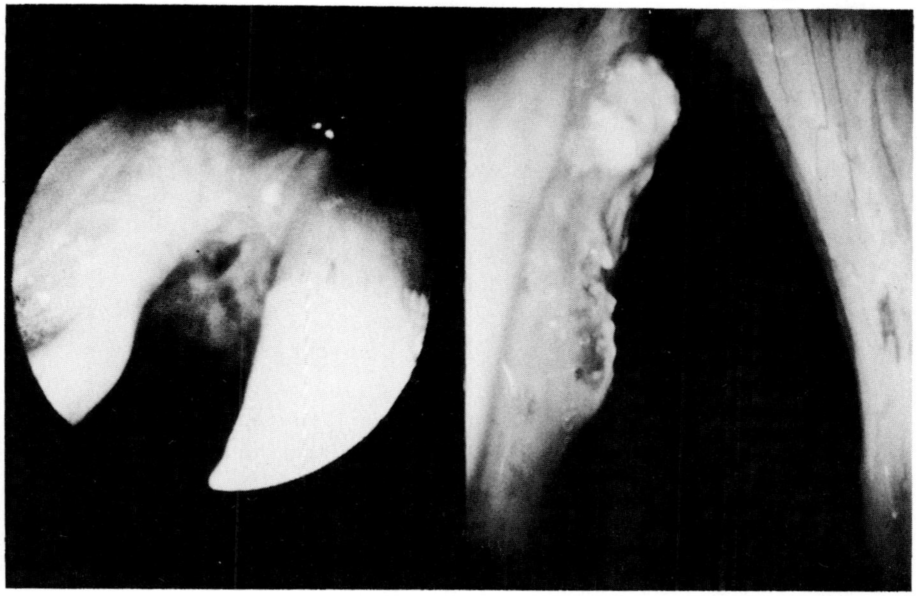

Fig. 1.
44 year old male. Carcinoma of larynx. T1a. (Right)
CO_2 LASER 15 20 watts C.W. super pulse. Tumor free 325 days after LASER operation. (Left)

New dimensions in otorhinolaryngology - head and neck surgery, vol. 2.
E. Myers, editor

SUPRACRICOID HEMILARYNGOPHARYNGECTOMY. SURGICAL TECHNIQUE, INDICATIONS, FUNCTIONNAL AND CARCINOLOGICAL RESULTS

J LACAU ST GUILY MD, D BRASNU MD, P CONTENCIN MD, A FABRE MD, H LACCOURREYE MD
Hopital Laennec, 42 rue de sèvres 75007 PARIS, FRANCE

Between 1964 and 1983, 240 patients with squamous cell carcinoma underwent a supracricoid hemilaryngopharyngectomy. The procedure was described in 1965 by Laccourreye and André. It consists in removal of supracricoid hemilarynx and entire ipsilateral pyriform sinus.

OPERATIVE TECHNIQUE

- Oral intubation.Tracheotomy performed just before resection
- L-shaped skin incision
- Ipsilateral radical neck dissection (RND). (NO patients : modified RND). In tumors of the pyriform sinus : ipsilateral total thyroid lobectomy and recurrent lymph chain dissection.

Exposure :

- Incision of the external thyroid perichondrium along the posterior border of the thyroid cartilage
- The musculoperichondrial flap, which is made up of the external thyroid perichondrium and attached strap muscles, is elevated and reflected medially.
- The hyoid bone is preserved or transected at the lesser horn depending on the location of the tumor.
- Disarticulation of the cricothyroid joint.

Excision

- Vertical medial incision of the cricothyroid membrane. Medial vertical thyrotomy.
- Vertical resection of the infra and suprahyoid epiglottis and of the preepiglottic space.
- Resection is continued across the ipsilateral vallecula above the hyoid bone.
- Horizontal resection of the cricothyroid membrane along the superior border of the cricoid cartilage.

- Vertical posterior resection : the incision of the lateral pharyngeal wall is extended downward. The size and location of the tumor determines the line of resection.
- Interarytenoid incision
- Disarticulation of the cricoarytenoid joint
- Release the lower part of the pyriform sinus from the cricoid
- The resected area is removed with the tumor

Closure

- mucosal suturing of the remaining arytenoid
- Suture of the lateral pharyngeal wall to the medial line and overlay suture of the musculo-perichondrial flap.
- The position of the oesopharyngeal inlet must be preserved
- Suction drains, closure of the skin incision, tracheotomy tube.

INDICATIONS

- Carcinoma of the upper part of pyriform sinus
- carcinoma of the lateral laryngeal margin with aryepiglottic fold involvement
- With normal vocal cord mobility.

CONTRAINDICATIONS are as following :

- Impaired vocal cord mobility.
- Extension to preepiglottic space, cartilage, lower part of the pyriform sinus, posterior tonsillar pillar, posterior pharyngeal wall, retrocricoid area, endolarynx.
- Age : 70 and over. Respiratory insufficiency.

MATERIALS

240 patients required the procedure between 1964 and 1983 : 150 had a pyriform sinus carcinoma, 90 had a lateral laryngeal margin carcinoma. Follow up of at least three years was available for 192 patients.

RESULTS

The post operative and functionnal results were as following

- there were 7 post operative deaths

- 222 patients had no airway impairment ; the average time of decannulation was 6 days. 11 patients had airway impairment : 6 definitive tracheotomies, 2 deaths by asphyxia, 3 temporary retracheotomies.

- 204 patients recovered a satisfactory deglutition ; the average time of removal of the feeding tube was 17 days. 15 patients underwent a definitive gastrostomy for deglutition impairment and aspiration. 11 patients underwent a secondary total laryngectomy for aspiration. 3 patients died from aspiration pneumonia.

10 local recurrences occured among 192 patients with a follow up of at least three years (5,2%).

These functionnal and carcinological results demonstrate the reliability fo the supracricoid hemilaryngopharyngectomy.

REFERENCES

1. André P, Pinel J, Laccourreye H (1965) : la chirurgie partielle verticale dans les cancers du sinus piriforme.
Ann. Otolaryngol. (Paris), 82 : 901-908.

2. Guerrier Y, Pinel J, Cachin Y, Laccourreye H, Dejean Y (1972) : la chirurgie conservatrice dans le traitement des cancers du vestibule laryngé et du sinus piriforme.
Rapport Congrès Français d'O.R.L. et de Chirurgie cervicofaciale. Arnette Paris.

3. Laccourreye H, Brasnu D, Beutter P (1983) : Carcinoma of the laryngeal margin.
Head and neck surgery 5 : 500-507.

4. Ogura JH, Spector GJ, Sessions DG (1975) : conservative surgery for epidermoid carcinoma of the laryngeal margin (aryepiglottic fold extension).
Laryngoscope 85 : 1801-1807.

New dimensions in otorhinolaryngology - head and neck surgery, vol. 2.
E. Myers, editor

HISTOLOGICAL EVALUATION OF CONTRALATERAL NECK METASTASIS OF PYRIFORM SINUS CANCER

YASUSHI MURAKAMI, TAKETSUGU IKARI, SHIGENORI HARAGUCHI, KOHJI OKADA, TAKESHI MARUYAMA AND SHIGEJI SAITO
Department of Otolaryngology, School of Medicine, Keio University, 35 Shinanomachi, Shinjuku-Ku, Tokyo (Japan)

INTRODUCTION

Each type of hypopharyngeal cancer, pyriform sinus cancer (PSC), posterior wall cancer (PWC) and postcricoid cancer (PCC) has a high incidence of neck metastasis, and radical surgery together with ipsilateral neck dissection has been the treatment of choice in most cases of advanced hypopharyngeal cancer. In spite of such radical extirpation followed by postoperative chemoradiotherapy, not a few recurrences in the contralateral neck was experienced in our department.

In order to decide the indication of prophylactic neck dissection in the contralateral neck, we studied on the incidence of neck metastasis of pyriform sinus cancer by means of histological evaluation of nodes obtained by bilateral neck dissection.

MATERIAL AND METHODS

In 86 patients with hypopharyngeal cancer that were treated before 1982, bilateral neck dissection was done only therapeutically in 12 cases of N_2. After 1982, on the contrary, bilateral neck dissection was routinely done in all 40 patients. They include 9 cases of N_0, 24 cases of N_1 and 7 cases of N_2.

Among these 52 cases that were treated by bilateral neck dissection, 37 cases of PSC were included.

Nodes obtained from these extirpated specimens were histologically evaluated by paraffin sections.

RESULTS

Among 37 cases of PSC, 26 (70%) cases showed histologically positive node in the ipsilateral neck and 10 (27%) cases in the contralateral. In all 10 cases that showed contralateral neck metastasis, positive node was histologically demonstrated also in the ipsilateral neck (Table 1).

TABLE 1
INCIDENCE OF NODE METASTASIS IN 37 CASES OF PSC
(Histologically evaluated)

	Ipsilateral	Contralateral
PSC (n= 37)	26/37 =70%	10/37 = 27%

These 37 cases of PSC contain 22 cases of well differentiated and 15 cases of moderately differentiated squamous carcinomas. Ipsilateral and contralateral neck metastases were histologically confirmed in 59% and 18% of well differentiated cases, and in 87% and 40% of moderately differentiated cases.

They are divided into 3 groups by T category; 11 cases of T_2, 22 cases of T_3 and 4 cases of T_4. Ipsilateral and contralateral neck metastases were demonstrated in 55% and 9% of T_2, 73% and 23% of T_3. Bilateral neck metastasis was found in all 4 cases of T_4.

Incidence of node metastasis related to a combination of histological differentiation and T classification is seen in Table 2.

TABLE 2
INCIDENCE OF NODE METASTASIS RELATED TO HISTOLOGICAL DIFFERENTIATION AND T CLASSIFICATION (Histologically evaluated)

		Ipsilateral	Contralateral
	T_2	1/5 = 25%	0/5 = 0
Well	T_3	10/15 = 67%	2/15 = 13%
(n= 22)	T_4	2/2 = 100%	2/2 = 100%
	T_2	5/6 = 83%	1/6 = 17%
Moderate	T_3	6/7 = 86%	3/7 = 43%
(n= 15)	T_4	2/2 = 100%	2/2 = 100%

As indicated in Table 2, contralateral neck metastasis was found in none of well differentiated T_2 lesion, and we conclude that ipsilateral neck dissection must be completed in all cases of PSC and bilateral neck dissection is advisable except for well defferentiated T_2 lesion.

© 1985 Elsevier Science Publishers B V. (Biomedical Division)
New dimensions in otorhinolaryngology - head and neck surgery, vol. 2.
E. Myers, editor

EXTENDED HEMIPHARYNGOLARYNGECTOMY IN PYRIFORM SINUS CANCER FOR VOICE PRESERVATION WITHOUT ASPIRATION - A MODIFIED TECHNIQUE

SANZO TAKEMIYA, FUMIYUKI SHIMADA, KEN OMURA & MASAHARU ICHINOSE
Department of Head & Neck Surgery, Chiba Cancer Center Hospital, 666-2 Nitonacho, Chiba 280, Japan

INTRODUCTION

Selection of a surgical technique of the partial laryngectomy with reconstruction procedure followed by minimal postoperative aspiration is demanded at the time of wide resection of the pharynx with voice preservation in pyriform sinus cancer. Extended hemilaryngectomy (near-total laryngectomy) with a dynamic speech tube, which was introduced by Pearson in 1980, has possible superiority as a surgical modality of the partial laryngectomy for voice preservation without aspiration not only in T3 glottic cancer, but also in pyriform sinus cancer. We modified his surgical technique in a point of reconstruction of the upper portion of a shunt airway.

CLINICAL MATERIALS AND SURGICAL MODALITY

Two cases of T4N1 and one of T3N0 pyriform sinus cancer were selected. Endoscopic observation localized extension of the primary tumor and it was inevitable to decide the excisional line. Preoperative radiotherapy was given in the total dose of 40 to 50 Gy in two cases and chemotherapy was performed in another case.

Radical neck dissection including prelaryngeal and paratracheal dissection on the affected side was performed before laryngopharyngeal exposure. The extent of resection of laryngeal tissues was almost identical to that in the original method. Wide pharyngectomy ranging from half to subtotal resection and including the vallecula, the base of the tongue, the lateral wall of thr mesopharynx, or the cervical esophagus was performed.

At producing the speech tube by rolling the preserved myomucosal segment of the larynx, a part of the skin paddle of the pectoralis major myocutaneous flap that took a share in supplementing the wall of the resected pharynx was utilized to resurface the gap at the upper part of the speech tube where the pharyngeal flap was brought over in the original method.

RESULTS

No complication related to surgery was seen. Food ingestion was possible in three weeks postoperatively. No postoperative aspiration was recognized. The preserved voice was excellent in two patients. Its sound pressure level was between 67 and 84 dB. The duration lasted from 7 to 18 seconds and subglottic pressure during phonation ranged from 0 to 30 cm in water. Three patients are free from local recurrence at the 6, 16 and 17-month-follow up.

DISCUSSION

This surgical modality can be applied to many cases of pyriform sinus cancer with oncological rationality of resection extent of the tumor, avoidance of postoperative aspiration and feasibility of the reconstruction procedure, and we agree with Dumich´s comment published in October, 1984 discussing factors of contraindication to this surgery; bilateral cord fixation, postcricoid involvement and extension across the interarytenoid area.

SUMMARY

We used a modified surgical technique of Pearson´s extended hemilaryngectomy and our key point was to use pectoralis major myocutaneous flap to reconstruct the airway in three cases of pyriform sinus cancer. Postoperative voice was satisfactorily preserved and no postoperative aspiration was recognized.

© 1985 Elsevier Science Publishers B.V. (Biomedical Division)
New dimensions in otorhinolaryngology - head and neck surgery, vol. 2.
E. Myers, editor

A SURGICAL TECHNIQUE FOR VOICE PRESERVATION IN POSTCRICOID CANCER BY CREATION OF SPEECH TUBE USING ANTERIOR HALF OF LARYNX

SANZO TAKEMIYA, FUMIYUKI SHIMADA, KEN OMURA & MASAHARU ICHINOSE
Department of Head & Neck Surgery, Chiba Cancer Center Hospital,
666-2 Nitonacho, Chiba 280, Japan

In this video movie authors demonstrated a technique of new surgical modality for voice preservation in a 58-year-old male patient with T2N1 postcricoid cancer. Oncologic rationality, surgical indication and postoperative laryngeal function of this surgical modality were discussed in our paper entitled "Voice Preservation in Postcricoid Cancer by Creation of Speech Tube Using Retained Anterior Half of Larynx" in this Congress.

SURGICAL TECHNIQUE

Operation was started under oral intubation and skin incision was T-shaped. The longitudinal segment was deviated laterally. Bilateral superior laryngeal neurovascular pedicles and unilateral inferior thyroid artery were preserved at pharyngolaryngeal exposure and paratracheal dissection. Lateral thyrotomy was done on both sides and the mucosa of the pyriform sinus was separated from the paraglottic space. The cricoid cartilage was divided in two parts to leave in situ one third of the anterior central portion. After tracheostomy at the third and fourth rings the trachea was reintubated from this stoma. Pharyngotomy was done bilaterally to traverse the lateral wall of the pharynx with 3 cm superior margin from the tumor. The lateral portion of the hyothyroid membrane was resected with preserving a superior laryngeal neurovascular pedicle. The aryepiglottic folds were transected at an appropriate height to preserve sensory innervation to the retained half of the larynx at least at one side. Supraglottic portion and vocal cords were divided anteriorly and posteriorly. Dividing the subglottic region on the frontal plane the incisional line reached the membranous portion of the trachea in a V-shape with a sufficient safety margin. The resection was completed by transecting the esophagus by 3 cm below the lower margin of the tumor after elevation of the laryngopharynx from the prevertebral fascia and by opening the esophagus at the posterior wall.

With confirmation of good blood supply to the preserved portion of the larynx and cervical trachea the mucosal tube was constructed to rehabilitate voice. The cut edge in a V-shape was reapproximated to form the longitudinal line. The mucosal edge was elevated from the laryngeal framework in case of occurrence of excessive tissue tension. The diameter of the constructed tube was no. 7 - 8 of a Nelaton catheter in size.

In this case the pharyngoesophagus was made by using the forearm flap. The anteromedial portion of the upper end of the skin tube was sutured to the orifice of the newly reconstructed vocal tract. The permanent tracheostoma was made.

RESULTS

No complication related to surgery was seen. Aspiration was clinically negligible and voice rehabilitation was satisfactory three weeks later postoperatively.

© 1985 Elsevier Science Publishers B.V. (Biomedical Division)
New dimensions in otorhinolaryngology - head and neck surgery, vol. 2.
E. Myers, editor

VOICE PRESERVATION IN POSTCRICOID CANCER BY CREATION OF SPEECH TUBE USING RETAINED ANTERIOR HALF OF LARYNX

SANZO TAKEMIYA, FUMIYUKI SHIMADA, KEN OMURA & MASAHARU ICHINOSE
Department of Head & Neck Surgery, Chiba Cancer Center Hospital,
666-2 Nitonacho, Chiba 280, Japan

INTRODUCTION

In patients with freedom from invasion to anterior half of the larynx and cervical trachea in postcricoid and cervical esophageal cancer, preservation of the anterior half of the part can be applied with oncologic rationality. In 1956 Som presented a surgical modality that contained preservation of the anterior half and primary closure of the pharyngeal defect using retained half as an autograft.

Our surgical modality is different from that of Som's in the point of creation of a vocal tract by using the preserved anterior half of the region and reconstruction of the digestive tract by using the skin flap.

CLINICAL MATERIALS AND SURGICAL MODALITY

Three cases of T2N1 postcricoid cancer and one of T1N0 cervical esophageal cancer were selected. Endoscopic observation localized extension of the primary tumor and it was inevitable to decide the excisional line. Preoperative radiotherapy was given in the total dose of 40 to 50 Gy.

Bilateral superior laryngeal neurovascular pedicles and unilateral inferior thyroid artery were preserved at pharyngolaryngeal exposure. Tracheostomy was placed at an appropriate level. Lateral pharyngotomy was performed on both sides with 3 cm superior margin from the tumor. Resection line was extended anteromedially to the upper portion of the pyriform sinus. Then the larynx and upper tracheal rings were divided into anterior and posterior halves on the frontal plane from the aryepiglottic folds to the sufficient margin of the membranous portion of the trachea. The anterior half was left in its original position associated with its blood supply and sensory innervation, whereas the posterior half was removed in continuity with the pharyngoesophagus. The mucosal edge of the cut surface of the preserved anterior half was elevated from the laryngeal framework and then longitudinally approximated to construct a mucosa-lined speech tube. The pharyngoesophagus was reestablished by means of a forearm flap or deltopectoral flap. The anteromedial portion of the upper end of the skin flap was sutured to the marginal zone of the orifice of the speech tube.

This surgical procedure was demonstrated in a T.V. video tape session of this Congress.

RESULTS

No complication related to surgery was seen. Primary reconstruction using the forearm flap in three cases made food ingestion possible in three weeks postoperatively. Postoperative aspiration was clinically negligible. The restored voice sounded slightly husky and its sound pressure level was between 67 and 75 dB. The duration lasted from 6 to 30 seconds and subglottic pressure ranged from 0 to 26 cm $H2O$. Two patients were free from disease for 18 months after surgery and the other two were unevaluable yet because of the immediate postoperative status.

DISCUSSION

This surgical procedure was indicated to cases of postcricoid and cervical esophageal cancer with its limited extension to the larynx and cervical trachea having unilateral neck metastases at the most. The second point is how to avoid postoperative aspiration in the conservation surgery and several significant factors can be itemized as follows: no peristalsis of the reconstructed pharyngoesophagus, wide luminal diameter, no stenotic suture to the esophagus and minimal contact of the food or excretion to the orifice of the vocal tract. Moreover the reconstructed pseudoglottis or preserved portion of the larynx is needed to concomitantly move with the suprahyoid muscles with swallowing, and has a function to prevent aspiration at the orifice, when sensorily innervated.

SUMMARY

In four cases of postcricoid and cervical esophageal cancer it was possible to leave safely the anterior half of the larynx and cervical trachea in situ and to reestablish vocal function without aspiration using the retained structure. Some factors mandatory to avoid aspiration were discussed.

© 1985 Elsevier Science Publishers B.V. (Biomedical Division)
New dimensions in otorhinolaryngology - head and neck surgery, vol. 2.
E. Myers, editor

HISTOPATHOLOGICAL STUDY OF THE PYRIFORM SINUS CANCER BY MEANS OF WHOLE-ORGAN SERIAL SECTION

MITSUTAKE TANI AND MUTSUO AMATSU
Dept. of Otorhinolaryngology, Kobe University School of Medicine, Kobe, Japan

INTRODUCTION

Hypopharyngeal cancer is one of the most dreaded and distressing diseases in the head and neck region. Increasing understanding of the histopathological modes of growth and spread of this tumor is needed for a better estimation of its prognosis. The present study is aimed at evaluation of detailed histopathological behavior of piriform sinus cancer by whole-organ serial sectioning.

MATERIAL AND METHODS

The material of this study consists of 20 surgical specimens removed at surgery between 1972 and 1983. All these 20 patients had surgery without previous radiotherapy. Each surgical specimen, that was opened along the posterior midline, was fixed in formalin, decalcified with dilute nitric acid, dehydrated, and then embedded in paraffin. Large sections were cut in the horizontal plane, and were stained with hematoxylin-eosin.

RESULTS AND COMMENTS

Lateral extension

The tumor frequently extended laterally outside the thyroid ala with invasion of the thyroid cartilage (25%) or around the thyroid cartilage without invasion (40%). Therefore, the thyroid cartilage did not seem to be a barrier against lateral extension of cancer.

Medial extension

When the tumor extended medially, the arytenoid cartilage was not invaded by tumor. After having reached the arytenoid cartilage, the tumor extended either anterior medially or posterior medially. In case of posterior medial extension, tumor often approached the crico-arytenoid joint, but actual invasion seldom took place, since tumor tended to spread along the crico-arytenoid muscle and/or the interarytenoid muscle.

When the tumor extended medially to invade laryngeal structures, vocal cord fixation occurred in 70%. Without extensive invasion of the intrinsic laryngeal muscles, there has been no vocal cord fixation subsequent merely to invasion of the crico-arytenoid joint or the recurrent laryngeal nerve trunk. Therefore, it is our conclusion that vocal cord fixation was due mainly to involvement of the intrinsic laryngeal muscles. Involvement of the arytenoid cartilage or the crico-arytenoid joint occurred after completion of fixation.

Superior extension

By superior medial extension, tumor invaded the aryepiglottic fold in 70%. By further superior medial extension, tumor extended to the lateral pre-epiglottic space or to the glosso-epiglottic fold, and resulted in invasion into the base of tongue in 25%. Superior growth was usually extensive because of the lack of any barrier. Invasion of the false vocal cord occurred by the direct retrograde submucosal route beyond the aryepiglottic fold in 40%. But invasion of the vocal cord occurred only in 10%.

Inferior extension

In case of inferior extension, tumor invaded the apex of the sinus in 70%. But this site located between the firm structures of the thyroid and cricoid cartilages restricted further superficial inferior extension. Therefore inferior spread into the cervical esophagus has not been the pattern in this material. Concerning further deep spread from the apex of the sinus, tumor escaped through the crico-thyroid space and reached the capsule of the superior lobe of the thyroid gland in 20%. But actual invasion was not found.

Primary site and direction of extension

Piriform sinus cancer arising primarily from its lateral wall had a different mode of extension as compared with that arising from its medial wall. Usually, the tumor arising primarily from its lateral wall had a tendency to extend laterally outside the thyroid ala, that meant that T_1 or T_2 changed directly into T_4 in the classification without being classified T_3. On the other hand, the tumor arising from its medial wall extended medially causing vocal cord fixation (T_3) without being classified T_2. This suggested that vocal cord fixation (T_3) in TNM classification of piriform sinus cancer remains still controversial.

Submucosal extension

My own study showed the maximum submucosal extension to be 16mm superiorly, 14mm inferiorly. A satisfactory margin of normal pharyngeal mucosa must be removed with the specimen at the time of operation. In piriform sinus cancer, at least 2 cm is thought to be necessary for safety margin, in view of the submucosal extension.

SUMMARY

In this study, the detailed histopathological behavior of the piriform sinus cancer was estimated by whole-organ serial sectioning. Our study was aimed at contributing the establishment of the true extent of this tumor and the determination of adequate treatment modalities.

New dimensions in otorhinolaryngology - head and neck surgery, vol. 2.
E. Myers, editor

DNA PLOIDY LEVEL IN RELATION TO IRRADIATION RESPONSE IN ORAL CAVITY CARCINOMAS

GUNNAR FRANZÉN, CLAES KLINTENBERG, JAN OLOFSSON, AND BJÖRN RISBERG
Departments of Oncology, Otolaryngology, and Pathology, University Hospital, S-581 85 Linköping, Sweden

INTRODUCTION

Radiotherapists know that tumours with apparently the same macro- and microscopic appearance respond differently to irradiation. An objective predictor for estimation of the response to radiotherapy should be of invaluable help for the clinician to select the most appropriate treatment for the patients.

Therefore, biopsies of squamous cell carcinomas from the oral cavity taken before and after preoperative radiotherapy (40-44 Gy) were investigated with the aim of evaluating the relation of the DNA ploidy level to irradiation response.

MATERIAL AND METHODS

Preparation

50 μm thick sections from diagnostic and surgical formalin-fixed and paraffin-embedded blocks from 24 squamous cell carcinomas of the oral cavity were prepared according to the method of Hedley et al. (1).

DNA measurements

Static cytofluorometry was performed using a Leitz MPV 3 cytophotometer. About 300 tumour nuclei and 10-20 lymphocytes were measured and the tumour stem line was determined using the lymphocytes as reference cells for DNA diploid value. The DNA ploidy level was compared with the T-classification and the histological findings in the surgical specimens.

RESULTS

The DNA histograms were classified into 3 groups: DNA diploid; DNA polyploid; and DNA aneuploid. A DNA diploid and a DNA aneuploid tumour are illustrated in Figs. 1 and 2. Five tumours were DNA diploid; 12 DNA polyploid; and 7 DNA aneuploid.

After irradiation 1 of the 5 DNA diploid tumours (all well differentiated) did not show any remaining tumour as did 2 of the 12 DNA polyploid and 5 of the 7 DNA aneuploid ones. In addition marked response was noted in 2 of the DNA polyploid and 1 of the DNA aneuploid tumours (see Table I).

No uniform pattern was found comparing histological differentiation and irradiation response.

There was no correlation between tumour size (T-classification) and response to radiotherapy as assessed histologically.

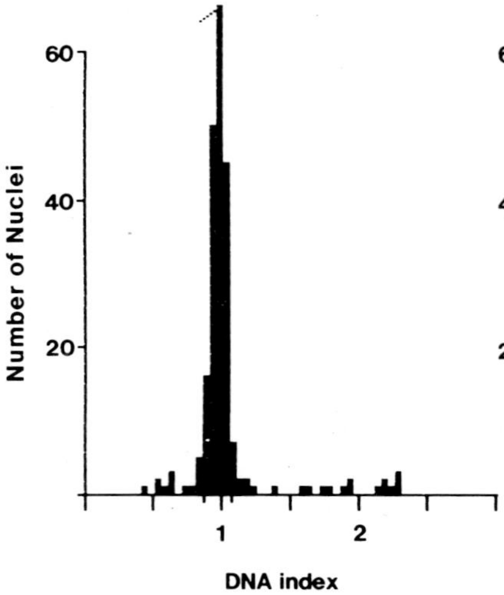

Fig. 1. DNA diploid tumour

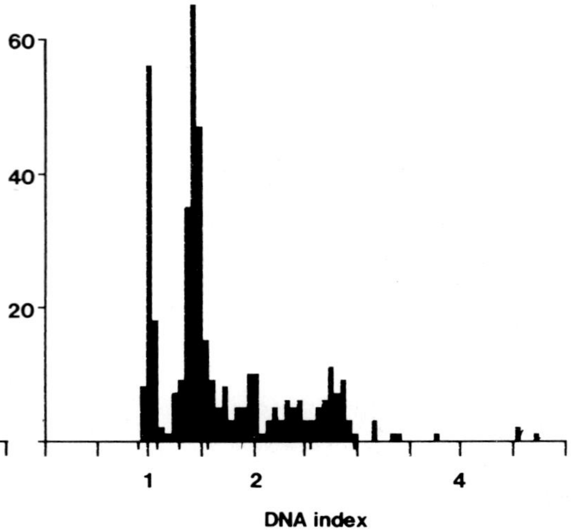

Fig. 2. DNA aneuploid tumour

TABLE I

RESPONSE TO RADIOTHERAPY IN RELATION TO DNA PATTERN

DNA Ploidy Pattern	Response to Radiotherapy as Assessed Histologically		
	No Remaining Tumour	Moderate Response	No Response
DNA Diploid (5)	1	0	4
DNA Polyploid (12)	2	2	8
DNA Aneuploid (7)	5	1	1

SUMMARY AND CONCLUSIONS

This pilot study indicates that DNA analysis may yield clinically applicable information concerning response to radiotherapy. DNA aneuploid tumours seem to respond better than DNA polyploid and DNA diploid ones. The size of the tumour does not seem to correlate with the histologically assessed response rate. An extended investigation on a larger series of oral cavity carcinomas is currently undertaken.

REFERENCES

1. Hedley DW, Friedlander ML, Taylor IW, Rugg CA, Musgrove EA (1983) Method for analysis of cellular DNA content of paraffin-embedded pathological material using flow cytometry. J Histochem Cytochem 31:1333-1335

© 1985 Elsevier Science Publishers B.V. (Biomedical Division)
New dimensions in otorhinolaryngology - head and neck surgery, vol. 2.
E. Myers, editor

SURGICAL ASPECTS OF MALIGNANT TUMOURS OF THE TONGUE

P. P. HAKIM, P. A. SHAH, R. P. SHAH
Dept. of Otolaryngology - JJ Hospital, Bombay, India

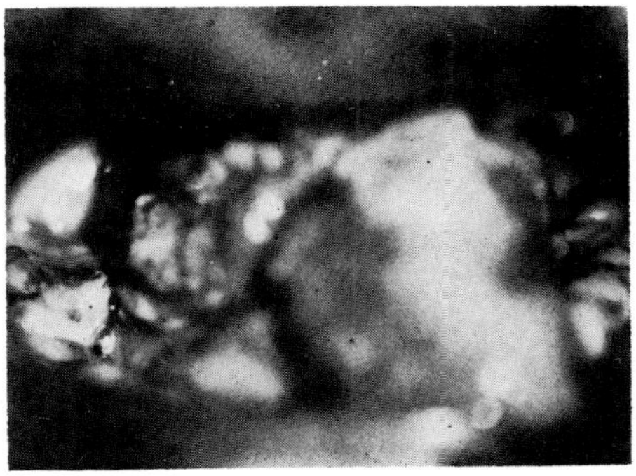

Fig. 1. Carc. foll. dental irritation

The tongue being a mobile organ attached to the floor of the oral cavity is surgically accessible. Hence malignant tumours related to it are amenable both to early detection and treatment. This paper stresses the importance of dental factors in the aetiology of carcinoma of the anterior 2/3 of the tongue. (Fig. 1)

This study also illustrates the feasibility of using a simple forehead flap for reconstruction of the tongue after partial or total glossectomy, especially in extensive lesions involving the base. It has a good blood supply and is quick and easy to perform. (Fig.2, & 3)

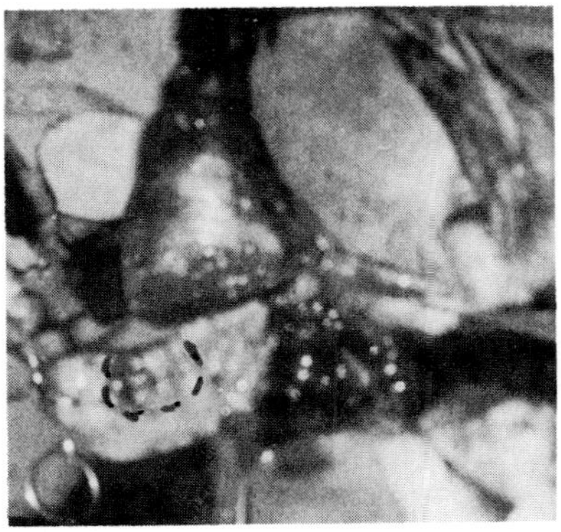

Fig. 2. Tumour being excised

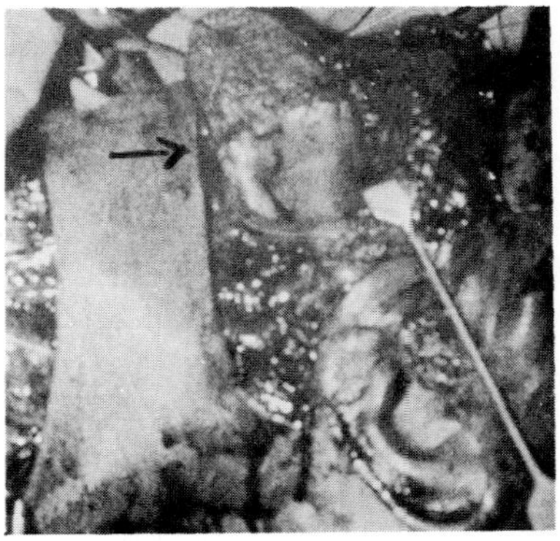

Fig. 3. Forehead flap sutured in position

MATERIAL AND METHODS

An analysis of cases of malignant tumours of the tongue seen over a period of 12 years, has been undertaken. In all, 98 cases were seen of which 75% were in an advanced stage of the disease. The maximum incidence was in the fifth decade while the M:F ratio was 3:1 which is comparable to that obtained by Rollo et al[2]. 85% of our cases were squamous cell carcinoma, dysphagia being the commonest symptom. The modalities of treatment used are shown in Table I.

(TABLE I) STAGING OF DISEASE TNM CLASSIFICATION WITH TREATMENT (98 CASES)

Stage	Total	Surg	Rad	Surg + Rad	Ch + Surg + Rad
I	6	3	1	2	-
II	26	6	9	11	-
III	34	11	7	16	-
IV	24	6	13	5	8

8 patients went DAMA prior to proper examination or treatment.

Surgery for base tongue tumours followed by radiation is advocated in well differentiated lesions, a five-year survival being 45% (Table II)

(TABLE II) OVERALL 5 YEARS SURVIVAL IN CARCINOMAS OF THE TONGUE

	Our series	Harrold	Whicker et al	Scanlon
Post. 1/3rd lesions 60	Radiation alone 20%. Surg.+Rad.45%	25% Surgery alone	42% Surgery + Radiation	25% Radiation alone
Ant 2/3rd lesions 38	Radiate alone 45% Surg.+Rad.70%		Rollo et al 50% overall	

Rollo et Al and Yarrington have also advocated surgery for base tongue carcinomas using local mucosal flaps to bridge the tongue defect. but we prefer the fore-head flap when a wide marginal excision is required

Our rate of complications has been higher - 20%, the Surgical Mortality being 10%, mainly due to poor nutrition & lack of post-operative facilities.

Though this paper stresses the need of surgery in cancers of the tongue, a combined approach with a radiotherapist, chemotherapist and a speech therapist is advised to achieve the best results.

REFERENCES

1. Yarrington C. Thomas Jr. (1980) Reconstruction of the Base of the tongue & Lateral Pharyngeal Wall, Seattle, Washington, Laryngscope 90 pp 202-206
2. Rollo et Al (1981) Squamous Carcinoma at the Base of the tongue. A clinico-pathological study of 81 cases. Cancer Jan 15 pp 333-342.
3. Harrold CC(1967)Surg.Treatment of Cancer of the tongue-Am J.Surg.pp 493-497

New dimensions in otorhinolaryngology - head and neck surgery, vol. 2.
E. Myers, editor

MANAGEMENT OF ADVANCED CANCER OF THE TONGUE BY TOTAL GLOSSECTOMY WITHOUT LARYNGECTOMY

P. GEHANNO, C. GUEDON, F. VEBER
Dept. of Head and Neck Surgery. Claude Bernard Hospital, 10 av de la Porte d'Aubervilliers, 75019 PARIS, FRANCE

INTRODUCTION

The treatment by radical surgical resection may provide good palliation of symptoms as well as long term survival for the patient afflicted by far advanced carcinoma of the tongue.

MATERIAL AND METHODS

Total glossectomy with preservation of the larynx was performed in 27 patients at Claude Bernard Hospital, Paris, from 1981 to 1983.
The mean age was 55 years. There were 25 male and 2 female patients.
The primary tumor was located at the base of tongue and extended beyond to involve the tonsil in 9 patients, both floor of mouth in 7 patients, vallecula and epiglottis in 6 patients and mandible in 4 patients.
Related symptoms included dysphagia, severe oral pain, speech impairment and in all cases non protrusive tongue.

RESULTS

Eighteen patients were operated on because of the failure of radiotherapy to control the primary tumor. Nine patients received planned postoperative radiotherapy. Larynx was retained in all 27 patients. A neck cissection in continuity with the tumor was performed in all patients. A jaw neck approach was required in 22 cases. Reconstruction was accomplished using the pectoralis major myocutaneous flap in 22 patients, the trapezius myocutaneous flap in 4 patients, the latissimus dorsi myocutaneous flap in 1 patient. Four of the 11 patients had controlled disease for 2 years, 2 for 3 years and 1 for 4 years.

COMMENT

Treatment of advanced tongue cancer is a very big challenge for both the patient and the surgeon. Most of tongue tumors are painfull and have produced a considerable degree of disability of speech and swallowing. Total glossectomy may offer the only chance for cure. Primary repair has lead in the past to major deformities and considerable disabilities stongly suggesting that total glossectomy was not a justifiable operation (1). Moroever total laryngectomy has been advocated as the only way to prevent chronic aspiration.

The use of myocutaneous flap has been proved a highly reliable method of tongue reconstruction providing adequate soft tissue to promote certain compensatory mechanisms. Theses include ; buldging of the posterior pharyngeal wall, lowering of the soft palate and elevation of the larynx (2, 3). Different surgical methods previously described to prevent aspiration (4, 5) have been found by the authors to interfere with compensatory mechanisms and were subsequently abandonned. Twenty patients had initial N0 neck status, 4 had N1, 3 had N3. Metastases in lymph nodes were found in 10 patients 3 of which had N0. Twelve of the 27 patients had regional recurrences after the initial surgical treatment all but two of which were manifest before the twelth month. A tumor that recurred in one of the 27 patients after initial surgery was controled by a subsequent surgical procedure. Survival data at 1 1/2 year revealed that 16 patients were dead and 11 patients were alive and free of disease. The severe pain was relieved in every patient. Rehabilitation of speech and swallowing was aided with active 'lip - tongue' exercise by a speech therapist. Four of the 11 patients with a follow-up from one and a half to four years maintained understandable voice but are still being fed by gastrostomy. Seven of the 11 patients with a follow-up of 1 1/2 to 4 years developed excellent speech and swallowing.

Eligibility for total glossectomy without laryngectomy include good physical condition with adequate pulmonary function and a highly motivated patient and family.

This series demonstrates that total glossectomy can provide excellent palliation of symptoms as well as an acceptable survival, and that, larynx preservation combined with selected reconstruction techniques can provide a successful rehabilitation.

REFERENCES

1. MARTIN H (1964) Surgery of Head and Neck Tumors. New York Hoeber-Harper pp 279

2. MYERS EN (1972) The role of total glossectomy in the management of cancer of the oral cavity. Otolaryng. Clin. N. Amer. 5 : 343-355

3. FLORES TC, WOOD BG, KOEGEL L, LEVINE HL, TUCKER HM (1982) Factors in successful deglutition following supraglottic laryngeal surgery. Ann. Oto. Rhinol. Laryngol. 91 : 579-583

4. EFFRON MZ, JOHNSON JT, MYERS EN, CURTIN H, BEERY Q, SIGLER B (1981) Advanced carcinoma of the tongue. Arch Oto. Laryngol. 107 : 694-697

5. KRESPI YP, SISSON GA (1983) Reconstruction after total or subtotal glossectomy. Am. J. Surg. 146 : 488-492

New dimensions in otorhinolaryngology - head and neck surgery, vol. 2.
E. Myers, editor

SEQUENTIAL INTRA-ARTERIAL CHEMOTHERAPY AND SURGERY-PRELIMINARY RESULTS OF A CLINICAL TRIAL

LUIZ PAULO KOWALSKI, ABRÃO RAPOPORT, JOSIAS DE ANDRADE SOBRINHO, ANTONIO SÉRGIO FAVA AND MARCOS BRASILINO DE CARVALHO

Head and Neck Service, Heliópolis Hospital, Rua Cônego Xavier 276, São Paulo-SP (Brazil)

INTRODUCTION

The treatment of patients with squamous cell carcinoma of the tongue and floor of the mouth has traditionally involved surgery and irradiation. Although the results of combining surgery and radiation therapy have produced improvement in local and regional control, there is an unaccetable high rate of local failure.

Chemotherapy has recently acquired a place of eminence in the management of head and neck cancer. It has been used as a palliative therapy and as an adjunct to radiotherapy or surgery.

On 1980 we started a randomized controlled trial for patients with operable squamous cell carcinoma of the tongue and floor of the mouth. This study is designed to compare standard treatment to intra-arterial chemotherapy followed by surgery and radiotherapy.

MATERIAL AND METHODS

This study began in January 1980 and will be concluded when one hundred patients have been treated. So far 49 patients have already been treated (24 in the group of study and 25 in the control group). There is no significant imbalance between the groups with respect to sex, age, race, histologic grading and extent of tumor (TNM-UICC).

The drug regimen was a combination fo Methotrexate (10mg/day X 5 days), Bleomycin (15mg/day X 5 days) and Vincristine (1mg - 1st and 6th days). Since 1981 Cisplatinum (50mg at the first day- 1 hour infusion) has been added to the scheme. Eight patients were treated with the first scheme ant 16 with the last one. The drugs were administered by a catheter insered in the superfitial temporal artery. Tumor regression was measured 5 days after completing chemotherapy and surgery performed 7 to 10 days after this. Only patients with histologically proved metastases on the neck were irradiated (5000 Rad).

RESULTS

Tumor regression were achieved in 37% of the patients treated with the first scheme (Methotrexate-Bleomycin-Vincristine) and in 47% of the patients treated with the last sheme (Methotrexate-Bleomycin-Vincristine-Cisplatinum).The only complete remission were seen in this last group. Major complications occurred in four patients(16%). Three patients died and one with cerebrovascular accident couldn't be operated on.These complications occurred among patients treated at the first two years of the study.

Fifty per cent of the patients submited to intra-arterial chemotherapy prior to surgery developed some form of postoperative complication. Forty per cent of the patients of the control group developed complications.These complications were more frequent and severe in the group of study (flap necrosis, mucous membrane necrosis, etc).

The preliminary results of this trial are shown in the following table:

	IAC + SURG.	SURG.
Postreatment death	3	1
Lost of follow up	2	0
Dead of unrelated disease	2	1
Dead of cancer	4	6
Alive	13(54%) (5-53 months)	17(68%) (4-38 months)

CONCLUSIONS

1-The preliminary results were similar in both groups. Till the present time intra-arterial chemotherapy did not enhance the survival rates.

2- The post intra-arterial chemotherapy mortality was one of the limitating items of these preliminary results.

3-There was no correlation between the degree of response to intra-arterial chemotherapy and survival rates.

4- Intra-arterial chemotherapy increased the number and gravity of postoperative complications.

© 1985 Elsevier Science Publishers B.V. (Biomedical Division)
New dimensions in otorhinolaryngology - head and neck surgery, vol. 2.
E. Myers, editor

AN UNUSUALLY AGGRESSIVE SQUAMOUS CELL CARCINOMA OF THE AERODIGESTIVE TRACT CORRELATING WITH IN VITRO ACTIVITY IN A SUBRENAL CAPSULE MOUSE MODEL

STEVEN M. PARNES, M.D., JAMES A. BENNETT, PH.D., GERALD COLMAN, M.D.,
Divisions of Otolaryngology, Thoracic Surgery, Plastic Surgery, The Albany Medical College, Albany, New York, USA

A 62-year-old white female presented to our service with a large squamous cell carcinoma of the left oral cavity. She was first treated for a squamous cell carcinoma of the right floor of the mouth in 1980 with local excision and radiation therapy. She developed a recurrence in 1982 in the right oral cavity and was treated with a right hemiglossectomy, hemimandibulectomy, and radical neck dissection. She remained tumor free until 3 weeks prior to admission when she noted a mass developing in the left side of her face.

On physical examination, there was a 10 cm necrotic, friable tumor mass completely replacing her remaining tongue and filling her oral cavity, adherent to the left buccal mucosa and extending to the base of the skull. She underwent palliative cryosurgery of which 95% of the tumor was removed. Within 3 weeks, the tumor had returned, several centimeters larger than the original size (Fig. 1). A second attempt was then made to remove the tumor. Specimens were removed for implant. There was massive bleeding during the extirpation of the tumor, and with 75% removed, the operation was terminated. The patient received minimal supportive care following surgery and expired one week later. The autopsy demonstrated local disease only.

Several specimens (average diameter 2 mm) were implanted as xenografts under the kidney capsule of immunosuppressed mice on the same day of surgery. Size changes, serially evaluated in the same 5 mice every week for 3 weeks, demonstrated an average growth in diameter of 2.2 mm $\pm$ .26 per week (> 100%). In addition, the exposure to two chemotherapeutic agents, Cis-platinum and 5-Flouauracil, did not impede tumor growth (Fig. 2). Tumor tissue architecture and differentiation of the xenografts were similar to that found in sections from the original tumor.

This finding is in marked contrast with our experience with other head and neck tumors where growth averaged about 10% per week and was often curtailed when the chemotherapeutic agents were employed.. This observation suggests that malignant tumors have intrinsic capacities for rapid growth, irrespective of the competency of the host immune system.

REFERENCE

Bennett J, McKneally M, Prevost L, Pilon V (1984) Accurate Prediction of the Chemosensitivity of Lewis Lung Carcinoma using a.Subrenal Capsule Assay (SRC) in Rats. Preclin. Pharmacol. Exp. Ther. AACR Abstract 1478.

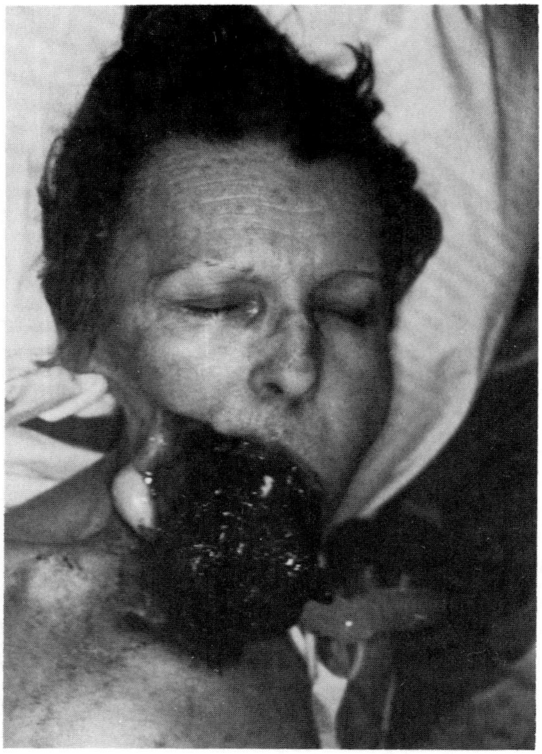

Figure 1: Recurrent tumor of the oral cavity.

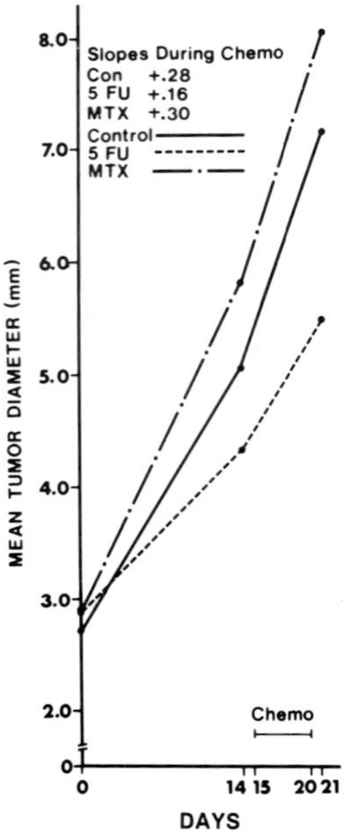

Figure 2: Tumor (xenograph) growth characteristics in the kidney capsule of mice.

© 1985 Elsevier Science Publishers B.V. (Biomedical Division)
New dimensions in otorhinolaryngology – head and neck surgery, vol. 2.
E. Myers, editor

SUPRACRICOID PARTIAL LARYNGECTOMY. SURGICAL TECHNIQUE, INDICATIONS, FUNCTIONNAL AND CARCINOLOGIC RESULTS

D. BRASNU MD, J. LACAU ST GUILY MD, M. MENARD MD, H. LACCOURREYE MD
Hopital Laennec, 42 rue de sèvres, 75007 PARIS

Supracricoid partial laryngectomy (SCPL) is a procedure for partial laryngectomy for treatment of vestibular, ventricular and glottic carcinoma which avoids having to perform a total laryngectomy.

In supracricoid partial laryngectomy, the thyroid cartilage is completely removed, whereas the hyoid bone, the cricoid cartilage and one or two arytenoids are conserved.

Depending on the location of the tumor, there are two variations of SCPL. The main difference between the two techniques is the preservation or excision of the suprahyoid epiglottis.

In the first variation, the entire epiglottis and the supra-glottic and glottic larynx are removed, and one or two arytenoids are preserved. Cricohyoidopexy is used for closure.

In the second technique, only the infrahyoid epiglottis is excised along with the supraglottic and glottic larynx, while the suprahyoid epiglottis and one or two arytenoids are preserved, cricohyoidoepiglottopexy is used for closure.

We systematically perform a bilateral neck dissection for supraglottic carcinoma even for clinically negative nodes (functionnal neck dissection). However, in cases of NO glottic carcinoma, we never perform any type of neck dissection.

The techniques used for ventilation during this procedure are particulary important and were designed to ensure maximal visualization during the laryngectomy and allow for accurate aligning of the skin and tracheal incisions. During laryngectomy, high frequency jet ventilation is employed through a small catheter previously inserted into the orotracheal tube. Once the larynx has been resected, the trachea is pulled upwards to the hyoid bone, and the tracheal incision for the tracheotomy is then aligned to the skin incision. Consequently tracheal ventilation is used during closure.

MATERIAL

61 patients underwent a supracricoid partial laryngectomy from 1972 through 1984. The first variation of SCPL was employed in 49 patients, two arytenoids were preserved in 7 patients. The second variation of this procedure was used in 12 patients and in most cases two arytenoids were preserved.

FUNCTIONNAL RESULTS

Decannulation ranged from 2 - 58 days and the average decannulation time was 6 days. 50 patients recovered normal deglutition. The nasogastric feeding tube was removed after an average time of 22 days with a range of 10 to 42 days. 9 patients underwent a temporary gastrostomy for aspiration pneumonia. No secondary total laryngectomy was required for any patient. 2 post operative deaths occured, one aspiration pneumonia and one ruptura of an aortic anevrysm.

CARCINOLOGIC RESULT

Follow up of at least 2 years was available for 37 patients. No local recurrence occurred in any patient. The 3 year-survival rate was 72% and the 5-year survival rate was 65%.

INDICATIONS FOR SCPL

The first variation of SCPL in which the epiglottis is completely removed is indicated for T2 vestibular carcinoma extended to the ventricle and/or the posterior third of the ventricular band as long as arytenoid and vocal cord mobility is normal. These tumor extensions are a contraindication to supraglottic surgery. In this variation of SCPL the preepiglottic space is totally removed. The second variation of SCPL which preserves the suprahyoid epiglottis is indicated for bilateral T1 glottic carcinoma and uni ou bilateral T2 glottic carcinoma as long as the arytenoid mobility is normal. It is important to emphasize that we no longer perform bilateral cordectomy, hemilaryngectomy and hemiglottectomy. This variation of SCPL involves the resection of the totality of the thyroarytenoid muscles including the anterior supracommissural area.

SCPL is also indicated for T1T2 ventricular carcinoma. A total laryngectomy is inapropriate since SCPL provides for the complete removal of the thyroid cartilage.

THE CONTRAINDICATIONS OF SCPL ARE :

- patient older than 70 years of age
- respiratory insufficiency
- arytenoid immobility

- subglottic invasion
- major preepiglottic space invasion.

IN CONCLUSION, supracricoid partial laryngectomy allows additionnal indication for partial laryngectomy in cases of vestibular, ventricular and glottic carcinoma.

REFERENCES

- Majer H, Rieder W. Technique de laryngectomie permettant de conserver la perméabilité respiratoire : la cricohyoïdopexie Ann. Otolaryng. 1959, 76, 677-687.

- Piquet JJ, Desaulty A, Decroix G. Cricohyoïdoepiglottopexie. Technique operatoire et resultats fonctionnels. Ann. Otolaryng. 1974, 91, 681_689

- Labayle J, Bismuth R. Laryngectomie totale avec reconstitution Ann. Otolaryng. 1971, 88, 219-228.

New dimensions in otorhinolaryngology - head and neck surgery, vol. 2.
E. Myers, editor

QUANTITATIVE EVALUATION OF ASPIRATION IN A NEW MODIFICATION OF NEOGLOTTIC RECONSTRUCTION

DANKO CERENKO, IVO PADOVAN
Department of Otolaringology, University Hospital "Dr. Mladen Stojanovic", Vinogradska 29, 41000 Zagreb,(Yugoslavia)

INTRODUCTION

The criteria used to evaluate quality of speech in neoglottic reconstruction have been well established. On the other hand, aspiration has not been evaluated equally well. Qualitative terms such as slight, tolerable, significant or intolerable aspiration are subjective, inprecise and unacceptable. We therefore aimed at resolving the following 2 problems: 1. To define the quantitative method of evaluation of aspiration, and 2. To determine the limits of acceptable and unacceptable aspiration.

MATERIAL AND METHODS

During last four years a total number of 41 patients undervent total laryngectomy with neoglottic reconstruction according to our new modification. It is the modified Staffieri's technique which differs from the original method in creating a very small fistula, about 2-3 mm in length. Such small fistula does not leak, but also does not allow phonation. During the course of postoperative radiotherapy repeated dilatation of the fistula is performed as a standard procedure, until fistula becomes functional.

1. Quantitative measurements of the aspiration range

Since swallowing of liquids is most likely to result in aspiration, we have chosen to use water for our measurements.Measuring is performed by placeing a tampon of known weight into the trachea. After swallowing the determined quantity of water, the tampon which absorbed the fluid which might have leaked through the fistula is weighed, and the difference in weight represents amount of aspirated fluid which is expressed in percents.In order to take into account as many variable factors which influence aspiration as possible, each patient was required to swallow 50 cc (or grams) of water 5 times over three different periods of time, 5, 15 and 30 seconds respectively.The range of aspiration as well as the mean value of aspiration was thus determined for each patient.

RESULTS

In defining the limits of acceptable and unacceptable aspiration not only numerical results of measurements performed, but also clinical manifestations of aspiration as well as patient's attitude had to be taken into consideration. Three groups of patients were differentiated:

1. The first group consisted of patients who did not have any clinical manifestations while drinking. Their mean value of aspiration was less than 2%.

2. The second group includes the patients in whom aspiration was a constant feature, but was well tolerated. In order to facilitate the definition of the upper limit of still acceptable aspiration, destinction had to be made between two subdivisions of this group with relatively acceptable aspiration: The II-A group is defined with the mean value of aspiration from 2-4%. The II-B group or transitional group towards the group with unacceptable aspiration requires attention. Patients are included in this group if their mean value of aspiration is between 4 and 5% only if they can maintain their minimal aspiration below 3%.

3. The third group included patients with unacceptable amount of aspiration with the mean value of aspiration more than 5%.

DISCUSSION

With the described surgical technique and the method of quantitative evaluation of aspiration we have shown that it is possible to offer an almost ideal result to 78% of the patients: nonprosthetic comfortable speech with acceptable aspiration less than 5%, with no need for continous medical help except for regular oncologic control

Out of 9 failures (22%), in 5 patients (12%) the mean value of aspiration was more than 5% and the fistula had to be closed. In 4 patients (10%) even prolonged dilatation of the fistula did not secure permanent speech. Two of these last 4 patients were rehabilitated by insertion of self-designed voice prosthesis

REFERENCES

1. Staffieri M, Serafini I (1976) La riabilitazione chirurgica della voce e della respirazione dopo laringectomia totale. In: Atti del XXIX Congresso Nazionale, Bologna, Ass.Otol.Osped.Ital. 28.Sett.,3.Ott.
2. Leipzig B, Griffiths CM, Shea JP (1980) Ann Otol 89:204-209

© 1985 Elsevier Science Publishers B.V. (Biomedical Division)
New dimensions in otorhinolaryngology - head and neck surgery, vol. 2.
E. Myers, editor

COMPARATIVE STUDY BY MEANS OF ELECTROGLOTTOGRAPHY AND SPECTROGRAPHY IN VOICE OF PATIENTS OPERATED BY CORDECTOMY OR TOTAL LARYNGECTOMY

G.MOTTA,U.CESARI,M.IENGO,G,VILLARI
2 nd Medical School-E.N.T. Dept.:Chief:Prof.G.Motta-Naples,Italy

INTRODUCTION

Electroglottography is normally employed for investigating the vibratory pattern of the vocal folds(1,2,3,4,5);in order to better understand the meaning of such a technique we decided to examinate those patients whose anatomic conditions were really far from the normal ones.

MATERIALS AND METHODS

Materials employed were an EG 830 Fabre electroglottograph(F-J electronics) and a Logica Serie 3 Spectrograph. 20 patients were observed(10 who underwent a cordectomy and 10 who underwent a total laryngectomy)by performing electroglottography and spectrography before and after logopedic treatment:electroglottography was executed looking for other vibrating structures substituting the vocal folds after radical operations of the larynx;spectrography for giving documentary evidence to any eventual recovery of a satisfactory voice after rehabilitation.

RESULTS

Concerning those patients who underwent cordectomy,our findings turned out as follows;

- before rehabilitation electroglottography gives an irregular trace without any possibility of finding out a vibratory cycle;spectrography is characterized by noise,given by the irregular blackening of the trace;
- after rehabilitation electroglottography gives a trace very similar to a normal one,even if a particularly sharp peak and a reduced amplitude are noticed;spectrography shows reduction of the noise,clear identification of the harmonics.

About whose who underwent total laryngectomy:

- before rehabilitation electroglottography gives a flat trace responding to the complete absence of phonation;spetrography only shows the noise due to explosive articulation of some phonema(grenouillage),without production of sound;
- after logopedic treatment electroglottography gives a trace resambling a normal one,even if a particularly sharp peak and a reduced amplitude are noticed; spectrography confirms production of sound,recovery of harmonics,assuring an intellegible message even if a compatible noise is observed.

CONCLUSIONS

Concerning electroglottography,the obtaining of regaular trace in patients operated by cordectomy and rehabilitated is explained by the vibration of the surviving vocal fold mucosa with the restoration tissue located where cordectomy was performed. A trace resembling a normal one in subjects operated by total laryngectomy and trained for esophageal voice is due to the vibratory pattern of the upper esophageal sphinter mucosa that,even for a very short time,produces a sound enough to be articulated along the "vocal tract" . So,glottic wave not only is vibratory cycle related,but it also may depend on other anatomic structures acting as a new glottis. Spectrography suggests that the setting up of a vibratory pattern after a radical operation of the larynx is responding to a satisfactory voice,confirmed by the recovery of the harmonics and their regular disposition.

REFERENCES

1)Beck J.D.(1967)Ueber funktionelle hypokinetische stimmstorungen Proefschrift In:Ludwig Maximilian Universität - München

2)Chevrie-Mueller(1967)Contribution a l'etude de traces glottographique chez l'adulte normal.Rev.Laryngol.(Bordeaux)88;227-243

3)Lecluse F.L.E.,Brocaar M.P,,Vershure J.(1975)The Electroglottography and its relation to glottal activity.Folia Phoniatrica 27:215-224

4)Loebell E.(1978)Ueber den klinischen Wert der EleKtroglottographie.Archiev. Oher USW,Hellsch,191:740-764

5)Van Michael C.(1967)Morphologie de la courve glottographique dans certains troubles tunctionnels du larynx.Folia Phoniatrica 19:192-202

© 1985 Elsevier Science Publishers B.V. (Biomedical Division)
New dimensions in otorhinolaryngology - head and neck surgery, vol. 2.
E. Myers, editor

A SIMPLE TECHNIQUE TO PREVENT TRACHEOSTOMAL STENOSIS FOLLOWING TOTAL LARYNGECTOMY

SHYUE-YIH CHANG, M.D.

Department of Otolaryngology, Veterans General Hospital, National Yang-Ming Medical College, Taipei, Taiwan, R.O.C.

INTRODUCTION

Tracheostomal stenosis is one of the major complications following total laryngectomy. Due to the probability of the causes of this complication arising, many preventive methods have been developed (1,2). However, these methods often complicating and increasing the difficulties of surgical procedures. Moreover, according to the literature, currently 4% - 42% of total laryngectomy patients still develop this type of complication (3,4). From this, it can be seen that this problem may not yet be adequately resolved.

PATIENTS AND METHODS

The total laryngectomy employs anterior neck apron incision. Its lowest point is connected by a U-shaped incision for the skin orifice of tracheostoma. Then take the skin and its surrounding soft tissue to create a skin orifice. The method of the trachea transection is to make a horizontal cut at the intercartilage space, preserving the soft tissue at the end of the trachea to avoid exposure of the outermost cartilage ring (Fig. 1). Finally the mucosa at the end of tracheal transection and the skin are precisely approximated with silk sutures. The suture should cross the intercartilage space. Besides this, the V-shaped suture should be used at the two connection points of the apron incision with the newly created tracheostoma. After the surgery, insertion of a tracheotomy tube is not necessary.

From February of 1982 through July of 1984, the author personally performed or directly supervised the performance of total laryngectomy on 62 patients, all of which used this type of method to create a tracheostoma. In the post-surgery follow-up period, aside from 2 patients who died within 6 months after surgery, all the other patients had at least 6 months of follow-up.

RESULTS

Of the 62 patients, only one developed tracheostomal stenosis. This patient was due to supraglottic cancer with preoperative radiotherapy and had a serious degree of post-operative wound infection. The other 59 patients who received at least 6 months of follow-up and the 2 other patients who died within 6 months after surgery, all had a tracheostoma of at least 10 x 8 mm or greater.

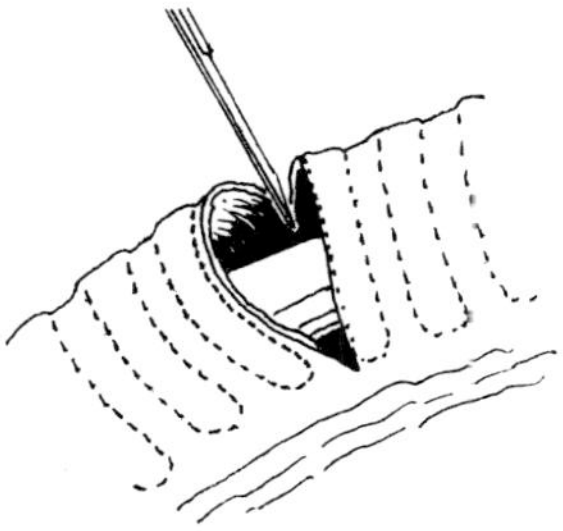

Fig. 1. The method of the trachea transection is to make a horizontal cut at the intercartilage space to avoid exposure of the outermost cartilage ring.

DISCUSSION

From the results discussed above, it can be seen that the development of tracheostoma stenosis appears to be mainly determined by surgical technique, and has no apparent meaningful relation with sex, location or size of tumor, surgical extent, radiotherapy, pre-surgical tracheotomy or post-operative development of pharyngocutaneous fistula.

The preventive methods that has been tried, aside from focussing on the possible causes, basically emphasize increasing the length of the circumference of the tracheostoma and altering the direction of scar constriction, such as oblique transection of the trachea (2,4) or varies types of Z-plasty (3,5). However, The author believes that these techniques easily causes cartilage exposure and can even induce stomal stenosis or complicating surgical procedures.

The simple and nature intercartilage transverse transection method used with this group of patients avoids cartilage exposure and infection, making the tracheal cartilage to serve as a natural stenting of the stoma. This is actually the basic principle of this method and has not been emphasized in previous literature. This tracheostoma construction method during laryngectomy should be able to ideally prevent the post-laryngectomy tracheostoma stenosis.

REFERENCES

1. 張學逸（1985）全喉切除術之併發症及其預防。中耳醫誌（附印中）

2. Griffith GR, Luce EA (1982) Tracheal stomal stenosis after laryngectomy. Plast Reconstr Surg 70:694-698

3. Lam KH, Wei WI, Wong J, et al (1983) Tracheostome construction during laryngectomy - a method to prevent stenosis. Laryngoscope 93:212-215

4. Yonkers AJ, Mercurio GA (1983) Tracheostomal stenosis following total laryngectomy. Otolaryngol Clin North Am 16:391-405

5. Myers EN, Gallia LJ (1982) Tracheostomal stenosis following total laryngectomy. Ann Otol Rhinol Laryngol 91:450-453

© 1985 Elsevier Science Publishers B.V. (Biomedical Division)
New dimensions in otorhinolaryngology - head and neck surgery, vol. 2.
E. Myers, editor

KERATOSIS OF THE LARYNX: HISTOLOGIC AND CLINIC CORRELATES

ANDREA GALLO*, MARCO DE VINCENTIIS*, PIETRO GALLO§ and DARIO MARCOTULLIO*

*2nd ENT Clinic and §Department of Pathology, University 'La Sapienza', Rome, Italy

The clinico-pathological definition of laryngeal keratosis is still controversial. In fact, the comparison among the series reported in the literature is made difficult by the existence of a lot of non-comparable histologic classifications. The main question to be solved is whether laryngeal keratosis is a unique entity or is a complex of different histological pictures, with different etiologies, evolutions and, as a consequence, different therapeutic approaches.

In order to solve such a problem, 72 patients with keratosis of the larynx, observed in the 2nd ENT Clinic of the University 'La Sapienza' of Rome, Italy, were studied.

The risk factors and clinical course were accounted for, the follow-up ranging from 10 months to 7 years (mean 3.4 years). The histologic diagnosis was performed on each patient according to a classification easy to be used and internationally agreed upon, like that proposed by the Armed Forces Institute of Pathology of Washington[1](DC, U.S.A.). The patients were accordingly subdivided into three groups: pachidermia laryngis, leukoplakia and Bowenoid dyskeratosis. Pachidermia laryngis corresponds to a form of keratosis lacking any displastic feature and characterized by acanthosis and hyperkeratosis. Leukoplakia is a keratosis with mild dysplasia: a chronic inflammatory infiltration underneath the epithelium is always evident and both papillomatosis and hyperplasia of the basal layer are present. Bowenoid dyskeratosis is characterized by moderate dysplasia involving the lower two thirds of the epithelium. Dyskeratosis, that is keratinization of isolated cells within the spinous layer is present, too. Most patients were male (91,7%), their ages ranging from 21 to 73 years (mean 52 years).

As regarding risk factors, a heavier exposure to tobacco smoking for patients with leukoplakia (average cigarettes consumption: 5.2×10^5) was noticed, as compared with the ones suffering from pachidermia laryngis (average cigarettes consumption 3.1×10^5). Such a difference is highly significant from a statistical standpoint ($p < 0.005$). On the contrary, Bowenoid dyskeratosis doesn't seem to be proportionally related to smoking habits.

Besides etiological differences, the distinction among 3 types of laryngeal keratosis is further substantiated by a different clinical evolution. All the patients, indeed, were alternatively treated by mucosal stripping or microlaryngoscopy chordectomy and the outcome after these treatments was different as related to the various types of keratosis. Pachidermia laryngis never recurred after chordectomy but rarely did it even after mucosal stripping (12%), accounting for the best prognosis. Leukoplakia did not also recur after chordectomy, but showed a higher recurrence rate (27%) after mucous stripping. No progression into cancer was observed in the period under examination for such a condition. Finally, Bowenoid dyskeratosis not only was noted to recur after mucous stripping, but also to show a frequent progression into infiltrating carcinoma (40%).

In conclusion, the histologic classification adopted revealed itself to be useful and reliable, in that it enables to differentiate risk factors, to predict the patients' outcome and to plan the most suitable surgical treatment. In the Authors' experience[2], laryngeal mucous stripping (together with life-style change and follow-up procedures) remains the choice therapy for both pachidermia laryngis and leukoplakia, whereas a prophylactic chordectomy must be performed in cases of Bowenoid dyskeratosis.

REFERENCES

1. Ash JE, Beck MR, Wilkes JD (1964) In: Atlas of tumor pathology. Armed Forces Institute of Pathology, Washington.

2. Gallo A, De Vincentiis M, Gallo P, Marcotullio D (1985) Acta Otorhinol. Ital. In press.

New dimensions in otorhinolaryngology - head and neck surgery, vol. 2.
E. Myers, editor

JEJUNAL GRAFT: USED AS RECONSTRUCTION OF THE UPPER DIGESTIVE TRACT AFTER EXTENSIVE LARYNGOPHARYNGECTOMY AND AS NEOGLOTTIS PHONATORIA AFTER LARYNGECTOMY

M.CH. GRASL*, K. EHRENBERGER*, W. WICKE*, H. SWOBODA*
H. PIZA**, R. ROKA**
*First Department of Otorhinolaryngology
**First Department of Plastic and Reconstructive Surgery
University of Vienna School of Medicine, Vienna Austria
A-I097 Vienna, Lazarettgasse I4

INTRODUCTION

Surgery for larger malignant laryngopharyngeal tumors requires aggressive managment, which is restricted by difficulties of reconstruction and rehabilitation (I). Sidenberg was the first in I959 using a revascularized isolated jejunal segment to reconstruct the cervical esophagus (2). Recent developments in microvascular surgery allows nowadays better implantation of free jejunal autografts (3).

We report about two applications of this method: I. reconstruction of the upper digestive tract after extensive laryngopharyngectomy (Group A); 2. creation of a Neoglottis Phonatoria after laryngectomy (Group B).

PATIENTS

Group A

Eleven patients with a T4 carcinoma, primary: larynx and hypopharynx each four and mesopharynx three cases; six had a local recurrence.

Group B

Seven patients with untreated T_I and T_2 carcinomas of the larynx without palpable regionar lymph nodes.

SURGICAL TECHNIQUE

During resection of the tumor (in two cases of mesopharynx tumor the larynx has been conserved) a second team of surgeons harvests the jejunal graft. Then the segment vessels are anastomosed to the external carotid artery and to the internal jugular vein or their branches. The graft is trimmed to size and anastomosed isoperistaltic to the pharynx and esophagus (Group A). In Group B we anastomosed the jejunal graft end to end to a tracheal stump, fixed it at the digastric muscles and after dorsal deflection again drawn downwards and inserted it into the reconstructed anterior wall of the hypopharynx.

RESULTS

Group A

Two patients died postoperative, one in a hepatic coma the other because of a carotid rupture after necrosis of the graft. Six patients had no problems with swallowing, one salivary fistula closed spontaneous. Aspiration was in those two cases where the larynx has been conserved. Three patients learned the esophageal speech. In three cases postoperative radiation was necessary and except one mild erosive inflammation of the jejunum well tolerated.

Group B

Healing occured withcut problems except one necrosis, which was resected; one transient aspiration was seen. Within a week a clear phonation through the voice generating tracheohypopharyngeal shunt was possible.

DISCUSSION

Although the increasing operating time is a disadvantage we believe that the use of the jejunal graft is justified in selected patients, but it requires the availability of an exsperienced microvascular surgeon (I). The advantages for patients of Group A are: one stage technique; no limit of resection of the tumor and left defect; fistulas occur rare because of the sufficient blood circulation of the margins, and therefore swallowing is already possible after two weeks; the cosmetic result is satisfactory; pre- and postoperative radiation is practicable and the esophageal speech is to be learned (3). In Group B a clear phonation, able to be modulated, resulted. The shunt needs no maintenance.

REFERENCES

I. Bailey BJ, Biller HF (I985) Surgery of the larynx WB Saunders Company

2. Sidenberg B et al. (I959) Immediate reconstruction of the cervical esophagus by a revascularized jejunal segment Ann Surg I49: I62-I7I

3. Sasaki TM et al. (I980) Free jejunal graft reconstruction after head neck surgery Am J Surg I39: 650-653

New dimensions in otorhinolaryngology - head and neck surgery, vol. 2.
E. Myers, editor

THE HEAD AND NECK CARCINOMA PATIENT WITH MULTIPLE PRIMARY TUMORS: A GROWING CHALLENGE

THOMAS W. GROSSMAN, M.D., FACS

INTRODUCTION

Billroth is generally credited with providing the initial report of a patient with multiple primary malignant neoplasms back in 1860. Since that time numerous authors have called attention to the relatively frequent occurence of multiple primary neoplasms, particularly in the upper aero-digestive tract.

METHODS AND MATERIALS

A retrospective review was conducted of all patients presenting with upper aero-digestive tract carcinoma at the Medical College of Wisconsin affiliated institutions for the ten year period from 1970 through 1979. A total of 790 such patients was identified.

RESULTS

Of the 790 patients studied, 132 ultimately developed additional primary neoplasms. Of these 132 patients, 104 developed a single additional primary, 22 developed two additional primaries, and 6 patients developed three or more additional primary neoplasms.

The majority of the index primary malignancies were fairly evenly distributed among the oral cavity, the larynx and the oropharynx. There was a lesser incidence of Index primaries in the hypopharynx, nose/nasopharynx and para-nasal sinuses.

About one third of the second primary tumors appeared in the lung. The incidence in all other areas was fairly evenly distributed.

Survival was markedly reduced in those patients who developed an additional primary cancer. At 24 months the single primary survival is 45% and the multiple primary survival is 19%. At 5 years the values are 27% and 3%.

There is no appreciable difference in survival after detection of the second primary neoplasm whether that neoplasm appears simultaneously that is (at the time of diagnosis of the index tumor), synchronously (within six months of index tumor diagnosis), or metachronously (more than 6 months after index tumor diagnosis).

In patient with an index primary of the larynx,the appearance of an additional primary had an even more disastrous effect upon survival. The 24 month survival in the single primary group was 64% compared to 3% in the multiple primary group.

In our group of patients with index laryngeal tumors, 113 were treated successfully. In this successfully treated group 2.7% developed a second primary tumor in the esophagus. This incidence does not differ significantly from the incidence of second primary esophageal lesions in the total patient population. All of these esophageal tumors appeared in the first two years following initial treatment.

In this same group of 113 successfully treated patients with index laryngeal tumors, 21 ultimately developed an additional primary neoplasm in the lung. The incidence is 18.6% - nearly one out of five patients. This is more than three times the incidence in our total group. Unlike esophageal second primaries, second primary lung tumors continue to appear even as long as seven or more years after initial diagnosis and treatment.

The patterns of treatment failure in the total patient population provide a graphic picture of this problem of second primary tumors. In the first year after initial treatment, failure at the primary site is the most common reason for failure. However, after 24 to 36 months the appearance of a second primary becomes more of a concern that failure of treatment of the index carcinoma.

DISCUSSION

Our data indicate that additional primary lesions continue to appear in relative ly constant numbers for many years after initial diagnosis and treatment. With the passage of time the total number surviving patients decreases. Thus, the actuarial incidence continues to rise and has been reported as high as 30% after five years.

The prevention, early detection, and effective treatment of these additional primary neoplasms is our challenge for the future.

© 1985 Elsevier Science Publishers B.V. (Biomedical Division)
New dimensions in otorhinolaryngology - head and neck surgery, vol. 2.
E. Myers, editor

MEDIASTINAL TRACHEOSTOMY FOR RECURRENT CANCER. USE OF A PERFORATED PECTORALIS MAJOR MYOCUTANEOUS ISLAND FLAP

M. HAMOIR *, N. CALTEUX **, T. ROBILLARD*, A.J. YOUSIF*, M. REMACLE*, A. DE CONINCK**, J. VAN DEN EECKHAUT*

* ENT. and ** PLASTIC SURGERY DEPTS. St. Luc Hospital, University of Louvain, 10, Av. Hippocrate, 1200 BRUXELLES

INTRODUCTION

First described for the treatment of stomal recurrence after laryngectomy by Sisson, (1). Mediastinal tracheostomy has been considered as a heavy intervention with major haemorrhagic risk. The use of a Pectoralis Major myocutaneous flap to carry out the tracheostomy has radically modified the postoperative picture (2,3).

OPERATIVE TECHNIQUE

We have adopted the principles according to Sisson (3) and Biller (2) . The excision of the tumour is large and confirmed by frozen section examination. The bone resection includes the manubrium as well as the sternal ends of the clavicles and the ends for the first two ribs.

The access to the superior mediastinum is large, permitting a mediastinal lymph node dissection. The trachea may be excised up to 2-3 centimeters from the carina. A Pectoralis Major myocutaneous island flap is used to conform the cervical skin defect and for the reconstruction of the stoma. The cutaneous paddle is rectangular in shape and is elevated from the parasternal region. It is larger in size than the area of the cervical skin loss, as it will be used for the stoma. An elliptical orifice is cut in the center of the paddle and fixed by sutures towards the trachea. The skin is invaginated towards the trachea without tension on the trachea. The basic principles stated by Sisson should be emphasised (3).

- The closure should be carried out without tension in order to avoid any breakdown or infection in the superior mediastinum.
- The thoracic duct must be repaired and ligated to prevent lymphorrhea.
- The hemostasis should be meticulous and drainage by suction catheter is necessary to avoid any hematoma forming a source of infection.

RESULTS

Between July 1982 and May 1984, we have carried out the operation on four cases. In each case, it consisted of salvage surgery for neoplastic recurrences. Neither necrosis of the flap nor arterial rupture occured. Two patients of the four are living in good health sixteen month later for one, and twelve months for the second,after the operation. The other two were unfortunate ; one died from hepatico-renal failure and the other from indeterminate cause, one and eight months after the operation respectivly.

DISCUSSION

Technique

The Pectoralis Major myocutaneous flap allows a one stage reconstruction of the mediastinum defect (2). This procedure permits us to obtain simultaneously a cervico-thoracic skin cover and to perform a stoma ; the muscle ensures an adequate cover for the great vessels by protecting them from the trachea and the resected bony edges. The dead space is therefore completely obliterated. The trachea may be transposed inferiorly and to the right of the innominate arterial and venous trunk to improve the mobility of the trachea and thus reduce the tension at the level of the stoma.

Indications

.Stomal recurrences following laryngectomy is the major indication.

.Laryngeal lesion T4 in which a preoperative tracheostomy cannot be avoided particularly in case of subglottic cancers and rare cases of primitive tracheal cancers. Harrison (4) proposed this intervention for subglottic cancers invading the cricoid cartilage.

.Cancers of the cervicothoracic esophagus and occasionally thyroid cancers with laryngo-tracheal invasion can justify this operation (5,6,7).

Prevention of stomal recurrence

The most effective measures for prevention are to avoid a preoperative tracheostomy; to carry out block dissection of the pre and paratracheal lymph nodes and to perform the resection on the healthy trachea controlled by frozen section. (8).

CONCLUSION

Mediastinal tracheostomy is a major surgical act. However, the use of the major pectoralis myocutaneous flap has radically

changed the postoperative picture.
The principal indication is stomal recurrence after laryngectomy. This intervention is better than any other therapeutic measure which can be offered to a patient who is condemned to suffer a bitter end. However, prognosis of these recurrences remains gloomy. Therefore, it is preferable to prevent recurrences as far as possible by adequate primary treatment.

REFERENCES

1. Sisson G.A., Straehley C.J. Jr, Johnson N.E. (1962). Mediastinal dissection for recurrent cancer after laryngectomy. Laryngoscope 72 : 1064-1077.
2. Biller H., Krespi Y., Lawson W. (1980) : A one stage flap reconstruction following resection for stoma recurrence. Otolar. Head Neck Surg. 88 : 357-360.
3. Sisson G.A., Goldman M.E. (1981) : Pectoral myocutaneous island flap for the reconstruction of stomal recurrence. Arch. Oto-Laryngol. 107 : 466-449.
4. Harrisson D.F.N., (1971) : The pathology and management of subglottic cancer. Ann. Otol. Rhinol. Laryngol. 80 : 6-12.
5. Grillo H.C. (1966) : Terminal or mural tracheostomy in the anterior mediastinum. J. Thoracic. Cardiovasc. Surg. 51 : 422-427.
6. Sisson G.A., Bytell D.E., Edison B.D., Yeh S. (1975) : Transsternal Radical Neck Dissection for control of stomal recurrences. End results. Laryngoscope 85 : 1504-1510.
7. Orringer M.B., Sloane H. (1979) : Anterior Mediastinal Tracheostomy. J. Thorac. Cardiovasc. Surg. 78 : 850-859.
8. Silver C.E. (1981) : Surgery for cancer of the larynx and related structures. Churchill Livingstone, New York.

New dimensions in otorhinolaryngology - head and neck surgery, vol. 2.
E. Myers, editor

ONCOGENE HYBRIDIZATION IN HEAD AND NECK CANCER

WILLIAM H. FRIEDMAN, BARRY ROSENBLUM, PAUL LOEWENSTEIN, HELEN THORNTON, GEORGE KATSANTONIS, MAURICE GREEN
Department of Otolaryngology-Head and Neck Surgery, St. Louis University Hospitals, 1325 S. Grand Blvd., St. Louis, Mo. 63104

INTRODUCTION

The authors have previously reported the presence of cellular transforming genes in human head and neck squamous cell carcinomas[1,2]. Using the NIH 3T3 transformation assay, putative oncogenes were first cloned and retransfected repetitively resulting in enhanced transformation efficiencies[3], i.e., NIH 3T3 mouse fibroblast cells were transformed into a malignant form at a greater rate with each serial passage. Human DNA was identified integrated into the DNA of the transformed mouse fibroblasts by hybridizing with human DNA from the Alu family of conserved human sequences. Since these reports, the authors have cross-hybridized the head and neck cancer putative oncogenes with known viral and human oncogenes yielding the first conclusive evidence of oncogenes in human head and neck squamous cell carcinomas. The known oncogenes, C-Myc and V-Myb were found to be clearly related but not identical to oncogenes extracted from squamous cancer cloned DNA of the nasopharynx, base of tongue and larynx.

MATERIALS AND METHODS

Head and neck squamous cell cancer DNA cloned in NIH 3T3 mouse fibroblast cells and isolated by the method of Graham, Blin and Stafford were hybridized against V-Myb avian viral oncogene and C-Myc human cell line oncogene under stringent and non-stringent conditions. The cloned human DNA was subjected to enzymatic digestion using either BamHl, BglII, or EcoRI prior to Southern Blot analysis. Hybridization was accomplished by probing the cloned human head and neck squamous cell DNA with nick translated plasmids containing retroviral and human oncogenes. These known oncogenes were obtained from the American Type Culture Institute. Southern Blot analyses were then performed by the method of Jeffreys and Flavell. Controls consisted of DNA obtained from NIH non-transformed fibroblasts.

RESULTS

Under stringent conditions (Tm-28 degrees Celsius) no hybridization between probe DNA and human DNA occurred. However, under nonstringent conditions (Tm-43 degrees Celsius) two oncogene probes did hybridize with cloned human DNA isolated from mouse fibroblast cells. This reveals that while human head and neck squamous cell cancer oncogenes are related to avian and human cell line oncogenes, they are not identical. Controls consisted of

DNA obtained from 3T3 nontransformed cells. There was no hybridization of control DNA with any probes under stringent or nonstringent conditions.

CONCLUSION

The presence of oncogenes in human head and neck cancers is confirmed by hybridization studies with previously identified oncogenes. Oncogenes isolated from human squamous cell carcinomas of the larynx, nasopharynx and base of tongue appear to be identical. This conclusion is based on a positive homology obtained with human and viral oncogene DNA probes using different enzymatic digestion processes. These oncogenes are related to the C-Myc human neuroblastoma cell line oncogene and to a lesser extent the V-Myb avian myeloblastoleukosis oncogene.

DISCUSSION

The precise role of oncogenes in human carcinogenesis remains unclear. However, it is widely believed that the oncogene is central to this process. Oncogenes have been identified in retrovirus DNA and certain retrovirus oncogenes are clearly involved in carcinogenesis in a variety of animal species. To-date no primate retroviruses are known to be clearly involved in carcinogenesis in humans. The presence or absence of oncogenes in normal head and neck epithelium has not been studied. To determine whether or not oncogenes exist in normal tissue and at what copy level, similar assay techniques of this tissue should be undertaken. Oncogenes may be unique to cancer DNA; however, these genes may exist in non-cancer DNA and become abnormally expressed through the mechanisms of gene expression, derepression or gene insertion. For example, the combination of alcohol and tobacco may be carcinogenic by a gene alteration or, in the presence of a virus, by gene insertion. If the head and neck oncogenes are not among those previously characterized, then sequencing and cloning experiments will be performed. It is hoped that biological assay techniques will yield the protein product of the head and neck oncogene and perhaps lead to the synthesis of specific peptide antibodies to the protein product. At this time the role of specific peptide antibodies in the treatment of squamous cell head and neck carcinomas is entirely speculative.If synthesized, these antibodies would be extremely useful in studying the role of oncogenes in head and neck cancers.

REFERENCES

1. Friedman WH, Rosenblum B, Loewenstein P, Thornton H, Katsantonis G, Green M (1983) Laryngoscope Vol 93:11 pp 1441-1444

2. Friedman WH, Rosenblum B, Loewenstein P, Thornton H, Katsantonis G, Green M (1984) Proceedings of the Fourth International Symposium Journal on Plastic and Reconstructive Surgery of the Head and Neck, C.V. Mosby Company, Chapter 172: September pp 1162-1166

3. Friedman WH, Rosenblum B, Loewenstein P, Thornton H, Katsantonis G, Green M, (1985) Laryngoscope Vol 95:3 pp 313-316

© 1985 Elsevier Science Publishers B.V. (Biomedical Division)
New dimensions in otorhinolaryngology - head and neck surgery, vol. 2.
E. Myers, editor

THE SELECTIVE ROLE OF CO2 LASER FOR THE TREATMENT OF LARYNGEAL CARCINOMA IN 1984 IN THE LASER SURGERY CENTER AT THE HOSPITAL OF SAINT RAPHAEL, NEW HAVEN, CONNECTICUT

EIJI YANAGISAWA, M.D., NRIPAL C. KAR, M.D., and KEAT-JIN LEE, M.D.
Section of Otolaryngology - Head and Neck Surgery, Hospital of Saint Raphael, New Haven, CT 06511 (USA)

INTRODUCTION

In the interest of being conservative, we feel that CO2 laser surgery should not replace radiotherapy or conventional surgery. However, in 1984, our feeling was that CO2 laser surgery can be a most useful alternative in the management of laryngeal carcinoma in carefully selected situations. Specific criteria in a center where laser surgery is used to treat laryngeal carcinoma include:

(1) patients under 30 years of age with T_1 N_0 M_0 or T_2 N_0 M_0 for whom radiation and disabling surgery is not advisable

(2) patients with T_1 N_0 M_0 or T_2 N_0 M_0 who absolutely refuse radiation or conventional surgery

(3) patients with recurrence after full course of radiation refusing total laryngectomy

In the first two groups of patients CO2 laser surgery was done as a curative measure whereas in the third group of post-radiation recurrent laryngeal carcinoma, it was a palliative measure.

PRINCIPLES AND METHODS

Clinical use of CO2 laser is gaining wide acceptance for its precise dissection, minimal postoperative edema, bleeding, scarring and short period of morbidity. We selectively chose the patients on the basis of their biopsy, clinical staging, age, physical status and patients' choice of his treatment.

First Group: Our clinical experience consists of selectively choosing patients for CO2 laser surgery from a younger age group who had T_1 N_0 M_0 or T_2 N_0 M_0 of laryngeal carcinoma. Selection of CO2 laser surgery over standard treatment modalities have been considered for patients in the younger age group to prevent the hazards of radiation exposure from radiotherapy in the long run since the patient will survive for another 40 or 60 years. Surgical intervention was also less acceptable due to its effects on voice production. For example, we had a young patient who was 23 years old having squamous cell carcinoma of right vocal cord extended from middle third to the anterior commissure. There was no evidence of recurrence of tumor at his last visit in March, 1985 which was 36 months after surgery.

Second Group: Patients in this group have early stage of laryngeal carcinoma ranging from T_1 N_0 M_0 to T_2 N_0 M_0. Patient denied treatment with radiotherapy or surgery and preferred the CO2 laser surgery for its precise dissection, less complications and short recovery period. For example, we had a 47 year old man having squamous cell carcinoma of middle third of the right vocal cord extending up to the right ventricle. The anterior and posterior commissures, false cords, pyriform sinuses, post-cricoid area and arytenoids were clear. Clinical stage was T_2 N_0 M_0. After a thorough discussion with the patient about the seriousness of his disease and different treatment modalities, the patient preferred CO2 laser surgery over surgery or radiation. The patient is doing well and there was no evidence of recurrence of carcinoma in his last visit on February 4, 1985.

Third Group: Our clinical experience with the third group of patients was with post-radiation recurrent laryngeal carcinoma. In this group, ages ranged from 50 years to 80 years. We selectively chose CO2 laser surgery for those patients who refused total laryngectomy as they were afraid of the resulting voice loss and morbidity of major surgery in their old age. The role of CO2 laser surgery as a palliative measure had already been explained to the patient. For example, in this group, a 65 year old man had post-radiation laryngeal carcinoma of the right vocal cord extending along the full length of the cord which was causing a mild degree of airway obstruction. Five years ago, the patient was classified as T_2 N_0 M_0 of the right vocal cord which was treated with 6400 rads of radiation in 47 days. Because of recurrent carcinoma and the desire of the patient to avoid laryngectomy, CO2 laser was used to excise the carcinoma. The patient did well after laser surgery. There was no evidence of further progression of the tumor in his last visit on February 25, 1985 which was 30 months after the laser surgery

REFERENCES

1. Lee KJ (ed) Essential Otolaryngology - Head & Neck Surgery, Third Edition, Medical Examination Publishing Co., Inc.

New dimensions in otorhinolaryngology - head and neck surgery, vol. 2.
E. Myers, editor

EXTRA-CAPSULAR SPREADING AS MORPHOLOGICAL PARAMETER OF PROGNOSTIC EVALUATION IN LARYNGEAL CARCINOMA

MOTTA G. JR., D'ANGELO L., VILLARI G., ANTONELLI C.
2nd Medical School-E.N.T. Dept.:Chief: Prof. G. Motta-Naples, Italy

INTRODUCTION

Several AA. (1,2,) reported that extra-capsular spread of latero-cervical lymphonodes in patients having neoplastic lesions of head and neck is a negative prognostic datum. It is well-known that the prognosis of these tumours is affected both by the extension and the grading of the primary lesion.

Taking into consideration the interest of the matter, we thought it right to evaluate, by an adequate follow-up, the prognostic significance of extra-capsular spread in metastatic nodes, in relation with extension and grading of the primary tumour.

MATERIALS AND METHODS

We observed 179 cases of T_2 and T_3 laryngeal carcinomas treated by total laryngectomy and bilateral neck dissection, with a three year follow-up. We did not consider as object of our study:

- patients preoperative irradiated;
- cases affected by verrucous and squamous cell carcinomas;
- subjects dead by no-neoplastic pathologies.

RESULTS

Our data show as follows:

1) Lymphonodal metastasis are more frequent in cases having a more extended and less differentiated primary lesion (Fig. 1);
2) more extended and less differentiated processes involve a higher rate of extra-capsular spread in latero-cervical metastasis (Fig. 2);

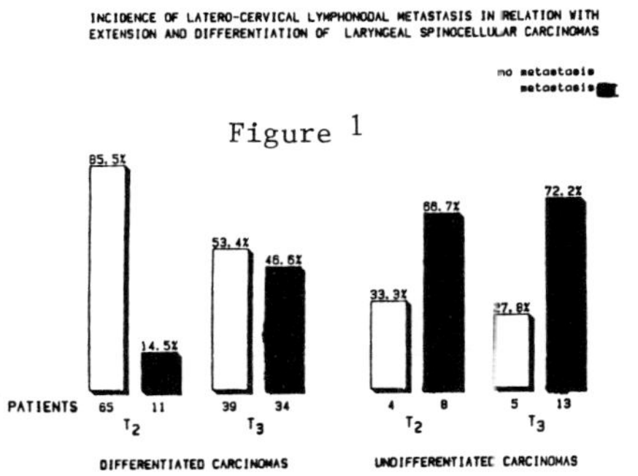

Figure 1

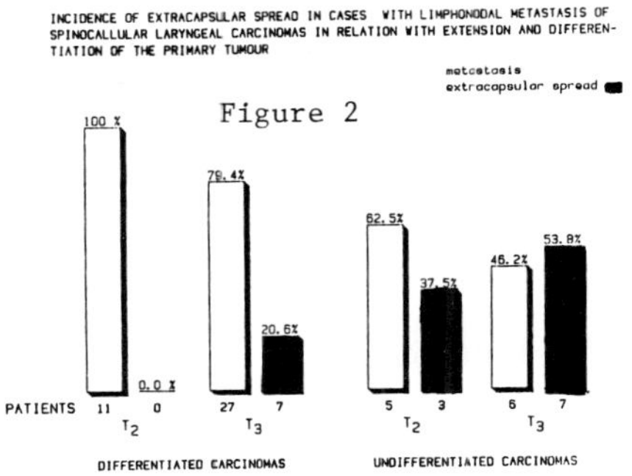

Figure 2

3) the presence of metastasis and extra-capsular-spread is indicative for worsening of the prognosis even if considering the survey taking into account both the extension and the **grading** of the primary tumour (Table 1);

	DIFFERENTIATED CARCINOMAS T_2		T_3		UNDIFFERENTIATED CARCINOMAS T_2		T_3		TOTAL	
	patients	dead patients %	patients	dead patients %	patients	dead patients %	patients	dead patients %	patients	dead patients %
N^+S^+	-	-	7	4 (57.1)	3	2 (66.7)	7	5 (71.4)	17	11 (64)
N^+S^-	11	2 (18.2)	27	8 (29.6)	5	1 (20.0)	6	2 (33.3)	49	13 (26)
N^-	65	2 (3.1)	39	2 (5.1)	4	-	5	1 (20.0)	113	5 (4)
TOTAL	76	4 (5.3)	73	14 (19.2)	12	3 (25.0)	18	8 (44.4)	179	28 (16)
			$p<0.005$		p NOT INDICATIVE		p NOT INDICATIVE		$p<0.0001$	

N^+ = METASTASIS
N^- = NO METASTASIS
S^+ = EXTRACAPSULAR SPREAD
S^- = NO EXTRACAPSULAR SPREAD

Table 1

4) death rate, on the other hand, is higher in more extended and less differentiated forms, especially if they occur together with limphonodal metastasis and, particularly, whenever metastasis show extracapsular spread (Fig. 3).

DEATH RATE IN CASES WITH NODAL EXTRACAPSULAR SPREAD IN RELATION WITH EXTENSION AND DIFFERENTIATION OF PRIMARY TUMOUR

Figure 3

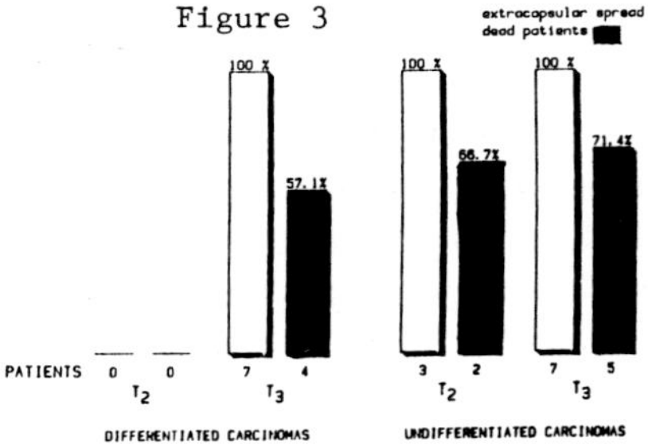

CONCLUSIONS

Our data support that extension of the primary tumour, grading, presence of metatastasis and, eventually, of extra-capsular spread are factors significantly correlated to the prognosis of neoplastic processes.

Moreover, our observations lead us to think that, in cases showing metastasis, especially is they occur together with extra-capsular spread, the prognosis is worse if the primary tumour is more extended and less differentiated.

REFERENCES

1)Cachin Y.(1977)Mecanisme de la metastase gannglionaire cervicale dans les carcinomes des voies aero-digestive superieures. Nuovo Arch. Ital.Otol.2:207-220.

2)Zoller M., Goodman M.L., Cummings C.W.(1978) Guidelines for prognosis in head and neck cancer with nodal metastasis. The laryngolscope 88:135-140.

New dimensions in otorhinolaryngology - head and neck surgery, vol. 2.
E. Myers, editor

HYPERTETRAPLOID CELLS IN DIFFERENT LARYNGEAL EPITHELIA - A PROGNOSTIC MARKER?

JAN OLOFSSON, GUNNAR FRANZEN, JAN LUNDGREN AND KAJ BJELKENKRANTZ
Departments of Otolaryngology, Oncology and Pathology, University Hospital, S-581 85 Linköping, Sweden

INTRODUCTION

The deviation from the normal DNA content shows the neoplastic nature of cells and carries diagnostic and prognostic information. Hypertetraploid cells occur normally in organs showing a facultative polyploidization but have not been reported in normal squamous epithelium.

In a microphotometric study of gallocyanin-chromalum stained tissue sections from laryngeal dysplastic and carcinomatous epithelia, Greisen[1] found the occurrence of hypertetraploid cells to be a negative prognostic factor.

The aim of the present study was to determine the ploidy, proliferative activity and occurrence of hypertetraploid cells in histopathologically verified vocal cord lesions and to evaluate the prognostic implications of these findings.

MATERIAL AND METHODS

Cytologic smears were obtained by scraping the vocal cords with a wooden pin at microlaryngoscopy. Biopsy material was then removed for histopathological examination. The material comprised 82 specimens removed from 71 patients.

The cytologic specimens were fixed and hydrolyzed and subsequently stained in 0.02% acriflavine-SO_2 solution. Cytofluorometry was performed using a Leitz MPV 3 cytophotometer[2].

The percentage of cells with DNA values outside the modal peak represented the proliferative activity. The fluorescence value should be at least 5c if the cells were considered hypertetraploid (HT).

RESULTS

The proliferative activity and number of HT cells are shown in Table 1. None of the patients with hyperplasia and mild dysplasia developed carcinoma but 2 had recurrent disease. In the group of 14 patients with moderate dysplasia 5 out of 7 with HT cells developed carcinoma. Only one of the seven patients without HT cells developed severe dysplasia. Of the 9 patients with severe dysplasia and with HT cells, 4 developed carcinoma and 4 had recurrent disease (see Fig. 1). Of the remaining 14 patients without HT cells only 1 developed a carcinoma and 3 had recurrent disease. There was a tendency for the 12 patients with carcinoma and HT cells to have a worse outcome than those 8 without HT cells, but the material is too small to allow further conclusions.

TABLE 1

PROLIFERATIVE ACTIVITY AND HYPERTETRAPLOID CELLS

Histopathology	Number	Per cent nuclei > 2c Range	Mean	Number of specimens with nuclei above 4c
Hyperplasia	14	1 - 7	2.1	0
Moderate dysplasia	17 (14)	1 - 10	3.0	7
Severe dysplasia	31 (23)	0 - 12	4.0	11 (9)
Squamous carcinoma	20	2 - 24	7.3	12

Figures in ( ) indicate number of patients

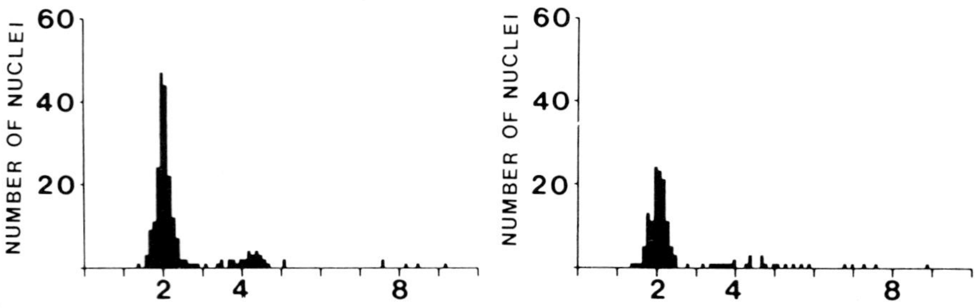

Fig. 1. Moderate dysplasia with HT cells (left). This patient later developed a carcinoma. Severe dysplasia with HT cells (right). This patient later developed a microinvasive carcinoma.

SUMMARY AND CONCLUSION

The proliferative activity increased the more severe the atypia. Hypertetraploid cells were only present in dysplastic and carcinomatous epithelia and seem to indicate a worse outcome for the patients.

REFERENCES

1. Greisen O (1975) Deoxyribonucleic adic content in the laryngeal mucosa with special reference to polyploid cell nuclei. Acta Pathol Microbiol Scand Sect A 83:704-708

2. Bjelkenkrantz K, Stål O, Gröntoft O (1983) A fast and reliable system for microcomputerized DNA cytofluorometry in tumour pathology. Histochemistry 79:145-155

© 1985 Elsevier Science Publishers B.V. (Biomedical Division)
New dimensions in otorhinolaryngology - head and neck surgery, vol. 2.
E. Myers, editor

ENDOLARYNGEAL CO_2 LASER SURGERY FOR RADIATION FAILURES

V. OSWAL

Department of Otolaryngology, North Riding Infirmary, Middlesbrough, Cleveland, United Kingdom

INTRODUCTION

A 48 year old male developed a T2 squamous cell carcinoma of his larynx. It is customary in the United Kingdom to offer radiation as a primary therapy for these types of lesions and reserve any surgery for radiation failures. This patient was therefore given a full course of radiation lasting over five weeks. The tumour showed an anticipated regression and clinically, no recurrence was detected for the next twelve months. There, however, persisted a fullness in the paraglottic region and eventually a biopsy showed a residual carcinoma. A total laryngectomy was advised but the patient turned it down even after repeated counselling. The patient had an additional problem of alcoholism. With the availability of the CO_2 Laser, an opportunity arose when one could offer him an endolaryngeal excision as an alternative, to which the patient agreed. This paper describes the technique, identifies the problems and discusses the application of the CO_2 Laser for radiation failure carcinoma of larynx.

METHOD AND MATERIAL

A flexible metal tube was used to maintain the anaesthesia. The tumour, along with the true cord, the false cord and the ventricle was excised with the CO_2 Laser beam, delivered endolaryngeally, through the operating microscope. The patient did not require pre or post-operative tracheostomy; and there was very little post-operative oedema or any significant pain. Apart from initial dysphagia, the patient recovered well. He remained hospitalised only for two days post-operatively. A check up six weeks later showed a good healing at the site of the operation. He, however, subsequently did show a recurrence and this time agreed and underwent total laryngectomy.

Several useful indices came out of this experience:

1. It is possible to use the CO_2 Laser endolaryngeally in irradiated cases without any serious complications.
2. The irradiated larynx, when laser excised, does not show any greater tendency to post-operative oedema requiring tracheostomy.
3. It does not show predilection to cartilage necrosis.
4. There is no greater risk of peri-operative or post-operative haemorrhage.

5. There is no undue risk of failure to heal normally.

6. Subsequent total laryngectomy, if and when undertaken, is not prejudiced in any way by the previous laser excision.

There were also some problems associated with laser surgery on an irradiated larynx:

1. The endoscopic anatomy is distorted due to radiation oedema or fibrosis.

2. The submucosal spread into the paraglottic region cannot be judged accuratelу due to carbonisation and inadequate view through the conventional laryngoscope.

These problems can be overcome to a certain extent by:

1. The surgeon using the laser on cadaveric larynx until proficient.

2. Excision of the lesion should include the true cord, the false cord, the ventricle with the aryepiglottic fold, with the subglottic mucosa of the affected side from the anterior to the posterior commissure, irrespective of the apparent tumour extension - in short a hemilaryngectomy.

3. In later stages of the operation, the metal tube should be removed and an anaesthetic maintained through jet ventilation.

4. Specially designed suction based microforceps and retractors should be used to deliver the paraglottic tissue into the larynx to ensure adequate excision.

5. The stortze expanding bivalve laryngoscope provides an excellent view.

RESULTS

A total of 10 endolaryngeal excisions have so far been carried out in radiation failure cases. In only two of these, the recurrence appeared to be completely localised and limited to the glottic surface of the true cord. Endolaryngeal excision was therefore advised and undertaken electively. One of these two patients remains disease free 18 months post-operatively with almost normal voice, the other patient developed a further tumour at the site of the operation and underwent total laryngectomy. In the remaining 8 patients, endolaryngeal excision was undertaken because of patient refusal or severe concurrent disease. In these patients, endolaryngeal excision provided a useful palliation avoiding tracheostomy. In some instances, laser excisions have been repeated several times.

In summary it is not the intention of the author to advocate endolaryngeal laser excision as an alternative to radical surgery in cases of recurrent disease or radiation failures. Total laryngectomy must remain the treatment of choice for these cases. Only in extremely selective cases of a localised recurrent disease, an endolaryngeal laser excision be offered and undertaken by surgeons fully conversant with laser techniques and its limitations.

New dimensions in otorhinolaryngology - head and neck surgery, vol. 2.
E. Myers, editor

PRESENCE AND DISTRIBUTION OF LANGERHANS CELLS IN NORMAL AND NEOPLASTIC LARYNGEAL MUCOSA

TAMPLENIZZA P (1), OTTAVIANI F (2)

Clinica Otorinolaringoiatrica I (1) e II (2)
Università degli Studi di Milano (Italy)

INTRODUCTION

Immunity accessory cells are lymphoid elements derived from a bone-marrow monocitic-macrophagic line, and they express Ia like surface antigens codified by the HLA DR/DP locus of the MHC. Langerhans' cells (LC) fall into the wider category of Ia positive cells and distinguish themselves by expressing the OKT6 antigen (1).

Our purpose was to ascertain if LC are present in the human larynx and to start a study about the possible involvement of these cells in neoplastic pathology of the larynx.

MATERIAL AND METHODS

We examined 53 biopsies from normal human laryngeal mucosa and 30 specimens of laryngeal carcinomas of different histological grade, in stages T2 and T3, and arising from various sites of the larynx. We used histochemical, immunohistochemical and immuno electron microscopy methods (2) (Fig. 1).

RESULTS

In normal laryngeal mucosa concentration of LC is directly proportional to the presence of pluristratified pavimentosus epithelium, and it greatly decreases passing in the transitional epithelium nearing zero as it sets closer to the respiratory epithelium.

We found a positive relation between the histological grade of the laryngeal squamous cell carcinomas and the presence of the mononuclear reactive infiltration: the latter is more conspicous within well differentiated carcinomas. Presence and distribution of LC are in positive relation to the histological grade of the tumor. Consequently there is a strong positive relation between the entity of the mononuclear infiltration and the number of LC within the same specimen. On border of the tumors, within small areas of *in situ* or microinvasive carcinomas, it has been possible to recognize a subepithelial layer not yet upset by tumoral or reactive infiltrations. In these cases LC appear often isolated within the subepithelial layer, an extremely rare finding in normal laryngeal mucosa.

Finally our data support the hypothesis that the host tries to counteract the neoplasia by means of a local immune response within which LC certainly play a rôle, as confirmed by their significant relations with the histological grade of the tumor and the entity of the mononuclear infiltrate.

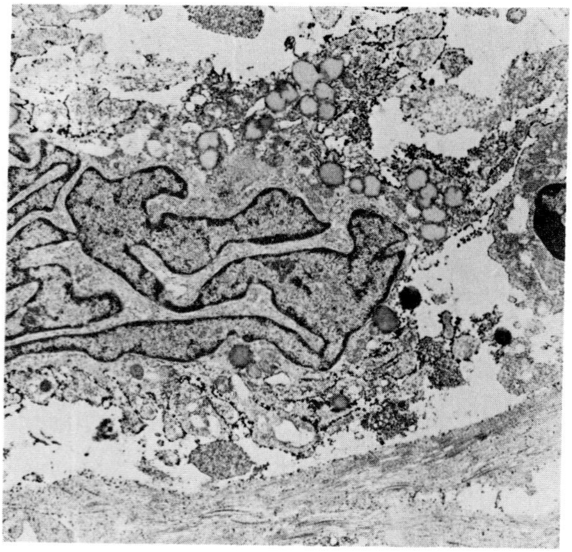

Fig 1. Langerhans cell as it appears after the immuno electron microscopy technique.

REFERENCES

1. Harrist TJ, Muhlbauer JE (1983) J Invest Dermatol 80: 100-103
2. Chu A, Eisinger M, Soo Lee J (1982) J Invest Dermatol 78: 177-180

New dimensions in otorhinolaryngology - head and neck surgery, vol. 2.
E. Myers, editor

CLINICAL T AND PATHOLOGICAL T IN THE SUPRAGLOTTIC CANCER

GIUSEPPE RIZZOTTO, GIORGIO CARLON, ITALO SERAFINI, TONI PAZZAIA

Dept. ORL , U.L.S. N. 12 " Sinistra Piave"Vittorio Veneto, Via Forlanini (Italy)

INTRODUCTION

The classification of supraglottic T by the TNM system has been criticized and discussed since the demonstration of its poor anatomic.

Clinical correlation and its limited prognostic valve. The T clinical evaluation is, still, the only tool to compare different cases and it is the most important consideration in programming the surgery, so that each attempt to improve the prognostic valve of this system shows a deep practical involvement materials and methods.

In the present work we analyzed 100 cases of supraglottic carcinoma, surgically operated as follows: a) supraglottic laryngectomy with mono or bilateral resection in monoblock (80 cases); b) total laryngectomy with mono or bilateral resection (10 cases); c) supraglottic laryngectomy without resection (10 cases), but without recurrene or metastasis after a minimal two years follow up.

The T clinical pre-surgical evaluation was based on the uicc rules.

In the pathological determination of T, made on serial hystologic sections of the surgical biopsy, the clinical consideration of the mobility was replaced by the morphologic element of the infiltration grade.

So that the terms "normal mobility" of T1 and "without fixation" of T2 have been replaced by the term "without deep infiltration", that means a neoplastic proliferation not going beyond the epiglottis on the front and the quadrangolar membrane on the side. For every case was available a 2-8 years follow up.

36 cases have been classified of poor prognosis, 32 with lymphonodal metastasis in the surgery, 2 with neck recurrence, 1 with tongue recurrence and 1 with spread metastasis in the follow up. The other 64 cases left without metastasis or recurrence, after a minimal two year follow-up, have been determined of good prognosis.

RESULTS

Table 1 shows the correlation between clinical and pathological T. The total equality is limited to 34 cases: 6Tla, 5Tlb, 7T3, 16T4.

In 5 cases are detectable "minor mistakes": 4 transposition Tla - Tlb and a double carcinoma (supraglottic Tla -glottic Tla) clinically classified T2. In 61 cases there wasn't any correspondence between T and pT. The most frequent"mistakes" were due to: 1) lack of identification of a deep invasion (53 cases) 2) lack of identification of the extralaringeal extension.

The most conflicting clinical category is the supraglottic T2. In fact none of the T2 classified 13 cases was in the pT2 category: a) two cases because of the negative glottic involvement; b) 1 case because the glottic lesion was distinct from the supraglottic lesion; c) 10 cases (6 of which also without cord involvement) because of a deep invasion of the paraglottic space (pT3). In the examined cases there aren't supraglottic tumors that spread on the glottic space without haveing deeply infiltered the larynx structures before. The prognostic meaning, valued as evidence of lymphonodal metastasis or recurrences in the follow-up, is explained in table 2 , where the frequency of poor prognosis. Cases are summarized for each class of T and pT.

Finally, the clinical valuation of T has a good correspondence with the pathologic valuation only when the spreading of the neoplasia is on the surface. On the contrary, the clinical evaluation of the mobility has a poor correlation with the morphologic evaluation of the deep invasion that is a better prognostic index.

The T2 clinical category, finally, doesnit seem to have an anatomical correspondent and even from the clinical point of view it seems to be more useful in the choice of the surgery rather than in the determination of a prognostic index.

Pathological T \ Clinical T	1a	1b	2	3	4	
1a	6	2		13		21
1b	2	5		30	5	42
2	2	1		10		13
3				7		7
4				1	16	17
	10	8	0	60	21	100

Tab. 1. Correlation between clinical and pathological T.

Fig. 2. Follow - up (2-8 years)

© 1985 Elsevier Science Publishers B.V. (Biomedical Division)
New dimensions in otorhinolaryngology - head and neck surgery, vol. 2.
E. Myers, editor

PRIMARY MALIGNANT MELANOMA OF THE LARYNX

THOMAS M. SCHRIMPF, M.D., ROBERT J. SCHRIMPF, M.D., THOMAS PANKE, M.D.

Departments of Surgery (Otolaryngology Section) and Pathology, Good Samaritan Hospital, Cincinnati, Ohio USA

INTRODUCTION: Mucosal melanomas of the head and neck are rare and aggressive tumors. Malignant melanoma of the larynx is even rarer and more lethal. To our knowledge, the world literature contains only 24 cases of primary laryngeal melanoma. Primary mucosal melanoma of the upper aerodigestive tract has several controversial features. These include: the etiology of the melanocytes; the proper treatment modality; and the prognosis. 19 of the 24 cases reported were in English language literature. Of these, 5 arose from the epiglottis, 6 from the ventricle-false cord, 4 from the true cord, and 2 from the pyriform sinus and 2 from the arytenoids. Melanoma arising from 2 separate sites in the larynx has not been reported. We recently treated a patient with primary laryngeal melanoma arising from multiple sites in the larynx with multiple "satellite" lesions of the larynx. This may represent the first reported case of such "field melanization" of the larynx.

CASE REPORT: A 67 y.o. W.F. presented with 4 weeks of hoarseness. Laryngoscopy revealed dark cystic lesions arising from the epiglottis, right FVC, and both A-E folds. Both necks were negative to palpation. Panendoscopy with biopsy revealed primary laryngeal malignant melanoma. A negative metastatic work up was obtained. She underwent total laryngectomy and right RND which was well tolerated. The pathology report described 2 exophytic, pigmented malignant melanomas, one arising from the midline of the epiglottic base and extending into the submucosal tissue. The second tumor arose from the right FVC. Sections from the epiglottis and supraglottic structures revealed multiple foci of malignant melanoma-in-situ. The neck specimen revealed 56 lymph nodes, all negative for neoplasm. At this time, she is 6 months post treatment and is doing well.

DISCUSSION: Head and neck melanomas arising from mucosa are less common than those of the skin, but their prognosis is poorer. Whether this is due to later diagnosis, quicker spread or a different etiology, is unknown. They are not related to junctional nevi and seldom occur in the pigmented olfactory area of the nasal cavity. Melanocytes do occur in the upper airway and are the probable source of these tumors, however, laryngeal melanocytes are rare, and, until recently their presence was debatable.

The scarcity of mucosal melanoma is illustrated by Conley's review of 772 head and neck melanomas over 37 years. This reported 601 cutaneous, 112 ocular, and 50 mucosal melanomas. Shah et al, in a 37 year review of 74 mucosal melanomas found 4 laryngeal melanomas.

Mucosal and cutaneous melanomas differ in several ways. Size is directly related to prognosis in cutaneous but not in mucosal melanomas. Satellitosis is frequently seen in cutaneous melanomas but not in mucosal melanomas. Lymph node metastases are more frequently associated with cutaneous than with mucosal melanomas and are more prognostic.

Mucosal melanomas occur oftener in an older population than do cutaneous melanomas, with 80% in patients over 50 and 43% of cutaneous melanoma in patients over 50. Cutaneous melanomas are rare in blacks but 16% of mucosal melanomas are found among them. Mucosal melanomas have an average survival of 2.6 years. The 5 year survival is 11% while the 10 year survival is .5%.

Controversy exists as to the etiology of these mucosal melanomas. The origin of melanocytes from neural crest tissue and their migration with ectoderm has been well established but not their movements to non-integumentary sites. Theories attempting to explain the presence of melanocytes at nonectodermal sites include: the migration of melanoblasts with mesoderm to versceral sites, the transformation of neural crest elements into melanocytes and metaplasia of squamous epithelium into melanocytes.

The origin of melanocytes in the larynx is even more of an enigma. Goldman et al studied adult larynges and found microscopic melanocytes in "an appreciable number." What the stimulus for the conversion of melanocytes into melanoma is, remains obscure. Goldman suggests that perhpas the same factors that cause squamous metaplasia cause malignant transformation of melanocytes. Conley, in his larger series, found no relationship between local irritation and melanoma.

There is little controversy as to the optimum treatment of the mucosal melanoma primary site, which is best done via surgery. Elective neck dissection, however, is controversial. In Conley's series of cutaneous and mucosal melanomas, negative necks treated with neck dissection had a 5 year survival rate of 55%, versus 38.5% for non-treated necks. However, in a review of mucous membrane melanomas, he doubted the benefit of elective neck dissection for those cases where there is low incidence of metastases. The anatomy of mucosal lymph channels affects this controversy. The lymphatics are large and easily penetrated. There are no obstructions in the form of lymph nodes, until the lymph has reached the parapharyngeal or lateral neck systems. This lymph anatomy resembles that of the scalp, however, the incidence of neck metastases is lower for mucous membrane melanoma than for the scalp. We were uncertain as to the efficacy of performing an elective neck dissection, however we felt that this added little additional morbidity. In summary, we have presented a case of laryngeal melanoma and compared it to other melanomas of the head and neck.

© 1985 Elsevier Science Publishers B.V. (Biomedical Division)
New dimensions in otorhinolaryngology – head and neck surgery, vol. 2.
E. Myers, editor

MODIFICATION IN T-E SHUNT(AMATSU'S TECHNIQUE) TO PREVENT ASPIRATION

SATOMI TANIGUCHI, TAKASHI FUKAZAWA, YUKAKO SHIMOMURA, FUMIHIDE OUMURA
Dept of Otolaryngology, Kobe Central Municipal Hospital, Kobe(Japan)

There have been numerous efforts to restore voice after total laryngectomy. Among them, the T-E shunt which Amatsu introduced in 1977 is technically easy, maintenance-free, and applicable to most cases of laryngeal cancer except for those in which the tumor extends to the trachea.

The voice produced by Amatsu's technique is usually fluent and intelligible. But because of the continuity of the esophagus, aspiration seems to be unavoidable and requires digital compression when patients swallow liquids.
In our experience with this method, the more fluent the patient, the more aspiration he has. To eliminate this, we folded the membranous portion of the trachea above the anastomosis and created a valve-like slit.

SURGICAL TECHNIQUE

After total laryngectomy is completed, the trachea is raised upward. The lower edge of the tracheal stoma(at the level of the fifth or sixth ring) and skin are sutured with several stitches on the sternum. A side-to-side anastomosis(Amatsu's technique) starts downward from exactly 1 cm below the distal end of the trachea. The length of the anastomosis is about 1 cm.

A U-shaped incision around the anastomosis is made. The first sutures of both inside margins of the U-shaped incision produce a small pocket covering the anastomosis. The raw surface of the pocket is covered by a second set of sutures with the outside margins of the U-shaped incision approximating the bilateral cartilagenous portions. Closure of the distal end of the membranous portion creates a valve-like slit in the midline(inner shunt). Both tracheal cartilages are disigned so as to cover the slit. For this, several shallow cuts are made bilaterally on the trimmed cartilagenous portions.

A long narrow Penrose stent is inserted through the anastomosis to ensure its remaining patent. This stent should be affixed at the top of the shunt by fine nylon suture through the skin. Otherwise, the stent often breaks down the lower sutures. The shunt is completed by closing both margins of the cartilages(outer shunt). The stent is removed at 2-3 weeks after the operation. At the same time, speech training starts.

MATERIALS AND RESULTS

Between September 1983 and January 1985, 15 patients with 14 laryngeal and one piriform carcinoma were operated upon with this method.

Aspiration could be classified into two groups. One is resting aspiration with small "beads" appearing when swallowing saliva and the other is swallowing aspiration requiring digital compression when swallowing liquids. At present, five out of 15 patients have swallowing aspiration(one moderate, four mild). Two have resting aspiration.

The voices of 12 patients are excellent and intelligible. Two are fair but intelligible. These two need some effort when they exale. One failed to obtain voice and will require revision.

COMMENT

The larynx has a valve movement to prevent aspiration. We create the valve by folding the membranous portion of the trachea at the midline, approximating both cartilages. Besides, the difference of the location of the outlet and the inlet of the inner shunt may prevent aspiration. These mechanical and anatomical conditions can considerably eliminate aspiration. Seven patients had postoperative rediation therapy. Of these, only one patient had stenosis of the shunt. Stenosis and swallowing aspiration were easily corrected by opening the outer shunt. Because of short-term observation, this comment must be limited. Further investigation will follow.

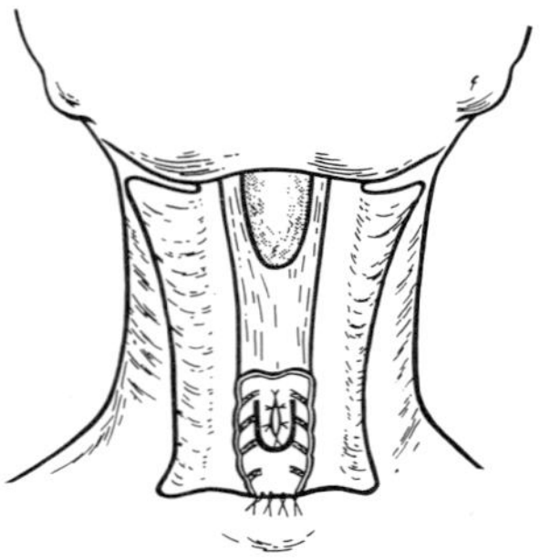

Fig.1. U-shaped incision line around the anastomosis.

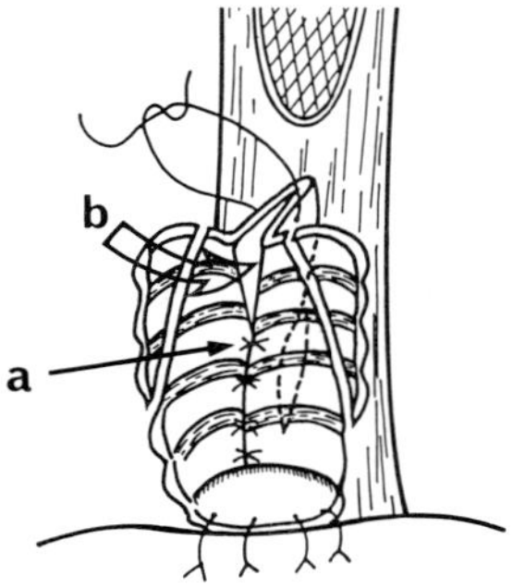

Fig.2. Both inside margins of the U-shaped incision have been sutured(a). b: Valve-like slit

REFERENCE

Amatsu,M.:J. Otolaryngol. Jpn. 80:779-785 1977

© 1985 Elsevier Science Publishers B.V. (Biomedical Division)
New dimensions in otorhinolaryngology - head and neck surgery, vol. 2.
E. Myers, editor

HEAD AND NECK CANCER IN NIGERIA
CLINICAL EVALUATION OF PATIENTS SEEN AT LAGOS UNIVERSITY TEACHING HOSPITAL 1973-1983

OLAWALE O. IDEWU, M.D., F.A.C.S., LYDIA MONYE, M.D., VICTOR MORDI, M.D., F. A. DUROSINMI-ETTI, M.D.

INTRODUCTION

Previously it was believed that cancer in general and head and neck cancer in particular are less common in black Africans than the Europeans and Americans. The incidence of cancer among black Africans has "increased" in the last two decades and is still on the rise. Three factors are responsible for this apparent increase: (1) The number one killer--infectious disease--among Africans has been to some extent curbed due to the availability of antibiotics; (2) the assessibility and availability of health-care facilities to more people; and (3) conscious efforts of the clinicians to look for and diagnose this ominous malady--cancer.

MATERIALS AND METHODS

A prospective study of patients with head and neck cancer seen in the Out-Patient Department of Lagos University Teaching Hospital, Lagos Nigeria, from 1973 to 1982 was conducted. The study was limited to the most commonly seen head and neck cancers--cancer of the upper aerodigestive system.

The history and physical examination are conducted, followed by an endoscopic or visual examination, usually under general anesthesia, and a biopsy to obtain tissue diagnosis. The patient's age, sex, symptoms, clinical and histological diagnosis were recorded. Patients whose ages could not be determined were automatically excluded from the study.

RESULTS

The total number of patients in the study is 251. Out of this, 105 (42%) had nasopharyngeal carcinoma; 63 (25%), cancer of the nose and paranasal sinuses; 43 (17%), cancer of the oral cavity; and 40 (16%), laryngeal carcinoma. Squamous cell carcinoma (differential and undifferential) was the predominant histological diagnosis. Generally, more males are affected than females. In nasopharyngeal carcinoma, the ratio of male to female was 2.5 to 1, while cancer of the nose and paranasal sinuses showed 1.5 to 1. The cancer of the oral cavity was strongly 2 to 1, while laryngeal cancer was practically the disease of the males. Nasopharyngeal carcinoma is more common among young adults with pick age between 20 and 30 years.

TABLE I.
THE PATIENTS WITH HEAD AND NECK CANCER SEEN AT LAGOS UNIVERSITY TEACHING HOSPITAL 1973-1982

	MALE	FEMALE	TOTAL
NASOPHARYNGEAL	74	31	105
NOSE AND PARANASAL SINUSES	38	25	63
ORAL CAVITY	29	14	43
LARYNX	36	4	40
TOTAL:	177	74	251

The cancer of the nose and paranasal sinuses, cancer of the oral cavity, and cancer of the larynx are more common in age group 41-60 years, with pick between 40 and 50 years. Cancer of the oral cavity was more frequent in the older group than in the other three groups. Very few head and neck cancer patients above 70 years were seen.

DISCUSSION

In the U.S.A. and Europe, cancer of the larynx and the oral cavity are generally associated with tobacco and alcohol. Among our patients only an infinitesimally small percentage smoked and/or drank. It has been suggested that environmental, dietary and genetic factors play a more important role in the etiology of cancer among black Africans. Research work to unveil the possible cause of head and neck cancer in Nigeria continues.

ACKNOWLEDGEMENTS

Sincere thanks to Mr. Harry Przekop who has done an excellent work in photographic reproductions and Ruth Shea who has kindly accepted the challenge of typing all the necessary tables and illustrations.

REFERENCES

1. Choa G: Nasopharyngeal Carcinoma. J. Laryngol. Otol., 88:145, 1974
2. Krajina Z: Epidemiology of Laryngeal Cancer. Laryngoscope, 85:1155, 1975
3. Martinson FD (1968) Cancer of Nasopharynx in Nigeria. J. of Laryng., 82:1119-1128.

© 1985 Elsevier Science Publishers B.V. (Biomedical Division)
New dimensions in otorhinolaryngology - head and neck surgery, vol. 2.
E. Myers, editor

"FURTHER EXPERIENCE WITH THE STYLOHAMULAR DISSECTION FOR MALIGNANCIES OF THE INFRATEMPORAL FOSSA". GEORGE P. KATSANTONIS, M.D., F.A.C.S., WILLIAM H. FRIEDMAN, M.D., F.A.C.S., BARRY N. ROSENBLUM, M.D., AND MARGARET H. COOPER, Ph.D., Department of Otolaryngology - Head and Neck Surgery, St. Louis University School of Medicine, 1402 South Grand Blvd, St. Louis, Missouri 63104

INTRODUCTION

Malignancies of the infratemporal fossa usually arise in the parotid gland. However, advanced carcinomas of the oropharynx and nasopharynx may also extend into this area. Until recently these tumors were often considered to be inoperable. Increased familiarity with the surgical anatomy of the base of the skull has refined techniques for en bloc resection of this area and palliation and occasional cure can now be offered to these patients.[1,2,3,4] The authors described a new technique for the en bloc resection of the infratemporal fossa in 1981 which was termed "stylohamular dissection".[5]

SELECTION OF PATIENTS AND TECHNIQUE

From 1977 to 1984 18 patients underwent stylohamular dissections by the authors. All patients had clinical and/or radiological evidence of infratemporal fossa invasion by malignant neoplasms, originating either in the parotid region or in the naso-oropharynx. Clinical signs in addition to grossly palpable or visible lesions include trismus and pain along V3. Facial paralysis may be present in parotid neoplasms. Bony invasion of the skull base is considered a contraindication for the procedure.

Mandibular osteotomy is utilized to gain access to the median boundaries of the masseteric sling (internal and external pterygoid musculature). Medially the dissection is facilitated by the loose areolar tissue between the internal pterygoid muscle and bucco-pharyngeal fascia. The internal carotid artery is dissected and exposed to the carotid foramen. Pterygoid osteotomy and disarticulation of the mandible are performed in approaching the skull base. Following ligation of the internal maxillary artery at the pterygomaxillary fissure, the contents of the infratemporal fossa are swept posteriorly. The mandibular nerve and the middle meningeal artery are resected at the foramen ovale and spinosum which are routinely exposed during this procedure. The technique is totally extra-oral for lesions of the parotid region. In pharyngeal malignancies a composite resection is performed along with the stylohamular dissection and the lateral pharyngeal and retropharyngeal space are included in the tumor bloc. A pectoralis major myocutaneous flap is usually utilized to close the surgical defect.

RESULTS AND DISCUSSION

Two CVAs in the immediate postoperative period resulted in one death and one patient recovering with resolving hemiparesis in the months following surgery. No other serious complications occurred in the 18 patients. Nine of the eighteen patients are alive with a postoperative range from one to seven years. Three patients died with uncontrolled local disease and two with distant metastases. Four patients are dead of unrelated causes. One of these patients had local recurrence at the time of his death. The palliation was excellent in sixteen patients.

In patients with infratemporal fossa malignancies without bony or intracranial invasion, en bloc surgical resection is the only possibility for cure or palliation. If a tumor bloc is not established the incidence of recurrence within two years of the initial treatment is approximately 95%.[1] The stylohamular dissection enables the surgeon to maintain a cancer bloc by utilizing surrounding planes of cleavage while sparing vital structures. The medial boundary of the dissection is the plane between the internal pterygoid muscle and buccopharyngeal fascia. This roughly corresponds with an imaginary line connecting the styloid process and the hamulus. The vessels at the base of the skull can be easily avoided as they lie medially and posterior to this plane. When the parapharyngeal space needs to be included in the tumor bloc the medial boundary of the dissection lies medial to the stylohamular plane. In these circumstances internal carotid visualization and protection is critical in avoiding injury to this vessel.

Stylohamular dissection, thus far, has offered a dependable systematic surgical approach to the recurrent tumors of this area. Surgical morbidity and mortality of the procedure is low, palliation is excellent and cure can be offered in some of the cases.

REFERENCES

1. Fairbanks-Barbosa, J (1961) Surgery of extensive cancer of the paranasal sinuses. Presentation of a new technique. Archives of Otolaryngology. 73:pp:129.

2. Eilber, FR and Zarem, HA (1977) Pterygoid dissection for extensive cancer. An old concept revisited. Plastic and Reconstructive Surgery. 59:pp:545-550.

3. Biller, HF, Sugar, JN, Krespi, YP (1981) A new technique for wide field exposure of the base of the skull. Archives of Otolaryngology. 107:pp: 698-702.

4. Krespi, YP, Sisson, GA (1982) Skull base surgery and composite resection. Archives of Otolaryngology. 108:pp:681-684.

5. Friedman, WH, Katsantonis, GP et al. (1981) Stylohamular dissection. A new method for en bloc resection of malignancies of the infratemporal fossa. Laryngoscope. 91(11):pp:1869-1879.

New dimensions in otorhinolaryngology - head and neck surgery, vol. 2.
E. Myers, editor

CARCINOEMBRYONAL ANTIGEN PRODUCTION OF TUMORS IN THE CEPHALIC-CERVICAL REGION

ISTVÁN LAMPÉ, MD; ÁGNES TÓTH, MD
Department of Ear-Nose-Throat (Director: István Lampé, MD, University Professor), Medical University, 4012 Debrecen, Hungary

The carcinoembryonal antigen (CEA) was first described by Gold and Freedman /2,3/ in 1965. The beta-glycoproteid of 180 000 molecular weight develops in the tissues of the embryonal alimentary canal, but in healthy adults it is not demonstrable any more. Under pathological conditions in the course of intensive cell proliferation and protein synthesis (e.g. tumors) the compound characteristic of an earlier phase of ontogenesis can develop in a large amount again, and with the cell-surface shedding it can come into the blood stream. According to our present knowledge we get elevated values not only in case of alimentary canal tumors but also in tumors of the bronchia, breast, gynaecological organs, testicle, thyroid gland and the head-neck region.

73 patients with planocellular carcinoma were examined using commercially available radioimmunassay kits (CIS-CEAK-PR), the tumors being in the larynx, hypopharynx, naso-pharynx or the oral cavity. The CEA value for the total number of patients was 19.83 ng/ml. Values from 0.0-4.9 ng/ml were considered negative - this was found in 8.2% of the patients; from 5.0-9.9 ng/ml moderate - detected in 22 patients, 30.1%. Values above 10 ng/ml, showing an expressed positivity were found in 45 patients, 61.6%.

As a control examination we determined CEA values in 63 healthy subjects. Here the mean value was 3.36 ng/ml. In three heavy smokers we found elevated, pathological values of 12-15 ng/ml.

Of the examinations by the firm Hoffmann - La Roche performed on 9000 patients /1/ 90% was positive in case of pancreas carcinoma, 61% in stomach c.c., 51% in head-neck c.c. and 31% in heavy smokers.

Our examinations show that the CEA is unsuitable for cancer screening or the early diagnosis of cancer /4/, but the elevated CEA values indicate more careful search of the carcinomatous process; decreasing or normal CEA values after surgery - on the basis of repeated and follow-up examinations - refer to the efficiency of the therapy; while recurrently increasing values are indicative of relapses and metastasis /5/.

Relying on our results we can say that the CEA kits have a place in the oto-rhino-laryngological laboratories and in the diagnosis and prognosis of malignant carcinomatous patients.

REFERENCES

1. CEA Roche Test. Basel: F. Hoffmann - La Roche A. G. in: Grossenbacher, R.: Arch. Otorhinolaryngol. 222, 23 (1979).

2. Gold, P., Freedman, S. O.: Demonstration of tumorspecific antigens in human colonic carcinoma by immunological tolerance and absorption techniques. J. Exp. Med. 121, 439 (1965).

3. Gold, P., Freedman, S. O.: Specific carcinoembryonic antigens of the human digestive system. J. Exp. Med. 122, 467 (1965).

4. Grossenbacher, R.: Stellenwert des CEA-Testes bei Malignomen im ORL-Bereich. Arch. Otorhinolaryngol. 222, 23 (1979).

5. Tóth, Á., Csarkó, P., Lampé, I., Udvardy, M., Juhász, E.: A fej-nyaki daganatok carcino-embryonalis antigén produkciójáról. Fül-Orr-Gégegyógyászat 30. 78-83. (1984).

New dimensions in otorhinolaryngology – head and neck surgery, vol. 2.
E. Myers, editor

INFANTILE CERVICAL NEUROBLASTOMA

O.L.MENDONÇA CRUZ, I.D.MIZIARA, V.ODONE FILHO, A.MINITI
Hospital das Clīnicas da Faculdade de Medicina da Universidade de São Paŭlo - Brasil, Rua Eneas de Carvalho Aguiar 255 - 6º andar
05403 - São Paulo - Brasil

INTRODUCTION

Neuroblastoma is one of the most common tumors in infancy. It belongs to a class of tumors that grow out of the sympathetic nervous system tissues. The sites of origin are, therefore, among the most diverse: adrenal gland (40%),paravertebral tissues in the torax (11%), pelvic nerves (6%), retroperitoneal sympathetic chain (5%), cervical chain (2%) (Gross, R.E.et al., 1959).

The case present shows a patient with primary Neuroblastoma of cervical ganglial chain, with local picture simulating cronic otomastoiditis. The rarety of the cervical localization and the peculiarity of the clinical expression in this case are the facts that taked us to present it.

PRESENTATION OF THE CASE

A 6 years old white female child, with a history or pain on the left ear since 6 months, preceded by facial paralysis and nodules in the retro and infra-auricular region. Since a week, otorrhea and fullfilment of external auditory canal by a polypoid formation. At physical examination, good general state, without fever. Presence of edema and hyperemia of the retro and infra-auricular region with a solid and immovable mass, painful and multilobulade at the palpation. Polypoid formation filling the external auditory canal. Periferic facial paralysis on the left side.

Planigrafic study of the temporal bone didn't show any bone involvement. This fact associated with a unsatisfactory clinical evolution revealed the necessity of a incisional biopsy of the cervical mass, that demonstrated the presence of Neuroblastoma. So, several complementary exams were made and all of them with normal results except the myelogram (cytologic chart compatible with Neuroblastoma) and high levels of urinary dosage of vanil-mandelic acid (VMA).

After that general evaluation, the tumor was classed Stage III-c (St. Jude Children's Research Hospital) or IV-S (Evans & D'Angio).

TREATMENT

Intensive chemotherapy with this following drugs association: A) Ciclofosfamida (150 mg/m^2/EV for 7 days) and Adriamicina (35 mg/m^2/EV in the 8th day); B) Cis-Platinum (90 mg/m^2/EV) and Vincristina (1,5 mg/m^2/EV, after 48 hours); C) Vincristina (same dose) and Dimetiltriazeno-Imidazol-Carboxamida (900 mg/m^2/EV, after 24 hours). Three courses of each association were made with 21 days of interval. We observed a good clinical evolution, with total regression of the peri-auricular swelling. A new biopsy of the region didn't shown presence of tumor.

DISCUSSION

The Neuroblastoma is a characteristic tumor of the childhood, and the cervical localization is very rare. In this case the simulation of chronic otomastoiditis induzed a initial mistreatment. The certain diagnostic is only possible through a anatomical-pathological study, and the preferential treatment is the chemotherapy. Surgery is only indicated for cases of localized tumors without metastases. The good evolution we had attends the good results reported in the literature with this type of treatment, although with a careful follow-up.

REFERENCES

1. Gross RE, et al (1959): Neuroblastoma Sympatheticum. A study and report of 217 cases. Pediatrics 23:1179-1191.
2. Evans AE, et al (1980): Staging and treatment of neuroblastoma. Cancer 45:1799-1802.
3. Breslow N, McCann B (1971): Statistical Estimation of Prognosis for children with neuroblastoma. Cancer Res 31:2098-2103.
4. Evans AE, et al (1980): A review of 17 IV-S neuroblastoma patients at the Children's Hospital of Philadelphia. Cancer 45:833-839.
5. Nitschke R, et al (1983): Neuroblastoma: Therapy for infants with good prognosis. Medical and Pediatric Oncology 11:154-158.
6. Pellerin D, et al (1983): Place de la Chirurgie dans le traitment du neuroblastome. Chir Pediatr 24:3-9.
7. Evans AE, et al (1971): A pratical aid in the diagnosis and management of children with neuroblastoma. Pediatrics 47:913-916.

© 1985 Elsevier Science Publishers B.V. (Biomedical Division)
New dimensions in otorhinolaryngology – head and neck surgery, vol. 2.
E. Myers, editor

S-100 PROTEIN AS AN AID TO THE IDENTIFICATION OF MELANOCYTIC TUMORS OF THE HEAD AND NECK

RALPH METSON, DUAN-REN WEN, ALISTAIR J. COCHRAN and MARTYN W. BURK
Divisions of Head & Neck Surgery, Surgical Oncology, and Surgical Pathology, UCLA School of Medicine, Los Angeles, California 90024

INTRODUCTION

S-100 protein is an acidic protein of unknown function recently identified in malignant melanoma cell lines[1]. It has been found to be a relatively specific marker for malignant melanomas with little cross-reactivity for the cells of non-neural, non-melanocytic tumors. We present a patient with multiple head and neck tumors in whom diagnosis was aided by detection of S-100 protein.

CASE PRESENTATION

A 69 year old white female presented with a three mm black lesion on her right temple and an inverted right nipple. A right modified radical mastectomy was performed for an infiltrating ductal carcinoma. A wide local excision of the temple lesion demonstrated nodules of amelanotic tumor cells in the dermis that were regarded as most consistent with a metastasis from the breast primary. One year later a one cm, mobile, nontender right parotid mass developed. A right superficial parotidectomy revealed an undifferentiated neoplasm that was also regarded as consistent with a metastasis from the breast primary. Electron microscopy demonstrated no melanosomes.

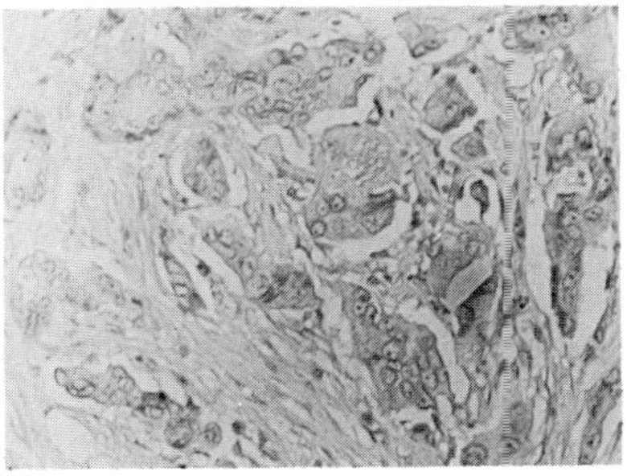

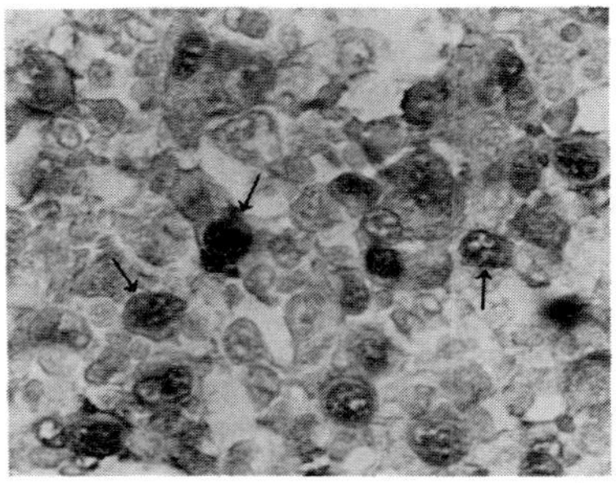

Fig. 1. Adenocarcinoma of breast shows no evidence of color development in tumor cells indicating the absence of S-100 protein
Fig. 2. Malignant melanoma of parotid shows dark cytoplasmic staining (arrows) of tumor cells indicating the presence of S-100 protein

At this time we became aware of of S-100 protein techniques. The patient's past surgical specimens were recut and stained for S-100 protein which was absent from the cells of the breast tumor (Fig. 1). The cells of the temple skin and parotid tumors, however, both contained readily detectable S-100 protein (Fig. 2). These findings were interpreted as showing that the right temple lesion was a primary malignant melanoma and the right parotid mass a metastasis from it. Therefore we were highly suspicious that the new right orbital mass was a metastasis from the melanoma rather than from breast. Subsequent therapy was planned accordingly.

DISCUSSION

S 100 protein is a nervous system-related cytoplasmic protein which was originally found in glial and Schwann cells but has recently been identified in human malignant melanoma cell lines. By application of immunoperoxidase techniques and aminoethyl carbazole as the indicator, S-100 protein stains a red color which is readily discernible from brown melanin pigments[2].

Over 60 cutaneous human malignant melanomas have been tested and all contained S-100 protein regardless of the organ from which they were derived. S-100 protein staining is not directly related to the amount of melanin present, making the technique especially useful in the diagnosis of amelanotic melanomas, as in the case described in this report. However, S-100 protein is not a marker for malignancy. In 33 benign skin nevi tested, all were found to contain some S-100 protein. With one exception in 51 non-neural non-melanocytic tumors studied so far, no S-100 protein has been found.

In the case presented conventional light and electron microscopy staining techniques failed to identify the tissure of origin for the tumors of the temporal skin and parotid gland. The clinical presentation led the patient's physicians to consider that these undifferentiated tumors were metastases from breast carcinoma. However, this assumption was proved false by the demonstration of S-100 protein in the skin and parotid lesions and absence of S-100 protein in the breast cancer. These findings led to the diagnosis of malignant melanoma originating in the temple and metastasizing to the parotid and orbit.

REFERENCES

1. Gaynor RB, Irie RF, Morton DL, Herschman HR (1970) Nature 286:400
2. Cochran AJ, Wen DR, Herschman HR, Gaynor RB (1982) Int J Cancer 30:295

© 1985 Elsevier Science Publishers B.V. (Biomedical Division)
New dimensions in otorhinolaryngology - head and neck surgery, vol. 2.
E. Myers, editor

CARCINOMA OF THE PAROTID DUCT

RALPH METSON, LARRY HOOVER, OTHELLA OWENS, PAUL H. WARD
Division of Head & Neck Surgery, UCLA School of Medicine, Los Angeles, California 90024

INTRODUCTION

Carcinoma of the parotid duct (Stensen's duct) ia a rare neoplasm usually providing the clinician with an unexpected diagnosis. Fifteen cases have been described in the English literature.[1,2] The pathology of these tumors is similar to that of primary parotid neoplasms. They usually present as anterior cheek masses; however, ductal compression may lead to intermitent swelling of the parotid gland which mimicks of sialolithiasis.

The purpose of this paper is to review the literature on parotid duct carcinomas and present a rational approach for treatment based upon two recent cases at our institution.

CASE PRESENTATIONS

Case 1. A 62 year old male presented with a slowly enlarging nontender four cm right cheek mass of three months duration A smaller 1.5 cm firm, nontender mass was palpable intraorally just lateral to Stensen's duct orifice. The facial nerve was intact. A superficial parotidectomy was performed in continuity with the parotid duct and a cuff of intraoral mucosa. (Figs 1 & 2). The larger intraparotid mass showed ductal dilatation and inflammation. The smaller mass in Stensen's duct, however, revealed a squamous cell carcinoma arising fron the ductal tissue, therefore the adjacent buccal branch of the facial nerve was resected. The patient received full course postoperative radiation therapy. He remains free of recurrent disease at five years. (Fig. 3a)

Case 2. An 82 year old female presented with a 20 year history of intermittent right parotid swelling. A one cm mass was palpable at the orifice of Stensen's duct. The facial nerve was intact. Biopsy under local anesthesia demonstrated a mucoepidermoid carcinoma. The patient underwent a right superficial parotidectomy with resection of the parotid duct, overlying buccal branch of the facial nerve, and a cuff of buccal mucosa. A right radical neck dissection was also performed for a positive submandibular node. She received full course radiation and remains disease free at two-and-a-half years.

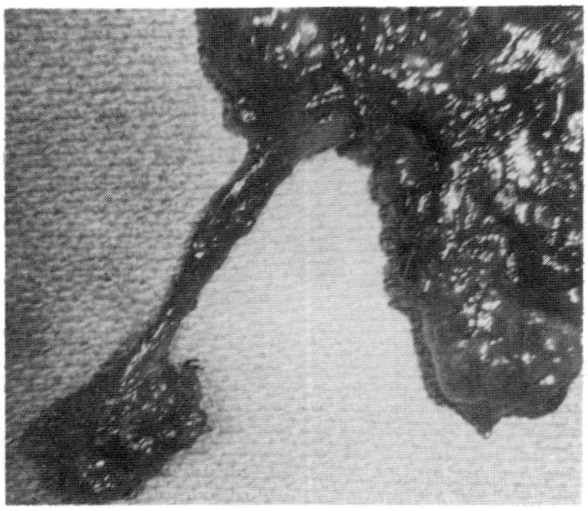

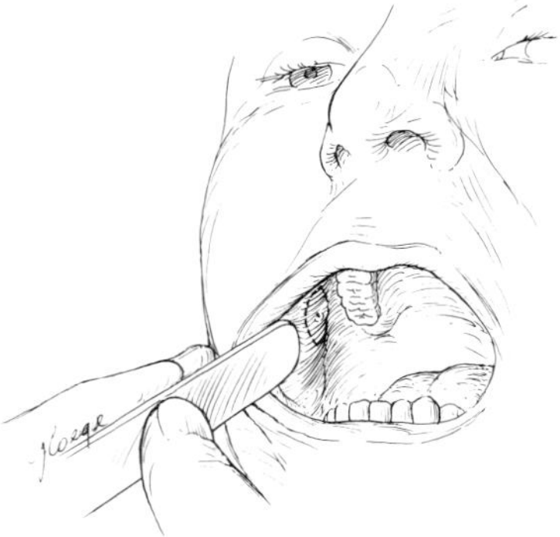

Fig. 1. Gross specimen showing superficial parotid, duct orifice tumor and connecting parotid duct.
Fig. 2. Dotted lines indicate appropriate cuff excision of buccal mucosa surrounding parotid duct.

DISCUSSION

Despite the rarity of Stensen's duct carcinoma, its behavior and treatment are not unlike that of primary parotid tumors. We report two cases of parotid duct carcinoma, one presenting as a mass, the other as recurrent parotid swelling. Of the 15 cases of primary parotid duct carcinoma in the English literature,[1,2] there were eight females and six males with a mean age of 48 years. The duration of a presenting mass varied from three months to two years. The pathology included five cases of squamous cell carcinoma, five mucoepidermoid carcinomas, two adenocarcinomas, two epidermoid carcinoms, and one sarcoma. Because of the unsuspected diagnosis at time of surgery, these cases were often treated by incomplete or local excision followed by radiation therapy. We feel this limited treatment results in the relatively high mortality rate described for this lesion.

It is our belief that this resection should include the superficial parotid lobe and the entire parotid duct with a cuff of normal appearing buccal mucosa, as well as any facial nerve branches overlying the tumor. There is no place for transoral local resection.

REFERENCES

1. Fayemi AO, Toker C (1974) Arch Otolaryngol 99:366
2. Owens OT, Fliegel A, Ward PH (1982) Otolar Head Neck Sur 90:671

© 1985 Elsevier Science Publishers B.V. (Biomedical Division)
New dimensions in otorhinolaryngology - head and neck surgery, vol. 2.
E. Myers, editor

FROM MACRO- TO MICRO-ENDOSCOPIC SURGERY WITH CO_2 LASER IN 400 PATIENTS WITH A HYPOPHARYNGEAL (ZENKER'S) DIVERTICULUM

Paul E. Hoeksema, M.D., J.J.M. van Overbeek, M.D., E.Th. Edens, M.D

Since 1964 over 350 patients with a hypopharyngeal diverticulum have been admitted to our clinic. Except for one case, who showed a carcinoma in the diverticulum, all these patients were treated endoscopically, regardless of the size of the pouch.
Up until 1981 we applied, in principle, Dohlman's technique whereby the septum, after electrocoagulation is divided with a diathermic knife.

In cases of a large diverticulum we often prefer to cleave the septum in several sessions.
Mostly we do not attempt to split the septum over its entire length Separation down to the bottom of the pouch increases the risk of mediastinitis. Moreover, our experience indicates that in dividing as far as the floor of the pouch, cicatricial tissue can give rise to stenosis. In this way many of our treated patients show more or less radiological evidence of a small residual pouch, but are usually quite free from symptoms. In only a few cases did we observe an obvious enlargement of a diverticulum remnant. Repetition of endoscopic treatment is always possible, but a small residual septum is not further cleaved when the patient has no discomfort.
Postoperatively the patient is put on a fluid diet and antibiotics and is normally discharged after four or five days.

In 1981 we modified the original technique by applying a micro-endoscopic procedure with a specially designed scope, an operating microscope and a CO_2 laser.
The scope has a broad opening and a split-end; it tapers down and has a total length of approximately 27 cm. Channels in both lateral walls serve for light conductors during introduction and for cannulae to remove, by continuous suction, steam and smoke associated with the use of the laser. The scope is adjusted and fixed to a chest support, resting on a frame mounted over the patient.

The microscope, with a 400 mm objective focus length, is connected by an adaptor with micromanipulator to a Sharplan CO_2 laser. An output of approximately 25 Watt is used for severance of the septum. Before using the laser a wet patty is placed in the esophagus to protect its ventral wall from laser impact.

The micro-endoscopic lasertechnique offers the possibility of a very precise and thin cutting of all the cricopharyngeal muscle-fibers. As advantages of laser treatment with regard to the conventional (Dohlmans's) technique can also be mentioned: less postoperative pain and less tissue necrosis, resulting in no stiff cicatrization.

From 1964 till 1984 378 patients with a hypopharynx diverticulum have been admitted to our clinic. With the exception of the case with a carcinoma, all patients were treated endoscopically, 69 of them with the laser technique.

In the 8 patients with a tendency to stenosis, the septum was split as fas as the bottom of the pouch. In our laser patients we have until now not noticed a stenosis.
Due to the good results which we have obtained, it can be stated that the micro-endoscopic technique with the CO_2 laser means an improvement on the original Dohlman's method.

Complications Endoscopic Treatment Hypopharyngeal Diverticula

	Electrocoagulation 308 pat.	CO_2 laser 69 pat.
Mortality	1 - 2 days postoperative	0
Mediastinitis	1 - cured by conservative therapy	3 - mediastinotomy 1 pat.
Haemorrhage	4 - endoscopically controlled	1 - stopped spontaneously
Esophageal fistula	1 - closed spontaneously	0
Tendency to stenosis	8 - endoscopically dilations gave satisfactory results	0

© 1985 Elsevier Science Publishers B.V. (Biomedical Division)
New dimensions in otorhinolaryngology - head and neck surgery, vol. 2.
E. Myers, editor

SILICONE TRACHEAL CANNULA - UPDATE

William G. Lavelle, M.D., William W. Montgomery, M.D. and Edward E. Jacobs, Jr., M.D.; Harvard Medical School, Boston, MA USA

The Montgomery® Silicone Tracheal Cannula,* developed in 1976, has now been used in a large number of patients. Various modifications of the cannula allowing for long term usage, use with obese necks and coincident use of valves have been developed. While certain complications such as granulation tissue, crusting, malrotation, wound infection and trauma do occur, careful attention to detail in the placement of the cannula along with careful wound management postoperatively can reduce the risk of these problems to a minimal level. Based on our experience, we recommend the following:

1) The use of the tracheal fenestrator to make the tracheotomy opening.

2) Proper placement of the cannula at the time of surgery. This should be confirmed by direct vision and routine lateral X-ray or xeroradiograph.

3) Removal of granulation tissue, administration of steroids and placement of long term cannula if indicated to prevent granulation tissue formation.

4) The wing-shaped faceplate is sutured in place and left for 7-10 days. The groove into which the plate has been inserted should be recorded to ensure the proper placement at a later time of the small silicone ring washer.

Available from: Boston Medical Products, 100 Charles River Plaza, Boston, MA USA 02114

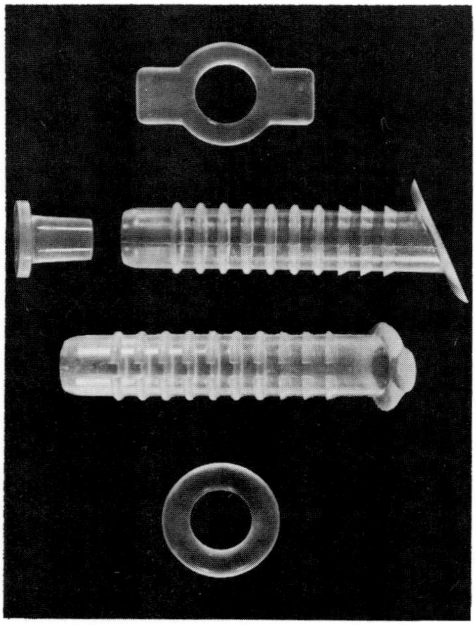

5) Use of an extralong cannula in those patients with obese necks.

6) Strict hygiene of the cannula should be maintained. The patient should be well educated regarding proper care and management of the cannula. Betadine should be applied to the wound edges during the procedure and on a daily basis postoperatively.

7) The use of humidity and/or Mucomyst, and cleaning of the cannula with a cotton-tipped applicator dipped in hydrogen peroxide to avoid crusting.

8) Avoidance of irritants such as smoking and mechanical trauma to the cannula.

9) Changing of the cannula at recommended intervals by a physician familiar with the procedure.

© 1985 Elsevier Science Publishers B.V. (Biomedical Division)
New dimensions in otorhinolaryngology - head and neck surgery, vol. 2.
E. Myers, editor

TYMPANOPLASTY UPON DEMAND. EXCLUSION OF THE ANTRUM. ELIMINATION OF THE ATTIC

DRS. F. OLAIZOLA, D. ALAMINOS, J.A. RODRIGUEZ-NUÑEZ
Proceedings Unit, Biomedical Division, Elsevier Science Publisher B.V., P.O. Box 1527 BM Amsterdam (The Netherlands)

INTRODUCTION

A controversy exists among the various schools. Some favor closed techniques while others advocate open techniques, the latter being disillusioned with the percentage of failures resulting from closed techniques.

As regards Cholesteatoma, tympanoplasty failures are due to 3 causes: Pocket Cholesteatoma, Residual Cholesteatoma and Metaplastic Cholesteatoma.

Several studies conducted by different schools show that the places where the greatest number of relapses occur are as follows: the anterosuperior portion of the attic and the anteroposterior portion of the middle eardrum in closed techniques, which portions we refer to as shaded areas due to the control and direct vision difficulties inherent to the abovementioned areas. Residual cholesteatoma.

Conservation or reconstruction of the walls of the duct without the presence of the ossicles promotes invagination and formation of Cholesteatoma pockets.

The formation of antromastoid cavities, of the attic and of the outer portion of the attic, increases penumatic space excessively, weakens tube functioning by causing it to be insufficient and promoting negative pneumatic pressure and Cholestatoma pockets.

To avoid these inconveniences, we have been following a series of techniques as of 1979 which endeavors to do away with such difficulties. Demand Technique (D.A.A.).

MATERIAL AND METHOD

In 1979 we began dealing with the initial cases, these being fully accounted for and having a controlled technique as of 1981. From 1979 thru 1984, we have registered a total of 123 cases, the follow-up period being from 7 months to 4 years.

The D.A.A. technique has 4 tenets: epytympanic access; direct arrival at the point of the lesion (D); exclusion of the antrum by way of a septum (A) and elimination of the attic by integrating it to the duct (A).

We conduct the following procedure as per existing lesions: I) Gain direct access to the attic through the upper wall and destroy the bone and middle eardrum for full control. Remove the cholesteatoma from the attic, as well as from the aditus and middle eardrum, if necessary. Perform bony septum on the aditus. Treat the plastic eardrum in the middle eardrum, together with the attic that was destroyed, incorporating it to the duct while continuing to cover same. II) Should lesions encroach upon the antrum, discard enough bone in order to have access to it, and once the lesion is removed, perform septum as indicated above, excluding the antrum. III) Should lesions encroach upon all of the mastoid, the antrum is reached as indicated in II), and access is continued through the mastoid for the purpose of eradicating the lesion in its entirety. The procedure is conluded in the same fashion as the previous ones, by performing a septum in the aditus and exclusion of the antromastoid cavity. The time required for the plastic and covering procedures of the duct is the same as in other cases. The bony septum is not absolute and has dehiscence which allows some control of possible complications.

RESULTS

Our surgical procedures have changed. From 1974 thru 1979 we performed as follows: Closed Tech.: 80%; Demand Tech.: 6.2%; Open Tech.: 5%; Open Obliterative Tech.: 8.8%. From 1979 thru 1984 we performed as follows: Closed Tech.: 12.5%; Demand Tech.: 43.7%; Open Tech.: 17.2%; Open Obliterative Tech.: 26.6%.

Failures: Cholesteatoma relapses: 4 cases, 4%. Continued Infections: 3 cases, 2% Mean percentage: 6.4%.

Epidermic pearls: 1 case, 1.07%.

These results improve upon taking into account the year 1984. Cholesteatoma Relapses: 0.5%; Infection: 1%; Pearl 0.9%; Mean Percentage: 2.4%; Present Healing Rate: 92.1%. Recovery of Hearing: Cases I) 83.3%; Cases II) 42.8% and Cases III) 38.5%. Mean Percentage: 54.8%.

CONCLUSIONS

Short postoperative period. Better control of the operating field...

than with closed techniques. Normal postoperative life. Reduction in cholesteatoma relapses. Functional results similar to those of other techniques. Oldest case to date: 6 years. To draw conclusions, we must wait until we have a large block of patients with this postoperative time.

New dimensions in otorhinolaryngology - head and neck surgery, vol. 2.
E. Myers, editor

DOES STATUS OF MIDDLE EAR INFLUENCE THE GRAFT TAKE RATE OF TYPE I TYMPANOPLASTY ?

YIM-WAH PANG, WING-KIN CHAN
Department of Otolaryngology, Veterans General Hospital, Taichung, Taiwan, ROC

Between Jan 1983 and June 1984, we performed 270 ears of type I tympanoplasty for the cases of chronic otitis media. All these surgeries were carried out with underlay technique under local anesthesia. We routinely utilized endaural incisions and the temporalis fascia was taken as graft material. Follow up period ranged from 6 months to 2 years. The overall graft take rate was 92.59%. Twenty cases failed after surgery. Table I,II and III showed the relationship between the status of middle ear and the graft take rate (GTR).

Table I
RELATIONSHIP BETWEEN STATUS OF MIDDLE EAR & GRAFT TAKE RATE(GTR)

Status of middle ear	Success/Total	GTR %	P
Middle ear discharge			
Dry	167/182	91.8	
Serous	12/12	100.0	
Mucoid	36/37	97.3	
Purulent	33/37	89.2	
Bloody	2/2	100.0	0.5374
Tympanosclerosis in membrane			
Absence	205/224	91.5	
Presence	45/46	97.8	0.2384
Status of middle ear mucosa			
Normal	204/222	91.9	
Polypoid	15/17	88.2	
Granulation	25/25	100.0	
Tympanosclerosis	6/6	100.0	0.3750
Eustachian tube function (Deflation-inflation test)			
Normal	208/223	93.3	
Functional obstruction	25/29	86.2	
Organic obstruction	17/18	94.4	0.3744

Table II
RELATIONSHIP BETWEEN THE SIZE OF PERFORATION & GRAFT TAKE RATE(GTR)

Perforation	Success/Total	GTR %	P
Central			
Large(larger than 75%)	129/145	89	
Medium (25 - 75 %)	76/78	97.4	
Small (less than 25 %)	39/41	95.1	
Marginal	5/5	100.0	
Attic	1/1	100.0	0.7823

Table III
GRAFT TAKE RATES OF TOTAL, MEDIUM AND SMALL PERFORATIONS

Perforation	Success/Total	GTR %	P
Total	27/35	77.1	
Medium	76/78	97.4	0.0016
Small	39/41	95.1	0.0488

We concluded that: 1.Discharging ears, presence of tympanosclerosis or abnormal mucosal change of middle ear would not influence the graft take rate of type I tympanoplasty. 2. Eustachian tube function assessed by deflation inflation test could not predict the outcome of graft healing. 3. There was no relationship between the size of tympanic membrane perforation and the graft successful rate. However, if we compared the result of total perforation to the graft take rates of small and medium perforations, we found that the former certainly had a much less excellent result than the latters.

New dimensions in otorhinolaryngology - head and neck surgery, vol. 2.
E. Myers, editor

INFLUENCE OF MIDDLE EAR PATHOLOGY TO CERAVITAL IMPLANTS

RALF RECK
Department of Otorhinolaryngology, University of Mainz, Germany

Since 1978 we have clinical experience with ossicular replacement prostheses, made from the bioactive glass ceramic Ceravital (1,2,3,4,5). From a total of about 3000 ear operations we reconstructed the sound conducting system in 950 patients with Ceravital prostheses. Our clinical trial bases on our experimental studies in animals (4). The bioactive glass ceramic Ceravital has the following composition: SiO_2 40-50; P_2O_5 10-15; Na_2O 5-10; CaO 30-35; K_2O 0.5-3.0 and MgO 2.5-5.0 percent per weight. It is obvious, that about 50% of the weight of the material is formed by calciumphosphate. Calciumphosphate is the common base of all bioactive ceramics.

Bioactivity of an implant presumes a chemical reaction of the implant with the implantation bed. In consequence, a certain change of the surface of all bioactive implants can be observed. The amount of degradation is one of the limitating factors for suitability of an artificial prosthesis.

Our semiquantitative studies on animals have shown, that in the rabbit's middle ear there is a progressive conversion of the implant's surface in the bony implantation bed as well as in the soft tissue supporting structure (4). These implant surface conversion processes are decisively determined by the tissue covering the implant.

When the implants are overlaid with a "varnish-like" avascular fibrous bone layer containing few cells, no manifestations of conversion processes reflecting a deeper than 20-60 µm breakdown of the implants were seen on the glass ceramic surface two years after implantation. When the implants were in complete contact with soft tissue (for instance scar tissue, granulation tissue), a degradation of the implant's surface up to 450 µm could occasionally be observed.

In 53 patients with Ceravital implants tympanoplasty revision operations were carried out. Clinical indications of the operations had been: recidive perforation 32%; recidive cholesteatoma 21%; conductive hearing loss 19%; severe adhesion 17%; fibrosis 11%.

The histological examination of the 53 retrieved implants confirmed the basic findings in animals (5). They allow a quite exact prediction of the fate of an implant in a human's middle ear, dependent on the middle ear pathology.

Figure I demonstrates the depth of lysis of the 53 retrieved implants. The indication of the diagramm confirmes that even within 15 months the implants may be dissolved to an extent of about 500 µm, on the other hand, they may be found completely unchanged 5 years after operation without any degradation.

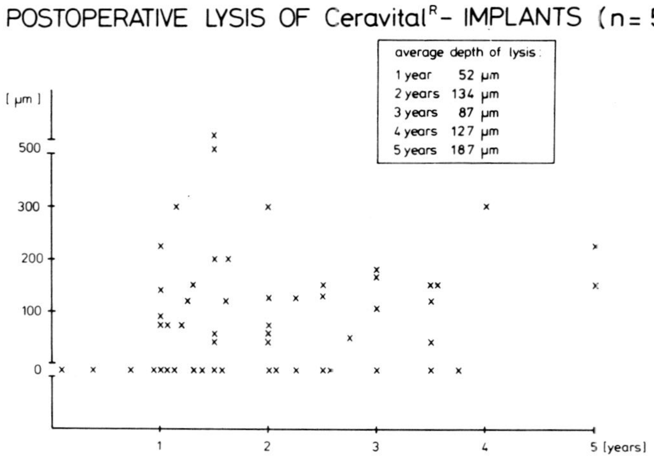

FIGURE I

The comparison of the depth of lysis and the middle ear pathology leads to the conclusion: in cases with permanent tympanic membrane perforations and mucositis with edema, granulation tissue or polyp formation the implants get dissolved. In dry ears with permanent perforations or ventilated ears and closed tympanic membranes, no remarkable lysis or degradation has been found in follow-ups to seven years.

REFERENCES

1. Reck R (1979) Arch Otorhinolaryngol 223:369-373
Erste tierexperimentelle und klinische Erfahrungen mit bioaktiver Glaskeramik in der rekonstruktiven Mittelohrchirurgie.
2. Reck R (1981) Clin Otolaryngol 6:63-65
Tissue reactions to glass ceramics in the middle ear.
3. Reck R (1983) Laryngoscope 93:196-199
Bioactive glass-ceramic: a new material in tympanoplasty.
4. Reck R, Helms J (1984) In: Grote J (ed) Biomaterials in Otology.
Fundamental aspects of bioglasses and surgery with bioactive glass ceramic implants.
5. Reck R (1984) Laryngoscope 94 Suppl 33:1-54
Bioactive glass ceramic in ear surgery. Animal studies and clinical results.

© 1985 Elsevier Science Publishers B.V. (Biomedical Division)
New dimensions in otorhinolaryngology - head and neck surgery, vol. 2.
E. Myers, editor

ABSENCE OF BLUNTING WITH MODIFIED OVERLAY TECHNIQUE

SUAREZ GUMERCINDO., SUAREZ G. SAUL., URIOL MIGUEL

From the Department of Otolaryngology of the Regional Medical Center of National University of Trujillo-Peru.

INTRODUCTION

Several surgical techniques for reconstruction of the middle ear have been described previously, with the "overlay" technique (1) (2) (3), and undesirable side efect, known as "blunting" has been reported (2).

When we began to use Farrior's technique (1), in which more than 95 per cent, of the skin of the ear canal is removed, and later replaced in its original place covering the temporal fascia graft. This blunting phenomenon was observed in some of our cases, so we introduced a modification to overlay technique with no blunting complication in 100 patients operated on at the university Regional Hospital of Trujillo, with a follow up period of 1 to 3 years.

MATERIAL AND METHODS

Procedure

Under local or general anesthesia, a retroauricular incision with a temporal fascia graft of 15 to 20 mm. and simple mastoidectomy was performed in all patients, followed by skin detachment, working from the outer to the inner portion of the external auditory canal, up to the perforation (Fig. 1. The skin of the anterior wall is detached 3 mm. from the annulus, in reverse fashion (Fig. 2).

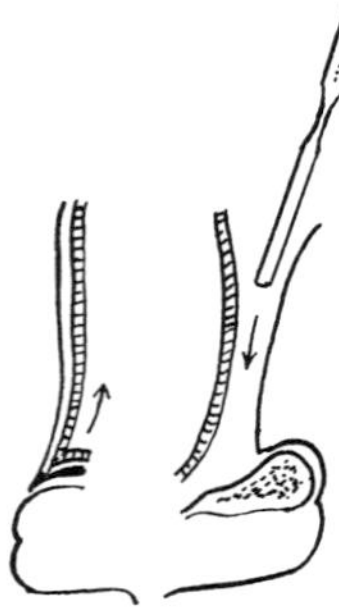

Figure 1

Elevation of the Canal Skin: Post. Sup. and Inferior walls.

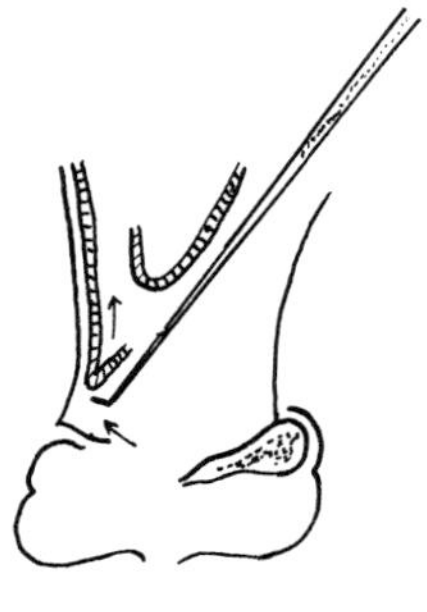

Figure 2

Elevation of the skin of the angle anterior wall.

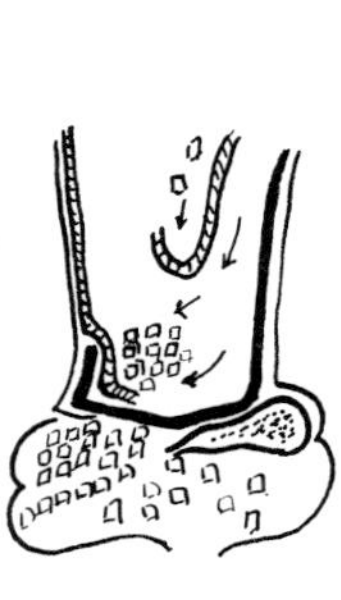

Figure 3

Fascia graft, is covered with anterior wall skin pressure with Absorbable Gelatin Sponge.

A small cotton ball impregnated with Xylocaine and Adrenalin is placed under the skin flap for hemostasis to facilitate the graft isertion, after removal, then the graft is implanted and external pressure with Absorbable Gelatin Sponge is applied against the anterior wall angle (Fig. 3). A second layer of Absorbable Gelatin Sponge plus Hydrocortisone Antibiotic is then applied, following the well known procedure of the overlay technique, and in the final stage the packing is left in place fo 8 to 10 days.

DISCUSSION

Blunting may be due to an accumulation and organization of blood deep to the skin graft or to a too liberal disposition of the fascial graft over the anterior canal wall with subsequent formation of an excessively thick subcutaneous layer, which fills in the angle between the canal wall and the drum (2).

With our modification of overlay technique, in which a satisfactory hemostasis and "hooking" of the graft with preservation of the growing border of the anterior wall skin are the main objetive, no "Blunting" was observed in 100 consecutive patients operated on and followed up for 1 to 3 years.

The lack of this complication could be due to new epithelial growing from the anterior wall angle to the posterior wall, in the same direction of the displacement which we observed with the drainage tube used in the treatment of the serous middle otitis.

Other factors which may contribute to the absence of blunting, are the use of a relative large temporal fascia graft and the external pressure with a gauze for to 8 to 10 days.

REFERENCES

1. Farrior B. (1968) Tympanoplasty in 3 - D 1: 21 - 101.
2. Gordon D.L. Smyth (1972) Tympanic Reconstruction 5: 115-117.
3. Shambaugh G. (1967) Surgery of the Ear. Tympanoplasty, pp 447-471.

New dimensions in otorhinolaryngology - head and neck surgery, vol. 2.
E. Myers, editor

EXPERIMENTAL STUDY AND CLINICAL APPLICATION OF HYDROXLAPATITE IN MIDDLE EAR SURGERY

ISAO TAKIMOTO, MASAHIKO HARA
Department of Otorhinolaryngology, Aichi Medical University.
Yazako, Nagakute-cho, Aichi, Japan

INTRODUCTION

Recently, the use of Hydroxylapatite (H.A.) for biomedical purposes has been increasing. In the area of otolaryngology, H.A. has been used for middle ear surgery such as reconstruction of the ossicular chain or posterior ear canal wall and mastoid obliteration.

We performed histological experiments on animals to study the affinity of H.A. with surrounding tissue and obtain fundamental data for clinical use. Then we used H.A. in 30 cases of middle ear surgery and observed that clinical process.

EXPERIMENTS ON ANIMALS

Method

To evaluate safety and usability, we embedded H.A. in a hole drilled in the tympanic bulla of adult guinea pig. One month later, the guinea pig was sacrificed and the tympanic bulla was examined in a non-decalcified and Hematoxylin-Eosin stained preparation.

Results

Macroscopically, the embedded H.A. was tightly connected to the surrounding tissue.

In microscopic findings, H.A. showed no absorption and no foreign body reactions, and had entered the connective tissue in H.A. pore. Though no bone formation on H.A. surface was observed but bone induction seemed to be promoted by H.A..

H.A. was well covered by fascia outside and by mucoperiosteum inside.

CLINICAL EVALUATION

Two kinds of H.A. were used: plate type for reconstruction of the posterior ear canal wall and separation between attic and antrum, and block type for obliteration of mastoid cavities.

Subjects

30 cases, age--from 5-72 years old (I2 subjects were under I5), disease--cholesteatoma I6, simple perforative otitis 3,reoperation 9, congenital meatal atresia I, after trauma I.

Operation

reconstruction of posterior ear canal wall- I0, mastoid obliteration-I6 (6 cases overlap with another group), separation between attic and mastoid antrum- I0.

Results

We observed the subjects for 6-27 month after operation and obtained positive results except for three cases of H.A. exposures from mastoid cavities. These three cases were all in the re-operation group and H.A. exposure occured because of the re-used skin which covered mastoid cavity in the former operation.

COMMENT

Analysis of the failure cases showed that there were no problem with the compatibility of H.A. material itself but it is necessary to check the surface and to stimulate blood circulation of the covered skin.

Plate type H.A. is easy to trimm to adapt to size of defect of the posterior ear canal wall but a more plastic character is required because of its fragility.

There did't observed bone formation on H.A. surface in this region which was seen on the mandible of dog or cervical bone of rabbit. This might be caused by a difference in blood circulation or the volume of bone marrow around H.A..

However, we can observe bone induction character near H.A..

Although there might be a little meaning of bone formation in the ear because of its immobility, we would like to study further to confirm whether new bones may form over the long term of subjects' lives.

REFERENCES

I. Grote JJ, Kuijpers W, de Groot K (I98I): Use of sintered hydroxylapatite in middle ear surgery. ORL,43:248-254

2. Blitterswijk CA, Grote JJ, Kuijpers W (I983): Macroporous and dense hydroxylapatite as middle ear implants. Fourth European Conference on Biomaterials. Leuven, Belgium

© 1985 Elsevier Science Publishers B.V. (Biomedical Division)
New dimensions in otorhinolaryngology - head and neck surgery, vol. 2.
E. Myers, editor

NEW CERAMIC IMPLANTS IN MIDDLE EAR SURGERY

ETSUO YAMAMOTO
Department of Otolaryngology, Faculty of Medicine, Kyoto University, Sakyo-ku, Kyoto, Japan

Various metal and plastic materials have been used as synthetic implant materials for ossicular reconstruction. They have partially or completely extruded in many cases because of poor biocompatibility.

Two different prototypes of columella materials made from alumina ceramics (Bioceram®, Kyocera, Japan) were designed by the author for ossicular reconstruction (Fig. 1). CORP-P (Ceramics Ossicular Replacement Prosthesis-Partial) is used as a columella to fit onto the stapes head, and CORP-T (Ceramics Ossicular Replacement Prosthesis-Total) is used as a columella placed onto the footplate of the stapes. Both prototypes of CORP consist of a head for contact with a fascia graft, a shaft and a base for the stapes. The heads of both types have the same convex and elliptic shape (4 mm X 2 mm) that permits smooth contact with the fascia graft and prevents extrusion of the CORP. The diameters of the columnar shafts differ between both types (1.2 mm for CORP-P, 0.8 mm for CORP-T). Three kinds of lengths are prepared for each prototype: 3, 4 and 5 mm for CORP-P and 5, 6 and 7 mm for CORP-T. Yttria (Y_2O_3) is added to CORP to increase its radiopaqueness.

In addition to the general properties of ceramic implants, CORP has these two characteristics: the unique shape of its head allows easy and smooth contact with the fascia graft, and the radiopaqueness makes it possible to confirm the position of the implants by X-ray examination.

The usual operative techniques using these implants are as follows. CORP-P can be utilized in cases in which the superstructure of the stapes is not affected by disease. The depression of the disc-shaped base is fitted onto the head of the stapes and the shaft of the columella is supported by a micro-sliced cartilage plate having a wedge-shaped cut. The convex-shaped head of the columella and the cartilage plate are covered by a fascia graft. CORP-T can be used in cases in which only the footplate of the stapes remains after complete removal of the diseased tissues. The disc-shaped base of CORP-T is placed on the footplate, and the columella is stabilized with a sliced cartilage plate in the same manner as described for CORP-P. The head of the prosthesis and the cartilage plate are covered by the fascial graft.

During the past 4 years, 162 CORPs have been implanted, and the postoperative results concerning hearing and stability of CORP were satisfactory. Hearing was examined in 98 ears followed for more than one year. Good hearing results (postoperative air-bone gap within 10dB) were obtained in 33 of 52 ears using CORP-P (63.5%) and in 22 of 46 ears using CORP-T (47.8%). In most cases implanted CORPs were stabilized in the middle ear. Exposure or extrusion of CORP from the middle ear occurred in 8 of 162 ears (4.9%) and dislocation of CORP in the middle ear in 6 (3.7%).

Application of CORP as a columella material for ossicular reconstruction may achieve the clinical importance of human ossicles.

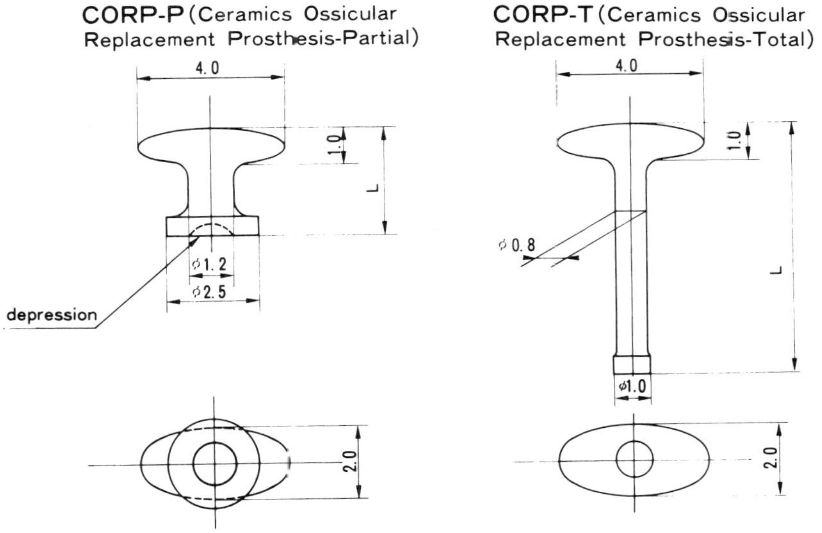

Fig. 1. Shape and dimension of CORP in milimeters.

New dimensions in otorhinolaryngology - head and neck surgery, vol. 2.
E. Myers, editor

SMITH-McGUKIN SPOT

Charles W. Smith

It is a continual source of amazement to me that despite describing the Smith-McGukin Spot in 1964, there is no reference to this in the voluminous literature and reports of lengthy meetings on the pathology of ear disease. I cannot pretend that the spot is of great importance, but it appears in some 10-20% of patients with the glue ear syndrome and apart from adding interest to the investigation of the many patients with this condition, may contribute something to the understanding of two problems which face us in such cases: (1) there is no reliable way of forcasting the prognosis, (2) there are still unanswered questions about the aetiology and pathology.

Simple, yet striking, pathological changes that can be seen with the naked eye might have been expected to interest the experts. Photographs of the tympanic membrane with good colour rendering and satisfactory depth of focus have been easily obtainable in recent years with the aid of a tympanoscope and strong flash manufactured by Karl Storz. The different appearances associated with the Smith-McGukin spot will be demonstrated by means of these.

A typical spot can be placed anywhere on the membrana tensa. It has a rose pinkish colour, a clear cut margin and is fed by one or two vessels running from the perimeter of the drum to the centre of the spot. Spots are sometimes multiple and occasionally seven or eight may surround the whole of the periphery of the drum like a necklace. They sometimes have an irregular outline rather than the typical oval appearance. Less frequently several spots may coelese to create an extensive pink opaque discolouration. Though initially of a homogeneous pink colour, they often change slowly over a period of time and areas of yellow, grey and white may appear.

Frank McGukin thought that they were probably the result of blood in the middle layer of the drum and precursors of tympanosclerosis. This mistake has recently been given further support by a colour picture in publicity material produced for Karl Storz. The spots are due to a spherical polyp arising from the mucosal surface of the drum and visible through it. It is possible to pick the polyps off the mucosa with the tip of a micro-sucker through a myringotomy incision when there is minimal bleeding as the polyps have an extremely fine and narrow pedicle.

As might be expected, section shows them to be simple chronic granulomas packed with histiocytes, polymorphs and lymphocytes. Occasionally they contain cholesterol crystals in common with much of the granulation tissue that has been obtained from patients with chronic otitis media unassociated with cholesteatoma. Alcuin blue staining may show some positive material suggesting that mucus-producing cells can be present.

Apart from giving clues to the aetiology and pathology of chronic sero-mucinous otitis media and by their presence confirming the diagnosis in cases where other tests have produced equivocal results, the SM spot can be used as a means of giving some indication of the prognosis in an individual case. Observed over many months it can slowly shrink and become more dense as the colour changes from rose pink to a darker red. These changes indicate that the otitis media is resolving and give added encouragement to those surgeons who wish to adopt a conservative approach to an individual case and to avoid one of the many unnecessary operations that are carried out throughout the world. All too often children are placed on the waiting list for surgery and by the time this is carried out the middle ear is fully aerated and free of any abnormal exudate. Such unnecessary surgery is undesirable for the patient and brings discredit to the speciality.

The polyps are susceptible to absence of fluid in the middle ear and will disappear very rapidly after myringotomy and insertion of a grommet. It seems very likely that either their nutrition is obtained partly from the middle ear effusion, or at least that like sea urchins they require a very wet climate to survive. Karmody has suggested that the polyps arise as a positive response to the infective element in sero-mucinous otitis media and provide a rapidly available source of white cells to combat this.

I hope that searching for the Smith-McGukin Spot will give Otologists added incentive to examine their patients carefully and that further investigations and research into this interesting pathological feature will add to our understanding of the aetiology and, therefore, proper treatment of sero-mucinous otitis media.

References: Smith, C (1964) Proceedings of the Royal Society of Medicine 57,776

Karmody, Colin S (1985) Personal communication

New dimensions in otorhinolaryngology – head and neck surgery, vol. 2.
E. Myers, editor

ACRIDINE ORANGE STAIN IS SUPERIOR TO GRAM STAIN IN THE BACTERIOLOGICAL EXAMINATION OF MIDDLE EAR EFFUSIONS

PAUL VAN CAUWENBERGE & MAGDA RYSSELAERE
Departments of Otorhinolaryngology and Ophthalmology, State University Hospital, B-9000 Gent (Belgium)

INTRODUCTION

The controversy about the role of bacteria in otitis media with effusion (OME) is mainly due to the variety of bacteriological techniques used, including sampling and transport, and to the fact that, even if bacteria are present in the middle ear effusions (MEE), their number is very often scant (1). There is, consequently, a need for the use of highly sensitive bacteriological techniques.

It was the purpose of this study to investigate the value of three different stains in the bacteriological examination of MEE in cases of OME.

MATERIAL AND METHODS

The material consists of 112 MEE from children, aged 1 to 6 years, with OME of at least 2 months duration, and in whom tympanostomy tubes were inserted.

In the standardized set-up that we use (2), three different stains (Gram, Acridine Orange and Giemsa) were used to get a maximum of information, not only about the possible involvement of bacteria in the effusion studied, but also about the condition of the bacteria present and the role of inflammatory cells. In addition, aerobic and anaerobic cultures were performed.

RESULTS

The over all results of the detection of bacteria by the different stains and cultures are subject of an other publication (3).

AOS was clearly superior in the detection of bacteria. In 52 % there was a concordance with the results of Gram stain : in 22 % the same bacteria were seen in both stains and in 30 % no bacteria were found. However, in the 48 % of the effusions where a discordance between both stains was noted, AOS was superior in detecting bacteria in 33 %, while Gram stain revealed in only

15 % bacteria which were not seen with AOS. This means that Gram stain was unable to show bacteria undoubtetly present in the effusions, because seen with AOS. The absolute number of failure of Gram stain to detect bacteria is even higher, because, when comparing the results of culturing with the findings of the direct microscopic examination, it was found that in 17 % of the effusions cultures were positive where Gram stain was negative ; for AOS this was 12 %. Giemsa stain had the worst scores with regard to the detection of bacteria : in 57 % there was a concordance with AOS, but in 40 % bacteria seen with AOS, were not found with Giemsa stain ; in only 4 % Giemsa revealed bacteria not seen with AOS. When comparing the results of Giemsa stain with those of culturing, Giemsa stain showed to be unable to show culturable bacteria in 27 % (this was only 17 % for Gram stain and 12 % for AOS).
When plotting the results of the entire direct microscopic examination against the results of culturing, and at the same time considering the microscopic aspect of the effusion, we noted that in glue and pure mucoid effusions direct microscopic examination never failed to show bacteria which could be cultured. In seromucoid and purulent effusions the failure was very low (resp. 4 % and 8 %), while in serous effusions this was 27 %. Dead microorganisms are colored red or orange with the AOS, while living bacteria take a green-fluorescent color. When plotting our results of bacterial detection by AOS against those of culturing, we noted that effusions yielding fluorescent green bacteria in AOS, had indeed a higher positive bacterial culture (49 %) than those where bacteria were colored red or orange (34 %).

DISCUSSION

Gram stain has always been considered as the most valuable stain in the detection of bacteria in all kinds of smears. However, another interesting staining technique, the fluorescent acridine orange staining, revealed its superiority in detecting bacteria in fluids, where inflammatory cells and cell debris are also present (4,5). However, in most instances the samples are fixed, e.g. by heat, so bacteria are killed and are colored red or orange, which make them very easily recognizable among the green-fluorescent epithelial and inflammatory cells (4,5).

In our study we did not use a fixation technique, but we mixed the fresh effusion with the acridine orange solution and observed the preparation without delay under a fluorescent microscope. In this way, we were able to identify green-fluorescent bacteria (alive) from red and orange bacteria (dead). This discrimination is, however, not an absolute one as was demonstrated by the fact that in the presence of fluorescent bacteria cultures remained sterile in 51 % and that in the presence of red or orange bacteria cultures turned out to be positive in 34 %. From our results we concluded that more than one stain should be performed in the bacteriological and cytological examination of MEE, to obtain a maximum of information.

REFERENCES

1. Van Cauwenberge P (1982) Acta otorhinolaryng belg 36:5-239
2. Van Cauwenberge P, Rysselaere M, Declercq G (1985) In : Marquet J (ed) Surgery and Pathology of the Middle Ear. Martinus Nijhoff Publishers, Boston-Dordrecht-Lancaster, pp 333-337
3. Van Cauwenberge P, Rysselaere M, Waelkens B, Aurus-Nasus-Larynx (in press).
4. Kronvall G, Myhre E (1977) Acta Pathol Microbiol Scand (B) 85 : 249-254
5. Kleiman MB, Reynolds JK, Watts NH, Schreiner RL, Smith JW (1984) J Pediatrics 104 : 401-404

© 1985 Elsevier Science Publishers B.V. (Biomedical Division)
New dimensions in otorhinolaryngology – head and neck surgery, vol. 2.
E. Myers, editor

SURGICAL TREATMENT OF DERMATOLOGICAL CARCINOMAS OF THE NOSE : 196 CASES OPERATED ON BETWEEN 1979 and 1984

C. BEAUVILLAIN de MONTREUIL, L. LELIEVRE, H. MASSOT and F. LEGENT
Department of ENT - C.H.U. - Nantes (France)

INTRODUCTION

Over a five-year period, in collaboration with the Nantes Dermatology Department, our surgical team operated on all dermatological epitheliomas of the nose greater than 1 cm diameter.

21 % of the carcinomas of the skin are situated on the nose (Thèse H. MERCIER) ; there were approximately 80 % basal cell carcinomas and 20 % squamous carcinomas.

Malignant melanomas as well as lentigo maligna are infrequent in the nose (two cases only).

Treatment of cervical nodes metastasis of squamous carcinomas was made as requested. No prophylactic node treatment was provided.

MATERIAL AND METHODS

During five years from 1979 to 1984, 196 dermatological carcinomas of the nose were operated on.

52 % of our patients were over 70 years of age and 5 % under than 40 (table).

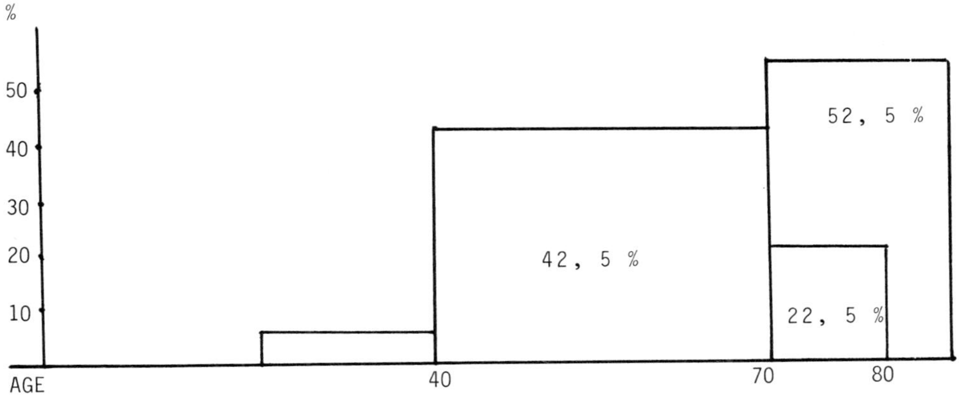

The different surgical acts performed are indicated in the following table.

SIMPLE SUTURE	13	GLABELLAR FLAP	39
TOTAL SKIN GRAFTS	15	FOREHEAD FLAP :	45
LLL PLASTY OF DUFOURMENTEL (near the Rhomboïd flap)	16	Median or Oblique 26 Island flap 19	
ROTATION FLAP (RIEGER-MARCHAC)	22	MISCELLANEOUS	4
NASOLABIAL FLAP	34	AMPUTATION	8

It is to be noted that there were only 15 total skin grafts (7, 5 % of cases), whereas there were a relatively large number of naso-labial flaps (20 %) and glabellar flaps (17 %), the two together constituting nearly 40 % of cases.

The glabellar flap is used for a very frequent form of carcinoma on the internal angle of the eye.

The nasolabial flap is used for carcinoma of the nasogenian groove or of the wing of the nose.

The forehead flap

There are two forms of forehead flap :

- First the median or oblique forehead flap which is essential in cases of extensive loss of substance from the bridge or wings of the nose or columella.
- The second form of frontal flap is the supraorbital island flap ; its offers the advantage of allowing surgery to be performed in a single operation without severing the pedicle of the flap.

The limits of the incision for surgical excision were usually 0, 5 cm from the macroscopic borders of the lesion on the surface, and in depth as far as the bony or cartilaginous level which was often preserved.

It is to be noted that difficulties were encountered in cases of recurrent carcinoma or fibrosing basal cell carcinoma due to the dissemination of their neoplastic cells which required a wider resection (greater than 1 cm). In these cases it was important to assess the quality of surgical escision, either by extemporaneous examination or by waiting 48 to 72 h for the histological results before attaching the surgical flap. The chemosurgery of Mohs may also be employed in these circumstances ; however, our team has had no experience with this procedure.

We cannot give a statistic of cure of these cancers ; indeed, the last cases were operated on one year ago.

DISCUSSION

If we consider the role of surgical treatment of dermatological carcinomas of the nose in comparison with other treatments, it may be noted that electrocoagulation is applied to tumors less than 5 mm in diameter and cryosurgery to those less than 1 cm in diameter.

The inconveniences of surgical treatment are an immediate, extensive and quite visible scar, and in 1 case out of 10 the need of a second operation of the scar under local anesthesia. Its advantages are numerous. In 80 % of cases, local anesthesia is possible, with hospitalization during 1 or 2 days. Surgery allows histological examination of the entire excised piece. Healing is rapid, and the scar is often barely visible or invisible a year later in subjects over 60 years of age.

CONCLUSION

Surgery of dermatologica carcinomas of the nose is an excellent therapeutic method ; it is the only treatment of the fibrosing basal cell carcinoma.

REFERENCES

1. Barre-Mercier H (1978) Epitheliomas cutanés de la région nasale : à propos de 120 cas. Thèse médecine, Nantes.

2. Beauvillain C, Litoux P, Lelièvre L, Massot H, Boutet JJ, Legent F (1984) Les lambeaux dans la chirurgie réparatrice des épithéliomas dermatologiques du nez (rhinopoièse exclue). A propos de 144 cas opérés. Ann Otolaryngol 101: 341-348

3. Cronin TD (1983) The VY rotational flap for nasal tip defects. Ann Plast. Surg 11:282-288

4. Dufourmentel C (1962) La fermeture des pertes de substances cutanées limitées. Le lambeau de rotation en L pour losange dit "LLL". Ann Chir Plast 7:61-66

5. Fleury P, Lacomme Y, Legent F, et al (1977) Les affections dermatologiques en ORL. Rapport de la Société Française d'ORL et de Chirurgie cervico-faciale

6. Jost G et al (1977) Réparations plastiques des pertes de substances cutanées de la face. Rapport de la Société Française d'ORL et de Chirurgie cervico-faciale

7. Marchac D (1970) Lambeau de rotation frontonasal. Ann Plast Surg 15:44-49

8. Marchac D, Duport G (1980) Résultats carcinologiques et esthétiques du traitement chirurgical de 138 épithéliomas basocellulaires. Ann Chir Plast 25:127-134

9. Morel-Fatio D Réparations des pertes de substance chirurgicales de la face. EMC Techniques Chirurgicales

10. Reynaud JP (1983) Le lambeau en hachette dans la réparation des exérèses cutanées de la pyramide nasale. Ann Chir Plast Esthet 28:369-375

New dimensions in otorhinolaryngology - head and neck surgery, vol. 2.
E. Myers, editor

RECONSTRUCTION OF LARGE TRACHEAL DEFECTS

JACK SIDI, MORDECHAI BACHAR, ARISTEDE AVRAHAM

Department of Otolaryngology and Head & Neck Surgery, Beilinson Medical Center, Petah Tiqva and Sackler School of Medicine, Tel Aviv University, Israel

1-2% of malignant tumors of the thyroid gland tend to invade the anterior and/or the anterolateral wall of the trachea. In some cases invasion is extensive and radical surgery results in large defects of the upper part of the cervical trachea and larynx. Reconstruction of such large, surgically produced laryngotracheal defects to achieve closure of the tracheostomy and to provide laryngeal speech may be done by using reversed and advanced cervical flaps. Musculocutaneous flaps have been most popular in recent years. Prosthetic graft materials of different kinds including plastics and metals have also been used in experimental and clinical work (Table 1).

TABLE I: EXPERIMENTAL GRAFT MATERIALS

A - Plastic (mesh or rings)		B - Metals (mesh or coils)
Polyethylene	Dacron	Stainless steel
Acrylic	Silicone	Tantalum
Teflon	Proplast	Vitalium

Titanium plates were used in two patients to reinforce cervical flaps with very satisfactory results.

Case No. 1 : A 50-year-old male, who was operated for an intraluminar invasive papillary adenocarcinoma of the thyroid. A total thyroidectomy with partial resection of the cricoid cartilage and 5 tracheal rings was performed, leaving a large defect. The left recurrent nerve was sacrificed and the patient had great difficulty in communication. The endotracheal lining was provided by rotating a circumferential cervical skin flap around the defect. A titanium plate was shaped and fitted to replace the cartilaginous defect and finally covered by an advancement flap. The flaps and implant were fixed using 4 stainless steel sutures and buttons.

Case No. 2 had a very large defect after resection of an intraluminar infiltrative tumor of the thyroid gland which was reconstructed two years after the first operation, using the same procedure for restoration of the anterolateral wall of the trachea.

In our experience titanium plates, which are innert, and baskets for the reconstruction of the tracheal wall and mandibular defects, have proved to be well tolerated as implants. They are very efficient as blood supply from both flaps is achieved through the holes of the plate, so that the fixation sutures may be removed early, within 3 to 4 weeks, and the tracheostomy closed.

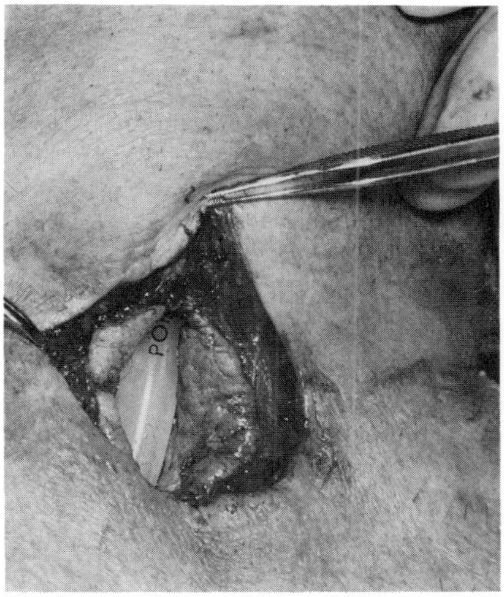

Fig.1a -A circumferential skin flap is reversed around the defect.

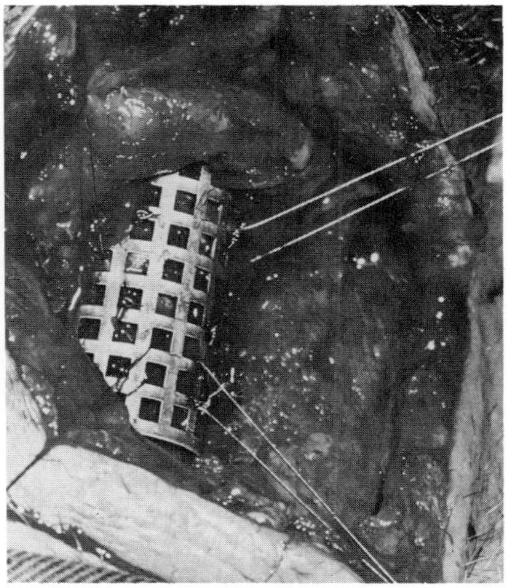

Fig.1b -The titanium plate is placed over the inverted flap.

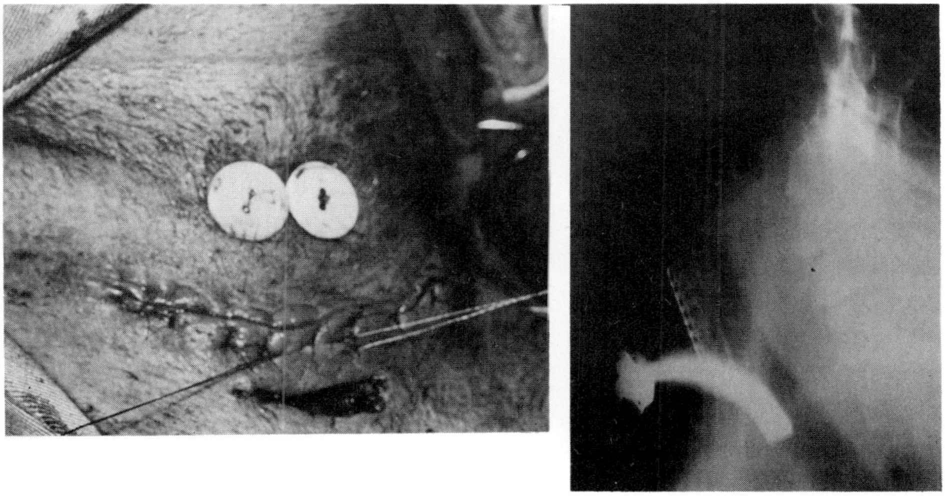

Fig.2 -Postoperative X-ray. The titanium plate in place provides patency of the tracheal lumen.

New dimensions in otorhinolaryngology – head and neck surgery, vol. 2.
E. Myers, editor

THE VERSATILE NASO-LABIAL FLAP

Thomas C. Tyler, M.D., Venice, Fl.

The naso-labial flap can replace tissue loss of the midface and intra-oral areas. When properly planned it gives excellent and reliable results. The flap is hairless in females and for the most part in males and gives excellent tissue match. It is a strong flap with rich subdermal anastomosis (Fig. 1).

Figure 1. Bilateral inferiorly based naso-labial flaps for total floor of mouth reconstruction without post-operative breakdown demonstrates its strength.

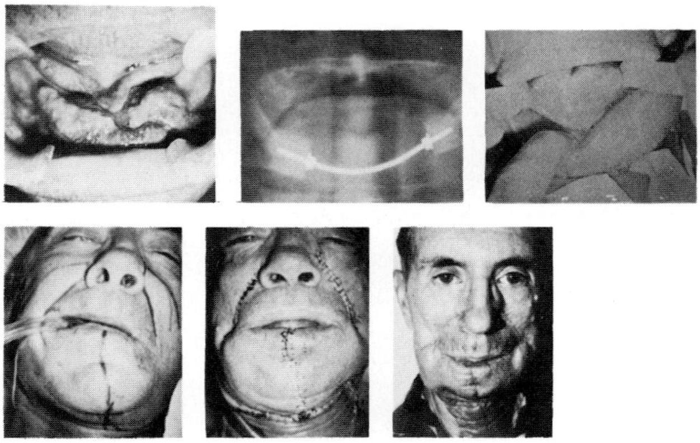

The donor site can give up to 3cms. in width with depth as needed. The scar falls within the naso-labial crease and becomes unnoticeable (Fig. 2).

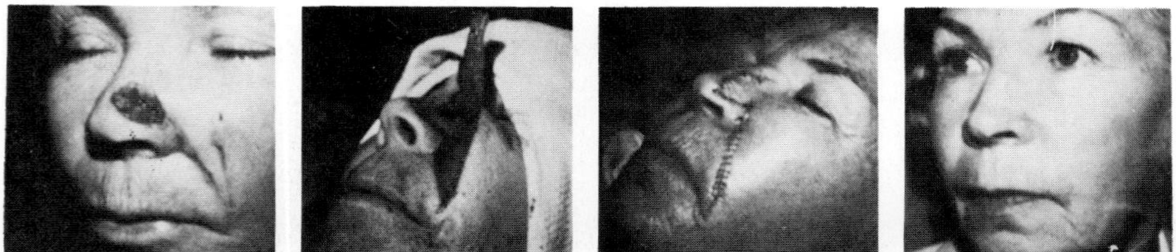

Figure 2. Large MOHS defect on nose. At three months no visible scar in naso-labial fold

Technique: The length of the flap is determined by the amount of tissue to be replaced. Its width depends upon the mobility of the patients cheek. The lateral borders should be kept as short as needed to give a greater base as well as safety and cosmesis. After undermining it is advanced to and matches its puzzlemate at the medial side. This is very important and should be the first maneuvre on rotating the NL flap (Fig. 3).

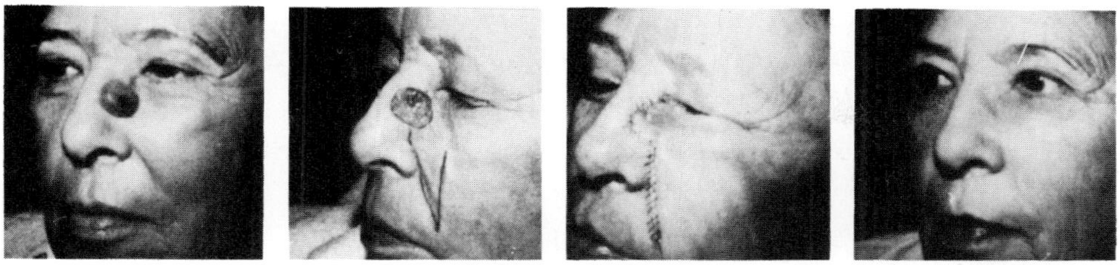

Figure 3. Large squamous cell excised. Lateral border rotated and meets medial puzzlemate with exact fit to prevent lateral bunching.

The medial area should be undermined as needed to give strong dermal-subdermal closure (5-0 Vicryl) and allow exact skin level match. A triangle above the defect may need to be excised to prevent buckling on rotating the flap. Once the lateral border is rotated and secured the donor site is closed. Remaining work is to match the trimming of the flap to the depth of the defect. Anchoring sutures of the deep tissue at the lateral borders of the flap secures the flap to the defect without comprising its vascularity and also prevents lateral bunching.

Figure 4. Large rim defect of nose from MOHS surgery. Flap is folded uner to provide good nasal rim and intranasal tissue.

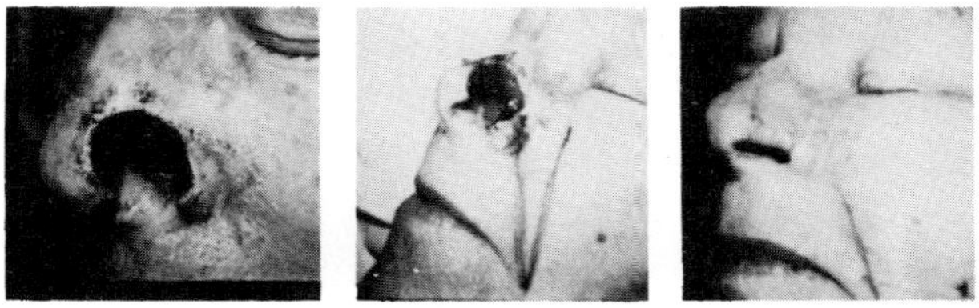

Figure 5. Patient with third recurrence of basal cell carcinoma with the entire tip and columella replaced by superiorly based naso-labial flap. Sectioned and set in at twelve days.

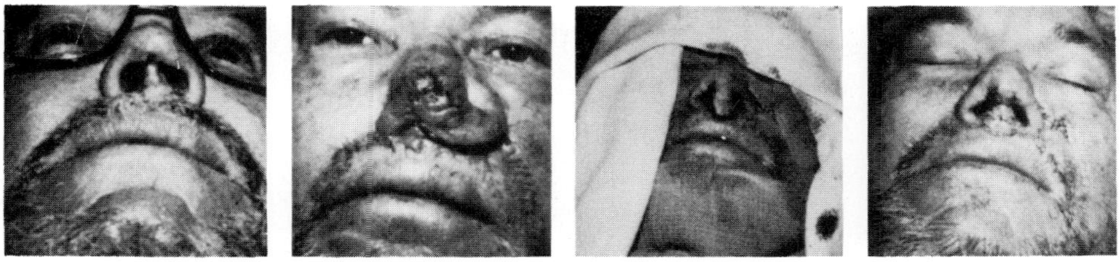

Figure 6. Patient with excision of a T2 squamous cell carcinoma of the right buccal mucosa with inferiorly based naso-labial flap used. The thickness of the defect in the buccal mucosa warranted a thick flap. The figure shows the post-operative appearance intra-orally and the only small residual dimple at the left labial commissure.

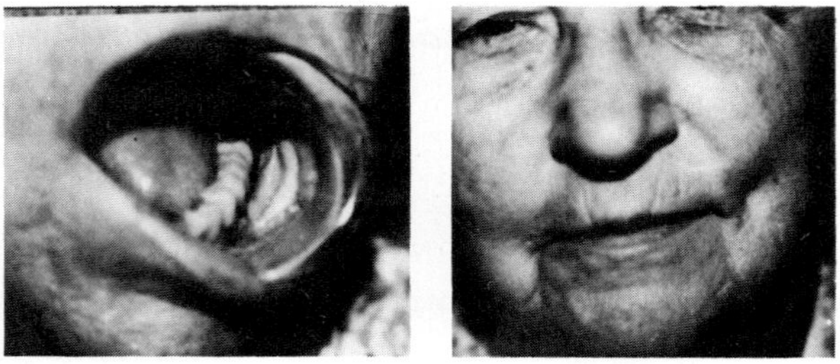

References:

1. Conley, John: Regional Flaps of the Head & Neck. W.B. Sanders Co., 1976.

New dimensions in otorhinolaryngology - head and neck surgery, vol. 2.
E. Myers, editor

DESIGN & CONSTRUCTION OF FACIAL FLAPS

Thomas C. Tyler, M.D., Venice, Fl.

Defects of the face (neck) are devastating to the patient and can be a perplexing challenge to the surgeon. Surgical goals after excision of lesions, should be reliability and cosmesis. At times when scars do not fall in corresponding crease lines, time, muscle, and gravity are all working in favor of the surgeon.

Langer's lines (natural crease lines) and the lines of maximum extension (LME), perpendicular to these, are the tools of facial flap reconstruction. Think of Langer's lines as the ribs of an accordion and the LME as the direction of the expansion of the accordion. The donor site is the most important expansion area in planning the flap. This is especially true with large flaps of the face. The LME's will change when dealing with a large area and this is the art connected with the science of flap construction (Fig.1).

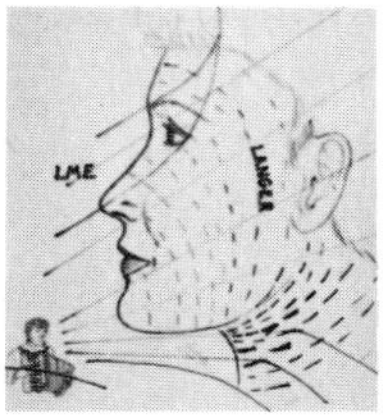

Fig. 1

The cervico-facial flap uses advancement and rotation of skin from the neck LME and the facial LME. Figure 2.

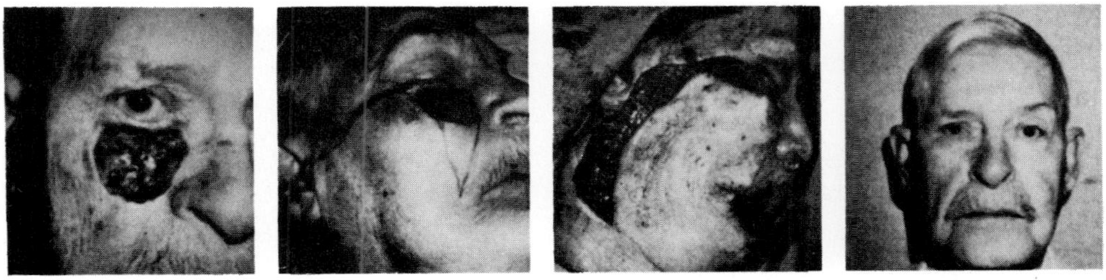

The Limberg or rhombic flap is a work-horse. The defect created is an equalateral parallelogram with angles of 60 & 120 degrees. The flap begins at one of the obtuse angles as an extension of and equal to the short diagonal of the defect. The third side is 60 degrees from this or parallel to the side of the defect and of the same length. It is usually directed at the LME of the defect unless because of the size to be covered it will be directed at the LME of the donor site (Fig. 4).

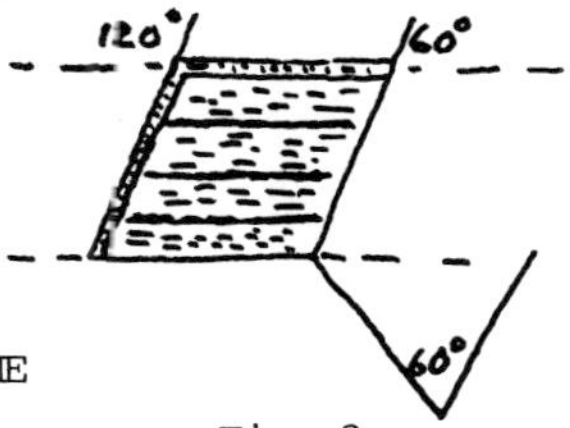

Fig. 3

Figure 4.
Large MOHS defect from recurrent basal cell carcinoma in scar.

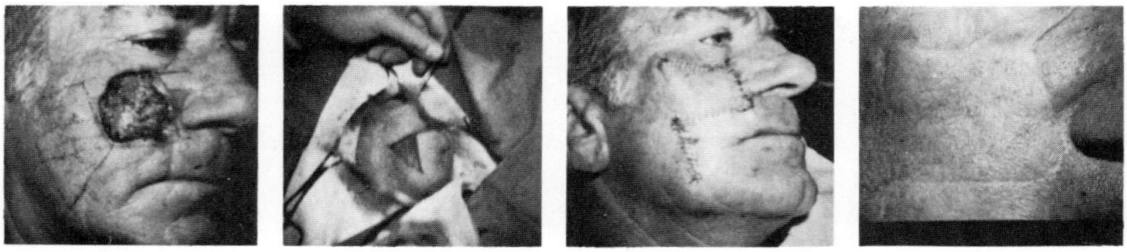

Figure 5.
For large lesions multiple rhombic flaps cane be developed using the same principle. Large bulky pushy squamous cell carcinoma of the right temple.

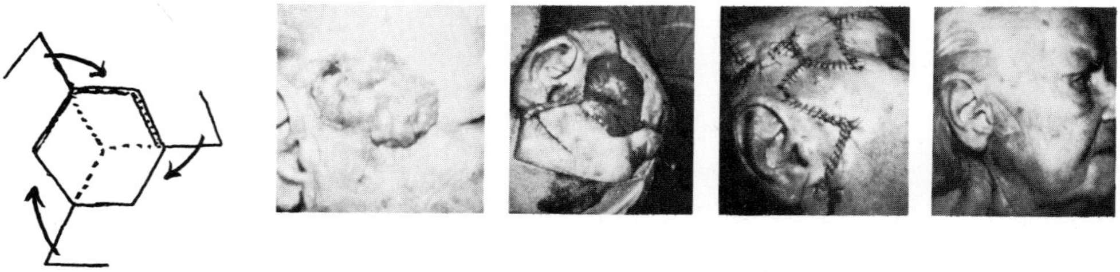

The Dufourmental Flap is used for rhombic defects of 60 to 90 degrees or more of a square. Orientation lines are drawn from the short diagonal of the defect and of the defect side of the donor flap. The third side is towards the LME drawn originally to the defect and parallel to the diagonal of the defect. Figure 6, shows both limberg and dufourmental approaches to the flap. Notice the flap is obtained from the donor area not the recipient area. This is a large infiltrated squamous cell carcinoma.

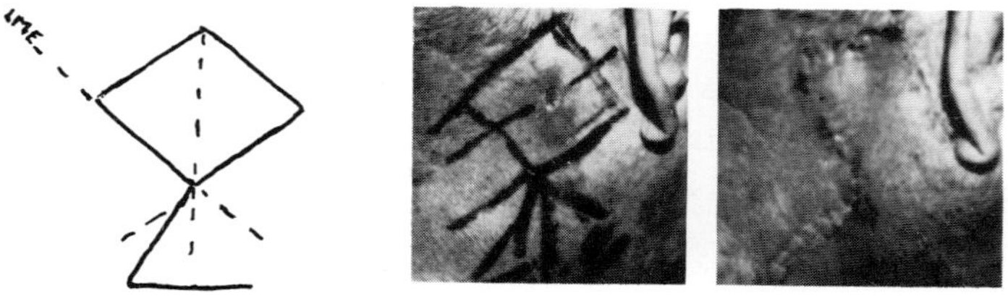

The rhombic to W flap can be used for areas where skin elasticity is less (nose, scalp, chin). It reduces scar contracture. The extensions for flap formation are equal to the long diagonal.

Figure 7.

Represents a large recurrent ulcerative basal cell.

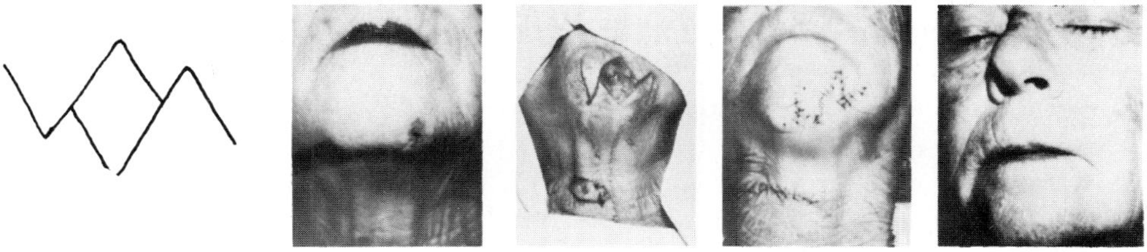

References:

1. Brobyn, T.J., et al: Facial Resurfacing with the Limberg Flap. Clinics in Plastic Surgery Vol. 3, No. 3, July 1976
2. Borges, A.F., The Rhombic Flap. Plast. Reconstr. Surg., Vol. 67 No. 4: 458, April 1981
3. Conley, John, Regional Flaps of the Head & Neck. W.B. Sanders Co. 1976.
4. Becker, H., The Rhomboid-20-W. Technique for Excision of Some Skin Lesions and Closure. Pl. Reconstr. Surg. 64.4:444, Oct. 79.

© 1985 Elsevier Science Publishers B.V. (Biomedical Division)
New dimensions in otorhinolaryngology - head and neck surgery, vol. 2.
E. Myers, editor

FIELD CANCERIZATION IN THE HYPOPHARYNX AND CERVICAL ESOPHAGUS

KATSUNORI UMATANI, TAKEO SATO, HIROSHI MIYAHARA, KUNITOSHI YOSHINO and YOSHIHIRO TSURUTA

Department of Otorhinolaryngology, The Center for Adult Diseases, Osaka, 3 Nakamichi 1-chome, Higashinari-ku, Osaka, 537 (Japan)

INTRODUCTION

The concept of multicentric cancer or field cancerization in the hypopharynx and cervical esophagus has not been accepted commonly, and a local recurrence may result from unrecognized multicentric cancer present at the time of the initial resection.

MATERIAL AND METHODS

11 cases of macroscopic field cancerization were found among 102 patients with squamous cell carcinoma of the hypopharynx and cervical esophagus from September, 1978 through November, 1983. Table I shows these 11 cases.

TABLE I

FIELD CANCERIZATION IN THE HYPOPHARYNX & CERVICAL ESOPHAGUS

Case No.	Age	Sex	B.I.	S.I.	Location	T N	Treatment	Follow-up
1	54	M	3400	330	PS	T2N1	RT	DOD, 1y4m
					Esophagus	T3N2	RT	
2	65	F	135	0	PC	T3N0	OP	NED, 6y1m
3	47	F	0	0	Hypopharynx	T4N1	OP	DOD, 1y6m
4	73	M	795	159	PS, Meso	T4N1	OP	NED, 4y1m, Local rec→RT
5	56	M	2880	108	PS	T3N3	RT→OP	DOD, 1y11m
					Floor of Mouth	T1N0	RT	
6	65	M	800	90	PC, PS	T2N1	OP→RT	DOD, 1y
7	56	M	1000	100	PS	T2N3	OP	AWD, 3y5m
					Esophagus	T3N0	RT	
8	87	M	3035	240	PS	T3N0	OP	DOD, 3y, Lung meta
					Ce	T1N0		
9	73	M	1590	135	PS	T2N3	OP→RT	DOD, 7m
10	58	M	925	135	Meso	T1N0	RT	DOD, 1y1m, Lung meta
					Ce	T3N0	RT	
11	58	M	950	84	PW	T2N3		
					Meso	T2N0	RT	NED, 1y9m
					Esophagus	T2N0		Local rec→OP

B.I.:Brinkman index, S.I.:Sake index, PS:Piriform sinus, PC:Postcricoid, PW:Posterior wall, Meso:Mesopharynx, Ce:Cervical esophagus, NED:No evidence of disease, AWD:Alive with disease, DOD:Dead of disease

RESULTS

The incidence of macroscopic field cancerization in the hypopharynx and cervical esophagus was high (10.8%). Typical cases of field cancerization are shown in Figure 1. Only one (Case 3) of the 11 cases of field cancerization was radiation-induced carcinoma, who developed squamous cell carcinoma of the hypopharynx and papillary adenocarcinoma of the thyroid 28 years after radiation therapy for tuberculous cervical adenitis. On the other hand, alcohol and tobacco abuse commonly coexisted in male patients developing field cancerization in the hypopharynx and cervical esophagus. It was suggested that the most significant carcinogen of the upper aerodigestive tract was alcohol and tobacco abuse and radiation. The esophagoscopy with Lugol's solution spraying method should be performed on cases of cancer of the hypopharynx and cervical esophagus, particularly if there was alcohol and tobacco abuse. Since unexpected local recurrences are mainly due to inadequate resection, the concept of field cancerization must be considered in surgical treatment.

We stressed the value of the esophagoscopy with Lugol's solution spraying method and the need for a careful long-term follow-up of these patients.

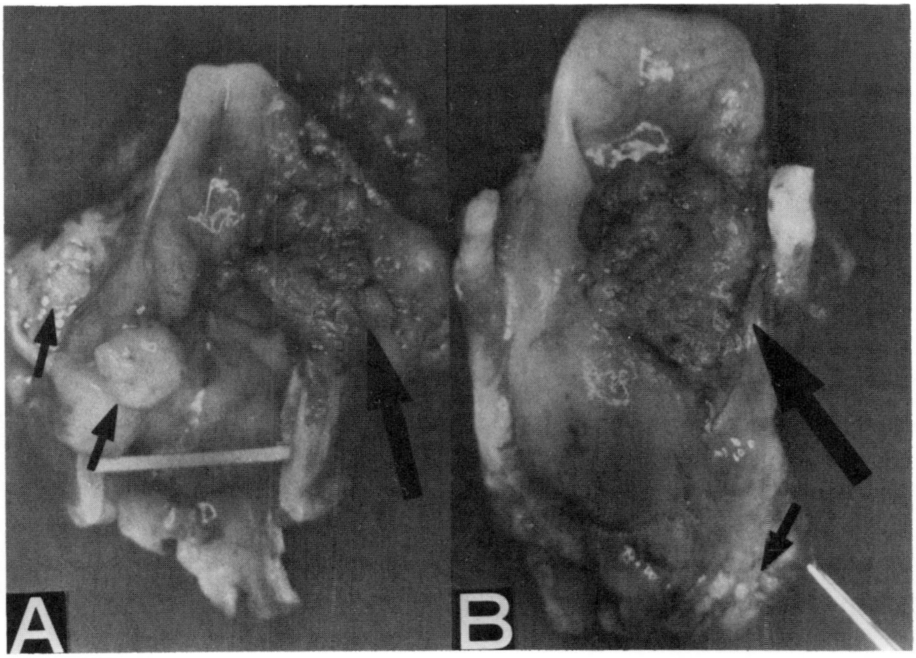

Fig. 1-A. Photograph of pharyngolaryngectomy specimen of Case 7. Note main tumor of the right piriform sinus (large arrow) and small tumors of the postcricoid and left piriform sinus (small arrow). B. Case 8. Note main tumor of the right piriform sinus (large arrow) and small tumor of the cervical esophagus (small arrow).

© 1985 Elsevier Science Publishers B.V. (Biomedical Division)
New dimensions in otorhinolaryngology - head and neck surgery, vol. 2.
E. Myers, editor

SQUAMOUS METAPLASIA OF THE SUPRAGLOTTIC REGION WITH REFERENCE TO SMOKING HABITS

KUNITOSHI YOSHINO, TAKEO SATO, HIROSHI MIYAHARA, KATSUNORI UMATANI and YOSHIHIRO TSURUTA
Department of Otolaryngology, The Center for Adult Diseases, Osaka, Japan

INTRODUCTION

Carcinoma arising in the supraglottic region of the larynx is almost always squamous cell type, although covered by ciliated pseudocolumnar epithelium (respiratory epithelium). Squamous metaplasia has been proposed to explain this apparent discrepancy. Cigarette smoking is considered to be one of the factors which may play a role in the potential malignant transformation. However, there are few clinical studies of a relationship between squamous metaplasia and cigarette smoking. In this study, the extent of squamous metaplasia of the supraglottic region was assessed and its relation to smoking was investigated.

MATERIALS AND METHODS

Larynges were obtained at autopsy or surgery. Larynges with carcinoma from subjects with history of irradiation were excluded. A total of 134 larynges were studied, 37 (24 males, 13 females) without and 97 (90 males, 7 females) with carcinoma. Eighteen non-smokers, who were all free from carcinoma, and 116 smokers were identified. The larynges were split in the sagittal plane posteriorly, fixed in 10% formal saline for more than one week, and stained by the pyronin Y method described by Stell (1,2).

RESULTS

According to the extent, the squamous metaplasia of the supraglottic region was classified macroscopically into the five types shown in Fig. 1.

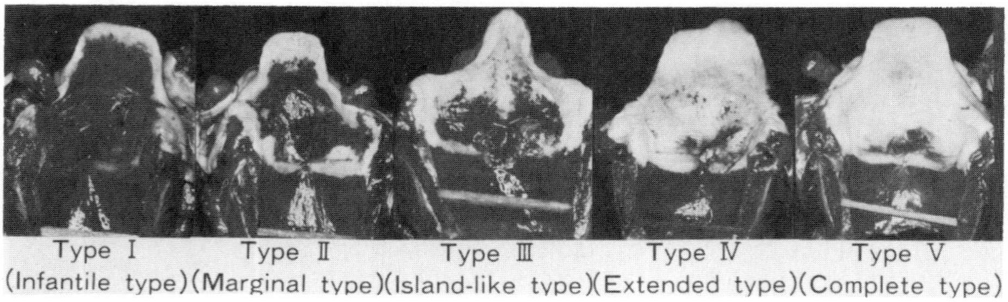

Fig. 1. Classification of squamous metaplasia of the supraglottic region.

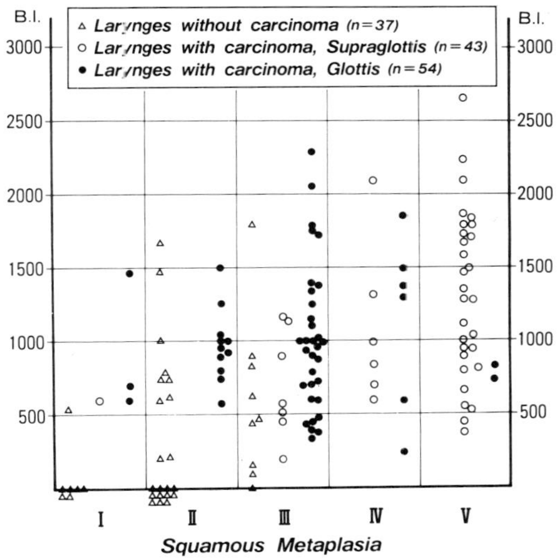

Fig. 2. A relationship between squamous metaplasia and Brinkman Index (B.I.).

The results are shown in Fig. 2.

Larynges without carcinoma

Their ages varied from 0 to 84 years. Eighteen non-smokers' larynges were examined to elucidate the effect of aging alone. With increasing age, the metaplasia tended to progress slightly; the representative metaplasia older than 40 years was type II. On the other hand, of the 19 smokers' specimens, 8 (42%) showed type III metaplasia, but no type IV or V. From these findings, it would appear that squamous metaplasia is progressed by aging to type II, and by addition of smoking habits to type III.

Larynges with carcinoma

All specimens were from smokers. Sixty-seven percent (29/43) of the supraglottis showed type V metaplasia. In contrast, 59% (32/54) of the glottis showed type III metaplasia. Brinkman Index of type V was significantly higher than that of type III ($P<0.001$). These results suggest that highly advanced squamous metaplasia of the supraglottic region should precede supraglottic carcinoma, and excessive smoking habits accelerate the metaplasia (squamous metaplasia as digestive tract) and cancerization.

REFERENCES

1. Stell PM, Gregory I and Watt J (1972) Techniques for demonstrating the epithelial lining of the larynx. J Laryngol Otol 86: 589-594
2. Watt J, Gregory I and Stell (1971) A simple method for the post-mortem demonstration of squamous metaplasia in the larynx. J Path 104: 149-151

New dimensions in otorhinolaryngology - head and neck surgery, vol. 2.
E. Myers, editor

SUSPENSION LARYNGOSCOPY : A RETROSPECTIVE STUDY

M. ENGLENDER, M. HARELL, J. HALEVI
Department of Otolaryngology, E. Wolfson Hospital, Holon 58100, Israel

INTRODUCTION

Suspension laryngoscopy which is nowadays a routine "minimal" surgical procedure all over the world, was described as such by Lynch in 1920 (1). Although Moore in 1921 (2) considers "intralaryngeal" removal of various growths as unsatisfactory procedures which "should be condemned", suspension laryngoscopy using the operation microscope is today widely accepted. This pioneer work is defined as "Naked Eye Laryngoscopy" since no microscope was available.

Despite today's widespread use of microlaryngoscopy there is a relative paucity of publication regarding its technique, results and complications. We only found one recent study (3) which deals with these topics. Most of the recent publications deal with laser (4) or even stroboscopic (5) microsurgery which are less commonly used techniques.

This is a retrospective study of 100 patients who underwent suspension microscopic laryngoscopy in our department, over the period of two years (1983-1984). Surprisingly, benign growths were found in almost equal numbers in male and female patients, while malignant and premalignant findings dominated in the male group (table 1).

TABLE I
LESIONS ACCORDING TO M/F DISTRIBUTION

	Males	Females	Total
Benign	33	37	70
Premalignant	9	4	13
Malignant	13	1	14
Total	55	42	97*

* 3 patients underwent suspension laryngoscopy for inspection only.

MATERIAL AND METHODS

One hundred patients underwent suspension microlaryngoscopy. Ninety-seven of them for organic lesions and only three for direct inspection of the larynx which was impossible on indirect examination. All of them had general anesthesia using the jet ventilation technique (6), which enables excellent relaxation and prevents interference of the endotracheal tube with the surgeon's view and access to the larynx. Fifty five patients were males and 45 were females. Their mean age was 46 years.

RESULTS

The most common clinical symptom was hoarsness (92%). One patient had hemoptysis, and one had a sensation of a foreign body. More than 60% were heavy smokers, or heavy users of alcohol. Vocal cord nodules were found in 30% of the patients, vocal polyps in 20%. There were 13 patients with premalignant lesions according to histological diagnosis. The only malignant histological diagnosis was squamous cell carcinoma of the larynx with a net male over female predominance (13:1).

DISCUSSION

In a retrospective analysis of 600 cases of microlaryngoscopy performed by Kleinsasser between 1964-1967, most of the patients were over 50 years old. Seventy five percent were males and 25% females (7). In our study the male to female ratio has diminished, with 55% males and 45% females. This correlates with the retrospective analysis of Pashcow and Mattucci (3). Patients mean age in our study was 46 years, i.e., four years younger than in Kleinsasser's study. This could be a reflection of the changes in social habits in modern society. We found a high incidence of cancer probably because all patients suspected of having chronic laryngitis or carcinoma underwent direct microlaryngoscopy and biopsy. Also our male to female ratio in cancer patients is twice as high as commonly reported (13 males and only one woman). This finding could be a result of the small number of cancer patients in this series.

REFERENCES

1. Lynch RC (1920) Trans Amer Laryngol Assn, pp 119-124
2. Moore I (1921) In: Intrinsic cancer of the larynx. London: University of London press, pp 13-18
3. Pashcow MS, Mattucci KF (1983) Int Surg, 68: 331-335
4. Ossoff RH, Karlan MS (1983) Otolaryngol Head & Neck Surg, 91: 456-460
5. Saito S, Fukuda H, Kitahara S (1975) Arch Otolaryngol 101: 196-201
6. Winerman I, Ezra S, Man A, Segal S (1982) Can Anaesth Soc K 29: 117-120
7. Kleinsasser O (1968) In: Microlaryngoscopy and endolaryngeal microsurgery 1st ed, Philadelphia, WB Saunders

New dimensions in otorhinolaryngology - head and neck surgery, vol. 2.
E. Myers, editor

FOREIGN BODIES IN THE AIRWAY AND FOOD PASSAGE STATISTICAL ANALYSIS OF 2,631 CASES

SHYH-FENG KO

Department of Otolaryngology, National Taiwan University Hospital, No. 1, Chang-Te Street, Taipei, Taiwan, Republic of China 100

INTRODUCTION

Gustav Killian removed a piece of bone from the human bronchus in 1897 and it was recognized as the first actual removal of a foreign body from the lower airway with a rigid endoscopic tube. He was credited as the one who first did successful work in bronchoscopy. Chevalier Jackson, on the other hand, contributed so much to the improvement of the instrumentation and development of bronchoesophagology to achieve the present high status of perfection. Though flexible fiber optic endoscopy has become safer and more comfortable procedure for diagnosis, rigid endoscopy still retains its place in the therapeutic bronchoesophagology for the removal of airway and esophageal foreign bodies by the otolaryngologist.

MATERIALS

This study comprises 2,631 cases of airway and esophageal foreign bodies treated at the Department of Otolaryngology, National Taiwan University Hospital from 1970 to 1984.

METHODS

All cases were reviewed in clinical data and course. The statistical analysis work was done and it showed an interesting and significant result.

RESULTS

Airway foreign bodies:

i. Total: 353 cases

ii. Annual average: 23.5 (353/15) cases

iii. Airway foreign bodies to total foreign bodies: 13.4% (353/2,631)

iv. Kinds of airway foreign bodies:

Peanut	173 cases	49.0%
Vegetable	103	29.2
Others	77	21.8

Esophageal foreign bodies:

i. Total: 2,278 cases

ii. Annual average: 151.9 (2,278/15) cases

iii. Esophageal foreign bodies to total foreign bodies: 86.6% (2,278/2,631)

iv. Kinds of esophageal foreign bodies:

Bone	999 cases	43.9%
Coin	591	25.9
Denture	67	2.9
Others	621	27.3

DISCUSSION

15-year period (1970-1984) at National Taiwan University Hospital:

i. Total endoscopies (laryngoscopy, bronchoscopy and esophagoscopy):8,158 cases

ii. Endoscopic removals of foreign body: 2,631 cases

Monthly distribution revealed two peaks:

The first: July-August

The second: December-January

Airway and esophageal foreign bodies nowadays can be safely removed through the rigid endoscope by a skilful otolaryngologist and the result is satisfactory. In this series, all cases were successfully treated and there was no mortality or severe complications.

CONCLUSION

The incidence of airway and esophageal foreign bodies was still high in Taiwan. Few complications were encountered. The contributory factors might include:

1. Undelayed seeking of medical help by the patient.
2. Skilful endoscopic removal and good care by the otolaryngologist.

REFERENCES

1. Jackson and Jackson (1950): Bronchoesophagology. W.B. Saunders Co., Philadelphia and London.
2. Hung WC (1953): Foreign bodies in airway and food passages. Arch Otolaryngol 57:603-612.
3. Kuo BWF (1971): Bronchoesophagology in Taiwan — a statistical study. JOSROC* 6:79-115.
4. Lee SY (1973): Endoscopy at ENT Department, 2 years' statistical report at NTUH. JOSROC* 8:49-60.
5. Kuo BWF (1965): Airway foreign bodies-a series of 85 cases. The Journal of the Formosan Medical Association 64:512-527.
6. Lee SY (1983): Peanut in the tracheobronchial tree. JOSROC* 18:39-45.

* JOSROC : The Journal of Otolaryngological Society of the Republic of China

© 1985 Elsevier Science Publishers B.V. (Biomedical Division)
New dimensions in otorhinolaryngology – head and neck surgery, vol. 2.
E. Myers, editor

HYDRON GEL IMPLANTS IN VOCAL CORDS

Z.KRESA, J.REMS AND O.WICHTERLE
From the Department of Otorhinolaryngology, Faculty of Medicine, Charles University, Plzeň, and the Institute of Macromolecular Chemistry, Czechoslovak Academy of Sciences, Prague, Czechoslovakia

In this communication we would like to describe a new operational method for vocal cord adjustment in the case of insufficient closure of the glottis.

The method consists in introducing a shaped implant of hydrophilic gel, dried to a glassy-hard state, into the vocal cord. The operation is performed in total endotracheal anaesthesia in direct laryngoscopy according to Kleinsasser. The mucosa of the upper surface of the vocal cord is incised transversally at the length of about 2 mm (about 2 mm in front of the insertion of the processus vocalis), all this being done under the operational microscope. With the help of special instruments a submucosal tunnel is made in the upper surface of the vocal cord, as near as possible to its free edge. The implant is then slid into this tunnel, swells within a short time and becomes a highly elastic soft matter. As the volume of the implant swells and becomes similar to the elasticity and other properties of the surrounding tissue, it is fixed in vocal cord. After swelling the implant permits the penetration of water and of small molecules and ions, disolved in the surrounding tissues and in body fluids. Nutrients and metabolites can then pass through the gel from one tissue into another. This merit makes this gel basically different from all other plastics.

Implants for vocal cords are made of modified Hydron with swelling capacity of 130 - 140% (for vocal muscle atrophy) and 200% (for recurrent nerve paralysis). Hydron was developed in the Institute of Macromolecular Chemistry the Czechoslovak Academy of Sciences Prague in 1955 for medical purposes. This biomedical material has been used since late 60th in opthalmological and other medical applications and approved for these applications by medical authorities in most countries (for example soft contact lenses are made of Hydron). By choosing specific conditions of synthesis the structure of this substance was intentionally made such as to allow of its long-term deposition in living tissue.

The implants can be used unilaterally (in patients with recurrent nerve paralysis or vocal muscle atrophy), or bilaterally (in patients with atrophy of the vocal muscle), exceptionally two or three implants in one vocal cord can be used (in patients with recurrent nerve paralysis at large insufficiency of the glottis).

On the whole 64 implantations in 50 patients have been carried out during the period of 14 years - in the Department of Otorhinolaryngology, Faculty of Medicine, Charles University, Plzeň (in 37 patients with the atrophy of the vocal muscle and in 13 patients with the paralysis of the recurrent nerve).

After the implantation of a hydrophilic gel (the implants are 6,7,8,9 and 10 mm long, with swelling capacity of 130 - 140% and 200%), a practically normal shape of the vocal cords was restituted anatomically in all cases. The edge of the vocal cords was reinforced, the excavation levelled, the mass increased and the closure of the glottis improved. These results were reflected objectively in a improved quality of the voice, an increase in the voice volume and in an extended phonation time; subjectively, the patients reported a decrease or even complete disappeareance of vocal fatiguability.

The vibration of the vocal cords remained preserved in all cases after the operation, but in patients with two or three implants in one vocal cord (in patients with recurrent nerve paralysis at large insufficiency of the glottis) were atypical and irregular vibrations. The sonagraphis examination performed both before and after operation detected objectively improved voice, disappeareance of secondary noise and better visualisation of the main formants of the vowel ("ah" in this case).

No complications could be observed after the operation. Up to present day, i.e. after more than 14 years time after the operation the vocal cords of all patients operated on have been completely calm and their function has been preserved within the range mentioned above.

References - at the first author:

Zdeněk KRESA, M.D., Head of the Phoniatric Department,
Faculty of Medicine, Charles University Plzeň,
Sokolovská Street 77, PLZEŇ , 323 14 Czechoslovakia

New dimensions in otorhinolaryngology - head and neck surgery, vol. 2.
E. Myers, editor

THE RELATIONSHIP BETWEEN XEROSTOMIA AND RADIOTHERAPY IN NPC PATIENTS

PING CHANG, JAU-EN CHERN
Department of Otolaryngology, Veteran General Hospital
Taipei, Taiwan, R.O.C.

INTRODUCTION

Nasopharyngeal carcinoma (NPC) is the most common malignant disease in Otolaryngology at VGH, Taipei. It constituted 57.03% of all Malignancies and was on the top in Otolaryngology. (TABLE I) Radiotherapy is the first choice for treatment of NPC. There are many complications in using radiotherapy for NPC patients; xerostomia is one of them and is a long-standing trouble for these patients.

TABLE I MALIGNANCIES OF OTOLARYNGOLOGY AT VGH TAIPEI

	1975	1976	1977	1978	1979	1980	1981	1982	Total	%
Ears	1	4	2	2	1	0	1	0	11	0.49
Nose	6	4	7	11	8	5	8	8	57	2.55
Sinuses	13	13	17	23	15	13	18	17	129	5.78
Tongue	14	13	15	18	19	26	17	21	143	6.41
Floor of M.	3	2	0	5	4	6	0	3	23	1.03
Oropharynx	10	13	20	25	25	22	20	31	166	7.44
Tonsil	7	5	4	6	6	11	7	13	64	2.87
Hypopharynx	2	7	3	11	11	11	11	18	68	3.05
Larynx	20	22	24	37	37	46	48	56	298	13.35
Nasopharynx	131	131	155	159	180	185	182	150	1273	57.03
Total	207	214	247	297	313	325	312	317	2232	

MATERIAL AND METHODS

Patients

From April to Sep. in 1983, we selected admitted patients for this study. They were divided into two gruops. Group I consisted of 8 NPC patients, they received radiotherapy by using Co 60, with a tumor dose of 200 rads per day, 5 days a week and a total of 7000 rads in 7 weeks. Saliva was collected pre-, intra-, and post-radiotherapy. Group II consisted of 7 patients with ear and nasal diseases, they were not treated by radiotherapy and used as control.

Methods

Using a series of larcrimal duct probes inserted into the orifices of Wharton's and Stensen's ducts and dilated gradually after surface anesthesia. And then two segments of polyethylene tubes, #3 or #4 were put into each duct. we dripped a few drops of 5% citric acid solution on the surface of the tongue every 5 minutes for 6 times to stimulate salivary secretion, and collected the saliva through the inserted tubes. If there was no saliva after 30 minutes that was considered as negative.

RESULT

The salivary flow of non-radiotherapy patients showed about 2-11.2 cc in 15 minutes. The initial salivary flow in NPC patients showed a little bit lower than the control. Successive salivary flows were checked after each 1000 rads irradiaation, but no more saliva could be collected since then after 1000 rads irradiation and 6 months after radiotherapy. (TABLE II)

TABLE II SALIVARY FLOW PRE-, INTRA-, POST-RADIOTHERAPY

Pts.	Pre-R/T	1000 rad	2000 rad	3000 rad	4000 rad	5000 rad	6000 rad	7000 rad	6 M. Post-R/T
1	-	-	-	0	0	0	0	0	0
2	-	0	0	0	0	0	0	0	0
3	1.5	0	0	-	-	0	0	0	0
4	1.4	0	0	0	F	0	0	0	-
5	2.0	0	0	0	0	0	0	0	0
6	F	0	0	-	0	0	0	0	-
7	2.1	0	0	-	0	0	0	0	-
8	3.2	0	0	0	-	-	0	0	0

F= failure of saliva collection

DISCUSSION AND CONCLUSION

We know the saliva has anticarriogenic function. If a patient with dental carries undergoes radiotherapy, this tooth gradually decays and this leads to osteoradionecrosis of the jaw. So we always suggest the proved NPC patient has his dental condition checked and all diseased teeth extracted prior to radiotherapy. Shannon and Cheng et al., their reports supported our result: the salivary glands will loss their function following irradiation. Pratt et al., used WR-2721 to protect salivary glands of rats with good result. But it is still too early to apply this to human-beings.

It is clear that salivary glands will produce no saliva after radiotherapy in NPC patients. Xerostomia is inevitalbe in their later days. Fortunately, Shannon formulated an artificial saliva to relieve the dryness of the mouth with encouraging results.

REFERENCES

1. Cheng VST et al (1981) The function of the parotid gland following radiation therapy for head and neck cancer. Int. J. Radiation Oncology Biol. Phys. 7: 253-258
2. Pratt, NE et al (1980) Radioprotection of the rat parotid gland by WR-2721. Int. J. Radiation Oncology Biol. Phys. 6:431-435
3. Shannon, IL et al (1977) A saliva substitute for use by xerostomic patients undergoing radiotherapy to the head and neck. Oral Surg. 44:656

New dimensions in otorhinolaryngology - head and neck surgery, vol. 2.
E. Myers, editor

CANCER OF THE NASOPHARYNX (N.P.C.)

GEORGE CHOA
Honorary Lecturer in E.N.T., Department of Surgery, University of Hong Kong.
Room 1608 Hang Seng Bank Building, Central, HK

INTRODUCTION

Cancer of the nasopharynx is a squamous carcinoma, common in the Southern Chinese, less common in Alaskan and Canadian Eskimos, Greenlanders, and certain groups in South East Asia and Southern Africa, but least common in Caucasians. It is one of the most difficult tumours to detect early. It arises in an area of the body which is notoriously difficult to examine. The lateral pharyngeal recess, for example, is often not visible because it can be slit-like, deep, and crossed by fibrous trabeculae. Cancer in situ arising from the depth of the recess will therefore escape detection by the examiner. Hence if one is to make an early diagnosis, that is, at Stage I (Tl NO) all physicians should be fully aware of the disease no matter how uncommon it may be in his community. In Hong Kong where there are over 12,000 cases on file in the Department of Radiotherapy and Oncology of the Queen Elizabeth Hospital, Kowloon, only about 10% of the cases examined and treated were at Stage I.

SYMPTOMS

(1) a foreign body sensation in the nasopharynx, this being due to a swollen area, not necessarily ulcerated. This discomfort makes the patient try to get rid of it by forcible sniffing (hawking).

(2) a sense of fullness in one ear, with or without tinnitus. This discomfort is due to blockage of the Eustachian tube (E.T.) by edema, a consequence of sepsis or the infiltration of tumour around the medial end of the E.T. The finding of fluid in the middle ear often follows. Actual invasion of the E.T. is extremely rare. The author has seen only one such case in a Caucasian and that was nearly 30 yeasrs ago while he was studying in London.

(3) blood in the post-nasal drip, no matter how little or intermittent, is significant. The blood is an indication of ulceration but the ulcer may be very small and difficult to detect on nasopharyngoscopy.

(4) morning cough with blood tinged sputum, the blood having trickled into the trachea in the course of the night.

Having obtained a history of one or more of the above symptoms, a thorough investigation into the possibility of the disease must be carried out. This must include a clinical examination and blood serology, the latter to study the titre of the patient's serum antibodies, especially IgA, against the Epstein Barr Virus (E.B.V.) antigens. Routine x-rays of the skull to include the naso-pharynx, base of skull and the chest are also carried out.

SIGNS

The nasopharynx is difficult to examine. Local anaesthesia and retraction of the soft palate may be required. Fiber-optic endoscopy is an added tool. A very careful search must be made for the following changes:

(1) swelling at the cartilaginous end of the Eustachian tube (TORUS) which forms the anterior boundary of the lateral pharyngeal recess,

(2) an elevated area in any part of the nasopharynx. Look carefully for changes especially in the vicinity of the lateral pharyngeal recess,

(3) presence of blood clots - this signifies ulceration,

(4) distortion of the normal pattern of the adenoids in young adults,

(5) fluid in the middle ear,

(6) signs of infection without nasal pathology,

(7) the actual presence of an ulcerated area.

VIROLOGY

The presence of IgA antibody against the viral antigens is an outstanding feature of N.P.C. These antibodies are detected in the serum from 95% of N.P.C. patients but rarely in healthy subjects or patients with other cancers. Such antibodies thus provide a convenient means, a marker, to assist in the diagnosis of the disease.

The following tests are routinely done:

IgA - VCA (viral capsid antigen)
95% positive in N.P.C.
5% in healthy subjects
1 : 10 diagnostic
IgA - E.A. (early antigen)
1 : 5 positive

RADIOLOGY

In suspected cases supporting evidence may be provided by radiology, routine x-ray views used are the lateral, submento-vertical, occipito-submental, 25° occipito-mental and 25° occipito-frontal.

The sub-mental vertical projection is particularly valuable in demonstrating any changes in the lateral pharyngeal recess.

If plain x-rays are not helpful, a C.T. Scan should be done. A scan has the following advantages:

(1) soft tissues can be well defined, especially the parapharyngeal spaces,

(2) asymetry can usually be seen,

(3) infiltration of the brain by tumour can be observed,

(4) sub-epithelial tumour tissue can be demonstrated, often more extensive than the naked eye can observe,

(5) there is better definition of bone at the base of the skull.

SUMMARY

Cancer of the nasopharynx is seldom diagnosed early for the following reasons:

(1) The lack of awareness of the disease amongst primary care physicians particularly in parts of the world where the disease is not common.

(2) The lack of concrete symptoms and signs of an early tumour.

This would be particularly so if the neoplasm is submucosal.

(3) Nasopharyngoscopy is a difficult procedure. In addition, there are anatomical barriers which prohibit a thorough examination of the nasopharynx, especially hidden areas like the lateral pharyngeal recess (Fossa of Roseumuller).

(4) The detection of EBV antigens in the serum of patients is helpful in making an early diagnosis,

(5) Supportive evidence by radiology is valuable.

REFERENCES

1) CHOA, G. Cancer of the Nasopharynx in Cancer of the Head and Neck, Chapter XVI, edited by James Y. Suen and Eugene N. Myers, Churchill Livingstone N.Y. Edinburgh, London and Melbourne 1981.

2) STEIN, W. Advances in Endoscopic Diagnosis of Nasopharyngeal Carcinomas. Grundmann et al. (eds): Cancer Campaign. Vol. 5 Naso-pharyngeal Carcinoma Gustav Fischer Verlag. Stuttgart. New York. 1981.

3) NG, M.H. Professor and Head, Department of Micro-biology, University of Hong Kong. Personal Communications.

New dimensions in otorhinolaryngology – head and neck surgery, vol. 2.
E. Myers, editor

INCIDENCE OF NASOPHARYNGEAL MALIGNANT GROWTH (N.P.M.) AND LOCK-JAW AS BIZARRE PRESENTATION

DR.S.K. DE.

INTRODUCTION

Nasopharynx is aptly called the "silent area of cancer".The bizarre presentations of N.P.M.are due to its hidden position,extensive lymphatic supply, anatomical relations and natural pathways of spread. In this paper the incidence and the significant aspects of N.P.M. in this sub-continent and lock-jaw trismus as bizarre presentation have been reported.

MATERIAL AND METHODS

The paper is based on clinicopathological study of 80 cases of N.P.M.seen between 1966 and 1984. Age incidence among the patients are particularly noted and various presenting features are recorded and grouped into various presentations. Symptomatology and features in lock-jaw cases in particular are recorded. Various investigations are carried out to arrive at the diagnosis in these bizarre presentations.

OBSERVATIONS

Total No.of N.P.M.observed during the period was 80 cases. Sex incidence shows : Male 68 cases (85%), Female 12 cases (15%).Age incidence is shown as per table No.1.

TABLE - 1
Age incidence in N.P.M.growth

Age Group	No.	Percentage
Below 30 years	37 cases	46.25%
Above 30 years	43 cases	53.75%

Various presentations of N.P.M.are shown in table No.2

TABLE - 2
Presenting features in N.P.M.(80 cases)

Presentations	No.of cases	Percentage
Cervical	45 cases	51.25%
Rhinological	20 "	25%
Otological	2 "	2.5%
Neurological	5 "	6.25%
Ophthalmological	2 "	2.5%
Lock-jaw	6 "	7.5%

Cervical presentation was observed in highest number of cases (51.25%). An uncommon bizarre presenting feature eg.lock-jaw was seen in 6 cases as primary and 3 cases as associated feature. The associated features in lock-jaw presentation were restricted mobility of the soft palate, facial pain,occasional epistaxis and cervical metastasis in some cases.

DISCUSSION

Incidence - It has long been recognised that the N.P.M. is prevalent among Mongolian races, but it is found that incidence of this malignant growth is quite common in this sub-continent. Several authors of different parts of India have presented series on N.P.M.-Rao (1966) reviewed 48 cases ; Sinha et al (1969) 49 cases ; Taneja et al (1963) 29 cases. This series (1985) presents 80 cases from Eastern India.

Age incidence - One significant aspect in this series is the large number of cases of N.P.M. in the lower age group (below 30 years) ie. 46.25%. Clifford et al (1963) reported 29 years as the average age. Reports from western countries, Ledermann (1961). Dawes(1969) Friedmann (1968) mentioned incidence of lower age group below 10%. From this it can be concluded that the N.P.M. in Afro-Asian countries is more common in younger age group than in West.

Presentations : N.P.M. may show different bizarre presentations, such as cervical, rhinological, ophthalmological, neurological and otological. Cervical presentation is the commonest presentation (51.25%) as shown in table No.1. In addition to the common presentations "Lock-jaw" as primary bizarre presentation has been seen in 6 cases and as associated feature in 3 cases. This is a comparatively new feature of N.P.M. reported by few authors as shown in table 3.

TABLE - 3

Lock-jaw as presenting feature in N.P.M.

Authors	Primary presentation	Associated feature
Clifford et al (1963)	Nil	4 cases
Sinha et al (1969)	1 case	4 "
This series	6 cases	3 "

Mode of spread in Lock-jaw cases : It spreads around the Eustachian tube from the primary site in the fossa of Rosenmuller and first involves the muscles of the soft palate causing restricted mobility and asymmetry of the soft palate. Then it involves the deep muscles of mastication (Med.pterygoid) and 3rd division of 5th cranial nerve resulting in trismus and hemifacial pain.

Diagnosis in Lock-jaw presentation : is confirmed by -

a) Nasopharyngoscopy, b) Cytology, c) Biopsy and histopathology.

REFERENCES :

1. Clifford P et al. Brit.Med.J. : 1, 1256, 1963.
2. Dawes J.D.K. et al. J.Laryng.Vol.83 211, 1969.
3. Digby K.H.,Ann.Roy.Col.Surg.Engl. 9, 253,1951.
4. Friedmann I. ; Proc.Can.Otolaryng.Soc., 22, 1968.
5. Lederman M.: Cancer of the Nasopharynx,Springfield, 111, 1961.
6. Rao P.B.: Cancer of the Nasopharynx. J.Laryng. 80, 151, 1966.
7. Sinha A.,Abrol B.M.,Gupta S.N.;Ind.J.Otolaryng. 21,17,1969.

New dimensions in otorhinolaryngology – head and neck surgery, vol. 2.
E. Myers, editor

EPSTEIN-BARR VIRUS EARLY ANTIGEN INDUCTION IN NASOPHARYNGEAL HYBRID CELLS BY CHINESE MEDICINAL HERBS

MITSURU FURUKAWA TAKASHI KOMORI RYOZO UMEDA
Department of Otorhinolaryngology, School of Medicine, Kanazawa University, 13-1 Takara-machi, Kanazawa 920 (Japan)

INTRODUCTION

Cancer of the nasopharynx(NPC) is one of the most important cancers in Chinese population. Zeng and coworkers(1) showed that the geometric mean titer of complement-fixing antibody to Epstein-Barr virus(EBV) in sera from persons aged 20 years and older in high-risk areas for NPC was significantly higher than that from persons of the same age group in NPC low-risk areas, and that the positive rate of IgA/VCA(viral capsid antigen) antibody to EBV from normal individuals in NPC high-risk areas increasing with increasing age. These data indicate that EBV is more active in persons living in NPC high-risk areas, as a result of the activation of EBV by internal and environmental factors.

Recently, we have described the establishment of EBV infection in epithelial cells derived from the nasopharynx by cell fusion of lymphoblastoid cell line originating from the adenoidal lymphocytes carring the EBV genomes(2). Using this cells we report herein the EBV activations in some of the Chinese medicinal herbs.

MATERIAL AND METHODS

Cells. Nasopharyngeal hybrid cell line, A2L/AH cells were cultured in Eagle's minimum essential medium supplemented with 10% fetal calf serum. The medium was removed and replaced with 5ml of Eagle's medium containing varied concentration of plant extraction.

Chinese medicinal herbs. Daphne genkwa, Wikstroemia indica and Croton oil were kindly supplyed from Dr. Yan Sun, Cancer Institute, Chinese Academy of Medical Sciences.

Plant extraction. The method for ether and water extraction was followed by Dr. Ito's method(3).

Immunofluorescent test. Induction of EBV-early antigen(EA) was assayed by indirected immunofluorescent test. EA-positive cells were detected by staining cell smears with EA(+), VCA(+) serum [anti EA-IgG antibody titer, 1 : 320, anti VCA-IgG antibody titer, 1 : 1280].

RESULTS

The EBV-EA inducing ability was found in both ether and water extracts from all of the test materials. Their activity was much greater in cells from ether extracts than in those from water extracts under the same experimental conditions. The EA-positive rate was from 18.2 to 42.2% in ether extracts and 1.0 to 3.8% in water extracts respectively at 10 μg/ml of the concentrations. The EA-positive rate of n-butyrate alone was about 40% , and it was the same as that found in 10 μg of the ether extract in Daphne genkwa which is commonly used as a purgative drug. The EA inducing ability of the water extract was considerably lower than that of n-butyrate. However, when a combined treatment of n-butyrate and water extract was examined, an increasing effect was seen (Table 1.)

TABLE I

EFFECT OF CHINESE MEDICINAL HERBS ON EBV-EA INDUCTION IN A2L/AH CELLS (percent of EA-positive cells)

	Ether extraction		Water extraction		
Medicinal herbs	10 μg/ml	1 μg/ml	10 μg/ml	5 μg/ml	10 μg/ml with SnB
Daphne genkwa	42.2	4.6	3.8	2.2	50.4
Wikstroemia indica	32.4	3.0	3.4	2.2	40.4
Croton oil	18.2	1.2	1.0	0.4	46.6
		< 0.1			
Control	4 mM SnB(Sodium n-Butyrate) alone showed a 40.2% positive rate				

Based on our current work, we conclude that nasopharyngeal carcinoma may be initiated by chronic EB-virus infections as a result of the activation of EB-virus genomes through the intake of promoter substances such as extracts from th Euphorbiaceae plants resulting in the appearance of cancerous cells. The resons for the appearance of tumors only in the nasopharynx are not yet clear.

REFERENCES

1. Zeng Y. Liu YX, Liu ZY, Zhen SW, Wei JN, Zhu JS, Zai HJ(1979) Chinese J Oncol 1: 2-7
2. Takimoto T, Furukawa M, Hatano M, Umeda R (1984) Annals of Otol Rhinol Laryngol 93: 166-169
3. Ito Y, Yanase S, Fujita J, Hirayama T, Takashima M, Imanaka H (1981) Cancer Lett 13: 29-37

© 1985 Elsevier Science Publishers B.V. (Biomedical Division)
New dimensions in otorhinolaryngology - head and neck surgery, vol. 2.
E. Myers, editor

EB VIRUS ANTIBODIES AND LYMPHOCYTE SUBSETS IN NASOPHARYNGEAL CARCINOMA BEFORE AND AFTER RADIATIONTHERAPY

TSONG-CHOU LYNN AND SHIH-MIEN TU
Department of Otolaryngology, National Taiwan University Hospital, Taipei, Taiwan, ROC

Epstein-Barr virus(EBV)-associated antibodies and lymphocyte subsets were studied in 108 patients with nasopharyngeal carcinoma(NPC) and 34 normal controls.

The EBV-associated antibodies were titrated by indirect fluorescent antibody (IFA) method using P3HR-1 cells as the source of viral capsid antigens(VCA) and Raji cells induced by IUdR as the source of early antigens(EA). Before radiationtherapy, mean antibody titers and seropositive rates were significantly increased in NPC patients than in controls; for anti-VCA/IgG, 1:502 vs 1:87, and 68.5% vs 5.9%, respectively, for anti-VCA/IgA, 1:40 vs 1:1.8, and 66.7% vs 2.9%, respectively, for anti-EA/IgG, 1:123 vs 1:2.2, and 64.8% vs 0%, for anti-EA/IgA, 1:12 vs 1:1.0, and 45.4% vs 0%, respectively. The increase in antibodies was positively correlated with disease extent of NPC, but was not correlated with the sex, age, total lymphocyte counts, helper/suppressor ratio, and WBC counts of NPC patients.

Lymphocyte subsets were identified with monoclonal antibodies (Ortho Co.) by IFA method, too. Before radiationtherapy, the helper T lymphocytes(OKT_4^+) in NPC patients comprised 38.2 ± 10.5% which was significantly different from 45.8 ± 8.0% in controls.

The helper/suppressor ratio in NPC patients was 1.33 ± 0.65 which was significantly different from 1.64 ± 0.48 in controls. But this ratio was not correlated with the disease extent, sex, age, total lymphocyte counts, WBC counts and EBV-associated antibodies of NPC patients.

The percentages of B lymphocytes($OKIa^+$, 12.8 ±4.6%), total T lymphocytes(OKT_3^+, 68.7 ± 9.6%), suppressor lymphocytes(OKT_8^+, 32.2 ± 8.6%), and total lymphocyte counts (2541 ± 905) and WBC counts (8385 ± 2811) in NPC patients were not significantly different from those of controls.

After radiationtherapy, the mean EBV-associated antibody titers in the four classes were decreased significantly to about half value of those before treatment (Table I). On the other hand, the helper cells decreased remarkably to 27.2 ± 9.6%, and the suppressor cells increased remarkably to 36.8 ± 13.0%, resulting in the significant decrease of helper/suppressor ratio to 0.88 ± 0.53 (Table II).

It is concluded that in NPC patients, EBV-associated antibody titers were significantly increased and helper cells were significantly decreased than normal controls before radiationtherapy. After radiationtherapy, both the EBV-associated antibody titers and helper cells decreased singificantly as compared with those before radiationtherapy. Therefore, the humoral antibody system and T lymphocyte system operated independently in NPC patients.

TABLE I

EBV ANTIBODIES IN NPC PATIENTS BEFORE AND AFTER RADIATIONTHERAPY

	No. of Patients	Anti-VCA antibodies				Anti-EA antibodies			
		IgG		IgA		IgG		IgA	
		GMT	% ≥1:640	GMT	% ≥1:40	GMT	% ≥1:160	GMT	% ≥1:40
Before R/T	51	1:382	62.7	1:30	64.7	1:95	62.7	1:8	39.2
After R/T	51	1:194	43.1	1:17	51.0	1:53	47.1	1:6	29.4
Control	34	1: 87	5.9	1:1.8	2.9	1:2.2	0	1:1	0

EBV: Epstein-Barr virus
NPC: nasopharyngeal carcinoma
VCA: viral capsid antigens(EBV)
EA : early antigens(EBV)
GMT: geometric mean titer
R/T: radiationtherapy

TABLE II

DISTRIBUTION OF OKT4^{+}/OKT8^{-} RATIO IN NPC PATIENTS BEFORE AND AFTER RADIATION-THERAPY

T4/T8 ratio	Patients with nasopharyngeal carcinoma(NPC)					
	Before R/T			After R/T		
	No.	%		No.	%	
0.10-0.20	0	0		3	4.3	
0.21-0.79	9	13.0		33	47.8	
0.80-1.19	23	33.3		20	29.0	
1.20-1.59	19	27.5	53.5	6	8.7	18.8
1.60-1.99	7	10.1		2	2.9	
2.0 -3.20	11	15.9		5	7.2	
Total	69	100.0		69	100.0	

© 1985 Elsevier Science Publishers B.V. (Biomedical Division)
New dimensions in otorhinolaryngology - head and neck surgery, vol. 2.
E. Myers, editor

SYSTEMATIZATION OF NASOPHARYNGEAL TISSUE

JOSE ROMEU

E.N.T. Department, University of Barcelona.
Dr. Roux Street, 127. 08017 Barcelona (Spain)

MATERIAL AND METHODS

This study was conducted on the entire nasopharynx tissue of 15 subjects whose ages ranged from 40 to 55 years, within 8 hours of their death.

The source of this tissue was topographically classified and the histological study was performed by the classic hematoxylin-eosin staining method with viewing by light microscope.

SYSTEMATIZATION OF NASOPHARYNGEAL TISSUE. HISTOLOGICAL CHARACTERISTICS.

The nasopharynx is lined with pseudostratified ciliated columnar epithelium of the respiratory type, containing some interspersed goblet cells. There may also be a smaller proportion of non-keratinized squamous epithelium of the digestive type, although it is not found in any given location but in a parcelled or focal way amidst the respiratory epithelium. Moreover, transition zones may be observed between these two types of epithelia.

The respiratory columnar epithelium has folds which penetrate deeply into the subepithelial connective tissue. These folds, called crypts, are usually rather shallow and unbranched, as opposed to the case with the tonsils (1).

Beneath both the respiratory and digestive epithelia, there is lax connective tissue and adipose tissue whose mass contains an abundance of mucous glands with excretory ducts.

In the most anterior area of the lateral wall, between the auditory tube cartilage and the choanae, the epithelium is always of the respiratory type. No lymphatic tissue is observed, but a fine layer of connective tissue and an abundant vascularization with veins of marked muscular wall (of the so-called vascular erectile tissue type) are viewed (2).

A fine layer of connective tissue and smooth muscle tissue is observed in the posterior wall beneath the epithelium.

The samples in which cartilage is observed come from the lateral wall of the nasopharynx. This cartilage is surrounded by mucous glands and lies very close to the epithelium, which is of the respiratory type.

A fundamental component of the nasopharynx is the subepithelial lymphatic tissue, which is found everywhere but in the anterior part of the lateral wall.

The lymphatic tissue is associated with both types of epithelia, but it is found in a higher proportion in areas lined with respiratory epithelium.

In the areas where there are crypts of respiratory epithelium, lymphatic tissue usually abounds and a migration of lymphoid elements toward the mass of the epithelium, between the epithelial cells, can frequently be observed.

CONCLUSIONS

1. Presence of islets of non-keratinized squamous digestive epithelium.
2. Absence of lymphatic tissue in the anterior part of the lateral wall of the nasopharynx, with the anterior part between the cartilage and the choanae.
3. The auditory tube cartilage is very close to the nasopharynx tissue epithelium, which is of the respiratory type.
4. Greater association of lymphatic tissue with respiratory epithelium than with digestive epithelium.
5. Invagination of respiratory epithelium within the mass of connective tissue.

REFERENCES

(1) Ham, Arthur W. (1975) Tratado de Histología, 7th Ed., Edt. Interamericana.

(2) Rhodin, Johannes A.G. (1974) Histology, New York Oxford University Press, London Toronto.

New dimensions in otorhinolaryngology - head and neck surgery, vol. 2.
E. Myers, editor

REVIEW OF NASOPHARYNGEAL CARCINOMAS AT GEISINGER MEDICAL CENTER - 1960 - 1979

DREW J. STETZ, D.O., DONALD P. VRABEC, M.D.

ABSTRACT

A twenty year retrospective analysis of nasopharyngeal malignancies is presented. The initial symptoms as well as the delay in diagnosis were investigated. Age and sexual predominance were noted. Radiation therapy and surgery of the malignant tumors of the nasopharynx along with complications of treatment were examined. Tumor type, staging, and nodal involvement were analyzed for prognostic indicators of survival.

A twenty-year analysis (between 1960 and 1979) of patients with nasopharyngeal carcinoma was performed at the Geisinger Medical Center, Danville, Pennsylvania. Due to our geographic area and somewhat skewed population, all patients were Caucasian. A total of 76 patients were evaluated. Eight patients were excluded. Patients were excluded due to a refusal of therapy (two), a wish to receive radiation therapy elsewhere (five), or were lost to follow-up (one).

Histopathologic slides were reviewed with the Department of Pathology.[2] The slides were grouped according to the World Health Organization Classification[3] with the modification used by Dickson[4] who combined the nonkeratinizing and undifferentiated carcinomas together. Keratinizing squamous cell carcinomas were also included in this category. Lymphoepithelial tumors were evaluated separately because previous reports that describe a better prognosis with this category.[5] The criteria used for diagnosing lymphoepitheliomas is described by Batsakis.[6] Sixty-five percent (44) were diagnosed as either squamous cell carcinoma (undifferentiated, nonkeratinized, or keratinized) epidermoid carcinoma or transitional cell carcinoma. Fifteen percent (10) had lymphoepitheliomas, and the remainder of patients included one rhabdomyosarcoma, ten lymphomas, two plasmocytomas, and one chordoma.

Seventy-five percent of the patients diagnosed as having squamous cell carcinoma of the nasopharynx were male and twenty-five percent were female. This represents a population ratio of 3:1. Of the patients with lymphoepitheliomas, 80 percent (8) were male and 20 percent (2) were female; a ratio of 4:1. The decade of greatest frequency of nasopharyngeal malignancies was the sixth. The average age at the time of diagnosis for men with squamous cell carcinoma was 55.38 years and women 50.73 years. The average age of males with lymphoepitheliomas was 43.28 years and the average age of females was 32.5 years. Presenting signs and symptoms relevant to nasopharyngeal carcinoma were evaluated. The initial sign in 32 percent (23) of the patients was a neck mass, followed by nasal obstruction in 31 percent (22), middle ear effusions 28 percent (20), epistaxis 17 percent (12), facial pain 7 percent (5), dysphagia 7 percent (5), sore throat 5.6 percent (4), jugular foramen syndrome 2.8 percent (2), and nasal drainage, confusion, tinnitus, and cord compression each representing 1.4 percent of the patient population.

The insidious nature of nasopharyngeal carcinoma was best demonstrated by reviewing the delay in diagnosis, assuming that the symptoms were related, and the stage of the disease when the diagnosis was obtained. The average delay from the onset of symptoms to the time of diagnosis was 6.4 months. The squamous cell carcinomas and lymphoepitheliomas were staged according to the TMN classification.[7] In order of increasing frequency, Stage I squamous cell carcinoma was diagnosed in 5 percent (2), Stage II in 9 percent (4), Stage III in 32 percent (14), and Stage IV in 55 percent (24). No lymphoepitheliomas were found in Stage I, 10 percent were found in Stage II and Stage III, and 80 percent in Stage IV.

The major mode of treatment for patients with nasopharyngeal carcinoma was radiation therapy. The most common early complication of radiation therapy was mucositis which was found in 67.6 percent (48) of the patients. This complication was followed by desquamation in 9.8 percent (7) of the patients, loss of taste in 8.4 percent (6), and choanal stenosis, generalized weakness, nasal crusting, hypopituitarism, and facial palsy each representing 1.4 percent of the patients with complications from radiation therapy.

A total of 12 percent (5) of the patients underwent unilateral neck dissections as a salvage procedure for squamous cell carcinoma (with neck nodes positive in all cases). One case represented recurrent disease, and the others radiation failure. Five-year survival in this small group of patients was 80 percent. Bilateral neck dissections were performed in two patients, both of whom expired within one year.

The survival time of each stage was then compared. The patients with Stage I disease squamous cell carcinoma had 100 percent three-year survival (2) as compared with Stage II who had 25 percent (1) three-year survival. Seventy-two percent (10) of the patients with Stage III and 30 percent (7) of the patients with Stage IV disease had a three-year survival. This represents an overall three-year survival of 46 percent. No patients with Stage I, II or III lymphoepitheliomas survived for three years. Twenty-eight percent (2) of the patients with Stage IV lymphoepitheliomas had a three-year survival. One patient was excluded due to death from myocardial infarction. The five-year survival of the patients with Stage I squamous cell carcinoma was 50 percent (1). Stage II had a 25 percent (1), Stage III 65 percent (9), and Stage IV 17 percent (4) five-year survivals. The overall five-year survival of patients with squamous cell carcinoma was 34 percent (15). The patients with lymphoepitheliomas had a zero percent five-year survival in all stages of disease. A three-year survivor succumbed to a cerebrovascular accident three years post-radiation therapy. Due to the small sample of patients diagnosed as having Stage I or Stage II disease, a fair comparison of survival cannot be drawn with Stage III or IV disease, and this most probably accounts for a better survival with Stage III disease.

The male patients surviving with squamous cell carcinoma had a 4.5 year survival average, and the female survival average was 3.67 years. This represents a combined 4.28 year survival for all stages of the disease. The male patients with lymphoepitheliomas had an average of 1.92 years survival while the females had a two-year survival time, representing a 1.94 year survival average time. The male patients in both groups combined had a better three and five-year survival. Nodal involvement was reviewed as a prognostic indicator and N-3 lesions were found to have the poorest five-year survival.

The remainder of survival statistics for patients with nasopharyngeal malignancies were as follows: The patients with lymphomas had a 25 percent five-year survival, the patients with chordoma and plasmocytoma had a 100 percent five-year survival, and the patient with rhabdomyosarcoma died two years after diagnosis.

In summary, 68 cases of nasopharyngeal malignancies were reviewed and histologically subdivided. It was found that the average age and survival was less in patients with lymphoepitheliomas as compared with the patients with squamous cell carcinoma. This contradicts previous studies indicating that lymphoepithelial disease is a prognostic indicator of better survival.[8] This may suggest that the lymphatic tissue is an innocent bystander for a host response and perhaps should not be classified as a separate lesion. The average time from the onset of symptoms to the time of diagnosis was 6.4 months. A neck mass was found to be the major presenting symptom in our study and is felt to herald the disease as in other studies reviewed.[9] There was a male predominance with slightly better survival rates noted in the male patients.

The majority of patients received radiation therapy from 6,000 to 7,000 rads and had mucositis as the most frequent early complication. Neck dissections were performed in four patients for salvage following radiation therapy and in one patient for recurrent disease. Survival following neck dissection is encouraging. The overall three-year survival of squamous cell carcinoma and lymphoepithelioma is 43.6 percent with the five-year survival of 33.3 percent in our study.

Unfortunately, the majority of patients were diagnosed as having the malignant process in Stage IV of the disease. Nasopharyngeal carcinoma was rarely diagnosed as a Stage I lesion. A thorough physical examination, relevant radiographic studies, and random nasopharyngeal biopsies are advocated when there is suspicion of nasopharyngeal carcinoma. As with other malignancies, a cure for the disease is felt to be dependent on early diagnosis and definitive therapy.

BIBLIOGRAPHY

1. Batsakis JG: Carcinoma of the nasopharynx. Tumors of the Head and Neck: Clinical and Pathological Considerations. 2nd ed., 1979, pp. 188-199.
2. Dr. Patrick Dorion and Dr. Peter Cera, Department of Pathology, Geisinger Medical Center.
3. Taxi, Hidvegi, Battifora: Nasopharyngeal carcinoma: Antikeratin immunohistochemistry and electron microscopy. Am J Clin Path 83(3):320-325, 1985.
4. Dickson, Flores: Nasopharyngeal carcinoma: An evaluation of 134 patients treated between 1971 and 1980. Laryngoscope 95(3):276-283, 1985.
5. Dickson RI: Nasopharyngeal carcinoma: An evaluation of 209 patients. Laryngoscope 91:333-354, 1981.
6. Batsakis JG: Carcinoma of the nasopharynx. Tumors of the Head and Neck: Clinical and Pathological Considerations. 2nd ed., 1979, pp. 188-199.
7. Rubin: Clinical Oncology, American Cancer Society, 1983. Chapter 19, Head and Neck Tumors, pp. 230-244.
8. Dickson, Flores: Nasopharyngeal carcinoma: An evaluation of 134 patients treated between 1971 and 1980. Laryngoscope 95(3):276-283, 1985.

New dimensions in otorhinolaryngology - head and neck surgery, vol. 2.
E. Myers, editor

THE VIENNA EXTRA- AND INTRACOCHLEAR PROSTHESIS : SPEECH-CODING AND SPEECH-UNDERSTANDING

I.J. HOCHMAIR-DESOYER, E.S.HOCHMAIR, K. BURIAN[x]
Dept. of Electr.Eng., Techn.Univ. of Vienna, A-1040 Vienna,
[x]II. ENT-Dept, Univ. of Vienna, A-1090 Vienna, AUSTRIA

INTRODUCTION

The Cochlear Implant project in Vienna has now gathered a total experience of 125 implant patient years with 24 patients who have received an extracochlear-implant prosthesis (now the "3M/Vienna multifrequency device") and 28 patients who have received an intracochlear implant prosthesis. The maximum implant duration is 80 months.

Independent of whether the implant comprises an electrode for intracochlear or for extracochlear placement, the sound processor always provides a processed analog broadband stimulation signal. It avoids the transformation of speech into pulses.

SOUND-CODING RATIONALES

For hearing induced by sinusoidal electrical stimulation the dynamic range is very restricted. The mean dynamic range for all patients averaged over the values measured at octave-stepped frequencies between 125 and 2000 Hz is 13.5 dB. Figure 1 includes threshold, most comfortable loudness and discomfort threshold traces for an extracochlear implant patient. In contrast to hearing aid wearers

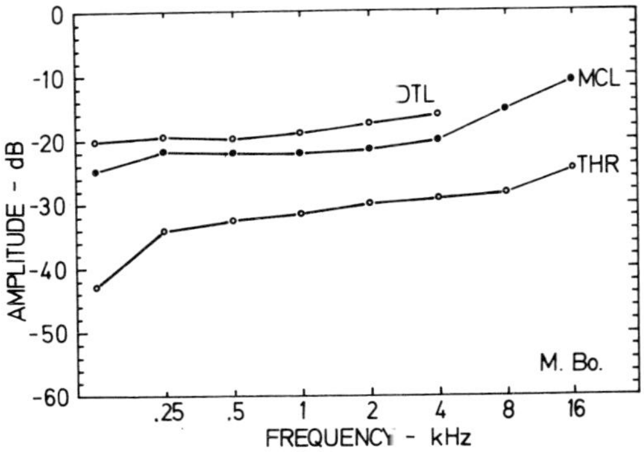

Fig. 1 : Threshold (THR) most comfortable loudness (MCL) and discomfort threshold (DTL) versus stimulation frequency for extracochlear-implant patient M.Bo., sinusoidal stimulation used.

cochlear implant patients with an intracochlear electrode or with an extracochlear electrode situated in the round window niche can perceive stimulation frequencies between 30 Hz and at least 15 kHz as hearing sensations and without discomfort.

. The range for electrical stimulus amplitude causing hearing sensations between threshold and discomfort threshold shows considerable variation among patients (Fig. 2).

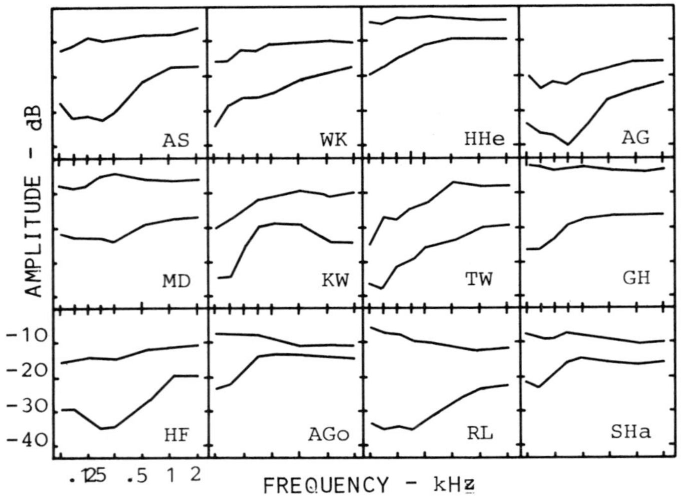

Fig. 2 : THR (lower) and DTL (upper) traces for sinusoidal stimulation for 12 extracochlear-implant patients.

. The patient's ability to discriminate frequencies gets very poor in the frequency range above 500 to 1000 Hz.

. Amplitude discrimination and temporal processing abilities, on the contrary, are comparable to the values for normal listeners in the majority of postlingually deafened patients.

The last 2 characteristics of electrically induced hearing suggest the use of a broadband analog coding scheme.

Several findings have confirmed the importance of the following 2 aspects of the broadband analog coding scheme :

a) The frequency response of the soundprocessor has to be adjusted such that it matches the patient's trace for most comfortable loudness for a continuous sinewave-sgianl whose frequency increases in small steps (1).
b) The bandwidth for the transmitted speech-signal should not be restricted (see below).

Since the soundprocessor comprises a syllabic compressor with the compression onset usually set to 60 dB SPL, proper frequency response adjustment results in aided free field audiograms with thresholds between 30 and 60 dB SPL, depending on the electrical dynamic range, with the lower values for the low frequencies. In most cases discomfort threshold cannot be reached up to 130 dB SPL.

Despite the poor frequency discrimination for frequencies above 1 kHz the implant patients can still make use of information contained in the high-frequency part of the speech-signal. Speech-tests in which speech signals low-pass filtered at 900 Hz and at 300 Hz and full bandwidth speech signals (approx. 100 Hz to 6 kHz) were used, showed that the full bandwidth signal results in the best speech comprehension (2).

Another study investigating final consonant cluster recognition in a computer-controlled 6-choice rhyme-test revealed that when the speech signal was lowpass filtered (Butterworth 42 dB/oct) at 4 kHz instead of 8 kHz the score decreased from 65 % to 55 % which, using the appropriate Wilcoxontest, is significant on the 2,5 % level.

The broadband analog coding scheme presents a large amount of information to the patient. The degree of speech recognition achievable and the improvements with time that have been found (Fig. 3) demonstrate that the auditory system of these patients can indeed use this information to a high degree.

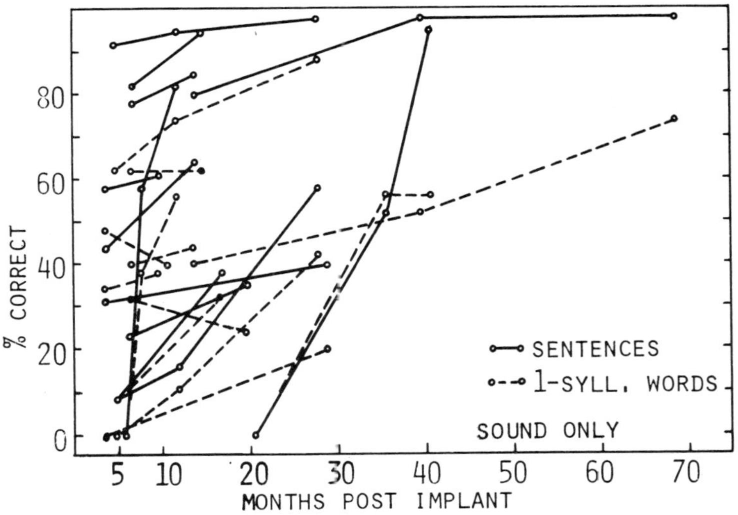

Fig. 3 : Recognition for open sets of single-syllable words and everyday sentences without lipreading versus time (5 extra-cochlear- and 7 intracochlear implant patients.

SPEECH UNDERSTANDING AND RELATED ABILITIES

Fig. 3 displays the development over time for results from open-set tests for single-syllable word and everyday sentence recognition without lipreading for taped material. In these tests a high percentage of the patients who ultimately reached some visually unaided recognition already showed some recognition in the first test conducted 3 - 5 months after implant surgery. There are two exceptions to this. For almost all patients improvements with time have been observed - even after many months of wearing the device.

The wide distribution of results from the open set word- and sentence-tests without lipreading is apparent from Fig. 4a. Approx. 50 % of the postlingually deafened patients have regained substantial amounts of understanding in quiet in the "sound only" condition. (Mean for single-syllable words : 30 %, mean for sentences : 45 %). The tests for word and sentence recognition were complemented by closed set identification tests for 16 consonants (mean : 46 %) and the 8 German long vowels (mean : 41 %), still without lipreading (Fig. 4b).

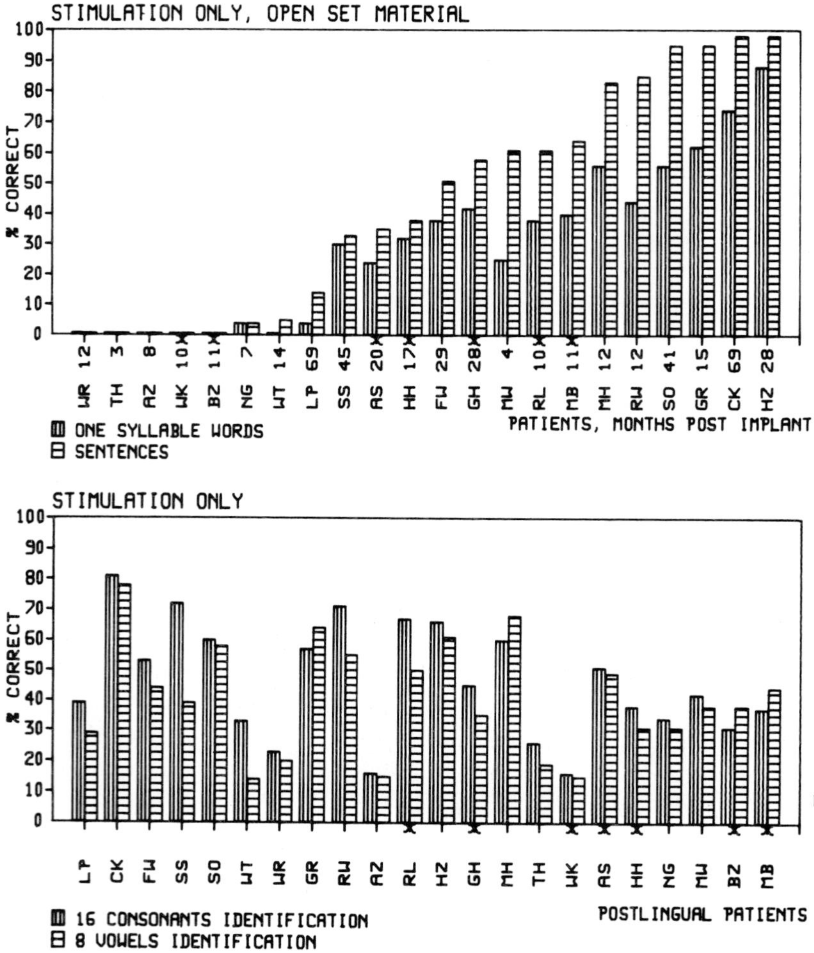

Fig. 4 : Recognition for open sets of single-syllable words and everyday sentences (a) and closed sets of 16 consonants and the 8 German long vowels (b) presented from tape (except for the consonants) and without lipreading. Data for all postlingually deafened implant patients with German mothertongue implanted for more than 3 months by Jan.85 are included. Patients who received extracochlear implants are marked by an x.

Correlations among all the results from these 4 tests were found to be significant on the 1 % level. They were also found to all inversely correlate with age.

In an attempt to investigate factors influencing the degree of speech recognition, 6 tests for temporal processing abilities including gap detection tasks, temporal difference limen determinations and periodic/aperiodic discrimination were also performed with all postlingually deafened patients.

The correlation found between the speech-test results and the temporal tests (3) confirm the importance of temporal processing abilities for speech understanding in these implant patients.

It was also found that none of the patients whose temporal difference limen were longer than 100 - 120 ms was able to understand single syllable words without lipreading (Fig. 5).

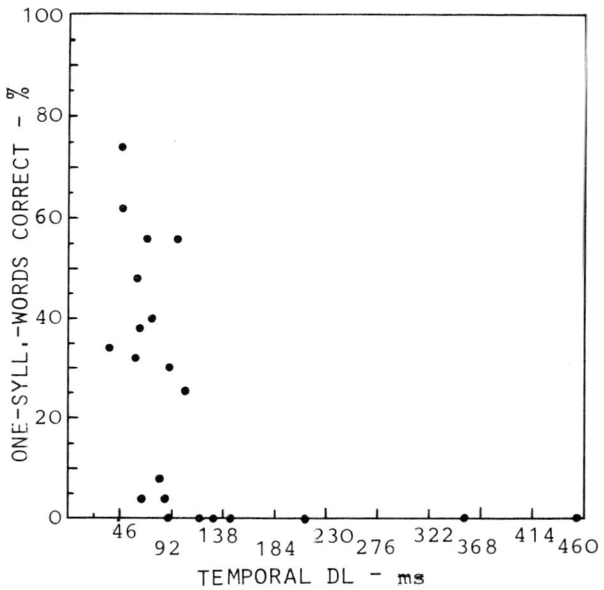

Fig. 5 :

Visually unaided single-syllable word understanding versus temporal difference limen.

A temporal difference limen below 100 - 120 ms is a prerequisite, and can be used for preoperative patient councelling but it does not guarantee visually unaided speech recognition. This is exemplified by patient B.Z. (Fig. 4a) who is the only patient we have seen so far who has a temporal difference limen of below 100 ms but is unable to perform in the periodic/aperiodic discrimination task which, in turn, correlates with voiced/unvoiced recognition.

ACKNOWLEDGEMENTS

This work is founded by the Austrian Science Research Fund under grants no. 4791 and 5680.

REFERENCES

1. Hochmair-Desoyer IJ British Journal of Audiology, in press.
2. Hochmair ES, Hochmair-Desoyer IJ (1985) In: Schindler RA, Merzenich MM (eds) Cochlear Implants. Raven Press, New York, pp.101-110.
3. Hochmair-Desoyer IJ, Hochmair ES, Stiglbrunner HK (1985) In : Schindler RA, Merzenich MM (eds) Cochlear Implants. Raven Press, New York, pp.291-304.

New dimensions in otorhinolaryngology - head and neck surgery, vol. 2.
E. Myers, editor

"COCHLEAR IMPLANT: COMPARATIVE STUDY OF THE MONO AND MULTICHANNEL IMPLANTATION"

J. BOSCH (1)   R. COLOMINA (2)

E.N.T. Department, Hospital de la Cruz Roja, Universidad Autónoma de Barcelona, Barcelona, Spain

INTRODUCTION

The best system for the replacement of a non-function cochlea and the hearing restore, is by "jumping" the intra-cochlear transduction mechanism and try to stimulate with electric and selective methods directly to the auditory nerve.
Our first experience in electrodes implantation in a patient totally deaf due to ototoxic drugs was perform in 1977, and we have done seven more cochlear implants. According to the results obtained we believe that the cochlear electrodes implantation still as a experimental surgery, which has not reached its fundamental goal; **the introduction of the total deaf in the world verbal communication.**
We show our experience results and the actual work to improve the verbal discrimination.

MATERIAL AND METHODS

In a cochlear implant research program there are six important aspects: 1) Patiens Selection. 2) The implant technical aspects. 3) The surgical technique. 4) The implanted system tolerance. 5) The stimulation and rehabilitation methods and 6) The results analisys to make suitable modifications in order to improve them.
1) Patients selection. We have eight patients, seven men and one woman.All of them totally deaf due to ototoxic drugs, except one due to otosclerosis. We select this group because we think that they have an important preserved nerve fibers.The quality obtained at rehabilitation will depend on the remaining fibers. The ages ranged from 24 to 46 years. Old patients are good lip reading and post-lingual deaf. Also important is to eveluate the intelectual level and the family environment.
2) The implant technical aspects. It has to transform an analogical sign into a digital sign in the nervous synapsis, doing the transduction work conditioning of signs, filtering and multiplexing to obtain the analogical-digital conversion. In our first experience the system had four platinum-iridium monopolar electrodes placed in four cochlear holes corresponding to the frequences 250, 500, 1300 and 4000. A fifth indifferent electrode was place in the temporal muscle. This system communicated with an external teflon connector.The stimulation unit had an integrated circuit which carried out the functions of an amplifier with a 110 dB. level on the sign supplied by the microphone. This can bring the continous use by the patient without danger of overstimulations, for an output sign a maximum variation

of 3 dB. in the input sign to 54 dB. For the second and third experiences four bipolar electrodes were implanted in the cochlear holes, the external connector was from nylon. In the fourth experience we used a new unwired stimulator, placing the receiver under the skin, to avoid the problems of the external connector. The set receiver has a resounding circuit composed of coil and tantalium condenser a diode detector an de-coupling condenser, each part sealed with silicone. The connection between the transmitter and receiver is effected by means of an inducer coil which is placed behind the ear, at the same level to the implanted coil of the receiver. Finally for the four last experiences a bicanal implant has been used through the round window with bipolar electrodes. The stimulator has a limitator-amplifier of active filters with a first canal ranging from 200 to 800 cycles and a second canal from 800 to 2500 cycles.

3) The surgical technique. In our 3 first experiences we did it by 4 holes at the promontory corresponding to frequencies 250, 500, 1300 and 4000.The fourth one was done by the introduction in the round window and subcutaneous connector. Our last four experiences was done by introduction of one bipolar electrode in the round window and subcutaneous connector.

4) The implanted system tolerance. We had not intolerance to the electrodes, but we have had problems with the external connector from hardened nylon of the third patient and was change for the subcutaneous receptor.

5) The stimulation and rehabilitation methods. This is carried out by a team which is formed by enginners who designed the system, phoniatrics and physiologists. The greater proportion of success in the words identification its ranging from 200 to 800 Hertz. The rehabilitation starts with groups of words and music. As those words are identified, little sentences are inserted, this process doesn't permit a correct identification of a conversation by the patient.

6) Results. Are satisfactory for the patient as he is able to re-join the sonorous world, they improve their vocalization, partial discrimination of groups of words, Which helps for verbal communication. To us the results are not satisfying, as we have not reached our aim, the reinsertion to the world of verbal communication.The mono and multichannel systems in our experience have similar results.

SUMMARY

After eight years from the first implantation did it for us, we can say that this patients recieve a lot of help bringing them back to the identification of music, noises, best voice regulation and discrimination of words groups after rehabilitation, we dit not have best results with multichannel implants. Actually with the incorporation of the microprocessors to the implant system we will improve the results of the verbal discrimination.

New dimensions in otorhinolaryngology - head and neck surgery, vol. 2.
E. Myers, editor

EVALUATION OF THE EXTRACOCHLEAR VIENNA/3 M IMPLANT - PATIENT SELECTION AND PRELIMINARY RESULTS

GÖRAN BREDBERG, BO LINDSTRÖM AND ARNE RISBERG

Department of Audiology, Södersjukhuset, S-100 64 Stockholm and Department of Speech Communication and Music Acoustics, Royal Institute of Technology, S-100 44 Stockholm (Sweden)

In order to evaluate the single channel extracochlear implant, it has been decided to operate 10 patients with the Vienna/3 M implant. A very careful patient selection program has been developed. After surgery the patients are followed at 1 month, 3 months, 6 months, 1 year and 2 years. After evaluation of these 10 patients a revised implant program will be discussed in Sweden.

PREOPERATIVE TESTING

After complete otological evaluation, audiometry and hearing aid testing is performed for evaluation of hearing remnants. A Swedish version of the MAC test battery is being prepared. Figure 1 demonstrates some tests that have been performed on five patients, four of which have been implanted. The last patient performs too well with hearing aid in several tests and was not included in the study. Vestibular testing, x-ray with tomography and electrical promontory stimulation are also included. Each patient went through a psychologic test battery including Defence Mecanism Test, Ravens matrix (Swedish version) and Q-sorting. A clinical interview was performed in order to establish a psychological profile for each patient and prepare him so that he has realistic expectations. The patients also had to perform, after a short training period, some additional tests with a vibro tactile device. The voices of the patients were recorded for specific evaluation postoperatively. The main criteria for inclusion in the program are; post lingual deafness, age between 20 and 60 years, no or very limited help with hearing aid or with vibro tactile device in the specific speech tests. Figure 2 shows some preoperative and postoperative results of electro stimulation.

POSTOPERATIVE TESTING AND RESULTS

In figure 3 the unaided hearing threshold and the threshold with implant from two patients are shown.

A specific training program has been designed where the patients after the fitting procedure train three times a week with additional home training for about 2 months and thereafter two times a week until 6 months. More and more of the training program is performed with a computer aided system which also will include most of the MAC test battery. Results of speechtracking from the two first patients are presented in figure 4. One patient is a very excellent lipreader and the other is a poor lipreader but both have good help with the implant as compared to their preoperative vibrator test. One patient ÅB with progressive hearing loss until deafness two years ago, performs so well that she scores almost 100% in the closed speech tests (figure 5). We have therefore started with open speech tests and for instance in one test she could make 8 out of 14 correct answers (57%).

In the training program an improvement over time has been very striking for all the patients and it seems as an important improvement has occured after six months of training. One patient four weeks after surgery developed twitches in the face, synchronous with the intensity of the stimulus but this symptom disappeared after three weeks of no stimulation and has not reappeared since. Two male patients have experienced problems with the loudness of their own voice. By changing the microphone position to the chest these problems are reduced. No other complications have occured. The selection of new patients is continued with the goal of 10 patients within 2 years.

PER CENT CORRECT ON PREOPERATIVE SPEECH TESTS

SUB-JECT	dB_M BEST EAR dB	USE OF HEARING AID	NUMBER OF SYLLABL. G = 33	THREE SPONDEE G = 33	TWELVE SPONDEE G = 8	QUESTION TEST	
						VISUAL	AUDIO-VISUAL
Å.B.	108	NO	94	67	17	85	95*
L.Å.	108	NO	78	44	N.R.	10	10*
R.L.	107	YES	100	83	50	10	60
B.J.	>120	NO	72	56	N.R.	55	40*
A.F.	95	YES	100	83	67	20	75

G = PER CENT CORRECT WITH GUESSING
* = RESULT WITH MINIVIBRATOR
78 = SIGNIFICANT P<.05

Fig. 1

DYNAMIC RANGE

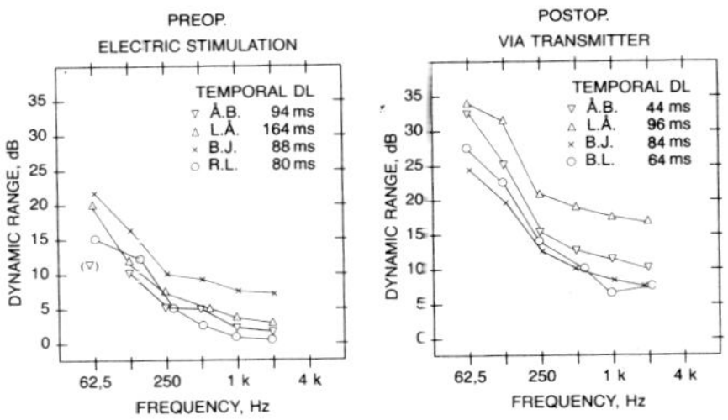

Fig. 2

AUDIOGRAM

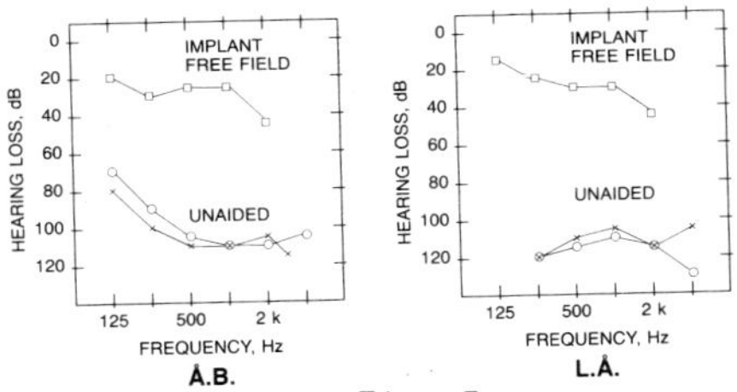

Fig. 3

SPEECH TRACKING

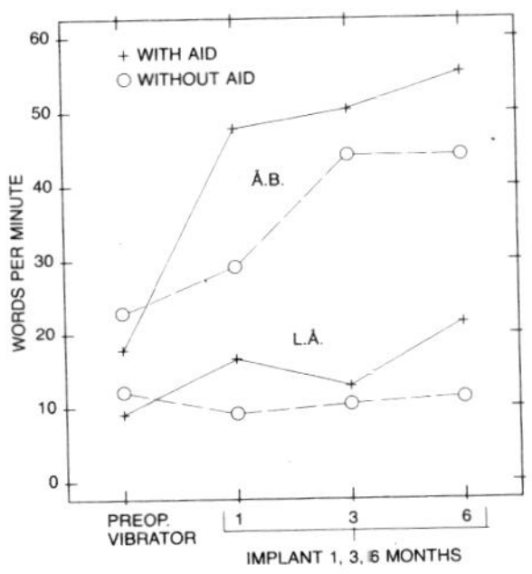

Fig. 4

RESULTS ON SPEECH TESTS

SUBJECT Å.B.

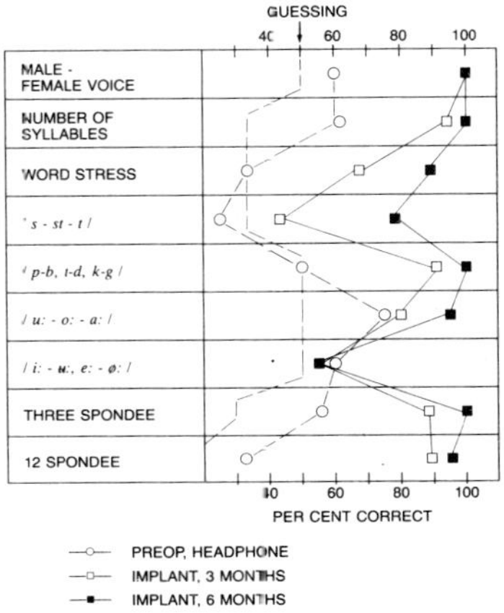

Fig. 5

© 1985 Elsevier Science Publishers B.V. (Biomedical Division)
New dimensions in otorhinolaryngology – head and neck surgery, vol. 2.
E. Myers, editor

RESPECTIVE INDICATIONS OF SINGLE AND MULTICHANNEL COCHLEAR IMPLANT IN CASE OF PRE-LINGUAL DEAFNESS

C.H. CHOUARD, C. FUGAIN, B. MEYER and F. CHABOLLE
E.N.T. Dpt.-CHU St-Antoine, 184 Rue du Fbg St-Antoine - F. 75012 - PARIS

INTRODUCTION

In our experience of 94 cases of implanted patients, the multichannel cochlear implant Chorimac-12 supplies the patient with a wide frequency information which is demonstrated by specific psychophysic tests. This rich information explains why all of our patients achieve hearing, have been able to make intensity differenciations between several sounds, and achieve different sound sensations by stimulating the different channels of the device. All our implanted and reeducated patients achieved psychoaffective improvement. But in case of pre lingual deafness (54 cases) the possibilities of speech discrimination without help of lip reading remains frequently low. In order to improve our indications for implanting we try to preoperatively know the clinical results of device use.

METHODS

We have studied the correlation between the preoperative status and the clinical results of our prelingual totally deaf patients. The preoperative status has been assessed by mean of : 1- the value of the threshold level of the round window electrical stimulation test (R.W.E.S.) ; 2- the features (coded in 3 types) of the electrical Tone Decay Test (TDT) performed during this test ; 3 - the patient's socialization level assessed by 5 parameters, each of them coded from 0 to 3 : motivation, intelligence quotient, schooling, quality of oral and written langage, and performances in lip reading. The clinical results have been assessed by the number of hours per days the patient actives its device, the percentage of good responses in closed lists of 2, 4 and 8 words without lip reading, and the difference between pre and postoperative percentages of good response in open list with help of lip reading. These 3 parameters allow to determine the auditory efficacity of the prosthesis.

RESULTS

Among various data which may influence the clinical results, only a few statistically significant correlations may be extracted between them an the prosthesis efficacity. This efficacity depends on the value of the socialization coefficient, the higher this value, the better the results will be. Thus this auditory efficacity may be regarded as the ratio of auditory performance/coefficient We have reported that there is a significant correlation between this prosthesis efficacity and the electrical threshold level obtained during the RWES.

Some clinical observations must here be reported although they have no statistical value because of the lack of cases studied.

The prosthesis efficiency will usually be better in case of TDT type I obtained during the pre-operative R.W.E.S., and good frequency discrimination at different intensity levels of the different pairs of electrodes. On the contrary the prosthesis efficacity will be unsatisfying in the case of partial or total ossification of the cochlea and lack of implanted and/or functioning electrodes.

Furthermore one must emphasize that associated handicaps make impossible a quantitative measurement of · the prosthesis efficacity. Nevertheless the clinical results we obtained, despite and even because of these handicaps, explain why blindness, autism, aphonia and paraplegia do not represent contraindications for implanting.

INDICATIONS

We think that cochlear implant must be as soon as possible, because our experiments on guinea-pigs demonstrated that chronic cochlear electric stimulation of totally deaf new born animals is able to prevent the brain stem auditory atrophy elicited by this deafness , and because in case of pre-lingual deafness, the younger our implanted patients are the better the clinical results obtained with the multichannel cochlear implant. For all these reasons one may think that totally deaf children must also benefit from an effective hearing aid, i,e, to be implanted as soon as possible. But today it is practically impossible to perform this implantation before the age of 5 years, because of the general opinion amoung otologists concerning this proposition, and over all because our device is actually too big to be offered to children younger than five years. Moreover one may ask if it is reasonable to supply a patient with 12 electrodes, when preoperative tests allow us to predict that his atrophied brain stem will not be able to use these 12 different frequency bands he will supplied with. It would be worthwile to only supply this patient with a single channel system, the coast of which is less expansive, even if its performances are less good. Moreover in very young children this single channel implant may be placed in an extra-cochlear position as long as the certitude of the total deafness cannot be assessed For all these reasons we can summarize our current indications in case of prelingually deaf patient in the table I.

AGE	PRONOSTIC VALUE	IMPLANT CHOICE
< 6 years	Good	Single channel Extra cochlear
	Bad	Single channel Extra cochlear
> 6 years	Good	12-Multichannel system
	Bad	Intra-cochlear Single channel

Table I - Choice of the implant in children as a fonction of the age and the pronostic value of the preoperative tests.

New dimensions in otorhinolaryngology - head and neck surgery, vol. 2.
E. Myers, editor

EVALUATION OF A 22-CHANNEL COCHLEAR IMPLANT

SUSAN B. WALTZMAN, PH. D. AND NOEL L. COHEN, M.D.

Department of Otolaryngology, New York University Medical Center,
550 First Avenue, New York, N.Y., U.S.A.

INTRODUCTION

A cochlear implant program, utilizing the Australian multichannel cochlear prosthesis, was initiated at New York University Medical Center and Bellevue Hospital Center in 1984. The device consists of a 22-electrode array inserted 25 mm into the scala tympani, and a receiver-stimulator, implanted behind the mastoid process. The external portion consists of a wearable speech processor and microphone headset. The microphone converts incoming auditory stimuli into electrical signals, which are encoded by the processor in digital form and transmitted to the implant via inductive coupling from the coil on the headset. Voice frequency is coded by pulse rate, and second formant frequency is coded by stimulating different electrodes along the scala tympani.[1]

SUBJECTS

Six patients received the device in 1984 and one patient was implanted in March, 1985. Pre-surgical evaluations included audiologic, otologic, radiologic, medical and psychological testing. All patients had a bilateral profound sensorineural hearing loss with the duration of deafness ranging from one to 54 years. Patients ranged in age from 21 to 62 years. All had lost hearing after acquiring speech and language and were unable to benefit from amplification.

RESULTS

Following the surgery, using a facial recess approach, and post-operative programming of the wearable speech processor, all patients showed a restoration of hearing sensation. All patients received weekly training and testing sessions[2] for a period of at least ten weeks. During these sessions, vowel recognition, consonant recognition and speech tracking data were collected. All of the testing was performed under three conditions: lipreading alone, lipreading, plus cochlear implant, and cochlear implant alone. For the six patients who have completed the training, the mean consonant recognition score for the lipreading alone condition was 43.5%. The lipreading, plus cochlear implant, mean score was 56.1%, and for the cochlear implant alone condition, the score was 22.0%. For the vowel recognition task, the mean scores were 80.7% - lipreading alone; 89.3% - lipreading, plus cochlear implant; and 31.9% - cochlear implant alone. Significant individual differences were evident. Speech tracking scores for all six patients showed an improvement when the cochlear implant was utilized in conjunction with lipreading. In addition, three of the seven patients have demonstrated open-set speech discrimination ability on a variety of word, sentence and tracking scores. It should be noted that Patient #1 is functioning with a single-channel system, due to an unforeseen obstruction in the scala tympani. He consistently performed the poorest on all tasks, under all conditions. See Fig. 1.

SUMMARY AND CONCLUSIONS

All patients using multichannel stimulation have shown: 1) a restoration of hearing sensation; 2) a recognition of a wide variety of environmental sounds; and 3) an increased ability to discriminate speech, when the cochlear implant is used in conjunction with lipreading. In addition, three of the six patients have shown an ability to discriminate speech, using the cochlear implant alone, without the benefit of lipreading: on Word-22 lists, two of the six patients obtained scores of 42% and 20%, respectively.

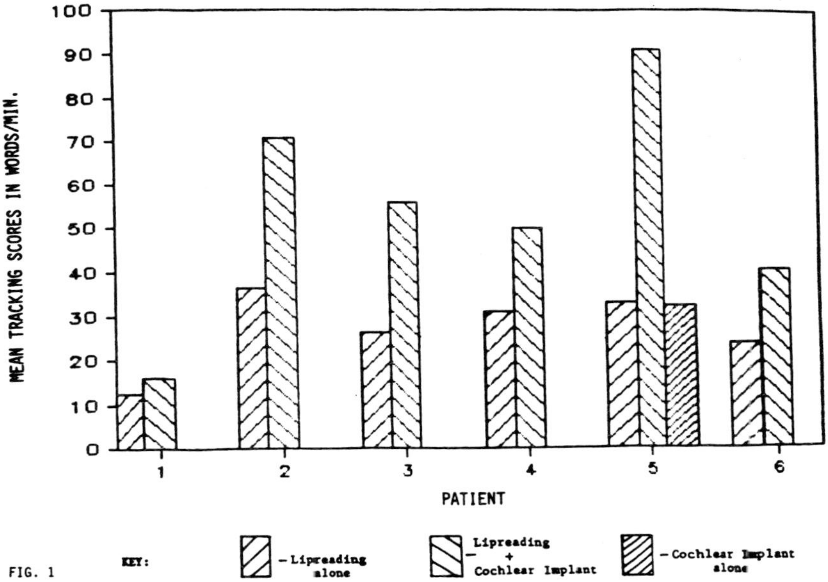

FIG. 1

REFERENCES

1. Clark, GM, Tong, YC, Patrick, JF, Seligman, PM, Crosby, PA, Kuzma, JA, Money, DK (1984) A Multichannel Hearing Prosthesis for Profound-To-Total Hearing Loss. Journal Medical Engineering & Technology, 8:1.

2. Nucleus Multichannel Implantable Prosthesis, Procedures and Protocols. Manuel (North America) Nucleus, Ltd. Copyright, November, 1983.

New dimensions in otorhinolaryngology - head and neck surgery, vol. 2.
E. Myers, editor

SOUND EXPERIENCE BY MULTICHANNEL COCHLEAR IMPLANT PATIENTS

JAMES L. PARKIN, M.D., M.S.
Professor of Surgery, Chairman Otolaryngology-Head and Neck Surgery, University of Utah School of Medicine, Salt Lake City, Utah 84132

INTRODUCTION: The history of the multichannel cochlear implantation program at the University of Utah dates back to the mid 1970's and has been detailed earlier.[1,2] Federal Drug Administration approval for additional implants was obtained in February 1984. Between April 1984 and March 1985, 13 additional patients have been implanted at the University of Utah. Two revision surgeries have been necessary. The early experience with these patients is reported.

MATERIAL AND METHODS: Implantation has been restricted to postlingually deafened adults who receive no significant speech benefit from hearing aids. The patients have extensive preoperative evaluations consisting of comprehensive audiologic evaluation, electronystagmography, complete medical and psychological assessment, biplaner temporal bone CT scanning and transtympanic electrical promontory stimulation. Educational video presentations, informational booklets, and counselling sessions enlighten the patient as to potential risks and benefits of implantation.

The wrapped bundle of intracochlear electrodes is inserted through the round window into the scala tympani via a mastoidectomy-facial recess approach. The indifferent electrode is placed in the temporalis muscle and a promontory electrode is seated in the anterior inferior promontory. The percutaneous pedestal is attached to the posterior inferior mastoid cortex with special bone screws. The electrical integrity of the implant is assessed multiple times intraoperatively. Five to six weeks postoperatively, the patient has electrical characterization of the implant electrodes and custom fitting of the sound processor.

Two patients have had implant replacement. One, B.G., had a single channel unit removed and replaced with the multichannel implant. She reported the sound experience difference as, the single channel aid "gave me noises, Ineraid gives me recognizable (with practice) sounds." The second, R.N., had replacement of his multichannel unit because of below expectation performance. A third patient had his second ear implanted because of cochlear space restrictions in the first ear.

RESULTS: A recent patient survey reviewed the postsurgical experience of this group of 13 patients. Three of the patients have experienced superficial infections around the pedestal successfully treated with antibiotics and no effect on implant performance. Twelve of the 13 patients reported tinnitus before implantation. Nine of these report improvement in their tinnitus when the sound processor is being used. Presurgical vertigo problems were reported by three patients. Four patients reported vertigo experiences in the first two weeks postoperatively. All of the patients reported daily use of their sound processors. The range was 5 to 16.5 hrs/day with an average of 12.5 hrs/day use.

The patients were asked if they experience continued improvement in performance with increased sound processor use. Twelve of the 13 answered yes. The husband of the patient who reported no, stated that he did see continued improvement as his wife used the unit more. Another question on the survey asked "Knowing what you now know, would you go through with implantation again?" All 13 patients responded yes.

The patients were requested to evaluate their own speech understanding performance. This was done with the awareness of a definite learning curve. The longer the patient uses the sound processor, the better their speech performance becomes. For example, our first patient in this group, S.S., received his sound processor 9/15/84. His first speech testing was performed 10/8/84. By auditory stimulation alone with open set, live voice testing, he scored 12% on a 25 Spondee wordlist and 24% on CID sentences. Subsequent testing showed progressive improvement. His performance of 2/4/85 was 100% performance with 25 Spondee wordlist and 94% and 100% with two CID sentence lists.

Eight of the 13 patients reported a positive ability to understand some conversational speech without lip reading and some use of the telephone. Three of those with negative responses had had their sound processors less than six weeks.

Formal speech performance testing has not been accomplished on all patients. Many patients live at a distance requiring our contact with them and their testing to occur at varying intervals. The following speech recognition results were obtained with open set lists, utilizing audio input only and live voice. The first patient, D.C., was from our earlier implantation experience group. He received his sound processor in 1983 as the first patient with a portable Ineraid device. The remaining five patients are part of the current group of 13.

Pt.	Weeks with Processor	Spondee 25 Wd.	CID Sentences
D.C.	94	88%	48%
S.S.	21	100%	100%
J.P.	29	48%	DNT
L.O.	16	44%	12%
B.H.	14	32%	6%
C.C.	9	44%	36%

SUMMARY: The early experience with the Ineraid multichannel cochlear implant is very encouraging. All 13 patients are currently using their implants on a daily basis. Speech recognition results indicate the ability to evaluate patients with more standard audiologic tests.

REFERENCES:

1. Eddington DK, Dobelle WH, Brackmann DE, Mladejousky MG, Parkin JL (1978) Ann Otol Rhinol Laryngol 87:Suppl 53:1-39

2. Parkin JL, Eddington DK, Orth JL, Brackmann DE (1984) Submitted for publication Otolaryngol Head Neck Surg. Presented Amer Acad Otolaryngol Head Neck Surg, Sept 1984.

New dimensions in otorhinolaryngology - head and neck surgery, vol. 2.
E. Myers, editor

EXTRACOCHLEAR CHRONIC ELECTRICAL STIMULATION IN DEAF PATIENTS

ERNST A.RICHTER
ENT-Dept., AKH Linz, A-4020 Linz (Austria)

INTRODUCTION

In this first series of 3 bilaterally profoundly deaf patients the Vienna Extracochlear Implant was used. The reason for this decision was the favorable risk/ benefit ratio of this device as compared to the intracochlear implant (1).

METHODS

Patient selection was mainly based on the results of psychoacoustic electrostimulation tests using a transtympanic needle electrode placed on the promontory. Tone identification and temporal resolution, as described elsewhere (2), were tested, since these abilities are key factors for a successful function of this particular prosthesis. Implantations were done under general anesthesia using a combined retroauricular-enaural approach. The active electrode was introduced via an antrotomy - under direct view after elevation of the tympanomeatal flap - into the tympanic cavity. The posterior lip of the round window niche was drilled down to view the membrane. The ball shaped active electrode was positioned on the membrane using the spring load effect of the electrode wire. Pieces of conchal cartilage served as wedges to keep both electrode and wire in place prior to readaption of the tympanomeatal flap. In a similar way the larger ground electrode was wedged into an antral cell. Finally a cavity of the shape of the receiver disk was drilled into the cortical bone. Sutures through small holes drilled into the edges of the cavity keep the disk in position. Packings and skin sutures were removed about ten days later. At that time the speech processor, employing the "multifrequency coding scheme" (1), was adjusted and rehabilitation could then start. The rehabilitation program, a modification of the Vienna program (3), is structured in a hierarchial way. First the patients are shown how to handle their prosthesis effectively, then they are trained to recognize simple sounds as e.g. closing a door, type writing, dog barking etc. The perception of suprasegmental features such as rhythm and intonation is followed by the perception of segmental features of increasing level of difficulty, and the recognition of phonemes and, finally, closed and open lists of words and sentences. The patients are also encouraged to practice with taped material spoken by familiar speakers. We are convinced that well-structured rehabilitation is an important part of a successful cochlear implant program.

PATIENTS

Two of the patients are postlingually and one is prelingually deafened.

TABLE 1

Patient	year of birth	age at onset of deafness	cause of deafness	time between surgery and test
1	39	2 1/2	meningitis	7 mos
2	55	9	mumps	3 mos
3	58	24	progressive loss, hereditary	3 mos

RESULTS

The postoperatively collected data on temporal processing abilities were comparable to the preoperatively measured values i.e. a temporal difference limen of 120, 32 and 54 milliseconds at 125 Hz for patients 1,2 and 3, respectively. The electrical dynamic ranges between threshold and discomfort threshold at 125 and 1000 Hz were 10 and 4 dB, 22 and 11 dB and 26 and 16 dB for patients 1,2 and 3.

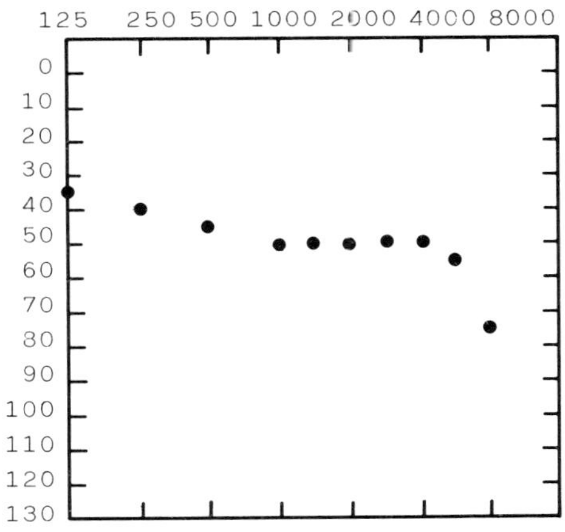

Fig. 1 :
Free field aided audiogram for patient 3 with the sound processor set to normal sensitivity. Discomfort threshold was not reached at any frequency up to 130 dB SPL.

Fig.1 is a free field audiogram for patient 3. This audiogram looks very similar for all 3 patients. Thresholds can be improved by 15 or increased by 5 dB using the "range control", which the patient can adjust himself. Patients 1 (R.G.) and 3 (M.K.) wear their device all day long, patient 2 only wears it at home.

Speech comprehension test were performed using an open list of 200 unknown every day sentences. Fig. 2 includes the scores. It should be noticed that all three

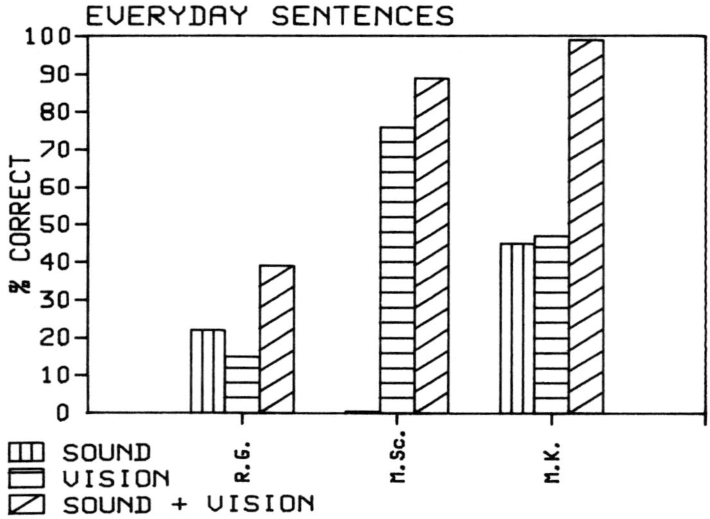

Fig. 2 : Recognition of unknown everyday sentences

patients had no acoustic sensations prior to implantation. Patients 1 and 3 demonstrated some understanding of sentences in the "sound only" condition. Patient 3 could recognize 45 % of the words after she had been wearing her device for only 2 1/2 months. With patient 2 identification of a closed set of 16 consonants was also tested and resulted in scores of 31, 69 and 94 % correct for the modalities "sound only", "lipreading only" and "lipreading + sound", respectively.

DISCUSSION

Implantation of the Vienna Extracochlear Prosthesis was successful in all cases. In these data collected soon after implant surgery an improvement in communication abilities for these 3 profoundly deaf implant patients is already apparent.

REFERENCES

1. Hochmair-Desoyer I.J., Hochmair E.S., Burian K., Stiglbrunner H.K. (1983) In : Ann. New York Academy of Sciences, Vol. 455 : pp. 295-306.
2. Bartosik H.F., Hochmair-Desoyer I.J., Fritze W. (1984) In : Life Support Systems, Vol.2, Suppl.1 : pp. 35-37.
3. Burian K., Eisenwort B., Hochmair E.S., Hochmair-Desoyer I.J. (1984) In : Adv. Audiol., Vol.2 : pp. 19-29.

ACKNOWLEDGEMENTS

The help of I.J. Hochmair-Desoyer in setting up the program is acknowledged. The work is funded by Hochschuljubiläumsstiftung der Stadt Wien.

New dimensions in otorhinolaryngology – head and neck surgery, vol. 2.
E. Myers, editor

COCHLEAR IMPLANT PRE AND POST LINGUAL CLINICAL EXPERIENCE

ARISTIDE ZUÑIGA C.
E.N.T. Dept. Hospital P.J. Quemada. Faculty of Medicine
University of Chile. Santiago-Chile.

INTRODUCTION

Pre-lingual bilaterally sensory neural profound deafness has been recovered to socially useful acoustical perception.

MATERIAL AND METHODS

Artificial prosthese specially designed gives physiological electrical stimulation with current range 0-100 micro A.,R.M.S., bandwidth 200-5 K Hz, F.M. pulses duration 1-35 microsec. Surgery is transcanal and retroauricular. Platinum wire in round window with reference in promontory. Transcutaneous external connection silicone isolated. Pre and post-operatory standard and free-field audiometry is used and so Brain Stem Evoked Response (B.S.E.R.). Implementation criteria under Helsinski norms.

RESULTS

Patient Y.P.T. (Fig. 1-2). Significant post-operatory threshold changes both B.S.E.R. and Audiometry left ear. Sociogram reveals progressive learning of elementary language. An improvement of the behavior and discrimination both in frequency and intensity. Diction from gutural to inteligible.

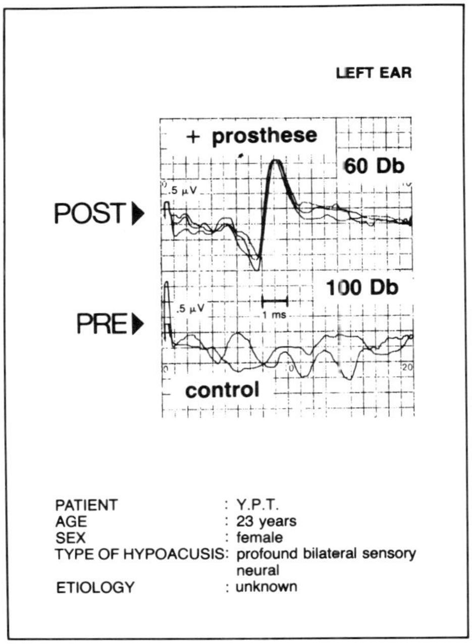

FIG. ① BRAIN STEM EVOKED RESPONSE (BSER)

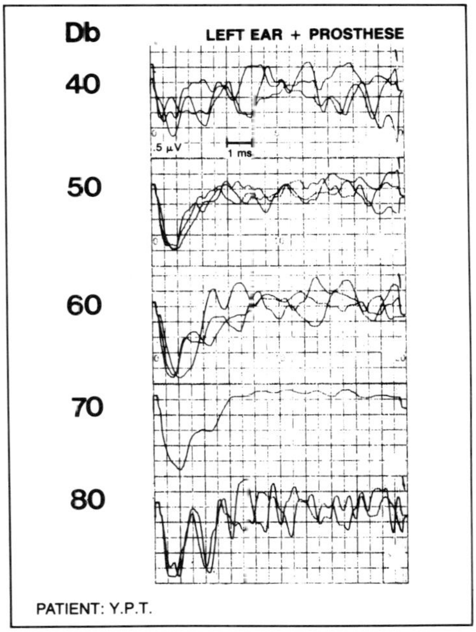

FIG. ② BRAIN STEM EVOKED RESPONSE (BSER)

Patient M.V.V. (Fig. 3). Similar responses as previous case. Was discontinued by oxidation of steel inox wires. At present ready to receive Pt electrodes.

Patient S.D.B. (Fig. 4). Intelligent energy transference is demonstrated in this post-lingual patient with unilateral severe hearing loss (Cho esteathoma surgery). Once implanted recover both audiometric threshold levels to normality and B.S.E.R. in early temporal relation. These experiences are evident in video-tape.

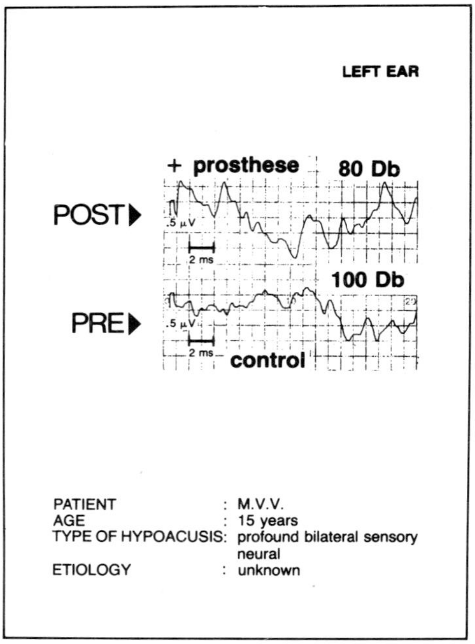

FIG. 3 BRAIN STEM EVOKED RESPONSE (BSER)

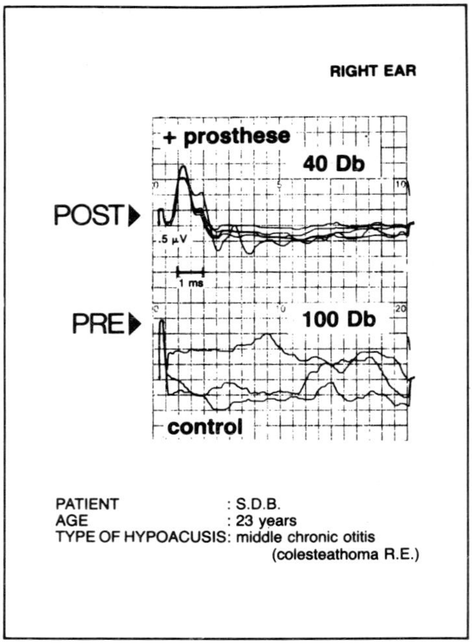

FIG. 4 BRAIN STEM EVOKED RESPONSE (BSER)

HYPOTHESES OF ENERGY TRANSFERENCE

(Fig. 5) Generator (single electrode) creates an electric field (vectorial) (1) in a closed volume conductor system (cochlea). Interaction with transmission line (nerve) is postulated through Ampere - Maxwell Law. Excitability and tonotopy as function of nerve fibers filter characteristics. (2).

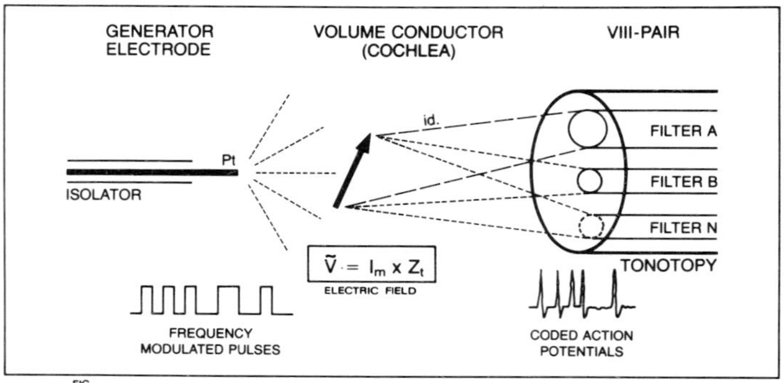

FIG. 5 **SINGLE ELECTROD ENERGY TRANSFERENCE HYPOTHESIS**

REFERENCES

1. Schmitt, O.H. Biological transducers and Coding. In A Study Program. J.L. Oncley Ed. Am. Physical Soc. Wiley. 1959.

2. Zúñiga, A. Conversión de Energía en el sistema auditivo. Modelo Analógico (In progress).

New dimensions in otorhinolaryngology - head and neck surgery, vol. 2.
E. Myers, editor

EVALUATION OF CANDIDATES FOR COCHLEAR IMPLANT SURGERY

F. O. BLACK, D. J. LILLY, L. P. FOWLER[1], and PAUL STYPULKOWSKI[2]
Good Samaritan Hospital and Medical Center, 1015 N.W. 22nd Avenue, Portland, Oregon USA[1], 3-M Corporation[2]

INTRODUCTION

In an attempt to determine the ability of an implant candidate to use electrical signals for detection and comprehension of speech, the Good Samaritan Hospital and Neurological Sciences Institute Cochlear Implant team perform a tympanotomy under local anesthesia and insert a temporary electrode onto the round window membrane of candidates as a pre-implant procedure.

BACKGROUND

In theory a multiple channel cochlear implant system should provide more auditory information to a patient than a single channel system. The theoretical advantage of a multi-channel system will be realized only when: 1) we better understand the neural coding system used by the abnormal human auditory system (Bilger, et al, 1977) and 2) we can estimate more accurately the number and distribution of surviving ganglion cells in an individual patient (Simmons and Smith, 1983). Until these goals are accomplished, the decision to use a given implant system for a given patient will remain somewhat arbitrary.

PATIENT SELECTION CRITERIA

Patients must have a profound bilateral sensorineural hearing loss, no medical contraindications, and little or no benefit from amplification. The hearing loss must have occurred post-lingually, and the patient must be at least 18 years of age. Candidates must undergo basic audiometrics, a hearing aid evaluation, a trial with amplification, a complete vestibular evaluation, a minimal auditory capabilities (MAC) test battery, and a lip reading ability assessment.

DIAGNOSTIC TYMPANOTOMY

The electrode is placed onto the round window membrane and left in place for two to three days. The following pre-implant evaluations are performed: 1) electrically evoked ABR'S, 2) electrical stimulation of the contralateral acoustic reflex, 3) the three octave pitch test, and 4) the temporal difference limen (DL) test.

ADVANTAGES OF THE PRE-IMPLANT INSPECTION OF THE MIDDLE EAR SPACE AND ROUND WINDOW STIMULATION (AS ADVOCATED BY SIMMONS)

Advantages to the direct evaluation of the middle ear space and direct electrical stimulation include: 1) anatomical inspection of the round window membrane and niche, 2) confirmation of a round window reflex, 3) round window stimulation requires less current than promontory stimulation, 4) round window stimulation provides a good approximation of patient performance with the 3-M Vienna extracochlear implant, 5) the round window platinum-irridium ball electrode may be left in place for several days, 6) round window stimulation permits evaluation of electrical thresholds, maximum comfort level, loudness discomfort level (LDL or UCL) and computation of dynamic range, 7) round window stimulation permits generation and evaluation of electrically evoked auditory brainstem response, 8) round window stimulation permits evaluation of the electrically evoked contralateral acoustic reflex (these reflexes provide indirect evidence of the ability of the system to respond to acoustic-like electrically evoked auditory percepts), and 9) round window stimulation permits evaluation of pre-surgical psycho-physical responses to electrical signals, which include the three octave pitch test and the temporal difference limen test. These tests provide indirect evidence of the ability of the subject to use electrical stimulation for identification of signals contained in speech.

Ultimately, pre-implant round window stimulation or a similar procedure will be required for the development of objective techniques for pre-implant evaluation of infants and young children. Many of these patients will not have the ability to perform the psycho-physical tests, consequently alternative methods must be established for obtaining the information necessary for selection of the appropriate implant system for the individual child.

In summary, the direct electrical stimulation of the round window membrane appears to hold great promise as a pre-operative evaluation technique for cochlear implant patients. Results from five patients to date indicate that patients with the better results from the above tests also perform better on speech tracking tests post-operatively. Companies providing cochlear implants are encouraged to provide processors which can be used with a temporary round window electrode in order to further refine pre-op diagnostic techniques for patients with cochlear implants.

REFERENCES

1. Bilger, R.C., (1977), Evaluation of Subjects Presently Fitted with Implanted Auditory Prostheses. Annals of Otology, Rhinology & Laryngology, Suppl. 38, Vol. 86.

2. Simmons, F.B. and Smith, L. (1983), Estimating Nerve Survival by Electrical ABR. Annals of the New York Academy of Sciences, 405:422-423.

© 1985 Elsevier Science Publishers B.V. (Biomedical Division)
New dimensions in otorhinolaryngology – head and neck surgery, vol. 2.
E. Myers, editor

CLINICAL IMPLICATIONS OF HISTOLOGICAL FINDINGS IN THE ANIMAL LABYRINTH EXPOSED TO COCHLEAR IMPLANT SURGERY

P.A. BURGIO
Otologic Products/Life Science Sector, 3M Center, St. Paul, MN 55144

INTRODUCTION

Histological changes in response to various surgical procedures similar to those employed clinically for human cochlear implants were evaluated in the cochlea of the dog, the cat and the chinchilla. Also assessed were the histological implications of damage to the cochlea resulting from surgery or electrode insertion. Previous studies have shown that mechanical damage to cochlear tissue results in sensorineural degeneration, growth of fibrous tissue and new bone.[1-3] Studies have reported significant damage to cochlear tissues by some types of electrodes inserted greater than 10 mm into the cochlea.[1,2,4] The histological evaluation is now in progress. Results to date are presented in this report.

MATERIALS AND METHODS

The cochleas of the dog, cat, and chinchilla were exposed using sterile surgical techniques. The cochleas were opened two ways. Some were opened by drilling through the otic capsule near the round window, others by puncturing the round window membrane. In some animals, platinum electrodes 2-3 mm long were implanted without electrical stimulation. Fascia was placed in the round window niche of four dog cochleas to enhance the formation of fibrous tissue and closure of the window after surgery. Absorbable gelatin sponge was used for a similar purpose in two dog cochleas. After 2-9 months, the dog and cat tissues were fixed by whole body perfusion in 10% formalin. The chinchilla tissues were fixed by transcochlear perfusion. The cochleas were decalcified, embedded in araldyte, and sectioned at 5 microns for microscopic assessment.

RESULTS

When there was no mechanical damage to cochlear tissues, opening the round window or drilling in the otic capsule caused only localized formation of fibrous tissue and new bone. Only a thin fibrous capsule surrounded the platinum electrode. All animals showed this response (dog cochleas, N=7; cat cochleas, N=3; chinchilla cochleas, N=7). (See Figure 1.)

In cases where mechanical damage to the cochlear duct or osseous spiral lamina occurred during the surgical procedure there was fibrous tissue and new bone formation in the area of damage. This response was seen in all specimens

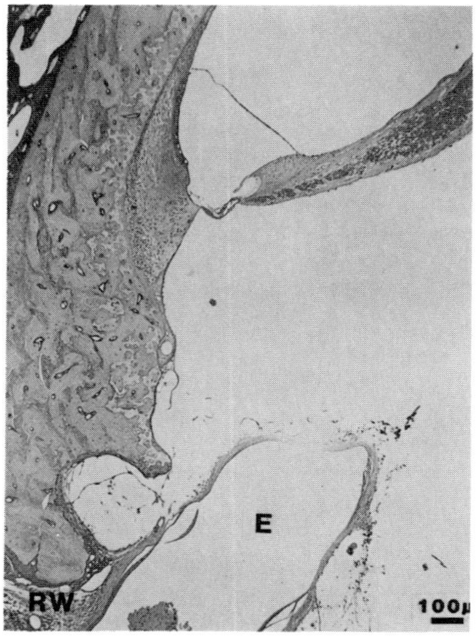

FIGURE 1: Cross-section of basal turn of dog cochlea implanted 6 months with short single wire electrode. Inner hair cells are present adjacent to electrode and round window. The tissue response to both surgery and electrode was localized to the round window (RW) and thin fibrous capsule around the silicone rubber insulation on the electrode (E). The round window was closed with fibrous tissue.

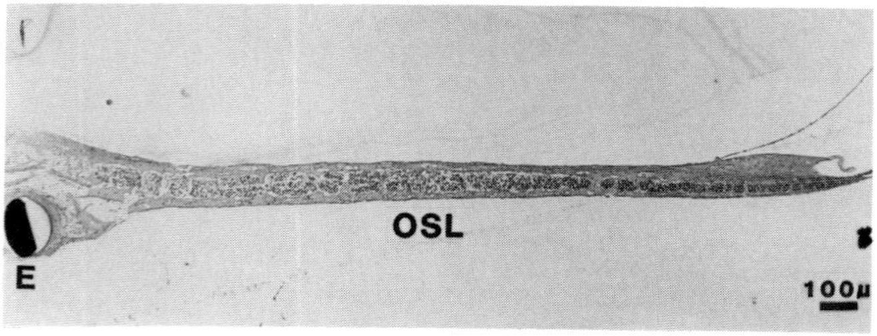

Figure 2: Cross-section of osseous spiral lamina (OSL) basal turn of dog cochlea implanted 6 months with single wire electrode (E) inserted through a hole in the otic capsule. Damage to spiral lamina occurred during installation. Nerve damage was severe next to electrode and extended apically about 1/4 turn. The upper basal turn was normal.

(dog cochleas, N=5; cat cochleas, N= 2; chinchilla cochleas, N=2). This tissue response occurred even without electrical stimulation of the tissues. In all cases where fascia was compared to absorbable gelatin sponge, the fascia showed less inflammatory response.

Mechanical injury to limited portions of the cochlear duct and osseous spiral lamina by the implant caused localized sensorineural degeneration. When the damage to the duct or lamina was severe, the degeneration extended outside the area of injury. (See Figure 2.)

DISCUSSION

Opening the cochlea and inserting an electrode produces a standard foreign-body response but little if any sensorineural degeneration when the cochlea is opened with minor mechanical damage to its tissues. However, the lack of reliable landmarks on the otic capsule makes it likely that drilling a hole in the otic capsule will cause damage to the cochlear duct or the osseous spiral lamina. This damage results in formation of fibrous tissue, new bone formation, and sensorineural degeneration. The round window entry to scala tympani results in less damage, especially because of the well-established landmarks.

The study indicates that the least traumatic entry into the cochlea (through the round window with minimal drilling) is preferred. More destructive entries may lead to adverse tissue reaction and sensorineural degeneration. Electrode designs that damage cochlear tissues during insertion can result in nerve degeneration and occlusion of scala tympani. These responses limit the insertion of electrodes of new designs.

REFERENCES

1. Galey FR (1984) Acta Otolaryngol (Stockh) Suppl 411, pp 33-44
2. Johnsson L-G, House WF, Linthicum FH (1982) In: Cochlear Implants: Progress Perspectives. Ann Otol Rhinol Larnygol, pp 74-89
3. Spoendlin H (1984) Ann Otol Rhinol Laryngol (Suppl) 112: 76-82
4. Sheppard RK, Clark GM, Pyman BC, Webb RL (1985 Ann Otol Rhinol Laryngol 94: 55-59

New dimensions in otorhinolaryngology - head and neck surgery, vol. 2.
E. Myers, editor

IOWA COCHLEAR IMPLANT COMPARISON PROJECT

BRUCE J. GANTZ, M.D.
Department of Otolaryngology-Head & Neck Surgery, University of Iowa, Iowa City, U.S.A.

The University of Iowa has developed a center to evaluate different cochlear implant designs in a uniform manner. Patients implanted here as well as those from research centers in the United States are being studied to determine the audiologic and other effects of the cochlear implant designs undergoing clinical trials in the United States. Two single channel and two multichannel devices have been evaluated in 13 postlingual profoundly deaf adults.

MATERIALS AND METHODS

The patient population consists of 4 patients with the the Los Angeles (LA) House implant[1]; 3 patients with the Vienna (V) Hochmair single channel intracochlear device[2]; 4 patients with the Melbourne (M) Clark multichannel implant[3]; and 2 patients with the the University of Utah (U) Eddington multichannel implant[4]. All but three patients have been using their devices for a year at the time of the evaluation.

The audiologic battery consists of selected tests from the Minimal Auditory Capabilities battery (MAC) of Owens et al[5] and tests developed at The University of Iowa (Iowa Cochlear Implant battery, Tyler et al)[6]. All tests are presented at 65 dB SPL in a sound field in a single-walled sound treatment room. Three randomizations of each of the tests are available. The order of presentation of the tests is randomized within and across subjects. The audiovisual tests are recorded on videotape and the sound version is presented before either the vision-only or sound-plus-vision tests. The remainder of the tests except one live voice test with a familiar speaker are recorded on audiotape. None of the test material is used for rehabilitation purposes or training prior to testing. Repetition of material is not allowed. Tests are organized into five categories: everyday sounds, prosody tests, closed-set and speech related tests, open-set speech, and audiovisual tests.

RESULTS

All patients were able to identify some environmental sounds in an open-set format. Three patients were able to distinguish 50% of the sounds. In a closed-set five-choice format 8 of 13 patients scored above 70%. Ability to process suprasegmental information such as alteration in fundamental frequency and amplitude is assessed with three tests designed to detect the prosody transitions. All four of the implant designs tested consistently process prosody information reflected by their rather uniform performance with this task.

All patients except two single channel patients were able to determine the difference between speech and an amplitude modulated white noise. Performance in a noisy environment was evaluated using a spondee four-choice test and a spondee four-choice word test with a multitalker noise at a signal-to-noise ratio of 10 dB (Fig. 1). The two patients with the Utah device performed better on this task than the other designs.

Three audiovisual tests and a monosyllable word test (NU-6) are used to assess open-set speech understanding with sound alone. The sentence test without-context (Fig. 2) presented simple sentences in the sound-only, vision-only, and sound-plus-vision conditions. The 6 multichannel implant patients were able to identify some words and complete sentences without visual cues. All patients demonstrated an improvement with their implant-plus-vision over vision-alone. If contextual material was available prior to sentence, all 4 implant designs provided some limited speech understanding in the sound-alone condition. In addition, if sentences are presented by a familiar speaker "live-voice", most patients identified more words than with strangers on tape.

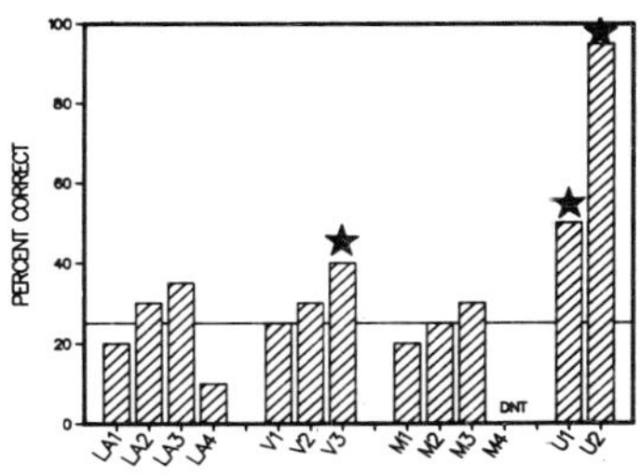

Fig. 1 * = p > .05 line = chance

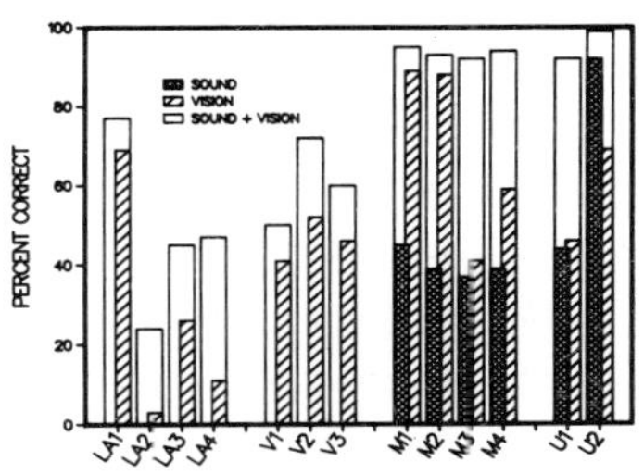

Fig. 2

DISCUSSION

The four cochlear implant designs evaluated in this study improve the communication skills of postlingual profoundly deafened adults. All patients obtained an improvement in their speechreading ability and received sufficient information to identify some environmental sounds. Both of these are important benefits for profoundly deaf patients. All patients are able to detect alterations in voicing frequency and amplitude of the speech signal. There appears to be no differences among devices on the prosody tasks even though the speech coding strategies are quite diverse. The results of the open-set speech tests demonstrate the consistent ability of the two multichannel implant designs to provide enough information to patients for them to recognize some speech without visual clues or contextual information. The addition of place information to the speech processing scheme appears to be a definite advantage for the patients evaluated.

The dramatic results obtained with patient U2 illustrate the potential benefit that multichannel cochlear implants can provide in select patients. The reasons for U2's exceptional performance, however, are unknown. Additional patients must be evaluated before any conclusions can be drawn regarding differences in multichannel speech processing schemes.

In summary, multichannel cochlear implants that provide place information in addition to fundamental frequency and amplitude changes are allowing profoundly deaf patients to recognize some words without visual cues. In our limited series, multichannel cochlear implant patients consistently out-perform single channel designs. All of the implants, as expected, do enhance lipreading ability and provide useful information about speech and non-speech sounds.

REFERENCES

1. House WF, et al. (1982) Ann Otol Rhinol Laryngol 91(Suppl.)
2. Hochmair-Desoyer IJ, Hochmair ER, Burian K, et al (1983) Ann NY Acad Sci 405:295-306
3. Clark GM, Tong YC, Dowell RC (1983) Ann NY Acad Sci 405:370-376
4. Eddington DK (1980) J Acoust Soc Am 68:885-891
5. Owens E, Kessler DK, Telleen CC, Schubert ED (1981) The minimal auditory capabilities battery. Auditec, St. Louis
6. Tyler RS, Preece JP, Lowder MW (1983) The Iowa cochlear implant tests. The University of Iowa, Iowa City

© 1985 Elsevier Science Publishers B.V. (Biomedical Division)
New dimensions in otorhinolaryngology - head and neck surgery, vol. 2.
E. Myers, editor

PITCH MATCH TEST FOR TINNITUS BY HEPTATONIC SCALE

KATSUICHIRO OHSAKI, MAMORU KIMURA, IKUO INOKUCHI, TOMOAKI SUGIURA,
SHINGO NAKAGIRI, TETSUYA FUJIMURA, AKIRA KIMURA, YU MASUDA & IKUO KOIDE
Division of Clinical Otology, University Hospital, Tokushima University,
School of Medicine, Tokushima (Japan)

In order to measure the pitch near the central frequency of subjective tinnitus (tinnitus), the pitch match test using heptachord on the basis of temperament musical scale was attempted to tinnitus.

We guessed that approximate frequency value(AFV) was measured as accurately as possible to the tinnitus because one octave is divided into seven steps and we are most accustomed to and familiar with heptatonic scale since childhood. And we manufactured parts of machinery of oscillator by way of experiment for practical use of this test.

MATERIAL & METHOD: From June 1983 to Jan. 1984, 30 tinnitus in 27 ears of 22 patients of various otologic diseases were tested. Age of patients was from 27 to 75 years old($\overline{x}$=50.5, S.D.=±13.2). Both male and female were 11.

First of all, we measured a rough frequency of tinnitus pitch at one octave interval, by bracketing method. Then we measured AFV of tinnitus by presenting pure tone frequencies of heptachord recorded on tape in conformity to ascending method of pure tone audiometry.

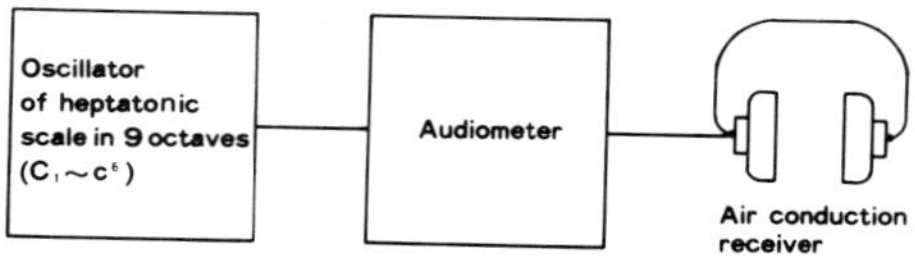

Fig. 1. Blockdiagram of experimental apparatus measering tinnitus using the pure tone heptachord frequency

The experimental apparatus aiming at the practical use of this test presents 63 tones in 9 octaves(C^1-c^6) and was designed so that pitch and loudness of tinnitus could be measured(Fig.1).

RESULTS & DISCUSSION: AFV of tinnitus could be measured in 19 patients(86.4%).

The lowest AFV of tinnitus was 98.00Hz=C(sol) in the patient of right chr. otitis media postop.. The highest AFV was 4186.08Hz=c^5(do) in the patient of left otosclerosis and right sensorineural hearing loss respectively.

Eight tinnitus(29.6%) out of measured 27 tinnitus belong to octave c and 7 tinnitus(25.9%) octave c^1 respectively. Three tinnitus(11.1%) belong to the octave c^2, c^3 and c^4 respectively, and 2 tinnitus to the octave c^5.

We discuss about the validity why heptachord pitch match test could accurately measure the pitch of tinnitus.

1) Relationship between relative interval ratio of heptatonic scale and frequency difference limen(FDL): From the historical review by Plomp(1), minimum

frequency difference to distinguish the two pitches between two simultaneous tones to the same ear is 50-100Hz in the 1000Hz.

Meurmann(2) measured $\Delta F/F \times 100\%$* in the diseased ear, presenting simultaneous two tones to the same ear - a pure tone and a modulation frequency pulsating tone. The relative FDL showed 1.0-3.0% in the sensorineural hearing loss and 1.5-5.0% in the Ménière's patients. Relative interval ratio is about 12% in the whole tone and about 6% in the semitone.

As we compared relative interval ratio in semitone with relative FDL between two simultaneous tones above-mentioned diseased, we noticed that relative interval ratio in semitone might be composed of a certain level, nearer to the minimal fractional difference in Ménierè's patients.

2) Psychoacoustical model(Fig.2): While pitch of sound, like mel scale, can be expressed one-dimentionally on the spiral curved line, described on the lateral surface of tonal bell devised by Ruckmick, the sense of tonality can be expressed three-dimentionally as a spiral change on the lateral surface of tonal bell. For example, we feel two tones of octave between "do" and one octave upper "do" nearer than two tones of narrow 2nd interval between "do" and "re": this phenomenon is called approximation of octave.

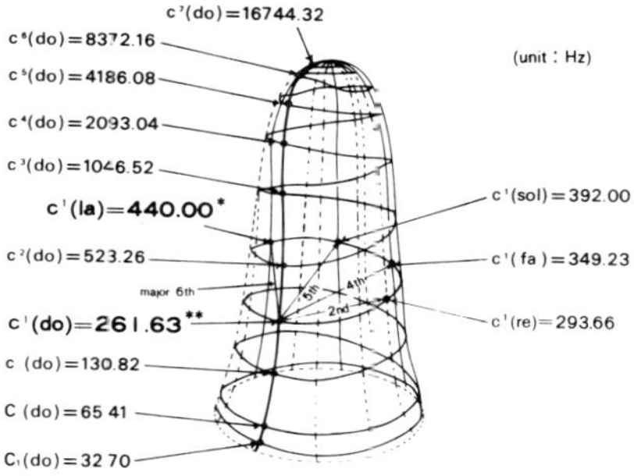

Fig. 2. Pitch and tonality of sound (Ruckmick: 1929)

* : Standard frequency ** : Center "do" in piano

Therefore, we think that FDL between neighbouring two tones on the heptachord could be discriminated easier than one octave interval on physical scale in standard pure tone audiometer if we referring to Ruckmick's model.

SUMMARY: 1) AFV of tinnitus could be measured in 19 cases(86.4%) by heptachord pitch match test in this series. 2) Experimental apparatus for the practical use of this test was devised and test tones were presented to the congress. 3) We discussed about validity why heptachord pitch match test could accurately measure the pitch of tinnitus.

REFERENCES: 1) Plomp R(1964):J Acoust Soc Am 36:1628-1636. 2) Meurmann OH(1954): Acta Otoloryngol.(Suppl)(Stockh) 118:114-155.

* $\Delta F/F \times 100\%$: Relative difference limen in frquency.

New dimensions in otorhinolaryngology – head and neck surgery, vol. 2.
E. Myers, editor

EXTERNAL ELECTRICAL STIMULATION - TINNITUS CONTROL - TINNITUS SUPPRESSION WITH PROLONGED STIMULATION

A. SHULMAN,M.D., Associate Professor
Division of Otolaryngology - Center Communication Sciences
Downstate Medical Center, SUNY, Brooklyn, New York

J. TONNDORF,M.D.,Professor Emeritus
Department of Otolaryngology, College of Physicians and Surgeons
Columbia University,New York, New York

INTRODUCTION

External Electrical Stimulation (EES) for Tinnitus Control (TC)-Tinnitus Suppression (TS) has produced significant results in selected tinnitus cases. The present report Stage IV, represents clinical observations in N-20 patients selected for ongoing prolonged EES of one month or longer from 10/84-4/30/85. Clinical research with prototypes have been ongoing since February, 1983, (Stages I-III)[1]. In Stage IV both patient selection and TC/TS have been tested for consistency of results and conclusions.

METHOD AND MATERIALS:- A definitive device - the Tinnitus Suppressor - was applied as a headset for EES on N-20 patients. The device was designed and was modified by Richard Dugot of the Audimax Corp. So. Hackensack, New Jersey. The device produces a constant voltage of 5v p-p; current at the skin electrode interface of 2-2.5ma; a low radio frequency carrier signal of 60KHz modulated by frequencies of 200-20,000Hz. The power delivered to the head is below 20 milliwatts. All patients completed a medical audiologic evaluation by a neurotologist and audiologist. Patient selection was based on maskability of the tinnitus; a peripheral site of lesion of the tinnitus; no active ear disease or vestibular asymmetry. The Electrical High Frequency Audiometer was used to determine threshold response from .5-20KHz before and following EES. All patients agreed to a trial period of EES for one month. The patients are reported in four GRPS. based upon the extent of completion of the one month trial period. An initial trial of one hour of EES was completed in the office by all patients. The duration of EES was individualized for each patient. A Maximum Tinnitus Intensity Comfort level was established. This is the maximum tinnitus comfort that can be achieved with the shortest duration of EES. Efficacy is based upon the effect(s) of EES on the tinnitus parameters of intensity, location, quality, duration. A Tinnitus Intensity Index for tinnitus intensity is recorded daily on a scale of 0-7 i.e. (7 is the poorest and 0 represents absence of tinnitus). Increased tinnitus intensity, ear blockage, rebound were followed by cessation of EES for 24-48 hrs.; followed by resumption of EES at half of the duration of stimulation.

RESULTS:- Significant tinnitus intensity reduction was experienced. In GRPS.1-4- overall, N-11/20 (55%). GRP 1 patients were stimulated for at least one month, reported transient TC-TS N-9/12 (75%); consistent TC/TS for 1-3 mo. - N-5/12 (41%); consistent TC/TS for all GRPs. -N-5/20 (25%). Improvement of tinnitus was reported for its quality, location and duration. Patients with successful EES for TC/TS were maskable; demonstrated a predominantly peripheral site of lesion; absence vestibular asymmetry; absence active ear disease.[2,3]. The Maximum Tinnitus Comfort Level is highly individual, and variable (1-5 Hrs.). GRP. 1 patients described adaptation; habituation. Significant rebound effect in all groups. GRP. 2 patients discontinued EES within 1-14 days due to increased intensity. GRP.3 patients declined EES, due to headset. GRP 4 patients had a vestibular asymmetry; discontinued EES after one hour trial due to increased tinnitus intensity. Subjective hearing improvement GRP.1 (N-3). Transient vertigo GRP 1 -(N-2); GRP 4 (N-1). Ear blockage GRP.1 (N-4); GRP.2 (N-2) GRP.3 (N-0); GRP 4- (N-1). The Electrical High Frequency Audiometer in GRP 1 (N-7) revealed fluctuation in threshold responses around the tinnitus frequency - maximum ± 15dB.

DISCUSSION, CONCLUSIONS:- Complications include increased tinnitus intensity; rebound, ear blockage. Original intensity levels followed cessation EES within 24-48 hrs. Maximum duration of stimulation should not exceed 5hrs. The Maximum Tinnitus Comfort Level is the most comfortable level of tinnitus intensity achieved with the shortest duration of stimulation. The present study supports the previous criteria of patient selection. The key elements for TC/TS using EES are patient selection, establishment and maintenance of a maximum tinnitus comfort level, development of monitoring systems to attempt to objectivize the subjective complaint of the tinnitus symptom.

REFERENCES

1. Shulman, A: External Electrical Stimulation In Tinnitus Control. Am. Jrl. Otol. Vol. 6, No.1 pp 110-115,1985.

2. Shulman,A: External Electrical Stimulation - Tinnitus Suppression - Hearing: Preliminary Results. Proceedings II Intl. Tinnitus Suppression - Laryngol Otol. Suppl. 9:141-144,1984.

3. Shulman,A; Seitz,M.: Central Tinnitus - Diagnosis and Treatment Observations Simultaneous Binaural Auditory Brainstem Responses with Monaural Stimulation in the Tinnitus Patient. The Laryngoscope Vol. XCI, No.12, pp 2025-2035, December, 1981.

New dimensions in otorhinolaryngology - head and neck surgery, vol. 2.
E. Myers, editor

ELECTROPHYSIOLOGICAL DIAGNOSIS OF PERIPHERAL FACIAL PALSY

AKIRA KIKUCHI
Department of Otorhinolaryngology, School of Medicine, Yamagata University, Yamagata, Japan

Electroneurography (ENoG) is an electrophysiological diagnostic method for predicting the prognosis of peripheral facial palsy. It provides an electric stimulation to the facial nerve from the stylomastoid foramen and records mainly the orbicularis oris muscle contraction by surface electrodes, and the prognosis is evaluated in terms of the ratio of the amplitude of the normal side to that of the lesion side (ENoG value).

In 175 patients with Bell's palsy seen within 2 weeks after the onset and given a conservative therapy in our Department, recovery of the facial movement (May's score modified by Hosomi) at 1, 2 and 6 months after the onset and the appearance of sequelae were examined. Diagnostic criteria of the prognosis were formulated on the basis of the ENoG values within 2 weeks after the onset.

The criteria indicated that patients with an ENoG value above 40% almost recovered within a month without any sequela, those with an ENoG value of 20-39% almost recovered within 2 months with a 1/10 incidence of sequela and those with an ENoG value of 5-19% recovered in many cases within 6 months. The incidence of sequela was 1/5 for those wih an ENoG value above 10% and 1/2 for those with an ENoG value below 10%. In patients with an ENoG value of 0-4%, the ENoG value was mostly 0% without sufficient recovery even after 6 months in whom the sequela amounted to 1/2.

The present criteria provide a larger advantage for precise evaluation than the conventional Esslen's criteria in that the former permits more patient distribution of cases, detailed assessment of the prognosis and quantification of the incidence of sequela. It was also found that 10-19% was a clinical critical limit below which a complete recovery was not expected.

To elucidate the pathology of paralyzed facial nerve of the corresponding severity, an experimenal rat model of facial palsy was prepared by compression of the nerve with a Pean's forceps for 30 seconds. The electrophysiological and histological changes of the facial nerve in this model were examined. ENoG was performed under general anesthesia 3, 5, 14, 28 and 56 days after induction of facial palsy. The buccinator ramus of the facial nerve immediately from the parotid gland was excised and fixed with glutaraldehyde and osmium tetrodoxide. After dehydration, it was embedded in epoxy resin for light and electron microscopy.

The mean ENoG value was 13% on the 3rd day, 18% on the 5th day, 27% on the 14th day, 32% on the 28th day and 78% on the 56th day, indicating recovery with time. Light microscopy revealed a reduction of residual myelinated nerve fibers in the beginning, which were reduced on the contralateral side to 33% on the 3rd day, to 16% on the 5th day and to 5% on the 14th day. But They were increased to 28% on the 28th day and 51% on the 56th day. Myelinated fibers' ratio increased parallel to ENoG value with 10 days delay. That delay came from the 10mm distance from electrical stimulated region to excised region. Electron microscopy revealed no distinct evidence of degeneration on the 3rd day, and appearance of high density area within the axis cylinder on the 5th day with progression of degenerative changes such as disappearance of microfilaments and microtubules. On the 14th day, the nerves were almost lost with the exception of only myelinated fibers and Schwann cells. The degenerative changes disappeared and myelinated fibers increased on the 28th day, and a number of myelinated fibers on the 56th day.

These findings indicated that this experimental facial palsy corresponding to approximately 13% ENoG is a pathology perfectly recoverable by reinnervation, because the surrounding connective tissue is preserved, despite Waller's degeneration.

REFERENCE

1 Esslen, E: Electromyography and electroneurography. In Facial Nerve Surgery, pp.93-100, Kugler Med.Pub. Amstelveen/Aesculapius Pib Co. Brimingham, 1977

2 Hosomi, H et al.: Critical examinations at healing of peripheral facial nerve palsy. Practica Otologica (Kyoto) 67: 351-358, 1974

© 1985 Elsevier Science Publishers B.V. (Biomedical Division)
New dimensions in otorhinolaryngology - head and neck surgery, vol. 2.
E. Myers, editor

RESULTS OF CALORIC TESTS AND VISUAL SUPPRESSION TESTS IN SEASICKNESS

TAKASHI MATSUNAGA*,M.D., NOBUYA FUJITA*,M.D., HISAMI KAKIUCHI*,M.D.,
HIROYUKI YAMAMOTO*,M.D., KATSUNARI YANE*,M.D. and SHINJI OHHIRA**,M.D.

* : Depts. of Otolaryngology, Nara Medical College, Shijo-cho 840, Kashihara, Nara, 634, JAPAN
**: Depts. of Otolaryngology, Municipal Hospital of Suita, Katayama-cho, Suita, Osaka, 564, JAPAN

INTRODUCTION

Seasickness is a physically ill state that is characterized by several kinds of uncomfortable autonomic nervous symptoms caused by a shake of a ship giving an abnormal acceleration stimulus to the vestibular labyrinth through the brain stem, but its details still remain unclear. Moreover, it has a problem of very great personal difference.

As a consistent clinical study of susceptible factors of seasickness, caloric tests and visual suppression tests were performed in both the seasickness group and the non-seasickness, and the relations were examined between seasickness and susceptibility of the vestibular labyrinth.

MATERIAL AND METHODS

During the 25th of Nov. and the 2nd of Dec., 1983, the habitual seasickness group of 22 men (44 ears) and the non-seasickness of 29 (57 ears) were selected in 124 students (from 19 to 20 years old) of Merchantile Marine College who practiced to sail on Miyazaki-Amami Islands and Amami Islands-Tokyo routes of the Japan Sea area aboard a training ship belonging to the navigation school of the Ministry of Transport. The habitual seasickness group was including the students who had seasickness in this voyage with an answer of usual seasickness to the questionnaire before the voyage.

Mean maximum slow phase eye velocity (mean max. SPEV) and visual suppression rates of nystagmus (Takemori's method) induced by caloric tests (15 sec irrigations of 50 ml water of 30°C and 44°C) were measured, and compared between both of the groups by a t-test.

RESULTS

There was no significant difference in each caloric irrigation between both the groups except the tendency of smaller mean max. SPEVs in the habitual seasickness groups. And there was also no significant difference between both of the groups in each caloric irrigation except the tendency of greater difference in mean max. SPEV between the right and the left in the habitual seasickness groups.

In the mean values between both of the groups there was no significantly difference except the significantly ($P < 0.05$) greater difference in the difference of fixation suppression rates in visual suppression tests between the right and the left in the seasickness groups (Table 1).

CONCLUSION AND COMMENTS

The previous reports describe that the seasickness groups has slightly longer durations of nystagmus and seasation of dizziness in the caloric tests. On the other hand, few of reports describe relations between seasickness and mean max. SPEVs of caloric nystagmus , and between seasickness and fixation suppression rates.

The results of this study were that the habitual seasickness groups tended to have a smaller mean max. SPEV and its greater difference between the right and the left than the non-seasickness without significence. This fact makes it considered that the seasickness groups tends to have vestibular functions of inner ears more lowered, unbalanced, and irritated to a motion stimulus. And the habitual seasickness group, compared with the non-seasickness, has a greater difference in fixation suppression rates of caloric nystragmus between the right and the left and this fact also makes it considered that the seasickness group has more unbalanced function of visual fixation including vestibular cerebelli and more lowered functions in dynamic pursuit of moving objects. Hereafter, these problems would be examined clinically in patients with seasickness.

REFERENCES

1. Matsunaga, T. (1964) : Correlation of susceptibility to seasickness to vestibular function. Jap. Jour. Otol. (Tokyo) 67 : 259-278 (in Japanese).
2. Takemori S. (1977) : Visual suppression test. Ann. Otol. 86 : 80-85.
3. Tutsumi M., Matsunaga, T. et al (1980) : Motion sickness. Q & A. Roppo Co. Tokyo pp426-429 (in Japanese).

TABLE I

A FIXATION SUPPRESSION RATES IN VISUAL SUPPRESSION RATES (M ± SD)

	Fixation suppression rates	
Subjects	Mean value (%)	Difference between Rt and Lt
Habitual seasickness group	47.1 ± 28.3 (N=8)	53.3 ± 35.9* (N=4)
Non-seasickness group	49.5 ± 21.3 (N=22)	22.0 ± 16.6* (N=11)

* : $P < 0.05$

New dimensions in otorhinolaryngology - head and neck surgery, vol. 2.
E. Myers, editor

NERVE EXCITABILITY TEST USING PERCUTANEOUS NEEDLE ELECTRODES

TAKEO KOBAYASHI, M.D. and KOSUKE ISHII, M.D.

Department of Otolaryngology, Central Hospital of Japanese National Railways, Yoyogi, Shibuya, Tokyo 151, Japan

Department of Otolaryngology, University of Tokyo, Hongo, Bunkyo, Tokyo 113, Japan

INTRODUCTION

One of the disadvantages of conventional NET using surface electrode is that it is occasionally unreliable. This may be due to the placement of the electrodes or to the electrical characteristics of the skin that vary with temperature, perspiration, tonus, and thickness of the soft parts covering the nerve. In order to eliminate the variability of skin resistance as a compounding variable, we chose instead to stimulate the facial nerve trunk using thin needle elctrodes inserted at the stylomastoid area.

METHOD

Stainless steel needles for acupuncture were used(diameter, 0.21mm; length 15mm). Two needles were inserted, so that the nerve should lie between two needles. A square wave electrical pulse of 1msec in duration was applied. A minimal threshold voltage for eliciting the contraction was then determined.

SUBJECTS

Thirty nine cases of unilateral acute facial palsy (Bell's palsy and Hunt's syndrome) were seen in our facial nerve clinic in 1984. All cases were of recent onset; and in all cases, conservative treatment was administered. Thirty four cases were studied with NET and EMG.

RESULTS

Thirty four cases were followed up with EMG examination two or three times. All cases which showed positive response with surface stimulation also had a positive response with needle stimulation. Cases were devided into four groups, A, B, C and D. Their recoveries were shown in the table.

COMMENT

We had 39 cases of Bell's palsy and Hunt's syndrome in 1984. In 5 cases(group D), NET was not done, because of good facial muscle movement at their first visit. Eventually, each of these five cases showed complete recovery within 4 weeks.

In this study, 34 cases were followed with NET and EMG. There were no cases which remained completely paralyzed. Twenty seven cases(group A and B) showed good recovery. Seven cases(group C) showed incomplete recovery.

From our study, 32 out of 39 cases(82%) showed complete recovery in their EMG pattern (Bell's palsy, 23 out of 26 cases(88%); Hunt's syndrome, 9 out of 13 cases(69%)).

CONCLUSION

NET using needle electrode is simple and useful. Children can easily tolerate the procedures. For prognostication it is more effective than conventional NET using surface electrodes.

TABLE

	cases			surface stimulation	needle stimulation	recovery in EMG
A	22	B	18	+	+	good
		H	4			
B	5	B	4	-	+	good
		H	1			
C	7	B	3	-	-	poor
		H	4			
D	5	B	1	NET not done (see text)		good
		H	4			

B: Bell's palsy H: Hunt's syndrome

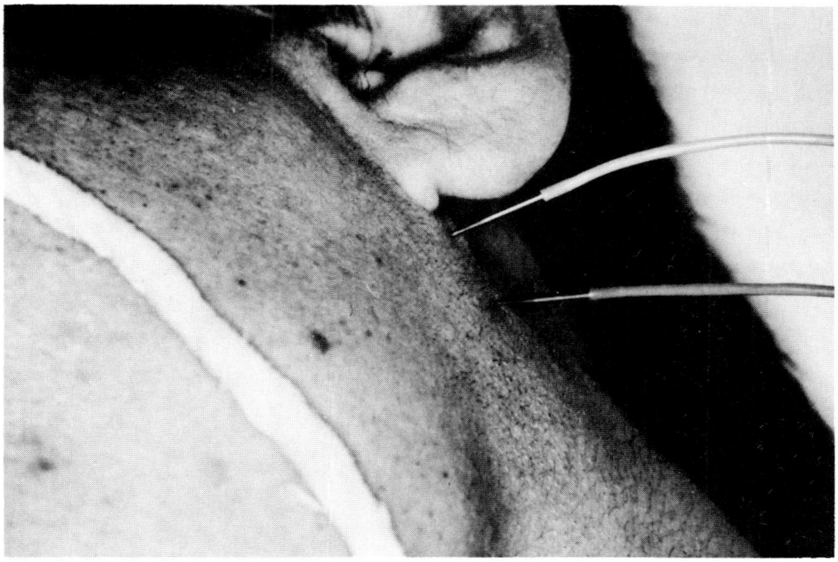

Fig. Stimulation needles inserted at the stylomastoid area.

© 1985 Elsevier Science Publishers B.V. (Biomedical Division)
New dimensions in otorhinolaryngology - head and neck surgery, vol. 2.
E. Myers, editor

"CONGENITAL CHOLESTEATOMA OF THE MIDDLE EAR: A SURGICAL APPROACH"

MARK J. LEVENSON, M.D., SIMON C. PARISIER, M.D., ERIC SMOUHA, M.D., SHULA WENIG, M.S.
CHILDREN'S HEARING INSTITUTE, MANHATTAN EYE, EAR & THROAT HOSPITAL, 210 E. 64th STREET, NEW YORK, NEW YORK 10021

INTRODUCTION

Over the past eight years, twenty-two children have presented with well defined cholesteatomas behind intact tympanic membranes. The majority of these children have had a prior episode of otitis media, and a white mass was discovered on routine examination by the child's pediatrician. Fifteen cases of these "congenital" cholesteatomas operated upon with a minimal follow-up of one year are reviewed.

Fifteen children ranging from two to eight years of age (mean 4.5 years) underwent surgery for the removal of cholesteatoma presenting behind an intact tympanic membrane. Follow-up ranged from one to eight years (3.2 yrs. mean). All cases were excluded with history or clinical evidence of prior tympanic membrane perforation, prior otorrhea, prior myringotomy, or otologic surgery. There were nine males, and six females. Lesions were classified pre-operatively with respect to the quadrant of the tympanic membrane where the mass was visible upon otoscopic exam.

Transcanal Approach:

1. Extended tympanomeatal flap of 280° based inferiorly.
2. Elevation of tympanic membrane off short process of malleus with micro-cup forceps.
3. Longitudinal periosteal incision along medio-lateral aspect of handle of malleus with tabb knife.
4. Elevation of periosteum off malleus, in continuity with tympanic membrane.
5. Severing attachments of tympanic membrane from umbo and reflection of flap inferiorly.

Results:

Of the nine anterior quadrant cases, seven were removed by a transcanal tympanotomy alone. Two were combined with an atticotomy. Lesions pre-operatively assigned to the posterior quadrant group, had increased ossicular involvement (4/6), and required tympanomastoidectomy (5/6) for adequate removal.* Recurrence occurred in 2/6 posterior quadrant lesions both of which had canal wall up, posterior tympanotomy approach procedures initially. Recurrent disease has not yet occurred in the anterior quadrant lesions. Anterior quadrant lesions uniformly appeared to rise medial to the malleus from the region of the tensor tympani tendon, and were limited laterally by the anterior malleolar ligament. Typically, these lesions were well defined pearls, not in continuity with the tympanic membrane. Of note is that 5/15 cases had minor or major associated congenital ab-

* Table 1

normalities.

Discussion:

Derlacki and Clemis's exclusion of cases as "congenital" on the basis of a prior episode of otitis media may not be realistic, since greater than 70% of all children have a documented episode of otitis media prior to two years of age.[1,2] The occurence of these lesions behind normal appearing tympanic membranes, medial to the malleus, in ears with normal middle ear mucosa, speaks against the lesions being of the primary or secondary acquired types. Their etiology may be due to an epithelial rest trapped medial to the tympanic ring during early development, or alternatively secondary to metaplasia of pleuripotential mucosal elements.[3,4]

Successful removal of anterior quadrant lesions can be accomplished by an extended transcanal tympanotomy in most cases.° Posterior lesions are more destructive and most require tympanomastoid surgery for adequate excision. Seven cases not reviewed in this report have been operated upon in the past year, and it appears to the authors, as well as others, that the incidence of these lesions is increasing.[5]

Table 1: Surgical Approach:

QUADRANT	NUMBER CASES	TRANSCANAL	TRANSCANAL ATTICOTOMY	TYMPANO-MASTOID
ANTERIOR	9	7	2	-
POSTERIOR	5	1	-	5
ANTERIOR/ POSTERIOR	1	-	-	1

REFERENCES:

1. Derlacki, EL, Clemis JD (1965) Ann. Otol, Rhinol. and Laryngol. 74:706-727.
2. Bluestone CD, Stool SE (1983) Pediatric Otolaryngology. W.B. Saunders, Philadelphia pp. 513-564.
3. Aimi K (1983) Laryngoscope 93:1140-1145.
4. Sade J, Babiacki A, Pinlous G (1983) Acta Otolaryngol 96:119-129.
5. Schwartz RH, Grandfast KM (1984) Pediatrics 74:No.2 236-239.

° See Transcanal Approach on prior page

© 1985 Elsevier Science Publishers B.V. (Biomedical Division)
New dimensions in otorhinolaryngology - head and neck surgery, vol. 2.
E. Myers, editor

EPITHELIAL MIGRATION ON THE TYMPANIC MEMBRANE AND EXTERNAL CANAL

KUNIHIKO MAKINO, MUTSUO AMATSU
Department of Otolaryngology, Kobe University School of Medicine, Kobe, Japan

INTRODUCTION

Although the pathogenesis of external auditory canal cholesteatoma(EACC) is still controversial, the common understanding concerning the etiology is based on the disturbance of epithelial migration. In this study, an ink-dot staining method was used to examine epithelial migration in normal ears, in the case of EACC and in pathologic tympanic membranes.

MATERIALS AND METHODS

Twenty-four normal ears, seventeen ears of EACC, 6 bilateral and 5 unilateral and eleven pathologic tympanic membranes, such as 5 atrophic membranes, 3 cloudy membranes and 2 OME, were examined in this series to clarify the pattern and the rate of epithelial migration. 0.5% India Ink was used as a marker dye, and was applied to the tympanic membrane and external canal by cotton-tipped applicators. The changes were examined at two-week intervals, using microscope and were recorded by photography and sketch.

RESULTS

Migratory pattern in normal ears. The migratory patterns in pars tensa were classified into three types (Fig.1). In pars flaccida they were classified into two types (Fig.2). In type 1, the marker dyes at the manubrium mallei crossed pars flaccida, and in type 2, they did not cross pars flaccida. In both areas, the migratory courses were in good accordance with that of the vessels.

Migratory rate in normal ears (Fig.3). The migratory rate on the tympanic membrane was the fastest in the anterior inferior quadrant and the slowest in the posterior superior quadrant. The migratory rate on the external canal was faster in the inferior wall and the posterior superior wall. It was approximately 142 μm/day.

Epithelial migration and findings of the tympanic membrane and external canal in EACC. Lowered migratory rate and desquamation were found in all cases. The abnormal pattern was found in one case. The findings of the tympanic membrane showed atrophy (14 ears), clouding (10 ears), retraction (3 ears) and adhesion (1 ear), which suggested avasucularization. The skin of the external canal showed the mixed status of congestion (14 ears) and avascularization (9 ears).

Epithelial migration in pathologic tympanic membranes. In all of these cases, lowered migratory rate and desquamation were found. The abnormal pattern was found in 4 atrophic membranes and 1 cloudy membrane.

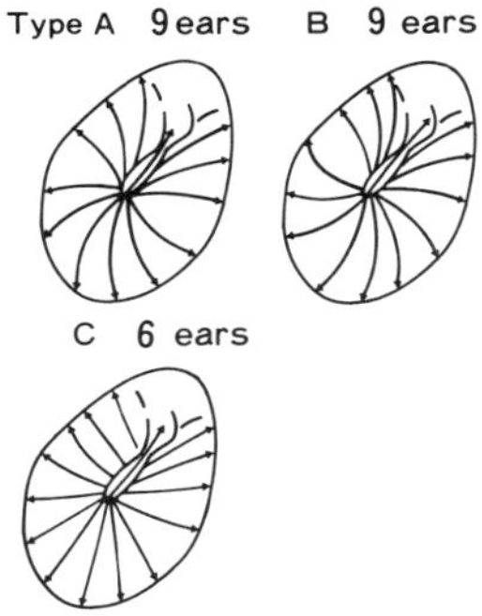

Fig.1. Migratory pattern in pars tensa.

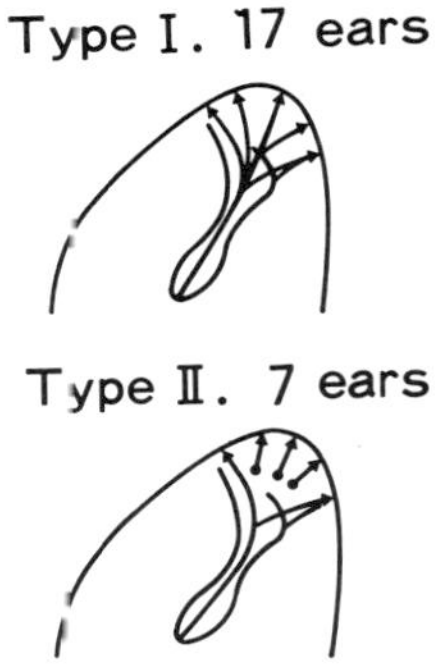

Fig.2. Migratory pattern in pars flaccida.

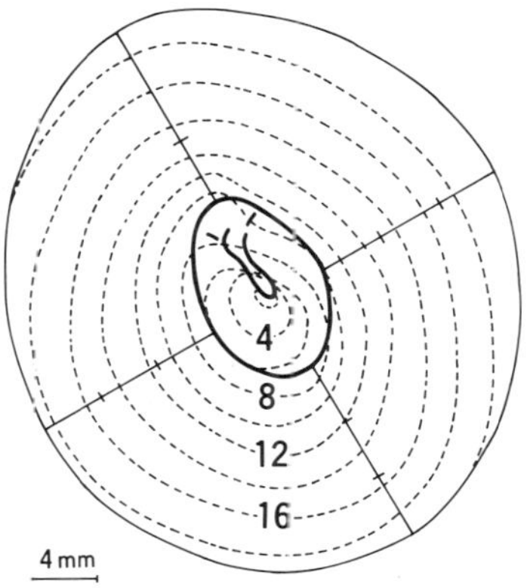

Fig.3. Migratory rate in normal ears. The dot lines show the migratory distance at two-week intervals.

DISCUSSION

In 1964, Alberti made clinical investigation of ink-dot migration pattern, and noted the umbo to be the center of migration. In 1968, Litton postulated that in the human there was the generation center at the umbo. However, the factors which determine the direction of epithelial migration are obscure up to date. In our study, the direction of epithelial migration was in good accordance with that of the vessels, and the Litton's generation center theory, the direction of epithelial migration may be controlled by the vessels nurishing the epidermal layer of the tympanic membrane. Therefore, in poor blood supply of the tympanic membrane and external canal, epithelial migration is considered to be disturbed. In fact, in our study using the avascularized tympanic membranes, such as atrophy, clouding and OME, epithelial migration was disturbed.

In EACC, the findings of tympanic membranes showed poor blood supply. Therefore epithelial migration in EACC is considered to be distrubed. This result in keratinization on the external canal in situ. Under the condition of keratinization, bone resorption will occur by some chemical mediators.

CONCLUSION

Epithelial migration was examined in normal ears, in the cases of EACC and in the pathologic tympanic membranes. The migratory course was in good accordance with the course of the vessels. In EACC and pathologic tympanic membranes, epithelial migration was disturbed. It was suggested that epithelial migration was disturbed in poor blood supply. The disturbance of epithelial migration was considered to be the pathogenesis of EACC.

New dimensions in otorhinolaryngology - head and neck surgery, vol. 2.
E. Myers, editor

STUDY OF EUSTACHIAN TUBE DRAINAGE FUNCTION WITH RADIOISOTOPE (99^m Tc)

SILVIO A.M. MARONE, M.D.; AROLDO MINITI, M.D.
Otorynolaryñgology Department of Faculty of Medicine of São Paulo University, São Paulo, Brazil

INTRODUCTION

The knowlege of the physiological condition of the Eustachian tube is of major significance to the understanding of the middle ear pathology as well as for the treatment of each case. This paper was made to study the drainage function of the Eustachian tube.

METHOD

Subjects

38 ears belonging to 31 patients presenting disacusis from the Otorynolaryngology Ambulatory of Hospital das Clinicas of the Faculty of Medicine of São Paulo University were studied; from these 18 were women, 13 men, 28 whites, 4 blacks, 1 yellow. During the clinical examination all patients presented eardrum perfurations, without any signs of reactivation of the original sickness (absence of pathological discharge) previously diagnosed through RXs and otomicroscopy. As to the diagnosis, 26 patients presented a chronic post-infection middle ear otites sequela, 3 presented a chronic media otites resulting from direct trauma in the eardrum, 1 patient presenting a surgical sequela following a mastoidectomy due to cholesteatoma, and 1 patient presenting a chronic medium otites caused by barotrauma.

Procedure

The choice of the Tecnetiun (99^m Tc) as tracer was based on its physical qualities-tracer perfectly adaptable to the detection sistem, pure gamma emissor, low energy and 6 hours half-life. We used a volume of 0,2 to 0,5 ml of 99^m Tc, dissolved in physiological solution with a activity of 500 µCi, wich was placed in the tympanic canty through the perforation, aided by a curved beveless needle and an otoscope.

The detection and analyses sistem was compose of a Cintilation Gamma Camera Ohio Nuclear, model Sigma 400, and a digital microprocessor model PDD 11/34. A high resolution collimater was also employed. To obtain a better image avoiding superpositions, after placing the radiofarmaco in the middle ear, the patient was placed in front of the cintilation camera with the head leaning on it and tilted to the opposite side 15 degrees so that the salpingo-atico-antral axis remais perpendicular to the Gamma Camera. The patient was asked to swallow every 30 seconds, initiating the recording of the images on the processor, beeing afterwords photografed and analysed.

RESULTS

The Lafaye et al. classification was adopted. We classified as:

A) Tubes with normal drainage (N) when the beggining of the tracer drainage starts between 2 and 3 minutes and the passage to the rhinoparynx occurs around 10 minutes.

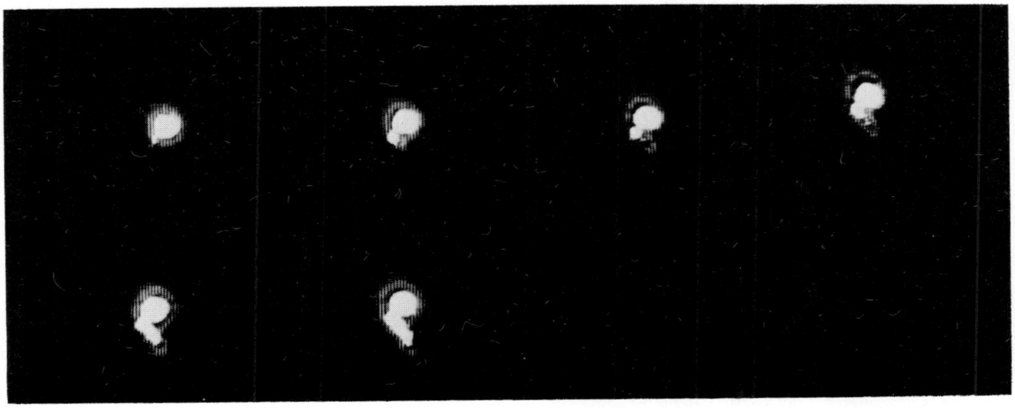

Fig. 1 - Sequential images showing the tracer passage at 1, 3, 8, 12, 16 and 20 minutes after its introdution, revealing a Eustachian tube with normal drainage function (N).

B) Tubes with delayed drainage (D) when the beggining of the tracer drainage starts around the 5th minute and its progression around the 15th minute.

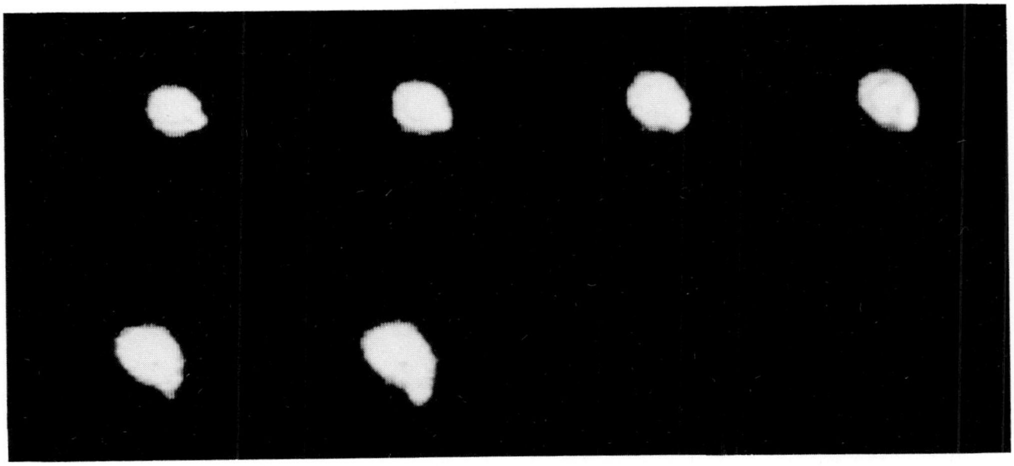

Fig. 2 - Sequential images showing the tracer passage at 1, 3, 5, 10, 15, 20 minutes after its introduction, revealing a Eustachian tube with delayed drainage function (D).

C) Tubes with accelerated flow (A) when the drainage occurs immediatly after the tracer introduction in the middle ear.

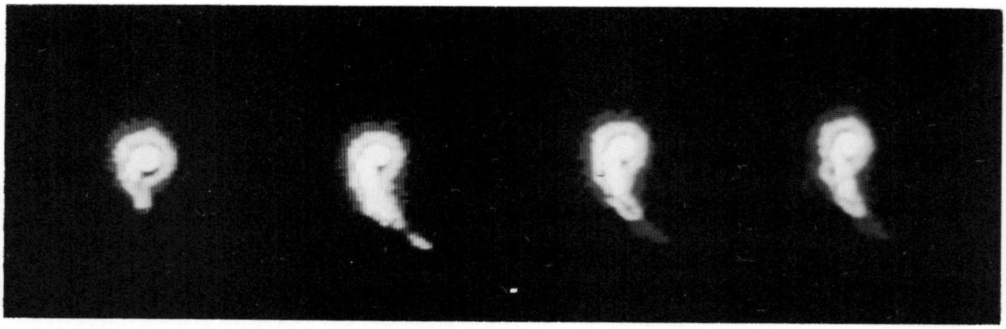

Fig. 3 - Sequential images showing the tracer passage at 1, 3, 5, 10 minutes after its introduction, revealing a Eustachian tube with accelerated drainage function (A).

D) Obstructed tubes (O) when the drainage is not done up to 20 minutes after the introduction of the tracer.

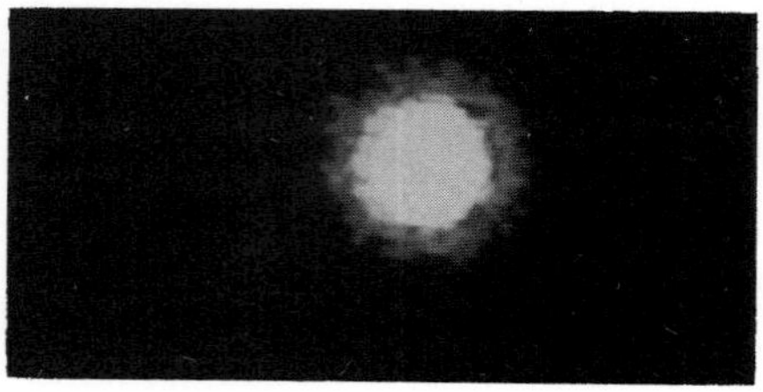

Fig. 4 - Image of the tracer after 20 minutes of its introduction, revealing a obstructed tube (O).

CONCLUSIONS

1 - The use of radioative isotope in the evaluation of the Eustachian tube drainage function is a very accurate method, being a very good test to evaluate this function.

2 - The use of a radioactive isotope diluted in physiological solution, is an entirely physiological method, to evaluate the tube drainage function, allowing a better evaluation of its physiology.

3 - The use of a radioactive isotope in the evaluation of the tube drainage function does not produces side effects reactions neather on the auditive or infection point of view.

NOTE: The references of this paper are related in the paper "Study of the Eustachian tube drainage function with radioisotope (99^m Tc), and the relationship with equipressive function".

© 1985 Elsevier Science Publishers B.V. (Biomedical Division)
New dimensions in otorhinolaryngology - head and neck surgery, vol. 2.
E. Myers, editor

STUDY OF THE EUSTACHIAN TUBE DRAINAGE FUNCTION WITH RADIOISOTOPE (99^m Tc), AND THE RELATIONS WITH THE EQUIPRESSIVE FUNCTION

SILVIO A.M. MARONE, M.D.; AROLDO MINITI, M.D.
Otorynolaringology Department of Faculty of Medicine of São Paulo Univertity, São Paulo, Brazil

INTRODUCTION

The perfect knowledge of the physiological condition of the Eustachian tube is of major significance to the otologist, to understending the middle ear pathology as well as for the treatment of each case. In the propedeutic methods of the Eustachian tube what is generaly evaluated is only the equipressive function, that its alone, could not identify its functional integrety, so that the specialist will be in doubt in witch therapeutic method will choose.

Because in the literature we do not have informations if the result that we obtain in the evaluation of the equipressive function has the same significance of those that we obtain in the evaluation of the drainage function, we undertaked this paper.

METHOD

Subjects

38 ears belonging to 31 patients presenting disacusis from the Otorynolaryngology Ambulatory of Hospital das Clinicas of the Faculty of Medicine of São Paulo University were studied; from these 18 were women, 13 men, 26 whites, 4 blacks, 1 yellow. During the clinical examination all patients presented eardrum perfurations, without any signs of reactivation of the original sickness (absence of pathological discharge) previously diagnosed through Rxs and otomicroscopy. As to the diagnosis, 26 patients presented a chronic post-infection middle ear otites sequela, 3 presented a chronic media otites resulting from direct trauma in the eardrum, 1 patient presenting a surgical sequela following a mastoidectomy due to cholesteatoma, and 1 patient presenting a chronic medium otites caused by barotrauma.

Procedure

In the evaluation of the equipressive function of the Eustachian tube, the inflation-deflation test as proposed by Bluestone (1972 and 1975) and Rock (1976) was used, employing the Damplex ZA21 impedanciometer pump-manometer of the eletroacustic impedance bridge.

The following classification were used:

A - Tubes presenting normal equipressive function (N) open themselves after deglutitions with pressure of 330 mm H_2O ± 70 mm H_2O, and equalize pressure of

-200 mm H_2O to pressures higher tham -100 mm H_2O.

B - Tubes with partial obstruction (P.O.) require pressures higher tham + 400 mm H_2O and equalize pressures of -200 mm H_2O to -100 mm H_2O.

C - Tubes with total obstruction (T.O.) do not equalizes pressures higher than + 400 mm H_2O neither pressure of -200 mm H_2O.

D - Open tubes (open) are not capable of sustaing any positive or negative pressure. One notices the presence of oscillations of the monometer's needle, with sincronize with respiration.

RESULTS

In the evaluation of the Eustachian tube drainage function we employed the classification used in our previous work "Study of Eustachian tube drainage function with radioisotope (99^m Tc).

Drainage function / Equipressive function	AC	N	D	O	T
Open	-	1 (2,6%)	-	-	1 (2,6%)
N	3 (7,9%)	7 (18,4%)	2 (5,3%)	1 (2,6%)	13 (34,2%)
P.O.	-	3 (7,9%)	2 (5,3%)	3 (7,9%)	8 (21,1%)
T.O.	-	4 (10,5%)	7 (18,4%)	5 (13,2%)	16 (42,1%)
T	3 (7,9%)	15 (39,5%)	11 (28,9%)	9 (23,7%)	38 (100%)

Table I - PO = partial obstruction; TO = total obstruction; O = obstructed; T = total; D = delayed; Ac = acellerated; N = normal.

The results presented on Table I were evaluated by the statistic Cohen Concordance test (1960) in order to verify the mutual relationship between the equipressive and drainage function. This study showed that the concordance is casual, and therefore the two methods of tube evaluation may be considerated independent among themselves.

It was also noticed in Table I that 13 cases (34,2%) were considerated normal regarding the equipressive function and 15 cases (39,5%) normals as to the drainage function. However since all the patients presented middle ear pathology these results apperantly normal should regarded as false normals. Using the two drainage function evaluation systems, the normal results are reduced to 7 cases (18,4%) almost half of them.

CONCLUSIONS

1 - The equipressive and drainage function tests are independents among themselves.

2 - The use of both testes reduces pratically 50% of the cases considerates as false normals.

3 - The two tests complete themselves; their association allows the obtainence of a better evaluation of the tube tympanic system.

REFERENCES

1. Bluestone CD, Paradise JL, Beery QC (1972) Laryngoscope 82:1654-70

2. Cohen J (1960) Educ Psychol Meas 20:37-46

3. Eckelman WC, Levenson SM (1979) In: Rocha FG, Herbert JC Bases de Medicina Nuclear. Guanabara Koogan, Rio de Janeiro, pp 145-173

4. Lafaye M, Gaillard de Collogny L, Jourde H, Plagne R, Callier J, Meynel G (1974) Ann Oto-laryng (Paris) 91:665-680

5. Poch Broto J, Valles Varela H (1983) Cah oto-rhino-laryng 18: 101-107

6. Rock EH (1976) In: Northern JL (ed) Selected Readings in Impedance Audiometry American Electromedics Corporation, New York, pp 328-333

7. Bluestone CD, Beery QC, Cantekin EI, Paradise JL (1975) Ann Otol (St.Louis) 84:333-338

8. Gaillard de Collogny L, Lafaye M, Jourde H, Plagne R, Callier J, Meyniel G (1974) J franç Oto-rhino-laryng 23:623-628

9. Gaillard de Collogny L, Lafaye M, Veyre A, Bruneaud D, Callier J, Mayniel G (1977) 94: 233-243

New dimensions in otorhinolaryngology - head and neck surgery, vol. 2.
E. Myers, editor

INNER EAR FUNCTION IN DIABETES MELLITUS WITH PERIPHERAL NEUROPATHIES

(1) Y.N. MEHRA (2) Y.K. SHARMA (3) S.B.S. MANN & (4) R.J. DASH
Department of Otorhinolaryngology
Postgraduate Institute of Medical Education & Research, Chandigarh, India.

The occurrence of neurological complications of diabetes mellitus has long been recognised. Diabetic peripheral neuropathy is the common one. Involvement of the cranial nerve has been reported occasionally. These are secondary to severe angiopathy. The hearing function of diabetics have been studied by other workers and 40-50% of the patients had sensori-neural hearing loss. Studies of vestibular system have been few.

We studied 102 diabetes mellitus patients with peripheral neuropathy to see, if such patients are more prone to dyfunction of inner ear.

Audiological tests were performed with puretone audiometery. Special tests were done, where necessary.

Vestibular tests with alternate hot & cold caloric stimulations was done. Resulting nystagmus was studied for the parameters of total duration, total beats and maximum speed of the slow component from the ENG record.

Only 26 gave history of hearing loss of mild degree. 17 had tinnitus as a symptom.

18 patients complained of vague giddiness.

AUDIOLOGICAL TESTS

51 out of 102 had sensorineural hearing loss in one or more frequency of more than 20 dB. The older age group patients had descending audiogram. Once the phenomenon of aging is excluded only 24 patients showed mild hearing loss of 20-30 dB.

VESTIBULAR TESTS

No patient showed any spontaneous or positional nystagmus.

11 patients out of 91 showed markedly diminished caloric responses which could not be explained in any other causes and are presumed to be the result of diabetes. All of these belonged to the older age group and had long history of diabetes. Six of these 11 patients had hearing loss. Dimmunition of vestibular

responses in old age was also seen, when comparison was made of the post caloric responses of patient below the age of 40 with those of above the age of 41 years.

Brain stem evoked response audiometery was performed in a group of 20 normals of 40-50 years. Results of these were compared with the results of a matched group of 20 diabetic patients.

There was no difference in the latency of wave I & wave II in diabetes & normal.

It was noticed that the latency of wave III, IV & V was delayed in diabetic patients. However, 3 patients of diabetes with peripheral neuropathy did not show any difference in the latency, from the diabetic group.

CONCLUSION

1. Peripheral neuropathy in diabetes can be seen in age group 10-80 years. In our series none of the cases showed involvement of any cranial nerve.

2. Vestibular functions tests reveal that there is no sponteneous or positional nystagmus in any case.

3. Diminished vestibular responses to caloric stimulation was met in 11 cases out of 91 (12%) for whom record is available and only 5 of these had hearing impairment. The vestibular impairment is met with more commonly in older age group.

4. The incidence of both cochlear and vestibular impairment in our study of diabetes with peripheral neuropathy is not higher than the comparative incidence in diabetes without neuropathy.

5. There is a delayed transmission of the auditory stimulus in the auditory pathway at the level of brainstem and midbrain in diabetes.

BIBLIOGRAPHY

1. Axelsson, A., and Fagerberg, S.E. (1969)-Acta Otolaryn. Stockholm. 66:49-64

2. Donald, M.W., Bird, C.E., Karnhuber, E.(1980)-Progress in Brain research, Vol. 54:516.

3. Friedmann, S.A., Schuman, R.H. & Wells, S.(1975)- Arc. of Int. Med. 135:573.

4. Jorgensen, M.B.(1961)-Arch. Otolaryng. 74-164.

5. Mehra, Y.N. and Moudgil, B.D.(1967)- Acta Otolaryng.63 :33

New dimensions in otorhinolaryngology – head and neck surgery, vol. 2.
E. Myers, editor

HEARING CONSERVATION SURGERY FOR ACOUSTIC TUMORS - A CLINICAL-PATHOLOGICAL CORRELATIVE STUDY

J. GAIL NEELY, M.D., F.A.C.S.

Professor and Head, Department of Otorhinolaryngology, University of Oklahoma Health Sciences Center, P.O. Box 26307, Oklahoma City, Oklahoma 73126.

ABSTRACT

It has been estimated that hearing conservation is possible in 50% of patients with tumors extending medial to the porus acusticus 1.5cm or less and who maintain speech discrimination scores of 80% or greater. Others have indicated that a hearing level of 30dB or less and 80% discrimination are ideal candidates for hearing preservation surgery.

The purpose of this paper is to review twenty-two cases of solitary schwannoma of the eighth nerve, in which adequate tissue was available for histologic fiber analysis, using the established preoperative predictive criteria for hearing preservation surgery. The objective of the review is to describe the histology found in patients meeting these preoperative criteria.

Ten cases were 1.5cm or less; five cases had a discrimination score of 80% or greater; and four cases had a puretone average of 30dB or less. Only three cases satisfied any two criteria and only one case satisfied all three criteria. All cases had significant fiber destruction and tumor infiltration. The one case that met all three criteria demonstrated severe tumor infiltration within the cochlear nerve and the trunk of the eighth nerve; in two of five subserial en block tumor-nerve cross-sections no fibers could be identified crossing the tumor.

In conclusion, histologic data suggests that complete tumor removal in attempts to preserve hearing may be beyond our surgical capabilities. They further suggest that the present preoperative criteria for selection of patients for hearing preservation are inadequate.

New dimensions in otorhinolaryngology - head and neck surgery, vol. 2.
E. Myers, editor

A SEM STUDY ON THE VASCULAR SYSTEM OF THE ENDOLYMPHATIC DUCT AND SAC

YOSHIO OGURA, RYUSUKE SAITO, KIYOSHI MATSUBARA, NORIAKI MATSUMOTO, MASAAKI FUJIMOTO, TAKUYA OHMICHI, AND KAZUTAKA TERAZAWA

Department of Otolaryngology, Okayama University Medical School
2-5-1 Shikata-cho, Okayama 700 (Japan)

INTRODUCTION

The vascular system of the endolymphatic duct and sac (ES) plays an important role in the occurrence of endolymphatic hydrops. The vascular structure of this area, however, has not been elucidated yet detailedly, even though there have been extensive studies on this structure[1]. In the present paper, a study was reported on the observation of the vascular corrosion casting from ES in a rat by scanning electron microscopy (SEM).

MATERIAL AND METHODS

Twenty healthy Wistar rats weighing 200 to 400 gram were used. The blood vessels were perfused with metacrylate resin (Mercox) to obtain vascular corrosion casts[2]. The bony tissue around the inner ear was macerated in 20% KOH, decalcified by Plank and Rychlo s method, and covered with gold. The specimen was examined in SEM.

RESULT AND DISCUSSION

The arterial supply of ES was derived chiefly from branches of the posterior meningeal artery[1] (PMA), which ran medially and also laterally to the sigmoid sinus (SS) (Fig. 1.). Any branch from the posterior vestibular artery was not identified as a supplying artery to ES. The vessels of ES consisted of triangular dense capillary nets with extensive vascular anastomoses with vessels in surrounding bony channels. The most prominent feature of the vessels surrounding ES was the capillaries of thin-walled irregular sinusoid type[3] (Fig. 2.). Small peculiar vessel was observed which ran between- and connected the capillary networks of the vestibule and ES. The vein of the vestibular aqueduct (VVA) collected venous drainage from ES and emptied into SS. This vein was sometimes divided into two or three small branches. VVA, which was present in most experimental mammals, was considered equivalent to the vein running through the paravestibular canaliculus (PVC) in man[4,5,6]. Inadequate venous drainage through PVC might be the cause of endolymphatic hydrops[7].

SUMMARY

The vascular corrosion castings of ES in a rat were observed by SEM. Fine vascular construction was elucidated on the supplying arteries, capillary network and venous drainage of ES and vicinity. Anatomy and function was discussed on the references.

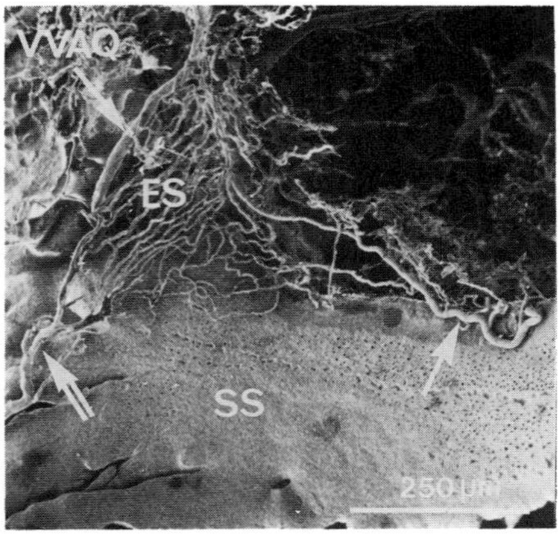

Fig. 1. Two branches of PMA. One runs medially (⇐), and the other runs laterally (←) to SS.

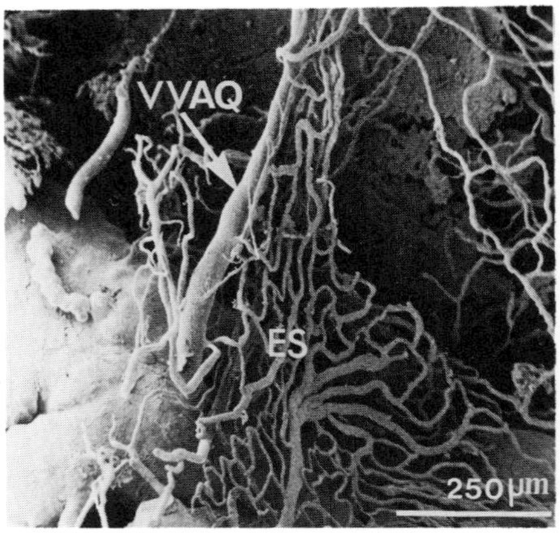

Fig. 2. Capillary network surrounding ES which shows thin-walled irregular sinusoid type.

REFERENCES

1. Bast TH, Anson BJ (1946) The Temporal Bone and the Ear. Charles C Thomas Publisher, Springfield Illinois US, pp 249-259

2. Matsubara K, Aoki T, Kawashima S, Saito R, Ogura Y (1979) Vascular anatomy of the inner ear of the guinea pig - A SEM study of the corrosion cast. Auris-Nasus-Larynx 6:1-11

3. Rask-Andersen H (1979) The vascular supply of the endolymphatic sac. Acta Otolaryngol 88:315-327

4. Ogura Y, Clemis JD (1971) A study of the gross anatomy of the human vestibularbular aqueduct. Ann Otol Rhinol Laryngol 80:813-825

5. Stahle J, Wilbrand HF (1974) The para-vestibular canaliculus. Can J Otolaryngol 3:262-270

6. Sando I, Egami T, Harada T (1980) Course and contents of the paravestibular canaliculus. Ann Otol Rhinol Laryngol 89:147-156

7. Gussen R (1982) Vascular mechanisms in Meniere's disease - Theoretical considerations. Arch Otolaryngol 108:544-549

© 1985 Elsevier Science Publishers B.V. (Biomedical Division)
New dimensions in otorhinolaryngology - head and neck surgery, vol. 2.
E. Myers, editor

TYPE II COLLAGEN IN THE HUMAN AND MONKEY EAR

T. ISHIBE[1], K. TOMODA[1], T. J. YOO[2], A. KANG[2], M. CREMER[2]

[1]Kansai Medical University, Osaka, Japan; [2]University of Tennessee and VAMC, Memphis, Tennessee, USA

INTRODUCTION

The presence of type II collagen autoimmunity in some cases of human ear disease has been proven (1). Temporal bone lesions were also induced by type II collagen autoimmunity in animals (2-4). This study examined type II collagen distribution in the human and monkey ear immunohistochemically by using monoclonal antibody to type II collagen.

MATERIALS AND METHODS

Healthy human temporal bones taken from autopsy and three temporal bones from macaca mulatta were used in this study. For immunological studies, indirect immunofluorescence and immunoperoxidase staining were performed. Temporal bones were fixed in 95% cold ethanol, decalcified with PH 7.4 5% EDTA, and embedded in 56°C melted paraffin. Sections 7μ thick were deparaffinized and treated with testicular hyaluronidase to extract proteoglycans that mask antigenic sites of type II collagen. Nonspecific background staining was reduced by incubating sections with normal goat serum in 1% bovine serum albumin. Endogenous peroxidase was blocked with 0.5% H_2O_2 in methanol. Monoclonal antibody to chick type II collagen (produced in mice by a hybridoma technique), which cross reacts to human and monkey type II collagen was used as the first antibody. Peroxidase conjugated goat anti-mouse IgG or FITC was used as the second antibody. Normal mouse serum, mouse monoclonal antibody against human type V collagen and mouse antistreptococcus M protein monoclonal antibody were used as negative controls and articular cartilage was used as a positive control.

RESULTS AND CONCLUSIONS

Positive staining to type II collagen in the human and monkey ear was observed in the following areas: 1) inner ear: enchondral layer and globuli interossei in the otic capsule, Rosenthal canal, Cribriform base, spiral ligament, osseous spiral lamina, subepithelial layer of endolymphatic ducts, macula sacculi, macula utricle and crista ampullaris, semicircular canal membrane. 2) middle ear: inter-ossicular joints, stapes footplate, eustachian tubal cartilage, tympanic membrane, fissula antefenestraim. 3) external ear: tympanic annulus, cartilage plate in the auricle and external ear meatus. Thus, type II collagen could be considered an important component of the ear tissue and these results suggest possible immune injury sites by the immunocytes or autoantibody to type II collagen.

ACKNOWLEDGEMENTS

This research was supported by grants from the Deafness Research Foundation, National Hearing Association, American Otological Society, and Veterans Administration

REFERENCES

1. Yoo TJ, Stuart JM, Kang AH, Townes AS, Tomoda K, Dixit S (1982) Type II Collagen Autoimmunity in Otosclerosis and Meniere's Disease. Science 217:1153-1155

2. Yoo TJ, Yazawa Y, Tomoda K, Floyd R (1983) Type II Collagen-Induced Autoimmune Endolymphatic Hydrops in Guinea Pig. Science 222:65-67

3. Yoo TJ, Tomoda K, Stuart JM, Kang AH, Townes AS Type II Collagen-Induced Autoimmune Otospongiosis: A Preliminary Report (1983) Ann Oto Rhino Laryn 92(2):103-8

4. Yoo TJ, Tomoda K, Stuart JM, Cremer MA, Townes AS, Kang AH (1983) Type II Collagen-Induced Autoimmune Sensorineural Hearing Loss and Vestibular Dysfunction in Rats. Ann Oto Rhino Laryn 92(3):267-271

© 1985 Elsevier Science Publishers B.V. (Biomedical Division)
New dimensions in otorhinolaryngology - head and neck surgery, vol. 2.
E. Myers, editor

T CELL SUBSETS OF COWDEN'S DISEASE –A REPORT OF 4 CASES–

TAKASHI KOMORI, MITSURU FURUKAWA AND RYOZO UMEDA

Department of Otolaryngology, School of Medicine, Kanazawa University, Kanazawa, Ishikawa, 920 Japan

INTRODUCTION

The first case of Cowden'disease was described in 1963 by Lloid and Dennis under the name of the family of the first propositus. Over 60 cases of Cowden's disease have now been reported. But, the etiology of Cowden's disease remaines uncelar. As we recently had the occasion to investigate about peripheral T cell subsets of four patients family members, we report these cases and the immunological features of this disease.

CASE REPORTS

Case 1: 55 year-old woman with cutaneous facial papules (CFP), oral mucosal papillomatosis (OMP), acral keratoses (AK), palmoplantar keratoses (PK), GI tract polyposis (GIP), fibroma of vocal cord, angiolipoma of breast and leiomyoma of uterus.

Case 2: 27 year-old man with CFP, OMP, AK, PK, and GIP.

Case 3: 30 year-old woman with CFP, OMP, AK, PK, GIP and goiter.

Case 4: 23 year-old woman with CFP, OMP, AK, PK, GIP, multiple adenomas of thyroid gland and hemangioma of thigh

MATERIAL AND METHOD

Peripheral blood mononuclear cells of four patients, their family members and control population were isolated by Ficoll-Hypaque gradient centrifugation. The monoclonal antibodies OKT3, OKT4, OKT8, OKT11, OKIal, OKB 1, and Leu7 were used for defining T cell subsets. The cells were analyzed on the fluorescence activated cell sorter. Sheep red-cell receptors were assesed according to E-rossete formation.

RESULTS

In the patients, OKT3+ cells and OKT4+ cells were decreased, whereas OKT8+ cells and OKT11+ cells were in the normal range. No abnormalities in other lymphocyte-subsets were detected.

TABLE 1

% REACTIVITY WITH MONOCLONAL ANTIBODIES IN COWDEN'S DISEASE

	OKT3	OKT4	OKT8	OKT11
patients	37.2±3.1*	18.6±2.7*	17.0±2.4	75.4±1.2
control	67.4±5.4	40.2±4.7	25.8±3.5	74.6±5.4

Reslts are expressed as mean ± 1 S.D.
* $P < 0.05$

DISCUSSION

The basic causative defect in Cowden's disease is unknown. Ruschak et al reported a case of this disease that showed impaired response to the T cell mitogens and they proposed the possibility of defects in T cell function. The development of monoclonal antisera able to recognize specific T cell subsets has provided fascinating information regarding abnormalities in T cell regulation. In our data, the patients had decreased number of helper T cells and mature T cells. These results suggest an immunoregulatory abnormality contributing to or associated with the pathogenesis of this unusual disease.

REFERENCES

1. Lloid KM, Dennis M (1963) Ann Intern Med 58: 136-142
2. Weary PE, Gorlin RJ, Gentry WC, et al (1972) Arch Dermatol 106: 682-690
3. Ruschak PJ, Kauh YC, Luscombe HA (1981) Arch Dermatol 117: 573-574
4. Salem OS, Steck WD (1983) J Amer Acad Dermatol 8: 686-696

New dimensions in otorhinolaryngology - head and neck surgery, vol. 2.
E. Myers, editor

IMMUNOHISTOLOGICAL ASPECTS OF FOCUS-TONSILS AND PUSTULOSIS PALMARIS ET PLANTARIS

KIYONORI KUKI

Depertment of Otorhinolaryngology, Wakayama Medical College, Wakayama (Japan)

INTRODUCTION

Pustulosis palmaris et plantaris (PPP) is a chronic dermatosis characterized by sterile pustules on the palms and soles.
At present, two methods of the treatment are employed; one is the use of corticosteroids, and the other is the removal of the foci based on the focal infection. However, they are neither reliable nor can be considered as established. Especially, we have found that the tonsillectomy to treat PPP results in a significantly high cure rate. The mechanism and why or how tonsillectomy exerts such an effect remains completely unknown. We have researched the pathogenesis of PPP by means of histological and immunohistological techniques.

MATERIAL AND METHODS

Experiment I: Histological and immunohistological identifications of tonsillar lymphocytes.

Tonsils. Tonsils with the recurrent tonsillitis and the focus-tonsils of PPP were surgically removed and immediately frozen at -80°C.

Histological examinations. Hematoxyline & Eosin staining was done.

Immunohistological examinations. Tonsils were sectioned at 4 μm on a cryostat and placed on glass slides, fixed with acetone.
The primary mouse monoclonal antibodies were used. As a secondary antibody, we used a biotynilated horse antimouse IgG. As a third layer we applied avidin-biotynilated peroxidase(ABC). The peroxidase activity was demonstrated with the 3',3'-diaminobenzidine tetrahydrochloride. α-Naphthyl esterase staining was used for the identification of macrophages.

Monoclonal antibodies. Twe types monoclonal antibodies of OKT and Lew series of T and B cell subsets were used.

Experiment II: In vitro sensitization of tonsils with tonsillar epithelial antigens.

Tonsillar epithelial antigens. These antigens were prepared as described previously by T.Enomoto et al. in 1983.

In vitro sensitization of tonsils. Small tonsil cubes were sensitized in vitro with RPMI medium containing tonsillar epithelial antigens and rapidly frozen at -80°C. The immunohistological examinations as described in the experiment I were done.

RESULTS

Experiment I

Histological examinations. At the tonsils with PPP, the infiltration of inflammatory cells into the crypts, thickening and thining of the lacunal epithelium, and modarate subepithelial inflammatory changes were observed.

Immunohistological examinations. These results are shown in the table. No differences were observed in the distributions of T and B cell subsets between the recurrent tonsillitis and focus-tonsils.

Experiment II

The S-IgD bearing lymphocytes predominantly increased in the mantle zones of focus-tonsils, though the tonsils of the recurrent tonsillitis were not affected. The other lymphocyte subsets demonstrated no characteristic defferences in focus-tonsls or in the recurrent tonsillitis.

Esterase positive cells, distinguishing macrophages, increased in the subepithelial areas of focus-tonsils, but not in the tonsils of recurrent tonsillitis.

Table

Distribution of Lymphocyte Subsets in the Tonsils.

	Habitual tonsillitis				P.P.P.			
	sub-epithelial	inter-follicular	mantle	germinal center	sub-epithelial	inter-follicular	mantle	germinal center
Leu-1 / Leu-4	+	+++	−	±	+	+++	−	±
Leu-2a	±	±	−	−	±	±	−	−
Leu-3a	+	+++	−	±	+	+++	−	±
Leu-7	±	−	−	+	±	−	−	+
OKT8	+	+	−	−	+	+	−	−
OKT10	++	+	−	−	++	+	−	−
IgM	±	−	+	+	±	−	+	+
IgA	±	±	−	−	±	±	−	−
IgE	±	−	±	−	±	−	±	−
IgD	−	−	++	−	−	−	++	−
HLA-DR	±	+	++	++	±	+	++	++
OKM_1	±	−	±	−	±	−	±	−
OKIa	±	±	++	+	±	±	++	+
Esterase	++	+	+	+	++	+	+	+

© 1985 Elsevier Science Publishers B.V. (Biomedical Division)
New dimensions in otorhinolaryngology - head and neck surgery, vol. 2.
E. Myers, editor

INFECTIOUS AND NEOPLASTIC ORAL MANIFESTATIONS OF THE ACQUIRED IMMUNODEFICIENCY SYNDROME

CARL A. PATOW, M.D.[1], DAVID M. LEWIS, D.D.S.[2], AND
ABE M. MACHER, M.D.[3]

1. Otolaryngology, Head and Neck Surgery, Walter Reed Army Medical Center, (WRAMC), Washington, D.C. 20307-5001 and the Uniformed Services University of the Health Sciences, Bethesda, MD 20205, 2. Oral Diagnosis, WRAMC, 3. Laboratory of Pathology, National Cancer Institute, National Institutes of Health, Bethesda, MD 20205

Since the first reports, in 1981, of the acquired immunodeficiency syndrome (AIDS) over 10,000 cases in the United States have been reported to the Centers for Disease Control. The syndrome is defined by strict clinical criteria: Kaposi's sarcoma or an opportunistic infection indicative of a defect in cell mediated immunity occuring in an individual with no known cause for underlying immunosuppression. Initially, homosexuals, bisexuals, intravenous drug users, and hemophiliacs were identified as groups at risk for AIDS. Recent reports, however, have documented vertical maternal-fetal transmission and horizontal transmission to sexual partners of opposite sex.

Patients with AIDS frequently present with oral complications, both infectious and neoplastic. The experience in treatment of oral manifestations of AIDS for patients referred to the National Institute of Health, Bethesda, MD and Walter Reed Army Medical Center, Washington, D.C. is reviewed.

Kaposi's sarcoma (KS) was seen in nearly every mucosal and cutaneous region of the head and neck[1]. Lesions varied from painless blue to brown pigmented macules to raised firm darkly pigmented masses. Large oral and pharyngeal KS lesions occassionally ulcerated and bled, causing dysphagia, pain, and inanition. Radiation therapy is effective for local control of symptomatic oral lesions[2]. For widespread KS, chemotherapy offers temporary palliation.

Oropharyngeal candidiasis and candida esophagitis in AIDS patients are relatively responsive to conventional antifungal therapy. Oral candida is treated with nystatin liquid and ketaconazole troches. If the infection persists oral ketaconazole or intravenous amphotericin B may be required. Recurrence of of oral candida is common after treatment is stopped and maintenance oral antifungals may be required.

Episodes of mucocutaneous herpes simple virus infection may be prolonged in AIDS patients. Painful oral ulcers frequently develop and recurrence is common. Episodes usually respond to a 7 to 10 day course of intravenous acyclovir.

Histoplasmosis capsulatum may present as an oral lesion, and may clinically be confused with squamous cell carcinoma. Diagnosis is made by special stains of biopsy material, culture and serologic studies. For patients with AIDS, treatment with amphotericin B and ketaconazole have not been curative[3].

Human T-lymphotrophic virus type III (HTLV-III), a possible causative agent for AIDS, has been demonstrated to be present in saliva from AIDS patients[4]. Physicians examining the oral cavity of AIDS patients should therefore take personal precautions to minimize exposure to HTLV-III, cytomegalovirus, and other AIDS associated salivary born infectious agents.

REFERENCES

1. Patow CA, Steis R, Longo DL, etal. (1984) Otolaryngol Head Neck Surg 92:255-60.

2. Patow CA, Stark TW, Findlay PA, etal. (1984) Otolaryngol Head Neck Surg 92: 713-6.

3. Wheat LJ, Slama TG, Zeckel ML (1985) Amer J Med 78:203-10.

4. Groopman JE, Sarngadharan MG, Salahuddin SZ, etal. (1985) Ann Int. Med 102:63-6.

The opinions or assertions contained herein are the private views of the authors and are not to be construed as official or as reflecting the views of the Department of the Army or Department of Defense.

© 1985 Elsevier Science Publishers B.V. (Biomedical Division)
New dimensions in otorhinolaryngology – head and neck surgery, vol. 2.
E. Myers, editor

PERIPHERAL BLOOD LYMPHOCYTE RESPONSE TO EXOGENOUS IL 2 ADMINISTRATION AND ENDOGENOUS IL 2 PRODUCTION IN PATIENTS WITH ADVANCED CANCER OF LARYNX +

ERNESTO PROTO•, PAOLO PUXEDDU•, FRANCESCO PANU•, GIUSEPPINA ORGIANA••, DANIELA DEGIOANNIS••, GIOVANNI MANTOVANI••
Dps of Otolaryngology•, Internal Medicine and Clinical Oncology••, Univ. of Cagliari Medical School, Cagliari, Italy

INTRODUCTION

The Interleukin 2 (IL 2) is a lymphokine produced by T lymphocytes which plays an unique role in various immunologic phenomena. The IL 2, which is able to maintain the long-term growth of normal T cells, is an antigen-nonspecific, genetically unrestricted mediator produced by T cells or T cell lines that have been stimulated with antigens, mitogens and alloantigens. Recent studies in animals demonstrated that IL 2 could augment Natural Killer (NK) cell activity, thus increasing cellular immune function in vivo.
Aim of the study. Study aims were (1) to assess response of peripheral blood lymphocytes (PBL) in patients with cancer of larynx to polyclonal mitogens, to exogenous IL 2 added in culture either on PHA-prestimulated or non PHA-prestimulated PBL; (2) to evaluate endogenous IL 2 activity induced in culture medium of PHA-prestimulated mononuclear cells (MNC) of the same pts, using either whole MNC or non-adherent cells.

MATERIAL AND METHODS

Patients

Twenty nine pts were studied for aim (1), six for aim (2), seven healthy subjects (age/sex matched) served as controls. The mean age of pts was 63 Yrs, the most common histologic type was highly differentiated epidermoid ca., the TNM staging was predominantly T1-T3, NO, MO. The pts underwent all surgical excision of the tumor (partial or total laringectomy) according to conventional techniques; nobody was given radio- or chemotherapy.

Lymphocyte cultures

PBL were cultured in microtitre plates, pulsed with ^3H thymidine and counted by liquid scintillation. 1.5 x 10^5 PBL were cultured per well. Endogenous IL 2 production was evaluated according to the method of Nakayama et al. (1983).

RESULTS

Our results provide evidence that laryngeal cancer pts have a T cell functional depression,due to a failure of IL 2-producing T cell subset,causing a markedly reduced or absent IL 2 production. This lack of IL 2 availability,directly demonstrated by endogenous IL 2 production assay,may explain some,if not all,other cancer re_ lated immune deficiencies such as impairment of gamma interferon production,of NK cells activity etc. The response of not previously PHA-stimulated PBL of pts to exogenous IL 2 suggests that NK cells impairment might not be primary but secondary to an imbalance of immunoregulatory factors in which the IL 2 seems to play an impor_ tant role. In over 50% of the pts addition of medium containing IL 2 caused DNA synthesis to rise very close to normal values,as in pts with primary immune deficiencies;this finding supports the hypothesis that the IL 2 administration in vivo might contribute to correct the cancer immune imbalance,so leading possibly to di_ sease cure. An aliquot of the pts,the so-called "low responders", show,besides or instead of reduced IL 2 production,also a reduction of IL 2 receptor expression,probably due to an impairment of IL 2-responding T cell subset. In the endogenous IL 2 production assay our data indicate also that the adherent cells have a suppressive effect on IL 2 production in cancer pts.

REFERENCES

1. Nakayama E,Asano S,Takuwa N,Yokota J,Miwa S (1983) Clin. Exp. Immunol. 51:511

+ This work was supported by C. N. R. Rome,PF "Oncologia",Grant N.84.00549.44.

© 1985 Elsevier Science Publishers B.V. (Biomedical Division)
New dimensions in otorhinolaryngology – head and neck surgery, vol. 2.
E. Myers, editor

SPECIFIC ANTIGENS ASSOCIATED TO SQUAMOUS CELL CARCINOMA, ISOLATED FROM MAXILLARY CANCER

S.SAITO, N.KOMATSU, M.SAKAI, H.MIYAKE, S.YAMAUCHI (1) K.KATO (2)
Dept. of Otolaryngology, Tokai University School of Medicine, Isehara, Kanagawa, Japan. (1)
Reseach Labolatories Pharmaceuticals, Nippon Kayaku Co., LTD., Tokyo, Japan (2)

INTRODUCTION

It is well known that tumor makers have been used in the immunological diagnosis or monitering for carcinoma of various organs. The initial porpose of this study was to prepare specific antibodies to squamous cell carcinoma. Isolation and specification of squamous cell carcinoma associated antigen have been attempted in our department since 1980, and we successfuly detected squamous cell carcinoma associated antigen (SCCAA) by new technique.

MATERIALS AND METHOD

MATERIALS

In this investigations we used tissue specimen of the maxillary bone that were pathologicaly identified as squamous cell carcinoma. A new technique was devised for isolation and characterization of SCCAA.

METHOD OF ISOLATION AND SPECIFICATION OF SCCAA

10 um thick of frozen sections of maxillary carcinoma were placed directly to an ampholine PAG-plate for isoelectricfocusing. After electropholesis, we could find more numerous bands in frozen section than the other samples. Specific component at around pH6.1 were determined on the PAG-plate.

Isolation of SCCAA was carried out by chromatofocusing. Their absorbance at 280nm was measured and specific component at around pH6.1 was collected. After immunization of rabbits by SCCAA, anti-SCCAA was obtained. Purification of anti-SCCAA was performed by using of Protain-A sepharose cl-4B. Thus we obtained purified IgG component of anti-SCCAA.

We examined the specificity of IgG component of anti-SCCAA by Ouchterlony immuno-diffusion test. The precipitin line of immunological identity was demonstrated of squamous cell carcinoma of maxillary sinus.

Molecular weight of SCCAA was investigated by using of SDS-PAG and immuno-blotting. There were two components (170K-225K), and other two components were 120K-136K, and minor component 76K.

RESULT

DETECTION OF SCCAA ON VARIOUS TISSUES

Detection of SCCAA on the tissues were investigated by indirect immunofluorescence and immunoperoxidase technique. Positive reaction was demonstrated on the cell membrane of squamous cell carcinoma. Twenty-nine specimens from squamous cell carcinoma of the various organs and metastatic lymph nodes were stained by same technique. Twenty-seven out of 29 (93%) were positive to SCCAA, while specimens from tissues other than squamous cell carcinoma were difinitively negative.

TABLE 1
DETECTION OF SCCAA ON SQUAMOUS CELL CARCINOMA OF THE VARIOUS ORGANS

Subjects	No. of tested	No. of positive (%)
Maxillary cancer	16	15 (94)
Esophageal cancer	3	2 (67)
Lung cancer	2	2 (100)
Cervical cancer	4	4 (100)
Metastatic lymph nodes		
Esophageal cancer	2	2 (100)
Cervical cancer	2	2 (100)
TOTAL	29	27 (93)

CONCLUSION

There are various kinds of tumor makers such as CEA, AFP, TPA, etc. and they have been used for screening, detection, diagnosis and differentiating of tumor, determined virulence and degree of malignancy, monitering for tumor during and after anti-cancer therapy.[1]

Our first aim was to prepare specific antibodies, as tumor maker, to squamous cell carcinoma for to diagnose early staged squamous cell carcinoma of the head and neck tumor. It was performed unique technique, and it is assumed that this new isolated SCCAA is specific to squamous cell carcinoma and quite useful for early diagnosis of this malignant tumor.

REFERENCE

1. Wendell D. Winters (1983) : New Technique for Detecting Tumor Makers: A Prospective. Cancer Detection and Prevention 6:21-31

New dimensions in otorhinolaryngology - head and neck surgery, vol. 2.
E. Myers, editor

TYPE II COLLAGEN-INDUCED AUTOIMMUNE SALPINGITIS IN THE RAT

N. SUDO[1], K. TOMODA[2], R. FLOYD[1], T. ISHIBE[2], T. J. YOO[1]

[1]University of Tennessee, Memphis, Tennessee, USA: [2]Kansai Medical University, Osaka, Japan

INTRODUCTION

The pathogenesis of otitis media with effusion is intimately related to eustachian tube dysfunction. In this study, we have further extended our original observations that type II collagen induced an autoimmune salpingitis (1,2) and also investigated whether or not type II collagen-induced salpingitis was transferable by immune sera.

METHODS AND MATERIALS

We examined 28 controls, 46 type II collagen immunized and 15 immune sera transferred Wistar rats. Immunized rats were injected with 200μg of native bovine type II collagen (BIIn) in the foot pad and boosted 1 week later. Twenty-five, 13 and 8 immunized rats were sacrificed 2 weeks, 8 weeks and 6 months after the last immunization, respectively. Fifteen rats were injected (I.V.) with 2.5 - 3ml of fourfold concentrated immune sera obtained from immunized rats and sacrificed 1 month later. The temporal bones were dissected en bloc, decalcified and stained with hemotoxylin and eosin, alcian blue or immunofluorescence staining. The temporal bones were also examined electromicroscopically using a standard technique. Sera samples collected from all animals were measured for antibody level by the ELISA method (3).

RESULTS AND CONCLUSION

The eustachian tubes of BIIn immunized animals were histologically characterized by infiltration of the mucosa and submucosa with mononuclear cells, goblet cell hyperplasia, sero-mucous effusion, chondrolysis, replacement with fibrous tissue and loss of the usual basophilic staining of the tubal cartilage. Salpingitis was observed in 12 of the 25 immunized rats 2 weeks post-immunization; in 10 of the 13 rats, 8 weeks post-immunization; and in 4 of the 8 rats at 6 months post-immunization. Chondritis was found in 3 of the 13 rats 8 weeks after immunization. In the serum transferred rats, salpingitis was found in 5 out of the 15 rats but chondritis was not observed (Table I). No control animal showed any ear degeneration.

The histopathological observations of salpingitis in the serum transferred rats were similar to those observed in the immunized rats but the degree of otopathological changes were less than that of the immunized rats. Both immunized and serum transferred rats which had salpingitis showed IgG and C_3 deposits in the perichondrium and intercellular matrix of the tubal cartilage. The antibody level is also elevated in these animals.

Electronmicroscopic findings indicate an increased permeability in the capillaries and intercellular space as well as cellular infiltration in the submucosa of the immunized rats.

The results suggest that type II collagen immunization induces autoimmune salpingitis in rats. These lesions were also observed in the rats which received immune sera. Thus type II autoimmune response might play a role in the pathogenesis of eustachian tube disease.

TABLE I

EUSTACHIAN TUBE DISEASE IN RATS

	No. of Animals	Salpingitis	Chondritis
Collagen Immunized Rats	46	27	3
2 weeks group	25	13	0
8 weeks group	13	10	3
6 months group	8	4	0
Control Rats	20	0	0
Serum Transferred Rats	15	5	0
Control Rats	8	0	0

ACKNOWLEDGEMENTS

This research was supported by grants from Deafness Research Foundation, National Hearing Association, American Otological Society, and Veterans Administration.

REFERENCES

1. Tomoda K, Yoo TJ (1984) Type II Collagen-Induced Autoimmune Salpingitis in Rats. In: Lim DJ, Bluestone CD, Klein JO, Nelson, JP (eds) Recent Advances in Otitis Media with Effusion. BC Decker Inc., New York, pp 220-232

2. Tomoda K, Yoo TJ (1985) Type II Collagen-Induced Autoimmune Salpingitis in Rats. Annals Oto Rhino Laryn 94(2):156-161

3. Yoo TJ, Tomoda K, Stuart JM, Cremer MA, Townes AA, Kang AH (1983) Type II Collagen-Induced Autoimmune Sensorineural Hearing Loss and Vestibular Dysfunction in Rats. Ann Oto Rhino Laryn 92(3):267-271

New dimensions in otorhinolaryngology - head and neck surgery, vol. 2.
E. Myers, editor

GENERATION OF MONOCLONAL ANTIBODY REACTIVE WITH HUMAN MAXILLARY SINUS CARCINOMA CELLS.

MITSUAKI TAKAHASHI, NAOKI KANAI AND MEGUMI KUMAI
Department of Otolaryngology, Asahikawa Medical College, Asahikawa, Japan

INTRODUCTION

Until now many monoclonal antibodies against a variety of human tumors have been reported and some of them have been used for their diagnosis and treatment. We report here an attempt to generate monoclonal antibodies reactive with human maxillary sinus carcinoma.

MATERIALS AND METHODS

Human cells

1) AT-MS-1 line was established from a patient KI with maxillary sinus carcinoma (moderately differentiated squamous cell carcinoma) by us.

2) Cell lines and peripheral lymphocytes.

Monolayer cell lines of various origins (see Table I), eight T cell lines, ten B cell lines, and two myeloid cell lines (see Table II) were used. Peripheral lymphocytes were obtained by Ficoll-Conray centrifugation.

Production and screening of hybridomas.

One $x10^7$ AT-MS-1 cells were inoculated into the peritoneal cavity of BALB/c mouse three times at 1 week interval. Three days after final immunization, spleen cells from immunized mouse were fused with P3/x63-Ag8-653 cells in the presence of polyethylene glycol. Hybrids were selected in a medium containing hypoxanthine/ aminopterin / thymidine by an established method. The supernatants were tested against a panel of acetone-alcohol fixed human cells by indirect immunofluorescence analysis using FITC-conjugated rabbit anti-mouse immunoglobulin (DAKO, Denmark). The positive supernatants were further selected on the basis of negative reactivity against T cell, B cell and myeloid cell lines or peripheral lymphocytes in the radioimmunoassay using ^{125}I-labeled $F(ab')_2$ fragments of goat anti-mouse IgG.

Immunoperoxidase assay.

To determine the localization of molecules detected by these monoclonal antibodies, deparaffined tissue sections incubated with the supernatants were stained with VECTASTAIN ABC Kit (Vector Laboratories, USA).

RESULTS

Table I shows the reactivity patterns of three monoclonal antibodies (1A2, 8B1 and 10B2) against a wide variety of cell types in indirect immunofluorescence analysis. All three monoclonal antibodies reacted with at least one of three cultured lines of epithelial origin (AT-MS-1, Hela or SK-Lu-1) but not with four non-epithelial cultured lines or peripheral lymphocytes from a maxillary sinus carcinoma patient KI. On cellular radioimmunoassay these three monoclonal antibodies did not bind to all the cultured T cell, B cell and myeloid cell lines tested (Table II) or normal peripheral lymphocytes from several individuals. From the examination on tissue sections using immunoperoxidase technique, it was shown that (1) monoclonal antibody 10B2 reacts with maxillary sinus carcinoma cells, but not with stroma cells and mucous epithelium, (2) 8B1 reacts not only with the carcinoma cells but all the other tissue components, and (3) 1A2 does not react with any components of the tissues examined. We, therefore, conclude that monoclonal antibody 10B2 is a useful antibody to discriminate maxillary sinus carcinoma cells from normal maxillary sinus cells.

TABLE I

REACTIVITIES OF THREE MONOCLONAL ANTIBODIES*

Cell line	Origin	1A2	8B1	10B2
AT-MS-1	maxillary sinus ca.	○	●	●
Hela	cervical ca.	-	-	●
SK-Lu-1	lung cancer	○	-	●
SK-MEL-33	melanoma	-	-	-
SK-MEL-37	melanoma	-	-	-
SK-RC-7	renal cell ca.	-	-	-
G-II	giant cell tumor, bone	-	-	-
OZa	Osteosarcoma	-	-	-
KOM	Osteosarcoma	-	-	-
Kushi	leiomyosarcoma	-	-	-
PBL from maxillary sinus ca. patient (KI)		-	-	-

* Determined by indirect immunofluorescence technique. ● positive ○ partially positive

TABLE II

CELL LINES NOT REACTIVE WITH 1A2, 8B1 AND 10B2 IN CELLULAR RADIOIMMUNOASSAY

T cell lines : Molt-4F, Jurkat-SKI, TALL-1, HSB-2, Peer, MT-1, MT-2 and Sommer.
B cell lines : BT-1, Raji, Ky, Sa, HO, Wa, HOR, SH, LG-2 and LG-10.
Myeloid cell lines : K562 and HL60.

ACKNOWLEDGEMENTS

We thank Dr Sasaki for the gift of the non-epithelial monolayer cell lines.

New dimensions in otorhinolaryngology - head and neck surgery, vol. 2.
E. Myers, editor

RECONSTRUCTION OF SUBGLOTTIC LARYNX: A CLINICAL AND EXPERIMENTAL STUDY

MICHAEL FRIEDMAN, M.D., VYTENIS GRYBAUSKAS, M.D.

Department of Otolaryngology, Head and Neck Surgery, University of Illinois, 1855 West Taylor Street, Chicago, Illinois 60612

INTRODUCTION

Subglottic and tracheal reconstruction or, more specifically, cricoid reconstruction, have plagued investigators for quite some time. The aim of reconstruction is to create a good airway and a normal voice by providing a permanent supportive framework over which the mucosa can regenerate. The large variety of reconstructive procedures described in the literature indicates the lack of a single reliable operative approach.

In our experiment, a sternocleidomastoid myoperiosteal flap was utilized for closure of cricoid defects. Periosteum was used because it is easily shaped to fill in the defect. It is a strong, fibrous elastic tissue that is capable of airtight closure. Early epithelization has been shown by several investigators who have used pedicled periosteal flaps for laryngotracheal repair.[1] The osteogenic capability of periosteum was first demonstrated by O'lier in 1867, and has been demonstrated many times since then.[2] There have been case reports of myoperiosteal flap reconstruction of the cricoid, but no study has shown the presence of bone growth in these patients.

EXPERIMENTAL STUDY

Six mongrel dogs underwent resection of the anterior body of the cricoid cartilage along with its underlying mucosa from one cricothyroid joint to the other after careful identification and preservation of both recurrent laryngeal nerves. In six other dogs, the cricoid was crushed and a tracheotomy performed. Subsequently the scarred subglottis was excised.

A superiorly based myoperiosteal flap was rotated medially and the periosteum of the manubrium sewn to the surrounding perichondrium and cartilage circumferentially with interrupted chromic sutures. Strap muscles, subcutaneous tissues, and skin were closed. No drains or tracheotomy tubes were used.

The dogs underwent direct laryngoscopy and bronchoscopy at one month and every three months thereafter postoperatively to evaluate the subglottic airway. At one month complete epithelialization of the myoperiosteal graft had taken place. An excellent airway was seen on endoscopy with little to no subglottic airway narrowing. At six months the airway was rigid and no collapsing of the airway was seen with the inspiratory-expiratory cycles.

Upon sacrifice of the dogs at nine months, the histologic sections of the larynx showed clear evidence of bone growth within the periosteum.

CLINICAL STUDY

Four patients had cricoid and tracheal reconstruction with a similar sternocleidomastoid periosteal flap. All patients underwent resection of scar tissue and necrotic tissue and reconstruction with our flap. A stent was placed in the subglottis for six weeks. The stent was then removed endoscopically. Within four weeks after stent removal, all patients were decannulated. None of the patients had any complaints of shortness of breath or stridor. CT scanning of the reconstructed area shows calcified areas offering solid support.

DISCUSSION

The need for cricoid reconstruction is a rare problem for which multiple procedures have already been described. The techniques for bone grafts or flaps are not ideal; although they all provide skeletal support, they do not conform well to the defect site in all cases and long term success rates are poor.

We and others have used the myoperiosteal flap for reconstruction of small defects of trachea and the cricoid in patients following resection. Prior to this study, however, we have not been able to assess the presence of definite skeletal support in these areas. This study has clearly shown the ability of the periosteal flaps to grow bone.

The myoperiosteal flap has definite advantages over other forms of reconstruction. Vascularity appeared to be excellent in all of our cases and we had no subsequent tissue loss. Airtight closure of the defect was accomplished in the experimental dogs and in our patients. The absence of bone at the time of reconstruction allows for the pliability necessary for adequate closure, whereas the subsequent growth of bone supplies the skeletal support needed for long term success. There is an absolute tension free suture line created that is not possible with other forms of laryngotracheal reconstruction.

CONCLUSIONS

Cricoid loss secondary to trauma or resection requires multiple options for reconstruction. Our study has shown the ability of a myoperiosteal flap to not only survive but create stable skeletal support for the subglottic area. The flap is ideal because its pliability allows it to conform to any defect; the availability, location, and ease of elevation all add to its convenience.

REFERENCES

1. Finkalsrud, EW, Plested, WG (1966) In: J Thorac Cardiovasc Surg 52. Tracheobronchial Reconstruction with Autologous Periosteum, pp.666-674

2. Ritsila, V, Alhopuro, S, Rintala, A (1972) In: Scond J Plast Reconstr Surg. Bone Formation with Free Periosteum - An Experimental Study, 6:51-56

© 1985 Elsevier Science Publishers B.V. (Biomedical Division)
New dimensions in otorhinolaryngology - head and neck surgery, vol. 2.
E. Myers, editor

THE USE OF A NASAL CARTILAGE GRAFT (HOMOGRAFT) FOR TREATMENT OF TRACHEAL STENOSIS IN A CHILD

A. WILDER, Y. FLATAU, G. ROSEN
Department of Otorhinolaryngology, Central Emek Hospital, Afula, Israel

INTRODUCTION

The most frequent causes of tracheal and laryngeal stenosis in children are tracheotomy or prolonged endotracheal intubation with artificial respiration. Attempts at treatment of this problem started at the beginning of the century by Terner (1916). Since then many materials have been used as grafts for dilation of the stenosis, including free fascia (Taphel 1940). Rib cartilage (Grafoord & Lindgren 1965) and auricle cartilage autograft (Caputo & Consiglio 1961), but most of them failed for various reasons, including excessive granulation tissue formation, fibrosis, and immunological rejection.

We report a case of an infant who suffered from post intubation tracheal stenosis and received a nasal cartilage homograft from his father, and we wish to describe and discuss the histological findings 2 months after the transplantation.

CASE REPORT

A 19-month-old infant was hospitalized for the fourth time because of stridor and suspicion of a foreign body in the trachea. An endotracheal tube was inserted, and was left in place for 1 month because repeated attempts of extubation failed. After 1 month the tube was removed and tracheotomy was performed, which was later replaced by T-Tube, since subglotic stenosis developed. Recurrent trials of extubation failed, so the T-Tube was left in place for 3 months. After 3 months a graft of cartilage with mucus membrane on one side removed from the nasal septum of the infant's father was implanted as a wedge between the two parts of the thyroid cartilage and the middle of the cricoid cartilage by laryngofissure procedure.

At first the T-Tube was left in place, but as the infant's condition gradually improved, two months later the T-Tube was closed, and then taken out. Unfortunately a short time later the child developed massive broncho-pneumonia, probably due to aspiration, and died. During resuscitation, bronchoscopy showed a good stable lumen of the glotis and trachea.

HISTOLOGICAL FINDINGS

At post mortem examination of the infant's larynx, the father's homograft was found to be intact, and the lumen of the larynx was macroscopically and microscopicaly (Fig. 1) patent. The histological and histochemical examination of the graft revealed that the nuclei had disappeared, which conclusively indicates its death. In addition, a narrow cuffings of lymphocytes was found around the graft with some irregularity of the border, but no lymphocytes were present within the cartilage (Fig.2). Small blood vessels were seen adjacent to the graft, but these appeared smaller than those adjacent to the child's cartilage.

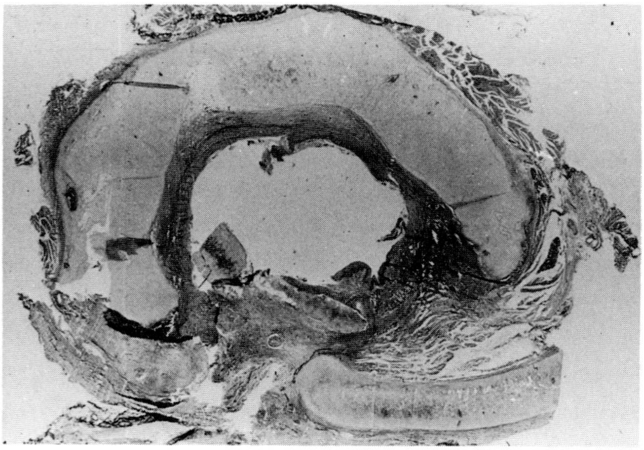

Fig. 1. Microscopic view of infant's larynx.
The lumen is patent.

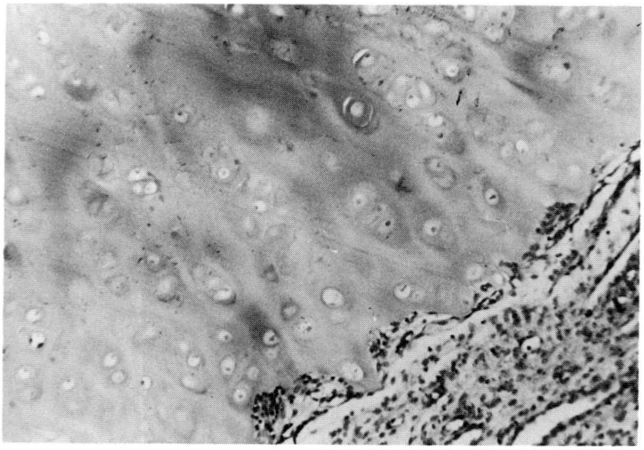

Fig. 2. Histological view of the graft demonstrates disappearance of nuclei and lymphocyte infiltration around the irregular border line.

PAS staining of the graft and the surrounding infant's cartilage showed that the graft stained stronger, indicating an increase in neutral mucopolysaccharides. The infant's cartilage stained positively by both Alcian Green and Alcian blue, while the graft gave negative results, indicating reduced levels of acid mucopolysacchrides in the graft. The polysaccharides are responsible for many of the important characteristics of the cartilage, such as toughness and resilience.

DISCUSSION

The incidence of tracheal stenosis after prolonged intubation or tracheotomy is 1%-10%. In the past many kinds of materials have been used as grafts for dilation of the stenosis, but most of them failed for various reasons.

Toohill (1981) performed auto-transplantation of nasal cartilage in adults. His clinical results were good, but no histological work up was made. In a survey of the literature we were unable to find any similar work describing the microscopic findings and the histochemical changes of a homograft cartilage transplant. The question arises as to the cause and mechanism of the failure of the graft to survive. The presence of blood vessels, although somewhat smaller than normal adjacent to the graft, would appear to make it unlikely that the failure to survive was due to inadequate diffusion. The presence of lymphocytes around the graft indicates an immune response. The absence of lymphocytes within the graft suggests that the mechanism of the failure was diffusion of antibodies into the graft. This suggestion requires further study for substantiation.

This is the first description of transplantation of cartilage from an adult to a child, and we believe that it is important to report the histological findings, since parents' nasal cartilages are easily available and although, histologically the cartilage graft was dead, its function was preserved and it kept the lumen of the airway patent.

REFERENCES

1. Turner AL (1916) J Laryngol Otol 31: 3-13
2. Taffel M (1940) Surgery 8: 56-63
3. Grafoord C, Lindgren AGH (1965) Acta Chir Scand 92: 481-506
4. Caputo V, Consiglio V (1961) J Thor Cardiov Surg 41: 594-595
5. Furstoss JA, Toohill RJ (1973) Ann Otol Rhinol Laryngol 82: 831-837
6. Toohill RJ (1979) Otolaryngol Clin N Am 12: 909-917
7. Drettner B, Lindholm CE (1970) Acta Otolaryngol 70: 401-407
8. Laurian N, Zohar Y (1981) Laryngoscope 91: 609-615

© 1985 Elsevier Science Publishers B.V. (Biomedical Division)
New dimensions in otorhinolaryngology - head and neck surgery, vol. 2.
E. Myers, editor

THE SAFETY OF NEONATAL INTUBATION

SK DANKLE, DE SCHULLER, RE MCCLEAD, J BUTLER

Departments of Otolaryngology and Pediatrics, Columbus Children's Hospital and The Ohio State University, Columbus, Ohio, (USA)

INTRODUCTION

A popular method of airway management in neonates requiring prolonged ventilatory support has been endotracheal intubation. Several investigators have suggested that neonates can tolerate intubation for extended periods of time.[1-3]

Recently, several reports have indicated a disturbingly high incidence of severe laryngeal injury resulting from prolonged intubation.[4-7] The purpose of this study was to review the experience of neonatal intubations at Columbus Children's Hospital.

SUBJECTS AND METHODS

Over a 3 year period (1977-1980), 508 patients admitted to the newborn intensive care unit required intubation and ventilatory support. The charts of the 343 patients who survived hospitalization were reviewed. The majority of these patients (89%) were less than 24 hours in age and 62% were pre-term. Birth weights and any antenatal complications were noted. In addition, the route, tube size, difficulty and duration of intubation were recorded for analysis. Complications following extubation were identified, as well as their respective treatment. Finally, it was recorded whether the patient was ultimately extubated successfully or whether tracheotomy was necessary.

RESULTS

Total Population:(N=343)

- Birth weights: 650-5696 grams; $\bar{x}$ = 2272g.
- Antenatal complications: 135 patients (39%).
- Duration of intubation: 1-104 days; $\bar{x}$ = 9.15 days.
- Successfully extubated: 334 patients (97.4%).
- Failed at least one extubation attempt: 71 patients (20%).

Extubation Failure: (N=71)

- Upper airway obstruction: 12 patients (17%).
- Lower respiratory tract or other: 59 patients (83%).
- Subsequently extubated successfully: 66 patients (93%).

Tracheotomies: (N=9)

Anticipated prolonged ventilation (no stenosis): 4.

Failed extubation (stenosis): 5.

Acquired Subglottic Stenosis: (N=5)

Birth weights: 820-2680 grams; $\bar{x}$ = 1409 grams.

Duration of intubation: 18-83 days; $\bar{x}$ = 56.2 days.

The overall incidence of acquired subglottic stenosis following prolonged intubation in this study is 1.5% (5/343). A comparison was made of those who were successfully extubated and those who developed significant subglottic stenosis and is shown in Table 1.

TABLE 1

SUCCESSFUL EXTUBATION		ACQUIRED STENOSIS
334 (97.4%)	N	5 (1.5%)
2282 grams	birth weight	1409 grams
5.3 %	$\geq$ 3 intubations	60 %
7.8 days	duration intubated	56.2 days

CONCLUSION

Endotracheal intubation in the neonate is safe even for prolonged periods. The overall incidence of significant subglottic stenosis resulting from neonatal intubation in this study is low (1.5%).

The risk of acquired subglottic stenosis following prolonged neonatal intubation appears to be related to very low birth weight ($<$ 1500 grams), multiple intubations, and protracted time of intubation.

REFERENCES

1. Hawkins DB (1978) Laryngoscope 88:201-224
2. Ratner I, Whitfield J (1983) Am J Dis Child 137:40-43
3. Conner GH, Bushey MJ, Maisels MJ (1980) Ann Otol Rhinol Laryngol 89:459-461
4. Fan EL, Flynn JW, Pathak DR (1983) Crit Care Med 11:431-433
5. Papisdero MJ, Pashley NRT (1980) Ann Otol Rhinol Laryngol 89:512-514
6. Jones R, Bodnar A, Roan Y, Johnson D (1981) Am J Dis Child 135:367-368
7. Fan ED, Flynn JW, Pathak DR, Madden WA (1982) Crit Care Med 10:453-455

New dimensions in otorhinolaryngology - head and neck surgery, vol. 2.
E. Myers, editor

THE ANTERIOR CRICOID SPLIT PROCEDURE AS AN ALTERNATIVE TO TRACHEOTOMY: FURTHER EXPERIENCE

JAMES A. STANKIEWICZ, M.D.

Department of Otolaryngology - Head and Neck Surgery, Loyola University Medical Center, 2160 S. First Avenue, Maywood, Illinois U.S.A.

INTRODUCTION

In 1980, Dr. Robin Cotton published a paper recommending the anterior splitting of the cricoid cartilage as an alternative to tracheotomy in selected neonates intubated with endotracheal tubes but unable to be extubated. He was successful in extubating 9 of 12 patients without needing tracheotomies. Using his criteria and technique in 10 patients who were unable to be extubated, nine were successfully extubated after the cricoid split procedure. The test results are presented and discussed.

TECHNIQUE (See Table I AND Reference 1)

DATA (See Table II)

The patients were intubated from 8 days to 2 years. (Trach tube). Neonates specifically were intubated from 8-16 weeks. Seven patients were neonates. Patient six had an encephalopathy with prolonged intubation. Tracheotomy was recommended but both parents who were pediatricians had read about the cricoid split and insisted it be tried. As predicted, it was unsuccessful and tracheotomy was performed. At surgery, the patient had glottic and subglottic stenoiis. Patient seven had had a tracheotomy in place with subglottic stenosis and could not be decannulated despite a number three endotracheal tube sized airway. A cricoid split performed with the assistance of Dr. Cotton allowed for extubation. Patient nine was a drug overdose who could not be extubated. She had 3 intubations in 8 days and had marked edema and granulation. Cricoid split was successful in her case. All seven neonates were evaluated and treated according to Dr. Cotton's protocol. Follow-up of 3-5 years in 6 neonates and 1 child shows no patient with any stridor, tracheotomy, or difficulty with intubation for other surgeries. Two patients died from other problems. All wounds have healed and are imperceptible.

DISCUSSION

The purpose of the cricoid split is to allow for anterior decompression of the cricoid and tracheal cartilages to reduce edema and inflammation. Adhering strictly to the criteria for neonates, seven out of seven patients were extubated. In older children, 2 out of 3 were extubated. Our neonatal unit handles the smallest babies in Chicago with over 500 admissions per year in a 30 bed unit where 50% of babies are intubated at any one time. Proper tube size, intubation techniques, and nursing care usually leads to uneventful extubation. However, in carefully selected extubation failures, the anterior cricoid split procedure can be successful in avoiding tracheotomy in the neonate and on occasion in older children.

TABLE I - TECHNIQUE

1. Evaluate airway utilizing endoscopy
   A. Minimal glottic pathology
   B. Subglottic pathology limited to edema, mucosal ulceration and/or granulation tissue
   C. Patient must be ready for extubation
2. Incise cricoid, tracheal rings 1 and 2 and cricothyroid membrane vertically in midline
3. Tissue layers closed loosely with small drain
4. Drain removed following day
5. Wound drainage occurs for 3-5 days. Post-op antibiotics are given.
6. Extubate in routine fashion in 1 week - steroids prior to extubation

TABLE II
CRICOID SPLIT

CASE	AGE (BIRTH)	INTUBATIONS	WT.	EXT.
1	30 wks.	3 (11 wks.)	1230	+
2	28 wks.	5 (12 wks.)	940	+
3	30 wks.	4 (16 wks.)	900	+
4	33 wks.	3 (12 wks.)	820	+
5	34 wks.	3 (8 wks.)	1000	+
6	18 mos.	3 (6 wks.)	-	-
7	24 mos.	Trach (2 yrs.)	-	+
8	26 wks.	3 (8 wks.)	1300	+
9	16 mos.	3 (8 days)	-	+
10	28 wks.	3 (8 wks.)	1100	+

REFERENCES

1. Cotton RT, Seid AB (1980) Ann Otol 89:508.

ACKNOWLEDGEMENT

Thanks to Mrs. Joan Findlay for her help in manuscript preparation.

New dimensions in otorhinolaryngology – head and neck surgery, vol. 2.
E. Myers, editor

ULTRASTRUCTURAL FINDINGS IN TRIGEMINAL NEURALGIA

JOSE MARIA SANCHEZ FERNANDEZ and MIGUEL ANGEL CROVETTO DE LA TORRE
Departments of Otolaryngology and Pathology. Civil Hospital of Bilbao. Spain

INTRODUCTION

The idiophatic Trigeminal neuralgia still remains as a Pathogenic enigma. The purpose of this paper is to study the Retrogasserian Root, as well as the Infraorbital nerve in several patients suffering symptomatic Trigeminal neuralgia.

MATERIAL AND METHODS

In this study we have employed the material proceeding from four patients, three males and one female, ranged between 52 and 72 years.

Patients nº 1 and 2 suffered a maxillary sinus cancer and a infraestructure Paget disease respectively, without any neurological symptoms. A total maxillectomy was performed in the first case and a partial maxillectomy in the second one.In both cases the Infraorbital nerve were isolated and inmersed, just after the surgical exeresis, in a 2% solution of glutaraldehyde in phosphate buffer at pH 7.4. Patient nº3 complains a nasopharynx cancer with a symptomatic Trigeminal neuralgia of the second and third roots. The patient nº4, a female 71 years old, suffers an Idiophathic Trigeminal neuralgia. In both patients a Retrogasserian neurectomy was performed after diverse unsuccesful medical treatmentes. The posterior root nerves were also fixed in glutaraldehyde and processed following our routine electron microscopy procedures[1].

RESULTS

The Infraorbital nerve of patients nº 1 and 2 is composed of numerous myelinated and unmyelinated fibers. The myelinated fibers is formed by the myelin sheath, the axon and the Schwann cell. The myelin sheath shows, as normaly occurs, a regular alternanting lamellae pattern of dense and lighert lines. In the unmyelinated fibers the axon may appear totally surrounded by the Schwann cell cytoplasm, but at times it may contact with the basement membrane through the mesaxon.

In the patient nº 3 some myelinated and unmyelinated fibers remain normal but others offer numerous alterations. In this patient the pathological nerve fibers may follow diverse sequences in the degeneration process. An hipermyelination with a normal axon appear in the first stage. In the second one, an axonal and cytoplasmic vacuolization can be observed in the myelinated and unmyelinated fibers. In the third one, numerous spherical lamellar elements proceeding from the myelin sheath breakdown appears. Also vacuolization and vesicles with needle-like structures are apparent.

In the forth case a segmental demyelination can be recognized. The myelin sheath dissapear in spherical areas that may contain myelin debris.The axon remains even normal, but containing vesicles with needle-like structures that can seen in the Schwann cell cytoplasm Fig. 1 In other areas myelin sheath breakdown is very important and coexist with an increment of vesicles with needle-like structures in the axon and in the Schwann cell cytoplasme

DISCUSSION

Beaver et al[2] and Kerr and Miller[3], studied the Trigeminal Garglion and the posterior Trigeminal Root from patients who had a Trigeminal neuralgia. Vacuolization, hipermyelination, segmental demyelination and hipertrofy of axis cylinders with microneuroma formation were their findings. Our observations, in the case 3 (symptomatic neuralgia) may corrspond to that seen in Wallerian secondary degeneration process.In the case 4 (idiopathic Trigeminal neuralgia) the presence of a segmental demyelination in some fibers remaining the axon intact may signify a primary myelin sheath disease. Nevertheless, the appearance of other nerve fibers with severe alteration of their axon and myelin sheath may express a further degeneration process who is taking place.

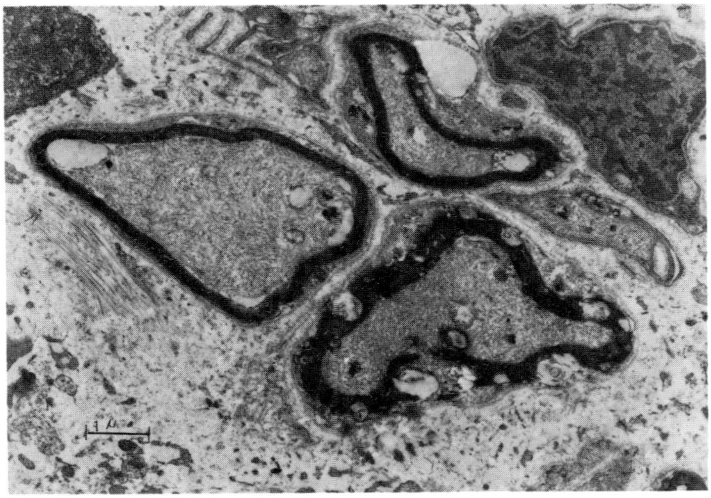

Fig. 1 Idiopathic Trigeminal neuralgia. Segmental demyelination and axoplasmic vacuolization can be observed.

REFERENCES

1.-Sanchez Fernandez J.M., Rivera Pomar J.M. 1983. A study of development of utricular and saccular maculae in man and in rat. Am. J. Otol. 5 : 44-45

2.-Beaver D.,Moses H.L., Ganote C. 1965: Electron microscopy of the Trigeminal Ganglion. Arch. Pathol. 79 : 471-582

3.- Kerr F,MillerR.1966. The Pathology of Trigem. neural. Arch. Neurol.15:308-319

New dimensions in otorhinolaryngology - head and neck surgery, vol. 2.
E. Myers, editor

THE ADVANTAGES OF CO_2 LASER IN TRANSORAL RESECTION OF CANCER OF THE ORAL CAVITY

JACK SIDI, ARISTEDE ABRAHAM, KARL SEGAL, GADI HAREL
Department of Otolaryngology and Head & Neck Surgery, Beilinson Medical Center, Petah Tiqva and Tel Aviv University Sackler School of Medicine, Israel

The use of CO_2 laser surgery, a most valuable and practical method for tissue ablation or excision, represents a significant advance in the management of benign and certain malignant lesions of the oral cavity. Its advantages for intraoral lesions are multiple: bleeding is practically absent during the procedure, permitting continuous observation during dissection and precise excision from safe margins. The ability to carry out effective and precise excisional surgery is the most important attribute of this method. The lack of tissue distortion is an advantage to the pathologist in determining adequate margins by frozen section examination.

Laser induced wounds are characterized by minimal postoperative edema; there is no need for a tracheostomy. There is remarkably little pain at the resection site. This fact may be explained by the minimal damage to the surrounding tissues and the sealing of the nerve endings. Patients may eat on the evening of the operation and are discharged on the following day. The wound may be left open and allowed to heal by re-epithelialisation in 2 or 3 weeks, depending on the size of the surface defect.

Generally speaking, most benign lesions of the oral cavity are resectable transorally. In dealing with carcinoma of the oral cavity, areas of leucoplakia, carcinoma in situ, verrucous carcinoma and superficial lesions up to 4 cm in diameter may be excised at the desired depth with laser. Stensen's duct will heal by secondary intention. As long as there is no bone involvement, tumors extending to the alveolar ridge may be resected with the periosteum.

T_1 and T_2 lesions of the anterior two-thirds of the tongue and noninfiltrating tumors of the floor of the mouth can be removed by laser excision with the following limitations: 1. Normal mobility of the tongue must be present; 2. Deep margins must be obviously accessible by palpation; 3. Lesions extending toward the posterolateral portion of the floor of the mouth are unsuitable for transoral resection; 4. Occasionally, transoral resection may be used in palliation of bulky tumors prior to radiation or chemotherapy.

Before resecting the lesion, the excision margins may be marked initially with the laser, using brief bursts of low power. The lesion is then put on tension by transfixion with one or two traction sutures and excised at the desired depth, on the basis of palpation and with the line of resection in constant view. If a deep margin shows tumor close to the resection edge, it may be assumed that further treatment is necessary by conventional surgery or a full course of irradiation therapy which can safely be implemented without waiting for complete healing. Transoral resection can only be expected to control primary tumors. Nodal disease requires neck dissection and eventual postoperative irradiation in addition.

Occasionally a patient may present with a metastatic node and a small accessible T_1 lesion of the tongue or of the buccal mucosa. Such a primary lesion may be managed by adequate transoral resection and the metastatic disease by discontinuous radical neck dissection and postoperative radiotherapy. Discontinuous radical neck dissection may well be indicated in some of the T_2 lesions without palpable nodes, since there is a high incidence of positive occult metastasis.

As stated by Strong et al., survival rates of the patients treated in this way will depend largely on the ability of the surgeon to deliver a specimen which can be found to have free margins on histologic examination, and will be greatly influenced by the presence or absence of metastases.

Thirty-five cases of malignant tumors of the oral cavity were removed by laser surgery. All of these tumors were classified as T_1 and T_2 lesions except for three cases which had consecutive neck dissection and radiotherapy in addition to transoral resection; 2 cases were given radiotherapy alone after intraoral excision; 1 of these had local and nodal recurrence and died 14 months after surgery; 1 presented with a second primary lesion which was resected by laser beam and is now free of disease. Postoperative follow-up is from 10 to 34 months. Three of the patients were classified as T_3 lesions, 2 of them, aged over 85 years, had positive nodes. The transoral excision was done to reduce the tumor mass prior to irradiation therapy. One had verrucous carcinoma and is free of disease 28 months after surgery. The other 2 died after 13 and 15 months.

Considering the tendency for less radical surgery in selected cases of cancer of the tongue and floor of the mouth, laser surgery is a most valuable tool for safe resection, offering short morbidity and greater comfort for the patient with practically no complications.

© 1985 Elsevier Science Publishers B.V. (Biomedical Division)
New dimensions in otorhinolaryngology - head and neck surgery, vol. 2.
E. Myers, editor

SURGICAL TREATMENT OF ADVANCED OR REGRESSED CANCERS FROM THE THYROID GLAND

DR. D.O. RODRIGUEZ-MORA

Surgical services of the Head, Neck and Otorhinolaryngology. Cancer Institute SOLCA Guayaquil - Ecuador

The advanced cancers or cancers regressed from the Thyroid Gland do not permit for much discussion on which therapeutic to choose. They always present great surgical problems even for the surgeons with sufficient training in the handling of voluminous cervical tumors or adhered to vital organs.

75 Cases of this type of tumors treated surgically of a total 408 during the period of May 1975 to 1984.

	CASES	PERCENTAGE
Differential Ephyteliomes	56	76.6 %
Medular Ephyteliomes	3	4 %
Indifferential Ephyteliomes	8	10.6 %
Mesenquimatics Sarcomas	5	6.6 %
Metaplasic Cancers	3	4 %

As we can appreciate, this pathology is frequent. All histological forms can be found. The advanced cancers can generally be accompanied by nodes, which once past the gland can filter the trachea, larynx, esophagus from which the recurrent paralysis is frequent. In occasions it can provoke acute tracheal compressions:

The surgical treatment has a triple interest:

A) The extended cervicotomy permits a precise study of the extension of the tumor.

B) To extirpate if possible, is the only chance for patient survival.

C) The precise knowledge of the histology permits orientation for the complementary treatment of the study of the total gland.

New dimensions in otorhinolaryngology - head and neck surgery, vol. 2.
E. Myers, editor

SINUS HISTIOCYTOSIS WITH MASSIVE CERVICAL LYMPHADENOPATHY: A CASE REPORT AND REVIEW OF THE LITERATURE

VANESSA G. SCHWEITZER, M.D.[1], GREGG D. BOBIER, D.D.S.[2], AND STEVEN V. WEILERT, M.D.[3]

Departments of [1]Otolaryngology, [2]Oral Surgery, and [3]Pathology, Henry Ford Hospital, Detroit, Michigan U.S.A.

Sinus histiocytosis with massive cervical lymphadenopathy (SHML) was originally described in 1969 as a benign clinicopathological entity characterized by massive bilateral cervical lymphadenopathy, fever, leukocytosis, elevated erythrocyte sedimentation rate, and hypergammaglobulinemia, usually occurring within the first two decades of life.[1] The etiology and pathogenesis of SHML are not known. The two most popular theories implicate either an infectious etiology or an impairment of cell mediated immunity. Diagnosis requires lymph node biopsy. Histologically, SHML should be differentiated from other diseases considered in the differential diagnosis of cervical lymphadenopathy: malignant lymphoma of histiocytic type, malignant histiocytosis, histiocytic medullary reticulosis, monocytic leukemia, familial hemagophagocytic reticulosis, storage diseases, eosinophilic granuloma, sarcoidosis, infectious mononucleosis, and common inflammatory reactive lymph node disorders such as cat scratch fever, tuberculosis lymphadenitis, or syphilitic lymphadenitis. The key microscopic features are massive sinus histiocytosis, lymphophagocytosis, proliferation of mature plasma cells in medullary cords, and prominent lymph node enlargement due to dilatation of the subcapsular and medullary sinuses, progressing to total effacement of the lymph node architecture. A distinguishing histological feature is "emperipolesis", i.e. the presence of numerous lymphocytes within the cytoplasm of sinus histiocytes, presumably representing phagocytosis (Figure 1).

Although no cases of SHML manifesting cytologic malignant transformation have been identified, the clinicopathological entity of SHML represents a spectrum of disease from isolated nodal enlargement (i.e. self-limiting cervical lymphadenopathy) on one end of the spectrum to diffuse organ involvement with SHML infiltrates associated with immunodeficiencies at the other end of the spectrum. Of the 215 registered cases, 97% have cervical lymphadenopathy, 30% have dissemination to other nodal (axillary, inguinal, paravertebral) and extranodal sites, and 30-43% have abnormal chest x-rays showing hilar or mediastinal involvement. Multiple sites of extensive extranodal infiltration have been described: 1)orbit and eyelids; 2)nasal cavity and paranasal sinuses; 3)oral cavity and tonsil; 4)salivary glands (usually submandibular); 5)trachea and bronchus; 6)skin; 7)abdominal viscera (kidney, liver, spleen, pancreas, duodenum); 8)testicles; 9)long bones; and 10)cerebrum and spinal cord.[2] The extranodal dissemination of SHML has been associated with tracheal or bronchial destruction, epidural infiltration and paraplegia, and cranial neuropathies with ptosis, deafness, tongue atrophy, and palatoplegia. Six cases of SHML accompanied by osseous involvement have been reported.[4] The osseous lesions are usually lytic with involvement of the medulla of long bones (usually affecting the epiphysis , diaphysis, and metaphysis) and other less common sites, the skull, vertebral bodies, pelvis, phalanges, metacarpals, and ribs.[3,4]

Fourteen of the 215 (7%) registered SHML cases had a fatal outcome due to central nervous system, renal, and pulmonary involvement with 71% of fatal cases demonstrating immune dysfunction, i.e. hematologic autoantibodies, inflammatory joint disease, and unusual infections as cryptococcal meningitis. Causes of death as a result of an immunodeficiency state include amyloidosis, Wiskott-Aldrich syndrome, exfoliative dermatitis, hemolytic crisis, glomerulonephritis,

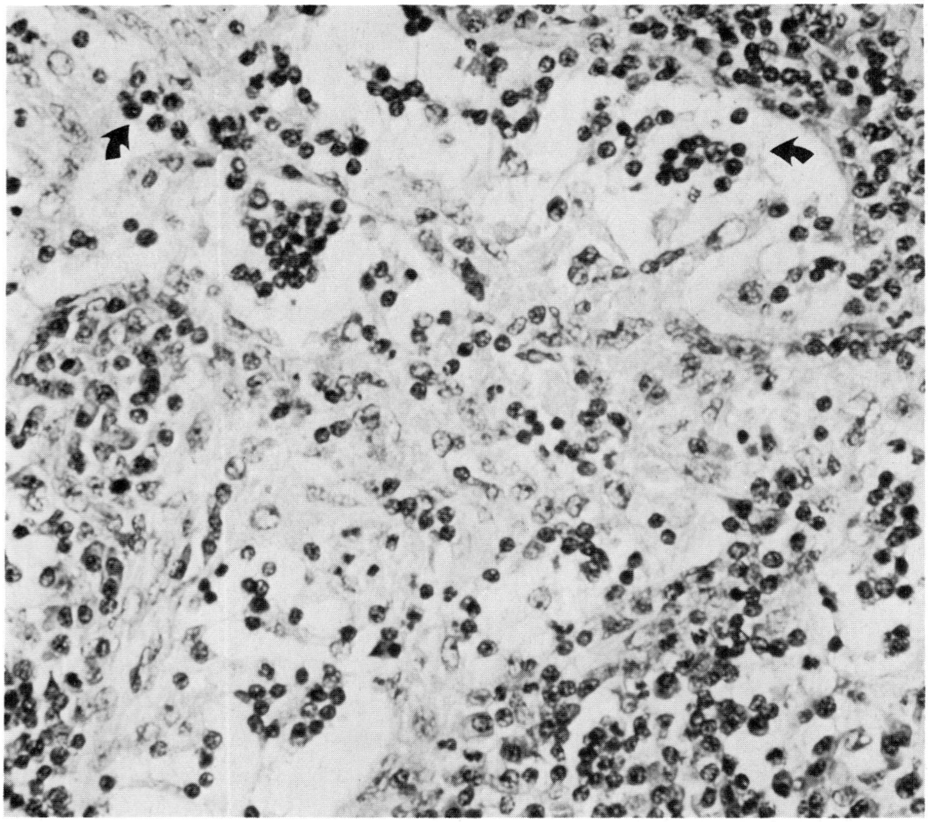

Figure 1 Photomicrograph of lymph node shows marked sinus dilatation by foamy or vacuolated histiocytes, mature plasma cells filling the medullary cords, histiocytic phagocytosis of small lymphocytes ("emperipolesis") (arrows). Hematoxylin and eosin, x157

pancytopenia, and exudative enteropathy.

Although no curative treatment is known, corticosteroids, radiation therapy, vinblastine and oral cyclophosphamide and surgery have been used to palliate constitutional symptoms and mechanical obstruction from massive lymphadenopathy.[5,6] Surgical therapy is indicated when nodal or extranodal deposits cause nasal or tracheal obstruction, or when epidural and vertebral involvement precipitate cranial neuropathies and paraplegia. Since one-third of SHML patients have evidence of disease for 5 years and a mortality rate of 7% exists with benign histologic disease, all patients with SHML should be carefully screened for evidence of immunodeficiencies that may precipitate a fatal outcome.

Presented is a case report of a 66 year old black female with a 2 year history of a 6 cm, multilobulated, rubbery, nontender submandibular neck mass with

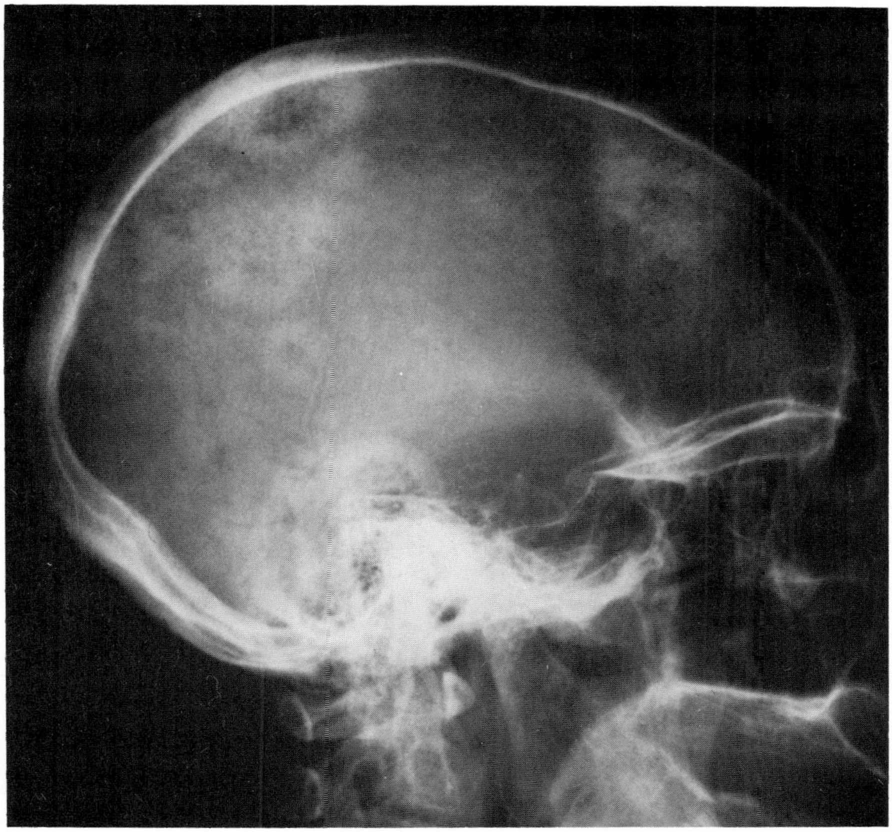

Figure 2 Osseous manifestations of sinus histiocytosis with massive cervical lymphadenopathy. Lateral skull view demonstrates multiple lytic areas with "fuzzy" borders and large areas of surrounding sclerosis.

bilateral cervical lymphadenopathy, lymphocytosis, elevated sedimentation rate, polyclonal hypergammaglobulinemia, and multiple lytic skull lesions (Figure 2). Left suprahyoid dissection and excisional biopsy of the neck mass was diagnostic for sinus histiocytosis of the cervical lymph nodes with extranodal involvement of the adjacent submandibular gland and extracapsular nodal extension.

REFERENCES

1. Sanchez R, Rosai J, Dorfman RF: Sinus histiocytosis with massive cervical lymphadenopathy: An analysis of 113 cases with special emphasis on extranodal manifestations. Lab Investig 36(3):349-350, 1977.

2. Foucar E, Rosai J, Dorfman RF: Sinus histiocytosis with massive lymphadenopathy: An analysis of 14 deaths occurring in a patient registry. Cancer 54:1834-1840, 1984.

3. Siegel MT, Shackelford GD, McAlister WH: Sinus histiocytosis: Some radiologic observations. AJR 132(5):783-785, May 1979.

4. Walker PD, Rosai J, Dorfman RF: The Osseous Manifestations of Sinus Histiocytosis with Massive Lymphadenopathy. Am J Clin Path 75(2):131-139, Feb. 1981.

5. Penneys NS, Ahn YS, McKinney SC, et al: Sinus histiocytosis with massive lymphadenopathy: A case with unusual skin involvement and a therapeutic response to Vinblastine-loaded platelets. Cancer 49:1994-1998, 1982.

6. Newman SB, Sweet DL, Vardiman JW: Sinus histiocytosis with massive cervical lymphadenopathy: Response to cyclophosphamide therapy. Cancer Treat Rep 68(6):901-901, June 1984.

© 1985 Elsevier Science Publishers B.V. (Biomedical Division)
New dimensions in otorhinolaryngology - head and neck surgery, vol. 2.
E. Myers, editor

FINE NEEDLE ASPIRATION IN THE INITIAL EVALUATION OF CERVICAL ADENOPATHY

ASHOK SHAHA, MD, CAROLYN WEBBER MD, JOSE MARTI FACS, Department of Surgery and Pathology, Downstate Medical Center, 450 Clarkson Avenue, Brooklyn, New York 11203

INTRODUCTION

Cervical adenopathy is related to variety of different pathologies amongst which metastatic carcinoma from the Head & Neck area is the most important. Amongst many investigations 'untimely lymph node biopsy' is best avoided from the earlier teachings of Hayes Martin (1). Often extensive work up is done to find that the patient has hyperplastic nodes, tuberculosis or lymphoma. Occasionally complete work up including CXR, Ba Swallow, GI series, Barium enema, CAT scan, ERCP etc is done before appropriate evaluation of the neck node for the fear of metastatic carcinoma. Is there any way to evaluate the pathology of the nodes without open biopsy? Most of the time the issue is, can we find out if the patient has metastatic carcinoma so that we can do appropriate work up for the search of the primary and treat the patient adequately without an untimely lymph node biopsy. We have used fine needle aspiration in the evaluation of suspicious cervical adenopathy routinely as the initial investigation.

MATERIAL AND METHODS

One hundred patients with suspicious cervical adenopathy were evaluated by FNA cytology. Ten or twenty cc syringe with 22 gauge needle was used. No local anesthesia was used. The specimen was obtained in the core of the needle which was spread on the slides. The slides were fixed most of the time in 95% alcohol or Cytoprep was occasionally used to spray on the slides. Few dry slides were routinely made for Wright Staining. Variety of staining methods were used - mainly Hematoxylin-Eosin like frozen section, Pap staining, and Wright stains. Special stains such as mucin stains were used in special circumstances. (2,3,4).

RESULTS

Adequate specimen was obtained in 98% of the cases. Malignant pathology was detected in 48 cases while 52 had benign lymph nodes. In patients where benign pathology was noted on FNA, open biopsy was done in many cases depending on the clinical suspicion regarding TB etc. In no patients where the FNA was reported as benign, malignancy was found by open biopsy or by clinical follow up. Patients in whom lymphoma was suspected open node biopsy was done for definitive type of lymphoma, electron microscopic studies and marker studies. FNA was very useful in patients presenting with neck nodes after their previous treatment of head & neck cancer. Open node biopsy was avoided in this group and proceeded with neck dissection based on the clinical and cytologic findings. Wherever the clinical findings did not correlate with FNA, importance was given to clinical evaluation in regards further work up or follow up. There were no complications in this group of patients. The diagnostic accuracy of FNA in this group was 96% .

DISCUSSION

A practical algorythm was used in this group of patients with cervical adenopathy. FNA was used as a definite guide however more importance was given to the clinical suspicion and findings. A detailed history and complete head & neck examination was done including the use of Storz fiberoptic scope when necessary. If no pathology noted in head & neck areas then FNA was used routinely. The findings of FNA can be divided in two groups, (A) benign or (B) suspected malignant. (A) Most of the patients reported benign had either hyperplastic nodes, chronic inflammation (drug abuse etc) or TB. Open biopsy after repeat thorough head and neck exam is done according to the clinical suspicion. (B) If FNA was suspicious of metastatic epidermoid carcinoma panendoscopy, multiple biopsies, open excisional biopsy followed by neck dissection was the usual practice. If FNA was suspicious of met adenocarcinoma a search was made for primary and treatment approached according to the findings. Open biopsy considered for final definitive diagnosis if no primary can be found. If FNA was suspicious of metastatic thyroid carcinoma appropriate thyroid workup (scan) and adequate surgery was done. Whenever FNA and clinical findings were suspicious of lymphoma and no lesion noted in the upper aero-digestive areas, open biopsy was done for definite histopathology.

We strongly feel using FNA, above algorythm and clinical correlation, the diagnostic accuracy can exceed 96%. It is the most effective diagnostic investigation and cost effective in the initial evaluation of cervical adenopathy (5,6).

TABLE I

Cervical Adenopathy-----------Adequate Specimen 98%

FNA-Total 100 Complications 0

Benign - 52	Malignant -	48
Hyperplasia	Lymphoma	10
TB etc.	Met Adeno Ca	5
	Met Thyroid Ca	6
	Met Sq. Ca.	21

REFERENCES

1. Martin H (1961) Untimely Lymph Node Biopsy. Am J Surg 1C2: 17-18.

2. Feldman PS et al (1983) Fine Needle Aspiration In Squamcus Cell Carcinoma of the Head & Neck. Arch Otolaryngeal 109: 735-742.

3. Young JEM, Archibald SD, Shier KJ (1981) Needle Aspiration Cytologic Biopsy in Head & Neck Masses. Am J Surg 142: 484-489.

4. Frable MAS, Frable WJ. (1982) Fine Needle Aspiration Biopsy Revisited. Laryngoscope 92: 1414-1418.

5. Smith TJ et al (1985) Accuracy and Cost Effectiveness of Fine Needle Aspiration Biopsy. Am J Surg 149: 540-545.

6. Weymuller EA, Kiviat NB, Duckert LG (1983) Aspiration Cytology: An Efficient and Cost Effective Modality. Latyngoscope 93: 561-564.

© 1985 Elsevier Science Publishers B.V. (Biomedical Division)
New dimensions in otorhinolaryngology - head and neck surgery, vol. 2.
E. Myers, editor

SIGNIFICANCE OF POSITIVE MARGINS IN BASAL CELL CARCINOMA

W W SHOCKLEY, MD and F J STUCKER, MD
Department of Otolaryngology/Head and Neck Surgery, LSU School of Medicine,
P. O. Box 33932, Shreveport, Louisiana 71130-3932

INTRODUCTION

Surgical excision is often utilized as primary treatment for basal cell carcinoma and for smaller lesions immediate histologic control is seldom employed. Occasionally the surgeon is faced with a pathology report which states that tumor extends to the surgical margin. At this point, the dilemma is whether to re-exise the area in question or to observe the patient for evidence of recurrence. In order to address this problem the literature was reviewed concerning the significance of positive margins following excision of basal cell carcinoma.

MARGINAL EXTENSION BY BCC

Few authors have published studies which evaluate the recurrence rates in patients with positive margins. Gooding, in a review of 1,197 excisions, found 66 excised lesions with marginal extension (1). Only 34.8% of these cases had recurrence of the tumor. Pascal and associates, reviewed 42 cases in which there was incomplete excision, 14 recurred for a frequency of 33% (2). Taylor and Barisoni noted a recurrence rate of 24% in those patients having had lesions excised with tumor found at the margin (3). However, many of the patients were followed for only two years.

The timing of recurrence is widely variable although in those patients with positive margins the mean interval from excision to recurrence is from 12 to 24 months (1,2,3,4). In Lauritzen's series of 101 BCC's, inadequately excised tumors manifested recurrence sooner with 70% seen by 2 years while those with "adequate" surgery had only 50% of the recurrences evident by 2 years (4).

"DISAPPEARANCE" OF RESIDUAL BCC

It has been shown by several authors that re-excised specimens often fail to demonstrate histologic evidence of neoplasm. Sarma and associates reviewed 43 cases of "inadequately excised" BCC in which re-excision was performed 2-4 weeks after the initial surgery (5). In only 3 cases (7%) was microscopic residual tumor identified. From our combined series we found that in only about 20% of the specimens could residual tumor be identified (1,2,5,6). Numerous ideas have been proposed explaining the "disappearance" of these tumor cells (5,7).

DISCUSSION

Based on our review of the literature, we would strongly recommend re-excision of those lesions which were 2cm or greater in diameter or of the morphea subtype. We also would consider the following locations as high risk for recurrence: ear, nose, malar, periorbital, and periauricular regions. Lesions with marginal extension which could be considered relatively safe for observation would be those of the nodular type, originally less than 2cm, and involving the cheek, forehead, and neck.

REFERENCES

1. Gooding C, et al (1965) New England J Med 273:923-924
2. Pascal R, et al (1968) Plast Reconstr Surg 41:328-332
3. Taylor A, Barisoni D (1973) Brit J Surg 60:522-525
4. Lauritzen R, et al (1965) Surgery 57:813-816
5. Sarma D, et al (1984) J Surg Oncol 25:79-80
6. Epstein E (1973) Brit J Derm 89:37-43
7. Goldwyn R, Kasdon E (1978) Ann Plast Surg 1:286-289

New dimensions in otorhinolaryngology - head and neck surgery, vol. 2.
E. Myers, editor

SEQUENTIAL CISPLATIN (DDP) AND 5-FLUOROURACIL (5-FU) IN ADVANCED SQUAMOUS CELL HEAD AND NECK CANCER

KASI S. SRIDHAR
Papanicolaou Comprehensive Cancer Center, University of Miami School of Medicine & V.A. Hospital, Miami, FL, USA

INTRODUCTION

A report from Wayne State indicated a high response rate in head and neck cancer for cisplatin followed in 4 hours by a 120 hour infusion of 5-FU (Weaver A, 1982). The toxicities consisted of vomiting, mucositis and leucopenia. The present study used a 24 hour interval between cisplatin and 5-FU, to permit adequate hydration and correction of electrolyte disturbances.

MATERIALS AND METHODS

Thirty-eight patients with measurable histologically proven advanced head and neck cancer with no prior chemotherapy and who were not amenable to curative therapy with surgery and or radiation therapy were selected for this study. Patients with impaired renal, hepatic or hematological dysfunction, were excluded. Twenty patients had recurrent cancer after prior surgery, radiation therapy or both. Eighteen patients with bulky inoperable stage IV tumors received neoadjuvant chemotherapy prior to definitive therapy. Patients with no prior radiation therapy were irradiated at the time of maximal response. There were 33 men and 5 women with a median age of 58 (range 28-75 years), Zubrod performance status was 0-2:31 patients; 3-4:7 patients.

Therapy began with at least 6 hours of prehydration followed by cisplatin 100 mg/m^2 IV at the rate of 1 mg/minute and 24 hours later by 5-FU IV infusion at the rate of 40 mg/m^2/hour until the appearance of mucositis or, in its absence, a maximum of 120 hours. In 30% of patients FU was stopped between 72 to 112 hours. In subsequent courses, mucositis was avoided in these patients by individually reducing the length of FU infusion by 2 to 4 hours. Multi-agent antiemesis was used prophylactically in all patients (1). The cycles were repeated every three weeks in responders.

RESULTS

All the 38 patients were evaluable for response and toxicity.

The results are summarized in Table 1.

TABLE 1

SEQUENTIAL CISPLATIN 5-FU CHEMOTHERAPY IN HEAD AND NECK CANCER.

	Recurrent Cancer	Stage IV Inoperable Cancer
Number of patients	20	18
Complete response rate (CR)	20%	17%
Partial response rate (PR)	60%	77%
Total response rate (RR)	80%	94%
Median response duration (CR)	52+weeks	30+weeks
Median response duration (PR)	16+weeks	18 weeks
Median survival	39 weeks	40 weeks
Median survival in CR patients	100+weeks	36+weeks

Median survival in patients with partial response was 22 weeks and in non-responders 10 weeks.

Toxicities were frequent but were well tolerated. Toxicities consisted of hypomagnesemia (47%), alopecia (44%), hyponatremia (37%), vomiting (25%), transient azotemia (11%), & mild/moderate leucopenia (10%). Moderate/severe mucositis, dermatitis, thrombocytopenia, and severe leucopenia (<2000/mm^3) were rare (5% each).

CONCLUSION

Cisplatin in combination with 120 hour 5-FU infusion can effectively palliate over three-fourths of patients with advanced head and neck cancer. It is disappointing that complete responses are uncommon in this patient population and response durations in partial responders are short. A 24 hour interval between cisplatin and beginning of 5-FU infusion may cause less myelosuppression. The lack of myelosupression in this sequence may permit newer combinations with other drugs to prolong the duration of response and increase complete remission rate, which are the critical determinants of long-term survival.

REFERENCES

1. Sridhar, K.S., Donnelly, E., Rosenfeld, C. Combination antiemetic regimen (BIRD) including diphenhydramine, droperidol, metoclopramide and dexamethasone in cisplatin based chemotherapy regimens. Proc. Amer. Soc. Clin. Onc. 3:100, 1984.

New dimensions in otorhinolaryngology – head and neck surgery, vol. 2.
E. Myers, editor

COMBINATION ANTIEMETIC PROPHYLAXIS IN CISPLATIN CHEMOTHERAPY OF ADVANCED HEAD AND NECK SQUAMOUS CELL CANCER

KASI S. SRIDHAR
Papanicolaou Comprehensive Cancer Center, University of Miami School of Medicine, and V.A. Hospital, Miami, FL, USA

INTRODUCTION

Chemotherapy with cisplatin combinations are widely used in palliating head and neck cancer. Nausea and vomiting have been universal with cisplatin chemotherapy (1). Metoclopramide and other single agent antiemetics eliminated nausea and vomiting in only a minority of patients (1).

MATERIAL AND METHODS

A four-drug antiemetic combination of diphenhydramine (Benadryl), droperidol (Inapsine), Metoclopramide (Reglan), and dexamethasone (Decadron) was used in prophylaxis in 111 courses of high dose (100 mg/m^2) or moderate dose (50 mg/m^2) cisplatin chemotherapy in 40 patients with advanced head and neck cancer.

Antiemetic prophylaxis was initiated one hour prior to the cisplatin therapy. Each drug was infused intravenously in 75 cc D5/W over 15 min. Prophylaxis was given in the following sequence: 10 mg dexamethasone 60 minutes, 50 mg diphenhydramine 45 minutes, 2 mg/kg metoclopramide 30 minutes and 1 mg droperidol 15 minutes prior to beginning cisplatin. Cisplatin was given at the rate of 1 mg/minute I.V. All patients received 2 mg/kg metoclopramide at 1 1/2 hours, 4 1/2 hours and 7 1/2 hours following the beginning of cisplatin. Cisplatin infusion was interrupted if necessary to administer the second dose of metoclopramide.

There were 34 men and 6 women with median age 57 (28 to 76) years. Eighty-eight percent of patients had a Zubrod performance status 0-2. Five had prior vomiting with other antiemetics. Thirty-three patients received cisplatin (100 mg/m^2) + 5-FU (960 mg/m^2/day x 5) and 7 other cisplatin regimens.

The patients received an average of 2.8 courses (range 1-10) of chemotherapy with 30% receiving only 1 course and 25% receiving more than 4 courses.

RESULTS

The majority of patients (31/40, 77.5%) experienced complete protection from symptoms of nausea and vomiting in their first course of treatment, and 60% experienced complete protection in all their courses of treatment (Table 1). The majority of patients who had any symptoms had both nausea and vomiting (14 of 16). Four patients had reportable side-effects (10%), but no patient terminated the study as a result of intolerable side-effects. Neither clinically significant sedation or diarrhea was observed. Tachyphylaxis was not observed.

TABLE 1

RESULTS

	Patients	**Courses**
Number	40	111
% With No Nausea*	60%	76%
% With No Vomiting*	60%	82%

*No correlation with age, sex, performance status, prior chemotherapy and prior vomiting.

Despite the small number of patients, it appears that older patients were more likely to have nausea than younger patients (Mann-Whitney U test: p=0.048). However, there was no significant difference in age between those who vomited and those who did not (p=.277). Although there appeared to be some differences between men and women, these differences were not significant using Fisher's exact test (nausea: p=0.602; vomiting: p=0.154).

CONCLUSION:

The combination of metoclopramide, droperidol, dexamethasone and diphenhydramine is well tolerated and highly effective in preventing nausea and vomiting in moderate ($\geq$ mg/m^2) and high dose ($\geq$ 100 mg/m^2) cisplatin chemotherapy regimens for head and neck cancer.

REFERENCES:

1. Seigel LJ and Longo DL. The control of chemotherapy induced emesis - Review. Ann. Int. Med. 95:352,1981.

New dimensions in otorhinolaryngology – head and neck surgery, vol. 2.
E. Myers, editor

MALIGNANT FIBROUS HISTIOCYTOMA OF THE HEAD AND NECK

DAVID L. WEBB, ROBERT SAWYER, DONALD J. WITTICH
Otolaryngology Service, Brooke Army Medical Center Fort Sam Houston, Texas 78234-6200

Atypical fibroxanthoma is an uncommonon tumor of fibrohistiocytic origin. The term atypical fibroxanthoma has been used by Helwig at the Armed Forces Institute of Pathology, since at least 1956; he subsequently described the disease in 1963 as a benign histiocytic process despite its malignant histology. The malignant counterpart to atypical fibroxanthoma is the malignant fibrous histiocytoma (MFH). When considered as a single entity, only 1% of these tumors are of the malignant variety, however, 23% of these malignancies occur in the head and neck[1].

CASE REPORTS

Case #1

A 65-year old white female presented with a 8 month history of painless mass over the right lower anterior cheek, which was excised in May, 1982. MFH was diagnosed and margins were noted to be positive. Tumor recurred within one month, and on 17 June 1982 the patient underwent a wide local excision of the thin mass with partial mandibulectomy and reconstruction utilizing a platysma myocutaneous rotation flap. There was no adenopathy found and frozen sections revealed margins free of tumor. The patient received 5000r of postoperative radiation. Two year followup reveals no evidence of disease.

Case #2

A 39 year old white female underwent biopsy of a nodule above the left eyebrow late in 1983 which was read as a reactive process with marked atypia. The nodule was excised on 26 Jan 1984 and read as atypical fibroxanthoma. A wide excision was done 2 Feb 1984 which revealed aggressive tumor extension into muscle. The AFIP now felt this tumor to be MFH. Re-excision on 16 Feb 85 down to periosteum revealed no residual. The wound was closed primarily and patient is free of disease at one year.

DISCUSSION

The age of presentation of MFH varies from the neonatal period to the 90's with a mean age of 43 years. There is a male predominance of 3:1. Symptoms depend on site of origin but generally consist of a slow growing mass with average duration of symptoms prior to diagnosis of 83 months. Pain has not been found to be predictive of malignant histology but those tumors arising in deep tissues usually are considered to be malignant. The tumor is locally aggressive with 22% metastasizing, the outlook is poor with 11 of 15 reported surviving only 13 months. Metastases occur equally in nodes, viscera and bone[2].

A variety of histiologic patterns may be seen to include histiocytes, spindle cells, giant cells and inflammatory cells. Mitoses vary greatly in number from as few a 0 to as many as 80 per high powered field. The degree of pleomorphism also varies. The histiocytes vary in size and number and contain nuclei which are round to irregular in shape. The chromation within the nuclei varies from delicate to clumped with prominent eosinophilic nucleoli. Cytoplasm of the histiocytes varies from a finely granular, acidophilic quality to extensively vacuolated cells are known as foam or xanthoma cells.

The fibroblastic cells are elongated with spindle shaped or ovoid shaped nuclei. Both the fibroblasts as well as the histiocytes show a varying degree or pleomorphism and mitotic activity. The presence of fibroblasts, with or without a storiform pattern, when combined with giant cell lesions may be malignant histologically. Light microscopy alone is usually sufficient to establish a diagnosis of malignant histiocytoma, though electromicroscopy may be a helpful adjunct[2,3].

Etiologic factors include solar exposure as well as radiation exposure and trauma; none were present in either of our cases[2,3].

Aggressive wide local excision remains the treatment of choice. Radiation therapy has not been established as effications, though it is still utilized in recurrent, unresectable or extremely aggressive lesion. Chemotherapy has not been a helpful adjunct[2,4].

REFERENCES

1. Brandenburg JH, Frank JW: Malignant fibrous xanthoma of the Lip. Otolaryng Head Neck Surg 88:154-156 1980.
2. Blitzer A, Lawson W, Biller HF: Malignant fibrous histiocytoma of the head and neck. Laryngoscope 87:1479-1499 (1977).
3. Batsakis JG: Histiocytic tumors (benign and malignant). Tumors of the Head and Neck Clinical and Pathological Considerations 2nd ed. 264-265(1979).
4. Ogura JH, Toomey JM, Stezen M, Sobol S: Malignant fibrohistiocytoma of the head and neck. Laryngoscope 90:1429-1440, (1980).

New dimensions in otorhinolaryngology - head and neck surgery, vol. 2.
E. Myers, editor

CLINICOPATHOLOGICAL STUDIES OF MALIGNANT MELANOMA

Toshikazu HIRANO (1), Yasuo HATTORI (2), Goro ASANO (3) and Kurata YUGE (4)
Dept. of Otorhinolaryngology (1,2,4) and 2nd Dept. of Pathology (3), Nippon Medical School, 1-1-5, Sendagi, Bunkyo-ku, Tokyo, 113 Japan

INTRODUCTION

Malignant melanoma is thought to be derived from the dopa positive melanocytes found in skin and also mucosa such as oral and nasal cavities, and maxillary sinuse. This tumor sometimes has a diagnostic problem in the abscence of typical histopathological features, such as amelanotic melanoma. And the assessment of its malignancy and prognosis is also another difficult problem. Although there are some histological classifications, they are not enough to assess the prognosis of malignant melanoma. Therefore, besides morphological characteristics, the authors investigated the immunohistochemical localization of S-100 protein and neuron specific enolase (NSE), which were useful tumor markers for malignant melanoma. The obtained morphological and immunohistochemical results were compared with patients' outcome.

MATERIALS AND METHODS

Materials: 32 primary malignant melanoma (11 mucosal lesions and 21 skin lesions).

Methods: 1. light microscopic observation (HE, Grimelius, Fontana-Masson stains), 2. electron microscopic observation, 3. immunohistochemical observation with ABC method (S-100 protein and NSE), 4. observation in vitro, 5. clinicopathological correlation.

RESULTS

Tumor tissues were classified into three cell types from the pure morphological stand point. These cell types were round, spindle and mixed-cell type.

From the immunohistochemical study, 31 out of 32 cases were positive for S-100 protein and 28 of 32 cases were positive for NSE. These immunoreactivities and melanin pigmentation in three histological cell types were as follows. Immunoreactivities of S-100 protein and degree of melanin pigmentation seemed not to correlate with three cell types. However, S-100 protein reactivities and amount of melanin pigmentation seemed to have inverse relationship. On the other hand, for immunoreactivities of NSE, round-cell types were intensely positive in general, spindle-cell types were weakly positive and mixed-cell types revealed the intermediate reactivities. And this tendency was also recognized only in mucosal lesions.

The relationship between staining intensity for NSE and McGovern's grading in 21 skin lesions seemed to exist a direct proportion. This revealed that histologically deeply invasive cases showed intense reactivity for NSE. The relationship was studied among tumor cell types, staining intensities for S-100 protein and NSE, and melanin pigmentation from selected cases, whose prognoses were known. According to this, it was evident that round-cell type showing strong reactivity for NSE had poorer prognosis. On the contrary, intensity for S-100 protein and melanin pigmentation seemed not to correlate with prognosis.

Electron microscopically, in round-cell type, tumor cell had few mitochondrie and several irregular sized melanosome formation from 150 mu till 800 mu in diameter. However, desmosome or basement membrane like structure were not recognized. In spindle-cell type, tumor cell had several regular sized melanosome formation from 100 mu till 300 mu in diameter. The cytoplasmic edge was very complicated and so it revealed tight attachment among tumor cells. In mixed-cell type, tumor cell had large vacuoles with polymorphic melanosmoes and collagenous fibers were seen in stroma.

In vitro, the cell-line from round-cell type showed more rapid growth than the cell-line from mixed-cell type.

DISCUSSION

In our study, most of cases showed positive staining for S-100 protein immunohistochemically. And staining intensity of S-100 protein showed inverse relationship with the extent of tissue melanin pigmentation. However, the amount of S-100 protein and melanin pigmentation seemed not to correlate with prognosis.

On the other hand, NSE is an enzyme in glycolytic pathway and an increase of immunohistochemical staining for NSE may reveal the metabolic activity of tumor cells. In this study, deeply invasive skin lesions and round-cell type melanoma showed intense reactivity for NSE. Furthermore, electron microscopically, tumor cell showed irregular sized melanosomes and incomplete formation of basement membrane like structure and cellular attachment apparatus in round-cell type, and the cell line from round-cell type showed more rapid growth in vitro.

Therefore, in malignant melanoma, round-cell type showing intense staining for NSE is considered to have poorer prognosis clinicopathologically.

© 1985 Elsevier Science Publishers B.V. (Biomedical Division)
New dimensions in otorhinolaryngology - head and neck surgery, vol. 2.
E. Myers, editor

A HISTOCHEMICAL EVALUATION OF EXPERIMENTALLY REINNERVATED CANINE LARYNGEAL MUSCLES

K.Brøndbo (1), C.Hall (2), H.A.Dahl (3), E.Teig (1) and K.M.Gujord (3).
Dep. of Otolaryngology (1) and Institute of Experimental Surgery (2), Rikshospitalet, and Anatomical Institute (3), University of Oslo, Norway.

Introduction

Several techniques of reinnervation of the posterior cricoarytenoid muscle (PCA) - the sole abductor of the vocal cords - have been tried (1,2,3). Histological and histochemical studies of the reinnervated muscles may be helpful in the evaluation of such experiments. In the present study PCA muscles subjected to different reinnervation procedures have been studied histochemically.

Material and methods

The PCA in 16 dogs were subjected to experimental denervation and reinnervation. The reinnervating nerve was the phrenic (n=5), the ansa cervicalis (n=5) or the recurrent nerve itself (selfreinnervation) (n=6). In all but three of the latter cases the adductor branch of the recurrent nerve was cut and ligated. In addition three animals served as denervation controls. Three to seven months postoperatively the two PCA muscles, experimental and control, were removed for histochemical evaluation. The muscles were mounted, cut and processed together for comparison. Cryostat sections, 10 µ thick, were incubated for actinomyosin ATPase, NADH-TR and α-GPDH. Using a morphometric technique the muscle fiber type composition was calculated in the different muscles. The absorbance values in a sample of muscle fibers in the three incubations were measured photometrically, thus obtaining a semiquantitative measure of oxydative and glycolytic capacity.

Results

Most of the muscle fibers in the denervated muscles were small and quite intensily stained. The reinnervated muscles, regardless of operation procedure, all looked reinnervated by histological and histochemical criteria. The muscle fiber type composition of the experimental and control muscles as revealed by ATPase incubations, is shown in Table 1. It will be seen that the reinnervated muscles contain a third fiber type with intermediate staining characteristics (IIi), which is lacking in the normal muscles. Incubations for the metabolic enzymes NADH-TR and α-GPDH showed reduced staining intensity for both enzymes in all the reinnervated muscles with the possible exception of some of the phrenic nerve reinnervated muscles incubated for α-GPDH.

TABLE 1 MUSCLE FIBER TYPE COMPOSITION IN PER CENT

LEFT SIDE (NORMAL)			RIGHT SIDE (EXPERIMENTAL)		
I	II	EXPERIMENTAL PROCEDURE	I	II	IIi
48	52	Selfreinnervation (n=6)	53	43	4
45	55	Phrenic nerve reinnervation (n=5)	40	57	3
49	51	Ansa cerv.nerve reinnervation (n=5)	39	56	5

Discussion

The histological and histochemical evaluation of the reinnervated PCA muscles showed that successful reinnervation had taken place. This is in accordance with the result of the functional analysis (4). The difference in fiber type composition between the reinnervated and control muscles is rather small and its functional significance is questionable. The reduced percentage of type I muscle fibers in the muscles reinnervated by the phrenic and ansa cervicalis nerve, however, may indicate a faster speed of contraction and reduced endurance. The reduced activity of mitochondrial NADH-TR may support this assumption.

References

1. Tucker HM (1976) Human laryngeal reinnervation. Laryngoscope 86:769-779
2. Rice DH (1982) Laryngeal reinnervation. Laryngoscope 92:1049-1059
3. Crumley RL (1982) Experiments in laryngeal reinnervation. Laryngoscope 92 (suppl):1-27
4. Brøndbo K, Hall C, Teig E & Dahl HA. Experimental reinnervation of the posterior cricoarytenoid muscle in dogs. Under preparation.

New dimensions in otorhinolaryngology - head and neck surgery, vol. 2.
E. Myers, editor

RESTORED ABDUCTION OF PARALYZED VOCAL CORDS FOLLOWING REINNERVATION OF ABDUCTOR MUSCLES BY PHRENIC MOTONEURONES IN THE CAT

F.BALDISSERA (1) G.CANTARELLA (2) G.MARINI (1) F.OTTAVIANI
Istituto di Fisiologia Umana II (1), Clinica Otorinolaringoiatrica (2)
Università di Milano,Italy

INTRODUCTION

Bilateral laryngeal paralysis is the cause of dyspnea and tirage, while phonation is left at a socially acceptable level. Surgical therapies such as arytenoidectomy and arytenoidopexy procure a stable glottic widening but impair phonation. Recent studies (1-2-3) have shown the possibility to re-establish inspiratory abduction of the vocal cord through selective reinnervation of the posterior cricoarytenoid (PCA) muscle. The aim of this work was to analyze how the respiratory function of the paralyzed larynx can be restored following reinnervation of the PCA muscle by phrenic motoneurones.

MATERIALS AND METHODS

In 8 adult cats under Nembutal anesthesia (40 mg/kg) the recurrent laryngeal nerve (RLN) was exposed in the larynx and the adductor branch was cut and ligated. The RLN was transected lower in the neck. In 5 cats the superior branch (C_4-C_5) of the phrenic nerve was anastomosed to the RLN distal stump. In 2 control cats a branch of the cervical plexus was sutured to the RLN in the same way. The occurrence of reinnervation was checked by one or more of the following criteria in the anesthetized animal: i) periodical direct laryngoscopies with a flexible endoscope; ii)electrical stimulation of the regenerated nerve; iii) recording of spontaneous and evoked EMG activity in the PCA muscle; iiii) labeling of the reinnervating motoneurones by Horseradish Peroxidase (HRP).

RESULTS

Animals with phrenic-recurrent anastomosis: In all these animals, a recovery of the respiratory abduction of the paralyzed vocal fold could be ascertained by laryngoscopy within 45-60 days from the phrenic anastomosis. The abduction was clearly detectable at each inspiratory act; it was somewhat delayed and sometimes wider in respect to the abduction of the contralateral fold. After the recovery was established, in each animal the PCA muscles and the RLN were surgically exposed. Electrical stimulation of the regenerated RLN produced a visible contraction of the PCA muscle and a wide abduction of the corresponding vocal cord. The integrated EMG activity of the reinnervated PCA muscle showed

(Fig.1) an inspiratory burst with the "triangular" configuration,peculiar to cat diaphragmatic activity (4), opposed to the "trapezoidal" shape of the laryngeal burst recorded from the contralateral PCA muscle. The phrenic driven EMG started with a 150-200 ms delay compared to the contralateral normal side.

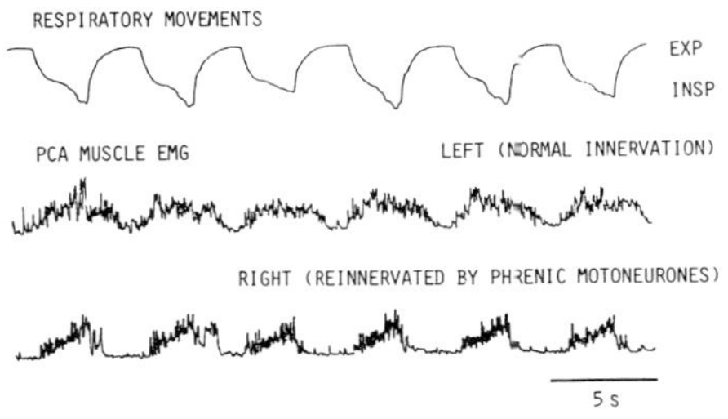

In 2 animals the localization of the reinnervating motoneurones was identified through HRP retrograde transport. About 200 motoneurones were labeled in lower C_4 and upper C_5 spinal segments, where the rostral part of phrenic nucleus is situated in the cat (5).

Control animals: In the 2 control cats the vocal fold paralysis still persisted 4 months postoperatively. However, electrical stimulation of the regenerated RLN elicited the contraction of the PCA muscle and the abduction of the vocal cord. Reinnervating motoneurones were identified through HRP labeling in the segments lower C_3 and upper C_4.

DISCUSSION

These results provide evidence that PCA muscles can be selectively reinnervated by a spinal motor nerve with a high rate of success. When the phrenic nerve is utilized, the abduction of the paralyzed vocal fold can be obtained during every inspiration. Since the unilateral phrenic nerve sacrifice is well tolerated, the use of this nerve for reinnervation of the PCA muscle may be a valuable means for improving the respiratory function in bilateral paralysis of the larynx.

REFERENCES

1. Crumley RL (1982) Laryngoscope 92 (Suppl.30): 1-27
2. Rice DH (1982) Laryngoscope 92:1049-1059
3. Rice DH,Burstein FD (1983) Arch Otolaryngol 109:480-481
4. Feldmann JL, Grillner S (1983) The Physiologist 26: 310-316
5. Duron B,Marlot D,Larnicol N, Jung-Caillol MC, Macron JM (1979) Neurosci Lett 14: 159-163

© 1985 Elsevier Science Publishers B.V. (Biomedical Division)
New dimensions in otorhinolaryngology - head and neck surgery, vol. 2.
E. Myers, editor

FUNCTIONAL RESULTS AFTER EXPERIMENTAL REINNERVATION OF THE POSTERIOR CRICOARYTENOID MUSCLE OF THE LARYNX IN DOGS

ERIK TEIG (1), KJELL BRØNDBO (1), CHRISTIAN HALL (2) AND HANS A DAHL (3)
Department of Otolaryngology (1) and Institute of Experimental Surgery (2), Rikshospitalet, and Anatomical Institute (3), University of Oslo, Norway

In cases of bilateral recurrent nerve paralysis, reinnervation procedures basically fall in 3 categories: 1) Recurrent nerve suture, ("self-reinnervation"), 2) Phrenic nerve anastomosis, 3) Ansa hypoglossi nerve anastomosis (including nerve muscle pedicle). The usefulness of such procedures is dependant both upon successful reinnervation of the posterior cricoarytenoid (PCA) muscle, and upon sifficient activity of the innervating nerve during the inspiratory phase of the respiratory cycle. We wanted to compare the functional results achieved in a series of dogs subjected to recurrent nerve sectioning and various forms of reinnervation.

MATERIAL AND METHODS

The right recurrent nerve was cut in 16 dogs. In 6 dogs the nerve was anastomosed to itself. In 3 of these the adductor branch of the recurrent nerve was cut and ligated. In 5 dogs the nerve was anastomosed to the sternothyroid branch of the ansa cervicalis nerve, and in 5 dogs the nerve was anastomosed to the phrenic nerve. In all these the adductor branch of the recurrent nerve was cut and ligated. After 3-7 months the dogs were anaesthetized with intravenous barbiturates and tracheostomized. The relevant nerves were surgically exposed in the neck, and the laryngeal function was examined through direct laryngoscopy with rigid fiber optics attached to a camera for photographic documentation. A histochemical examination of the PCA muscles is presented in a separate report. The movements of the vocal cords were observed and photographed during quiet inspiration, during forced inspiration, i.e. after the tracheal tube had been obstructed for 30 seconds, and during supramaximal electrical stimulation.

RESULTS

The maximal vocal cord movements are shown in table 1.

TABLE 1 MEAN VOCAL CORD EXCURSIONS IN MM

TYPE OF REINNERVATION		QUIET INSPIR.		FORCED INSPIR.		ELECTR.STIM.	
		Left	Right	Left	Right	Left	Right
Recurrent nerve							
- Adductor br.intact,	n=3	0.6	0.2	4.6	1.4*	6.1	4.9**
- Adductor br.cut,	n=3	0.5	0.3	4.4	2.0	6.0	3.3
Ansa cerv.nerve,	n=5	0.4	0.0	3.9	0.1	6.3	5.4
Phrenic nerve,	n=5	1.2	1.7	3.7	2.7	5.4	4.9

* Medial bowing of the vocal cord ** Adductor branch sectioned

DISCUSSION

The findings of Murakami and Kirchner (1) that the adductor branch of the reinnervated recurrent nerve must be cut to obtain adequate abduction, was confirmed. The lack of visible inspiratory abduction after selective PCA reinnervation with the ansa cervicalis nerve was unexpected and surprising, since the sternothyroid muscle in the dog shows EMG activity during inspiration (2). We must conclude that this activity was not sufficient to cause visible contraction under the present experimental conditions. Crumley (3) and Rice (4) found that the nerve muscle pedicle implantation advocated by Tucker (5) failed to reinnervate the PCA muscle in dogs. The present findings further question the rationale of using this nerve with or without donor muscle attached. An increased vocal cord abduction was seen during quiet inspiration on the left intact side after the right phrenic nerve was cut and anastomosed to the right recurrent nerve. This is thought to be caused by a lack of inhibitory vagal Heering-Breuer reflex impulses due to inadequate expansion of the lung on the experimental side. If this theory is correct, the resulting increase in the nervous drive of the inspiratory muscles further enhances the usefulness of the phrenic nerve as a source for PCA reinnervation.

REFERENCES

1. Murakami Y & Kirchner JA (1971) Vocal cord abduction by regenerated recurrent laryngeal nerve. Arch Otolaryngol 94:64-68
2. Andrew BL (1955) The respiratory displacement of the larynx. A study of the innervation of accessory respiratory muscles. J Physiol 130:474-487
3. Crumley RL (1982) Experiments in laryngeal reinnervation. Laryngoscope (suppl 30) 92:1-27
4. Rice DH, Owens O, Burnstein F, Verity A (1983) The nerve nuscle pedicle. Arch Otolaryng 109:233-234
5. Tucker HM (1976) Human laryngeal reinnervation. Laryngoscope 86:769-779

© 1985 Elsevier Science Publishers B.V. (Biomedical Division)
New dimensions in otorhinolaryngology - head and neck surgery, vol. 2.
E. Myers, editor

INTUBATION DAMAGE AND RECURRENT NERVE PARALYSIS AFTER THYROIDECTOMIES

R. HOFFMANN, V. BARTH, W. SCHAETZLE
Universitaet des Saarlandes, ENT clinic Prof. Dr. W. Schaetzle, Homburg/Saar, West Germany

During the period between January 1984 and April 1985 we examined 214 patients in the phoniatrics section of the E.N.T. University Clinic Homburg/Saar. We had 52 male patients and 162 female patients. The patients were between 18 to 80 years. The preoperative examinations were done 4 days before the operation. On the average, the control examinations were done 4 days after the thyroidectomy. The curriculum of the medical examination was: E.N.T. examination, direct laryngoscopy, zoom-laryngoscopy and stroboscopy. The examinations revealed small endotracheal traumas and nerve damages of the larynx. We found 4 various groups of larynx trauma:

1) 38 patients with soft thickening at the vocal process of the arytenoid
2) 9 patients with intubation granuloma
3) 7 patients with laryngeal edema
4) 7 patients with hematoma of the larynx

The traumatic change disappeared completely within 2-3 weeks with the aid of medicinal therapy and voice restriction. We have treated the patients with antibiotics (e.g. aerosol therapy-locabiosol-fusafungin), with antiphlogistics (e.g. Alph-intern-chymotrypsin) and with mucous membrane therapeutics (e.g. Gelomyrtol-myrtol).

Postoperatively we found 10% nerve damage of the larynx. After 214 thyroidectomies, we saw 19 recurrent laryngeal nerve paralyses (14 in (14 in paramedian position, 3 in intermedian position, 2 bilateral recurrent nerve paralyses).

After a clean closed wound (within 2 weeks) we began therapy with exponential current impulses and with simultaneous voice therapy.

Voice stimulation is of great importance in conjunction with vocal-consonant combinations, e.g. PA or PO. This therapy is only successful if the patient speaks with a middle pitch of voice. The voice exercises should be supported by effective diaphragmatic respiration. This treatment took on the average 5 months (3 times per week).

After this treatment we had the following therapeutical results:

1) 7 recurrent nerve paralysis: Restitutio ad integrum
2) 10 full compensation of the paralyses
3) 2 bilateral paralysis (arytenoidectomy)
4) 3 full compensation of superior laryngeal nerve paralysis with added conservative voice therapy.

CONCLUSIONS

1. early postoperative larynx control is necessary
2. laryngeal intubation damages can be treated successfully
3. teflon injections are not necessary if recurrent nerve paralysis is treated by early electrical stimulation and conservative voice therapy

REFERENCES

1. F. Martin, Th. H. WiH (1983) elektrodiagnostische und histometrische Untersuchungen über den Einfluss von Reizstrom auf die Atrophie der denervierten eılkopfmuskulatur im Tierexperiment, Laryng. Rhinol. Otol. 62, pp 590 - 596.
2. Ritchie, A.E. (1954) Electrical diagnosis of peripheral nerve injury, H.M. Stationery office, London.

New dimensions in otorhinolaryngology – head and neck surgery, vol. 2.
E. Myers, editor

ELECTRODIAGNOSIS OF MOTORIC DISORDERS OF BRAIN NERVES (COMPUTER AIDED EMG AND NMG *

WALTER F.THUMFART
ENT-Department, University of Erlangen - Nuremberg (West-Germany)

INTRODUCTION

Electrodiagnosis of the brain nerves, especially electromyography and neurography are the most reliable tools for diagnosis of brain nerve disorders. The method is well established for investigations of the facial nerve,extensive use of laryngeal electromyography was not established until 1976,with the introduction of transoral zoom-endoscopic electrode application in the awake patient (fig.1). A well trained electromyographer was necessary up to now, to detect the different potentials visually and acousticallly. Analysis has been limited therefore to a few simple parameters of voluntary and spontaneous activity. So there is need for computer based techniques of EMG signal analysis.

MATERIAL AND METHODS

The EMG unit consisted of a Medelec SDS 6. The EMG and NMG signals were recorded with bipolar needle or hooked wire electrodes. NMG was performed using a computer aided method of electrostimulation with trains of 10, 20, and 50 pps. In addition, a delayed last stimulus of the train was used at intervals from 10 ms down to 1 ms. For EMG analysis the signals were sampled at a rate of 10 kHz in 10 segments consisting of 512 sampling points each. The power spectra from all segments were added to give an average spectrum that was displayed using a logarithmic power scale with a range of 40 dB. Four parameters characterizing the spectrum were computed from the average spectrum: Root-Mean-Square, Center Frequency, Zero Crossing Density, and Equivalent Bandwith (LINDSTRØM).

RESULTS

In nonparetic muscles the computer aided EMG-spectrum showed at rest only a small peak in the low frequency region and a very low overall power, expressed by the RMS value, and no contribution from closer fibres, reflected in the low value of the equivalent bandwith. The spectrum recorded during voluntary activity on the other hand resulted in higher RMS and center frequency values, as well as equivalent bandwith. Where the signal exhibited an interference pattern, the zero crossing density was even higher (fig.2).

* Supported by the Deutsche Forschungsgemeinschaft

In cases of denervation the spectrum at rest had a peak in the lower to mid frequency region, indicating that there is electrical activity in the fibres close to the recording electrode. The spectrum recorded under voluntary activity in these denervation cases did not differ very much from the spectrum at rest, particularly the RMS value did not rise very much compared to non-paretic cases.

The NMG investigation in normal subjects showed a decrease of the amplitudes of the muscle action potential after the 5th or 6th stimulus with increase of train frequency, that is 20 or 50 pps. The narrowing of a single stimulus to a stimulus train led to the result, that with the low delay of 6.8 ms the second response was diminished. Below this delay this second response could not be distinguished. This makes evident, that other indices of conduction functions of the nerve fibres may prove to be useful in the diagnosis of axonal conduction disorders.

CONCLUSIONS

The application of computer-aided electromyography with varied stimulation may allow a better classification of the motor fibre involvement in brain nerve neuropathies and can increase the traditional diagnostic potentials. Future development of the methods will allow more and more of the EMG and NMG to be automatically evaluated, and more fruitful clinical diagnosis and physiology will be possible.

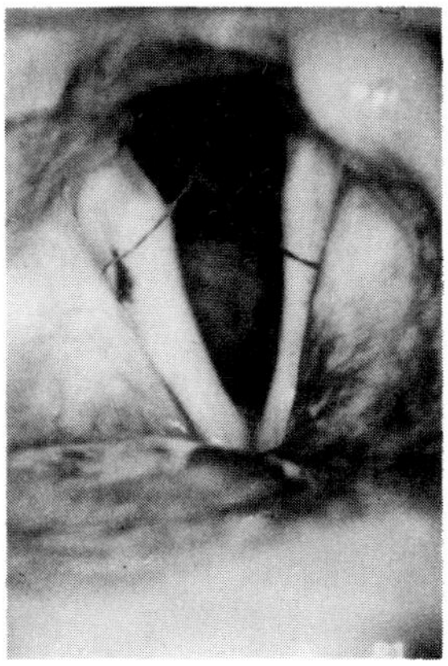

Fig.1 Laryngeal electromyography with 80 μ hooked wire electrodes after zoom-endoscopic application in the awake patient.

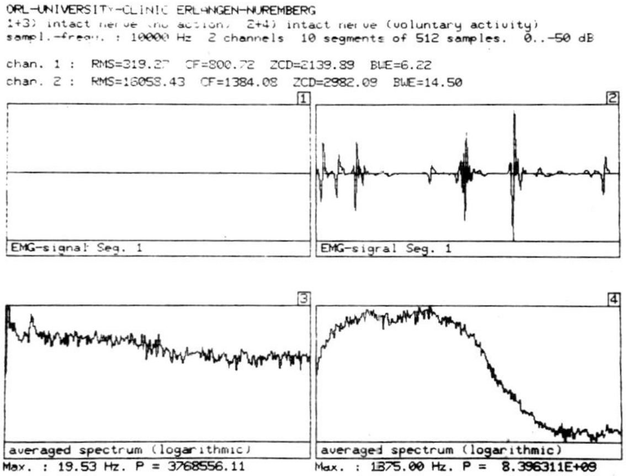

Fig.2 Average power spectrum of intact nerve electromyograms with (trace 2 and 4), and without (trace 1 and 3) voluntary activity.

New dimensions in otorhinolaryngology - head and neck surgery, vol. 2.
E. Myers, editor

NECROTIZING CHONDRITIS OF THE LARYNX IN A DIABETIC PRESENTING AS A SUBGLOTTIC CARCINOMA

ROSS NEVIN CLARK

Department Otolaryngology - Head & Neck Surgery, Humana Hospital Biscayne, North Miami, Florida (USA)

INTRODUCTION

Malignant otitis externa or necrotizing otitis externa is a well established clinical entity. The medical as well as surgical treatment has been well documented. The degree of cartilaginous and/or boney involvement of the infection is directly related to the gravity of the prognosis in these patients.

This paper will present a case of necrotizing chondritis of the larynx caused by pseudomonas aeruginosa in a diabetic female maskerading as a subglottic carcinoma of the larynx. Once the clinical diagnosis was determined, successful surgical and medical treatment were instituted following the basic treatment plan that would be used in malignant otitis externa.

CASE REPORT

A 73 year old diabetic female, well controlled on insulin, presented to the office with a 4 week history of progressive hoarseness without odynophagia. Just preceeding the onset of the hoarseness the patient related a mild upper respiratory infection. Also noted by the patient was a tendency for aspiration of liquids with a mild productive cough. Treatment with 1 gram of Keflex per day for 2 weeks by her internist was unsuccessful in alleviating her symptoms. The patient had no history of alcohol consumption and had not smoked cigarettes for over 30 years.

Physical examination revealed a severly hoarse white female in no respiratory distress. Indirect laryngoscopy revealed a keratotic as well as granular subglottic mass with a polypoid left vocal cord having limited movement. There were no palpable cervical nodes or masses, however, there was mild tenderness over the thyroid cartilage.

The patient was admitted to the hospital for direct laryngoscopy and biopsy. CBC was normal except for a WBC of 11,800. Chest films were normal. Temperature was 99.2 orally. Multiple biopsies revealed only granulation tissue. A CT Scan of the larynx after the initial biopsy showed a large subglottic mass markedly distorting the larynx and narrowing the airway (figures 1A-1D). Marked destruction of the thyroid lamina was also evident on the scan. The patient was placed on IV Mandol 2 grams each 6 hours.

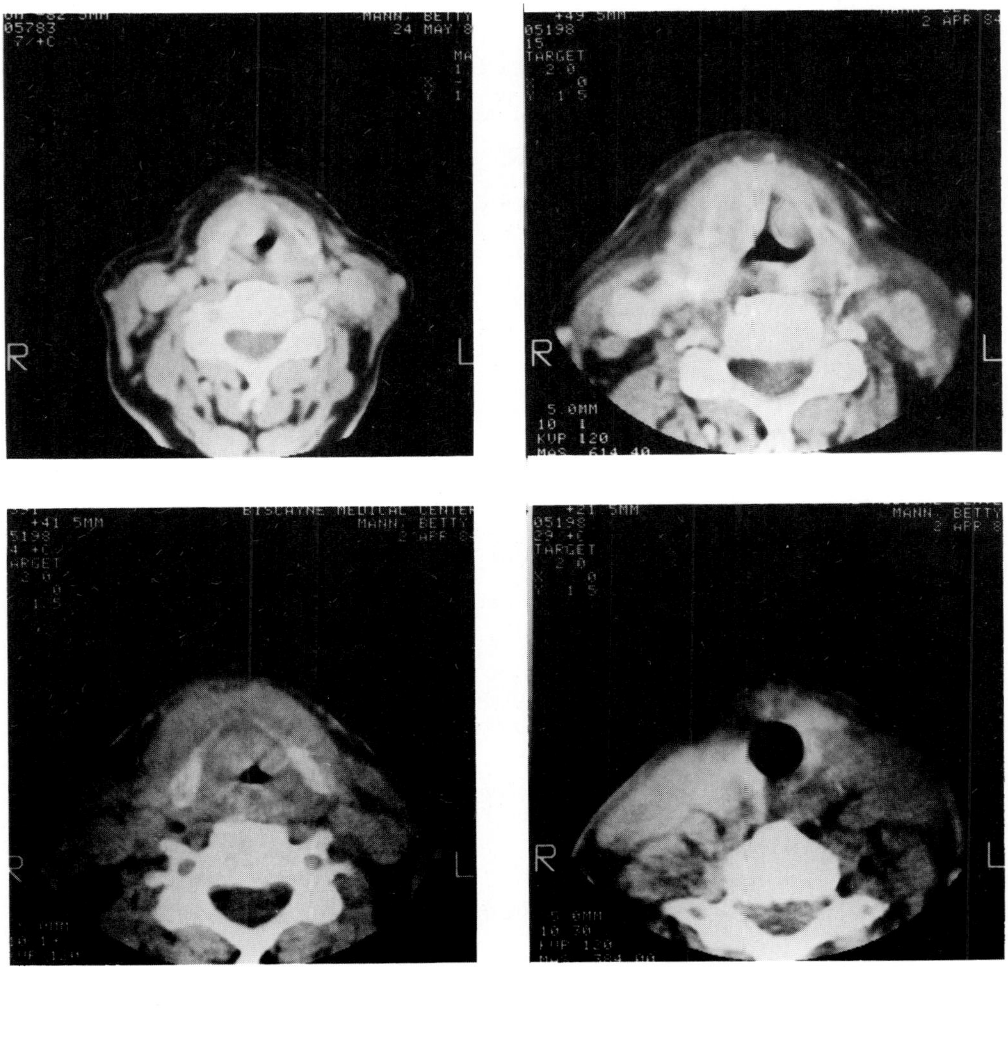

Despite parenteral antibiotics the patient experienced progressive stridor and was again taken to the operating room. A tracheostomy was performed followed by a thyrotomy. The majority of the thyroid cartilage was gone. The larynx was full of granulation tissue and purulent material. The larynx was thoroughly debrided down to relatively normal tissue. This procedure necessitated removing both true and false cords to the arytenoids with the adjacent perichondrium and any remaining cartilage. The cricoid was left intact as well as the majority of the epiglottis. The larynx was reconstructed using the preserved strap muscles to produce an anterior airway. Gram negative bacilli were seen on initial smear of the laryngeal material followed by a positive culture for pseudomonas aeruginosa. The patient was started on IV Tobramycin and Ticarcillin which was maintained for 6 weeks with appropriate monitoring. The patient had an uneventful post-op course and was essentially symptom free for the duration of her antibiotic therapy. She was successfully decannulated 4 months after her surgery and has done well since with no stridor. Her voice is hoarse but strong and intelligible.

SUMMARY

This is the first known documented case of necrotizing chondritis of the larynx although multiple cases of fungal laryngeal infections have been described. The initial diagnosis was delayed due to the clinical appearance of a subglottic carcinoma. The successful management consisted of radical debridement of the larynx with 6 weeks of parenteral Ticarcillin and Tobramycin.

BIBLIOGRAPHY

Chandler, J.R. (1972) Annals of Otology Rhinology and Laryngology, 81,648-58
Pathogenesis and Treatment of Facial Paralysis Due to Malignant External Otitis

Donegan, J.O., Wood, M.D. (1984)
Histoplasmosis of the Larynx, Laryngoscope 94:206-9

Klein, S.M., Flint, A., Moss, J.A. (1983)
Primary Aspergillosis of the Larynx Simulating Carcinoma
Hum. Pathol. 14:184-6

Payne, J., Koopmann, C.F. (1984)
Laryngeal Carcinoma - Or is it Laryngeal Blastomycosis, Laryngoscope 94:608-11

© 1985 Elsevier Science Publishers B.V. (Biomedical Division)
New dimensions in otorhinolaryngology - head and neck surgery, vol. 2.
E. Myers, editor

EARLY AND LATE MANAGEMENT OF GUNSHOT WOUNDS TO THE FACE AND NECK

PAUL J. DONALD, M.D, University of California Davis

Although the management of gunshot wounds was once considered to be mainly the province of the military surgeon, the alarming increase in urban violent crime and the absence of handgun control, coupled with the "wild west" mentality of the public make these injuries not an uncommon occurrence in contemporary America. A system of management of these wounds is incomplete without an understanding of wound ballistics.

The transfer of kinetic energy from the speeding missile, shot from a gun to the target tissue, is the principal determinant of injury severity. Since $KE = \frac{\text{mass X velocity}^2}{2}$, the muzzle velocity of the weapon is the most crucial factor. Guns are roughly divided into low and high velocity types, with the former having a muzzle velocity less than 2,000 ft/sec, and the latter greater than this. In civilian practice, most gunshot wounds are the result of handguns, which are of the low velocity type. As the missile travels through the target tissue, it creates a shock wave forming a "temporary cavity." This produces an area of tissue damage surrounding the path of the bullet that varies in size directly with muzzle velocity. High velocity weapons create large temporary cavities, whereas those of low velocity are usually only slightly larger than the permanent cavity or track left by the bullet. The specific gravity of the target tissue is also an important determinant of injury. Tissues of high specific gravity such as bone are shattered, creating secondary missiles, each with its own specific track of damage. Tissues and organs with a low specific gravity, such as lung, experience far less injury. Other factors related to the character of the bullet are important in wounding. The composition of the bullet will determine whether it will fragment as in the case of a lead bullet, or simply pass through the target as a copper jacketed one will. If the bullet is hollow pointed or, worse still, deeply scored on its tip, the fragmentation is more extensive. The ogive or "pointedness" of the bullet will affect both flight and penetration, as will its tumble, pitch, yaw and spin.

Shotgun injuries are a special consideration. Within 6 meters, a shotgun is a high velocity weapon. Self inflicted shotgun wounds and those delivered by assailants at close range are devastating in extent, blasting facial tissues apart with pellets, often lodging in the brain.

The principles of early management are directed at cleansing the wound and ensuring primary and secondary healing of the defect. The wound is copiously irrigated with sterile saline or Ringer's lactate, preferrably in a pulsatile fashion. All foreign material driven into the wound such as clothing or wadding from the load (in the instance of a shotgun injury) is removed. The concept of "hot lead" sterilizing the wound tract is a myth. All such wounds must be considered as contaminated, mandating the use of tetanun prophylaxis and prophylactic antibiotics, especially if the upper aerodigestive tract is entered.

All devitalized tissue is removed. In a high velocity wound, this means that an extensive area of dead avascular tissue extending around the permanent tract may require debridement. Muscle is particularly susceptable to damage, is purplish in color, and does not bleed. However, debridement in the neck and face is usually far less extensive than that carried on for truncal or extremity wounds caused by the same weapon.

Reconstructive efforts are limited to the best restoration of occlusion possible, repair of facial fractures, and closure of soft tissues. Occlusion is the keystone of the face; and teeth are approximated by eyelet wires or arch bars. Facial fractures are wired together, but bone grafts are avoided except in the case of a blowout fracture of the orbital floor. In the mandible, extensive bone grafting, plating or the use of trays is contraindicated. The position of mandibular fragments is maintained by a Morris biphase apparatus. Definitive primary reconstructive efforts of soft tissue are limited to repairs of the facial nerve, parotid duct, lacrimal apparatus and eyelids. Continuity of mucosa and skin is essential. Bare areas of soft tissue should not be reconstructed with flaps at this time, because of the danger of infection which to varying degrees affects all gunshot wounds. Where missing epithelium and exposed soft tissue or bone exists, a skin to mucosal closure or coverage with a split thickness skin graft is done.

Late reconstruction involves the use of oversized musculocutaneous flaps for missing soft tissue and the judicious use of bone grafts for absent bone. A large flap can always be trimmed once the reconstructive work has finally been completed. An inadequately sized flap may necessitate a complete redo of the entire effort. Onlay and interpositional rib and illiac crest grafts are used for rebuilding the maxilla. Onlays of irradiated cartilage are also used to reconstruct the nasal skeletal framework and as an onlay for the zygoma. Mandibular reconstruction utilizes illiac crest bone and rib grafts. Cancellous bone, taken usually from the posterior illiac crest where it is more plentiful, is packed into tantalum or Dacron trays. Immobilization is achieved with intermaxillary fixation, the Morris biphase appliance, or in some cases even the long term use of a modified Barton bandage.

© 1985 Elsevier Science Publishers B.V (Biomedical Division)
New dimensions in otorhinolaryngology – head and neck surgery, vol. 2.
E. Myers, editor

CARDIAC ARRHYTMIAS IN OTOLARYNGOLOGIC SURGERY

RICARDO EPPRECHT, PATRICIO VIDAL AND MARIA DEL PILAR GONZALEZ

Clínica del Norte, Otorrinolaringología, Antofagasta, Chile.

INTRODUCTION:

Since 1978 we are using routinely cardiac monitoring during surgery. From the beginning we found a high rate of cardiac arrhytmias. This study was designed to evaluate this problem.

MATERIAL AND METHODS:

806 consecutives surgeries were analyzed in a prospective way. They were performed from February 1981 to November 1983. All operations were performed by the same surgeon (R.E.) and the anestesiologist was present in all of them. All arrhytmias were grafically registered and analyzed after with a cardiologist.

RESULTS:

There were 73 cardiac arrhytmias in 806 surgeries. This showed a general incidence of 9,0 % of arrhytmias in otolaryngologic surgery.

Depending from type of anesthesia, the incidence of arrhytmias was:

- 0.5% in local anesthesia
- 18.1% in conventional general anesthesia (including Succinil Choline and normal concentration of Fluothane)
- 8,9% in general anesthesia without Succinil Choline and low concentration of Fluothane.
- 3,5% in neuroleptoanesthesia (50% of arrhytmias appeared during infiltration with Adrenalin solution)

Analyzing incidence of arrhytmias in different types of Surgery. We found this incidence of arrhytmias:

- 30,5% in Laryngotracheal Surgery (Laryngeal Microsurgery and Tracheostomies)
- 15,2% in Tonsil and Adenoid Surgery
- 3,2% in Nasomaxilar Surgery (Septoplasties, Rhynoplasties,etc.)
- 0.4% in Ear Surgery (Tinpanoplasties, Stapedectomies,etc.)

0% in ten Head and Neck procedures (Laringectomies, Radical Neck Dissection, etc.)

51 of 73 Arrhytmias were potentially hazardous:

17 of them were complex in nature (association of 2 or more types of arrhytmia)

16 Ventricular Extrasystoles

13 serious Bradicardia and

5 polifocal Ventricular Extrasystoles

Arrhytmias appeared associated with:

Intubation or Extubation, 23 Arrhytmias

Adenoidectomy in 14

Tonsil Manipulation in 7

Vigorous treatment, including endovenous Lidocain in 22 cases. Additional Atropin in 2 cases.

53 of the 73 cases of Cardiac Arrhytmias were in children from 3 to 12 years old.

CONCLUSIONS:

1. A high incidence of cardiac arrhytmia was found in this series, specially in surgery around the respiratory tract: Laryngeal Microsurgery, Tracheostomies, Adenoidectomies and Tonsillectomies.

2. This incidence was dramatically decreased in replacing Succinil Choline and using a low dose of Fluothane.

New dimensions in otorhinolaryngology - head and neck surgery, vol. 2.
E. Myers, editor

MYCOSIS IN RECURRENT PURULENT TONSILITIS

M. FRADIS,* L. PODOSHIN,* R. GERTNER,* M. GRUSHKA,* I. BOSS** G. WELLISCH*** and Z. CAHANA***

Depts. of Otolaryngology*, Pathology** and Microbiology***, Haifa Medical Center (Rothschild), Faculty of Medicine, Technion, Haifa, Israel

INTRODUCTION

Infections caused by mycotic agents pose a challenging problem for the otolaryngologist. Since some of these organisms can exist as saprophytes in the human mouth and pharynx, their role as an etiologic factor of mycotic diseases is uncertain. To the best of our knowledge, no prospective study which analysed the mycotic tonsillar flora before and after long time penicillin treatment has been performed. In this prospective double-blind study we tried to analyse the mycotic tonsillar flora in patients suffering from acute recurrent purulent tonsillitis (A.R.P.T.) with or without prophylactic treatment by phenoxymethyl penicillin (PH.M.P.), comparing these findings with the corresponding flora of normal subjects.

MATERIAL AND METHODS

Ninety-seven patients, aged 3-31, suffering from A.R.P.T. were investigated during a two year period (1981-1983). The patients were randomly divided into two groups: Group I - 47 patients, treated by PH.M.P. prophylactic doses (750 mg/day for adults, 50 mg/kg a day for children). Group II - 50 patients that did not receive any treatment between the attacks of A.R.P.T. A control group of 24 patients, that underwent tonsillectomy because of the sleep apnea syndrome, were investigated in the same way. All patients were operated.

For bacteriological examination throat and tonsil swabs were cultivated on blood agar. After the tonsillectomy, smears were taken from the surface of the tonsils and after that the tonsils were homogenated and cultured on the same media. For fungal investigation, tonsillar and throat swabs were cultured on Sabourand agar and on selective agar - Sabourand - Cycloheximide Chloramphenicol. For actinomyces, thioglycolate broth was used.

For pathologic investigation the tonsillectomy specimens were fixed in formalin. They were cut serially at 0.5 cm intervals. The sections were stained with hematoxylin and eosin, Gramm, Periodic Acid-Schiff reaction, Gridley and Grocott techniques.

RESULTS

We found 15% fungi in the A.R.P.T. patients compared with 12.5% in the control group. Special attention was given to the actinomyces which is considered as an "opportunistic microbe" [1]. We found 11% actinomyces in the tonsils and 12% in the oral cavity. There was only a slight difference between the bacterial and myocotic flora when we compared the results obtained from the surface of tonsils and the homogenizate.

The following was found regarding the influence of long term prophylactic treatment with phenoxymethyl penicillin on the mycotic flora. There was a slight increase in the mycotic flora of the tonsils and oral cavity but the difference was not statistically significant. In histological examination, actinomyces granules were found in 11.3% of the 194 tonsils. Except for actinomyces, no fungi were found on histological examination.

DISCUSSION

Jokinen in 1976 found 64% fungi [2], Maher in 1982 found 21%, but lower figures have been reported by others [3;4]. In spite of their isolation in culture, neither moulds nor yeasts were demonstrated histologically in our cases. We agree with the opinion of Maher [3] that the fungus colonies in the tonsillar cripts reported by Jokinen [2] are more suggestive of the "ray fungus" of actinomyces granules. In our study, actinomyces were found in 11% in cultures and 11.3% in histological specimens. Those findings are compatible with the figures reported by Gruner [5]. Our findings indicate that patients suffering from A.R.P.T. may develop an increased mycotic flora and suffer later from respiratory allergies as suggested by Bernard in 1962 [6]. This is a point in favor of deciding for a tonsillectomy in an allergic patient, a decision that today is still contraversial. Our findings indicate that prophylactic penicillin treatment by phenoxymethyl penicillin does not increase significantly the mycotic flora of the tonsils and it is safe from this point of view.

REFERENCES

1. Peabody J, Seabury J (1960) J of Medicine 28:99-105
2. Jokinen K, Pajarre S, Palva A, Sipila P (1976) J.L.O. 90:945-952
3. Maher A (1982) J Laryngol Otol 96:229-240
4. Bertholf ME, Stafford MJ (1983) J Family Prod 16:919-924
5. Grüner O (1971) Acta Pathologica Mic Scan Sec A, 79:77-78
6. Bernard J (1962) JAMA 181:255-257

© 1985 Elsevier Science Publishers B.V. (Biomedical Division)
New dimensions in otorhinolaryngology – head and neck surgery, vol. 2.
E. Myers, editor

THE LARYNX IN PULMONARY TUBERCULOSIS

M. H. A. BEG, S. MARFANI
K. V. Site Hospital
Manghopir Road, Karachi,
Pakistan

INTRODUCTION.

Pulmonary Tuberculosis even today remains "Captain of all men of death" on a world wide basis. 80% or more of deaths are in developing nations.

In almost all cases Tuberculous Laryngitis is the direct result of Pulmonary Tuberculosis. The incidence of this disease is low in the West. In Pakistan though most of the chemotherapeutic agents are available, nutritional & preventive factors which combine to bring down the incidence of the disease are lacking How tuberculous Laryngitis has behaved in these local circumstances ? This survey was done to asses the involvement of the Larynx in Pulmonary Tuberculosis under local conditions.

MATERIAL & METHOD.

One Hundred unselected patients suffering from Pulmonary Tuberculosis and admitted in Ojha Institute of Chest diseases were subjected to examination of Larynx under local anaesthetic by an Olympus Nasopharyngoscope.

Results.

Larynx of 20 patients showed swelling & pale oedematous mucosa on arytanoids and interarytenoid region. This includes. 8 patients were in addition to arytenoids, epiglottis & one or both cords were also oedematous. Five patients showed oedematous cord only. Epiglottis was swollen and oedematous in three. One patient showed granuloma of left vocal cord.

False cords were hypertrophied in three. Arytenoid were granular in two patients and whole glottis was involved in three patients.

Discussion.

Tubercular involvement of Larynx is the commonest extra pulmonary manifestation of the disease involving respiratory system.[1] Thirty seven patients out of one hundred had lesion in their larynx. Tubercular involvement in our series are higher than in reported series as nowadays only advanced cases of Pulmonary tuberculosis not responding to treatment at home are admitted in the hospital, in our series 85 of our patients were suffering from advanced chest disease, Examination of larynx was done under local anaesthetic with a fibrescope which allowed detailed examination as compared to a quick look through a mirror and thus increased the number of cases.

The commonest pathologies found were in posterior part of larynx. This is well accepted lesion. This was followed by lesion in epiglottis.

Compared to symptoms lesions were seen in more patients. Thomson & Negus[2] have also noticed signs of Laryngitis in many patients before any symptoms may develop.

Examination of one hundred patients for the series did not reveal any ulcerative lesion in larynx or perichondritis. We further examined 10 patients with hoarseness among the rest of the patients in the hospital trying to locate any ulcerative lesions or perichondritis but no such lesion were found. This appears to be a definite & only change in the clinical pattern of Tubercular Laryngitis we noticed from prechemotherapeutic days.

REFERENCES.

1. SINHA, A (1981) in Textbook of Tuberculosis (RAO, K.M. etall Eds) Vikas Publishing House Pvt Ltd, New Delhi, PP 493-498.

2. Thomson, Sir Stclair and Negus, V.E. (1948) as quoted in Scott Browns Diseases of Ear Nose & Throat (Ballantyne J and Groves J eds) 4th Edition, Vol 4, 404 op, Butterworths, London.

© 1985 Elsevier Science Publishers B V. (Biomedical Division)
New dimensions in otorhinolaryngology - head and neck surgery, vol. 2.
E. Myers, editor

LIFTING OF THE VOCAL CORDS FOR REINKE'S SPACE OEDEMA

Dr. Jean Abitbol Chief of E.N.T. Department, Hopital De Passy, 75016 Paris, France
Dr. Robert J. Feder, Cedars-Sinai Medical Tower, Los Angeles, California, U.S.A.

Techniques for the removal of polyps have varied little since MacKenzie, basically calling for avulsion or stripping of all polypoid tissue from the vocal cords. Within Reinke's space, myxomatous, gelatinous matter is deposited in polyps; vascularity is increased if the pseudomyxoma is old. The more fluid material noted is likewise contained in this space. Conventional techniques involve stripping a single cord at one sitting with a second procedure approximately 5 or 6 months thereafter to avoid denuding approximating surfaces at the anterior commissure, thereby reducing the likelihood of web formation. With such techniques, mucosa is removed almost entirely on the free edge of the vocal fold, the waves take a very long time to come back.

TECHNIQUES OF LIFTING OF THE VOCAL CORDS

Standard microsurgical laryngoscope under suspension for endolaryngeal exposure is used. Reinke's space oedeme size does not appear to be a contraindication to this procedure. CO_2 *laser is employed to bloodlessly incise the superior surface of the vocal cord, just at 1 mm of the edge of the ventricular band. Section with laser stops 2 mm before the anterior and the posterior commissure. We observe after this incision a bubbling of the polypoid content. Power used is 10 watts, time is 1/10 second. A small suction tip is inserted into the incision and material within the Reinke's space gently aspirated. By careful dissection, the vocal ligament is delineated. A small cotton with naphtazoline-xylocain is put on the surgery bed which allows suction of the entire Reinke's space, then we pull out the cotton. Once evacuation is complete, an empty epithelial sac remains. Tension of the redundant epithelium is gently applied. This flap is lifted as like face-lift. The excess epithelium from the sac is trimmed with the laser if necessary. The reconstructed layer of epithelium is noted to completely conver the anterior commissure, the bed of the ventricule. We leave free of any traumatism the free edge of the vocal cords with that technique.*

Discussion

We operated 49 females and 16 males between 39-64. This technique allows bilateral polypoid surgery without fear of web formation, since the region of anterior commissure is not violated. Post operative healing in 65 operations thus far performed reveals epithelializations in 10 to 21 days. Video fiberstrobolaryngoscopy gave us a perfect objective result of the lifting of the vocal cords, pitch is higher and on the phone, ladies are no longer called "sir".

New dimensions in otorhinolaryngology - head and neck surgery, vol. 2.
E. Myers, editor

TREATMENT OPTIONS FOR OBSTRUCTIVE SLEEP APNEA PATIENTS

C.W. GEHRIS, JR., M.D. FACS

The Johns Hopkins University School of Medicine, Department of Otolaryngology-Head and Neck Surgery.

In the past five years, more than two dozen articles concerning surgical management of Obstructive Sleep Apnea have appeared in the Otolaryngology Literature. Following the appearance of Dr. Fugita's original description of the uvulopalatopharyngoplasty (1), a great acceleration of interest in both the obstructive Sleep Apnea Syndrome and its treatment arose.

Mandibular advancement (2), hyoidplasty (3) and tracheostomy modifications have been described (4). However, a clear understanding of other options is essential to providing informed consent for surgery.

The basis for any treatment is diagnosis. No sleep patient can be treated in the best manner without the benefit of polysomnography (PSG). Without the PSG we simply have no idea whether we're dealing with obstructive, central, or mixed apneas, or whether oxygen desaturation or arrhythmias are occurring. The syndrome is properly viewed as a chronic condition with slow progression over a period of years from a state of simple nuisance to potential life-threatening condition. The same treatment is not appropriate to each of these stages.

Based on history, physical, and polysomnographic data, one should form an impression of the stage and degree of severity of the disease. The staging of Simmons, etal (5) is simple and should be adopted by all workers in the field to improve comparability of results. One should also state where the basis of obstruction is likely to be. The Modified Mueller Maneuver can substantially increase the number of satisfactory responders selected for the UPP.

Weight loss, while difficult to achieve and maintain, remains effective and essential to the cure of the condition. Failure to maintain weight control is probably responsible for at least some UPP failures. Weight loss alone, in our series was as effective for some patients as UPP and must not be ignored.

Acetazolamide, Medroxyprogesterone, and Protriptyline are all effective for certain categories of patient. Otolaryngologists must be aware that many patients will be satisfactorily treated by these modalities and may not require surgery. This fact is essential to the provision of informed consent prior to airway surgery.

Continuous positive airway pressure (CPAP) is extremely effective, provided the patient can tolerate mask and apparatus. Most of the tubes, rigid stents, and shocking devices are either intolerable to the patient or ineffective. With regard to the surgical procedures available at this time, it is clear that tracheostomy is curative, and that for properly selected patients, UPP is highly effective. Excellent reviews suggest that, if the exact locus of the obstruction is determined, even morbid obesity is not a contraindication to UPP, whereas, if the obstructive site is not determined, UPP failure will result. The role of nasal obstruction remains to be determined but, the work of Olsen at the Mayo Clinic (6) suggested clearly that nasal obstruction can be highly adjunctive and perhaps even causative of airway collapse during sleep.

Our series of 81 patients demonstrates efficacy of weight loss with drug therapy; of CPAP, and tracheostomy as well as UPP. The 30 UPP patients were unselected with regard to morbid obesity or severity of condition, so that some of these patients were included in the tracheostomy group. It seems clear that nasal surgery is a useful adjunct with UPP.

Three deaths occurred in our series. All three patients had trachs of long standing (or had had trachs previously of long standing) and the deaths seemed unrelated to Obstructive Sleep Apnea. One death immediately post-op UPP is known to me. In this case, autopsy revealed hippocampal infarcts interpreted by the pathologist as compatible with hypoxia.

References:

1. Fugita, S., Conway, W., Zorick, F., et al., "Surgical Correction of Anatomic Abnormalities in Obstructive Sleep Apnea Syndrome: Uvulopalatopharyngoplasty", Otolaryngol Head Neck Surg. 89, 923-934 (1981).

2. Powell N., Guilkminault, C. Riley R., Smith L., "Mandibular Advancement and Obstructive Sleep Apnea Syndrome" Bull. Eur. Physiopathol, Respir. 19, 607-610, 1983

3. Patton, Timothy, M.D., Stanley E. Thanley, M.D., Robert C. Waters, M.D., Peter J. Vandermeer, M.D., and Joseph H. Ogura, M.D. "Expansion Hyoidplasty - A Potential Surgical Procedure Designed for Selected Patients with Obstructive Sleep Apnea Syndrome and Experimental Canine Results". Laryngoscope, Vol. 93, Nov. 1983, pp. 1387-1396.

4. Simmon, F.B., M.D. "Tracheostomy in Obstructive Sleep Apnea Patients", Laryngoscope 80, 1979, pp. 1702-1703.

5. Riley, R., M.D. DDS, C. Guilleminault, M.D., N. Powell, M.D.,DDS and F. Blair Simmons, M.D. "Palatopharyngoplasty failure, Cephalometric, Roentgenograms, and Obstructive Sleep Apnea", Otolaryngology-Head and Neck Surgery, Vol. 93, #2, April 1985, pp. 240-243.

6. Olsen, K., "Sleep Disturbances Secondary to Nasal Obstruction" Audio-Digest, Otorhinolaryngology V. 14, #3, Feb. 12,1981.

New dimensions in otorhinolaryngology - head and neck surgery, vol. 2.
E. Myers, editor

TEMPOROMANDIBULAR JOINT ANKYLOSIS IN CHILDREN

OP GUPTA

Professor of Otolaryngology, Institute of Medical Sciences,
Banaras Hindu University, Varanasi, India

INTRODUCTION

Whilst temporomandibular joint ankylosis is now an uncommon condition in the developed countries, it is still a common problem in developing countries like India. The condition is usually seen in children causing speech disorders (dysglossias), difficulties in mastication resulting in under-nourishment, potential dangers of airway obstruction, problems in the administration of general anesthesia and dental treatment and a progressive facial deformity with its associated psychological and social effects.

MATERIAL

From 1964 to 1984 inclusive, 17 children in the age range of 1-9 years with true temporomandibular ankylosis of different etiologies were treated. All the cases had a progressive intracapsular fixation of the joint with bony and fibrous fusion between joint surfaces. Cases of false ankylosis due to progressive extra-capsular fixation of the joint, pseudo-ankylosis due to pathological process restricting joint movement and trismus have been excluded[1].

ETIOLOGY

Causes of true ankylosis included trauma in 9 cases, mastoiditis 3 cases, osteomyelitis 1 case, hematogenous infection following measles and chicken pox in 2 cases and congenital/idiopathic 2 cases. Trauma is common in children who often fall on their chin with resultant damage to condylar head and degeneration of articular surface and eventual fibrosis and ankylosis[2]. Sometimes it results in intracapsular comminuted fracture with thin condylar cortex comminuting followed by haemarthrosis which becomes filled with osteogenic material[1]. Other causes of trauma are penetrating wounds (1 case) and birth injury following forceps delivery (1 case). The congenital type of ankylosis is caused by prenatal maldevelopment or intrauterine injury. It is often more severe, the condyle, sigmoid notch, coronoid process and zygomatic arch may be synostosed into an indistinguishable solid block of bone[2].

CLINICAL FEATURES

Bilateral involvement, not always symmetrical, was present in 12 cases. Many cases had severe mandibular retrognathia with shortening of both rami, antegonial notching and often an anterior open bite. Amongst unilateral cases lack of growth of the mandible on affected side was seen in 2 cases with gross deviation of chin by normal growth of the mandible on unaffected side.

TREATMENT AND RESULTS

Surgery comprised bilateral one-stage gap arthroplasty through horizontal/endaural incision with resection of adequate bone including condylar remnants, fused bone mass and in some cases, superior aspect of the ramus above lingula and coronoid process under general anesthesia through blind intubation or nasopharyngeal route. Interposition arthroplasty and lengthening of affected ramus by bone graft were not attempted because postoperative infection tends to extrude any substance previously inserted. Instead the wound was kept open for granulations to grow between bone ends followed by secondary suturing. Bilateral surgery as a staged procedure in 2 cases failed. Postoperative physiotherapy and speech therapy produced good results in 14 cases without relapse. Rajgopal et al.[3] also reported similar experience.

CONCLUSION

Adequate gap arthroplasty with early and sustained postoperative physiotherapy using a screw-in type of wooden dilating appliance and speech therapy gives good results, though appearance and occlusion may not be as good.

ACKNOWLEDGEMENTS

This study was partly supported by P.L. 480 Research Projects 01-0762 and 01-0772.

REFERENCES

1. Rowe NL (1982) J Roy Coll Surg Edin 27:67-79 & 167-173
2. Georgiade NG (1977) In: Converse MJ (ed) Reconstructive and Plastic Surgery. W.B. Saunders Co. Philadelphia, pp 1521-1539
3. Rajgopal A, Banerji PK, Batura V, Sural A (1983) J Maxillo-Facial Surg 11:37-41

© 1985 Elsevier Science Publishers B.V. (Biomedical Division)
New dimensions in otorhinolaryngology - head and neck surgery, vol. 2.
E. Myers, editor

LINGUAL TONSILLITIS--A COMMONLY OVERLOOKED DIAGNOSIS

D. WILSON HALES, M. D.
The Ogden Clinic, Ogden, Utah, USA

Lingual tonsillitis is a neglected and often overlooked diagnosis. Despite their location and ease of examination, the lingual tonsils too often are ignored as a source of upper airway and throat symptoms.

Review of 70 patient charts with this diagnosis shows several interesting patterns. Females comprise 80 percent of the patients. Eighty-five percent of the patients had previous tonsillectomy. Age of patients ranged from 14 to 83 years with a fairly uniform distribution in each decade between 20 and 80 years of age. Multiple episodes are reported with the same frequency as adult (palatine) tonsillitis. Symptoms had been present less than one month in 21 percent, two to six months in 43 percent and over six months in 34 percent, suggesting delay in diagnosis in most patients.

Symptoms in the acute case are typical and diagnostic. Complaints in the chronic case range from localized to diffuse, nonspecific symptoms and include such complaints as: sore throat, pain in throat, lump (something) in throat, pain in ears, hoarseness, pain on swallowing, cough, "plugged ears," "can't swallow a pill," "have to clear throat," swollen neck nodes, etc. Findings include large, bumpy lingual tonsils that often fill the valleculae and crowd the epiglottis. The laryngeal mirror is necessary and important. In both the acute and chronic stages crypts, fissures, and pits often filled with exudate can be seen. Cervical lymph node enlargement was found in 25 percent of patients. Palpation should always be done as part of the diagnostic exam. Other instruments can be used to visualize the base of tongue (fiberoptic laryngoscope, optical laryngoscope, etc.) but the mirror is faster, cheaper, available and effective.

Differential diagnosis with an enlarged mass at the base of the tongue includes: malignancies, specific disease (tuberculosis, lues, etc.), lingual thyroid, lingual cyst, thyroglossal duct cyst or abscess, lingual tonsils abscess, etc.

In my experience the acute symptoms respond to antibiotic treatment more slowly than the usual tonsillitis. Treatment for two or three weeks is the usual plan. Chronic lingual tonsillitis may require treatment for four to five weeks. Change in antibiotic or dosage schedule will often help. Lozenges, gargles, etc. can be used to relieve pharyngeal symptoms. Recent investigations into the role of immunologic defense mechanism have been conducted with no definite conclusion yet reached. Serum immunoglobulin levels are elevated with chronic infections and drop with satisfactory surgery.

Surgical removal is indicated for: treatment failures, recurrent acute attacks, enlargement that causes persistent troublesome symptoms, etc. This is best done under general endotracheal anesthesia to facilitate exposure and removal. In some patients traction on the tongue will bring the base of the tongue into view. Most commonly the lingual tonsils can be visualized with a curved tongue blade (as in a self-retaining tonsillectomy mouth gag with an angled tongue blade) and/or a mirror. In others the base of the tongue must be visualized using a direct laryngoscope. In cases where the tissue is exuberant enough, it is possible to remove the tissue by sharp or blunt dissection. The commonly available suction-coagulation (or insulated suction) tip used with the electro-surgical generator can be used to control bleeding or destroy tissue. Other techniques that have been used are: electric snare and punch, cryosurgery and CO_2 laser. Care must be taken to avoid extensive removal of tonsil tissue. This could lead to widespread cicatrix formation and possible stenosis. Surgery was done on nine percent of these 70 patients. In these cases sharp dissection was used, but the electrocoagulation tip was used in all the cases for control of bleeding and destruction of residual tissue. Results of surgery show improvement in symptoms in 83 percent of cases.

The postoperative course is painful because of: referred pain, the relatively slow healing of this area, the adult population, extensive scarring, involvement of the muscles of the base of the tongue, etc. Healing is usually complete in three weeks, but may take four to five weeks. The most common complication reported is bleeding. Antibiotics during the first ten to 14 days will minimize this possibility. I have not seen any complications in this series. Steroids were not found necessary. Change in voice, prolonged dysphagia, stenosis, etc. were not seen.

In summary, vague throat symptoms should be investigated more often and these symptoms can often be explained by lingual tonsil disease. The laryngeal mirror is an easy, effective way of making the diagnosis of lingual tonsillitis. Medical management is usually effective, but slow. Surgery can be difficult, convalescence can be prolonged, but the results are gratifying.

New dimensions in otorhinolaryngology - head and neck surgery, vol. 2.
E. Myers, editor

RHINOPLASTY IN IDENTICAL TWINS. A CASE REPORT

KHALIL AZEM M.D. FACS

Department of Otolaryngology, Damascus University School Medicine, Damascus (Syria)

Aesthetic rhinoplasty remains one of the most challenging and difficult surgical procedures in plastic surgery.

A successful result is a beautiful and natural apearing nose that functions normally and well. in identical twins a third factor is added that is to keep the patients as identical as possible and in another word to duplicate the results of surgery.

Rhinoplasty on identical twins is uncommon, in our search in the currrent texts and available literature we were unable to find any reported. From 1970 to 1984 we have encountered and performed one case of sub-mucous resection rhinoplasty on one identical twins in a total of over 3000 rhinoplasties.

The patients were 22 y/o Syrian females who requested having nasal plastic surgery that alters their nasal appearance while keeping them as identical as possible. although the patients were identical twins, there were few differences in their features as from the photographs. patient "A"(on the right screen) had a slightly larger nose with a mild right deviation of the nasal pyramide causing a degree of asymmetry. Her nasolabial angle measured 85° with a droopy tip and moderate columellar show. Intra-nasal examination revealed left caudal deflection with a large maxillary crest on the left side. As for patient "B"(on the left screen), her nose had a lesser external asymmetry with a straight dorsum inside. Her nasolabial angle measured 90° and her nose had a stronger projection of the tip. There were few noticeable differences in the overall appearance of the patients mostly around the mouth and chin areas. The height,weight and head circumference were identical. The patients requested no external incisions in any case.

Faced with this situation we were forced to plan the procedure in a careful manner. Although we use a cartilage spliting incision as a routine in our daily practice we found that it is inadequate in this case. We felt that a controled technique is needed, one that supplies both the exposure and the symmetrical conservative excision of bone and cartilage, and that changes tip projection and rotation in a measurable way. Our choice was a modification of the LIPSETT technique for tip plasty to be followed by the application of modern techniques of rhinoplasty preserving mucosa and minimizing osteotomies.

Under local anesthesia with I.V. sedation, we operated on the patients on the same day. On patient "A" using a bipedicle delivery of the alar cartilage, resecting one forth of their cephalic margins and cross hatching the remaining intact strip in an interdigitating fashion thus reshaping the contour of cartilage and maintaining its continuity at the same time. Both medial crus were sutured together close to the dome using an absorbable suture thus narrowing the tip and gaining some needed projection by borrowing few millimeters from the lateral crus and adding it to the medial crus. The septum was corrected applying the swinging door technique after elevating mucosa on the concave side only, allowing the septal cartilage to be brought to the midline. The scrolls of the lateral cartilages as well as the osteocartilagenous hump were removed in a sub-mucosal or extra mucosal fashion as discribed in Europe. Slight septal shortening was done with repositioning of the nasal spine. Oblique medial and high to low to high lateral osteotomy were carried allowing infracture with minimal pressure. Closure of the wounds with absorbable sutures with a dorsal transfixion suture over the dorsal margin of the septal cartilage was done as we believe it helps maintain tip support. A plastic splint was used to hold the repositioned septum in place followed by mini packing and tapping. A plaster of Paris splint was applied externally. Patient "B" was operated in the same fashion exactly without doing any septal work. Postoperatively the splints were removed in one week and the patients had an equal amount of swelling. They were satisfied with the results and have been followed up for one year. The post operative results were correlated to the preoperative differences specially septal deviation, tip droop and columellar show in patient "A".

The dilemma of operating on identical twins could face any surgeon at any time. A reliable technique that permits adquate exposure, controled consertative resection and monitored osteotomy is presented for use in that case to obtain close to duplicate results in occasionaly none duplicate nasal anatomy that might be present during surgery. We believe that this technique allows minimal resection with reshaping of the nasal elements to the desired form without sacrificing important structures. The slight differences between the two patients remained visible. We also recommend this technique for use in daily rhinoplasty practice in bulbous tip, tip asymmetry and over and under projecting tips. Its excellent results can not be surpassed.

New dimensions in otorhinolaryngology - head and neck surgery, vol. 2.
E. Myers, editor

THE BLACK NOSE: 1985 AN ANATOMIC AND PROFILE ANALYSIS

HERBERT L. BAKER, M.D.
Department of Otolaryngology, Veterans Administration Medical Center and Oregon Health Sciences University, Portland, Oregon, USA

An anatomic and profile analysis of 200 black American noses was performed at the University of Michigan Outpatient Clinic in 1979 and at Emanuel Hospital Clinic from 1979 through 1985. Cadaver dissections were used to determine external surface measurements and to develop a classification system for the black nose. Results of this survey will be presented and a profile analysis of the different types of black American noses will be described. It is anticipated that this classification system will provide a better understanding of anatomic characteristics of normal variations of Negroid nose, and thus improve the surgeons ability to evaluate the black patient for rhinoplasty[1].

METHODS AND MATERIALS

To determine the nasal bone characteristics between the black American cadavers versus Caucasian cadavers, ten black American cadaver specimens were dissected at Wayne State University. Measurements included the thickness of nasal skin, lower lateral cartilage, nasal bones and upper lateral cartilage. Internal measurements were carried out to compare Negroid and Caucasian skulls obtained from the Department of Anthropology at the University of Michigan. The measurements included nasal bone height, thickness of the nasal bone, upper piriform aperture, nasal spine, and the obtuse angle between the nasal bones and the frontal process of the maxilla.

In a review of the literature, several authors were of the opinion that the majority of black patients seeking a rhinoplasty wanted a Caucasian-like nose[2]. To determine the validity of this impression and answer other questions about the preference of black Americans seeking rhinoplasty, a survey of over 200 employees and outpatients at the University of Michigan, as well as Emanuel Hospital in Portland, Oregon, was conducted from 1979 through 1985. Eight external surface measurements were done on each of these patients.

The results of this study indicate:

1. It was very apparent there were only minor differences between the Caucasian and Negroid skulls measured
2. Thickness of the nasal bone was not significant
3. Variable upper and lower lateral cartilage thickness

4. Piriform aperture width was not statistically significant
5. There was a shorter nasal spine

Results of the survey of 200 employees very clearly illustrated that contrary to the literature, the vast majority of black Americans studied did not want Caucasian-like noses.

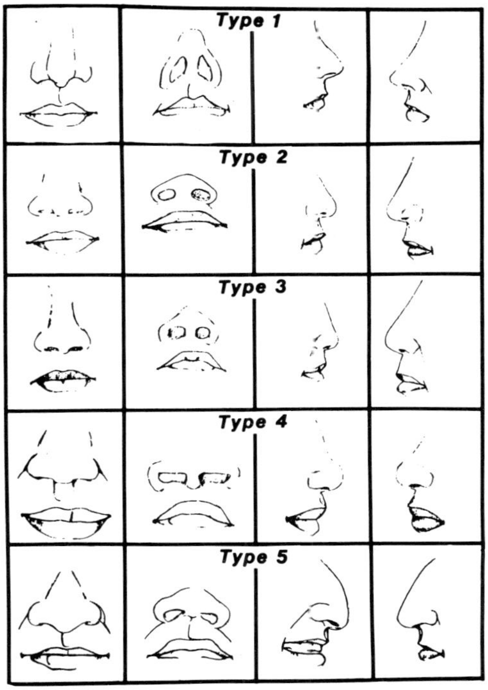

The purpose of this classification system (See Figure 1) is to help the rhinoplastic surgeon more accurately assess the black American nose preoperatively and thus encourage a more conservative approach in modifying specific features of the patient's nose. This ensures a closer resemblance to the more common, normal American Negroid nose as illustrated in this study. In hopes that this profile will help the rhinoplastic surgeon gain a more ethnic idea that will allow him to more accurately assess and evaluate the black American nose.

REFERENCES

1. Baker HL (1983) In: 4th Intl Symp on Facial Plastaic & Recon Surgery of the Head and Neck, pp 85-93, Los Angeles, Calif, USA

2. Schultz AH (1913) Am J Phys Anthrop 1:329

New dimensions in otorhinolaryngology - head and neck surgery, vol. 2.
E. Myers, editor

CLASSIC SEPTORHINOPLASTY WITH MODIFICATIONS

DAVID BERNSTEIN
Clinical Professor of Otolaryngology (Plastic Surgery),New York University Medical Center. Chief, Otolaryngology, Maimonides Medical Center. 1342 51St.,Brooklyn, NY 11219-3526, USA

INTRODUCTION

The development of rhinoplasty from its active beginnings in Otolaryngology-Head and Neck Surgery to the present has been fascinating and constitutes an important phase of a golden era in this field. This presentation is devoted to the effects of various modifications of the classic approach in which we have had the good fortune to be personally involved. Included are the concepts of septorhinoplasty, the supracolumellar transfixion, the homologous nasal hump implant and the effects of the occlusal film and later the axial submental x-ray. Preferential osteotomies, management of the twisted nose and tip reconstruction are closely connected matters which are discussed in relation to the various changes. A comprehensive correlated approach is stressed and personal experience is drawn upon based on involvement in residency training programs and practice for almost half a century.

SEPTORHINOPLASTY

To the otolaryngologist-head and neck surgeon the nasal septum is of special interest particularly from a functional standpoint. At first the submucous resection was performed as a separate procedure, then "as needed". It soon became evident to us that it was almost always necessary not only to correct pre-existing obstruction but also to compensate for the narrowing created by the lateral oseotomies. The concept of the submucous resection and rhinoplasty as a one stage procedure was then developed and named "septorhinoplasty" (1).

SUPRACOLUMELLAR TRANSFIXION

To gain access to the septum the classic transfixion incision was initially employed but this sometimes produced an unpleasant columellar retraction and an additional incision was usually needed to expose the caudal cartilaginous septum. The supracolumellar transfixion was therefore devised to minimize both difficulties. It was

2 mm. cephalad to the caudal septal margin, base down, and directly connected to the intercartilaginous incisions(2). The need for retrograde dissection often required in the high transfixion incision was also obviated.

HOMOLOGOUS NASAL HUMP IMPLANT

The supracolumellar transfixion did not impede access to the bridge required for the homologous hump implant and other implants utilized in nasal augmentation. The homologous nasal hump implant (3) which we employ a great deal is easily preserved, survives well on implantation and has greatly facilitated this type of nasal reconstruction.

AXIAL SUBMENTAL NASAL FILM

Nasal saddling is not infrequently related to trauma whose evaluation, prior to the occlusal film, was often difficult since the lateral and Water's exposures showed fewer than one half of the fractures. The occlusal film required intraoral placement and prolonged exposure since it was not screened. The axial submental approach was therefore devised (4), the screened film being placed under the chin. Better than 95% of the fractures were readily demonstrated and analysis of the various osteotomy angles for correction of the crooked nose was facilitated.

REFERENCES

1. Bernstein, D. (1956) Submucous Resection and Nasal Plastic Operation:Septorhinoplasty. NY State J. Med. 56:1936-39.
2. Bernstein, D. (1984) Supracolumellar Transfixion Incision in Septorhinoplasty. Proceedings 4th Int. Symposium on Plastic and Reconstructive Surgery of the Head and Neck, Vol.1, Chapter 11, C.V. Mosby, St. Louis.
3. Bernstein, D. (1973) Homologous Nasal Hump Implant. Arch. Otolaryngology, 98:385-6.
4. Bernstein, D. (1965) Axial Submental Nasal Film. Arch. Otolaryngology, 82:430-32.

New dimensions in otorhinolaryngology – head and neck surgery, vol. 2.
E. Myers, editor

THE VALUE OF THE SEPTAL CORRECTION IN THE TREATMENT OF TWISTED OR SADDLED NOSES

L. GOMULINSKI
Centre Hospitalier de Longjumeau, FRANCE

INTRODUCTION

In a large number of major deformities of the nose requiring rhinoplasty, be they twisted or saddled noses, the aesthetic abnormality is directly related to a complex deflection of the septum; this shows that there are no deviated noses without deviated septum and that only by reducing the deflected septum will the resulting aesthetic abnormality be corrected. These rhinoplasties will therefore require a long and meticulous period of septal correction and any attempt to avoid this process will inevitably result in failure.

ANALYSIS OF DEFLECTIONS

We will outline several cases:

1) The fracture line is in a perpendicular or oblique position to the incisive crest: there are three possible directions: (fig.1)

- A low fracture line : only the tip of the nose may be slightly twisted,the columella raised, with the upper lip appearing too high; in certain cases, the tip of the nose may be widened. (fig.3)

- A fracture line ending under the upper lateral cartilage : the nose is twisted laterally; there is a characteristic convexus on the upper lateral cartilage; only septoplasty can correct these abnormalities.

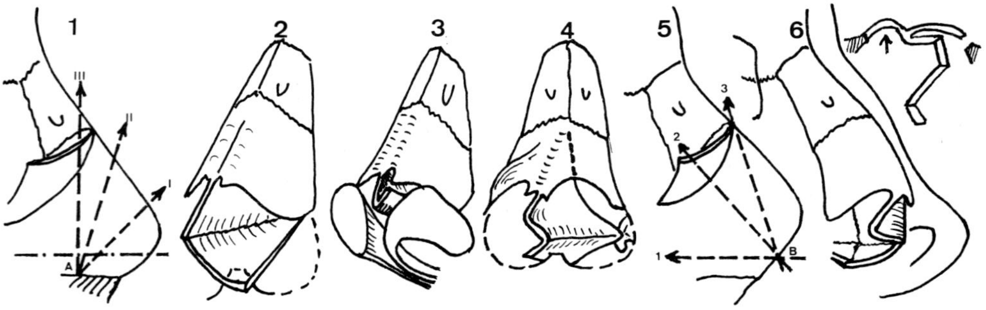

Fig.1.5. Possibles vertical or horizontal fractures lines.
Fig.2. Horizontal fracture.
Fig.3. Folding over of the antero-inferior edge: columella raised; the tip can be widened.
Fig.4. Vertical and horizontal fracture: summit of septal pyramid lowering the threshold of the nares if in anterior position.
Fig.6. Folding over of the antero-superior edge leading to a saddled nose.

- A fracture line ending under the nasal bone : the nose is bent from a high point; apart from septoplasty which is still essential in order to prevent the tip of the nose from being deviated in a lateral direction, it will be necessary to perform an osteotomy.

2) The fracture line is more or less parallel to the incisive crest: (fig.2-5) this sometimes leads to saddling if the angle is very small, but otherwise this deflection does not in itself lead to any aesthetic abnormality. It does, however, provide and added element of difficulty in operating and thus is of major importance, even more so as an osteo-cartilaginous block is formed at this place, precisely under the fracture line, as if the cartilage were impacted into the incisive block; the complete resection of this osteo-cartilaginous block is, as we shall see, one of the essential elements in the correction of all other abnormalities.

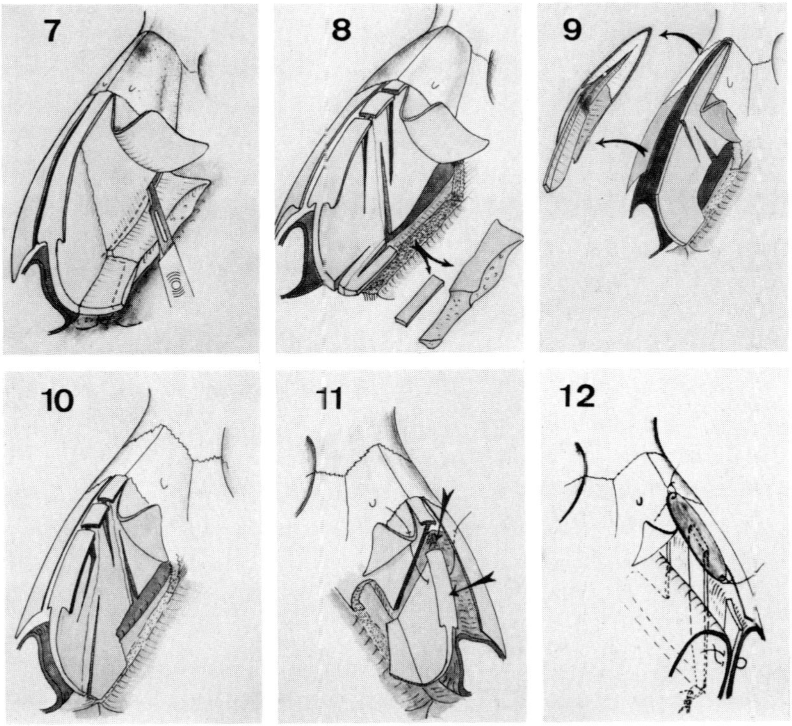

Fig.7. Resection of the osteo-cartilaginous block.
Fig.8.10. Several staggered incisions leading to correction of the saddled defect and straightening of the nose.
Fig.9. The resection of the hump may simplifie the septal correction.
Fig.11. Using the rectilinears fragments as simple graft.
Fig.12. The complete septal separation may lead to the collapse of the anterior septum.

3) Frequently there is both a vertical fracture as well as a horizontal fracture: This results in the formation of a "pyramid" which can sometimes deform or lower the nostril margin. (fig.4)

4) When the fracture line is near the antero-superior edge, it leads to a veritable folding over of this edge, resulting in the formation of a saddled defect with the appearance of a false hump next to it. (fig.6)

TREATMENT

Only by correcting the septal deflection, will its associated aesthetic abnormality disappear. First we perform a complete sub-perichondral elevation of the entire septum. It is then imperative that the osteo-cartilaginous block be resected from the base of the septum (fig.7). We subsequently make staggered incisions thereby creating "bridges" of cartilage which are extremely effective in preventing a collapse of the septum and in keeping it in its anatomical position. Due to these incisions, all desired rotary movements can be made. (fig.8-10).

In most cases, this same type of incisions allows for an antero-inferior or antero-superior overfold to be straightened out, thus correcting the saddle.

In certain cases, when there is a real osteo-cartilaginous hump, the septal correction may be simplified by resecting the hump. (fig.9)

There is one exception: in certain cases of serious shattering, the fractures are so close together that any attempt to rebuild the septum leads to instability. We therefore perform a simple graft, using the most rectilinears fragments, so that a vertical fragment directly supports another graft which is used to rebuild the dorsum. (fig.12)

In cases in which the nasal bone is no longer present, we are forced to use a "T" shaped graft in which the vertical section is osteo-synthesed to the nasal spine.

Apart from these exceptions, we prefer the staggered incision method which allows all movements while keeping the cartilage in right position.

The final support for the now highly wraken cartilage is provided by a layer of X-Ray film attached to both sides of the septum by transfixional stitches.

CONCLUSION

This meticulous treatment of septal deflections yields satisfactory and lasting aesthetic results, as no recurrence of these deflections has been observed in over five years. Furthermore, it is the only method which ensures the total restoration of the nasal airway.

© 1985 Elsevier Science Publishers B.V. (Biomedical Division)
New dimensions in otorhinolaryngology - head and neck surgery, vol. 2.
E. Myers, editor

EXTERNAL RHINOPLASTY FOR THE TWISTED NOSES

HASSAN MOUSTAFA & WALAE H. ABOUSHELEB
ENT DEP. OF TANTA FACULTY OF MEDICINE TANTA EGYPT.
P.O.Box 181 Orman Cairo Egypt

The nose is considered twisted when there is external assymetry of the dorsal nasal components to one or the other side of a mid vertical line passing through the mid nasion and the mid nasal filtrum points. Most of cases were due to neglected management of a side to side nasal trauma. Developmental deviation may be due to birth injury or forgotten mild trauma during childhood (Lawson 78) (1). The combined nasoseptal deviation causes clinical symptoms as alternating nasal obstruction, postnasal discharge and/or paranasal sinus infections or vacuum headaches.

Goodman 1974 (2) & 1982 (3) described the external Rhinoplasty approache. Write & Kridel 1981 (4) extended the indications and needs for the operation and mentioned its advantages in certain cases.

MATERIAL AND METHODS

Twenty case were operated upon during the years 1982-1984.

12 cases gave frank history of direct trauma. Eight cases were considered developmental or due to forgotten trauma during childhood.

15 cases had a C shaped deformity and 5 cases had an S shaped one. All cases had a variable degree of septal deviation to the opposite side of the deformity.

The cases were operated upon under general aneasthesia with a local infilteration of adrenaline 1/200000.

A mid collumellar inverted V incision joined on both sides by two marginal incisions along the lateral margin of the medial crura and the inferior margin of the lateral crura of the LLC. Elevation of the skin started at these incisions and carried upwards till complete exposure of the nasal skeleton. Proper inspection of the nasal bones and ULC enabled the surgeon to diagnose the exact site of the deformity which was almost always a fracture of the nasal bones extending to the deformed ULC. The latter was found in most of the cases fractured and included in adhesions and fibrosis. Cleaning of the subcutaneous tissues and

Perichondrium was completed. The septal cartilage was dissected between the ULC & LLC and delt with to correct any deformity present. The ULC and LLC are replaced by sutures. Hump removal and tip remodeling was done at this stage if needed. The bony replacement was done by the medial and lateral osteotomies as usual.

DISCUSSION

The direct inspection of this approach facilitated the dissection, freeing the cartilages of any adhesions and the replacement of sutures. The ULC is the one most commonly affected, and the one most difficult to inspect and replace in the closed technique. Keeping the cartilages in place by fine catgut sututes is essential for proper correction specially if bony or cartilagenous grafting is needed for augmentation. The inverted V shaped incision practically disappears after few months.

The advantages of External Rhinoplasty can be summerized as follows:-

1- Direct vision ensures the proper diagnosis and dynamics.
2- Proper dissection of both soft and bony tissues.
3- Subcutaneous tissue removal and thinning of the skin.
4- Control of bleeding ensures less edema and smooth postoperative.
5- Fixation of structures with sutures keeps the skeleton in place specially if grafting for augmentation is needed.
6- Correction of the ULC and nasal septum is effecient.
7- No intranasal incisions are used which may affect the nasal functions and may cause stenosis and adhesions.
8- The difficult cases as perforated nasal septum and the severly damaged crooked noses became comparatively easier operations.
9- It gives a better way for teaching and learning.

REFERENCES

1. Lawson V.G. J.Otolaryngology 1978 Feb Vol 7 P 56-66
2. Goodman W.S. Laryngoscope 1974 December Vol 84 (12)P 2195
3. Goodman W.S. Laryngoscope 1982 Feb Vol 92 (2) P 121-4
4. Wright W.K. & Kridel R.W. Laryngoscope 1981 June Vol 91 (6) P 945.

© 1985 Elsevier Science Publishers B.V. (Biomedical Division)
New dimensions in otorhinolaryngology - head and neck surgery, vol. 2.
E. Myers, editor

DECORTICATION (EXTERNAL) RHINOPLASTY

IVO F. PADOVAN and SLOBODAN B. JUGO
Depts. of Otolaryngology, University of Zagreb, YUGOSLAVIA, and
Muhlenberg Community Hospital, Greenville, Kentucky, USA

INTRODUCTION

the concept of performing rhinoseptoplasties under direct visual control after temporary elevation of the nasal skin is called decortication or external rhinoplasty. It was originated by Sercer from Zagreb (Yugoslavia) (1), and fully developed by his succesor Padovan in 1966 (2). The history of decortication rhinoplasty includes also Rethi from Budapest who was first to describe trans-columellar incision for correction of tip deformities (3), and Goodman from Toronto who popularized technique in North America (4). Initially the decortication rhinoplasty was used only for correction of severely deformed noses, congenital anomalies and revisions but gradually over the years the indications were extended to practically include all candidates for nasal reconstruction. In this article the authors wish to present the latest improvements in the technique of decortication rhinoplasty.

SURGICAL TECHNIQUE

A circumferential incision along the caudal border of the lower lateral cartilage is made on both sides and connected with a V-shaped transcolumellar incision. By careful sharp dissection the skin is elevated over the lower lateral cartilages. The skeletonization is extended up to the nasofrontal angle, and laterally as far as it is neccessary to obtain good exposure.The first step in performing rhinoplasty is to develop a periosteoperichondral flap. Incision is made on the right side of the frontal process of the maxilla a few mm laterally to the junction with the nasal bone just caudal from the synostosis of the maxilla and the frontal bone. The incision is extended caudally, gently curving over the upper lateral cartilage ending at the tip of the septum. The periosteo-perichondral flap is elevated using Cottle's knife over the midline to the corresponding line on the other side. The nasal septum is approached in between lower lateral cartilages and neccessary corrections are made in usual manner. The tip work is performed sub-perichondrally. The perichondrium of the lateral crus of the lower lateral cartilage is incised approximatelly 3 mm cranially to the planned line of resection and the perichondrium is elevated caudally. After resection of the cartilage, the perichondrium is replaced covering the cut edge of the cartilage. This prevents sharp marks on the skin of the nasal tip. Kyphectomy and paramedian osteotomies are performed next in usual manner under direct visual control. A small web of the bone in the nasal root in between the nasal bone and the nasal septum is removed with a fine straight chisel to provide room for the nasal bones to be moved medially. The lateral osteotomies are performed through separate vestibular incisions. The entire nose is evaluated by replacing the nasal skin and finishing touches are made as neccessary. The periosteoperichondral flap is replaced in its original position and sutured with 4-o dexon. The lower lateral cartilages are sutured in a desirable position and the skin incisions are meticulously sutured with 5-o nylon.

DISCUSSION

The most important advantage of the decortication approach is that periosteum and perichondrium of the nasal dorsum can be raised as a continous flap and preserved till the end of the reconstruction when it is used a cover for the new nasal dorsum. Secondly, the tip work can be performed in a precise and predictable manner. The septal work is facilitated especially if total reconstruction is needed. Kyphectomy and median osteotomies can be done under direct visual control. The main disadvantages of decortication rhinoplasty are prolonged operative time and more extensive surgical trauma to the nose. The columellar scar is virtually invisible and is very well accepted by the patients. Based on personal experiences on over 2ooo patients the authors conclude that decortication rhinoplasty is a valuable alternative to the endonasal techniques.

REFERENCES

1. Sercer A. (1957) Rev. Laryngol. Otol. Rhinol. 3-4: 161-168
2. Padovan I. (1966) Symp. Orl. Iug. 3-4: 354-36o
3. Rethi A.C. (1934) Rev. Chir. Plast. 2: 85-1o6.
4. Goodman W.S. (1973) Can. J. Otolaryngol. 2: 2o7-21o.

© 1985 Elsevier Science Publishers B V. (Biomedical Division)
New dimensions in otorhinolaryngology - head and neck surgery, vol. 2.
E. Myers, editor

SKULL BASE AND NECK APPROACH TO LARGE GLOMUS TUMOR SURGERY

DIAMANTE V., BARBON L., HAEDO G., MONTES S. AND ORFILA D.

Otorhinolaryngology Service of the Spanish Hospital, 2975 Belgrano Ave. 1209 Buenos Aires, Argentina.

INTRODUCTION

The authors believe that the only radical treatment for large glomus tumors is surgery. Here they describe a one-stage surgical technique and postoperative follow-up in a series of 15 patients.

Classification

To classify glomus tumors, the following scheme was adopted: 1-Tympanic, divided in A- Pure tympanic; B- Tympano-mastoid. 2 - Jugular, divided in A- Jugulo- tympanic; B- Jugulo-tympano-mastoid; C- Jugulo-infrapetrosal. B and C may or may not invade the endocranium.

MATERIAL AND METHODS

In our series of 15 patients, 5 male and 10 female, tumors were broken down as below: Jugulo-tympano-mastoid 4 cases; jugulo-infrapetrosal without endocranial invasion 9 cases; and with endocranial invasion 2 cases.

Surgical Technique

To start with, a retroauricular incision is made and extended towards the neck. The facial nerve is identified from the stylomastoid foramen. An approach is then made to the neurovascular area of the neck to ligate the external carotid above the lingual artery and the internal jugular vein. Radical antromastoidectomy with liberation of the third portion of the facial nerve is made. The tympanic bone is removed fully, exposing the sigmoid sinus.

The tumor's posterior pole is then approached and a satisfactory cleavage plane us usually found between the medial wall spared by the tumor and the involved lateral wall. The superior pole is freed from the otic capsule with extreme care to avoid a fistula.

The VII-th. nerve is cautiously detached from the neoplasia and its sheath escinded in case of tumor invasion. The anterior pole must be freed, seeking a cleavage plane between the adventitia of the carotid artery and the tumor.

To approach the inferior pole, the internal jugular vein must be severed in the neck, raising it to the skull base, in order to detach the tumor's medial surface. Having reached this point, the surgeon is then able to remove the sigmoid sinus, jugular bulb and vein, together with the neoplasia. The lower petrosal sinus is tamped down.

Following meatoplasty or external canal obliterative suture, the surgical site is then closed stepwise.

RESULTS

Barring a single death at 8 days postsurgery due to septicemia, our patients made satisfactory recovery. All preserved facial nerve function,except two with facial palsy prior to tumor removal. Four had postoperative paresia of the jugular foramen nerve, but three of them recovered normal deglutition. There were two cases of intradural invasion, less than 2 cm in diameter, which were resolved during the same procedure. No meningitis was observed. One patient had a CSF leak which remitted after medical treatment.

There has been no recurrence to date.

CONCLUSIONS

Radiotherapy application should be restricted to inoperable tumors. We indicate it after surgery in cases of tumors highly attached to the carotid artery or in case of uncertainty regarding total removal.

This procedure is indicated for all tumors involving the jugular bulb, no matter their extension or direction of growth.

REFERENCES

1. Fisch, U.: Infratemporal fossa approach for extensive tumors of the temporal bone and base of the skull. J. Laryngol. Otol. 92,949-967, 1978.
2. Fisch, U.: Infratemporal fossa approach for glomus tumors or the temporal bone. Ann. Otol. Rhinol. Layngol. 91: 474-479, 1982.
3. Gardner, G., et al.: Combined approach surgery for removal of glomus jugulare tumors. Laryngoscope, 87: 665-688, 1977.
4. Malcom D. Graham, Guest Editor. Sku base surgery, Otolaryn. Clinics of North America. August 1984.
5. Farrior. Infratemporal approach to skull base for glomus tumors. Otorrinolaringology 93: 1984.
6. Diamante V.; Barbon L.; Sachetti R.: Sistematización de los tiempos quirúrgicos de los tumores glómicos. Sociedad Argentina de O.R.L. 14-7-1976.
7. Herman; Jenkins; Fisch: Glomus tumor of the temporal regions. Archives of Otolaryngology, 107:209-214. 1981.
8. Glasscock, Harris: Glomus tumors: Diagnosis and treatment. The Laryngoscop, 84-11: 2007-2032. 1974.
9. Brammer, R.: Glomus tumors of the temporal bone: contemporary evaluation and therapy. Otolaryngology Chnics of North America. Number 5. 1984
10. Cantrell, R. et al: Catecholamine. Secreating infratemporal fossa paraganglioma. Ann Otolrhinolaryngol. 93: 1984.
11. Diamante,V.; Barbón, L.; Montes, S.; Haedo, G y Orfila, D.: Abordaje convinado de base de cráneo y cuello para la cirugía de los grandes tumores glómicos. Revista de la Fundación Otorrinolaringológica, N° 3, Pag. 51-61. 1982. Argentina.

© 1985 Elsevier Science Publishers B.V. (Biomedical Division)
New dimensions in otorhinolaryngology - head and neck surgery, vol. 2.
E. Myers, editor

MIDDLE EAR ADENOMA

JOHN S. LEWIS M.D. and MONTE KEEN M.D.

Considerable interest is present in the pathology and natural history of glandular tumors of the middle ear. Tumors reported in the middle ear have been labeled as adenomatous neoplasms, adenomas, ceruminomas, ceruminous adenomas, adenocarcinomas and carcinoid tumors. Glandular tumors arising in the middle ear generally run a benign clinical course, have cytologic uniformity and have been designated as middle ear adenomas. (1) These must be differentiated histologically from paragangliomas (glomus tumors), ceruminoma, adenocarcinoma, plasmacytoma or neuroendocrine tumors to avoid radical surgical treatment.

Fifty-one cases of middle ear adenoma have been reported in the English language literature. (2,3,4,5,6,7) Middle ear adenomas occur over a wide age range affecting teenagers and the lederly alike. The median age is in the fourth decade. There is no sexual bias. Symptoms are generally non specific and have often been present for several years. The tumors are interpreted clinically as glomus tumors, otitis media or cholesteatoma. Tomograms occasionally delineate a middle ear mass. Operative findings reflect a hypo-vascular or avascular lesion without boney invasion. Treatment is simple surgical excision, either transcanal or via post-auricular incision with mastoidectomy only if it enhances surgical exposure. The facial nerve is spared. Ossicles may have to be sacrificed for surgical removal. Radiotherapy in two cases had no therapeutic effect. Local recurrence occured in five out of forty-eight cases and only in those where tumor had been left behind. The overall recurrence rate of those completely resected was four percent.

Histologically middle ear adenomas demonstrate a variable adenomatous pattern. The neoplasm is granular in appearance, with the lumen staining positive for mucin and the granular cytoplasm often staining positive for neurosecretory granules. All middle ear adenomas stain positive for lysozyne which is considered to be a tumor marked for this disease. (2)

Case Report: A 23 year old asymptomatic whie male who sought employment with the F.A.A. and on physical examination was found to have a grayish-white mass protruding through the superior half of the tympanic membrane. Both audiogram and tympanogram were normal. Excisional biopsy was initially diagnosed as carcinoid tumor of the middle ear, but slide review both at the A.F.I.P. and Memorial Hospital called the tumor "middle ear adenoma". A CAT scan of the temporal bones showed a middle ear mass without bone destruction or mastoid invasion. An exploratory transcanal approach gave an excellant exposure with tumor filling the middle ear, involving incus and malleolar articulation. The tumor was removed piecemeal with sacrifice of incus, a portion of malleus and drumhead, and a fascia tympanoplasty carried out. Healing was without event, but patient has a marked mixed type of deafness.

In the previous 51 cases reported, the age varied from 14 to 80 years with a median age of 37 years. There was an even sex distribution. The most common symptoms were conductive hearing loss 64%, tinnitus 29%, fullness or blockage in the ear 18%, pain 14%, facial weakness 14%, One fourth of cases were completely asymptomatic and tumor visualized on routine otoscopy. Vertigo 11%, and chronic otitis media 7% were uncommon. CT scan of the temporal bones failed to demonstrate bone erosion in 95% of cases. More frequently cloudy or sclerotic mastoid cells with otitis media were diagnosed. Angiography was performed in 10% of cases without positive findings.

At surgery the tumor was found to be lobulated with involvement of the eustachian tube orifice, attic, and frequently encases the ossicular chain or portions thereof. None of the surgeons suspected a middle ear adenoma. The surgical procedures performed were (1) Transcanal or postauricular transtympanic excision 45% of cases, (2) Tympanomastoidectomy, 50%, (3) Temproal bone resection 5%. Mills and Fechner (2) reported a mean follow up of 4 years on 48 patients and stated that no patient died of unresected tumor. 80% were cured by the primary surgical procedure. 20% required a secondary procedure for recurrent disease. One patient required 3 surgical procedures. All cases resected were found to be free of tumor up to 4 years.

CONCLUSION

The middle ear adenomas is a rare distinctive tumor that behaves in a benign fashion. The origin is more likely from the epithelial lining cells or middle ear space and is often confused with more malignant tumors that are more common in this area and are treated erroneously by radical surgery. The purpose of this review is to present a typical case of middle ear adenoma and to abstract the recent reviews that document the benign noninvasive nature of this tumor. The importance of this case report is to alert the head and neck surgeon to the unusual diagnostic entity and to recommend simple local excision with close follow up as the primary modality of treatment or therapy.

REFERENCES

1. Batsakis, Tumors of the Head and Neck, 2nd Edition, Williams & Wilkins, pp 378-79, 428-429, 1981.

2. Mills & Fechner, "Middle Ear Adenoma," American Journal of Surgical Pathology, Vol. 8 #9, Sept. 1984.

3. Hyams & Michael, "Benign Adenomatous Neoplasms, (adenoma of the middle ear)", Clinical Otolarynology 1976 I pgs. 17-26.

4. Murphy et al, "Carcinoid Tumor of the Middle Ear." American Journal Clinical Pathology 73, Pg. 816-823, 1980.

5. Wetli, "Tumors of Ceruminous Gland," Cancer 29, Pg. 1169-1178, 1972

6. Jackson & Glascock, "Primary Adenoma of the Middle Ear," American Journal Otology 2, Pg. 105-107, 1980.

7. Jahsdoerfer, Fechner, "Adenomas of the Middle Ear," Laryngoscope, 93 pgs. 1041-1044, 1983.

© 1985 Elsevier Science Publishers B.V. (Biomedical Division)
New dimensions in otorhinolaryngology - head and neck surgery, vol. 2.
E. Myers, editor

TOTAL TEMPORAL BONE RESECTION FOR OSTEOGENIC SARCOMA: A PRELIMINARY REPORT

ROBERT T. SATALOFF, DONALD L. MYERS, B.R. ROBERTS, STEVEN TELIAN

Osteogenic sarcoma is a rare neoplasm that carries the worst prognosis of all temporal bone malignancies. For this reason, total, en bloc resection of the temporal bone as described by Graham, Sataloff, Kemink, et al[1] was used for the first time in an attempt to cure the disease.

T.H. is a thirty-seven year old female who developed a painful external auditory canal polyp. Biopsy revealed osteogenic sarcoma. CT Scan confirmed malignant destruction of the temporal bone. Metastatic work-up revealed no evidence of the lesion outside the primary site.

The patient underwent total temporal bone resection in May, 1984. Her postoperative course was complicated by cerebrospinal fluid rhinorrhea which required secondary surgery, meningitis which responded to medical therapy, and stroke which resulted in left arm weakness. While it is too early to report on the efficacy of her surgery, at the time of the preparation of this manuscript, (eleven months post-operatively) she is still free of disease, doing well and able to perform all her normal functions of daily living.

PROCEDURE

Total temporal bone resection is performed routinely in two stages. The first stage involves placement of a Silverstone or Kindt clamp (or similar occlusive device) around the carotid artery for gradual occlusion of the carotid artery over three to seven days, with the patient awake and alert.

The second stage is the definitive procedure. It is performed within one week of carotid occlusion and involves total en bloc resection of the temporal bone, internal carotid artery and cranial nerves VI through XII. The operation proceeds as follows:

1. Adequate padding to protect against *decubitus* ulceration, complete monitoring, drains, phlebitis protection, eye protection, large preparation.
2. Steroids and antibiotics are given prior to surgery.
3. A tracheotomy is performed and anesthesia is administered through it.
4. The patient's head is shaved and placed in Mayfield Tongs.
5. The incision is designed carefully to optimize blood *supply* to the flaps, allow adequate excision of the lesion, and facilitate primary closure.
6. With the carotid artery already having been occluded in the neck by the Silverstone clamp, we recommend occlusion of the distal end of the carotid artery early in the operation, intracranially between the cavernous sinus and the origin of the Ophthalmic artery, contrary to our original report.
7. The facial flap is elevated, and is carried forward in the fashion of a facelift flap. The facial nerve is transected peripherally and tagged for nerve grafting. The rest of the parotid gland and the main trunk of the facial

nerve are transected and taken with the bloc.

8. The internal carotid artery, and cranial nerves IX, X and XI, as well as the jugular vein, are elevated and resected with the bloc, along with the ascending ramus of the mandible and the condyle. The deep neck musculature is incised and the skull base is exposed just lateral to C-1, deep to the mastoid tip. The pterygoid muscles are divided and left attached to the skull base. The mandibular division of the trigeminal nerve is identified and preserved. It is followed *to* the foramen rotundum which is partially preserved.
9. A craniotomy is performed, raising a large bone flap that provides good suboccipital anterior middle fossa exposure. The temporal lobe is elevated and an incision is made in tentorium just medial to the superior petrosal sinus.
10. The transverse sinus is ligated.
11. The superior petrosal sinus is occluded with bi-polar cautery.
12. The brainstem is retracted and the inferior petrosal sinus, jugular bulb and foramen magnum are visualized. The placement of the inferior incision between the jugular bulb and the foramen magnum is visually confirmed and the area is assessed for tumor extent. Extreme care must be taken to avoid excessive retractor tension.
13. The anterior lateral bone cut is made through the superior petrosal sinus, carotid canal just proximal to the cavernous sinus, and through the skull base and lateral skull wall. This connects the anterior petrous apex with the neck and frees the anterior middle fossa floor. The medial extent of this cut stops approximately five millimeters above Dorello's canal.
14. The lateral posterior bone cut is completed using a drill, or chisel. It stops posteromedial to the mastoid tip, about one centimeter posterior to the jugular foramen.
15. The final bone cuts are made with a curved chisel. They start posteriorly and curve from the posterior lateral bone cut medial to the jugular foramen and a few millimeters lateral to the rim of the foramen magnum.
16. The facial nerve may be grafted to the brainstem.
17. If possible, the wound is closed primarily using a scalp flap.
18. Postoperative care is as important to the survival of these patients as is good surgery.

REFERENCE

1. Graham, M.D., Sataloff, R.T., Kemink, J.L., Wolf, G.T., McGillicuddy, J.E.: Total En Bloc Resection of the Temporal Bone and Carotid Artery for Malignant Tumors of the Ear and Temporal Bone. Laryngoscope, Vol. 94, No.4, 528-533, April 1984.

New dimensions in otorhinolaryngology - head and neck surgery, vol. 2.
E. Myers, editor

CANCER OF THE MIDDLE EAR

ESTEBAN SCOLA and BARTOLOME SCOLA
Servicio O.R.L. Hospital Provincial.Madrid

Cancer of the middle ear is a very rare condition, and is generally diagnosed late in the course of the disease.

The author´s personal experience with the management of 22 patients with primary carcinoma of ear form the basis of this paper.

EPIDEMIOLOGY AND ETIOLOGY.-

The proportion of cancer of the middle ear to all pathologic conditions is 1/5.000 to 1/20.000.

The cancer of the middle ear represents 7% of all cancers of the ear treated in our Service.

The median age was 58 years, and the span being 42 to 84 years.

Cancer of the middle ear has aproximatelly the same sex incidence, and in our cases, 13 were males and 9 females.

30% of our patients had an chronic otitis media for many years, but there is no hard data to support the theory that the chronic drainaje es the etiologic factor.

PATHOLOGY.-

-Squamous cell carcinoma............ 16 cases
-Basal cell carcinoma............... 3 "
-Adenocarcinoma..................... 3 "

The 3 basal cell carcinoma were present as a rodent ulcer on the retroauricular area with erosion into the mastoid process.

PATIENT EVALUATION.-

The patient usually presents with a chronic otitis media, with a bloody discharge and pain, that are one of the erlier signs. Vertigo and facial paralysis may occur (9 of our cases) and the symptoms usually indicate advanced cancer. Occasionally cancer of the middle ear may invade the parotid glande (4 cases) and the nasopharynx by the Eustachian tube (2 cases). 17% of our patients had cervical metastasis in the upper jugular nodes by the moment of the first examination.

On physical examination, the middle ear and auditory canal may be filled with a friable bleeding mass, and the biopsy of the mass must be carried out in order to establish the diagnosis.

One of our patients, the middle ear tumor wass associated with cholesteatoma, and at the time of surgery the middle ear and mastoid was found to be filled with friable bleeding tumor tissue and the patologic confirmation of cancer was returned after the surgery.

Routine mastoid x-rays are helpful, since approximately 40% of cases demonstrate bone destruction. Polytomography is a much more valuable technique in detecting bone destruction and the extent of the disease in the auditory canal and middle ear. If signs and symptoms suggest extension beyond the ear, CT scans is of inestimable value.

TREATMENT.RESULTS.-

There is no rules in the treatment of carcinoma of the middle ear. In the table we can see the procedures in our patients.

TABLE I.-TREATMENTS.-

-RADICAL MASTOIDECTOMY................................	5	cases
-RADICAL MASTOIDECTOMY+NECK DISSECTION+Co60........	2	"
-RADICAL MASTOIDECTOMY+Co60..........................	5	"
-SUBTOTAL RESECTION OF THE TEMPORAL BONE...........	1	"
-Co60...	5	"
-PALLIATIVE TREATMENT...............................	4	"

In our patients the 5 year cure rate is 28%, all of them treated by surgery or surgery plus radiotherapy.

The radical mastoidectomy amplified to the extension of the lesions is the treatment we made as the routine. The quality fo the exeresis does not satisfied the roules of the surgical oncology, so the complementary radiation therapy is absolutely necesary.

We have used the radiation therapy only as palliation for unresectable or recurrent lesions or as an adjunt to surgery.

The subtotal resection of the temporal bone we have carried out only once, with good result, but according to all published reports, this aggresive surgical resection does not increase the cure rate.

New dimensions in otorhinolaryngology - head and neck surgery, vol. 2.
E. Myers, editor

NECROTIZING OTITIS EXTERNA OCCURRING CONCURRENTLY WITH EPIDERMOID CARCINOMA

Mattucci, Kenneth F., M.D., Setzen, Michael, M.D., Galantich, Peter, M.D., Susin, Myron, M.D.

INTRODUCTION

Malignant external otitis (necrotizing otitis externa) is a disease entity first described in 1959 by Meltzer and Keleman[1] and later by Chandler[2] in 1968. It is characterized as primarily affecting middle aged and elderly diabetics. It most commonly involves the floor of the external auditory canal and frequently there are granulations at the junction of the bony and cartilaginous portion of the canal. The infection may progress to chondritis, osteitis, osteomyelitis and death[3,4]. The majority of cases are caused by Pseudomonas aeruginosa although other organisms can be involved. The diagnosis of necrotizing otitis externa is confirmed by the clinical history, the classical physical findings, isolation of appropriate microorganisms, and by microscopic tissue findings.

Squamous cell carcinoma is the most common malignancy affecting the external auditory canal. The appearance of such lesions may range from a simple polyp to ulceration. Symptoms may include purulent or bloody otorrhea, pain, hearing loss or cranial nerve palsy.

The signs and symptoms of necrotizing otitis externa and squamous cell carcinoma of the external auditory canal may appear the same. Chandler[5] mentions briefly that one case in his series of "malignant" external otitis died of a squamous cell carcinoma believed to be of external auditory canal origin. "Infections" resistant to conventional, aggressive medical therapy and masses of granulation tissue or ulcers of the external canal must be biopsied to either confirm the inflammatory process and/or to rule out the possibility of an underlying neoplastic process.

CASE PRESENTATION

A 55 year old diabetic female presented with right ear pain and purulent otorrhea of 3 weeks duration. Examination of the right external auditory canal revealed marked edema and hyperemia and granulation tissue on the floor of the canal at the junction of the cartilagenous and bony portion. Cultures revealed pseudomonas and proteus. Audiometric testing demonstrated a mixed hearing loss. The patient was admitted to the hospital for debridement, biopsy and institution of intravenous therapy (Moxalactam). Mastoid x-rays depicted clouding of the mastoid air cells AD. Facial nerve paralysis suddenly developed. Biopsy of the granulation tissue initially revealed chronic inflammation and necrotic tissue in areas of focal vasculitis. The patient's pain persisted and a second biopsy of this granulation tissue revealed a poorly differentiated squamous cell carcinoma.

A CT Scan revealed extensive destruction of the bony external canal and base of skull. Due to the clinical and radiographic extent of disease, the patient was treated with 5000 Rads of Radiation therapy of 8 weeks and received several courses of Bleomycin and methotrexate. Her medical state contirued to deteriorate and the patient expired from a massive myocardial infarction six months following the onset of her symptoms.

DISCUSSION

The similarity of symptoms of necrotizing otitis externa and squamous cell carcinoma of the external auditory canal can lead to confusion in the treatment of this disease. Clinically, this patient revealed the classical findings of necrotizing otitis externa established by Chandler in 1968[2]. The endaritis, common in diabetics and the vasculitis caused by the Pseudomonas organism leads to a progressive coagulation necrosis of tissue and spread along the base of the skull, leading to osteitis and osteomyelitis, occassionally progressive cranial nerve palsies, and may result in death.

Progressive pain and progression of disease in the face of appropriate medical treatment requires further inspection, examination under anesthesia with a debridement and incision and drainage of pockets of infection with repeat cultures and sensitivities and repeat microscopic tissue examinations. The differentiation of these two entities can only be made by microscopic tissue examination.

In view of this documented case of a true malignant process in the face of an infection, is it now not time to abandon the term "malignant otitis externa"? To avoid confusion in the communication of this disease process, which pathophysiologically is an inflammatory condition and not a neoplastic disorder, we agree with the more descriptive term necrotizing otitis externa.

CONCLUSION

A case of epidermoid carcinoma of the external ear canal occurring with necrotizing otitis externa is documented. Only biopsy and microscopic tissue examination can differentiate the two. The term "malignant external otitis" must be abandoned in favor of the more descriptive and less confusing term "necrotizing otitis externa".

BIBLIOGRAPHY

1. Meltzer PE, Kelemen: Pyocyanous Osteomyelitis Of Temporal Bone, Mandible and Zygoma Laryngoscope 69:1300-1316 1959.
2. Chandler, JR: Malignant External Otitis, Laryngoscopy 78:1257-1294 1968.
3. Paparella MM, Shumrick DA: Otolaryngology Vol. II, The Ear, W.B. Sanders Co., Phila., 2nd Edition 1980.
4. Jesse RH, et al: Cancer Of The Head and Neck, McCoomb & Fletcher; Williams & Wilkins Co. 1967 p412.
5. Chandler JR: Pathogenesis & Treatment of Facial Paralysis Due to Malignant External Otitis, Annals Otol. Rhino, Laryngoscopy 81:648-658 1972.

© 1985 Elsevier Science Publishers B.V. (Biomedical Division)
New dimensions in otorhinolaryngology - head and neck surgery, vol. 2.
E. Myers, editor

MALIGNANT NASOETHMOIDAL TERATOMA

RICARDO EPPRECHT*, GUSTAVO VALDES[x1], ANTONIO SOLA[x2] AND MARIA DEL PILAR GONZALEZ*

* Clínica del Norte, Otorrinolaringología, Antofagasta, Chile

x1 Departamento de Anatomía Patológica, Hospital Regional de Antofagasta, Chile

x2 Departamento de Radioterapia, Hospital Regional de Antofagasta, Chile

INTRODUCTION

This is a case report of a Malignant Nasoethmoidal Teratoma. There are 24 previous cases reported in the English Literature. Only 6 of them were cured.

CASE REPORT

J.G.C., a caucasian female 62 years old, was seen for the first time August 22, 1980, giving a history of 1 month with hemopurulent nasal discharge and right nasal obstruction. Right nasal cavity was occupied with a large tumor. Radiologic study revealed total cloudiness of right paranasal cavities. Biopsy showed a well differentiated carcinoma. September 16, 1980, a lateral rhinotomy approach was performed and a large tumor was removed. The tumor destroyed the anterior sphenoidal wall, external walls of nasal cavity and ethmoid cells and right nasal bones. This osseus bones were included in the resected specimen.

October 4, 1980, the pathologist informed a malignant nasoethmoidal teratoma: variegated embrionaric types of tissue were recognized in this tumor. Rabromioblastic differentiation and neurofibrillar tendency. High cellularity with mitosis and sarcomatoid aspect. Islands of epithelial tissue, with small hiperchromatic nucleii, with neuroepithelial aspect. Also, well differentiated epithelium with irregular cysts, with squamous, transitional and respiratory epithelium, with queratin focci and some regions with active proliferation.

5.000 Rads were given after surgery. Radiotherapy was stopped because of radioepithelitis and oral mucositis.

Last control April 1985 showed no evidence of disease.

© 1985 Elsevier Science Publishers B.V. (Biomedical Division)
New dimensions in otorhinolaryngology - head and neck surgery, vol. 2.
E. Myers, editor

CONSERVATION SURGERY FOR INVASIVE ETHMOID TUMORS

CHARLES N. FORD, M.D., ROGER C. MIXTER, M.D., RICHARD K. DORTZBACH, M.D.,
MANUCHER J. JAVID, M.D., LANNING W. HOUSTON, M.D.

Appropriate surgical management of invasive ethmoid neoplasms requires careful preoperative assessment of tumor location and appreciation of the proclivity of these lesions to spread to adjacent areas. The proximity of the anterior cranial fossa renders intracranial spread as likely to occur as invasion of the more surgically accessible nose, maxilla, and orbit. Adequate exposure may require a combined craniofacial approach to provide exposure for en bloc removal and repair. The extent of tumor involvement should determine the margins of resection rather than adherence to standard techniques of maxillectomy and orbital exenteration.

MATERIALS AND METHODS

Four cases are presented demonstrating our methods of evaluation, operative techniques of en bloc resection and repair. All patients had ethmoid invasive tumors. The pathology included an adenocarcinoma, mucoepidermoid carcinoma, malignant hemangiopericytoma, and osteogenic sarcoma arising in a field previously irradiated for retinoblastoma.

TECHNIQUES AND DISCUSSION

Accurate preoperative evaluation is the key to determining our surgical approach. Plain radiographs, tomography, ultrasonography, and vascular studies may be helpful in some instances, but we found computerized axial tomography (CAT) scan and magnetic resonance imaging (MRI) studies to be most valuable. The MRI technique clearly distinguishes tumor mass from other densities. In one patient, a large hemangiopericytoma of the medial orbit invaded the ethmoid labyrinth causing a secondary mucocele. Radiographic studies including a CAT scan revealed a mass of uniform density but the resonance characteristics of the contiguous lesions allowed differentiation. In several patients with ethmoid cancer, we observed densities in adjacent maxillary, frontal and sphenoid sinuses which could have been interpreted as extension of the primary tumor requiring more extensive surgery. MRI studies delineate the extent of the primary tumor as distinguished from other soft tissue and fluid densities.

Based on the preoperative evaluation, it is often possible to encompass an ethmoid lesion without total maxillectomy or orbital exenteration. The critical area of extension is intracranially into the anterior cranial fossa; it is not logical to extend the inferior margin of resection to include uninvolved dental and palatal structures while cutting tumor cells at the superior margin and achieving piece-meal extirpation. The entire orbit need not be exenterated to secure a margin where tumor encroaches on the periorbita. Subconjunctival dissection permits careful assessment of involvement of the periorbital structures and it is possible to achieve en bloc resections while preserving a visually-intact globe. Depending upon the extent of involvement, the preserved eye with good vision may be nonfunctional due to ptosis, enophthalmos, or ophthalmoplegia; but even in these instances, this eye is an important reserve in the event that the contralateral eye should fail.

Adequate exposure is essential to surgically define the limits of the tumor, afford en bloc resection, and for effective repair of the resultant defect. An extended mid-saggital incision, splitting the lip and extending along the alar facial groove to the scalp where it can continue as a hemicoronal incision, has proven versatile in this group of patients. Wide frontal craniotomy is aided by removal of a superior orbital rim-glabella bone window which affords excellent visualization of the floor of the anterior cranial fossa. This bone flap can be removed if involved with tumor or repositioned and wired in place following extirpation of the lesion. Midline exposure for the cribriform invading lesion that extends across the nasal cavity is facilitated by performing bilateral lateral osteotomies and cutting the nasal septum to allow lateral reflection of the external nose.

It is essential to be aggressive about en bloc resection of these lesions as they invade the anterior cranial fossa. This entails a craniofacial approach with adequate resection of skull base, dura, and frontal lobe where necessary. The challenge of repair of the resultant defect entails achieving a cerebrospinal fluid-tight seal and separation of the extradural space from the contaminated nose, nasopharynx, paranasal sinuses, and oral cavity. In this series, we have employed a combination of pericranial, temporalis, galeal, and frontalis muscle flaps to achieve closure.

SUMMARY

Ethmoid invading tumors present a difficult management problem for the combined efforts of the head and neck surgeon, plastic surgeon, neurosurgeon, and ophthalmic plastic surgeon. Careful preoperative assessment with CAT scans and MRI studies permit proper operative planning. Complete tumor removal is the primary surgical goal. En bloc resection should be achieved by adequate craniofacial exposure when the tumor invades the anterior skull base, but uninvolved structures should not be sacrificed unnecessarily.

© 1985 Elsevier Science Publishers B.V. (Biomedical Division)
New dimensions in otorhinolaryngology - head and neck surgery, vol. 2.
E. Myers, editor

BALLOON OCCLUDED ARTERIAL INFUSION WITH DIRECT HEMOPERFUSION FOR HEAD AND NECK CANCER

YASUHIRO HAYASHI
Depertment of Otorhinolaryngology, Wakayama Medical College, Wakayama, Japan

INTRODUCTION

In order to minimize side effects of the anticancer agents and enable local administration at large doses, we have developed a new method by combining balloon occluded arterial infusion with direct hemoperfusion by the use of activated charcoal for the treatment of the malignant tumors at the head and neck. In this method, the feeding artery to a cancerous organ is occluded with a balloon catheter and anticancer agents are injected on the peripheral side of the occluded part. Therefore, the concentration of anticancer agents in a local tumor area is high. Immediately after the local area is perfused, discharged anticancer agents are absorbed by an activated charcoal column for the purpose of relieving side effects.

MATERIAL AND METHODS

From 1981 to 1984, this method have been performed on 20 patients with malignant tumors of maxilla (13 cases) and tongue (7 cases). There were 13 males and 7 females, aged between 46 and 81 years. The anticancer agents we used in principle are 5Fluorouracil, Mitomycin C, Peplomycin, or Mitomycin C only. In a small number of patients, Adriamycin was combined.

RESULTS

The tumor reducing rate was calculated and the effectiveness was assessed. Out of 20 patients, 3 were assessed as marked responders and 11, responders. 3 patients were classified as no change and in 3 patients, assessment was impossible. The obtained response rate was 82.4%. As for the drug concentrations in the tissue, the levels of anticancer agents were significantly high. After the direct hemoperfusion was performed, the drug concentrations in the vein rapidly decreased. Furthermore, in spite of the anticancer agents at large doses, severe side effects such as bone marrow inhibition were rarely observed.

The therapeutic results are favorable as shown by a response rate of 82.4%. As far as the prognosis is concerned, we have not experienced enough observation time and the prognosis should be followed-up from now on. At present, we can say, at least that the current method can reduce a tumor size and subsequently, the operative area will be reduced. We consider that the present method has a possibility of being further advanced and applied to an extensive scope.

CONCLUSIONS

(1) The balloon occluded arterial infusion with direct hemoperfusion was performed on the patients with malignant tumors at the head and neck.

(2) The present method enabled anticancer agents to move into the cancerous organs at a high concentration.

(3) The direct hemoperfusion with activated charcoal well absorbed the discharged anticancer agents to the whole body.

(4) The therapeutic results in 20 patients are as follows: marked response in 3, response in 11, no change in 3, and unassessable in 3. The obtained response rate, 82.4%, was satisfactory.

(5) In spite of the anticancer agents at large doses, systemic side effects due to the present method were hardly observed.

New dimensions in otorhinolaryngology – head and neck surgery, vol. 2.
E. Myers, editor

MALIGNANT MELANOMA OF THE NASAL CAVITY TREATED BY CRYOSURGERY WITH LIQUID NITROGEN

B.OLARIU,D.OLARIU,V.CIUCHI,D.RADUCANU,V.ALBASTROIU
Dept.of Otolaryngology,Hospital of Tg.Jiu - and D.LAKY
"V.Babeş"Institute - Bucharest(Romania)

The malignant melanoma(MM),the worst of all neoplasms,is a rarity in the strictly otolaryngology field,especially in its mucous primitive location.

We present a case of achromatic primitive MM of the nasal cavity at a 69 years old woman,who was hospitalized in the Dept.of Otolaryngology,in November 1981.It was an unpigmented tumor,inserted in the left superior 1/3 of the septum,developed in the nasal fossa and vestibule,without clinical signs of node or visceral affectation and manifested through 2 major symptoms:progressive unilateral left nasal obstruction and repeated epistaxis.Clinically suspected of a carcinoma,it was excised by the cryosurgical technique with liquid N;the histopathological diagnosis being:Slightly differentiated carcinoma.

The patient is again hospitalized in September 1984,because of the reappearance,a month before,of the 2 previous symptoms, after about 3 years without any sign of disease.This time,a tumor is discovered,a bit larger than the first one,with the same site and characters,but having a very discreet bluish hue, from place to place,which suggests the possibility of a MM. Absence of clinical metastases.Excision is performed by the same cryosurgical technique,followed after 2' by a new cryoapplication on the insertion area and a security zone around and 3 more cryoapplications,postoperatively,at intervals of 3 weeks.Histopathological examination,using besides the common colors(H.E.,Van Gieson)a special color for melanine(also applied at the lamellae from the primitive tumor)shows granulations of melanic pigment in some tumoral zones,establishing the diagnosis:Achromatic endonasal MM,both of the primary tumor and of the recurrence.

REASONS for presenting this case are the following:
1.Rarity of endonasa site of MM.In the world literature,MM

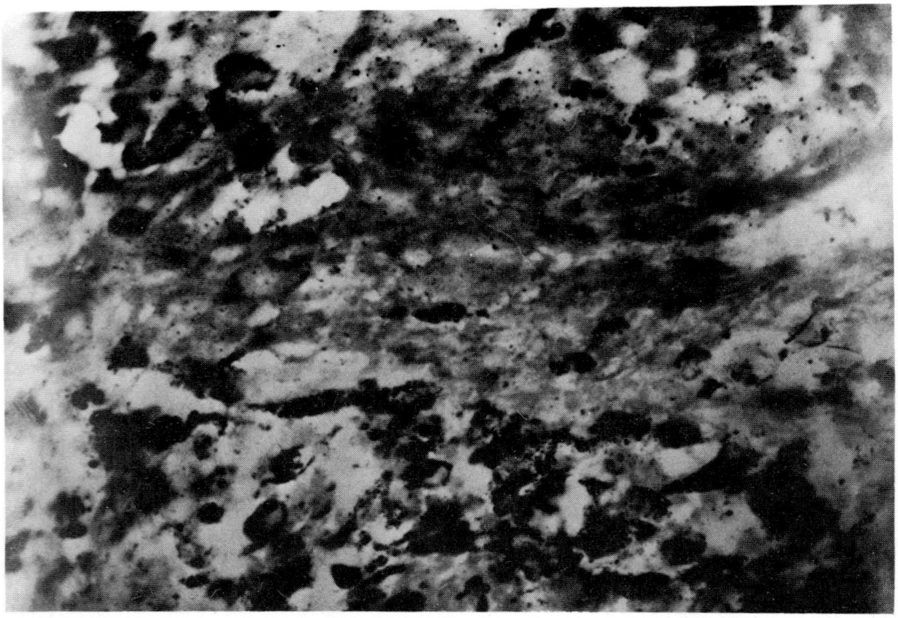

Figure 1 Histological section through the tumoral mass - 400 x
Color for melanine
Presence of melanic pigment into cells and stroma.

cases in such place are estimated at 1.8% of the head and neck MMs and at 3.6% of the total nasal and paranasal sinuses neoplasms.Three cases have been reported in Romania in the last 40 years,our case being the fourth one.

2.Difficulties of clinical and histopathological diagnosis.
Uncharacteristic symptoms just as the absence -at the primary tumor- of one or several polypectomies or of some poypi associated with the tumor or of some activating factors,could not show the possibility of a recurrent malignancy of MM type;especially,the absence of pigmentation constituted the major diagnosis difficulty.This was also reflected in the erroneous histopathological diagnosis of the primary tumor.At usual colours,there were heterogeneous images either of anaplazic carcinoma,slightly differentiated or of epidermoid type(sketches of keratozic globes)or images of sarcomatous tumor.It is only the specific color for melanine(clinically suggested by the discreet pigmentation of the recurrent tumor)that made the diagnosis precise.

3.Evolution modality.Our case is characterized by 2 elements: a/local recurrence of the tumor after a rather long time since the first intervention;b/absence of an extension,close to close and of a node or visceral dissemination.

4.Option for the cryosurgical treatment.The large surgical excision is admitted by all authors both as a method of unique treatment of the MM Ist stage and some types of 2nd stage(e.g. local recurrence)and as a bioptical method.Agreeng with this excision,we opted for the cryoexcisional technique with liquid N,considering that it has a series of advantages compared with the classical one,namely:-easier access to a rather complicated anatomical region;-lack of bleeding;-barring action in the intraoperative neoplasic dissemination;-perfect cicatrization; -possibility and even necessity to repeat local cryoapplication at certain postoperative intervals in order to consolidate the operation act;-simple,painless method,easily accepted by the patient;-possible immunological action of the cryotherapy to prevent metastases.

We have not applied the profilactic recional node dissection considering the conclusions of some authors who -through comparative studies on series of patients treated with/or without this method- proved its inefficiency and consequently its uselessness.

© 1985 Elsevier Science Publishers B.V. (Biomedical Division)
New dimensions in otorhinolaryngology - head and neck surgery, vol. 2.
E. Myers, editor

ADENOCARCINOMA OF THE ETHMOID SINUSES

JAN OLOFSSON, CLAES KLINTENBERG, HENRIK HELLQUIST AND HANNIBAL SÖKJER
Departments of Otolaryngology, Oncology, Pathology and Diagnostic Radiology,
University Hospital, S-581 85 Linköping, Sweden

INTRODUCTION

The incidence of nasal and paranasal sinus carcinomas is less than 1.0 per 100.000 per year in most reports[1]. Adenocarcinoma makes up only a few per cent of these carcinomas, and is most frequently found in the ethmoid sinuses, and has been associated with exposure to dust from hardwood[2].

MATERIAL

Thirty-five patients (31 men and 4 women - mean age 67 and 56 years respectively) were collected mainly during the last 15 years and derive from a region with about 900.000 inhabitants and a lot of furniture industries.

The clinical examination included radiography in all patients. Computed tomography was performed in 18 (Figs. 1,2).

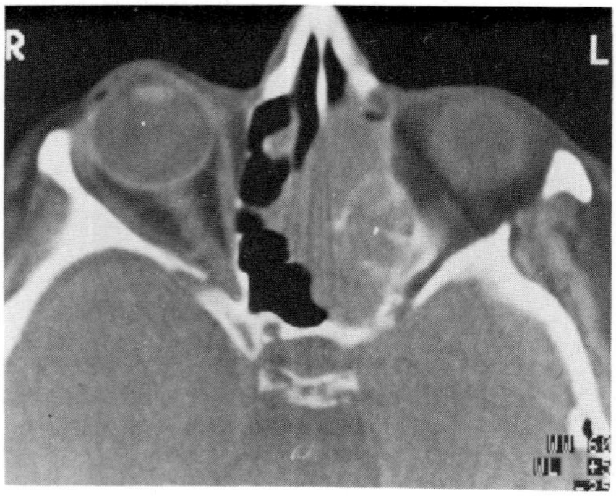

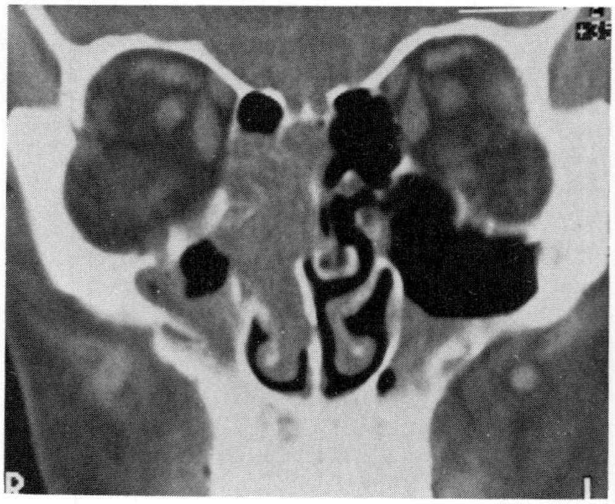

Fig. 1 (Left). Tumor filling the left nasal cavity, ethmoids, left sphenoidal sinus and bulging over the midline. No orbital invasion.

Fig. 2 (Right). Tumor involving the right ethmoids with destruction of the medial wall of the maxillary sinus. No orbital invasion.

CLINICAL DATA

Nasal obstruction (33), discharge (20) and bleeding (23) were the most common symptoms. Pain occurred in 9 patients and hearing loss and neurological symptoms in a single case each. Duration of symptoms varied between 1 - 36 months.

Radiography showed destruction outside the ethmoids in 28 and intraorbital extension in 10. Extension intracranially occurred in 4 and retromaxillary involvement was present in 4.

Twenty-five of the men were exposed to dust from hardwood for 17 - 65 years; 16 were furniture makers, 4 french polishers, 2 boat builders, 2 wood machinists, and one a wood worker teacher.

Two types of adenocarcinoma were recognized histologically; one with a papillary pattern (20) and one with an alveolar (15). Seventeen of the wood dust exposed patients had the papillary type of adenocarcinoma and 8 the alveolar type.

THERAPY

Twenty-four patients received preoperative radiotherapy followed by surgery 4 - 6 weeks later. Four patients had surgery alone and 5 received palliative radiotherapy. Two patients were not treated. External ethmoidectomy was performed in one patient; transmaxillary ethmoidectomy in 27 patients and combined with a neurosurgical approach in 2 patients and with an orbital exenteration in one.

FOLLOW-UP

Thirty patients were followed for 2 years; 24 were alive and 19 with NED. Twenty-four patients were followed for 5 years; 10 were alive and 8 with NED. Twenty-one of the 24 patients who received preoperative radiotherapy were followed for 2 years; 18 were alive and 15 with NED. Sixteen were followed for 5 years; 8 were alive and 6 with NED. None of the 6 patients with no remaining tumor in the surgical specimen after preoperative radiotherapy developed any recurrence.

SUMMARY AND CONCLUSION

Adenocarcinoma of the ethmoids are associated with exposure to dust from hardwood. Radiological examination and preferably computed tomography is necessary to correctly assess the tumor extent. A combination of surgery and radiotherapy is considered the treatment of choice in most reports. A 50 per cent 5 year survival was achieved with combined therapy.

REFERENCES

1. Robin PE, Powell DJ, Stansbie JM (1979) Carcinoma of the nasal cavity and paranasal sinuses: Incidence and presentation of different histological types. Clin Otolaryngol 4:431-456
2. Acheson ED, Hadfield EH, Macbeth RG (1967) Carcinoma of the nasal cavity and accessory sinuses in woodworkers. Lancet 1:311-312

© 1985 Elsevier Science Publishers B.V. (Biomedical Division)
New dimensions in otorhinolaryngology – head and neck surgery, vol. 2.
E. Myers, editor

CLINICAL TRIALS WITH UFT IN HEAD AND NECK CANCER

T. TAKAOKA, Y. INUYAMA AND J. TANAKA

Dept. of Otorhinolaryngology, School of Medicine, Keio University,
Tokyo (Japan)

INTRODUCTION

UFT is a new anticancer agent consisting of a mixture of 1-(2-tetrahydrofuryl)-5-fluorouracil, known as futraful, and uracil in a molar ratio of 1:4. Futraful is a masked compound of 5-FU, that is 5-fluorouracil, and shows its anticancer activity when it is converted to 5-FU by metabolic enzymes of the microsomes in the liver. The concentration of 5-FU which is converted from futraful retains its level in blood and cancer tissues much longer than when 5-FU is administered singly. Uracil is one of the chemical compounds from which DNA is constructed and shows no pharmacological activity and toxicity by itself. In 1978, Dr. S. Fujii of Japan found that when futraful and uracil were administered orally in a molar ratio of 1:4, the concentration of 5-FU in cancer tissue increased markedly and maintained its level for a very long time, whereas 5-FU in blood remained at a low concentration. This phenomenon is thought to result from the fact that 5-FU is converted from futraful by thymidine phosphorylase in cancer tissue as well as in liver microsomes and that uracil which is highly accumulated in cancer tissue inhibits degradation of 5-FU. The development of UFT was based on these findings with the expectation that it would reinforce anti-cancer activity of 5-FU without increasing its toxicity.

MATERIALS AND METHODS

From January 1981 to August 1984, 48 patients took part in this study, of whom 43 were evaluable. Their ages ranged from 23 to 83 years, of which 26 were male and 17 female. Primary sites of cancer which arose in these patients were mainly in the nose and paranasal sinuses, the oral cavity and the oropharynx. Histological findings revealed squamous cell carcinoma in most of the evaluable patients. However other histological types of cancer such as adenocarcinoma, adenoid cystic carcinoma etc. were also found. In the 43 evaluable patients, 7 had received no prior treatment and 36 had already had various treatments. A capsule of UFT contains 100 mg of futraful. Six capsules were administered orally to each patient everyday for at least four consecutive weeks before we evaluated the response of the drug, the administration being continued for as long as the patient showed a partial or complete response.

RESULTS

The results of UFT therapy in the 43 evaluable patients were as follows. Eight patients achieved a complete response and 8 patients had a partial response. The overall response rate was 37.2% which is fairly high for a single agent in the treatment of head and neck cancer. In these 16 responders to UFT, 12 patients could be followed up with UFT therapy alone. Among these patients UFT retained its effectiveness for 5.2 months on average. The longest disease-free interval was 18 months.

When we look into the response rate for UFT according to histology, UFT showed a 32.4% response rate in patients with squamous cell carcinoma. We also think that it might be noteworthy that UFT also showed a high response rate in patients with adenocarcinoma which is usually resistant to any type of anticancer agent, although there were not so many of these cases.

With regard to response rate according to primary sites, UFT revealed a 57.1% response rate in the nose and paranasal sinuses, 50.0% in the oropharynx, and 30.0% in the oral cavity. It was not effective in the treatment of nasopharynx cancer with only a 12.5% response rate.

In patients with no prior treatment, the response rate for UFT was 42.9%. Previously treated patients achieved a 36.1% response rate. There was no statistical significance between them. This suggests that UFT is effective even against cancer tissue which recurred after exposure to irradiation and/or other anticancer agents. We therefore think that UFT is a good candidate for neo-adjuvant chemotherapy, judging from the high response rate of 42.9% in patients with no prior treatment.

Of the 43 patients, 8 experienced some toxic effects of UFT which were mild evaluable and acceptable on the whole. These included anorexia, nausea, stomatitis and so on. Patients were able to continue taking the drug by reducing the dosage. Bone marrow suppression was also seen in several patients, but this was also mild and recovered soon after interruption of treatment.

CONCLUSION

We concluded that UFT was quite effective in the treatment of head and neck cancer with its high response rate as a single agent, good response of adenocarcinoma as well as squamous cell carcinoma, good response of recurrent cancer that had already been exposed to irradiation and/or other anticancer agents, and with its mild toxicity.

New dimensions in otorhinolaryngology - head and neck surgery, vol. 2.
E. Myers, editor

CALCIFYING EPITHELIAL ODONTOGENIC TUMOR: PINDBORG TUMOR A CASE REPORT

JOSE V. QUIROZ M.D. AND JOSE BELLASAI M.D.

From Head and Neck Surgery and Pathology Departments. Clinical Hospital of the National University, Asunción-Paraguay

INTRODUCTION

The Calcifying Epithelial Odontogenic Tumor was first described by Pindborg in 1956. At the present time, about 120 cases has been reported. It comparative rarity makes the diagnosis difficult for the pathologists and errors in diagnosis are occasionally made and may results in needless mutilation.

This case shows a typical error in diagnosis of malignacy with later confirmation of a Pindborg tumor.

CASE REPORT

A 22 year old man admitted to our service in March 1984, had developed a swelling on the cheek and buccal aspect of the left maxillar molar region, 8 months earlier. Roentgenograms revealed a unerupted 2nd molar desplaced upper, and sourrounded by both, radiopac and rarefacted tumor. The 3ed molar was desplaced forward.The aspirative biopsy and the frozen study showed a squamous cell carcinoma grade I. We performed total hemimaxillectomy with preservation of the orbit contents. Further examination of the specimen revealed to be a Calcifying Epithelial Odontogenic Tumor. At 15 months, the patient is doing well without evidence of recurrence.(Fig. 1)

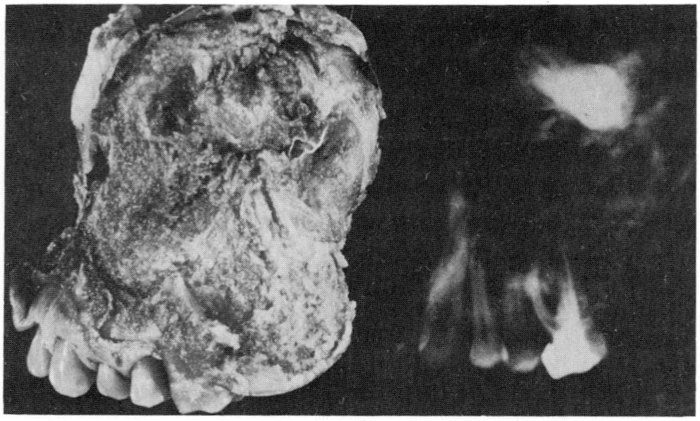

Fig. 1. Shows a cut section of the specimen and it roentgenogram with the unerupted teeth included in the tumor.

DISCUSSION

The rarity of this tumor does that fews pathologists have occasion to see many odontogenics tumors others than ameloblastomas. Many clinical features can be taken of literature. Like ameloblastomas, it ocurrs in the medial age of life, without predilection for sexes

There is a mandibular and premolar predilection. The tumor is found often in association with a unerupted tooth. Roentgenograms reveal a unilocular or multilocular cystic lesion with numerous scatered islands of irregular calcifications. Early, however, the tumor is characterizated by a well defined radiolucent area around the coronal aspect of a fully formed unerupted tooth. The striking features of this neoplasm are the cellular pleomorphims, a curious extracellular matrix and calcification. The tumor often appears as sheets of relativaly large, polhyedral epithelial cells separated by a scant connective tissues stroma. It can be confounded with carcinoma, but mitoses are rare. A distintive feature is an homogeneus eosinophilic amyloid-like bodies in and among the epithelial masses or in the stroma. The ultrastructural features of the cells are comparable to the cells of the stratum intermedium of the enamel organ.

Local aggressiveness is variable and no metastases have been reported. The tumor should be treated like an ameloblastoma.-

SUMMARY

The autors repor a typical case of Pindborg Tumor, analizying the clinical an histological aspect of the diagnosis of this rare tumor.

REFERENCES

1. Pindborg JJ (1956) Calcifying Epithelial Odontogenic tumor.Acta Path. Microbiol. Scand. (Suppl.) 111: 71
2. Pindborg JJ (1958) A Calcifying Epithelial Odontogenic tumor. Cancer 11: 838-843
3. Shafer WG, Hine MK and Levy BM (1963) A teexbook of Oral Pathology, 2nd ed. Philadelpia WB Saunders Company, pag.217
4. Vap DR, Dahlin DC and Turlington EG (1970) Pindborg Tumor, the so called calcifying epithelial odontogenic tumor, Cancer 25,629-636
5. Gorlin RJ, Chaudhry AP, and Pindborg JJ (1961) Odontogenic Tumors Classification, Histophatology, and Clinical Behavior in Man and Domestical Animals
6. Batsakis JG (1979) Tumors of the Head and Neck, 2nd ed. Baltimore The Williams and Wilkins Company, Vol II pag 537
7. Ai-Ru L, Zen L and Jian S (1982) Calcifying Epithelial Odontogenic tumors: A clinicopathologic study of nine cases. J.Oral Pathol. 11 (5) 399-405

© 1985 Elsevier Science Publishers B.V. (Biomedical Division)
New dimensions in otorhinolaryngology - head and neck surgery, vol. 2.
E. Myers, editor

CASE REPORT OF A BRANCHIAL CLEFT CYST FROM THE VALLECULA

YING P. HSIEH

Department of Otolaryngology Veterans Administration Hospital, Temple, Texas

Branchial cleft cysts are commonly found on the lateral aspect of the neck, which were thought to arise from the remnant of the branchial apparatus.

It is very unlikely, from this pathogenesis point of view, that the branchial cyst would occur in the oral cavity, however, we recently encountered a very unusual case, which was diagnosed pathologically as a branchial cyst arising from the vallecula.

The following case report would represent a different point of view of pathogenesis of branchial cleft cyst.

Case Report

A 62 year old male was seen in my clinic with chief complaints of a 10-year history of dysphagia and a 2-year history of progressive dyspnea. Thorough ENT examination disclosed a big cyst, estimated as about 5 x 5 cm, arised from the left vallecula almost obstructing the piriform sinus. The CT scan of the neck also confirmed the clinical finding. (Fig. 1)

He underwent a complete panendoscopic examination, which didn't reveal any other abnormality. Biopsy taken from the other sites were also negative. A few days later, under general anesthesia, excision of the cyst through left pharyngotomy approach (Fig. 2) was accomplished very successfully.

He was discharged two weeks after surgery without any previous symptoms. Follow-up in 4 months showed no evidence of recurrence.

The pathological report (Fig. 3) showed it was a branchial cyst, lined with stratified squamous epithelium surrounded by lymphoid tissue showing germinal centers.

Discussion

The occurrence of the branchial cleft cyst originating from the oral cavity is very unusual. It is very difficult to justify based upon the common concept that it arises from the remnant of the branchial arch. Dr. Bhaskar [1], after reviewing the pathological findings from 468 cases of branchial cleft cysts of the neck, found that 97% of the cysts were lined with stratified squamous epithelium surrounded by lymphoid tissue with germinal centers. He called it the lymphoepithelial cyst. Dr. Deane[2] also stated that the branchial cleft cysts are characterized by the dual structures, the stratified squamous or sometimes columnar epithelium, and also the lymphoid tissue.

Dr. Bhaskar postulated, from the histopathological point of view, that the branchial cleft cyst does not originate from the branchial arch. It actually represents a cyst in the lymph nodes, which develops from the ectopic epithelium entrapped in the lymph nodes during the embryological development.

Reviewing all the literatures, there are totally about 28 cases of branchial cleft cysts which arise from the oral cavity[3-6]. It seems to me, from the histopathological point of view, that the lymphoepithelial cyst is an appropriate term instead of the branchial cleft cyst.

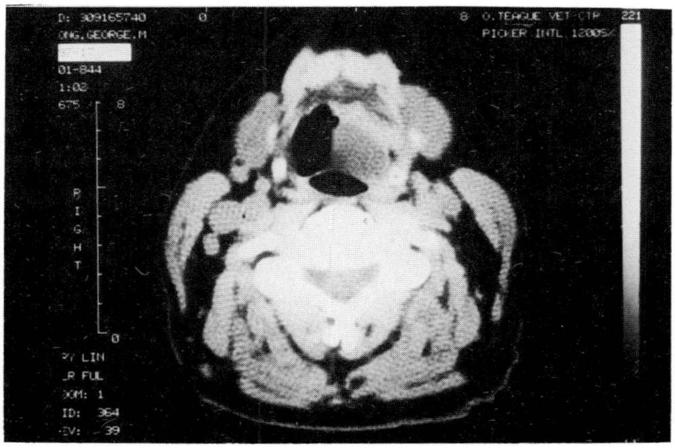

Fig. 1 The cyst encompasses the left vallecula and piriform sinus.

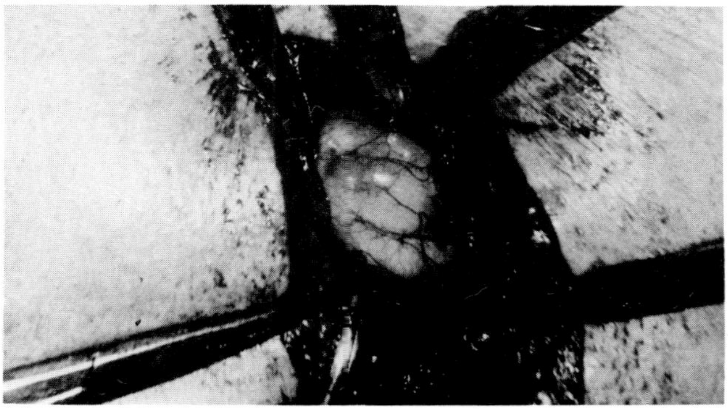

Fig. 2 The cyst was found to arise from the vallecula through the pharyngotomy approach.

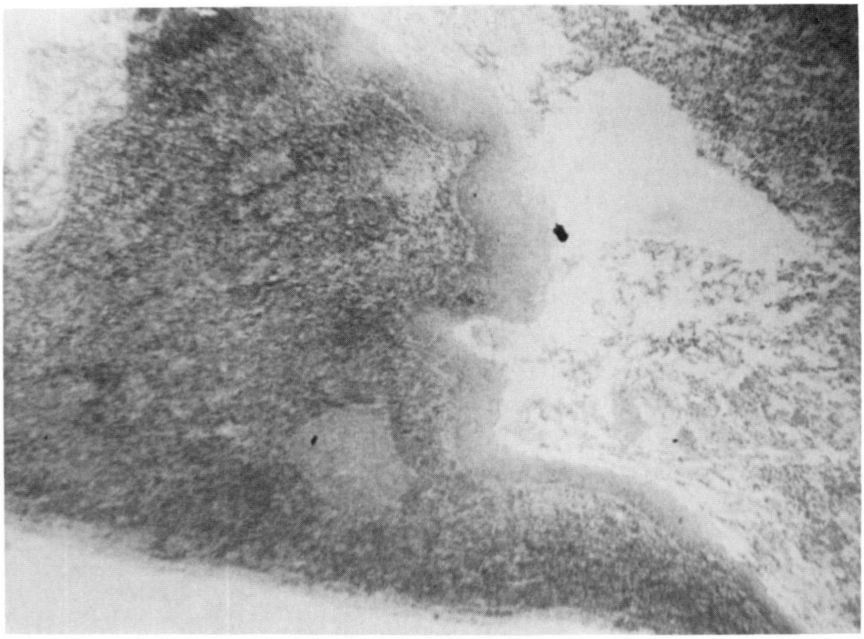

Fig. 3 The cyst is lined with stratified squamous epithelium surrounded by lymphoid tissue.

References

1. Bhaskar, S. N., and Bernier, J. L.: Histogenesis of Branchial Cysts: A Report of 468 Cases Am. J. Path. 35: 407-423, 1958.
2. Deane, S. A., and Telander, R. L.: Surgery of Thyroglossal Duct and Branchial Cleft Anomalies. Am. J. Surgery 136:348-353, 1978.
3. Calman, H. I.: Sublingual Branchiogenic Cyst; Report of a Case, Oral Surg., Mral Med. & Oral Path. 16: 333-338, 1963.
4. Gold, C.: Branchial Cleft Cyst Located in the Floor of the Mouth, Oral Surg., Oral Med., & Oral Path. 15:1118-1120, 1962
5. Vickers, R. A.: Lymphoepithelial Lesions of the Oral Cavity; Report of Four Cases, Oral Surg., Oral Med., Oral Path. 16:1214-1221, 1963.
6. Bhaskar, S. N.: Lymphoepithelial Cysts of the Oral Cavity. Oral Surg., Oral Med., Oral Path. 21:120-128, 1966.

New dimensions in otorhinolaryngology – head and neck surgery, vol. 2.
E. Myers, editor

SURGICAL TREATMENT FOR CONGENITAL MIDDLE EAR ANOMALIES

YOSHIO OGURA, YU MASUDA, SHUICHI WATANABE, KAZUNORI NISHIZAKI,
MICHIO SUEHIRO, AND KINYA UNO

Department of Otolaryngology, Okayama University Medical School
2-5-1 Shikata-cho, Okayama 700 (Japan)

INTRODUCTION

In view of the changes and improvement of the surgical techniques for congenital middle ear anomalies (MEA) and their results in the recent decades, a long-term statistical study was conducted on the surgically treated anomalous cases.

MATERIAL AND METHODS

On 218 ears with MEA operated in the University Hospital of Okayama from 1955 to 1983, chronological changes of the frequency of operative techniques in use and their results were investigated.

RESULTS AND DISCUSSION

Setting the criteria of the surgically successful case as the postoperative shortening of A-B gap more than 10 dB or hearing level less than 30 dB in the average of the speech range, the rates of success in each technique and period were shown on Table I. In the former group with the period of 1955-1978, the use of classical fenestration operation (CF) was predominant, and, on the contrary, tympanoplasty (TP) and stapes surgery (SS) were less frequent with poorer results. In the latter group of 1979-1983, no CF appeared on the table, and the

TABLE I
RESULTS IN RESPECTIVE PERIODS AND OPERATIVE TECHNIQUES

	1955-1978	1979-1983	Total
Canalplasty	5/ 18 (27.8%)	1/ 7 (14.3%)	6/ 25 (24.0%)
Tympanoplasty	15/ 31 (48.4)	26/28 (92.9)	41/ 59 (69.5)
Stapes surgery	8/ 12 (66.7)	12/14 (85.7)	20/ 26 (76.9)
Fenestration operation			83/108 (76.9)
classical	83/107 (77.6)		
oval window		0/ 1 (0.0)	
Total	111/168 (66.1)	39/50 (78.0)	150/218 (68.8%)

use of TP and SS were getting dominant with remarkably improved results.

The difference of the results by TP between the two groups seemed to be derived by the introduction of modified types of TP with the use of autograft ossicles and cartilage, polyethylene tube and plastipore PORP as the ossicular replacement.

In the discussion of SS, it would be convenient to divide the former group of the Table I into two groups as shown on the Table II. Since 1975, partial stapedectomy, especially, small fenestra technique using Teflon wire piston, was most frequently used and the results grew up excellently. The reason of the good results by this technique was considered to be its minor ill effect to the inner ear.

TABLE II

CHANGES OF TECHNIQUES AND RESULTS IN STAPES SURGERY

	Number of successful ears		
	1955-1974	1975-1978	1979-1983
Rosen	0/1		
Goodhill	0/1		
Shea	3/5		
House	1/1	1/1	
Partial stapedectomy		3/3	12/14
Total	4/8 (50%)	16/18 (88.9%)	

CONCLUSIONS AND SUMMARY

Operated 218 ears with MEA were statistically investigated.

Modified type techniques were more recommendable to improve hearing by TP.

Partial stapedectomy using Teflon wire piston was the most effective and harmless procedure in SS.

REFERENCES

1. Jahrsdoerfer RA (1978) Congenital atresia of the ear. Laryngoscope Vol 88, Suppl 13:1-48

2. Ogura Y (1979) Malformations of the sound conducting apparatus - Their fundamentals and surgical management. Oto-Rhino-Laryngol Tokyo Vol 22, Suppl 2:1-178

3. Nager GT, Levin LS (1980) Congenital aural atresia: Embryology, pathology, classification, genetics, and surgical management. In: Paparella MM, Shumrick DA (eds) Otolaryngology, 2nd ed, WB Saunders, Philadelphia, Vol 2, pp 1303-1344

© 1985 Elsevier Science Publishers B.V. (Biomedical Division)
New dimensions in otorhinolaryngology - head and neck surgery, vol. 2.
E. Myers, editor

THE INFLUENCE OF A NASAL DECONGESTANT. A SONOTUBOMETRIC STUDY

LARS OLÉN MD. BO FRIBERG BSc, INGEMAR MELÉN MD. LARS WÅHLANDER MSc, ENT Department, Kärnsjukhuset, 541 85 Skövde (Sweden)

INTRODUCTION

Impaired tubal function is considered a main factor in acute and secretory otitis media. Naturally there has been much research in trying to find effective treatments - pharmacotherapeutic and others - to promote the ET function in cases of upper respiratory infections (URI).

AIM

The aim of this investigation was to study the effects on the muscular opening function of the ET of a beta-adrenoreceptorstimulating agent, applied as a solutin sprayed into the nasal cavities (Xylometazoline, Otrivin ^{R})/

METHOD

The muscular opening function was recorded by using the sonotubometric method described by Virtanen (1977) with some modifications.

SUBJECTS

Altogether 156 young military servicemen suffering from acute common cold symptoms for two days as an average took part in the study. It was a prerequisite for the test procedure that the subject was not able to open at least one tube when in recumbency.

Another prerequisite was that the subject should be able to open both or one earlier closed tube when sitting in upright position or after a short physical exercise. These criteria were fulfilled by 34 subjects. These 34 persons were randomly divided into two parallel groups. Xylometazoline and placebo were administered in a double blind fashion. After spraying the nasal cavities twice the tubal opening was tested. If the tube did not open a cross-over trial was made and the tubal opening function was again tested.

STATISTICAL METHODS

In the statistical analysis we have used t-test, Fisher's exact probability test and sign test.

RESULTS

The results in summary

Position change. Sitting to lying - closing of ET $p<0.001$. Lying to half-sitting - opening of ET $p<0.002$.

Recumbency. Xylometazoline - opening of ET $p<0.005$. Placebo - NS.

DISCUSSION

The results show a significantly larger number of tubal openings after application of Xylometazoline compared to placebo. Improvement of tubal function in an elevated body position of 30 degrees has earlier been reported by Rundcrantz (1969).

CONCLUSIONS

Xylometazoline applied to the nasal cavities in persons suffering from acute common cold infection improves the muscular opening function of the ET> Since a good opening function is believed to prevent middle ear inflammation it is indicated to recommend the prescription of Xylometazoline for common cold.

Sonotubometry is a simple and useful method for studies of the tubal function qualitatively under strict criteria. The method can be safer by using coded test sound.

The investigation implies that further studies on pharmacotherapeutic effects on the ET may be performed using a modified sonotubometric method.

REFERENCES

1. Andreasson L, Ivarsson A, Luttrup S, Mollerstrom B, Tjernstrom O: Ekustachian tube function measured as pressure equilibration and sound transmission capacity. A comparison in healthy ears. ORL I Otorhinolaryngol Relat Spec 1984; 46(2): 74-83

2. Holmquist j, Olen L: Measurement of eustachian tube function. J Otolaryngol 1980; 94,16

3. Virtanen H: Eustachian tube sound conduction. Helsinki 1977

CHILDHOOD SEVERE-PROFOUND SENSORINEURAL DEAFNESS

LUCIO A. CASTAGNO,MD
M. LUCIA CARVALHAL,MD
Department of Otolaryngology,Federal University of Pelotas School of Medicine. Rua General Osorio,1585. Pelotas,96100,Brazil

INTRODUCTION

Childhood deafness is a disease with several etiologies.Prevalence vary from 0.5 to 49 per 1000.In our region it seems to be 2.23 per 1000.This study was designed to investigate deafness in children of a specialize school in Pelotas and to correlate the clinical data of this population with the normal ones.

MATERIAL AND METHODS

Fifty seven hearing impaired children were studied.Five (8.8%) had associated mental retardation.Data were obtained from interviews with the mothers.Pure tone audiometry and/or impedance audiometry were done in all children.Some were submited to electrocochleography.All had pure tone average at 0.5,¯ and 2 kHz higher than 70 dB in both ears.

Data were fed into a computer and statistical correlations (Chi square,Student's T test and linear regression curve) were done.

RESULTS

Sex distribution was unremarkable.Average age was 9.18 (3-18 years).Etiological diagnosis was achieved in 30(61.2%) children and was unknown in 19(38.8%).

TABLE I: Childhood deafness etiologies (n=49)

Group	CONGENITAL		POST-NATAL	
Etiology	Unknown	16	Unknown	3
	Genetic	6	Seizures	6
	Rubella	2	Meningitis	3
	Toxemia	1	Measles	1
	Neonatal asphyxia	9		
	Prematurity	2		
Total(%)	36 (75.5%)		13 (26.5%)	

An evasion of 22 children in socioeconomic class D (the poorest one) was calculated by linear regression applyed to classes A-B-C and most probably is secundary to the cultural and economic marginalization of their families.Analysis was done in relation to the normal children population in schools of the 5th Educational Region (Pelotas and neighborhood).As two sets of data were merged with some discrepancies in criteria of classes distribution,we grouped classes A-B and C-D to prevent serious errors.No significant difference between prevalence of deafness in the wealthier classes (A-B) and in the poorer ones (C-D) was found.

A higher prevalence of deafness in children with low birth weight (less than 2500 g) was found at a significance level of p=0.0024.There was no significant relationship between prematurity in the deaf population and in the normal ones.

Psychomotor development was assessed and related to normal populations.Significant correlations were observed in all criteria ($p < 0.005$),except "stand up", indicating a retarded development in the deaf children population.

DISCUSSION

Etiological diagnosis of severe-profound hearing loss in children may be a hard task,since it is difficult to distinguish between congenital deafness and the post-natal ones.Diagnosis was done in our population just with clinical exam and history.No serological tests were used,so one may presume a higher number of rubella cases as well as other infections.

No correlation was found between deafness and socio-economic level.It seems that the higher number of deaf children in the poorer classes is just because of the higher population in these classes in Brazil.

An important relationship was estabilished between severe-profound hearing loss and low birth weight newborns.It seems that low birth weight children have a higher risk of deafness.

Psychomotor development were retarded in the deaf children population.We emphasize the early diagnosis of childhood deafness as a way to better treatment and prevention of retarded development.

REFERENCES

1. Barros F et al (1984) Rev Saude Publ,Sao Paulo,18:301-312.
2. Carter C (1982) Dev Med Child Neurol 24:525-526.
3. Davis G (1979) Laryngoscope 89:1681-1688.
4. D'Souza S et al (1981) Arch Dis Child 56:245-252.
5. Nance W (1980) Birth Defects Origin Artic Ser 16:35-46.
6. Parving A (1980) Acta Otolaryngol 90:262-266.
7. Ruben R at al (1982) Laryngoscope 92:38-46.
8. Senecal J at al (1979) Sem Hop Paris 55:2008-2019.

New dimensions in otorhinolaryngology - head and neck surgery, vol. 2.
E. Myers, editor

EFFECTS OF IN UTERO ULTRASOUND ON FETAL HEARING: A PRELIMINARY REPORT

LEONARD W. BROWN, ROBERT SAWYER, KENNETH P. ASPINALL

Otolaryngology Service, Brooke Army Medical Center, Fort Sam Houston, Texas 78234-6200

Ultrasonography may be considered as a form of high frequency in utero noise exposure. There is known fetal response to acoustic stimulus as demonstrated by physiological changes with noise exposure, especially in the third trimester[1,2]. Possible in utero injury could therefore be caused by cavitation, thermal effects, or direct injury[3,4,5].

MATERIALS AND METHODS

Of one hundred and thirty two children ages four to six years old, thirteen were suitable as controls and thirteen as study patients. The remaining children were excluded based upon a history of prior ear disease or physical findings at the time of the study. The study group received from one to ten ultrasound exposures in utero; mean 2.6 per study patient.

Audiometrics, to include pure tone thresholds from 500 through 12,000 Hertz, SRTs, tympanograms and acoustic reflexes were performed on each patient using a GSI-10 audiometer.

FINDINGS

The study and control data were compared to evaluate differences between right and left ears, total ears of each group, trimester of exposure and number of exposures. There was found to be no significant difference (T 0.95) between the control ears and study ears as a whole. Additionally, no difference was noted between subgroups comparing exposure during first, second and third trimester.

A third subgroup, consisting of four patients with three or more in utero ultrasonographies, revealed a significant difference (T 0.95) at 12 KHz when the control ears tested were evaluated individually and compared to the total number of ears which received three or more in utero ultrasound. The mean value at 12 KHz of the control group was 18.1 decibels and of the study group 27.5 decibels. Among this subgroup, patients with the greatest exposure exhibited the greatest hearing loss.

DISCUSSION

Several points need to be considered to evaluate our data. First, although our population is small, the possibility of additional hearing loss with each ultrasonographic exposure in utero is of concern. Second, while not statistically significant with this patient number, the greatest change in hearing levels between 8 and 12 KHz appeared to be in patients who received ultrasonography during the third trimester. Third, if heairng loss is present secondary to ultrasound exposure, what anatomical changes have been induced?

CONCLUSION

Our data suggests two risk factors to be of concern during ultrasonogrpahy: (1) exposure during the third trimester and (2) multiple exposures.

REFERENCES

1. Taylor KJW: Experimental ultrasound damage of revelance of ultrasonography. Proceedings of British Institute of Radiology July 1971, page 563.
2. Szmeja Z, Slomako Z, Silorski K: The risk of hearing impairment in children from others exposed to noise during pregnancy. Intl J of Ped-Otorhinolaryngology (1971) pp 221-229.
3. Baker ML, Darilrymple GV: Biological effects of diagnostic ultrasound: A review. Ultrasound Feb 1978, pp 479-483.
4. Fry FJ, Kossoff G: Threshold ultrasoundic dosages for structural changes in the mannium brain. J of Acoustical Society of America. Vol 48 No.6, Part 2, 1970.
5. Birnholz JC, Benacerraf BR: The development of human fetal hearing. Science Nov 83, pp. 516-518.

© 1985 Elsevier Science Publishers B.V. (Biomedical Division)
New dimensions in otorhinolaryngology - head and neck surgery, vol. 2.
E. Myers, editor

TYMPANOMEATAL INDEX IN PERMEATAL SURGERY

A SINHA

Chairman, Department of Otolaryngology, Patna Medical College, Road 6/B, Rajendra Nagar, Patna 800016, Bihar (India)

During the past three decades permeatal surgery has been increasingly performed. The chief indications for this surgery are stapedectomy, tympanotomy and tympaoplasty of various types.

In permeatal approach the Surgeon encounters varying degrees of posterior bony meatal canal overhang. The overhang have to be removed to adequate degree to allow view of desired middle ear structures.

OBSERVATIONS

The author studied the various degrees of posterior meatal overhang and could identify three types: A, B & C.

Type A. In this type after the canal incision and elevation of the tympanomeatal flap, from its sulcus the entire oval window structures lay exposed. One could see lower part of Incus, incudo stapedial joint, stapes super-structure and oval window areas, including a part of fallopion canal, pyramid and stapedius tendon.

In these cases no bone of the meatal overhang has to be removed. The operation becomes simplified further when the otsclerotic focus is thin and bluish.

Type 'A' overhang were thus associated with wide, straight canal and thin otosclerotic focus.

Type B. These were cases with external canal moderately wide, slightly curved and some bony overhang. So that after elevation of the drum from the annulus and opening the middle ear one could visualize the lower part of incus, incudostapedial joint, parts of stapes crura and part of oval window. It was only after removing small amount of bony overhang that the entire oval window, part of fallopion canal and the pyramid with stapedius tendon could be brought into view. The otosclerotic focus in this type varied from thin blue to mild obliterative type, often sending band of thick stripes across the footplate, but they were comparatively easy to remove.

Type C. In this group the external canal was relatively narrow, and had a hump in the floor, making the canal rather curved. After incision and elevation of the annulus the middle ear was opened but one could not see the oval window structures, but visualize only part of lower end of incus and incudo-stapedial joint. By meticulous effort sufficient bony overhang had to be removed exposing the fallopion canal and pyramidal process. The otosclerotic focus in this type was thick and obliterative filling the oval window,partly or wholly. This required drilling and manipulation at the window.

The Types A,B & C as related to canal overhang and visualization of middle ear structures has been refered to as the "Tymponomeatal Index".

The observations on the 3-types of overhang in a series of 1680 cases subjected to stapedectomy during the period 1970-84 are given in Table:

Type of overhang (No. of ears)	External meatus	View on elevation of tympanomeatal flap	Curetting of post-meatal wall
Type A 650 (39%)	wide and straight	Stapes,oval window incus long pr, and pyramid.	Not required
Type B 700 (41%)	wide and curved	Partly Incus long pr.Crura of stapes.	Required partly
Type C 330 (20%)	Narrow and curved	Only lower part of Incus.	Required greatly

DEVELOPMENTAL AND CLINICAL SIGNIFICANCE OF BONY OVERHANG

Developmentally the lower arched part of the tympanic ring becomes ankylosed with the floor of the tympanum, while its posterior and upper end unites with the squamosal (Bast and Anson,1959).

It appears that in course of development and ossification,the tympanic ring flange undergoes alterations. This eventually influences as to how much the external bony canal be wide or narrow, straight or curved. They also bear certain relationship to the developing oval window structures. These in the adult and those suffering from otosclerosis hold a state refered to by the term 'Tympanomeatal Index' with overhang of Types A, B & C.

The clinical significance of the Index are:

(a)Helps in anticipating difficulties at operation:'to be forearned is to be forearmed'.

(b)Prognostic value in not expecting excellent result in Type C overhang with obliterative focus of otosclerosis.

(c)An additional paramater for caserecord evaluated with other dates clinical and audiological.

(d)Type A case be initially selected for specialists-in-training,like Residents.

(e)Also of value in Tympanotomy and Tympanoplasty.

© 1985 Elsevier Science Publishers B.V. (Biomedical Division)
New dimensions in otorhinolaryngology - head and neck surgery, vol. 2.
E. Myers, editor

IMPROVEMENTS IN THE SURGICAL TREATMENT OF CONGENITAL EAR DYSPLASIAS

L.S. MANOLIDES, P.D. MICHAILIDES

Dept. of Otorhinolaryngology and Neck Surgery, Aristotelian University of Thessaloniki, AHEPA Hospital, Thessaloniki (Greece)

INTRODUCTION

External, middle and inner ear congenital dysplasias are quite frequent mounting to rate of 1:3,800 child births out of which 10% are bilateral. However, the proportion of moderate or severe dysplasias combined with partial or total atresia of the auditory meatus is 1:15,000 child births; children suffering unilateral dysplasias are four times as many as those suffering bilateral ones. According to the modern conception, dysplasias are distinguished into minor and major. The treatment of minor dysplasias belongs to the surgery of the middle ear cavity aiming to the management of the conductive hearing loss, where, the diagnosis and treatment of major dysplasias are more complex, functionally and aesthetically.

MATERIAL AND METHODS

We studied 92 children suffering congenital ear dysplasias. Our study included children suffering lesions such as: dysplasias, partial or total abesence of the auricle, atresia of the external auditory meatus and dysplasias of the middle ear cavity (tympanic membrane and auditory ossicles).

Diagnostic Problems - Preoperative Estimation

Surgical treatment aims to: 1) the functional, 2) the aesthetic rehabilitation. Although both of them are significantly important, in cases of bilateral lesions the functional rehabilitation preceds the aesthetic one. Preoperative audiological examination establishes the functional status of the cochlea and the presence of conductive hearing loss. The test battery of the audiological examination includes all the routine tests of audiology. Nevertheless, it is from the radiological investigation that we obtain detailed information concerning the lesions existing in the ear. On clinical examination, the dysplasic degree of the auricle gives us a rough estimation of the middle ear condition. The larger the developmental lesion of the auricle, the greater the deformity that should be expected in the middle ear. In our opinion, the age of the patient undertaking such an operation arises from: a) the social and environmental condition of the child, b) the maldevelopment of the mastoid process and the middle ear cavity and c) the kind of lesion (unilateral or bilateral).

Operative technique

Attempting better postoperative results, we proceeded to a new surgical technique, much more promising then the previous one. We operated children suffering from: maldeveloped auricle, atresia of the external auditory meatus, absence of the tympanic membrane and the ossicles. The purpose of the surgical proceedure is: 1) the creation of external auditory meatus (functional and aesthetical), 2) the functional rehabilitation of the middle ear cavity, 3) the development of the auricle (aesthetic rehabilitation).

Initially we obtain a skin and cartilage graft which is to be used at a later stage for the formation of the external auditory meatus. In cases of bilateral defects, we use preserved cartilage. Though, a classical postauricular incision androtomy is performed. The andrum is sufficiently drilled anteriorly until we get ample surgical field. Keeping the entrance to the andrum as a landmark, we drill out the atritic plate overhanging the middle ear cavity until the hypoplastic mucosa replacing the tympanic membrane is revealed. We keep on drilling until we find remnants of the annulus fibrosus which compromises the limit of drilling inferiorly, thus avoiding traumatism of the temperomandibular joint. We decide about the type of tympanoplasty to be performed relying on the overall condition of the stapes as whole and particularly the base of it. Despite the size of the maleus and the incus which are unusually small and firmly attached to each other, the movement of the ossicular chain is normal, therefore there is no need to be removed. The preparation of a tympanic membrane homograft follows. The homograft is placed in the usual tympanic membrane site being loosely attached to the maleus. The annulus fibrosus of the homograft is fixed by Fibrin-Glue as well as the free skin graft used to cover the bone of the external auditory meatus. Now we prepare the cartilaginous homograft in such a way that it can take a tube-like form for replacing the missing cartilaginous part of the external auditory meatus. Performing the proper incisions, we remove the useless tissues and remnants of the cartilage of the hypoplastic auricle and the cartilaginous homograft is placed with its inferior rim being in contact with the underlying bony structures and its superior rim with the lateral surface of the auricle.

RESULTS

The early postoperative results can be seen ten days later. An external auditory meatus has been created, compromising normal anatomical features: there is no shrinking danger, it can be easily inspected, cleaned or self-cleaned; it always allows us the chances of a later cosmetic proceedure. Postoperative hearing ability is more than satisfactory.

© 1985 Elsevier Science Publishers B.V. (Biomedical Division)
New dimensions in otorhinolaryngology – head and neck surgery, vol. 2.
E. Myers, editor

SOME OBSERVATIONS ON DISCHARGING MASTOID CAVITIES

R.N.SRIVASTAVA, D.KUMAR, P.K. VARSHNEY, M. PANDEY
DEPTT. OF OTOLARYNGOLOGY, G.S.V.M. MEDICAL COLLEGE, KANPUR, U.P. INDIA.

INTRODUCTION

Inspite of great advancement in the field of otolaryngology, persistent otorrhoea after mastoidectomy is a burning problem to the otolaryngologists as well as quite annoying to the suffering patients. It has been a general belief of many otolaryngologists (Bois 1945)(1), Arora & Singh 1977 (2) that tubal infection due to chronic tonsillitis adenoids and sinus infection may cause recurrent and persistent infection to the middle ear. Other authors did not find benefit in discharge on removal of tonsils and adenoids in otitis media(Griffith 1937,(3),(Bluestone 1977,(4). It is also commonly observed that in attico-antral type of otitis media, with large adenoids and tonsils, who undergo mastoidectomy and in whome, the perforation has not been closed, continue to discharge. In these patients, persistence of ear discharge may be due to constant tubal infection, or due to remnant of disease (Kaiser,1930)(5), McKee & Portman (1963)(6), or due to effect of gap in the tympanic membrane which is allowing the infection in middle ear from exterior (Scenturia & Alferd, 1954)(7), Dalton & English(1962)(8).

In the light of such conflicting opinions, cases of post mastoidectomy discharging middle ear with dry mastoid cavities were re-explored, with the view to find out remnance of disease and grafting was done in the middle ear to avoid air born infection from external auditory canal. Condition of tonsils, adenoids and sinuses were also assessed.

MATERIAL AND METHODS

25 cases of 'post mastoidectomy discharging middle ear' with dry mastoid cavities were admitted in Ear Nose Throat ward, at L.L.R. Hospital, Kanpur in U.P. India. These cases were subjected for detailed clinical history and examination and relevant investigations, such as swabs from middle ear for bacteriological and mycological culture. Re-exploration of middle ear was done by end-aural or post aural route under general anaesthesia. In 20 cases, grafting was done and in rest 5 cases, disease from middle ear was removed after re-exploration.

RESULTS

In the present series of 25 post mastoidectomy discharging ears, predeliction was noticed towards females and 2nd decade.

'Post radical mastoidectomy' otorrhoea was due to repeated infections from external auditory canal or due to reformation of cholesteotoma or granulations. Out of these 16 cases, only 7 cases had a spain of few days with dry ear, rest 9 cases never had a dry ear post-operatively.

'Post modified radical mastoidectomy'otorrhoea may be due to remnant of disease during previous surgery or to persistent infection via external auditory canal. This variety was accounting for 5 cases.

4 cases of this series were of simple mastoidectomy with myringoplasty. 2 of them passed few days with dry ear, after surgery, while other 2 never had a dry ear. Failure to take up the graft subsequently leading to an open door for infection was again the cause of otorrhoea.

Proteus and staphylococcus accounted for 60% cases. Aspergillus niger was noticed in 4 cases. Absence of proteus normally, from the upper respiratory tract and their emergence in chronic infection of middle ear contradicts the view of spread of infection through eustachian tube.

On re-exploration, remnant of disease was present in 80% cases, most common site was epitympanum. Graft was applied in 20 cases.The cases were followed for the period of 1-9 months. In 12 cases, graft was accepted and ears were absolutely dry. In 5 cases graft was rejected but ear remained dry. In 3 cases, failure was noticed.

These observations suggest that, the tubal pathology may play a very minimal role in post mastoidectomy otorrhoea as only one of these 25 cases, was having adenoids, and 5 eustachian blockage. Thorough removal of the middle ear disease, prevention of infection via external auditory canal by grafting and regular cleaning may play vital role in curing otorrhoea.

REFERENCES

1.Bois LR (1945) Chronic Otitis Media, Ann. Oto. Laryngology,54.
2.Singh A & Arora MML (1977) Relationship between adenoids CSOM I.J.L.O. Vol. 29, No. 2, 69-71.
3.Griffith SE (1973) Lancet. 2:723.
4.Bluestone CD (1977) Status of T & A,Laryngoscope. 87:1240.
5.Kaiser (1930) Ann. Oto. Rhino. Laryngology. 84 Suppl. 19,44:48.
6.McKee WJE (1963) A controlled study of T & A Br. J. PSM 17,49-69.

© 1985 Elsevier Science Publishers B.V. (Biomedical Division)
New dimensions in otorhinolaryngology - head and neck surgery, vol. 2.
E. Myers, editor

ACUTE SENSORINEURAL HEARING LOSS DUE TO EXPOSURE TO LOUD SOUNDS IN ROCK CONCERTS AND DISCOS

YUKIO TODA, ISAMU TAKEYAMA, KUMI NAKAJIMA
Dept. of Otolaryngology, St. Marianna University School of Medicine, Kawasaki, Kanagawa, Japan

INTRODUCTION

Studies about the danger of auditory damage caused by rockn' roll music have been carried out in western countries, and we are also concerned about this problem in my country. But rock concerts as well as discos are still very popular among young adults, and cases of acute sensorineural hearing loss remain quite common. Moreover, its clinical features and causative factors are as yet unknown. So, we have tried to clarify the nature of the problem in order to prevent further auditory damage.

CLINICAL DIFFERENCES

For the past 4 years, we have been collecting data on this problem and TABLE I summarizes the clinical differences between the effects of rock concerts and discos. Surprisingly, more cases of unilaterally impaired hearing can be seen in the disco group than in the concert group. This fact didn't agree with our expectations because people move about far more in discos than at concerts. The poorer prognosis for the disco group indicates that the damage is generally more severe and consequently, more difficult to treat.

TABLE I
CLINICAL DIFFERENCES BETWEEN THE EFFECTS OF ROCK CONCERTS AND DISCOS.

	impaired hearing	severity	Audiogram	prognosis
Concerts 8 cases	unilateral 4 bilateral 4	severe 3 mild 5	dip 5 flat 3	poor 3 moderate 1 good 4
Discos 8 cases	unilateral 7 bilateral 1	severe 5 mild 3	dip 1 flat 4 others 3	poor 5 moderate 2 good 1

CAUSATIVE FACTORS

Rock concerts. 128 persons who attended a concert were asked to fill out a questionnaire describing any cochlear symptoms and their duration. They were also asked about their proximity to the speakers, physical fatigue, mental fatigue, excitement during concerts and the extent to which they were exposed to loud sounds in daily life. Excluding proximity, as far as the relationship between cochlear symptoms and causative factors goes, we found that only mental fatigue was statistically significant. Also, a statistical analysis showed that those who complained of cochlear symptoms tended to be located nearer the speakers than those who didn't complain. We concluded that proximity to the speakers as well as mental fatigue were the primary factors responsible for the onset of hearing impairment.

Discos. A spectral analysis of the sounds in a disco showed a high energy peak in the lower frequency range around 500Hz. Since we know that the acoustic reflex is prominent when the level of stimulation is below 1500Hz, we performed an experiment with 20 young adults to determine whether or not the acoustic reflex had a tendency to diminish after the consumption of alcohol. The intake of whiskey was equivalent to 1.4 ml of ethyl alcohol per kilogram of body weight. We measured the alcohol level in the blood and the threshold and amplitude of both the contralateral and ipsilateral acoustic reflex, when stimulated at 500Hz. For contralateral stimulation, a statistically significant decrease in the amplitude could be observed only immediately after consumption, while for ipsilateral stimulation, a significant increase in the threshold was observed for a period of up to an hour after consumption. The acoustic reflex seems to have a tendency to decrease due to the consumption of alcohol, and as a result, people will have a greater chance of suffering hearing damage if they are exposed to loud sounds while drinking alcohol in places like discos.

CONCLUSION

Further detailed study of the causative factors must be carried out before we can determine positively the warning signs of possible hearing impairment and thus caution people who have them about the risks they face in going to places with loud music.

New dimensions in otorhinolaryngology - head and neck surgery, vol. 2.
E. Myers, editor

ACOUSTIC REFLECTIVITY FOR DIAGNOSIS OF MIDDLE EAR EFFUSIONS: COMPARISON WITH RESULTS OF MYRINGOTOMY

MARVIN FRIED (1), JAMES KELLY (2), HOWARD ZUBICK* (3), DAVID VERNICK (4), AND MARSHALL STROME (5)
Joint Center for Otolaryngology, Harvard Medical School, 398A Brookline Avenue, Boston, MA 02215
*Speech & Hearing, Brigham & Women's Hospital, 75 Francis Street, Boston, MA 02115

ABSTRACT: The acoustic reflectometer (Acoustic Otoscope) is a new hand-held portable instrument that uses reflected sound from the tympanic membrane surface to assess the presence of a middle ear effusion (MEE). An accurate reading can be attained with up to 90% of the external auditory canal obstructed and in a crying infant. It is presumed that the greater the reflectivity of the sound stimulus, the more likely a MEE is present.

The predictive value of an acoustic reflectometer (Acoustic Otoscope) in determining the presence of a middle ear effusion was assessed in 59 children (118 ears) undergoing myringotomy and ventilation tube insertion (Table I). The instrument is 90% accurate in predicting the presence of fluid or air in the middle ear and is less accurate (55%) in predicting the presence of a partially fluid-filled mesotympanum.

MATERIALS AND METHODS: Fifty-nine children, 1-13 years of age were studied after informed consent was obtained. All children were studied pre and post-operatively on the day they were to undergo bilateral myringotomy and ventilation tube insertion.

Pneumatic otoscopy was performed by the surgeon (MF, JK or MS) just prior to the procedure to assess the presence of middle ear effusion. Degree of canal obstruction (none, partial, total) and agitation of the patient were documented. The acoustic reflectometer was then used bilaterally. Two readings were obtained from each ear - the highest reflectivity being taken as the correct measurement.

With the child fully anesthetized, repeat acoustic reflectometer readings were obtained prior to myringotomy.

CONCLUSION: Our present study demonstrates the accuracy of the acoustic reflectometer in diagnosing either the presence of a fluid-filled or air fluid middle ear. In the case of a partially fluid-filled ear, its utility is yet to be delineated. The effect of anesthesia on the middle ear effusion awaits further clarification.

REFERENCES

1. Shurin PA, Pelton SI. Tympanometry in the diagnosis of middle ear effusion. N Eng J Med. 296:412-417, 1977.

2. Cantekin EI, Bluestone CD, Fria TJ, Stool SE, Berry QC, Sabo DL. Identification of otitis media with effusion in children. Ann Otol Rhinol Laryngol (Suppl 68) 89:190-195, 1980.

3. Teele DW, Klein JO, Rosner B, Bratton L, Fisch GR, Mathieu OR, Porter PJ, Starobin SG, Tarlin LD, Younes RP. Middle ear disease and the practice of pediatrics - burden during the first five years of life. JAMA 249:1036-1029, 1983.

4. Teele DW, Teele JH. Detection of middle ear effusion by acoustic reflectometry. J Pediatr 104:832-838, 1984.

5. Matz, GJ, Rattenborg CG, Holaday DA. Effects of nitrous oxide on middle ear pressure. Anesthesiology 28:948-950, 1967.

6. Davis J, Moore, JRM, Lahiri SK. Nitrous oxide and the middle ear. Anaesthesia 34:147-151, 1979.

TABLE I

Correlation Between Reading from Acoustic Otoscope and Surgical Determination of Presence or Absence of MEE

Surgical Findings

	Acoustic Otoscope Reading	Amount of MEE at the time of surgery: Full	Greater than 2/3 Full	1/3-2/3 full	Less than 1/3 full	None
	0	1	1	2	1	14
Clear	1	1	0	1	0	4
	2	0	0	1	2	6
	3	1	0	1	1	6
cut-off*	4	0	0	3	2	6
	5	4	3	2	2	3
MEE	6	4	1	5	2	1
	7	8	2	0	0	0
	8	10	0	1	0	0
	9	0	0	0	0	0
	Total	29	7	16	10	40
	No. Correct	26	6	8	4	36
	% Correct	90%	86%	50%	40%	90%
	Average Reflectivity	6.3	5.0	4.1	3.7	2.0

Summary: Sensitivity (Full effusion) = 32/36 = 90%
Sensitivity (Partial effusion) = 12/26 = 55%
Sensitivity (Clear ear) = 36/40 = 90%

*Manufacturer's suggested cut-off point

New dimensions in otorhinolaryngology - head and neck surgery, vol. 2.
E. Myers, editor

DIABETES MELLITUS AND COCLEOVESTIBULAR DISTURBANCE

A.G. PIRAS, L.C. OLIVEIRA, E. LOCKHART, P. BRANDI, H.E. GUAITA, M.B. SAHAGUN

HOSPITAL ITALIANO - BUENOS AIRES, ARGENTINA

INTRODUCTION

Diabetes Mellitus is a complex disturbance produced by a lack of insulin activity.

Microvasculopathy is actually the pathognomonic expression of this illness.

It consists initially in a thicking of the basel membranes due to deposits of glucoproteic substances. This fact is probably linked to the modern concept of profeic-glycocilation which is most evidently expressed in the glycociled haemoglobine.

Jorgensen studied (1963) the temporal bone of 30 diabetic patients and found a thickening of the capillar walls by PAS positive substances at the stria vascularis, modiolus and inner ear canal. According to different authors, Schuknent, Edgar, Harril, Mangabeira Albernaz, main causes could be resumed; principaly the vascular origin, neuval degeneration, toxic alterations produced by substances of altered metabolism and desequilibrium of ionic relation in the endolymph.

In this paper, we intend to compare 30 diabetics with 30 non-diabetic patients, all of them with cocleovestibular symtoms, trying to find out whether there is any difference beteen both groups.

MATERIAL AND METHODS

Two groups of 30 patients each, were included in these studies. The first group formed by 30 diabetics, 16 female and 14 male, ages between 45 and 82 years old. The second group (control group) included non-diabetic patients of same sex and age of the first group.

All the diabetic patients were studied in the Nutritional Clinic of the Italian Hospital following criterion extablished by the "National Diabetic Date Group" in 1979.

The duration of the illness varied between 1 and 24 years (average age 10.4 years); three patients were insulin dependent and 27, insulin independent. Eight of these patients showed vascular lessions inherent to diabetics.

The control group was formed with otoneurological patients of the same age and sex like the diabetic group.

Symptomotology of both groups:

	NON-DIABETICS (30)	DIABETICS (30)
SICKNESS	14	11
VERTIGO	13	18
VERTIGO & NEUROVEGATATIVE SIGNS	5	0
INSTABILITY	14	18
LATERO-PULSION	8	10
UNILATERAL HIPOACUSIA	4	2
BILATERAL HIPOACUSIA	15	11
TINITUS	3	2

All the patients were examined and were tested by tone audimetric and veslibular study with electronistagmographic (Mingograph 34). The vestibular investigation was made based on the the comparison of the mean average of the speed of the slow component of the nystagmus checked in the response of the Hallpike test. The measure was obtained every 30 seconds. The results were analyzed by traditional statistical methods.

DISCUSSION

Our goal was to determine whether there could be any influence of diabetes in the genisis of cocleovestibular signs specifically related to age. The comparison of the results of the diabetic group, with those of the control group, demonstrated the influence of this illness is almost nonexistant and the cocleovestibular response quite similar in both groups.

The audiometric curves obtained are very much alike and show the typical pattern of presbyacusis. These suggest the cause of the hearing loss among the diabetics are the same as the control group. What the veslibular function concerns we have found, is a predominance of the nyslagmus of the peripheral type. This being the percentage of central alteration which is very low. The caloric test response supports the conclusion mentioned above. In this way we conclude the primary cause of the cocleovesibular damage of the diabetics, as well as the control group, is due the vascular alteration and the toxic factor or the ionic changes that don't play an important etiologic action on the chronic process that appears in older people.

© 1985 Elsevier Science Publishers B.V. (Biomedical Division)
New dimensions in otorhinolaryngology - head and neck surgery, vol. 2.
E. Myers, editor

THE APPLICATION OF HUMAN AND ANIMAL TISSUE FOR TESTING HUMORAL ANTIBODIES IN INNER EAR DISEASE

WEI N-R, GIEBEL W, KAUPP H, PLESTER D
University E.N.T.-Clinic, Silcherstraße 5, D-7400 Tübingen, GFR

INTRODUCTION

In some inner ear diseases as Morbus Menière, sudden hearing loss and progressive hearing loss the humoral antibodies against tissue were found to be more frequent in the serum of patients as in a normal collective without inner ear disorders (2,3,4). The assay by immunhistological techniques were up to now carried out mainly on fresh heterolog tissue or fixated and decalcified human temporal bones (3,4). Fresh human tissue promises to be more sensitive then after fixation and decalcification. The present study was performed to evaluate the differences between human and animal tissue as well as between fresh and fixated tissue in respect to their sensitivity in demonstrating humoral antibodies.

MATERIAL AND METHODS

The main test object was kidney tissue from mice anc human. The latter was obtained be nephrectomy in hyponephrcma. The tissue specimen were divided into three groups. 1. fresh tissue kept frozen all the time, 2. fresh tissue defrosted and frozen again and 3. tissue fixated with formaldehyde and frozen again. The six different tissue specimens were mounted on one block and cut, transferred to a coverslide und incubated simultaneously. Incubation was performed with a "positive" and a "negative" patient's serum and without serum as a control.

RESULTS

Mouse tissue shows a high degree of unspecific reaction with the FITC-marked antiserum irrespectively whether it was fixed or not. Human tissue proved to be relatively insensitive when it was fixed before use. The only exception is the perivascular connective tissue which shows similar reaction with humoral

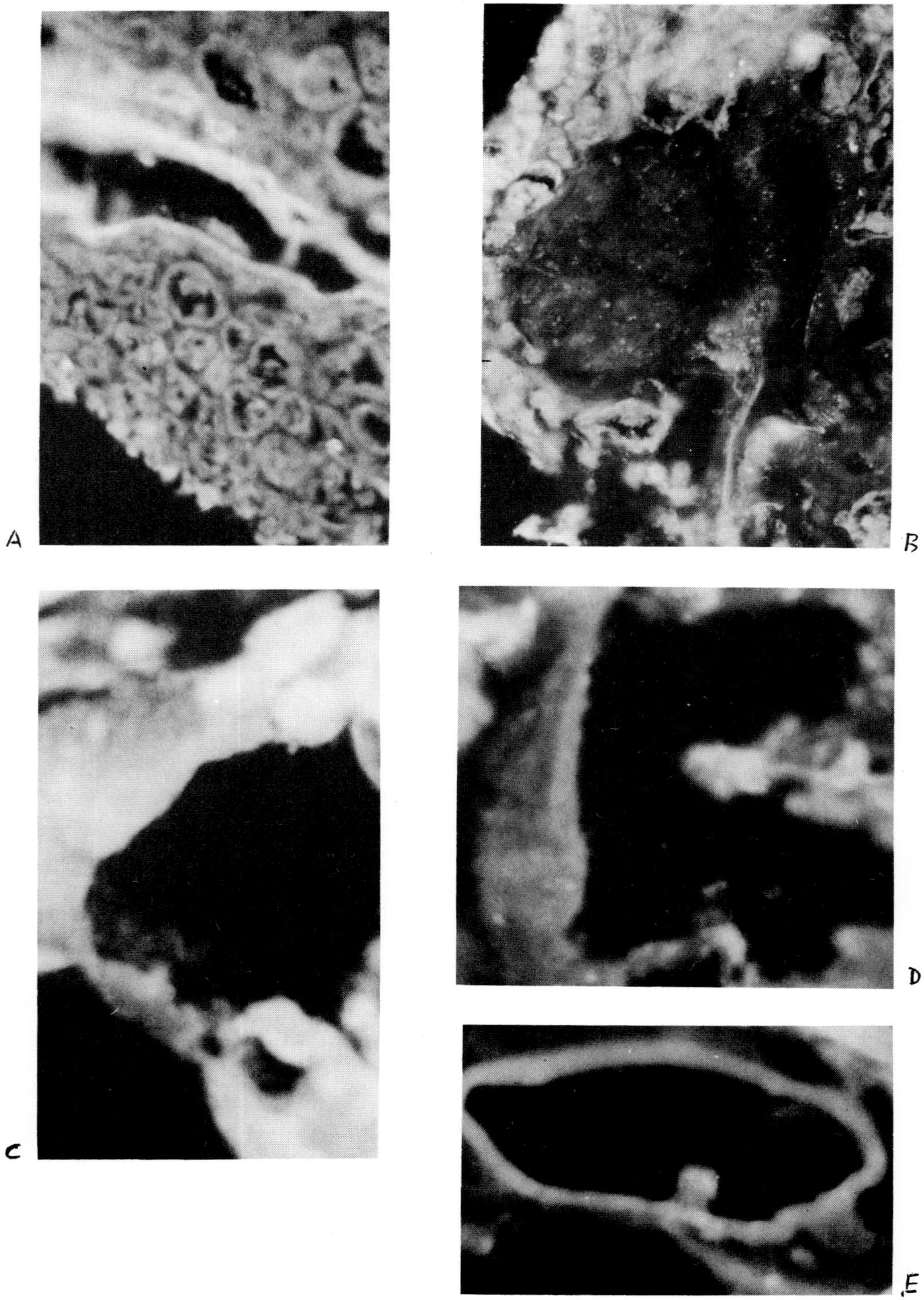
A
B
C
D
E

antibodies whether fixed or not. Human inner ear tissue shows similar reactions as human kidney tissue.

CONCLUSIONS

From the findings presented we can draw the following conclusions: Fresh human kidney tissue is most suitable for testing humoral antibodies in serum of patients with inner ear diseases.
Human kidney gives better differentiation than mouse kidney.
Fresh tissue is more sensitive than fixated tissue. Fresh human kidney tissue is easier to obtain and to handle than fresh human inner ear tissue.
Fresh human kidney tissue is recommended for studies on humoral antibodies in inner ear diseases.

REFERENCES

1. Arnold W (1984): Möglichkeiten der immunfluoreszensmikroskopischen Diagnostik am entkalkten menschlichen Felsenbein. Laryng.Rhinol. 63:260-265
2. Elies W (1983): Ein Fall von erfolgreicher Dexa-Methason-Behandlung bei beidseitiger chronisch-progredienter Innenohrschwerhörigkeit. HNO 31:443-444
3. Elies W (1983): Beiträge zur Ätiologie und Pathogenese ein- und doppelseitiger cochlear-vestibulärer Strömungen. Habilitationsschrift, Aachen
4. Giebel W, Kaupp H, Plester D (1985): Testing autoimmune reactions in inner ear diseases using fresh human inner ear and kidney tissue. Arch Otorhinolaryng (in press)

This study was supported by Breuninger-Stiftung, Stuttgart

Legend to figure:

Human kidney incubated with negative (A) and positive (B) serum.

Hamster cochlea incubated with negative (C) and positive (D) serum.

Hamster ampulla incubated with positive serum (D).

New dimensions in otorhinolaryngology - head and neck surgery, vol. 2.
E. Myers, editor

DETECTION OF VESTIBULAR ASYMMETRY BY DYNAMIC CHARACTERISTICS OF THE VESTIBULO-OCULAR SYSTEM

Y.SHIBATA, T.TOKITA, H.MIYATA AND Y.ITO
Dept.of Otolaryngology, Gifu University School of Medicine, Gifu, Japan

INTRODUCTION

To detect unilateral labyrinthine lesions, the dynamic characteristics of right and left vestibulo-ocular systems were displayed separately.

EXAMINATIONS SYSTEM

An examinee was seated on a rotating chair, the head and trunk fixed, and a sinusoidal pendular rotation was administered with eyes open in the dark, amplitude within ±10° and frequencies less than 3 Hz. Chair rotation was as rondom as possible. The head movement and eye movement data were stored on a computer disc at a sampling rate of 10 Hz for 120 sec. For data processing, saccadic eye movements were eliminated from eye movements, and the eye velocity curve was resolved into right and left directed eye movements. The transfer function was calculated using an autoregressive analysis, taking head movements as input data, and eye movements and right and left directed eye movements respectively, as output data. The results were displayed as Bode plots.

SUBJECTS

Ten normal subjects and 8 patients with unilateral labyrinthine disturbance were examined. Patients received examinations 2 weeks to 15 years after onset, and unilateral labyrinthine disturbance was diagnosed by caloric test.

RESULTS

(1) In a normal subject (Fig.1), gains for the vestibulo-ocular system increased at a rate of 5 dB / decade as the frequency was increased from 0.01 Hz to 3 Hz, indicating frequency dependent gain enhancement. Phases were about -180°. In the right and left directed vestibulo-ocular systems, gains were decreased below the level of the vestibulo-ocular system by about 4 dB at 0.1 Hz.

(2) In a patient with left labyrinthine disturbance (Fig.2), who was examined third week after onset, gains for the right vestibulo-ocular system were lower than the normal level. Phases were about 180°. Gains for the right directed vestibulo-ocular system were lower than those for the left directed vestibulo-ocular system. The gain decrease was 5.7 dB at 0.01 Hz, and 1.4 dB at 0.1 Hz, indicating the differences in gain were more remarkable at low frequencies.

(3) In another patient with right labyrinthine disturbance, who was examined

1 year and 4 months after onset, gains for the left vestibulo-ocular system were almost equivalent to the normal level. Phases were about -180°. Gains for the right directed vestibulo-ocular system were not distinctly different from those for the left directed vestibulo-ocular system. Eye movements towards healthy side were compensated. The differences in gain between right and left directed vestibulo-ocular systems were not detected in patients who received examinations more than 3 months after onset.

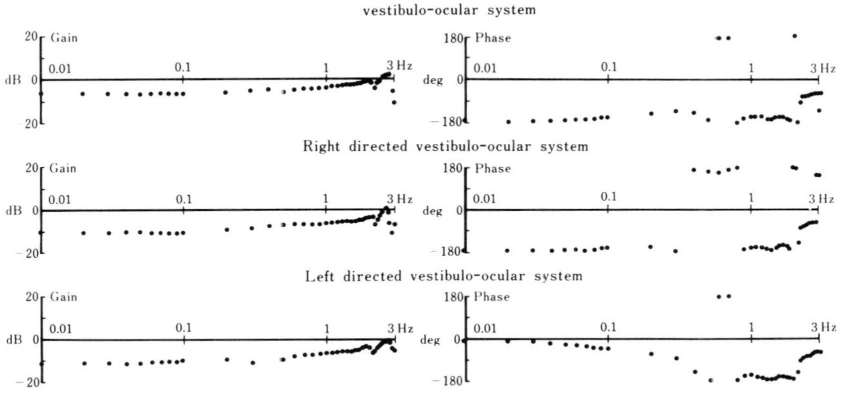

Fig. 1. Bode plots of the transfer function in a normal subject

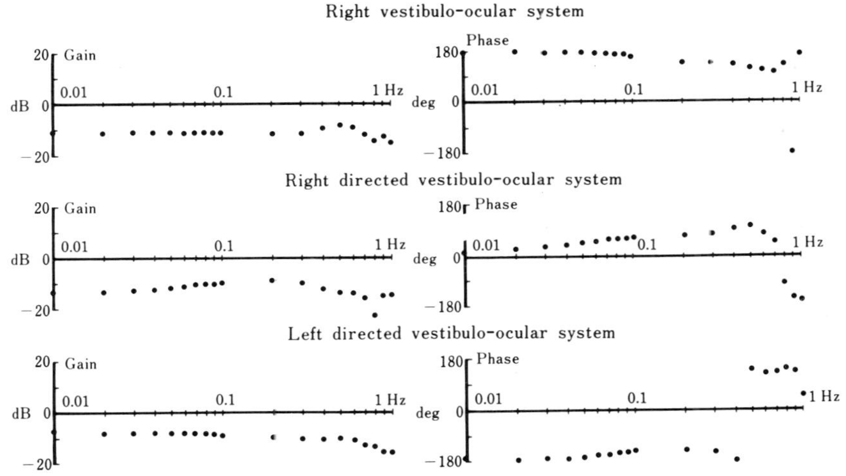

Fig. 2. Bode plots of the transfer function in a patient with left labyrinthine disturbance

© 1985 Elsevier Science Publishers B.V. (Biomedical Division)
New dimensions in otorhinolaryngology - head and neck surgery, vol. 2.
E. Myers, editor

CT RADIOLOGIC CRITERIA IN THE MANAGEMENT OF FRONTAL SINUS FRACTURE

PHILIP G. LIU,M.D.* JOSEPH B. JACOBS,M.D.* DEBORAH L. REEDE,M.D.**
WENDY A. COHEN,M.D.** HOWARD M. BERG,M.D.* NOEL L. COHEN, M.D.*

NYU Medical Center, Department of Otolaryngology* and Department of Radiology**, 550 First Avenue, New York, New York 10016

INTRODUCTION

The evaluation of frontal sinus fracture (FSF) requires more than physical examination and plain radiographs.[1] Over the last three decades complex motion tomography (CMT) has been the principal modality in assessing for posterior table, sinus floor, fronto-nasal duct (FND) and difficult anterior table fracture (fx). However, high resolution computed tomography (HRCT) is now widely recognized to be superior to CMT in the evaluation of FSF.[2,3] Because of its simplicity, speed, amount of information supplied and its superiority in delineating soft tissue and bony details, HRCT is now the predominant diagnostic modality utilized in the assessment of FSF in most centers. Since HRCT has been used in the evaluation of facial trauma only recently, to date studies in the management of FSF have been based on CMT. This report derives from the NYU-Bellevue Medical Center's experience with the management of FSF based on HRCT.

MATERIALS AND METHODS

Charts and radiographs of 16 patients with CT demonstrable FSF admitted to the NYU-Bellevue Medical Centers between June 1980 to December 1984 were analyzed with emphasis on clinical presentation, CT findings, therapeutic modality utilized, intra-operative findings and post-op follow-up. Non-contrast axial and coronal CT scans utilizing 5 mm cuts with 5 mm intervals were performed through the sinuses. Scans were performed with extended bone window and soft tissue settings. Based on HRCT and clinical findings, these patients were categorized preoperatively into groups requiring observation only, simple reduction in those requiring sinus obliteration or combined neurosurgical management. (Table 1)

RESULTS

Six patients required observation only; 6 patients required reduction of anterior table fx and 4 patients required sinus obliteration. Ages varied between 22 and 64 years with a male to female ratio of 15:1. The mechanism of injury were 11 due to assault, 4 due to vehicular accident and 1 due to domestic accident.

Edema over the site of injury was the most common physical finding regardless of the extent of anterior wall displacement. Two of 6 patients with significant displacement had no palpable deformity. All patients that underwent reduction and obliteration had intra-operative findings justifying the therapeutic modality chosen. The location and nature of both anterior and posterior wall fx by HRCT correlated well with the intra-operative findings. Anterior ethmoid cell injury regarded as CT evidence of FND injury was present in 5 patients. FND obstruction was confirmed intra-operatively by sinus peroxide irrigation failing to communicate with the nasal cavity in 3 of 4 patients. Pneumocephalus noted in 3 of 4 patients was accompanied by CT evidence of significant posterior wall fx. Thirteen of 16 patients had follow-up varying between 0-4 years. To date there has been no complication.

TABLE 1

FSF CLASSIFICATION BASED ON MANAGEMENT MODALITY

MANAGEMENT GROUP	TYPE OF FRACTURE
OBSERVATION (6)	Minimal/non-displaced ant. wall fx (6)
	Non-displaced post. wall fx (1)
	Non-obstructive FND injury (1)
REDUCTION (6)	Displaced/comminuted ant. wall fx (6)
OBLITERATION/EXENTERATION (4)	Displaced/communicating post. wall fx (4)
Combined neurosurgical repair	Sinus floor fx (1)
	FND injury with obstruction (3)

DISCUSSION

Prior to HRCT; due to the limitation of CMT indications for mandatory exploration of FSF have ranged from all posterior wall fx regardless of degree of displacement to routine exploration of all types of FSF because of the high incidence of occult FND injury. However, as HRCT can precisely define FSF relating to displacement of anterior, posterior wall, or sinus floor fx and suggest FND injury, we feel that management can now be based on the anatomic pathology as delineated by HRCT.

Non-displaced fx without FND obstruction regardless of which sinus wall involved requires observation only. FND patency can be assessed by serial sinus x-rays in non-surgical cases. Anterior table fx with CT showing significant displacement with or without gross palpable deformity requires reduction. Sinus obliteration is the recommended treatment for FND obstruction, significant cranial-sinus communication and floor fx because FND obstruction is known to be associated with mucocele and suppurative complications, while communicating posterior wall fx with CNS complications.[4,5]

REFERENCES

1. Bordley JE, Farrior JB (1981) Frontal Sinus Fractures and Complications, In English (ED): Otolaryngology Vol III, Chap 28 p 1-22, Harper & Row, Baltimore.

2. Rowe LD, Miller E, Brandt-Zawidksi A (1981) CT in Maxillo-facial Trauma. Laryngoscope 91:745-757.

3. Noyek AM, Cooper PE, et al (1982) Sophisticated CT in Complex Maxillo-facial Trauma. Laryngoscope 92: Supplement 27, p1-17.

4. Hybel RL, Newman MS (1977) Posterior Table Fractures of the Frontal Sinus: 1: An Experimental Study, II Clinical Aspects. Laryngoscope 87:171-179, 1740-1745.

5. May M, Ogura H, et al (1970) Fronto-nasal Duct Injury In Frontal Sinus Fractures. Arch Otolaryngol 92:534-538.

New dimensions in otorhinolaryngology - head and neck surgery, vol. 2.
E. Myers, editor

ULTRASONOGRAPHY OF THE PARANASAL SINUSES - A SCREENING METHOD IN CLINICAL ROUTINE

MAGNUS JANNERT AND LARS ANDREASSON
Dept of Otorhinolaryngology, University of Lund, Malmö General Hospital, S-214 01 Malmö (Sweden)

INTRODUCTION

Ultrasound for medical use has got an increased importance within different fields during the last decades. Keidel[1] already in 1947 indicated the possibility to use ultrasound in diagnosing diseases of the paranasal sinuses, but it was not until the middle of the seventies that Mann et al.[2] started to test the method clinically. The results presented were satisfactory but no suitable equipment to make the method more commonly used was available.

METHODS

Initiated by Professor Sven Ingelstedt our group in 1978 developed a simplified mobile diagnostic ultrasound equipment (Sinuson 810). After experimental and clinical tests of the equipment[3] the method has been in regular use since 1981 at the ENT-clinic in Malmö, Sweden.

RESULTS

The reduction in number of radiographic examinations is seen in Fig. 1. During 1978, just before the ultrasonic equipment was introduced in Malmö, 2 522 patients were subjected to X-ray examination at our Hospital. Already in 1979 the number of sinus X-rays had decreased to 1 830, and in 1982 1 026 radiographic investigations only were performed, i.e. a reduction by more than 50 % since 1978. This decrease means a considerable reduction in ionizing radiation and also saving of money and time. Furthermore, the diagnostic reliability increases and the therapy effect can be controlled[3].

CONCLUSIONS

Ultrasonic investigation of the paranasal sinuses is a new application of a method, some decades old, which gives a high diagnostic reliability without any loss of time and in a harmless way. This makes the method suitable as screening test in separating healthy air-containing sinuses from diseased ones. Of course, X-ray examination is of great value, e.g. in diagnostically uncertain cases and always when sinus surgery is planned.

REFERENCES

1. Keidel W (1947): Über die Verwendung des Ultraschalls in der klinischen Diagnostik, Ärztliche Forschung 1:349
2. Mann W, Beck Chl, Apostolidis Th (1977): Liability of ultrasound in maxillary sinus disease. Arch Otorhinolaryngol 215:67-74
3. Jannert M, Andréasson L, Holmer NG, Lörinc P (1982): Ultrasonic examination of the paranasal sinuses. Acta Otolaryngol (Stockh) Suppl 389

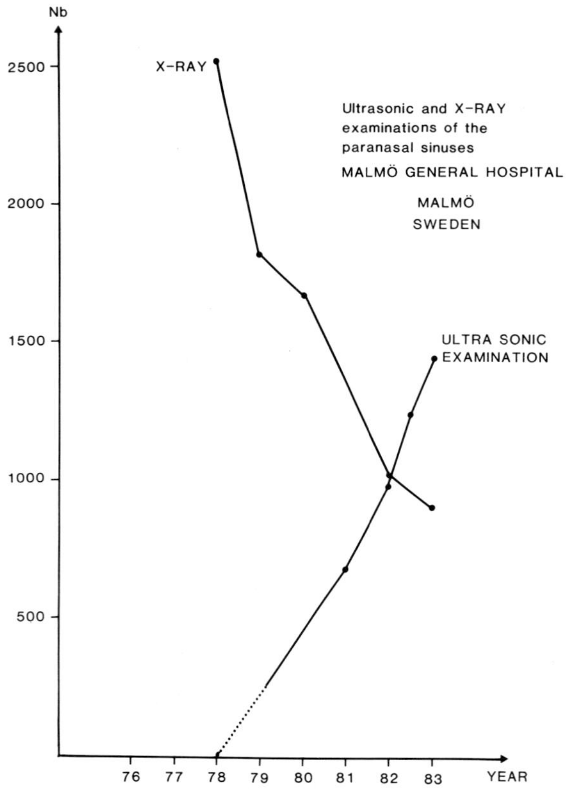

Fig. 1. Number of radiographic and ultrasonic examinations during 1978-1983 in Malmö.

New dimensions in otorhinolaryngology - head and neck surgery, vol. 2.
E. Myers, editor

TRANSMISSION ELECTRON MICROSCOPIC STUDY OF THE NOSE CILIA IN CHILDREN WITH CHRONIC AND RECURRENT AIRWAY INFECTIONS OF UNKNOWN ORIGIN : DIAGNOSIS OF IMMOTILE-CILIA SYNDROME

J BYLOOS*, J RAMET**, N ROM**, A MALFROOT**, PAR CLEMENT*
Depts. of Otolaryngology*, Pediatrics** and Anatomopathology, Free University of Brussels, AZ - VUB, Belgium

INTRODUCTION

This study deals with transmission electron microscopic examination of the nose cilia. Dyskinetic or dysfunctional cilia clinically result in the "immotile-cilia syndrome". It is a hereditary disorder characterized by recurrent chronic infections of the respiratory tract, and by a reduced fertility. In half of the patients, a situs inversus is encountered[1 2 3]

PURPOSE OF THE STUDY

The purpose of this study was to screen patients presenting recurrent airway infections for which typical etiologies had been ruled out, and to study the ultrastructure of their cilia with the help of a transmission electron microscope (TEM).

MATERIAL AND METHODS

Fifty-four children, aged 0 to 14 years, were investigated from 1980 through 1984 : 3 patients with nasal polyps; 39 patients with chronic infections of the respiratory tract. In addition, in one of them a sample was taken during a healthy period; 6 patients with Kartagener's triad (situs inversus, sinusitis, bronchiectasis); 1 neonate with situs inversus and respiratory distress syndrome; 1 patient with dextrocardia and bronchopulmonary problems; 1 patient with sinobronchial complaints, who has a brother and a sister presenting the Kartagener's triad; 1 healthy sister of a Kartagener, and finally, one healthy neonate was included as control. A nasal biopsy specimen of 2 mm^3 was taken from the concha inferior, using a microcurette. After staining, those tissue samples were ready for TEM examination.

RESULTS

Eighteen of the preparations from the 39 sinobronchitis patients could not be used because they included too few or no cilia. Five patients showed a normal ciliary ultrastructure. In 3/4 of the sinobronchitis patients, in 5 patients with the Kartagener syndrome and in the neonate with situs inversus, complete or partial loose of the dynein arms was a prominent feature, as well as ciliary disorientation. In one patient with situs inversus, absence of spokes was noted, while the dynein arms were normally present. Compound cilia were noted in all patients with nasal polyps, in 11 out of the 21 patients with chronic airway infection, in 5 out of the 6 Kartageners, in the patient with dextrocardia, and in the neonate with situs inversus. Supernumerary microtubules were found in 9 patients with sinobronchitis, in all the Kartageners, in one patient with nasal polyps and in the neonate with situs inversus. The patient on whom the biopsy was performed during a healthy period, showed the same ultrastructural anomalies as in the episodes of complaints. The brother of the two patients with the Kartagener syndrome, presented the same anomalies as the Kartagener children. The healthy sister of a Kartagener showed partial loose of the dynein arms and ciliary disorientation in certain cilia only. The ciliary ultrastructure was found to be normal in the control neonate.

DISCUSSION

It is important to establish a distinction between congenital and acquired anomalies. As congenital anomalies, we will note the complete or partial loose of the dynein arms and the ciliary disorientation, as well as anomalies of the spokes[4 5]. This is in contrast to the compound cilia and supernumerary microtubules which have already been described in the literature in cases of previous infectious diseases[6]. A second important point is the need for an early diagnosis as part of the therapeutic approach : from that very moment at least, symptomatic treatment can be instituted, as well as prevention in the form of physiotherapy and postural drainage, with the hope that this type of management will prevent bronchiectasis and ensure a life-long, almost normal, existence for these patients.

We feel it would be highly recommended to subject the nasal mucosa of all children who belong to that risk group to an early examination.

REFERENCES

1. White BL, Catlin FI, Stenback WA, Hawkins ED, Seil Heimer DK (1980) The immotile-cilia syndrome, one cause of persistent upper respiratory tract infections. Int J Pediatr Otorhinolaryngol 2 : 337-346
2. Goldman AS, Schochet SS Jr, Howell JT (1980) The discovery of defects in respiratory cilia in the immotile-cilia syndrome. J Pediatr 96 : 244-247
3. Afzelius B, Mossberg B (1983) In : Mc Graw-Hill (eds) The metabolic basis of inherited disease : the immotile-cilia syndrome including Kartagener's syndrome. Stanbury
4. Sturgess JM, Chao J, Wong J, Aspin N, Turner JAP (1979) Cilia with defective radial disease. New Engl J Med 300 : 53-56
5. Antonelli M, Modesti A, De Angelis M, Marcolini P, Lucarelli N, Crifo S (1981) Immotile-cilia syndrome : radial spokes deficiency in a patient with Kartagener's triad. Acta Pediatr Scand 70 : 571-573
6. Takasaka T, Sato M, Onodera A (1980) Atypical cilia of the human nasal mucosa. Ann Otol 89 : 37-45

© 1985 Elsevier Science Publishers B.V. (Biomedical Division)
New dimensions in otorhinolaryngology - head and neck surgery, vol. 2.
E. Myers, editor

MIDLINE PALATAL SPLIT FOR ACCESS TO THE CENTRAL SKULL BASE, CERVICAL SPINE, BRAINSTEM AND DEEPER NEUROLOGIC STRUCTURES

CHARLES M. JOHNSON, III, M.D., STEPHEN HARGETT, M.D.,
*T.S. PARK, M.D. AND *CHARLES HAWORTH, M.D.
Department of Otolaryngology - Head and Neck Surgery
*Department of Neurosurgery, The University of Virginia Medical Center, Charlottesville, Virginia 22908 (USA)

Multiple surgical approaches to the central skull base have been developed to allow removal of lesions while minimizing morbidity and maximizing exposure, including the transcervical subtemporal craniotomy, infratemporal fossa, rhinoseptal transphenoidal, and transpalatal approaches. One of the most versatile and technically least complicated has been the transpalatal, first reported by Brunk in 1909,[1] with either a midline palatal split or horizontal section based on both greater palatine vessels.[2,3]

The midline split operation for tumors of the cranio vertebral junction has been previously reported in adults, but not in children. We have successfully employed this technique for removal of an extradural clivus chordoma of the central skull base, ventral brainstem, and lateral gutters in a child.

SURGICAL TECHNIQUE

The uvula is incised into halves and the incision carried along the length of the soft palate through the median raphe, basing blood supply on the greater palatine vessels, and terminating in a "y" on the hard palate, allowing full flap retraction. The hard palate is resected in a posteroanterior direction until sufficient exposure is gained. The posterior pharyngeal wall is incised and resection of the anterior body of C_1 or of the clivus may be done with the high speed drill and tumor resected. Layered closure of the prevertebral fascia, pharyneal musculure, and mucus membrane of the posterior pharyngeal wall, followed by a three layer closure of the palate starting with the nasopharyngeal surface is done. A preformed acrylic obturator may be inserted after closure to maintain flap approximation. A tracheotomy has not been necessary; however, if extensive exposure of c-spine is made, it may be considered.

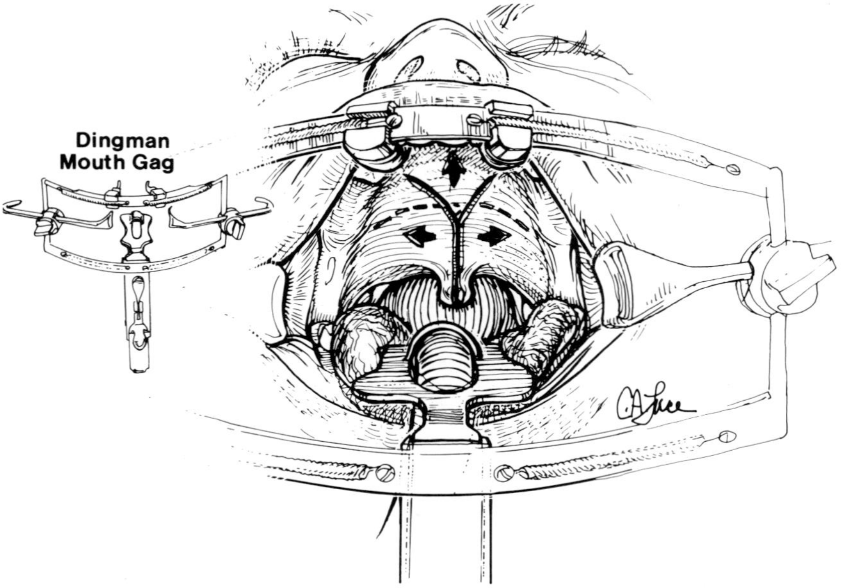

Fig. 1 Outline of Palatal Incision.

Speech has not been affected nor has necrosis of the palate lesion been noted. Infection has not been a problem, however, dural entry may be associated with morbidity not evidenced in our extradural resection.

This approach in children has allowed safe removal of large extradural lesions of the skull base. We feel it is a procedure of choice for the midline skull base in the pediatric population.

REFERENCES

1. Brunk A: A new case of unilateral osseous choanal occlusion: An operation through the palate. 2 Ohrenk 59:221-224, 1909.

2. Ruddy LW: A transpalatine operation for congenital atresia of the choana in the small child or infant. Arch Otolaryngol 41:432-438, 1945.

3. Alonso W, Black P, Connor G, and Uematsu S: Transoral transpalatal approach for resection of the clival chordoma. Laryngoscope 81:1626-1631, 1971.

New dimensions in otorhinolaryngology - head and neck surgery, vol. 2.
E. Myers, editor

INDICATIONS AND SURGICAL TECHNIQUES FOR LESIONS OF THE FACIAL NERVE DUE TEMPORAL BONE FRACTURES

R.F.Bento; A.Miniti and A.J.Tedesco-Marchese. Facial Nerve Group, Depts of Otolaryngology, Neurology and Neurosurgery, University of Sao Paulo, Medical School, Sao Paulo, Brazil

INTRODUCTION

Due to our emergence service our statistcs of Traumatic Peripheral Facial Palsy is bigger than of others ethiologies of facial paralysis. We studied for this paper 87 patients with traumatic facial palsys who were cared on in our service, from 1978 to 1982.

We found 87% of longitudinal fractures, 75% of transversal fractures and 6% of shattered ones. The motorcycle and motorcar accidents was the first incidence, followed by agressions and accidental falls.

Because of the very high incidence of the false positive in the site-diagnose of a lesion of the facial nerve in temporal bone trauma, (Bento R.F. (1)), and due to the some special characteristcs of a temporal bone trauma, we developped some criteriais to there management. We did not included, firearm projectil injuries in this series.

DIAGNOSIS AND SURGICAL INDICATIONS

The diagnose of a fracture of the temporal bone is made by history, physical examination and X-Ray (multidirecional tomography). We found C.T. Scan worse than convencional tomography to determine the local of fracture.

Once stablished that we have a fracture, the transversal and shattered ones was submitted to a imediate surgical exploration, because of the worse prognosis in our statistcs, Bento R.F. (1). In the longitudinal ones we use the same indication used to a idiophatic palsy patients. (Miniti A. (4)).

Eletrophisiologic evaluation and surgical exploration if we have a axioniotmese (more thant 90% of Damaged fibres). (Fisch U. (3)).

SURGICAL TECHNIQUES

The used approaches was:

a) Middle cranial fossa - 3 cases

b) Transmastoid - 11 cases

c) Total (Middle cranial fossa and Transmastoid) - 12 cases

We used the technique described by Fisch U. (3) for the middle fossa, and the classical transmastoid decompression, with the second and third portion exposion of the facial nerve.

In all cases we openned the facial nerve sheat.

RESULTS

Clinical Treatment: (61 cases 70,1%)

Evaluation in %

	Doctor	Patient
Excelent	68,8	54,1
Good	21,3	34,3
Regular	6,6	8,2
Bad	3,3	3,4

Surgical Treatment: (26 cases 29,9%)

Evaluation in %	Middle cranial fossa		Transmastoid		Total decompression	
	Doctor	Patient	Doctor	Patient	Doctor	Patient
Excelent	0	0	9	0	66,6	58,4
Good	33,3	0	45,5	27,2	25	41,6
Regular	33,3	66,6	27,2	54,5	8,4	-
Bad	33,3	33,3	18,3	18,3	-	-

COMENTS

As we can see above we have the best results in the group of clinical treatment, because we are in front of a neurotmesis of the nerve, and in the total nerve decompression group, because on trauma of the temporal bone maybe the fallopium canal is injuried in several places and is statistical significant, the better surgical results in these cases.

So, in facial paralysis due to fractures of the temporal bone if a surgical exploration is indicated the approach of choice is the total facial nerve decompression by the means of a middle cranial fossa approach and transmastoid approach.

REFERENCES

1 - Bento R.F.; Miniti A.; Ruocco J.R.:(1985) Traumatic Peripheral Facial Palsy, Diagnosis, Etiology and Treatment in: Preceedings of the V International Symposiumm in the facial nerve. Masson Paris.

2 - Fisch U.:(1977) Total facial nerve compression and electrical neuroniography in: Neurological Surgery of the ear. Birgmingham, Alabama, Aesculapius Publishing Company.

3 - Fisch U.; Esslen E.:(1972) Total intratemporal exposure of the facial nerve. Arch. Otolaryngol. 95:335-341-

4 - Miniti A.; Bento R.F.; Silveira J.A.M.:(1985) Bell's Palsy, Treatment and results in: Preceedings of the V Int. Simposiumm on the facial nerve. Masson Paris.

5 - Potter J.M.:(1964) Facial Palsy following head injury. Journal of Laryngology 78:645-657.

6 - Turner J.M.:(1944) Facial Palsy in head injuries. Lancet 246:756-767.

New dimensions in otorhinolaryngology - head and neck surgery, vol. 2.
E. Myers, editor

"PREDICTION OF OUTCOME OF UVULOPALATOPHARYNGOPLASTY USING PREOPERATIVE SOMNO-FLUOROSCOPY". *GEORGE P. KATSANTONIS, M.D., F.A.C.S., **JAMES K. WALSH, Ph.D., AND ***FESTUS J. KREBS, M.D. (*-***) Department of Otolaryngology - Head and Neck Surgery, St. Louis University School of Medicine, 1402 South Grand Blvd., St. Louis, Missouri 63104. **Sleep Disorders Center, Deaconess Hospital, 6150 Oakland, St. Louis, Missouri 63139

INTRODUCTION

Although uvulopalatopharyrgoplasty (UPPP) is beneficial to 50% to 60% of unselected patients with obstructive sleep apnea (OSA), the individual response to this operation remains unpredictable.[1,2] In a previous study by the authors it was reported that somnofluoroscopy (a lateral fluoroscopic study of the upper airway with synchronous polysomnography) provides valuable information about the dymanic function of the upper airway in patients with OSA.[3] We propose that individuals with occlusive episodes occurring in the oropharynx as demonstrated by somnofluoroscopy are expected to be good candidates for UPPP.

PATIENTS AND METHODS

Somnofluoroscopy was performed preoperatively on 34 consecutive patients undergoing UPPP for moderate to severe OSA. The somnofluoroscopy videotapes were scored either oropharynx or hypopharynx for: 1) the narrowest level of the airway during unobstructed breathing and 2) the level(s) of the airway at which occlusion occurred during apnea episodes. The patients were also categorized with respect to the degree of postoperative improvement in the apnea hypopnea index (A+HI) and severity index (SI: number of times oxygen saturation decreased below 85% per hour of sleep) into three groups, good responders (> 50% decrease in A+HI and > 85% decrease in SI), poor responders (∠ 50% decrease in both A+HI and SI) and mild responders (any other results).

RESULTS AND DISCUSSION

There were 13 (38.2%) good, 10 (29.4%) moderate and 11 (32.3%) poor responders in this series of patients. The various somnofluoroscopic patterns in relation to postoperative improvement are seen in the following table:

NARROWEST AIRWAY LEVEL	LEVEL(s) TO OCCLUDE	RESPONSE TO UPPP (N=34) GOOD	MODERATE	POOR	TOTAL NO:
O	O	12	4	3	19
O	O,H	0	2	2	4
O,H	O,H	0	3	3	6
H	H or O	1	1	3	5
		13	10	11	34

O=OROPHARYNX
H=HYPOPHARYNX

It is obvious that the majority of patients whose oropharynx was the narrowest level of the airway and the only level to occlude during an obstructive episode (favorable pattern) were good or moderate responders (85%). All other somnofluoroscopic patterns (unfavorable) were associated with much less favorable results. When statistically compared to all other patterns combined the

0,0 pattern was more frequently associated with a good UPPP response (X^2 = 22.67, DF = 2, P< .01).

Fiberoptic endoscopy and fluoroscopy have been utilized to visually examine the upper airway of OSA patients during sleep.[4] Somnofluoroscopy unlike fiberoptic pharyngoscopy provides visualization of the entire length of the upper airway prior to and during obstruction. The most interesting observation made during this procedure was the consistency of apnea dynamics (site and mechanism of obstruction) within an individual and the variability across OSA patients.[3] This variability may be related to CNS, anatomical or evolutionary factors and may account for the erratic response to the UPPP in our series and those of others.

In this series of patients 65% of the individuals with the favorable somnofluoroscopic pattern were good responders. This represents a 23% increase from the 42% good responder rate seen in the entire sample. Patients displaying unfavorable somnofluoroscopic patterns demonstrated only a 6.6% good and 26.6% moderate response rate to UPPP. It is therefore recommended that other treatment modalities be utilized when possible for OSA patients with significant hypopharyngeal involvement as seen during somnofluoroscopy (e.g. nasal c-pap, weight loss, tracheostomy). However, there was a small number of patients who did not respond well to UPPP in spite of a favorable somnofluoroscopic result. In addition, a few patients demonstrated a moderate response to UPPP although the somnofluoroscopic patterns were unfavorable. A number of coexistent and interactive factors that cannot be completely accounted for by somnofluoroscopy may be related to this small false-positive/negative rate. This may include position and sleep stage during somnofluoroscopy. In addition, some difficulty in the interpretation in obese individulas may contribute. Nevertheless, given the low morbidity risk of somnofluoroscopy, it appears to be a helpful procedure for selection of appropriate OSA candidates for UPPP.

REFERENCES.

1. Katsantonis GP, Walsh JK, Schweitzer PK, and Friedman, WH (1985) Further evaluation of uvulopalatopharyngoplasty in the treatment of obstructive sleep apnea. Otolaryngology Head & Neck Surgery. 93:(2)pp:244-250.

2. Fujita AS, Zorick, FJ, Conway W (1985) Evaluation of the effectiveness of uvulopalatopharyngoplasty. Laryngoscope. 95(1)pp:70-74.

3. Walsh, JK, Katsantonis, GP et al (1985) Somnofluoroscopy: A descriptive study of obstructive sleep apnea. Sleep. (In press).

4. Weitzman, DE, Pollack PC., et al (1978) The hypersomnia-sleep apnea syndrome: Site and mechanism of upper airway obstruction. Sleep Apnea Syndrome. pp:235-248. Alan R. Liss Corporation, New York.

New dimensions in otorhinolaryngology – head and neck surgery, vol. 2.
E. Myers, editor

THE CARBON DIOXIDE LASER PHOTOTHERMAL PEEL

RONALD ALLEN KIRSCHNER, B.C. McDonnell, R. Giuliano

The Institute For Applied Laser Surgery

Suite IL-17, Two Bala Plaza, Bala Cynwyd, Pa. 19004, U.S.A.

We currently use the term "Photothermal Peel" to describe a procedure which is very similar in nature to conventional dermabrasion. This technique has previously been called Laser Dermabrasion and Laserbrasion by a number of workers.

The Photothermal Peel may be used in place of conventional dermabrasion methods and chemical peels. If a lesion is being removed, the surgeon may obtain a tissue specimen by using a shave biopsy technique. This will provide confirmation of his clinical impression. It is, however, a limited specimen and should not be used for any problematic type of lesion. There should be no question in the operator's mind as to the benign nature of the lesion.

The changes that are wrought to tissue by any form of laser radiation are dependent upon several factors:

1. Power Setting
2. Spot Size
3. Duration of Exposure to the Laser Radiation

In nature, light is always accompanied by some degree of heat. It is both the light and the heat energies that create their resultant effect on tissue.

Procedure

The area to be treated is prepped with 70% alcohol. This is carefully washed from the operative field, with sterile saline, to eliminate any remaining vestiges of this combustible substance. The area is then draped with sterile wet towels. The patient's eyes must be protected with sterile wet eye pads or metal contact lenses, when one is working on the face. When working on other areas, the eyes may be protected by the same protective goggles that are worn by the O.R. staff.

The surgical site may be cooled by topical ice before the surgery progresses. This serves to decrease the effects of the thermal component of the beam. A small amount of local anesthetic in injected superficially to raise the are to be biopsied slightly from the surface. A shave biopsy is then obtained with a number 15 blade.

The Carbon Dioxide Laser is employed in a focussed or a slightly defocussed attitude over the lesioned area. The surgeon's hand will move in an oscillating fashion passing rapidly back and forth over the operative area in an even fashion. Between applications of the laser the operator will sequentially debride the treated superficial layer with a wet sponge. Following surgery the area appears much as tissue following a chemical peel. The patient will use a topical application of an antibiotic ointment several times daily. The wattage settings will vary with each surgeon. In our hands low settings ranging between 4-10 watts are usually employed.

This procedure is most effective for areas of lentigo senilis, flat keratoses and superficial scarring. As with all procedures of this type, the best results are obtained with fair skinned individuals with good skin trophicity.

New dimensions in otorhinolaryngology – head and neck surgery, vol. 2.
E. Myers, editor

PITUITARY TUMORS: DIAGNOSIS AND TREATMENT IN THE 1980's

ISAAC GOODRICH, M.D. and KEAT-JIN LEE, M.D.
Sections of Neurosurgery and Otolaryngology, Hospital of St. Raphael, New Haven, CT 06511 (USA)

INTRODUCTION

The diagnosis and treatment of pituitary tumors has changed dramatically over the past 15 years. This era has seen the initiation of radioimmunoassays of hypophyseal hormones, immunohistochemical tumor classification of secretory lesions, computerized tomography (CT), magnetic resonance imaging (MRI), digital intravenous subtraction angiography (DISA), the widespread acceptance of the transseptal, transsphenoidal (TSTS) microsurgical approach, and the use of bromocriptine for medical management of prolactinomas.

DIAGNOSIS

The most important aspect of diagnosis remains obtaining a careful history and physical examination. The major symptoms and signs are headache, visual difficulties, and endocrinopathy. Endocrine malfunction may present as either hypo- or hypersecretion. The majority of cases seen today are functional tumors[1], usually microadenomas (lesions less than 10 mm in diameter). Most cases of hypopituitarism present as prolactinomas, acromegaly, or Cushing's disease. Nonfunctional tumors are usually seen as macroadenomas with secondary symptoms of neural compression and/or hypopituitarism.

Once the clinical impression of a pituitary tumor is made, a series of endocrine screening studies are available. These include serum cortisol, ACTH, growth hormone, thyroid function tests, prolactin, FSH, and LH. More specific studies may be indicated, including TRH stimulation, oral glucose loading, and dexamethasone suppression testing.

The definitive diagnostic imaging study currently is CT scanning. CT scans are now accurate in diagnosing tumors as small as 2 to 3 mm in diameter. MRI has recently become available. It has several potential advantages over CT. No ionizing radiation is involved, nor are contrast agents used. Bone artifacts are not present. Visualization of the cavernous sinus and its contents, and the optic chiasm and nerves, is superior.[2,3] MRI is accurate in delineating the extent of macroadenomas, as well as localization of adjacent major vascular structures. Its degree of accuracy with microadenomas has yet to be determined. Difficulties with MRI include time duration required for the study[3] and a sense of claustrophobia with some patients.

If further visualization of vascular structures of the parasellar region is indicated, DISA will usually suffice. This involves computer enhanced visualization of appropriate vessels after venous injection, usually on an outpatient basis. Its morbity is extremely low.

TREATMENT

Medical therapy of nonsecreting tumors which present with hypopituitarism includes replacement cortisone and thyroid. Bromocriptine, a dopaminergic agent, has been extremely successful in treating prolactinomas. However, if this medication is stopped, tumor recurrence ensues. It has not been reliably successful in treating other pituitary tumors.

The TSTS approach is the preferable surgical approach to the pituitary in the vast majority of patients requiring surgery. It is considered the treatment of choice for patients with Cushing's disease, and is the preferred surgical approach for most patients with acromegaly, nonsecreting tumors, and prolactinomas who are surgical candidates. In experienced hands, TSTS surgery can obtain normal hormonal levels in over 70% of functional microadenomas, but in less than 50% of macroadenomas.[4] Craniotomy remains indicated in occasional selected cases.

Radiotherapy continues as an important therapeutic modality in some cases. This includes postoperative nonfunctional macroadenomas, functional tumors (micro- or macroadenomas) in which a persistently elevated hormone level exists after surgery and/or medical therapy, recurrent tumors, and poor surgical risk patients. The majority of cases (over 70%) will respond. In functional tumors, the maximal effect on excess hormone secretion may take several years. There is a delayed onset of hypopituitarism in about 20% of cases with previously normal endocrine function. Heavy particle radiation - proton beam or alpha particle therapy - may be employed with a similar success rate, usually in functional microadenomas without significant suprasellar extension.

REFERENCES

1. Wilson, CB (1984) J Neurosurg 61:814-833
2. Daniels, DL, Pojunas, KW, Pech, P, Haughton, VM (1984) Magnetic Resonance Imaging of the Sella and Justasellar Region. General Electric Company, Medical Systems Group, Milwaukee, p 2
3. Spetzler, RF, Zabramski, JM, Kaufman, B (1985) Neurosurg 16:511-524
4. Zervas, NT (1984) In: Black, PM, Zervas, NT, Ridgway, EC, Martin, JB (eds) Secretory Tumors of the Pituitary Gland. Raven Press, New York pp 378-380

© 1985 Elsevier Science Publishers B.V. (Biomedical Division)
New dimensions in otorhinolaryngology - head and neck surgery, vol. 2.
E. Myers, editor

SOME ANATOMICAL DATA RELATED TO THE TRANSNASO-SPHENOIDAL RESECTION OF THE PITUITARY FOSSA TUMORS

SHANGZE LING

Dept. of Otorhinolaryngology, The Affiliated Hospital of Guiyang Medical College, Guiyang, Guizhou Province, China

INTRODUCTION

Since the beginning of this century, the transnaso-sphenoidal resection of the pituitary fossa tumors has vastly been used in clinic. It has many merits than other routes used before. In China, it has been adopted since 1959. In order to afford some relevant anatomical data, we have measured 137 adult sagittal plane skulls.

MATERIAL AND METHODS

The measuring tools, including compasses, angulometer, set-square and ruler, take cm and degrees of angle as their unit.

According to the relationship between the sphenoid sinus and the sella turnica, we divided the developmental type of sinus into 6 groups. 1. Occipital sella(well developed). 2. Whole sella turnica. 3. Half sella. 4. Ante-sella. 5. Concha type(badly developed). and 6. Non-developed.

Then we measured the following 6 data. I. The shortest distance between the anterior nasal spine and the anterior wall of the sphenoid sinus. II. The shortest distance between the anterior nasal spine and the sella wall. III. The angle between the horizontal line and the line which joins the anterior nasal spine and the midpoint of the sella. IV. The shortest distance between the inferior margin of the nasal bone and the anterior wall of the sphenoid sinus. V. The shortest distance between the inferior margin of the nasal bone and the sella. VI. The depth of the sphenoid sinus along the line between the anterior nasal spine and the midpoint of the sella.(Figs 1 and 2).

RESULTS

The developmental type of the sphenoid sinus in this series are as follows: Occipital sella 12.4%, Whole sella 46%, Half sella 22.6%, Ante-sella 13.8%, Concha type 4.4% and Non-developed 0.8%.

The values of the 6 measured data are as follows: I. 5.49±0.44cm(4.7-7.0), II. 6.92±0.47cm(5.9-8.2), III. 31.16±4.75 degrees(20-44), IV. 4.97±0.42cm(4.1-6.3), V. 6.40±0.38cm(5.3-7.6), VI. 1.51±0.41cm

(0.3-2.4).

DISCUSSION

The different type of the sphenoid sinus in this series show that the status of pneumatization is poorer than other literature reported. It is probably influenced by the nationality and locality etc.

There are very few literature reports about the anatomical data of the transnaso-sphenoidal route. Hu et al reported the measuring data of 99 adult skulls, found that the distance between the anterior nasal spine and the anterior wall of the sphenoid sinus was 5.58± 0.045cm(4.8-7.0). Lee stated that this distance varied with the cranial contour and age. Our data show that the acquired values vary with the developmental type of the sphenoid sinus in positive proportion. Pu et al pointed out that the patients with occipital sella and whole sella are more suitable for the transnaso-sphenoidal operative route.

Our data might be useful for the transnaso-sphenoidal resection of the pituitary fossa tumors.

REFERENCES

1. Sen HC (1959) Surgery of the Ear, Nose and Throat. People's Publishers, Beijing, pp 211
2. Hu ML et al (1957) Chinese Journal of Otorhinolaryngology 5:257
3. Lee PS (1977) Rhinology. People's Publishers of Shanghai, Shanghai, pp 50
4. Pu GS et al (1964) Chinese Journal of Otorhinolaryngology 10:324

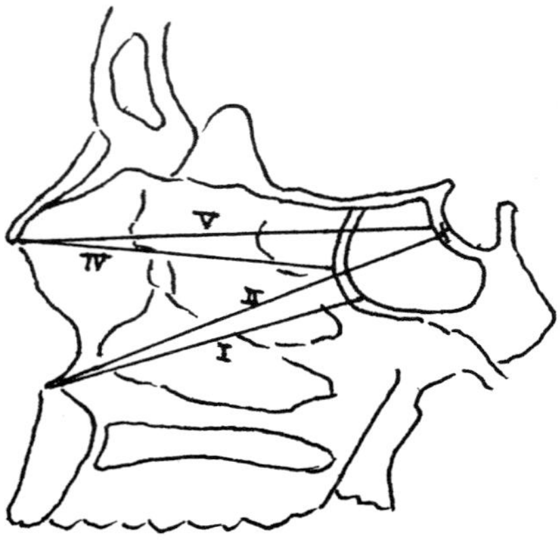

Fig. 1 Diagram of the measuring data

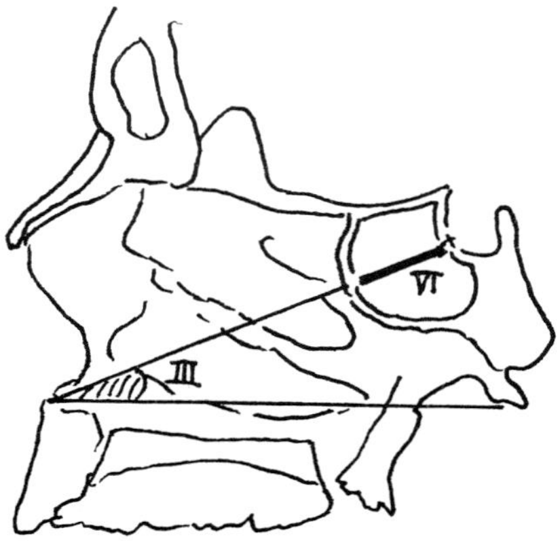

Fig. 2 Diagram of the measuring data

© 1985 Elsevier Science Publishers B.V. (Biomedical Division)
New dimensions in otorhinolaryngology - head and neck surgery, vol. 2.
E. Myers, editor

DISAGREEMENT BETWEEN METHODS OF NUTRITIONAL ASSESSMENT IN HEAD AND NECK CANCER

BERNARD S. LINN, DAVID S. ROBINSON

Veterans Administration Medical Center and University of Miami School of Medicine, 1201 N.W. 16th Street, Miami, Florida 33125 (USA)

INTRODUCTION

A major problem in assessing protein energy malnutrition (PEM) has been identification of patients for whom nutritional intervention was warranted. The prevalence of PEM in hospitalized patients has been found to be high, ranging from 20% to 40% depending on how PEM was assessed (1,2). The rate of PEM would be expected to be higher in head and neck cancer patients because of the symptoms of the disease. The diagnosis of PEM is often based on objective assessments of laboratory and anthropometric measurements. Although these areas are useful and often correlated with outcomes, no single measurement is consistently accurate in individual patients. Clinical assessment is the oldest and simplest way to assess malnutrition, but it is rarely used along with objective tests. To determine the relationship among anthropometric, clinical, and laboratory methods of measuring nutritional status, patients with head and neck cancer were studied.

MATERIALS AND METHODS

Immediately after admission to the surgical service in a VA Hospital, 80 men with head and neck cancer were evaluated with a 23-item Protein Energy Malnutrition Scale (PEMS) (3). Items rated on 4-point scales provide subscores for anthropometric, clinical, and laboratory areas. There are 4 anthropometric items (percent ideal body weight, percent weight loss, triceps skinfold, and midarm muscle circumference). The clinical covers 4 history items (inadequate intake, excessive nutrient losses, increased metabolic needs, and catabolic medications), and 6 physical examination items (cachexia, hair/nails, hepatomegaly/ascites, muscle atrophy, and skin change). The laboratory score is derived from 9 items (serum albumin, hemoglobin, lymphocytes, transferrin, retinol-binding protein, prealbumin, nitrogen balance, skin tests, and creatinine/height index). Scores in the 3 areas were averaged (range 1-4) so that areas were comparable. Scores of 2.5 or over indicate malnutrition. For this study, agreement between at least two areas was defined as true nutritional status. The 80 subjects were classified by number with malnutrition, number where all 3 areas agreed, and areas and directions of disagreement. The 3 subscores and total PEMS scores were also intercorrelated (Pearson Product Moment Correlations).

RESULTS

Table 1 shows that 50% had a total PEMS score of 2.5 or above. There was complete agreement of the 3 areas in 70% of the patients. For the 24 patients where one subscore disagreed, this happened 4 times for anthropometric, 5 times for clinical, and 15 times for laboratory scores. Direction of disagreement showed 1 out of 4 anthropometric, 2 out of 5 clinical, and 12 out of 15 laboratory scores pointed to malnutrition. Therefore, disagreement was 3 times as high for laboratory data and usually indicated malnutrition. Further, laboratory scores were correlated at somewhat lower levels with the other scores.

TABLE 1: AGREEMENT OF ANTHROPOMETRIC, CLINICAL, AND LABORATORY AREAS

AGREEMENT AND DISAGREEMENT	NUMBER	PERCENT
Agreement of All 3 Areas (above or below 2.5)	56	70
Number Malnourished	40	50
Areas of Disagreement (24 cases)		
Anthropometric	4	17
Clinical	5	20
Laboratory	15	63
Direction of Disagreement Toward Malnutrition		
Anthropometric	1	25
Clinical	2	40
Laboratory	12	80

CONCLUSIONS

Firstly, 70% agreement can be considered rather high between methods. This does not mean that any one area can as yet be used alone in evaluating patients. The study shows that clinical methods correlated highly with anthropometrics and significantly with laboratory data. Thus, a careful history and physical is an important part of assessment. Laboratory data can be misleading in that reduced serum proteins could imply hepatic disease, nephrosis, or protein losing enteropathy rather than malnutrition. Depressed cellular immunity can be related to infection, trauma, alcoholism, or age and not nutritional status alone. Because laboratory tests most often disagreed with other areas, these limitations need to be considered. False positive results from laboratory data alone could lead to nutritional intervention that would increase cost of care and possible patient discomfort.

REFERENCES

1. Bistrian BR, Blackburn GL, Hallowell E, et al (1974) JAMA 230:858.
2. Linn BS (1984 Am J Clin Nutr 39:66
3. Linn BS (1984) Ann Surg 200:747.

© 1985 Elsevier Science Publishers B.V. (Biomedical Division)
New dimensions in otorhinolaryngology - head and neck surgery, vol. 2.
E. Myers, editor

ECTOPIC THYROID TISSUE IN THE HEAD AND NECK

I. W. S. Mair, S. Økstad, T. J. Eide, J. A. Sundsfjord
University of Tromsø, 9000 Tromsø (Norway)

INTRODUCTION

The migration of the thyroid anlage along the course of the thyroglossal duct creates the opportunity for the occurrence of ectopic tissue at different sites from the foramen caecum to as far caudally as the diaphragm. Thyroid ectopia in the head and neck has been occasionally described in the tongue, the perihyoid region, larynx and trachea, esophagus, strap muscles, cervical lymph nodes and as far laterally in the neck as the submandibular region and carotid sheath (1).

Total thyroid ectopia is a rare condition, occurring approximately once for every 4.000-8.000 cases of thyroid pathology (2). The majority of these, 90%, have been sited in the tongue, with a female to male ratio of 5:1. In approximately 60% of these cases the ectopic lingual gland represents the patient's sole complement of functioning thyroid tissue.

Ectopic thyroid tissue has been most often reported in the walls of thyroglossal cysts, although the frequency has varied considerably, from 6 to 62% (3), presumably reflecting the thoroughness of the histological examination.

METHODS AND RESULTS

We have reviewed the cases of thyroid ectopia seen at our department during the ten-year-period 1974-1983.

41 thyroglossal cysts have been removed surgically after technetium scintigraphy had revealed a normally sited and otherwise unremarkable thyroid gland, and no uptake from the cyst or any other region in the head and neck. The literature contains very few reports of the results of scanning studies in thyroglossal cysts, and our negative findings indicate that the ectopic thyroid tissue is non-functioning.

Thyroid tissue was found in the walls of 17 cysts, this frequency of 41% being in agreement with the majority of earlier reports. Interestingly, this was age-dependent, being highest in the oldest age-group. We have found no other reports of a similar age-distribution, nor have we an acceptable explanation for our observation.

During the same ten-year-period we have managed 5 patients with total thyroid ectopia in the head and neck. Technetium scintigraphy revealed in all cases uptake only at the ectopic location. This is a surprisingly high frequency of ectopia in a population of only 250.000. None of our patients presented symptoms of clinical thyroid dysfunction.

Two of the lingual thyroid cases, a boy of 7 years and a 61-year-old female, were referred for hearing loss, and the ectopic gland was discovered during routine clinical work-up. In the third case, a girl, the tongue mass was noted at her first school examination. None had symptoms locally in the throat. The boy had slightly elevated TSH levels, and has been treated with low dosage thyroxin. Hormonal suppression therapy is also recommended for patients with symptoms locally, and is preferable to both surgical removal and translocation of the lingual gland to the neck.

The patient with perihyoid ectopia was a 5-year-old boy admitted for surgery with the clinical diagnosis of a thyroglossal cyst. Technetium scintigraphy showed uptake only in the latter, and surgery was therefore not performed. The relative frequency of thyroglossal cyst and total perihyoid ectopia is, therefore, 41:1, which is in agreement with the literature. In our opinion, these figures indicate that thyroid scintigraphy should be performed whenever the diagnosis of thyroglossal cyst is entertained, or the possibility of ectopic thyroid gland cannot be excluded with certainty.

The final case of total ectopia was a 32-year-old female who had accidentally discovered a swelling in the right neck three months previously. The mass was 3 cm in diameter, sited below the tip of the greater horn of the hyoid bone, with which it moved on swallowing. Hormone levels were normal, and the condition is unchanged two years later. This is, therefore, not an example of lateral aberrant thyroid with the attendant implications of malignancy.

Total thyroid ectopia is seen rarely, and most reports are of one or two patients. Our experience demonstrates that ectopic glands may be encountered relatively often, even in a department which serves a population of only a few hundred thousand individuals. A constant awareness of this possibility is, therefore, necessary, and liberal indications for scintigraphy should be employed.

REFERENCES

1. Willis RA (1958) The Borderland of Embryology and Pathology. Butterworth and Co., London, pp 311-313
2. Weider DJ, Parker W (1977) Ann Otol Rhinol Laryngol 86: 841-848
3. Allard RHB (1982) Head Neck Surg 5: 134-146

New dimensions in otorhinolaryngology - head and neck surgery, vol. 2.
E. Myers, editor

GLOTTIC RECONSTRUCTION BY THYROID CARTILAGE - EXTERNAL PERICHONDRAL FLAP

André PECH, Jean-Marc THOMASSIN, Michel ZANARET, Catherine SCAVENNEC, Maurice CANNONI
Clinique O.R.L. - CHU TIMONE 13385 MARSEILLE (FRANCE)

ABSTRACT

Laryngoplasty was performed using the perichondrium of the thyroïd cartilage. Techniques and results are described using this method, applied for glottic reconstruction after vertical partial laryngectomy of the frontolateral type after cordectomy. Anatomic and functionnal results in 22 cases are described.

Functionnal results after vertical partial laryngectomies of the cordectomy or frontolateral type are often uncertain. Indeed, after simple cordectomy, the voice is often satisfactory, the phonatory results after frontolateral laryngectomy are, in most cases, mediocre despite good phoniatric re-education.

MATERIAL AND METHODS

The clinical material for this study consisted of 22 cases : 14 cases for a frontolateral laryngectomy and 8 cases for a simple cordectomy.

There were 20 males and 2 females ranging in age from 36 to 75 years.

Surgical technique

1 - Skin incision : The superior incision is at the cricothyroïd junction. The inferior one is at the level of the third tracheal ring.

2 - Elevation of external perichondrium of thyroid cartilage : The external perichondrium is elevated from the thyroid cartilage ala on the healthy side with as wide a pedicle flap as possible on the side of the lesion.

3 - Thyrotomy : This is performed by means of the usual technique, either by medial thyrotomy or by exeresis of a cartilaginous triangle according to the principle of the frontolateral laryngectomy.

4 - Flap plication : The widest anterior extremity of the flap is folded over and, depending on the width, one can often, at this level, form a triple thickness. We use fibrin glue which gives the flap a certain rigidity. (Fig. 1)

5 - Intralaryngeal wound : The intralaryngeal wound is made through the thyroid ala on the side of the exeresis, with an orifice of approximately 5 mm to 6 mm in diameter.

6 - Laryngoplasty technique : The perichondrial flap is inserted into the intralaryngeal wound. The end of the flap is sutured to the posterior wall of the arytenoid. The anterior end of the flap is then anchored by one or two stitches transfixing the anterior thyroid cartilage. Fibrin glue is used to attach the

flap at its superior and inferior parts. Postoperatively, a low pressure tracheotomy tube is left in place for 3 to 5 days. The tube is then removed and the opening is allowed to heal over. (Fig. 2)

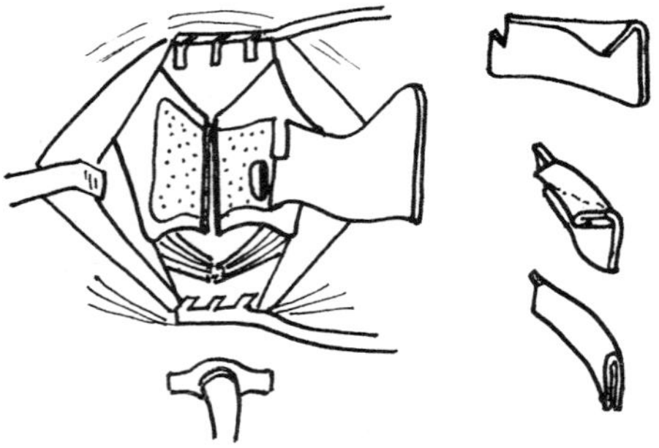

Fig.1 - Folding of perichondrial flap

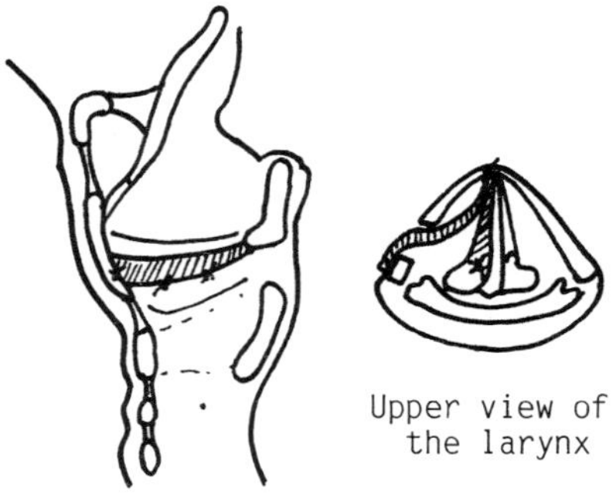

Fig.2 - Anchoring of flap

RESULTS

They could be considered on several levels :

a - Anatomic results

This flap has been reliable with a good vitality in all of our cases. We have noted that toward the 4th week there can be granulation tissue but without preferential position on the new cord. They require a secondary exeresis by direct CO_2 laser laryngoscopy. We have observed this phenomenon in approximately 45 % of our cases.

b - Phonatory function results

. Voice highness after the fundamental tone is normal : Male 125 Hertz, female 250 Hertz.

. Timbre : These voices are generally poor in high harmonic overtones. There are no harmonics above 3000 Hertz. As for timbre clarity, we obtained a clear timbre objectified on the sonogram by an almost complete absence of spikes on the line spectrum ; this condition was found in approximately 80 %.

. Intensity : The intensity of these patients is generally below normal.

. And finally, vocal effort is very discrete and phono-respiratory coupling is, in general, quite good.

During the postoperative period, it is important for the patient to avoid a vocal effort which would often involve a false cord voice.

DISCUSSION

Glottic reconstruction raises fears of insufficient follow-up and detection of a possible recurrence. We believe that recurrence will be as evident on this new cord as on the spontaneous cicatricial look. This laryngoplasty technique does not greatly complicate the surgical act in inself or the surgical follow up as in all of the cases the tracheostoma was closed after a maximum of 4 days.

© 1985 Elsevier Science Publishers B.V. (Biomedical Division)
New dimensions in otorhinolaryngology - head and neck surgery, vol. 2.
E. Myers, editor

FUNCTIONAL NECK DISSECTION IN CANCER OF THE LARYNX

M TOMAS, C GAVILAN, J GAVILAN.
ENT Dept. La Paz Hospital. Univ. Autónoma. Madrid. SPAIN

INTRODUCTION

Radical Neck Dissection (RND) vs Functional Neck Dissection (FND) controversy is arriving to an end. Nowadays most of authors agree that both procedures are oncologically radical while functional and cosmetic advantages of the functional dissection are evident and bilateral block dissection may be effected with no untoward consequences whenever indicated[1].

In the period 1969-1984, 948 patients suffering from cancer of the larynx underwent surgery in our Hospital. In 538 of them 702 FND have been performed.

The results of a 5 years period, with a minimum follow up of 5 years are presented.

MATERIAL AND METHODS

Neck dissection was carried out in 303 cases out of 390 (78%) patients suffering from cancer of the larynx (T_1 glottic cases excluded).

RND was performed on 30 (10%) patients, FND on 260 (86%) and a combined dissection on 13 (4%). In 120 cases FND was bilateral, being unilateral in 140 patients. Altogether 393 FND.

FND was performed on N_0,N_1 and N_2 patients (table I and II)

TABLE I

Treatment	Patients	FND	RND
Supraglottic laryngectomy	107	154	7
Total laryngectomy	193	236	36
Hemilaryngectomy	3	3	--
Total	303	393	43

FND was done according to the technique first described by Suárez [2].

RESULTS

231 (88.9%) patients out of 260 were free of disease in the neck at 5 years since the FND was performed.

The pathololological study of nodes was as shown in table II.

TABLE II

Staging	Patients	Neck Dissection	+ Nodes
N_0	224	FND	20%
N_1N_2	36	FND	42%
N_3	43	RND or combined	83%

Neck recurrences (nodes or primary tumor and cervical nodes) in a 5 years follow up were: contralateral to the unilateral FND 12%, ipsilateral to the FND 2.7%, and in RND 28%.

CONCLUSIONS

A wider adoption of FND would be desirable in order to improve cancerological safety. Bilateral approach to regional lymph nodes in cancer of the larynx is made possible routinely by FND which avoids the problems of unnecesary mutilation.

REFERENCES

1. Bocca E et al. (1984) Laryngoscope 94:942-945
2. Suárez O (1962) Les Ann. d'Otolaryngol. 79:22-34
3. Gavilán C et al. (1972) Acta Otorrinolaringol Ibero Am 23: 703-817

New dimensions in otorhinolaryngology - head and neck surgery, vol. 2.
E. Myers, editor

DIAGNOSTIC FEASIBILITY AND ASSESSMENT OF PROGNOSTIC FACTORS IN LARYNGEAL CANCER

M.F.VEGA, B.SCOLA, A. ALONSO, A.SANTOS, M.LOZANO Y M. DESCO
Instituto Oncológico. Hospital Provincial. Madrid. ESPAÑA

INTRODUCTION

The purpose of this retrospective study is to asses the role cf exploration methods in the diagnosis of extension of laryngeal carcinoma, as well that of different pronostic factors.

MATERIAL AND METHODS

In the period 1962-1982, we had 2000 patients (pts) with laryrgeal carcinoma treated, among them, 790 filled up the following conditions: histological proof, no prior antineoplastic therapy and a minimun 1 year follow-up.

The actuarial survival rate at ten years was studied with the following parameters; age, delay, histological differentation degree, T and N stages according to UICC, N stage according to AJC and clinical stage.

The statistical study for the assessment of the results was made by M. Desco, using the Kaplan-Meier and Cutler-Ederer methods, 1958, with Breslow and Mantel-Cox test to find the statistical significance according to the University of California 1983, BMDP program.

RESULTS

Prognostic factors: There isnt relation between age and survival. Time of delay has not prognostic value. As for celular differentation degree (G) there is a difference between the grade I (75%) groups and the grade III (67%), but this difference does not becomes statistically significative, but it is possible than with a larger number of cases there will be significance.

In midline afectation by clinical exploration, we find that when it is affected the survival is of 65%, but if it is not the survival reaches 73%, presenting - those two groups a statiscally y signigicativa difference with a p = 0.05.

As for value T, N and UICC stage:there is not significative cifference between T1A (80%), T1B (77%) and T2 (77%).There is significative difference in T1-T2 vs. T3(62%) T4 (50%). There is also in T3 vs. T4.

There is also in No (73%) vs. N1 (52%)-N2 (67%)-N3 (30%). There is a significative difference in N1 vs. N2-N3; and in N2 vs. N3.

There is a significative difference in stage I (80%)-stage II(77%) vs. stage-III (65%) stage IV (50%) and there is also in stage III vs. stage IV.

Diagnostic fiability:Routinely and with the purpose of classifying the clinical

T we perform direct and/or indirect laryngoscopic exploration and the usual radiology to find this data with a combination of both (always the worse one).

CORRELATION T CLINIC VS. pT (Nº 353)

		COINCIDE	INFRAVALUED	OVERVALUED
T1	SUPRAGL.(80)	36 (45%)	44 (55%)	
Nº 91	GLOTTIC (11)	9 (82%)	2 (18%)	
T2 Nº 50		17 (34%)	23 (46%)	20 (20%)
T3 Nº 129		77 (60%)	25 (19%)	27 (21%)
T4 Nº 83		47 (56%)		36 (44%)

Except for those in glottic T1 were the fiability index reaches 82%, in the other cases there is not a good clinic-pathological correlation, not surpassing the fiability index in 60%.

AFECTATION IN DEEPNESS	CONCORDANCES		
	RX	CLINICAL	BOTH
NO AFECTATION (121)	94%	100%	100%
PRE-EPIGLOT. SPACE (112)	20%	12%	23%
PARAGLOTT. SPACE (118)	56%	47%	75%

As we see in the table, the standard clinical and radiologic exploration represents a scarce fiability in the deepness afectation diagnosis.

N CLINICAL	SIMILAR pN	UNDER pN	OVER pN
No	83% (144)	17% (29)	
N1	49% (23)	15% (7)	36% (17)
N3	82.5% (23)		17.5% (5)

As to the adenopathies, the diagnosis fiability is of more than 80% in No or N3 cases: However in N1 cases the fiability decreases to 50%.

CONCLUSIONS

A low index of fiability in the loco-regional extension with standard methods of clinical exploration.

The presence of adenopathies is a significative obvious prognostic factor. The worse prognosis of the lesions that cross the mid-line could be attributed to a higher lateralization of the metastasic risk.

New dimensions in otorhinolaryngology – head and neck surgery, vol. 2.
E. Myers, editor

FAILURES OF SURGERY AND/OR RADIOTHERAPY IN LARYNGEAL CANCER

M.VEGA, B.SCOLA, A.ALONSO, A.SANTOS, M.LOZANO Y M.DESCO
Instituto Ocológico. Hospital Provincial. Madrid. ESPAÑA

INTRODUCTION

Going on with the retrospective study we assess the different therapies as the cause of the failures in the management of laryngeal cancer. We introduce the T and N concept of the recurrence, (Tr-Nr) using the UICC criteria in TNM.

RESULTS

Recurrences : 225/790 pts. (28.5%)- Local : 126 (16%) - Ganglionar : 70 (10%) Local+ganglionar : 20 (2.5%).

LOCAL RECURRENCES (Tr) AND SURVIVAL RATIO WITH CLINICAL T (Nº = 790 PTS).

Tr	Nº OF PTS.	Tr SURVIVAL	T SURVIVAL
Tr1A	13 (9%)	67%	80%
Tr1B	10 (7%)	57%	77%
Tr2	16 (11%)	47%	77%
Tr3	21 (14%)	17%	62%
Tr4	86 (59%)	5%	50%

Those who recurred as Tr1A and Tr1B, did not presented significative differences with T1A and T1B. Nevertheless, there was a difference in Tr2 vs. T2, p=0.05; in Tr3 vs. T3, p=0.0002; and Tr4 vs. T4, p=0.00001.

REGIONAL RECURRENCES (Nr) AND SURVIVAL RATIO WITH CLINICAL N (Nº = 790 PTS.)

Nr	Nº OF PTS.	Nr SURVIVAL	N SURVIVAL
Nr1	27 (27.5%)	52%	52%
Nr2	7 (7%)	27%	67%
Nr3	65 (65.5%)	12%	30%

Concerning the ganglionar recurrence, Nr1 and Nr2 did not presented a statistically significative difference with N1-N2; unlike Nr3 that presented a worse survival than N3, p=0.003.

LOCAL RECURRENCES IN pT FUNCTION AND ASSOCIATED OR NOT RADIOTHERAPY (550 PTS)

pT	SURGERY	SURGERY + RTX
pT1A	3/59 (5%)	4/30 (13%)
pT1B	4/52 (7.5%)	1/32 (3%)
pT2	2/33 (6%)	5/25 (20%)
pT3	16/146 (11%)	11/75 (14.5%)
pT4	6/52 (11.5%)	9/46 (19.5%)

In patients treated by surgery alone or by surgery plus RTX the percentage of recurrences is not significative in any of the stages, accordingly it seems than the complementary irradiation over the surgical bed does not improve the local control of the lesion.

pT	VERTICAL	HORIZONTAL	TOTAL
pT1s	0% (0/15)		
pT1A	8.5% (4/48)	8% (3/36)	0% (0/5)
pT1B	16% (2/12)	6% (3/49)	0% (0/23)
pT2	31.5% (6/19)	0% (0/6)	3% (1/35)
pT3	17.5% (4/23)	7% (7/92	15% (16/106)
pT4	0.0% (0/3)	23% (7/25)	11.5% (8/70)

Concerning the surgical technique used, the differences are only statistically significative if compared to the partial or total L. in favor of the later in pT2 and pT4.

No RECURRENCES IN FUNCTION OF TREATMENT

		RECURRENCE N			
TREATMENT	RECURRENCES Nº	N1	N2	N3	SURVIVAL
ABSTENTION	29/134 (21.5%)	13	4	12	82%
IRRADIATION	21/240 (8.75%)	3	0	18	87%
VFGC+RTX	19/180 (10.5%)	5	0	14	92%

In No cases there is not significative differences in therapeutical abstention vs. surgery and/or radiotherapy.

N+ RECURRENCES IN FUNCTION OF TREATMENT AND CAPSULA STATUS

TREATMENT	RECURRENCES Nº	TREATMENT	RECURRENCES Nº
VFGC	6/11 (54.5%)	RADICAL NECK	8/20 (40%)
VFGC + RTX	3/16 (18.75%)	RAD. NECK+RTX	3/14 (12.5%)

In N+ cases the complementary irradiation after a functional or radical dissection, permits a better control of regional spread. There is a significative difference in favor of RTX association, p=0.05.

CONCLUSIONS

Tr and Nr are valid factors of salvage possibilities, so a close follow up is mandatory during the first years.

With a good selection of cases Partial Surgery represents the same control index than Total L.

We find complementary irradiation effective only in N+ cases.

It is essential to introduce a randomized study in No treatment

New dimensions in otorhinolaryngology - head and neck surgery, vol. 2.
E. Myers, editor

RESULTS WITH SURGERY AND/OR RADIOTHERAPY IN LARYNGEAL CANCER

M.F.VEGA, B.SCOLA, A.ALONSO, A.SANTOS, M.LOZANO Y M.DESCO
Instituto Oncológico. Hospital Provincial. Madrid. ESPAÑA

INTRODUCTION

The purpose of this paper is to value the results on carcinoma of the larynx according to the therapy used.

RESULTS

The actuarial global survival has been of 78% and 68% at 5 and 10 years respectively. By stages: I (80%); II (77%); III (65%); and IV (50%).

Nº 760 PTS	I GLOTTIC	I SUPRAGLOTTIC	STAGE II
SURGERY	85.5% (41)	82% (76)	82% (81)
RADIOTHERAPY	87.5% (12)	57% (24)	62% (28)
SURGERY + RTX	60% (24)	85% (54)	77% (46)
	N.S.	p=0.0002	N.S.

In glottic stage I there is not a significative difference in the different therapies, as the smaller percentage in surgery plus radiotherapy is due to a late recurrence (at 8 years), what does not represent statistical significance.

The apparent failure of RTX in the supraglottic stage I, could be due to the incorrect diagnosis of invasion in deepness (pre-epiglottic-space) who would change those early stages in stage III, what does not invalidate RTX when there is conviction of the no invasion of the pre-epiglottic space (vegetative lesions confined to the suprahioid epiglottis).

In stage II, the lower survival percentage is due to the same causes than those of the former paragraph.

The worse results of radiosurgical association seems to be due to the inclusion in the group , of patients with a worse prognosis.

It is convenient in stage IV without adenopathies to differentiate clearly the group with limited extralaryngeal extension; capable to undergo a radical surgery with security, from the group of patients with massive extralaryngeal extension, in which the irradiation alone obtains poor results, than improve slightly when it is possible to associate both therapies.

In stage IV with nodes we can appreciate the need to complement with RTX, in cases of cervical nodes metastasis, and also the bad rpognosis of non resectable tumors.

© 1985 Elsevier Science Publishers B.V. (Biomedical Division)
New dimensions in otorhinolaryngology – head and neck surgery, vol. 2.
E. Myers, editor

ADVANCED RELAPSES IN THE TRACHEOSTOMA AFTER TOTAL LARYNGOTOMY. CLINICAL RESEARCH.

J.J.ALVAREZ VICENT M.D. AND BRUZON CARDIEL M.D.
Hospital Primero de Octubre. Madrid. Spain.

INTRODUCTION

The relative frecuency with which relapses appear in the tracheostoma of patients who had required an emergency tracheostomy prior to a later radical operation led us to make the following observations: 1. The relapse appeared in patient who had undergone an emergency tracheotomy 15 or 20 days before the total laryngotomy. 2. The location of the original tumor had no solution of continuity with the tracheostoma. 3. The relapse appeared 2 or 3 months after the surgical treatment had been performed, this appearance being earlier than normal relapses. 4. In identical circumstances, other patients did not suffer relapses, which we can explain by: predisposition, receptivity, personal inmunology, etc. 5. The relapse was not logical by limphatic tracts nor blood passages, and only the tumorous multicentricity remained (improbable because the tumor relapse towards below the skin, but never the opposite) or a true cellular implant in the wound of the tracheostoma.

MATERIAL AND METHODS

The study is carried out on the following patients:

- Six relapses in the tracheostoma with the following points in common: a) Glottic or vestibular tumors with paralysis which permit the passage of secretions to the trachea. b) Exophytic, ulcerated tumors which produce cellular scaling. c) Emergency tracheotomy. d) Relapse between 3 and 5 months. e) No relation with ganglionary metastasis.
- 15 totally laryngotomized patients who had undergone inmediate tracheotomy.
- 15 Supraglottic laryngotomized patients with previous inmediate tracheotomy.
- 15 supraglottic laryngotomized patients who had undergone tracheotomy 20 days before the definitive operation.

The progress of all these patients was followed for three years. In order to demonstrate cellular implantation,four points are necessary: Cell production. Scaling power. Possibility of woundbathing secretions. Positivity of neoplasic cells both in pharynx and trachea, for which we took following points: Papanicolauś stain in sputun is carried out before the operation. Papanicolau's stain in the tracheostoma during the previous tracheotomy. Mobility of the glottis. Macroscopic characteristics of the tumor. Localization of the tumor. Histological study of the tracheostoma. Histological study of the part. Study of postlaryngotomy secretion in supraglottic patients. Ample resection margins.

RESULTS

A.- Total laryngotomized patients. With greater ulceration, positive Papanicolau in sputum, which because of chord mobility in 33% in the tracheal stoma and which decrease as the tumor is less ulcerated and the glottic mobility is greater.

B.- Supraglotic laryngotomized patients, with previous tracheotomy. In this group, there were no relapses even when maintaining the tracheostoma for months. With 50% of positive Papanicolau in sputum and a 90% ulceration of the tumor, in the absence of glottic paralysis, the Papanicolau in the traceal stoma fell to 5%.

C.- Supraglottic laryngotomized patients with previous tracheotomy. The results were similar to the preceding group.

DISCUSSION AND CONCLUSION

Positive Papanicolau in sputum in ulcerated tumors. Negative Papanicolau in non-ulcerated tumors. Tracheal Papan.+ in laryngeal paralysis. Tracheal Papan. - in cords mobility. Delayed relapse in deep tissues with exteriorization to the tracheostome. Inmediate relapse (months) in those of the group studied, in skin with later invasion totrachea and deep tissues. No relapse in supraglotis patients. We have drawn the conclusion that this must be a hypothetical implantation in the wound of the tracheostoma, the cells being conveyed by the secretion when scaling is still produced due to persistence of the tumor, and which is favored by the microtrauma of the cannula in the tracheostoma. Something which does not occur in the supragl. patients.

New dimensions in otorhinolaryngology – head and neck surgery, vol. 2.
E. Myers, editor

MALIGNANCY PROCESS IN PRECANCEROUS LARYNX LESIONS. STATISTICAL-CLINICAL CONSEQUENCES. ALVAREZ VICENT M.D. AND COLLAB. Hospital 1º de Octubbre. Madrid. Spain

INTRODUCTION

For us, and as a conclusion of the conceptions of the malignancy process as expressed by diferent authors, we have arrived at the following transformative table:

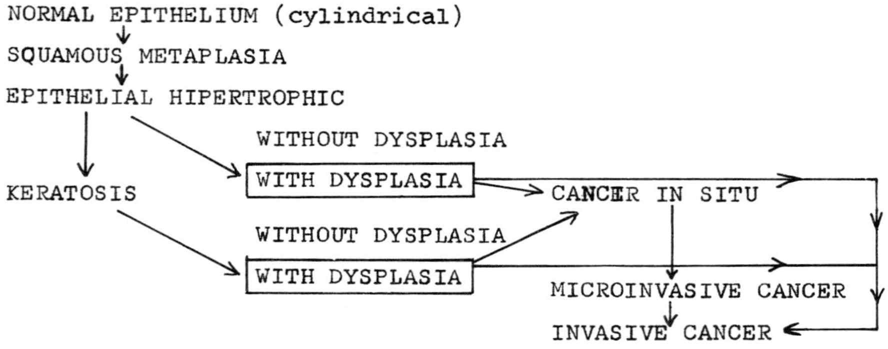

To sumarize: 1/ The malignancy process unfailingly goes through the transformation of the cylindrical epithelium into squamous. 2/ The concept of the malignancy process and its potential is solely in relation to the degree of dysplasia, and we should the follo - wing three groups: slight, moderate and severe. 3/ The concept of keratosis is but step in the transformation, wich may define the tumor but which does not transmi a malingnant potential. 4/ The reversibility of these processes is a fact when the irritating factors are absent, although it is disputable beginning form the CIS. 5/ It seems logical to suppose that the transformative pro - cess, from the normal epithelium up to the invasive cancer, must, in a high percentage of cases, go through all the steps; the fact this has not been proved out is owing to an error of space and time.

MATERIAL AND METHODS

Two groups have been chosen, of 50 patients each, suffering from white and red chronic laryngitis, as well as 20 patients with papillomatosis.

The protocol followed was that of performing a microscopy biopsy by extensive intraoperatory excision, and then proced in the follo wing way: No dysplasia, observation. Slight dysplasia, stripping. Moderate dysplasia, cordectomy and/or stripping. Severe dysplasia, cordectomy.

With this method, we have obtained the following parameters: 1.- Lesions which at no time were dysplasic (White L. 52%, Red L. 44%). 2.- Lesions which did not arrive at the malignancy stage (White L. 50%, Red L. 56%). 3.- Paracancerosis, lesions which although not being carcinomatous during the biopsy, did show the existence of cancer in the surgical part when the cordectomy was performed at the same time (White L. 20%, Red L. 20%, Papillomatosis 45%). 4.- Lesions which degenerated in relation to the number of total laryngitis (White L. 22%, Red L. 20%, Papill. 66%). 5.- Total number of C. finally arrived at by laryngitis in their malignancy process and paracancerosis (White L. 43%, Red L. 28%, Papill. 55%). 6.- Slight or moderate dysplasia is similar inthe two laryngitis (16%) 7.- Severe dysplasia (White L. 18%, Red L. 28%).

CONCLUSIONS

The malignancy process of chronic laryngitis is clearly proportional to dysplasia; this proportion ranges from 7% to 70% in fa - vor of slight, moderate and severe dysplasias compared with 1% in non-dysplasic.- White L. become malignantin a higher percentage.- Paracancerosis is a fact which must always be considered, and is found at 28% for white and red laryngitis, if we add on papillomatosis, this figure reaches 45%.- Polyps do not degenerate; however, adult papillomatosis reaches a degenerative power of 66%.- The total percentage of degeneration of the Chronic L. is 21%, this figure rising to 36% if we add on papillomatosis.- In those cases which led to exitus, stripping had been performed only on slight or moderate lesions.- Geater concomitance of CIS in Red L. (28%) than in White L. (18%).

© 1985 Elsevier Science Publishers B.V. (Biomedical Division)
New dimensions in otorhinolaryngology – head and neck surgery, vol. 2.
E. Myers, editor

FUNCTIONAL LARYNGECTOMY (BY THE EMPTYING OF THE LARYNX TECHNIQUE) REVISION OF 60 cases.

BRONCHALO BUTRAGUENO M.D.. and ALVAREZ VICENT M.D.
Hospital 1º de Octubre. Madrid. SPAIN

INTRODUCTION

Since ALVAREZ VICENT presented he FUNCTIONAL LARYNGECTOMY in 1971 which was publicate later (Ac.ORL Iber.XXIII-4-538-600-1972, Barcelona) and (Ann. Oto. Paris 1975, T.92, Num. 1-2,pag 61-72),we have been useing this method in a big number of patients.

This comunication try to make a investigation about 60 ills who have been treated regulary since 1971, and to present the results we have obtained in relation with a succession of parameters that was protocolated in 1972 in the first introduction of cases. We report to the decannulation, swallowing, fonation and relapses.

We considered that this method is indicated in the followings locations: 1.- Supraglottis tumors with detachment of the internal pericondrium, and the vestibular tumor extirpation. 2.- Cords tumors with supraglottic invasion. 3.- Cords tumors which invade arytenoids and supraglottis. 4.- Cords tumors with supraglottis, arytenoid and a litle pyriform sinus invasion. 5.- Tumors which invade both cords. In all cases it is always necessary to find the cartilage free from neoplasia.

At present we have lightly changed the newglottis reconstructive part, that we make through the formatiom with aproximation points whit the external pericondrium and covering the bloody zone, with all of these the fonation function has notably improved; the possible narrowness formation too.

Now we are going to analyse the obteined results of these 60 ills that we have got.

A.- OPERATED PATIENTS

Checked in 1985	54	90%
Died	6	10%

B.- TIME SINCE THE INTERVENTION

more than 5 years.......	27	45%
" " 4 "	15	25%
" " 3 "	18	30%

C.- SWALLOWING

good swallowing	56	93%
bad "	4	7%

This patients was operated afterwards the total laryngectomy

D.- DECANULATION

The decanulation time changed between 17 days the most precocious and 4 months the latest. In this series we have 7 patients we couldn´t closed the tracheostoma.

decanullated...........	53	88%
without decanullate....	7	11%

Reasons of the non-decanullation:

web-footed formation.........	3
Inflamation post-radioterapy.	3
child larynx (woman).........	1

E.- FONATION

The voice in these patients is good in those cases in which only one cord was extirpated and aphonic, which improves with time in cases of complete removal.

F.- RELAPSES

In this patients we have found, 6 relapses distributes in the time in this way:

Total Laryngectomy

3 months later......................	1	
7 " "	1	
1 year "	3	
3 years "	1	
All relapses........................	6	12%

CONCLUSIONS

a.- The care of postoperate do not defer of the a Supraglottic Laryngectomy and the middle time of hospitalize was 27 days. b.- The fonation and swallowing functions were returned to all the patients. c.- The decanullation and breathing for natural way get the 86% of the ills. d.- The relapses. We can consider like a good. We must think that these patients have been very selectioned.

© 1985 Elsevier Science Publishers B.V. (Biomedical Division)
New dimensions in otorhinolaryngology - head and neck surgery, vol. 2.
E. Myers, editor

'T' LARYNGECTOMY

MARCO DE VINCENTIIS, ANDREA GALLO, ROSARIA TURCHETTA
2nd ENT Clinic, University "La Sapienza", Rome, Italy

INTRODUCTION

For a long time total laryngectomies have been the surgical treatment of choice for glottic tumors. However, the so-called conservative surgery encounters more difficulties when approaching cordal tumors invading the anterior commissure[1]. The full involvement of this area requires such surgical techniques as a total laryngectomy or the more radical subtotal methods such as the Labayle procedure. In the Authors' opinion , lesions of one vocal cord invading the opposite side via anterior commissure (i.e. 'horse-shoe' lesions) may be treated by 'T' laryngectomy[2].

'T' laryngectomy is the result of the combination of the fronto-lateral laryngectomy[3] with horizontal glottectomy[4].

OPERATIVE TECHNIQUE

'U' shaped cutaneous incision of the Labayle-Guerrier type. Tracheotomy at 3th - 4th tracheal ring. Incision and separation of prelaryngeal muscles on the median line and partial disconnection of them from the hyoid bone, to increase the exposition of the larynx. After having freed the thyroid cartilage from the anterior muscolar connection, proceed to the identification of the upper horn, which must be separated bilaterally from the hyoid bone. We advise locating the vascular peduncle and binding it bilaterally. The larynx thus mobilised is rotated on one side and on the other in order to proceed to thyro-cricoid disarticulation, taking care at this stage, not to damage the recurrent nerves. The external perichondrium is incised, following a line parallel to the lower margin of the thyroid cartilage and turned upwards to expose completely the cartilagineous anterior commissure. Proceed to the first horizontal incision, sectioning the cricothyroid membrane and draw the line of cartilage resection to use as a guide for the cutting blade. The 'T' shaped incision is two vertical lines which imitate those of the 'fronto-lateral' at the top, but which, joined at the lower 2/3 of the cartilage, continue horizontally, parallel to the inferior margin of the thyroid cartilage, tracing the horizontal lines of section of the 'horizontal glottectomy'. The section is then taken from top to bottom. In this phase the surgeon can follow the section of the vocal cords under direct vision, gradually turning the 'T' over, forwards. The section internally will include the anterior commissure in full extension, the glottic plane and the anterior 3rd of the false vocal cords. The Morgagni ventricles are saved in the posterior 2/3, as the section is at a tangent to their lower limit. Once the exeresis is terminated, one must proceed to the 'pexy' between the two upper stumps corresponding to the upper 2/3 of the cartilagineous alae, and the cricoid with 3 points of suture in chromic catgut no. 3 (cricothyropexy). The cricothyropexy completed, proceed to the suture of the perichondrium previously cut away. The introduction of a soft stent is advisable for 3-4 days in the laryngeal lumen to act as a support in the initial stages of scarring. The nasal-gastric probe, for the feeding of the patient, must be maintained for at least 7 days.

RESULTS

The recent introduction of this operation, in the therapeutic protocol we carried out in our treatment of tumors in the glottic plane, has allowed the application of this method in only two cases which have come under our observation in the last 6 months. The two cases we have treated have shown a good, early recovery of laryngeal functions. Both patients were decannulised quickly for the wide opening of respiratory lumen.

REFERENCES

1. Guerrier J (1979) ORL 41:262-272
2. De Vincentiis M, Gallo A (1984) Acta Otorhinol. Ital. 4:395-405
3. Calearo CV, Teatini GP (1978) Laryngoscope 88:1929-35
4. Leroux-Robert J (1967) Mém. Acad. Chir. 93:349-361

© 1985 Elsevier Science Publishers B.V. (Biomedical Division)
New dimensions in otorhinolaryngology – head and neck surgery, vol. 2.
E. Myers, editor

PAROTID FASCIA : ANATOMICAL AND HISTOLOGICAL STUDIES AND SURGICAL IMPLICATIONS

GUY JOST, YANN LEVET, MICHEL WASSEF
Lariboisiere Hospital, 2 rue Ambroise Pare, 75010, PARIS, FRANCE

This report is the result of surgical, anatomical, histological and embryological studies, with particular attention to the findings of comparative anatomy. In it, we seek to correct an anatomical error wich has given rise to a dangerous surgical myth : - the error, held by the majority of anatomists for the past century (with the exception of the French anatomist Truffert) : that the parotid fascia is continuous with the deep cervical fascia. We state it is in reality none other than the upper part of the platysma muscle. - The myth : the "Superficial musculo aponeurotic system" (S.M.A.S.), is a veritable surgical chimera, based on a false anatomical concept, and of particular danger to the inexperienced surgeon.

When, in the course of a sub-platysma face-lifting, the parotid fascia is dissected to reinforce the flap, the parotid gland is exposed and the plane created at the lower end of the flap is in direct anatomical continuation with the platysma muscle. In addition, there are horizontal muscle fibers in the fascia, running parallel to the fibers of the plastysma.

COMPARATIVE ANATOMY

Studies of comparative anatomy remove all doubt that the parotid fascia is the upper part of the platysma muscle. In monkeys (where the platysma muscle is more developed than in man) the muscle fibers of the platysma adhere directly to the lobules of the parotid gland. There is no intermediate structure between the muscle and the gland the external wall of the parotid fossa is formed by the platysma muscle. During the course of evolution, the muscle became a fibro-muscular structure.

The evidence is indisputable : the parotid fascia is one and the same as the large muscular sheet well-known to specialists of comparative anatomy as the platysma. We have called this the "primitive platysma" to distinguish it from the platysma muscle. This "primitive platysma" consists of : the platysma muscle, the risorius muscle, the triangularis oris muscle, the anterior and posterior auricularis muscles, the parotid fascia.

EMBRYOLOGY

The "primitive plastysma" is in fact a single system, the remnants of a single muscle wich has undergone fibrous degeneration, and like its precursor, it has non bony insertions. All the others cutaneous muscles of the head and neck arise from a different embryologic origin, the "sphincter colli profundus". Their fibers run longitudinally, their plane is deeper, and they have bony attachements;

DISCUSSION

The SMAS described in 1976 is both anatomical and embryological impossibility. Indeed, it was claimed : 1- that the "system is independant of the parotid fascia" (wich is in reality the muscular plane) ; the SMAS, a muscular system, would thus be independant of muscle ! 2- that the SMAS is above all like and "intermediary tendon" between the frontalis and the platysma muscles. However, these two muscles cannot be joined in this way beacause they are not aligned, but run in opposing directions ; they lie in different planes ; and their embryologic origins are entirely different. Perhaps most important, the SMAS is dangerous. If the parotid fascia is not dissected in a sub-platysma face-lifting, the surgeon is necessarily obliged to pass under the plane of the platysma to tighten it ; He thus changes the planes. Furthermore, he must do this without any visible reference to the facial nerve, since the parotid gland is at no time visible. He therefore runs a great risk of cutting a branch of this nerve.

On the other hand, if it is decided to dissect below the parotid fascia, the parotid gland becomes visible, its anterior edge and inferior pole can be located. The solid flap thereby created is based upon anatomical reality, since it is continuous with the platysma ; it is firmly attached to the zygomatic arch and to the mastoid periosteum posteriorly. The superiority of this method is incontestable for the neck, although it may be difficult to appreciate for the face. In addition, it is anatomically sound and much surer for the VII than the so-called "sub-SMAS" dissection.

REFERENCES

1. G. JOST and Y. LEVET (1984) Parotid Fascia and Face Lifting : a critical evaluation of the S.M.A.S. concept. Plast. Reconstr. Surg 74, 1 : 42 - 51.

2. Y. LEVET, P. MENARD, G. JOST et M. WASSEF (1983) Le Fascia Parotidien. Bull Assoc. Anat. 67, 199 : 475 - 484.

New dimensions in otorhinolaryngology – head and neck surgery, vol. 2.
E. Myers, editor

FACELIFT AND LIPO-SUCTION

Thomas C. Tyler, M.D., Venice, Fl.

Cosmetic surgery has witnessed a positive progression of ideas and techniques for the rhytidectomy procedure in the past few years. The incisions, Sub-SMAS technique, the exact rotations of the facial and cervical flaps with preservation of the hairlines and the concept of as good a result with less radical surgery have given a consistent approach.

Suction lipectomy of the cervico-facial area allows maximum results with minimal complications. It bridges the gap between radical and conservative rhytidectomies allowing fat removal equal to or at times superior to total undermining and neck defatting. Areas that were considered unreachable and troublesome can be defatted within the realms of safety and without danger to cutaneous viability. Areas below the hyoid bone, along the platysmal bands, the sternocleidomastoid muscle to the clavicles, the mento-labial folds and the naso-labial folds along with the jowl areas are now approachable. Figure 1, shows the safe areas of lipo-suction in rhytidectomies.

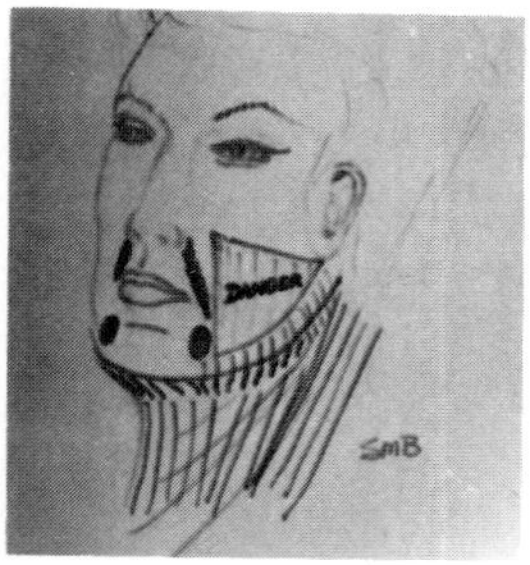

Fig. 1

Lipo-suction as a technique is relatively simple. Its technique can be learned by attending one of the many workshops offered throughout the country on lipo-suction surgery. It is almost amazing that the fat can be removed with almost no to minimal bleeding while maintaining good skin viability. Figure 2, shows the suctioned fat from a neck and jowl defatting. Cannulas of 15cm. x 4 mms. to 6mms., can easily handle the head and neck area. More fat absorption and tightening of the skin goes on two to three months after the surgery.

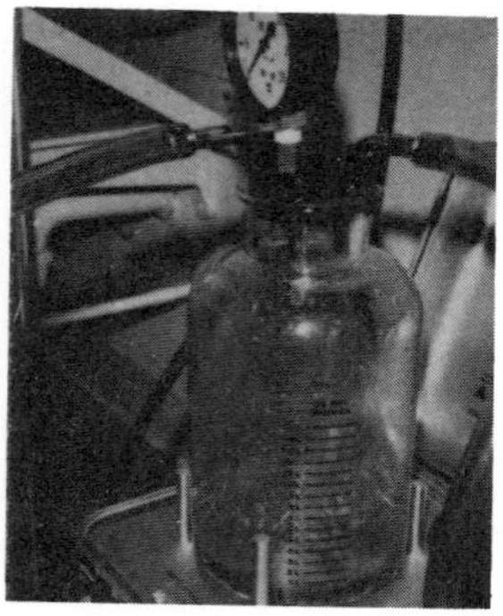

Fig. 2

Patients are marked (Fig. 3) in the sitting position prior to anesthesia, which in most cases is local with KV sedation. The lipo-suction is carried out in a criss cross fashion in the neck through 1 cm. incisions in the submental area and at both earlobes (Fig. 4 & 5). Jowl reductions to no more than 1cm. to 2cms. above the mandibular rim. Any higher than this can cause irregularities of the cheek. A smooth mandibular line is achieved after the SMAS procedure is performed and the cheek tissue raised. The naso-labial and labio-mental folds can be reached through intra-nasal vestibular incisions.

Figures 3-6

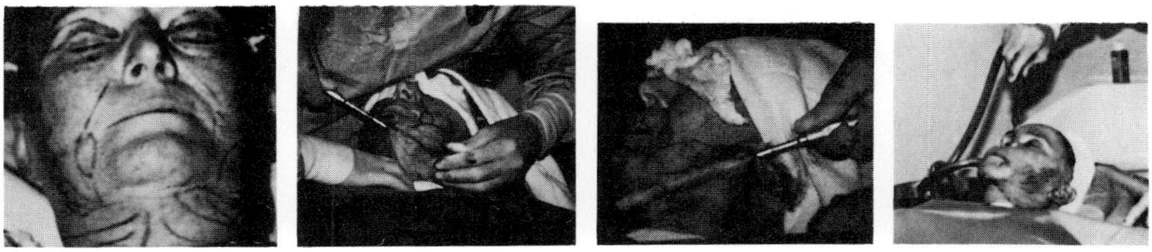

With experience lipo-suction greatly aids in the speed and safety of the patient with fatty fallen neck and heavy jowls. In the above type patient the two stage concept of rhytidectomy with a secondary tuck at the temporal area at six to eight months is a rewarding procedure.

No undermining is done with the lipo-suction cannulas in the temporal or cheek areas for it can leave tracking spores of the surgeon. The healing process seems to be the same without taping the neck and jowls as has been advocated by others. Lipo-suction is faster, safer and gives less complications and as good results or superior to conventional measure defatting of the neck and jowls. The patient with the fatty fallen neck and heavy jowls most of all no longer becomes a monumental challenge.

Figure 7.

Patient with heavy jowling with lipo-suction 1cm. to 2cms. above the mandible, followed by sub-SMAS technique, removes the heavy jowls and gives a rounded appearance to a square face.

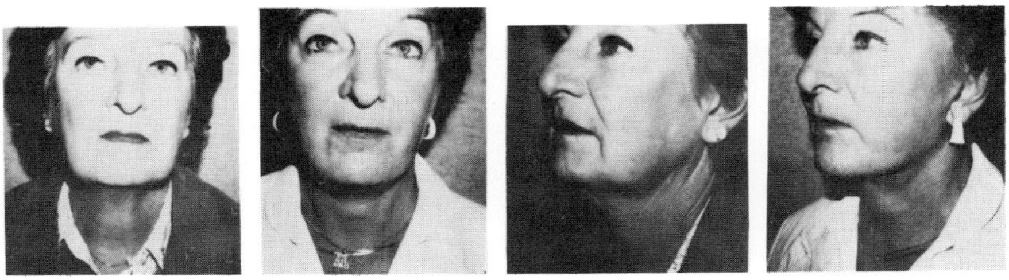

Figure 8.

A 75 year old patient who has had forehead lift, upper and lower blepharoplasties, rhytidectomy and lipo-suction. Notice the thinness of the fat over the platysma as well as the definition of the sternocleidomastoid down to the clavicles. Also the obvious removal of the jowl.

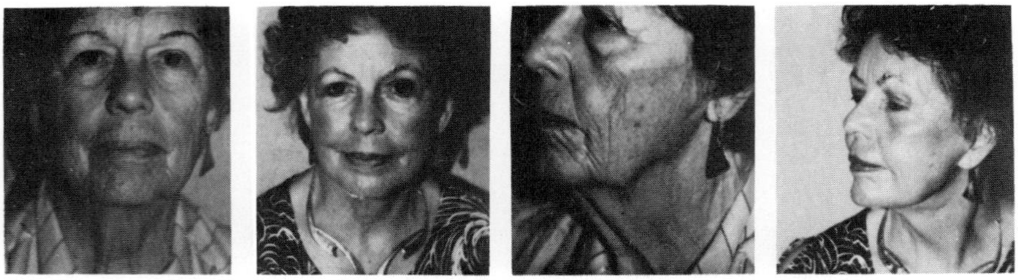

References:

Webster, R.C., et al: Face-Lift: Better results with safer surgery. In Ward, P.H., and Berman, W.E., Editors: Plastic and Reconstructive Surgery of the Head & Neck., proceedings of the Fourth International Symposium (Los Angeles, Ca.) June, 83. C.V. Mosby Co.

Kamer, F.M. Two-Stage Concept of Rhytidectomy. Otolaryngo Head & Neck Surgery 87:915-918 (Nov.-Dec.) 1979

Lipo-Suction Surgery Workshop, 1984 Garry Fenno, M.D., Houston, Texas.

New dimensions in otorhinolaryngology - head and neck surgery, vol. 2.
E. Myers, editor

THE CORONAL FOREHEAD LIFT

Thomas C. Tyler, M.D., Venice, Fl.

The peri-orbital area is the most expressive part of the face. Aging with ptosis and tonic muscle contractions of the frontalis-corrugator-procerus muscle complex cause a narrowing of the eyes along with a stern and unfriendly look to the face. The forehead lift, either alone or in conjunction with other cosmetic procedures brightens the face, softens the furrowed brow and gives a much more harmonius look.

Four cases are presented with different problems and the obvious benefits from the procedure.

Figure A. - Severe ptosis of the brow with actual functional benefit (lower blepharoplasty also performed). Patient post-op at one year.

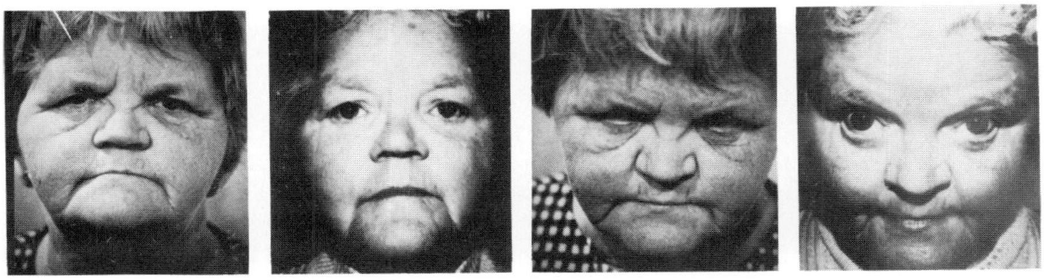

Figure B. - Patient with thickened corrugated and stressful forehead (upper and lower blepharoplasties also performed). Patient post-op at one year.

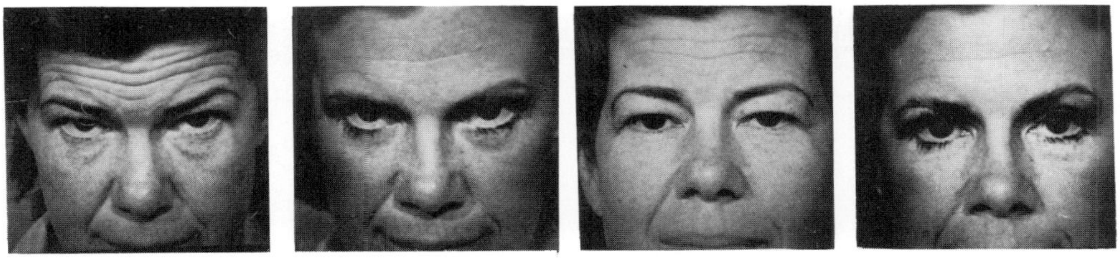

Figure C. - Two patients with stern faces needing softening. Patients post-op at one year.

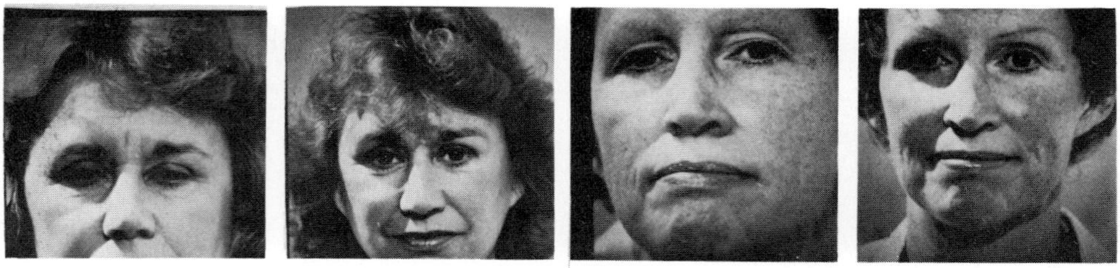

Figure D. - Patient who the total cosmetic look could not have been obtained without the forehead lift (rhytidectomy and blepharoplasties also performed).

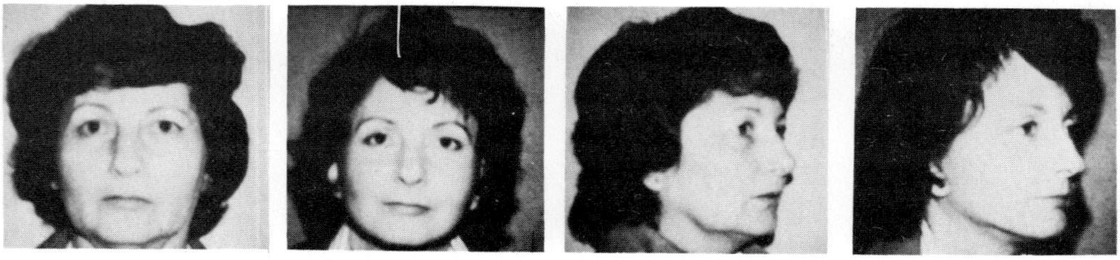

The methodology of the forehead lift is well established, fast, safe and has few complications. Bevelled incisions are made (Fig. 1A), and Raney clamps are used. The almost avascular subgaleal dissection (Fig. 1B), is carried down to the orbital rims, the tip of the nose (Fig. 1C), and the zygomatic arches (Fig. 1D).

The corrugator muscles are found by blunt dissection just medial to the neruo-vascular bundles then cut with cautery (Fig. 2A). Cautery section of the frontalis-procerus-corrugator aponeurosis just to the subdermal fat is performed under finger tension from the outside of the flap (Fig. 2B). Identical cuts are made on all large wrinkle sites over the frontalis skin (Fig. 2C) and also laterally above the eyebrows. Advancement and closure (Fig. 2D) after hemostasis is performed with skin staples to prevent hair loss (Fig. 2E). Approximately 2cms. of skin or more is usually taken, no drains are used.

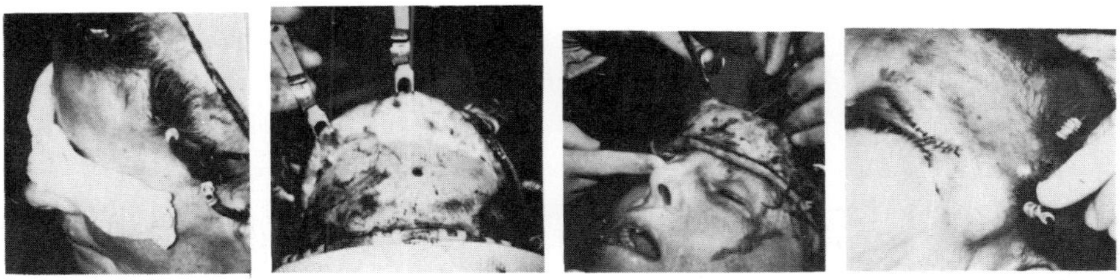

1 Fig. A Fig. B Fig. C Fig. D

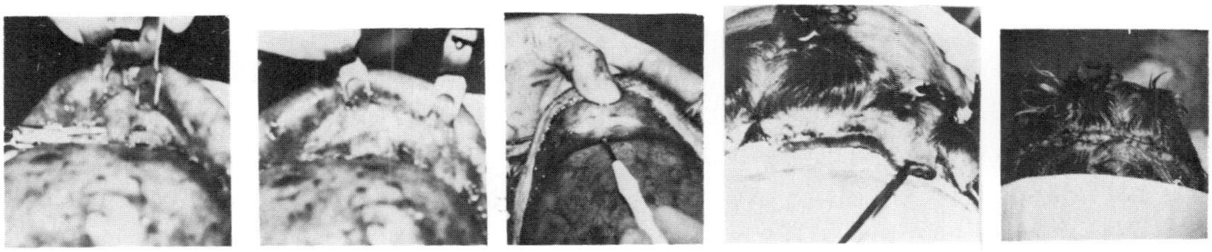

2 Fig. A Fig. B Fig. C Fig. D Fig. E

The complications of the forehead lift are minimal using the above procedure, no hematomas have occurred, drains are not used. With the stainless steel staples hair loss is not a problem. Approximately 20% of patients have post-operative headaches for one or two days, easily controlled with medications, rarely a neuralgia along the neuro-vascular area can occur post-op, probably from trauma of retraction.

The forehead lift probably should be considered on all secondary rhytidectomies.

References:

1. Pitanguy, l., Section of the Frontalis-Procerus-Corrugator Aponeurosis in the Correction of Frontal and Globellar Wrinkles. Annals of Pl. Surg. Vol. 2, No. 5, May '79.
2. Brennan, G.H.: The Forehead Lift: Symposium of the Aging Face. Otolaryngo. Clin. North Am. 1980, 13:209-223

© 1985 Elsevier Science Publishers B.V. (Biomedical Division)
New dimensions in otorhinolaryngology - head and neck surgery, vol. 2.
E. Myers, editor

OUR EXPERIENCES IN TOTAL AURICULAR RECONSTRUCTION

YOSHIHIKO NISHIMURA*, TAKEO KUMOI*, JUNPEI KIMURA** & NOBORU TAMURA**

* Department of Otorhinolaryngology, Hyogo College of Medicine, 1-1 Mukogawa-cho, Nishinomiya, 663 Hyogo (JAPAN)
** Department of Plastic & Reconstructive Surgery, Ashiya Municipal Hospital, 39 Asahigaoka-cho, Ashiya, 659 Hyogo (JAPAN)

INTODUCTION

In the total auricular reconstructive surgery, unfavourable results are not so rarely seen but one of the most disappointing results is the collapse or partial loss of the reconstructed auricle. To reduce it, for nine years we have tried to device a method by which the rib cartilage can be assembled and fabricated.

The microtic auricle is frequently associated with the air conductive dysfunction resulting from the atresia of the external auditory canal and or the structural defect of the middle ear. We have operated on just three microtic ear malformations by transplanting the allograft tympanic membrane with ossicles in order to improve the hearing loss.

METHODS AND RESULTS

Auricular reconstruction

To minimize the absorption of the grafted cartilaginous tissue, we carved and shaved as much as possible one plane of the rib block, in which an ample amount of proliferative cells existed in the subperichondrial layer. These cells are important for the cartilaginous tissue to live and support the shape for a long time. To prevent the collapse of the herical component, we fixed the 9th or 10th rib with almost all of its original width to the side surface of the base unit with mattress sutures of fine steel wire. This procedure has proved not only to retain its shape but to make the herical prominence higher (Figs. 1-3).

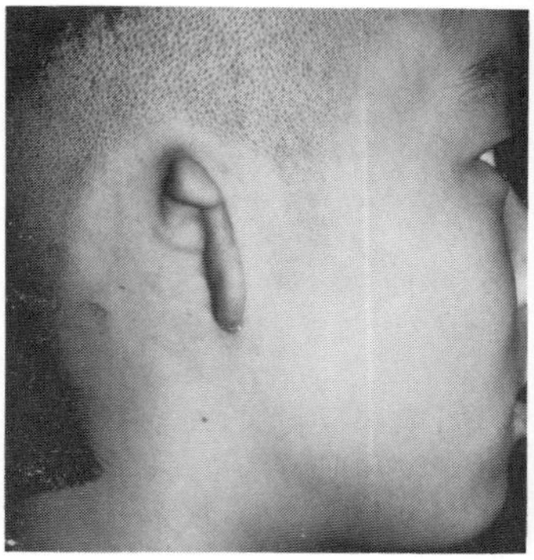

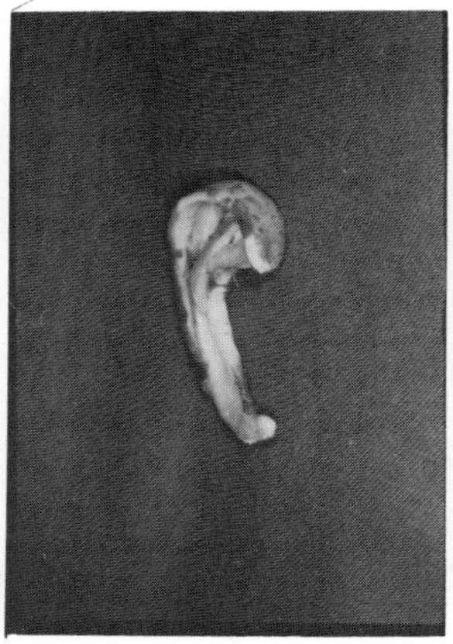

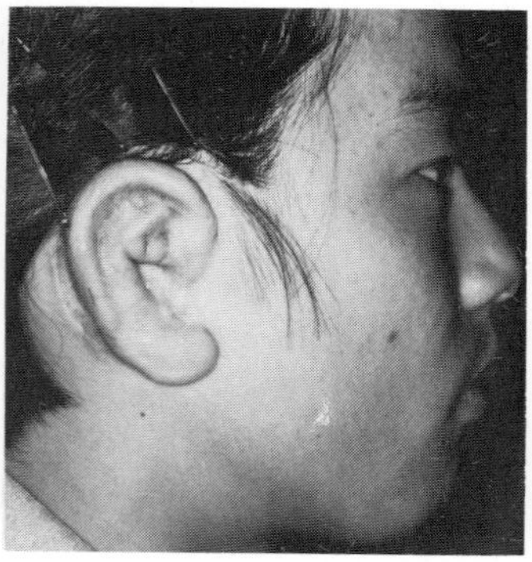

Fig. 1. 8-year-old male, right microtia, peanut type (grade III after Marx)
Fig. 2. Oblique front view of the completed framework, note over 7 mm in height herical component fixed lateral surface of the base unit.
Fig. 3. Six and half years' reconstructed auricle after the final operation.

Middle ear surgery.

General opinions on middle ear surgery for microtic ear are discouraged because of the disadvantages of the auricular reconstructive surgery and the complications for the surgery itself, but we are attempted to improve the hearing deficits by the allografting of the tympanic membrane with ossicles proffering from Hyogo Ear Bank. Our experience has been with just three cases, one bilateral microtia and two unilateral ones with congenital cholesteatomas. Operation was indicated after the comprehenssive findings on the middle ear and its surroundings were obtained by the C.T. images such as the presence or abscence and location of T.M. joint, middle ear structure, pneumatization, facial nerve, eustachian tube and inner ear structure and completed audiometry.

We reached the deformed middle ear cavity which was packed with a lot of tinny bonny pieces and removed them, creating a cavity. We confirmed the deformed stapes taking care not to damage facial nerve and dura. After digging a cavity and carving a shelf for setting an annulus, we put the allograft tympanic membrane with a malleus handle on the shelf and the stapes head. The autogenous temporal fascia was overlayed on the grafted drum. An autogenous free skin graft in shape of a tube was connected to it in order to build the external auditory canal. *We have not yet experienced a case of middle ear surgery with auricular reconstructive surgery.*

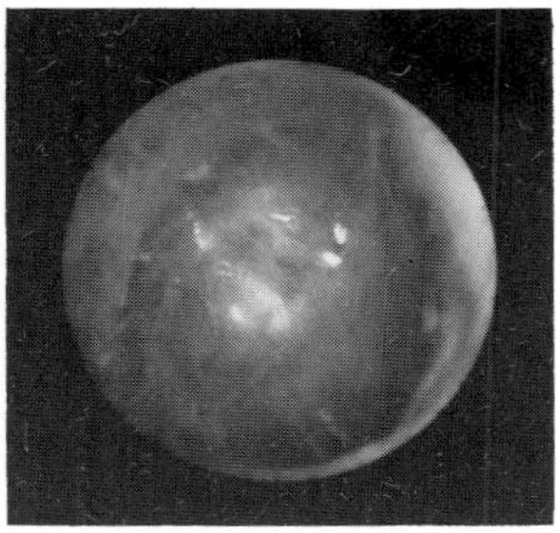

Fig. 4. Note the well vascularized allograted tympanic membrane after 15 postoperative months on 4-year-old boy, unilateral microtia (grade I). His external auditory canal was very shallow like as a pit and he had suffered from congenital cholesteatoma in the residual primary aural canal behind the bony obstructive plate. The membrane is still somewhat opaque but the malleus handle is slightly noticeable and two postoperative years' audiogram shows 15-20 dB average gain.

ACKNOWLEDGEMENTS

We gratefully acknowledge Hyogo Ear Bank (Chirman, Emert. Prof. R. Asai) which kindly proffered several precious lyophilized homografts and Associate Prof. T. Minatogawa who helped our middle ear surgery.

New dimensions in otorhinolaryngology - head and neck surgery, vol. 2.
E. Myers, editor

CORRECTIVE COSMETICS ADJUNCTIVE TO THE FIELD OF DERMATOLOGY AND COSMETIC SURGERY

N. CRAIG ROBERTS, M.D., M.S., F.A.C.S.
Director, Department of Research, Dermablend Corrective Cosmetics, Medical Division, P.O. Box 601, Farmingdale, New Jersey 07727

There has been a tremendous need for an effective concealer for patients who are not amenable to medical or surgical therapy. In 1981, at the instigation of fellow physicians and three universities, we were asked to produce a cover cosmetic that did not have the drawbacks of those marketed. After one year of research we produced Dermablend, a superior, versatile, effective concealer.

The original research was done with a pool of fifty-two patients referred by dermatologists, plastic, otolaryngology physicians and patients. The case studies consisted of vitiligo, lupus, scars, pigmentation disturbances, port wine lesions, pre/post operative conditions, dermabrasion and carcinoma after radiation.

Historically speaking, the cosmetic industry is mostly involved in the selling of its products based on the marketing tools of hope and beauty. A small neglected segment has been devoted to cover cosmetics. Dermatologists have been at the forefront of the meager use of camouflage cosmetics. They became involved because of their interest in the side effects, allergies and the dermatologic implications of cosmetics. Even though vitiligo has existed for thousands of years, there has never been an effective concealer. Physicians who were connected with a university government vitiligo program asked us to get involved.

In order to produce a superior product, it was decided that the following criteria should be inherent in the product: (a) Skin matching (shades, natural look); (b) Good coverage (opaque); (c) Greaseless (must not stain clothes); (d) Ease of application; (e) Waterproof; (f) Lasting qualities; (g) 100% fragrance free; (h) Applicable to all skin types (dry and oily). I believe this has been attained in Dermablend. Sensitivity, comedogenic and blocking tests were excellent. The sensitivity tests were done on Caucasians, Hispanics and Blacks, and included product and photosensitivity testing. There were no adverse effects. The comedogenicity tests were done on rabbits. There was no thickening or edema. The tests revealed that the Dermablend cover material was non-comedogenic. There is a 50 to 70% blocking effect, depending on the shade.

We, as physicians, know that there are many things that we can treat medically and surgically. We know that there have been many advances, new medicines, chemicals, biogenetics, lasers and prosthesis. The state of the art of treatment has rapidly advanced in all specialties. However, we are all confronted by situations where we are not entirely satisfied with what we have accomplished or we have a patient who we think we can offer nothing. This is the so-called "dead-end" patient. However, in dermatological situations and after you have become better acquainted with cover cosmetics, I would hope that you would add this entity to your armamentarium of treatment. This is especially applicable to dermatology, plastic surgery which includes otorhinolaryngology, and to the burn patient.

There is no question that patients with skin disfigurements suffer psychologically and are in need of rehabilitation. The conditions may be genetic or acquired. They may be present in burn victims and they may occur in patients pre or post surgery. Surgery may not be the answer. Adjunctive cosmetic applications may be the quickest, surest acceptable solution to visible correction. When this is attained, the disfigured patient may exhibit a rapid psychological reversal of symptoms and return quickly to a more secure, productive life. As of now, there is a vast pool of confused, unhappy people with severe emotional problems waiting for a helping hand and some small solution to what they feel is insurmountable. Now that we have an excellent camouflage system, we can serve as a vehicle to deliver this care to the disfigured patient.

Dermablend has been available domestically and in foreign countries for two years. I have lectured and demonstrated at many universities, and have helped to set up teaching and training sessions. I believe we now have a concealer that is more effective than any product available in the United States or overseas.

N. CRAIG ROBERTS, M.D.

1. Director, Department of Ophthalmology, Monmouth Medical Center, Long Branch, New Jersey

2. Clinical Associate Professor, Hahnemann University, Philadelphia, Pennsylvania

New dimensions in otorhinolaryngology – head and neck surgery, vol. 2.
E. Myers, editor

EXTUBATION IN ACUTE EPIGLOTITTIS USING FLEXIBLE FIBEROPTIC LARYNGOSCOPY

KEVIN BROWNE and KEITH CLARK

Department of Otorhinolaryngology, University of Oklahoma Health Sciences Center, P.O. Box 26307, South Pavilion, Oklahoma City, Oklahoma 73126, USA

INTRODUCTION

Endotracheal intubation has been widely accepted as a means of managing the airway in children with acute epiglottitis. This paper describes our experience with transnasal flexible fiberoptic laryngoscopy to aid the process of extubation. There is controversy regarding the timing of extubation. Some authors support the concept that the duration of the airway obstruction is limited and extubation should occur after an arbitrary time period of 24-36 hours.[3,4] Others believe that extubation should occur after defervescence of symptoms.[2,4] Direct observation for the return of the appearance of the supraglottic structures to near normal size is utilized by many.[1,5]

MATERIALS AND METHODS

Seventeen cases of acute epiglottitis at Oklahoma Children's Memorial Hospital from 1979 to 1984 were reviewed. Management included immediate control of the airway by endotracheal intubation under general anesthesia. Bedside examination was performed daily by the Otorhinolaryngology service using the Olympus ENF nasopharyngoscope transnasally. Patients were always extubated in the morning hours after the supraglottic structures were judged to be near normal size and character.

RESULTS

Group I consisted of individuals who were extubated after an arbitrary time period of 48-60 hours. Patients in group II were extubated after examination revealed near total resolution of the erythema and edema.

The six patients in group I were extubated after being observed for an arbitrary intubation period of 48-60 hours. Two patients in this group were self extubated prior to 48 hours. The average intubation time for group I was 76 hours.

Eleven patients in Group II were extubated after direct assessment of the supraglottis. Three patients were extubated after laryngoscopy under anesthesia with an average time of intubation of 64 hours. The average duration of intubation for eight patients assessed by serial fiberoptic exams was 58 hours. Two patients were self extubated prior to 48 hours in this group and were not reintubated. The average duration of intubation Group II was 61 hours. Six of the eleven patients in group II were judged to have significant edema of the supraglottis at 48 hours to warrant further intubation despite resolution of the signs and symptoms of the acute infection.

DISCUSSION

Vernon[3] reports a series of patients managed by nasotracheal intubation and spontaneous extubation after 36-48 hours. He feels that this is a very reliable technique and does not feel that adding a subjective assessment of the epiglottis to the criteria is necessary. Berry[4] does not advocate direct visualization of the epiglottis secondary to the impracticality of general anesthesia and the increased cost of hospitalization that would accompany the procedure. He further states that objective criteria for extubation, based on the appearance of the supraglottis, have not been established.

Rothstein and Lister[1] have studied the relationship between presence or absence of fever and the appearance of the supraglottic structures. These authors also agree that there is no correlation between the physical findings of the supraglottis and the absence of fever and advocate using direct visualization (direct laryngoscopy) as a means to determine the patients readiness for extubation.

Nussbaum[5] has reported the use of the flexible pediatric bronchoscope transnasally to assess the supraglottic condition at the bedside. Sixteen children were evaluated and a majority were extubated within 24 to 48 hours based on resolution of the edema of the supraglottis. We have not experienced the rapid resolution (e.g. within 12-24 hours) of the supraglottic edema and inflammation reported by Nussbaum.

Rothstein and Lister[1] provide the only objective criteria, delaying extubation until the proximal epiglottis became 3-4 mm in width. The lack of objective criteria as guidelines for extubation is manifest by the range of intubation periods reported in the literature. Development of objective criteria utilizing a consistent visible improvement is necessary to optimize the use of direct visualization.

A majority of our patients remained intubated beyond 48 hours as a result direct visualization. Our guidelines for extubation may be too strict. Support for this is given by the patients who were inadvertently self extubated early and did not require reintubation. Extubation was also delayed by the practice of not extubating patients during the afternoon or evening hours.

Although direct visualization did not significantly shorten the duration of intubation in our subjects, serial examinations with the flexible fiberoptic laryngoscope in our patients provided a simple means of viewing the supraglottis. More objective parameters concerning the condition of the supraglottis could shorten the time period of intubation. For those who utilize visual methods of determining when these patients should be extubated, this technique is as effective as direct laryngoscopy in the operating room but avoids the need for anesthesia and can be performed at the bedside.

REFERENCES

1. Rothstein P, Lister S (1984) Anesth and Analgesia 62:785-787
2. Faden HS (1979) Pediatrics 63:3
3. Vernon DD, Sarnaik AP (1984) Anesth and Analgesia 63:469
4. Berry FA (1984) Anesth and Analgesia 63:469-470
5. Nussbaum E (1983) J Pediatrics 102:2

© 1985 Elsevier Science Publishers B.V. (Biomedical Division)
New dimensions in otorhinolaryngology - head and neck surgery, vol. 2.
E. Myers, editor

FIBEROPTIC MANIPULATION OF THE UPPER AIRWAY & THE PREOPERATIVE ASSESSMENT FOR UVULOPALATOPHARYNGOPLASTY

JEFFREY N. HAUSFELD, M.D.
Proceedings Unit, Biomedical Division, Elsevier Science Publishers B.V.,
P.O. Box 1527, 1000 BM Amsterdam (The Netherlands)

INTRODUCTION

The preoperative evaluation of patients for correction of severe snoring or obstructive sleep apnea syndrome should include a careful history and physical examination, polysomnography to determine the percentage of peripheral obstruction versus central apnea and cephalometric radiographs when deemed necessary.

In addition to this, I am performing a fiberoptic nasopharyngoscopy and laryngoscopy in order to rule out any obstructive lesions of the upper respiratory tract. While examining the patient with the fiberscope, the physician is also able to obtain an idea of the dynamics of the patient's nasopharyngeal port during quiet and forceful inspiration (snoring).

The fiberscope is then used to manipulate the posterior portion of the soft palate to determine if this maneuver causes any alteration in the sound produced during forceful inspiration. This manipulation of the patient's upper airway has proven very useful in allowing the patient to more fully understand the pathophysiology of his condition and how the planned surgical procedure would be of benefit in alleviating his partial airway obstruction.

In addition, it aids the physician in the preoperative counseling of such patients after determining that alteration of the patient's velopharyngeal port would most likely eliminate the problem of snoring.

TECHNIQUE

First, the patient's nose is anesthetized with a topical anesthetic solution (5% cocaine or 4% Lidocaine). A flexible nasopharyngoscope is then placed through the patient's nose and is used to examine the nasopharynx, velopharyngeal port, hypopharynx and larynx. Once the examiner has determined that there are no other obstructing lesions of the upper respiratory tract, the nasopharyngoscope is then placed in the nasopharynx so that a view of the nasal side of the soft palate is obtained. The patient is then put in a reclining position with use of a motorized examining chair. The patient is then asked to simulate his snoring. It is helpful to have a spouse present during this examination to verify that this is similar to the patient's usual snoring problem. At this time, the tip of the fiberscope is maneuvered in such a way as to push the uvula and soft palate forward. The patient is then again asked to attempt to snore. If the source of the upper airway noise during sleep is coming from fluttering of the uvula and soft palate, then this maneuver will preclude the patient from snoring. The fiberscope is then placed back into the posterior nasal cavity and the patient is again asked to snore which he is usually able to do without any difficulty.

DISCUSSION

Fiberoptic examination of the upper respiratory tract is an important adjunct to the preoperative evaluation for the uvulopalatopharyngoplasty. The maneuver described above has proven to be very helpful in allowing the patient to understand how the surgery will help eliminate his snoring. When done on a large series of patients, this maneuver may prove to be of predictive value in determining whether the UPPP will be successful for any given patient. This in conjunction with other work which is now being investigated will help in the careful preoperative selection of patients as well as aiding their understanding and acceptance of this procedure.

REFERENCES

1. Borowiecki, B. and Sassin, J.: Surgical Treatment of Sleep Apnea. Arch Otolaryngology, Aug; 109: 508, 1983

2. Cotton, R.: Uvulopalatopharyngoplasty. Arch Otolaryngology, Aug; 109:502, 1983

New dimensions in otorhinolaryngology - head and neck surgery, vol. 2.
E. Myers, editor

TRANSCUTANEOUS OXYGEN AND CARBON DIOXIDE TENSIONS IN CHRONIC UPPER AIRWAYS OBSTRUCTION AND THE EFFECT OF TONSILLECTOMY AND ADENOIDECTOMY

A.G. TUCKER Department of Otorhinolaryngology
C.J. REYNOLDS Department of Child Health
The University of Liverpool, Liverpool, U.K.

INTRODUCTION

Case reports of children with chronic upper airways obstruction due to hypertrophy of the tonsils and adenoids have appeared with increasing frequency since Noonan (1) described two severely affected children with pulmonary hypertension. Measurement of arterial oxygen and carbon dioxide tensions (paO_2 and $paCO_2$) has been possible only by invasive methods and has been justifiable only in severely affected patients. Transcutaneous gas tensions measurements ($ptcO_2$ and $ptcCO_2$) have been possible recently (2).

MATERIALS AND METHODS

Transcutaneous oxygen and carbon dioxide levels have been measured in sleeping children using a mass spectrometer (Medishield MS2) and disposable surface probe to determine the levels before and after tonsillectomy and adenoidectomy. Respiration was monitored using a Pye MR10 recorder.

40 children were studied over a period of 8 months. Measurements were obtained after 9 p.m. when it was expected that most children would usually be asleep.

RESULTS

The normal level of $paCO_2$ in children is between 4 - 4.8 Kpa (3) and rises to the adult level of 5.3 - 5.9 during later childhood. We took the upper limit of normal to be 6.0 Kpa. 18 children had a $ptcCO_2$ within these limits ($\leqslant$ 6 Kpa) and 22 had a $ptcCO_2 >$ 6.1 Kpa.

The children were further differentiated into those with a normal transcutaneous oxygen and those who were hypoxic during sleep. Four groups of children were thus defined on their pre-operative levels: Group 1 were considered to have normal transcutaneous gases and group 4 were considered to be the most severely affected individuals.

Group	No.	$ptcO_2$	$ptcCO_2$
1	14	>10.7	<6.1
2	4	<10.7	<6.1
3	12	>10.7	>6.1
4	10	<10.7	>6.1

Following surgery, in groups 1 and 2 there is no significant change in either gas. In group 3, there is a significant fall in the $ptcCO_2$ to within the normal range. In group 4, there is a significant improvement in both gases although neither returned to within the normal range.

Group	Transcutaneous pO_2 (Kpa)			Transcutaneous pCO_2 (Kpa)		
	Pre-op	Post-op	P	Pre-op	Post-op	P
1	12.45	11.85	n.s.	5.50	5.20	n.s.
2	9.9	11.85	n.s.	6.07	5.06	n.s.
3	11.85	11.40	n.s.	6.45	5.90	0.02
4	8.40	10.20	0.04	7.60	6.81	0.02

DISCUSSION

The children of group 1 did not have chronic upper airway obstruction and their profiles have not changed. The transcutaneous gas profiles of children in group 2 are similar to those obtained from children with chronic lower respiratory tract disease (e.g. cystic fibrosis) and also do not benefit from E.N.T. surgery.

Group 3 do have chronic sleeping hypoventilation but without compromising $ptcO_2$. There is no evidence that chronic hypercapnoea alone without hypoxia is harmful. These children may grow out of their abnormality as the tonsils and adenoids involute.

Of more concern are the children of group 4. Although there is a significant improvement in both O_2 and CO_2, their gas profiles remain abnormal which may suggest other cardio-respiratory disease, secondary to their chronic upper airway obstruction, which is not immediately reversed by surgery.

REFERENCES

1. NOONAN J.A. Reversible Cor Pulmonale due to hypertrophied tonsils and adenoids: Studies in two cases. Circulation 32 supp., 16+ - 168 1965
2. GOODWIN B., MAKIN R.P., REYNOLDS C.J., COWEN J., HARRIS F. Transcutaneous blood gas measurements using a mass spectrometer and disposable surface probe. In: Frigerio A, McCamish M. (eds) Recent developments in biochemistry and medicin, vol. 3. New York: Plenum Publishing Co. 1979
3. BRADLEY A., SHIPFEL M., SEVERINGHAUS J.W. Effect of temperature on pCO_2 and pO_2 of blood in vitro J. Applied Physiology 9, 210 - 204 1956

New dimensions in otorhinolaryngology - head and neck surgery, vol. 2.
E. Myers, editor

BRONCHOSCOPY BY OTOLARYNGOLOGISTS IN SMALL HOSPITALS

BENGT G OLLMAN, GUNBJØRN AASAND
Departments of Otolaryngology, Visby County Hospital Sweden and
Kongsberg Hospital Norway

INTRODUCTION

The sad fact that treatment of bronchial carcinoma still gives very poor results should not refrain from the use of flexible bronchoscopy even in small hospitals. On the contrary it will be of great value to be able to omit, with the best certainty available, the presence of malignancy in cases where pulmonary disease has to be diagnosed. Periferal hospitals serving a population of about 50.000 people are often regarded as outpatient institutions with the aim of collecting and sorting patients and to forward the complicated cases to large and more sophisticated clinics. High efficiency in diagnosis is therefore cost saving for the small clinic, and should therefore be interesting for hospital boards and health politicians.

When it comes to bronchoscopy the indications for this procedure have increased so much during the last decades with the arrival of the flexible instruments that it is no longer a procedure only for advanced clinics in otolaryngology but also is used by many other specialities. To keep up training for foreign body removal however otolaryngologists should be keen in performing as many bronchoscopies as possible in the small hospital.

MATERIAL AND METHODS

Over an 11 years period 544 bronchoscopies in 536 patients have been performed in a population of 55.000 people. 207 of these patients have died, but only 86 of them have died from a disease diagnosed through the bronchoscopy, as can be seen from Table I.

The remaining 121 deaths have been attributed to diseases not diagnosed through the bronchoscope, but where bronchoscopy was used to evaluate the bronchial condition as to the presence of metastasies or airway compression. Included are also 17 patients who underwent therapeutic bronchoscopy during terminal care in the ICU. The cause of death for these 121 patients have been malignant diseases from the stomach, the genito-urinary tract or the blood, as well as emphysema, neurological disorders or cardiac failures. Only those patients where malignant disease has been diagnosed primarily through the bronchoscope have been referred from our department to an oncologic centre.

TABLE I
DEATHS FROM BRONCHOSCOPICALLY DIAGNOSED AIRWAY DISEASE
May 1st 1974 - April 30th 1985

Diagnosis	Deaths
Squamous cell bronchial carcinoma	40
Small cell and oat cell bronchial carcinoma	15
Adenocarcinoma	9
Undifferentiated bronchial carcinoma	4
Squmaous cell laryngeal carcinoma	4
Unspecified or other malignant tumours	14
Total	86

Of the bronchoscopically examined 329 patients are still alive. In 6 of these malignant bronchial disease has been found early and they have been treated succesfully at the oncologic or thoracic centre.

The remaining 323 have had diagnoses such as chronic bronchitis, middle lobe atelectasis, sarcoidosis, laryngitis, post-tuberculous bronchial strictures, foreign bodies and postoperative check-ups, and could all be treated in the local hospital with good result.

RESULTS

In small hospitals such as Visby in Sweden or Kongsberg in Norway, with long distances to oncologic centers and thoracic surgery, a high technical standard in diagnosing malignant bronchial disease is necessary. With a charged cost of 2.500 SEK pr day and a minimum stay of 3 days in the oncolocig, or big hospital clinic the 323 patients would have cost 2.4 million SEK and the travel expenses would have raised up to 1 million SEK, had these patients been referred.The loss of labour income and the social expenses would have added another 2 millions to the bill. Thus 5.4 million SEK have been saved by performing the bronchoscopies in the local hospital. Had the 121 patients, who died from other diseases also been referred from our clinic an extra cost of 4 million SEK would have occured. This equals nearly 1 million US dollars, saved by performing bronchoscopy in the small hospital.

We therefore claim that flexible bronchoscopy should be performed in small periferal hospitals by otolaryngologists on the following grounds:

1. Improved diagnosis in malignant bronchial diseases will be secured.
2. Proper skill in removing foreign bodies from the airways is maintained.
3. Unnecessary and discomfortable transportation is saved for hundreds of patients.
4. Large sums of money will be saved by the small hospital clinic.

New dimensions in otorhinolaryngology - head and neck surgery, vol. 2.
E. Myers, editor

SYNCHRONOUS SECOND PRIMARY TUMORS OF THE UPPER AERO-DIGESTIVE TRACT

ASHOK SHAHA, M.D. EDDIE HOOVER, F.A.C.S., NEAL HAMMERMAN, M.D., JOSE MARTI, F.A.C.S., Dept. Of Surgery, Brooklyn V.A. Hospital, 800 Poly Place, Brooklyn New York 11209

INTRODUCTION

The incidence of synchronous second primary tumors of the upper aerodigestive tract reported in the literature varies from 5 to 15% (Table 1). Since the original description of field cancerization by Slaughter, clinicians have always been looking for the second tumor in the head-neck area (1). Since the two main carcinogenic agents - smoking and alcohol have the deleterious effect on all of the upper aerodigestive tract it is not surprising to find the high incidence of synchronous and metachronous tumors in the head-neck areas. However it is of paramount importance to detect these tumors early enough so that appropriate therapy can be offered to these patients. The high incidence of synchronous tumors in the esophagus, and lung was initially reported by Cahan et al (2).

Variety of different methods have been used by various investigators to search for synchronous second primaries. Routine triple endoscopy with bronchial washings have been considered as important step in investigation of these patients by some authors (3,4,5,6).

MATERIAL AND METHODS

This is a prospective study of 100 patients over two year period. The search for second primary was made by clinical examination, routine chest XRay and Barium Swallow when indicated. More importance was given to repeat head & neck examination. Storz fiberoptic scope was used where nasopharynx and laryngopharynx were difficult to evaluate. Barium swallow was done only when there was suspicious history or weight loss. There were 99 males and one female. Their ages ranged from 40 to 88 years. All the patients were followed from 1 to 3 years.

RESULTS

In this prospective study the incidence of synchronous second primary tumors was 14%. Of this there were seven with second tumor in the head-neck region while four and three patients had tumors of the lung and esophagus respectively. One patient had 3 synchronous primaries. All these tumors were diagnosed by thorough head and neck examination, CXR and Barium study as indicated. Routine triple endoscopy was not done. Esophagoscopy was done only if the patient was to be anesthetised for evaluation of extent of tumor of the laryngopharynx or for biopsy. Bronchoscopy and bronchial washings were not done routinely in the presence of normal CXR. There were eight patients with the primary tumors in oropharynx while four and two patients had their primary tumors in the larynx or hypopharynx. The sites of synchronous second tumors in the head & neck area were as follows: soft palate-4; uvula, post pharyngeal wall and epiglottis, one each. There were 3 other patients with synchronous second primary of the rectum and one patient had carcinoma of the prostate. During the follow up period only one patient with Stage III transglottic cancer developed pleural effusion, lung masses and died 7 months after initial laryngectomy .

DISCUSSION

This study emphasizes the high incidence of synchronous second primary tumors of the upper aerodigestive tract (14%). The need for thorough examination can not be over emphasized. We have used endoscopy and esophagoscopy if the patient is to be anesthetised for evaluation of extent of the tumor in the laryngopharynx and for biopsy purpose. A suspicious history and history of weight loss is a definite indication of Barium swallow. A routine rigid or fiberoptic bronchoscopy and bronchial cytology is questioned in the absence of abnormal CXR. The value of positive bronchial cytology in the presence of another tumor in the upper aerodigestive tract and normal CXR is always questioned. We are not sure if the yield of routine bronchoscopy and bronchial washing is cost effective. It does involve two intubations for laryngoscopy and flexible bronchoscopy. However a routine esophagoscopy after evaluation of laryngopharynx does not involve increased time factor. We strongly feel the need to evaluate the patient for second primary tumor in the upper aerodigestive tract and outside. (Colon & prostate especially since most of these are elderly patients).

TABLE 1

SYNCHRONOUS SECOND PRIMARIES		
Gluckman	1979	9%
Shapshay et al	1980	14%
Maisel et al	1981	8%
McGuirt	1982	16%
Leipzig et al	1984	10%
Shaha et al	1985	14%

TABLE 2

SITES OF SECOND PRIMARIES		
Head & Neck	-	7%
Esophagus	-	3%
Lung	-	4%
Total	-	14%
Rectum	-	3%
Prostate	-	1%

REFERENCES

1. Slaughter DP, Southwick HW, Smejkal W (1953) "Field Cancerization" in Oral Stratified Squamous Epithelium. Cancer 6:963-968.

2. Cahan WG, Castro EB, Rosen PP, Strong EW (1976) Separate Primary Carcinomas of the Esophagus and Head & Neck Region in the Same Patient. Cancer 37:85-89.

3. Shapshay SM et al (1980) Simultaneous Carcinomas of the Esophagus and Upper Aerodigestive Tract. Otolaryngol Head & Neck Surgery 88:373-377.

4. Atkinson D, Fleming S, Weaver A (1982) Triple Endoscopy-A Valuable Procedure in Head & Neck Surgery. Am J Surg 144: 416-419.

5. McGuirt WF (1982) Panendoscopy as a Screening Examination for Simultaneous Primary Tumors in the Head & Neck Cancer: A prospective sequential study and review of the literature. Laryngoscope 92: 569-576.

6. Leipzig B et al (1984) Panendoscopy in Patients With Squamous Carcinoma of the Head & Neck. Exhibition at the International Head & Neck Conference. Baltimore.

© 1985 Elsevier Science Publishers B.V. (Biomedical Division)
New dimensions in otorhinolaryngology - head and neck surgery, vol. 2.
E. Myers, editor

MANAGMENT OF FOREIGN BODIES IN THE BRONCHI

WALAE H. ABOU-SHELEB, HASSAN M. MOUSTAFA.
FROM THE E.N.T DEPARTMENT TANTA UNIVERSITY, EGYPT

REVIEW OF LITREATURE

Inhaled F.B. usually happens in early childhood before the age of 6 years. Rothmanns et al. (1980), reported that about 80% of the F.B. were lodged in the right bronchus and that of vegetable nature consisted of a precentage of 70%. Aytac et al. (1977), concluded that a past history of F.B. aspiration is in itself an indication for bronchoscopic examination of the airways.

The sequela of this serious condition depends upon the nature of F.B., age of the victim, time of presentation and the gentle bronchoscopic technique. Good anatomical knowledge of the tracheobronchial tree, proper instrumentation and skilful anaesthetist are important factors for safe extraction of F.B. bronchi.

Kanata et al, (1979), concluded that in a series of 36 children under the age of 3 years with inhaled non contrast F.B., obstructive emphysema was found on the affected side in most of the cases.

Rothmann et al; (1980), reported no mortality in 225 children with inhaled F.B. Aytac (1977), in 500 cases reported 1.4% postbronchoscopy tracheotomy and 1.8% as a total mortality rate.

CASE MATERIAL

In this work 100 cases of inhaled F.B. had been done. Out of this group 90 cases were inhaled vegetable F.B. The commonest were water melon seeds, sun flower seeds, peanuts and soft food remnants. The other 10 cases were screw nails, hair pin, thumb tack, stainless steel and plastic balls, sea snail, broken inner tracheotomy tube and, tip of atropin glass vial. The youngest patient was aged 7 months and the oldest one was 25 years. Sixty five cases were found in the right bronchial tree.

CLINICAL PRESENTATION

Respiratory distress and stridor. Attacks of cough and cyanosis. Diminished air entry on the affected side with prolonged expiratory phase. Chest infection manifested by moist rales and bronchospasm. Impaired percussion note and atelectasis. Radiological examination revealed the non vegetable F.B.

PROCEDURE FOR F.B. EXTRACTION BY BRONCHESCOPY

Preoperative hydrocortisone and bronchodilator were given to minimise post bronchoscopy laryngeal oedema and to decrease bronchospasm. All cases were done under general anaesthesia using Hopkins optical bronchscope with suitable forceps for the inhaled object was used. All the patients were hospitalised for 1-4 days and put under antibiotics. Radiography was done before their discharge.

DISCUSSION

History is usually suggestive and bronchoscopy is an indication. Radiography of the chest declares the radio opaque F.B. but most of the vegetable F.B. are radiolucent, other data as atelectasis, collaps and emphysema are usually the main clue for the presence of F.B. In this work we used the optical Hopkins bronchoscope which has many advanteges over the old Jakson one. It allows excellent fibre optic illumination, magnifying lens and special channels for the malleable forceps and the anaesthetics.

Extraction of the F.B. by this optical bronchoscope was under vision wihtout interruption; suction can be achieved at the same time. Non of these cases needed post operative tracheostomy. The only mortality recorded in this group was the case of broken tip glass vial, from the present trauma and oedema of the tracheobroncheal mucous membrane in repeated trials in another center. Eight cases were bronchosoped for the unresolved chest infection in spite of promote treatment. Plant F.B. was found in the bronchi of these patients in spite of no history of inhaled F.B. Four cases of this group were found to have multiple F.B.,re-examination by bronchoscopy is essential not to miss another F.B.

REFERENCES

1- Aytac et., Inhalation of foreign bodies in children report of 500 cases. J. Thorac. cardiovase. Surge. 1977 74/1 (145-151).

2- Kanata J. and Kolihova E-Detsk, The problems of radiological diagnosis of non contrast Foreign bodies in Lower respiratory pathways in children. CESK Pediatr 1979 34/7 (396-398).

3- Rothman B.F. and Boeckman. Foreign bodies in the laryns and tracheibroncial tree in children-ANB. Otolarryngolog 1980 8915 (434-436).

© 1985 Elsevier Science Publishers B.V. (Biomedical Division)
New dimensions in otorhinolaryngolcgy - head and neck surgery, vol. 2.
E. Myers, editor

VIDEOFIBERSTROBOSCOPY - A METHOD FOR THE DIAGNOSIS OF LARYNXCANCER AT AN EARLY STAGE.

B. TOMMERUP (1), S. PRYTZ (2), and S. TELMER (3)
University Dept. of ENT, Rigshospitalet, Copenhagen, Denmark.

INTRODUCTION

It has been known for a number of years that reduced travelling wave of the mucosa indicates incipient malignancy. However, no measurings of the mucosal wave have ever been made; neither has it been attempted to compare T_1-cancer (carcinoma being localized to one vocal fold) to dysplasia/precancrose - concerning difference in mobility, mucosal wave, and vibratory cycle.
The aim of this investigation has been the finding of a clinical method for the purpose of a better, and more quick diagnosis of larynxcancer than has been known so far.

METHOD

All cases have been directly laryngoscopated using the Olympus fiberoptic laryngoscope type ENF-P. This fiberscope has been connected to the Brüel & Kjær rhino-larynx-stroboscope type 4914, and a Olympus 0 microcamera, and the Sony U-matic video-recorder with single frame. The shots have been taken with, and without stroboscopic lightning.

MATERIAL

35 patients, 32 men (91,4%), and 3 women (8,6%) were examined by means of videostroboscopy. 13 patients suffering from chronical laryngitis (CL), 11 patients from dysplasia (D), and 11 patients from T_1-cancer (T_1). 6 cases had to be omitted.

RESULTS

On looking at the videotape the mobility of the vocal folds has been assesed as well as mucosal wave, vibration cycle, phase displacement, and irregular vibration. After this the travelling wave of the mucosa has been measured, and regarding D, and T_1, significant difference was found between left, and right vocal fold, whereas there was no difference regarding CL. (Wilcoxon´s Test)
Table 1 shows the mean values of open quotient, speed quotient, and speed index - no significant difference was found. (Mann-Witney´s Test) (1,2)

	OQ	SQ	SI
CL	0,626	1,34	0,132
D	0,619	1,18	-0,055
T_1	0,650	1,36	0,161

Table 1 - The mean values of OQ, SQ, and SI

DISCUSSION

As expected a significant difference between left, and right vocal fold was discovered at measuring the travelling wave of the mucosa at patients suffering from T_1, and D. No difference, however, was found when calculating SI, which we think will have to be ascribed to the process itself, as the sharpness of image is not always of the best quality. Therefore certain difficulties may occur at stating the exact duration of the phases of one vibratory cycle. The glottal closure turned out to be inadequate. The same uncertainty is present in the measuring of the mucosal wave.

It is our oppinion, however, that the process is practicable when diagnosing larynxcancer at an early stage - especially when the signals are digitalized.

SUMMARY

35 cases were examined by means of videostroboscopy. 13 patients suffering from chronical laryngitis, 11 patients from dysplasia, and 11 patients from T_1-cancer. The mucosal wave was calculated as a result of which no significant difference was found between left, and right vocal fold regarding dysplasia, and T_1-cancer, as well as there was no difference as to speed index. The process is practicable when diagnosing larynxcancer at an early stage - especially when digitalizing the signals.

REFERENCES

1. Hirano, M: Clinical Examination of Voice. Springer Verlag, 1981.
2. Timcke, R., von Leden, H., and Moore, P.: Laryngeal Vibrations: Measurements of the Glottic Wave. A.M.A. Arch. Otolaryng. 68: 1-19, 1958.

© 1985 Elsevier Science Publishers B.V. (Biomedical Division)
New dimensions in otorhinolaryngology - head and neck surgery, vol. 2.
E. Myers, editor

ACOUSTIC NEUROMA - THE PATIENT'S PERSPECTIVE

DAVID A. WIEGAND, M.D.

Division of Otolaryngology and Head and Neck Surgery, The Milton S. Hershey College of Medicine of The Pennsylvania State University, Hershey, Pa. 17033

VIRGINIA FICKEL, M.S.

The Acoustic Neuroma Association, Carlisle, Pa. 17013

CRAIG ZIERDT B.S.

Carlisle. Pa. 17013

INTRODUCTION

While several large series of treatment results for acoustic neuroma patients have been published, no large study has gathered the results from many institutions or from the patient's perspective. This paper presents part of the data obtained from a questionnaire completed by 528 patients treated for acoustic neuroma in the United States and Canada. Emphasis is placed on the analysis of facial nerve function as assessed by these patients, who are members of The Acoustic Neuroma Association (A.N.A.), a non-profit patient self-help group.

METHOD

A detailed questionnaire was designed to elicit retrospective data concerning diagnosis, treatment, and sequelae of acoustic neuroma. The questionnaire was sent to each A.N.A. member. Responses were hand-scored and entered into a computer data bank, from which the data presented here were abstracted.

RESULTS

528 questionnaires were returned, a response of 64%. This includes 172 men and 356 women, ages ranging from 8 to 84 years. Date of surgery ranged from 1949 to 1984. Neuromas affected left and right sides equally. 85% reported hearing loss, 60% reported dysequilibrium, and 56% reported tinnitus as early symptoms. 20% reported symptom onset more than 6 years before diagnosis, which was made by an otolaryngologist in 68% of cases. 81 patients estimated tumor diameter as less than 2 cm., 236 estimated diameter between 2 and 4 cm., 158 estimated diameter greater than 4 cm., 53 were uncertain. 362 patients had a translabyrinthine approach, 52 had a posterior fossa approach, and 33 had a middle fossa approach for tumor excision.

Surgical results are shown below:

TUMOR DIAMETER LESS THAN 2 CM.	Number	75% Or Better Facial Nerve Function
Translabyrinthine	55	76%
Middle Fossa	3	66%
Posterior Fossa	6	100%

TUMOR DIAMETER 2 - 4 CM.	Number	75% Or Better Facial Nerve Function
Translabyrinthine	158	46%
Middle Fossa	14	64%
Posterior Fossa	20	40%

TUMOR DIAMETER GREATER THAN 4 CM.	Number	75% Or Better Facial Nerve Function
Translabyrinthine	83	38%
Middle Fossa	6	33%
Posterior Fossa	15	40%

While postoperative facial nerve function worsened with increasing tumor size, no clear advantage was shown for any surgical approach by this criterion when tumors of equal size were compared.

Overall, 75% of patients reported residual facial nerve deficit. 61% of those with deficit assess their facial nerve function as less than 50% of normal. 14% of those with deficit underwent a neural anastomosis procedure which improved facial nerve function.

CONCLUSION

This paper presents the first large sample of acoustic neuroma patients giving the patient's assessment of outcome for a variety of surgical approaches performed at institutions throughout the United States and Canada. While suffering from the limitations of all retrospective and subjective evaluations, it demonstrates that 75% of this group experience continued facial nerve deficit, and that different surgical approaches gave comparable results.

New dimensions in otorhinolaryngology – head and neck surgery, vol. 2.
E. Myers, editor

TRANSTEMPORAL REMOVAL OF ACOUSTIC NEUROMAS FROM THE CPA WITH PRESERVATION OF HEARING

MALTE ERIK WIGAND, TONI HAID, MICHAEL BERG, GERHARD RETTINGER
University of Erlangen-Nuremberg, Department of Otorhinolaryngology,
Waldstr. 1, 8520 Erlangen (Germany)

Since, in 1961, William House had designed the middle fossa approach to the internal auditory canal this operation has gained merits for the complete removal of small acoustic neuromas with safe preservation of the facial nerve, with occasional preservation of auditory function, and with an extremely low complication rate. The own good experiences with this transpetrosal access to the cerebello-pontine angle (CPA) from above have stimulated us to systematically modify this technique into a standard procedure for several indications of otologic surgery within the petrous pyramid and at the CPA (Wigand 1982). Among those even the management of large acoustic neuromas with preservation of hearing has become a goal.

SURGICAL TECHNIQUE

The main features of our surgical technique consist of:

- the extradural dissection of the middle cerebral fossa,
- extensive bone resection behind and in front of the internal auditory canal (CAI) almost to the tip of the pyramid. Figure 1 depicts the areas of bone resection schematically.
- resection of the superior petrosal sinus if necessary,
- broad exposure of the cerebello-pontine angle.

Facing the acoustic neuroma from above the facial nerve could be identified, and dissected from the beginning of the tumour removal. A consequent intracapsular tumour reduction by morcellation enabled the surgeon to stepwise bring the tumour capsule into vision, and to dissect the adherent vessels in contiguity. Also the blunt dissection of the tumour from the cerebellum and the brainstem was realized by direct visualization of these sites by the described superior transpetrosal - not translabyrinthine ! - approach. According to the modalities of the particular tumour growth also the dissection and preservation of the cochlear nerve was possible in many cases. All operations were carried out on patients in a reclined position as described by W. House earlier.

CLINICAL MATERIAL AND RESULTS

Out of a series of 163 acoustic neuromas operated in our department 96 (51 males, 45 females) underwent the enlarged middle fossa operation. Since 1981 this procedure was our method of choice. Table 1 gives our results with regard to the completeness of the tumour removal, the functional results and our complication rates. A certain transitory facial nerve impairment was frequent, due to the surgical trauma or postoperative swelling. It was not put down as complication.

Fig. 1 Extensive bone resection (hatched area) behind and in front of the internal auditory canal for the superior transpetrosal approach to the cerebello-pontine angle (schematic sketch after Valvassori)

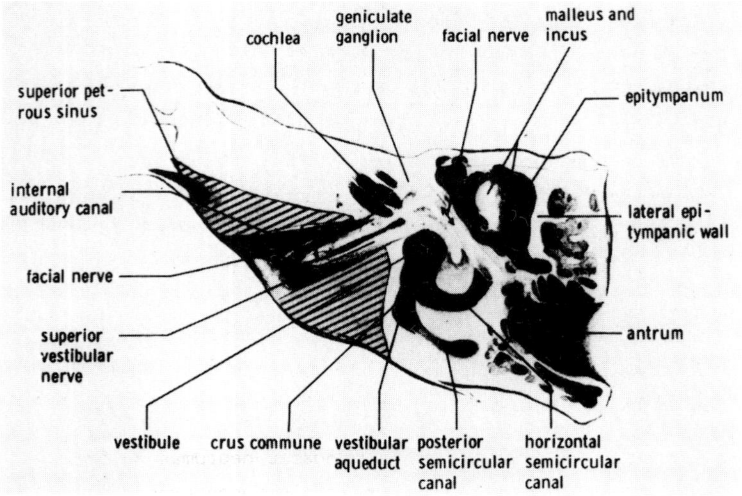

From the data we may conclude that the described surgical technique offers good chances for a safe and complete removal of acoustic neuromas of up to 3.5 cm diameter. Its slightly greater expenditure of surgical efforts to expose the CPA, in comparison to the suboccipital approach, is compensated by the lower incidence of complications and a higher rate of preserved auditory function. Another argument is the unrestricted visualization of the meatal fundus which remains unexposed by the suboccipital access.
The translabyrinthine approach to the cerebello-pontine angle, which is preferred by many otoneurosurgeons but always induces total deafness, is contraindicated for all ears which are considered as appropriate for hearing preservation or for the application of a cochlear implant. This procedure, therefore, was replaced by the above mentioned superior trans-petrosal (enlarged middle fossa) approach to the cerebello-pontine angle.

TABLE 1

ONCOLOGICAL AND FUNCTIONAL RESULTS AND COMPLICATION RATES OF 96 ACOUSTIC NEUROMA OPERATIONS BY THE ENLARGED MIDDLE FOSSA APPROACH

	total	tumour sizes A	B	C
middle fossa operations	96	16	33	47
complete tumour removal	79	16	29	34
planned subtotal resection (last hearing ear, palliation etc.)	11	0	2	9
resection subtotal for topographical or other reasons	6	0	2*	4
ears with preop. serviceable hearing	71	14	25	32
cochlear nerve preserved	67	14	24	29
postoperatively hearing ears	36	9	14	13
postop. / preop. hearing ears	51%	64%	56%	41%
postop. hearing with compl. tumour removal	49%	64%	56%	38%
facial nerve preserved	92	15	33	44
n.VII function well preserved	50	15	17	18
n.VII function slightly disturbed	34	-	16	18
n.VII function severely disturbed	12	1	2	9
transitory meningism/-itis	7	2	1	4
transitory neurological symptoms	7	0	1	6
permanent neurological deficit	0	0	0	0
letal exit	0	0	0	0
severe intra-/postop. hemorrhage	2	0	0	2
secondary wound healing	4	0	3	1
second operation for csf-fistula	1	0	1	0

Especially for cases with bilateral growth of acoustic neuromas or for tumours of the "last hearing ear" the enlarged middle fossa exposure of the CPA offers a fair chance to identify the facial nerve already at the onset of the tumour resection. From the sometimes considerably displaced position of the facial nerve the surgeon may gain a clearer idea of where to find and to preserve the cochlear nerve than with a suboccipital access to the CPA. In this typically neurosurgical exposure both the facial and the cochlear nerves can only be identified after tumour removal with a higher risk of unwanted total deafness. For the "last ear" and for giant neurinomas with good auditory function a two-stage procedure may be the indication of choice.

REFERENCES

House WF (1961) Surgical exposure of the internal auditory canal and its contents through the middle cranial fossa. Laryngoscope 71:1363-1385

Wigand ME, Haid T, Berg M, Rettinger G (1982) The enlarged transtemporal approach to the cerebello-pontine angle. Technique and indications. Acta Otorhinolaryngol Ital 2:571-582

Wigand ME, Rettinger G, Haid T, Berg M (1985) The removal of VIIIth-nerve neurinomas from the cerebello-pontine angle by an enlarged middle fossa approach. HNO 33:11-16

New dimensions in otorhinolaryngology - head and neck surgery, vol. 2.
E. Myers, editor

HEARING AFTER TRANSLABYRINTHINE RESECTION OF AN ACOUSTIC NEUROMA

ROBERT SAWYER, MD

Division of Otolaryngology, Department of Surgery, Uniformed Services University of the Health Sciences, Bethesda, MD USA

INTRODUCTION

Only eighteen cases have been reported in which destruction of a portion of the labyrinth has not been associated with inevitable loss of hearing. A patient, who underwent a translabyrinthine resection of an acoustic neuroma with preservation of the cochlear nerve, is presented as a thought provoking addition to this small series of cases.

CASE REPORT

A 67 year old white woman had a one month history of right sided headache when she awoke with diplopia, vertigo, tinnitis, and right ear pressure. Her family also noted some slurring of speech and questionable weakness of the corner of the mouth. Shortly after admission to the neurology service, pertinent examination of this frail appearing patient, was normal except for mild weakness of the right corner of the mouth and obvious right hearing loss. There was no nystagmus. Her symptoms rapidly cleared, except for right hearing loss and the weakness of the corner of the mouth. Her original audiogram revealed an assymetrical sensorineural hearing loss with very poor discrimination. A thorough workup was performed to evaluate what was thought to be a transient ischemic episode, but the only positive finding was a right acoustic tumor shown on air contrast CT scan.

TREATMENT AND EVALUATION

Ultimately a translabyrinthine excision of the 1 1/2 cm acoustic neuroma was performed. The tumor was unusually free of the facial and cochlear nerves and was easily removed intact, saving those nerves (normally only the facial nerve is preserved). Postoperatively, the patient did well, but from the second postoperative day onward she reported hearing "echoes" in the operated ear. Numerous audiograms were performed by serveral highly experienced audiologists. Each time using adequate masking, residual hearing with maximum conductive loss was found in the operated ear. Bone conduction levels in that ear at 250, 500, 1000 and 2000 Hz were 20, 40, 40, and 70 dB respectively. Finally bone conduction auditory brainstem evoked responses[1] revealed definite, repeatable waves 1 and 2 from the operated ear. The non-operated ear showed moderate high frequency sensorineural hearing loss but was otherwise normal in every evaluation.

DISCUSSION

In 1955, Sade-Sadowsky[2] reviewed the six cases in the literature in which the membranous labyrinth was damaged but with preservation of hearing and added three additional cases, all related to injury at fenestration operation. Shambaugh[3] and Pedersen[4] each reported one such case involving removal of the lateral semicircular canal. In 1969, Phelps[5] reported three cases in which hearing was preserved, despite labyrinthine invasion by cholesteatoma. He proposed that slow destruction by cholesteatoma may allow a protective wall of granulation tissue to be laid down walling off the adjacent labyrinth and thus allowing it to retain its function. To these fourteen cases, Bumstead, et al[6] added four additional cases, including one "pars superior labyrinthectomy" for recurrent cholesteatoma into the petrous apex for which all three semicircular canals (which were not involved with disease) were removed. They speculated that an acute inflammatory process might occasionally wall off the cochlea, preserving its function. They mentioned four narrowed areas of the membranous labyrinth as possible places for this to occur: 1) the ductus reuniens, 2) the saccular duct, 3) the utricular duct, and 4) the utriculoendolymphatic valve, focusing upon the utriculoendolymphatic valve as being the most likely, citing Schuknecht and Belal[7].

The case presented had surgical removal of all semicircular canals, the utricle and all but a tattered remnant of the saccule. It remained open for over an hour while the internal auditory canal was being drilled out and the tumor was being resected, then a plug of fat was placed. Using the "duct-inflammatory wall" theory, the site would have had to be at the ductus reuniens. An alternative would be that the torn membranous labyrinth was pinched closed by the fat until healing took place. In view of this case and clinical experience with preserved hearing in cochleosacculotomy surgery, in which a deliberate opening is created into the the membranous labyrinth, one must question the necessity for any inflammatory wall to theoretically explain hearing preservation with labyrinthine injury.

REFERENCES

1. Mauldin L, Jerger J (1979) Arch Otolaryngol 105:656-661
2. Sade-Sadosky N (1955) J Laryngol Otol 69:753-756
3. Shambaugh G (1967) In: Surgery of the Ear, W B Saunders, Philadelphia, p354
4. Pedersen C (1969) J Laryngol Otol 83:929-832
5. Phelps P (1969) J Laryngol Otol 83:1111-1114
6. Bumstead RM, Sade J, Dolan KD, McCabe BF (1977) Ann Otol 86:131-137
7. Schuknecht HF, Delal A (1975) J Laryngol Otol 89:985-996

New dimensions in otorhinolaryngology - head and neck surgery, vol. 2.
E. Myers, editor

CONSERVATIVE MANAGEMENT OF ACOUSTIC NEUROMA IN THE ELDERLY PATIENT

HERBERT SILVERSTEIN, M.D., ALAN McDANIEL, M.D., HORACE NORRELL, M.D.
Ear Research Foundation, 1921 Floyd Street, Sarasota, FL 33579

INTRODUCTION

Reports of acoustic neuroma surgery in the elderly patient are rarely encountered. Standard acoustic neuroma surgery with total removal, either through the translabyrinthine or suboccipital routes, produces significant morbidity in older patients, with a substantial risk of facial paralysis. In 1971, we began conservative treatment of acoustic neuroma in patients over the age of 65 (1).

METHOD

In this age group, patients suspected of having acoustic neuromas are completely investigated (with the exception of CT air contrast studies). If the patient has a small tumor with only symptoms of tinnitus and hearing loss, no surgery is immediately recommended. This tumor may not cause brainstem compression during the patient's lifetime. He is followed at yearly intervals with a CT scan. In patients with larger tumors, suffering from symptoms of brainstem compression, radical sub-total excision through the translabyrinthine approach is accomplished. Only a small amount of tumor capsule attached to the facial nerve is allowed to remain. Tumor removal is estimated at 90%. Operating time is greatly reduced and the patient's postoperative course is usually benign. Postoperatively their progress is followed clinically and yearly with CT scans. Should significant regrowth occur, a second procedure may be performed through the bony defect created by the original operation.

RESULTS

Since 1971, 15 patients with symptomatic acoustic neuromas measuring between 2.5 and 4cm have undergone radical sub-total resection. There were eleven women and four men aged 66 to 86 (average 74). Postoperatively, all patients were able to resume their previous lifestyles. There have been no deaths. Complications included meningitis (2), steroid psychosis (2), wound infection (2), and facial paralysis (1).

Two patients had rapid regrowth of the tumor. One became symptomatic, underwent a total resection elsewhere, and died of complications. The second patient is asymptomatic. A third patient has slow regrowth (0.2cm/yr) and remains asymptomatic. Four patients have died of unrelated causes. Eight patients are alive and asymptomatic with no regrowth of tumor.

Seven patients in the non-operative group had smaller tumors (0.8 to 2.5cm). The growth rate has been 0.2cm/yr in most cases. In three, there is no growth after one, three and six years. One patient recently developed progressive ataxia and headache and underwent subtotal resection. His tumor was 2.5cm, and his ataxia and headache improved after surgery.

DISCUSSION

In fifteen patients undergoing subtotal resection, there have been no deaths and few complications. Facial nerve function was normal in all but one case (94%). This rate is superior to those reported in other series of large acoustic tumors. The facial nerve is preserved by allowing a portion of tumor capsule adherent to the facial to remain undisturbed. In all other places the tumor is removed aggressively. The Silverstein Nerve Stimulator/Monitor* helps locate and preserve the facial nerve. Neurological signs rapidly and invariably improve after operation.

In the elderly, there appears to be a significantly slower growth rate in residual tumor following surgery. While 80% of non-operated patients have growth at 0.2cm per year (3), tumor remnants following sub-total resection show no growth in 80%.

SUMMARY

Total acoustic neuroma removal remains the treatment of choice in young, healthy patients. In the elderly patient with a large tumor a long procedure is not justifiable. When subtotal resection enables the older patient to live his remaining life without distressing neurological symptoms, we have accomplished our goal.

* WR Medical Electronics, St. Paul, MN.

REFERENCES

1. Silverstein H, Norrell H (1979) In: Silverstein H, Norrell H (eds) Subtotal Resection of Acoustic Neuroma in the Aged Patient. Neurological Surgery of the Ear, Vol II. Birmingham, AL, pp 262-268

2. Silverstein H, McDaniel AB, Norrell H (1985) Conservative Management of Acoustic Neuroma in the Elderly Patient. Laryngoscope (in press)

3. Wazen J, Silverstein H, Norrell H, Besse B (1985) Growth Rates in Acoustic Neuroma Documented with CT Scanning. Otolaryngol Head Neck Surg, 93:151-155

New dimensions in otorhinolaryngology - head and neck surgery, vol. 2.
E. Myers, editor

HEARING PRESERVATION AFTER ACOUSTIC NEUROMA SURGERY USING INTRAOPERATIVE DIRECT EIGHTH CRANIAL NERVE MONITORING

HERBERT SILVERSTEIN, M.D., ALAN B. McDANIEL, M.D., HORACE NORRELL, M.D.
Ear Research Foundation, 1921 Floyd Street, Sarasota, FL 33579

INTRODUCTION

With improved diagnostic techniques, small acoustic neuromas are more frequently found. Often the involved ear has retained useful hearing. The preservation of hearing, while accomplishing total tumor removal and preservation of the facial nerve function, has become a realistic objective in patients with small tumors.

METHOD

Both brain stem auditory evoked responses (BAER) and direct eighth nerve evoked action potentials (8NP) are recorded intraoperatively to help preserve hearing. A broadband click generator is fitted onto an ear mold in the patient's ear. A Nicolet Pathfinder II computer is employed (1,2).

The operation is performed through a retrosigmoid approach with the patient in a lateral supine position. Complete tumor removal is accomplished in all cases (3).

RESULTS

Since May, 1978, fourteen patients have undergone operation with a goal of hearing preservation. The tumor size varied from intracanalicular to more than 3cm medial to the porus. A CO_2 laser was used in four cases. Hearing was preserved in six cases (43%). All four patients with tumors larger than 2cm lost their hearing.

Tumors were removed from eight patients without 8NP monitoring and six were monitored. In the first group, 25% retained their hearing and in the second, 67%. The use of the CO_2 laser was not found to be advantageous.

Five patients had preoperative pure tone averages (PTA) of 30dB or better with at least 70% speech discrimination (SD). Hearing was preserved in 3, unchanged in 2. In the 10 patients with poorer scores, hearing was conserved in 3, but none was unchanged, having more than 30% loss of speech discrimination. Four patients had a history of sudden hearing loss before surgery and hearing was saved in none.

Poor reproducibility or absence of BAER waves or inability to record 8NP waves intraoperatively was associated with loss of hearing in six of eight patients. Conversely, good BAER repeatability and good 8NP were seen in three patients, two of whom had good outcomes.

Complications occurred equally in both monitored and non-monitored patients: transient facial weakness (3), CSF rhinorrhea (2), and tinnitus (2).

DISCUSSION

Hearing in the affected ear should be at least 50dB PTA with 50% SD scores before attempting preservation of hearing except in bilateral tumors. We have saved hearing in six of ten small tumors but have failed to preserve hearing in all four patients with tumors 2cm or larger.

Changes in intraoperative evoked potential wave form and latency appear to be correlated with the patient's hearing results. Due to advantageous signal-to-noise ratio, the 8NP is a more sensitive monitor of nerve trauma than the BAER. Good preservation of the 8NP is associated with good hearing results.

SUMMARY

While maintaining the major objectives of total tumor removal and facial preservation, hearing conservation is possible in 60% of patients with small acoustic neuromas (1.5cm or less). Monitoring the 8NP has proven a valuable tool during surgery to help preserve hearing.

REFERENCES

1. Silverstein H, Norrell H, Hyman SM (1984) Simultaneous Use of CO2 Laser With Continuous Monitoring of Eighth Cranial Nerve Action Potential During Acoustic Neuroma Surgery. Otolaryngol Head Neck Surg 92:80-84

2. Silverstein H, McDaniel AB, Wazen J, Norrell H (1985) Retrolabyrinthine Vestibular Neurectomy With Simultaneous Monitoring of Eighth Nerve and Brain Stem Auditory Evoked Potentials. (In press)

3. Silverstein H, McDaniel AB, Norrell H (1985) Hearing Preservation After Acoustic Neuroma Surgery Using Intraoperative Direct Eighth Cranial Nerve Monitoring. Am J Otol (In press)

© 1985 Elsevier Science Publishers B.V. (Biomedical Division)
New dimensions in otorhinolaryngology - head and neck surgery, vol. 2.
E. Myers, editor

NEURO-OTOLOGICAL FINDINGS IN CEREBELLAR TUMOURS

C.MORALES-GARCIA, E.RIOS, O.HOPPE and H.FANTUZZI

From the Departments of Neuro-Otology, The Barros Luco-Trudeau Hospital and Neurosurgery Institute, Santiago, Chile

MATERIAL AND RESULTS

The present paper is based on the clinical analysis of a group of 81 patients with cerebellar tumours examined over a period of 10 years. In all of these cases diagnosis was confirmed by means of surgical operation and/or necropsy. All patients were subjected to a complete neuro-otological and neurological assessments.

Neuro-otological findings generally accepted as suggesting cerebellar involvement seldom appeared. In fact, these signs were present in only 22 out of 81 patients with cerebellar tumours (27.16%); of them the most frequently observed was the dysrhythmia in postcaloric nystagmus (found in 18 cases or 22.22%). Only 3 cases (3.70%) showed vestibular hyperexcitability or rebound nystagmus and in only one patient (1.23%) it was possible to demonstrate the presence of ocular dysmetria.

Spontaneous nystagmus was present in 56 out of 81 patients (69.14%). In the majority of the cases (24 patients or 29.63%) it was unidirectional, either of first, second or third degree. In a little more than half of the patients there was positional nystagmus (41 cases or 50.62%), which was of the central or intermediate type (that is to say, with central and peripheral mixed characters).

The caloric tests were carried out in 79 patients, according to Fitzgerald and Hallpike's technique (1). In 39 of these patients (49.37%) the caloric tests were normal and in the remaining 40 cases (50.63%) different types of abnormalities of caloric responses were found. The most frequent abnormality was a unilateral canal paresis or paralysis (present in 14 cases or 35%).

A comparative study between those cases (24 patients) in which the lesion was limited to the vermis and those cases (24 patients) where involvement was confined to the cerebellar hemispheres showed that in 12 out of 15 patients with vermis lesions spontaneous nystagmus was bi-or multidirectional. On the contrary, in the majority of cases with cerebellar hemisphe res lesions (11 out of 17) spontaneous nystagmus was unidirec tional.

DISCUSSION

Nylén (2) has stated that, in cerebellar tumours, it becomes impossible to make a neuro-otological localization diagnosis between a tumour of the hemispheres and one of the vermis. Although it can be said that in general terms this statement seems to be a correct one, the clinical analysis of our pa tients demonstrated that different signs do exist either neurological or neuro-otological, whose presence strongly suggests localization of one type or the other. Thus, if in a patient with increased intracranial pressure symptoms the neurological examination shows lateralized neocerebellar signs (dysmetria, asynergia, or dysdiadochokinesia), peripheral cranial nerves in volvement (with the exception of sixth nerve paresis) or pyrami dal tract involvement, and in which neuro-otological examination shows unidirectional spontaneous nystagmus (specially if it is a second or third degree horizontal nystagmus), together with a unilateral canal paresis or paralysis or a unilateral cochleo-vestibular paresis, it is most probable that it is a cerebellar hemisphere tumour. On the other hand, in a tumour of the vermis, the neurological examination will only reveal non-lateralized neocerebellar signs and probably truncal ataxia; but in the majority of cases neither pyramidal tract nor cranial nerves involvement (different to the sixth nerve) will be found; neuro-otological examination will generally show bi-or multidirectional spontaneous nystagmus and most probably no unilateral canal paresis will be found in the caloric tests, nor either an eighth nerve peripheral involvement.

REFERENCES

1. Fitzgerald G., Hallpike C.S. (1942) Studies in human vestibular function: I. Observations on directional preponderance (Nystagmusbereitschaft) resulting from cerebral lesions. Brain 65:115.
2. Nylen C.O. (1939) The otoneurological diagnosis of tumours of the brain. Acta Otolaryng (Stockh), Suppl 33.

New dimensions in otorhinolaryngology – head and neck surgery, vol. 2.
E. Myers, editor

THE ENDOSCOPY OF THE CEREBELLOPONTINE ANGEL - INDICATION, TECHNIQUE AND RESULTS

MICHAEL HANDROCK, FALK OPPEL

ENT-Department and Departmert of Neurosurgery, Klinikum Steglitz, Hindenburgdamm 30, D-1000 Berlin 45 (FRG)

INTRODUCTION

The endoscopy of the cerebellopontine angle (CPA) is an important complement to the surgery of CPA or the internal auditory meatus. This technique was already presented in 1974 by Prott on the basis of anatomical studies. In 1977, we started on a further development and standardization of CPA endoscopy for clinical application.

INDICATION

Diagnostic endoscopy is indicated when a CPA tumor is suspected but cannot be clearly confirmed by radiological methods. With the improvement of computerized tomography, however, diagnostic endoscopy lost in importance. Therapeutic endoscopy either serves the neurotomy of sensory cranial nerves in cases of therapy-resistant pain (branches of the trigeminal nerve, glossopharyngeal nerve) or the neurotomy performed on the vestibular nerve in cases of Menière's disease and also on the cochlear nerve in cases of deafness and severe tinritus.

OPERATIVE PROCEDURE

Placement of a lumbar liquor drainage is followed by the mastoidectomy with exposure of the dura of the posterior cranial fossa. After incision of the dura, the liquor drainage is opened which leads to a backward displacement of the cerebellum and allows view into the CPA. Endoscopy or neurotomy is followed by dura occlusion with lyophilized dura for support, dura suture and oblieration of the mastoid antrum with abdominal fat.

RESULTS

From 1978 to 1984, we performed a total of 61 CPA endoscopies (20 diagnostic and 41 therapeutic endosccpies). In 6 of the 20 diagnostic endoscopies performed, no tumors could be found although the air-CT had not shown any filling of the internal acoustic meatus. Of the 41 therapeutic endoscopies, 31 were carried out due to therapy-resistant pain, especially trigeminal neuralgia, and 10 due to Menière's disease (Table). The follow-up results were very encouraging: of 16 patients with therapy-resistant pain who are still alive, 10 patients were completely pain-free and 2 had improved considerably. In particular, tumor patients in the terminal stage with most violent pains were pain-free immediately after the performance of neurotomy. The results in cases of Menière's disease were also excellent. In only 1 of 10 patients, attacks of vertigo recurred after a 1-year interval without vertigo. Postoperative audition was unchanged in 7 patients, improved in 2 patients and deteriorated in 1 patient. The tinnitus could be stopped or reduced in 6 patients. No patient evidenced the sensation of pressure in his ear any longer.

COMPLICATIONS

Severe complications such as intracranial bleeding, facial nerve paresis and so on could not be observed in any of the cases. 5 patients developed a liquor fistula postoperatively, which resulted in a slight meningitis in 3 cases. Other complications were insignificant and rare. Since the improvement of the occlusion technique (1982), liquor fistulae have no longer been observed.

SUMMARY

The endoscopy of the cerebellopontine angle constitutes a significant enrichment of the therapeutic possibilities available, especially in cases of Menière's disease and severe therapy-resistant conditions of pain in the head and face area. The carefully directed neurotomy performed on the specific cranial nerves yielded excellent long-term results and showed no severe complications.

Follow-up results in neuralgia and MENIERE's disease after endoscopic neurotomy

	neuralgia	MENIERE's disease
total	31	10
follow-up examined	16	10
dead	10	0
good results (no pains, no vertigo)	10	7
moderate results	2	2
poor results	4	1
postoperative interval	1-6 years	4 month – 3 years

References provided by authors on request.

© 1985 Elsevier Science Publishers B.V. (Biomedical Division)
New dimensions in otorhinolaryngology - head and neck surgery, vol. 2.
E. Myers, editor

DEXTRAN THERAPY FOR SUDDEN SENSORINEURAL HEARING LOSS

JANG JENQ-CHYUAN
CHANGHUA CHRISTIAN HOSPITAL, TAIPEI VETERANS GENERAL HOSPITAL

INTRODUCTION

Those cases that have sudden sensorineural hearing loss have had no previous ear disease. It is never easy to discover the reason, but the virovascular theory has been recognized widely as etiology. Fowler first proposed that temporary vascular occlusion could not as the result of vascular spasma but from a phenomenon of "blood sludging". Jaffe in 1970 discovered that there is a possible intravascular plugs in the stria vasculris and in the spiral ligment. Viruses are known to attach to erythrocytes and cause hemagglutination (in the test tube);viremia can cause swelling of capillary endothelial cells and viral infection can induce a state of mild hypercoaulation. Williams and Saunders in 1972 they believed the viral or vascular origin is the same thing. Various methods have reported some hearing improvement but previous treatment results had been similar to Mattox & Simmons that is equally to the spontaneous recovery rate 65%. Dextran is known to expand plasma volume, improve blood flow and play a thromprophylactic effect. Dextran action mechanism is suitable for viro-vascular problem and therefore should be considered in the treatment of sudden sensorineural hearing loss.

MATERIAL AND METHODS

From May 1981 to Jan. 1982, 90 cases of sudden snsorineural hearing loss were seen at Taipei Veterans General Hospital. They received complete examination and detailed history taking. Those 90 cases were injected with Dextran (500ml) during a 2-hour time period on daily basis for 10-15 days. The injection was done by author. The hearing test was repeated after each 5 bottles injection. The hearing acuity was evaluated at 0.5kHz, 1kHz, and 2kHz at average dB. Mild hearing loss was defined at 30-50 dB loss; 51-70 dB was considered as moderate hearing loss; 71-90 dB was severe hearing loss;and 90 or more dB loss was considered to be profound hearing loss. Post-injection results were put in four categories. Complete recovery: the average dB loss was less than 10 dB or equalled the univolved ear; good: the average dB loss was less than 40 dB or more than 50 dB but at least 30 dB improvement; poor: all other results.

RESULTS

On the 80 patients in study, 70 had unilateral diease (45 right, 25 left) and 10 cases involved both ears (bilateral). Fifty nine cases were male 21 were female. Age distribution ranged from 14 to 70 years (mean 49). Of the 35 cases that injection of Dextran within 5 days of onset, 28 (80%) of those cases were in the "complete" or "good" recovery caterory. Of the 61 cases that received injection of Dextran within 10 days of onset, 47 (77%) were in the "complete" or "good" recovery caterory. Table 1 shows the hearing result and the days of onset was significant difference. The subjective improvement of tinnitus was 74% (61/90). Finally it was learn that the patient with following conditions had a better prognosis: They received treatment early they had less hearing loss. They had upward sloping or flat audiogram. Table 2 shows threshold contour and the hearing recovery. Patient with severed hearing loss or 8kHx loss had a poor prognosis. Hearing recovery was not related to age or prescence or vertigo.

TABLE I

DAYS OF ONSET AND HEARING RECOVERY

Days	No. of ears	Recovery Type			
		Complete	Good	Fair	Poor
0-5 (a)	35	24	4	3	4
6-10 (b)	26	4	7	5	10
11-30 (c)	23	1	7	3	12
31-60 (d)	4	0	0	1	3
61-90 (e)	2	0	0	1	1
Total	90	29	18	13	30

$X^2 = 41.43$, $P<0.005$; $a>b$, $P<0.005$; $b>c$, $P>0.10$; $a>c$, $P<0.005$

TABLE II

THRESHOLD CONTOUR AND HEARING RECOVERY

Type	No. of ears	Recovery Type			
		Complete	Good	Fair	Poor
Upward Slope (a)	19	12	4	2	1
Flat Contour (b)	18	6	6	4	2
Down Slope (c)	10	4	4	1	1
Total Loss (d)	12	1	1	3	7
Unclassify (e)	10	6	2	1	1
8 kHz=N.R (f)	21	0	1	2	18
Total	90	29	18	13	30

$a>f$, $P<0.005$; $b>f$, $P<0.05$; $c>d$, $P<0.05$; $c>f$, $P<0.05$; $e>f$, $P<0.05$

© 1985 Elsevier Science Publishers B.V. (Biomedical Division)
New dimensions in otorhinolaryngology - head and neck surgery, vol. 2.
E. Myers, editor

BILATERAL SENSORINEURAL HEARING IMPAIRMENT ASSOCIATED WITH BILATERAL INTERNAL AUDITORY CANAL ENLARGEMENT

KEN KITAMURA
Department of Otolaryngology, Jichi Medical School, Yakushiji, Kawachi-gun, Tochigi, 329-04, JAPAN

INTRODUCTION

The purpose of this report is to demonstrate the neuroradiological findings of two cases with a long-standing history of bilateral sensorineural hearing loss.

CASE REPORTS

Case 1

A 69-year-old man had a long history of bilateral progressive hearing loss. Audiometry showed a sensorineural hearing loss of sloping type (Fig. 1). Ice water caloric tests (10 ml) revealed a decreased response in both ears. There were no other positive findings on neurological evaluation. A skull radiography showed an enlarged sella turcica in addition to bilateral enlarged internal auditory canals (Fig. 2). The lateral and third ventricles were also dilated on a CT scan. However, no tumor was demonstrated in either ventricle, sella or cerebellopontine angles.

At the age of 73 audiometry showed increased hearing loss for high tones in both ears. However, there was no significant change on neuroradiological examinations.

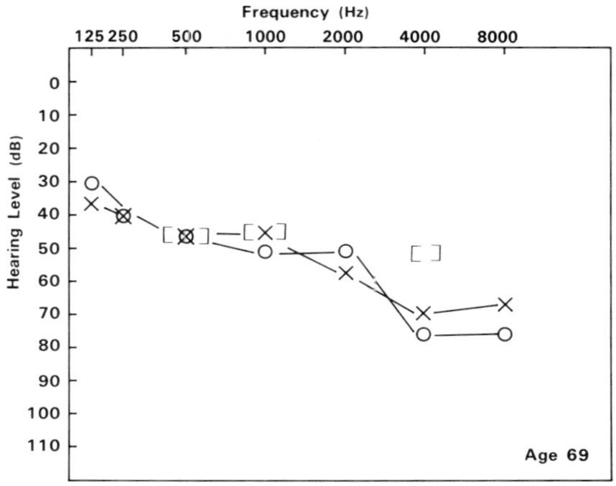

Fig. 1. (Case 1) Audiogram.

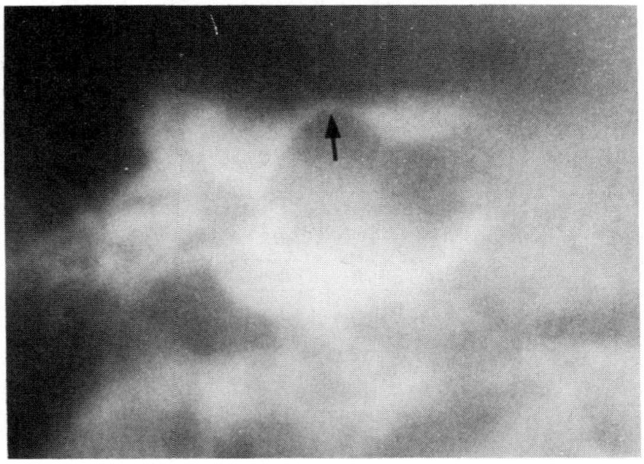

Fig. 2.(Case 1) Polytomography of the right ear shows wide internal auditory canal (arrow).

Case 2

A 39-year-old man with a complaint of bilateral hearing loss of 6 years' history was examined. Audiometry showed a sensorineural hearing loss in both ears (Fig. 3). Caloric tests (5 ml at 18°C) gave a good response. Maximum speed of slow phase was 23 °/s in the right ear and 20°/s in the left ear. General neurological examinations were negative. On polytomographic study both ears showed enlarged internal auditory canals. An air CT scan demonstrated no filling defect in either internal auditory canal (Fig. 4).

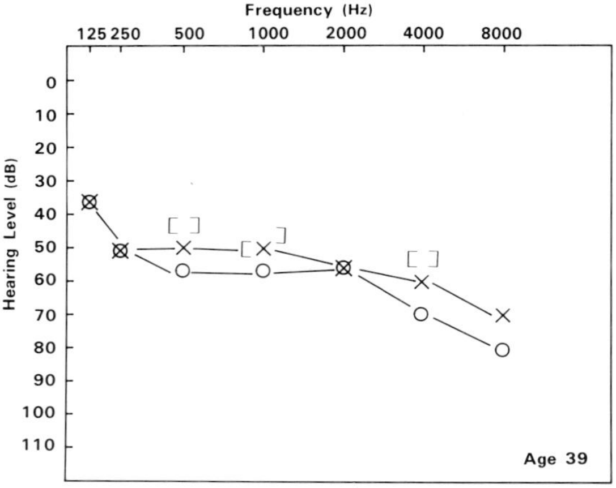

Fig. 3. (Case 2) Audiogram.

DISCUSSION

Both cases showed a bilateral sensorineural hearing loss without any history of vestibular symptom. On polytomographic study bilateral internal auditory canals were extremely enlarged in both cases. Although Davis and Rumbaugh have reported similar radiological findings as patulous canals, the causal relationship between sensorineural hearing loss and enlarged internal auditory canals has not been established (1). Since subclinical intracranial hypertension was demonstrated in the first case, it is suggested that CSF pressure plays a role in the enlargement of internal auditory canals as well as sensorineural hearing loss.

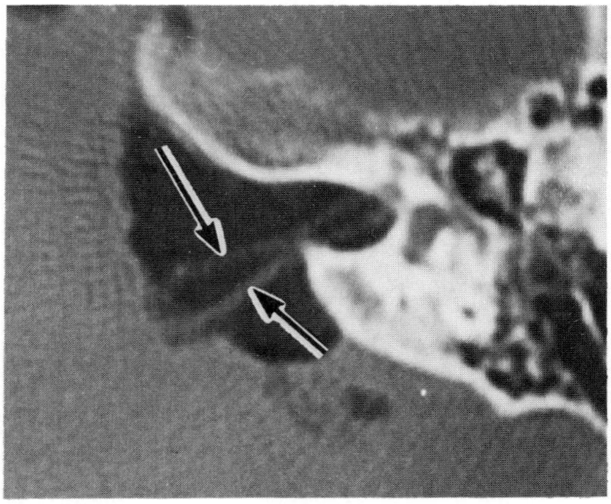

Fig. 4. (Case 2) Air CT scan of the right ear shows no evidence of tumor and normal cranial nerves (arrows).

REFERENCE

1. Davis DO, Rumbaugh CL (1979) In: Newton TH, Potts DG (eds) Radiology of the Skull and Brain. Mosby, St. Louis, p 445

© 1985 Elsevier Science Publishers B.V. (Biomedical Division)
New dimensions in otorhinolaryngolcgy - head and neck surgery, vol. 2.
E. Myers, editor

IS PROSTACYCLIN A COCHLEOPROTECTIVE SUBSTANCE?

O. MICHEL, R. MATTHIAS
ENT-Dept., Universitätsklinikum Steglitz, Berlin, West Germany

Prostacyclin (PGI_2) is a highly effective non-circulating hormone ameliorating the blood supply of tissues by vasodilatory action. Particularly similar properties have been described for PGE_2-derivate (Sulproston) in higher concentrations.

MATERIAL AND METHODS

1. Experiments in animals

White guinea pigs were poisoned with aspirin (350 mg L-ASA/kg bw i.v.), 8 hours later bolus injection of 500 ng/kg bw Prostacyclin was given and the hearing loss was measured by click-evoked compound action potentials. Guinea pigs were kept in an echoic room with an energy-equivalent noise stress of 106.2 db(A). Before, after 16 and 48 hours, prostacyclin-like activity was detected by bioassay in inner ears, cerebellum and kidney.

2. Experiments in man

In an open clinical trial, a high performance infusion pump was used to infuse Sulproston (120 ng/kg bw/min) in patients with Menière's disease and Prostacyclin (Epoprostenol, 6-10 ng/kg bw/min for 6 h) in patients with sudden hearing loss. Hearing thresholds were determined before and after treatment with pure tone and speech audiometry. In case of Menière's disease, results have been compared with the furosemide test (12 mg/kg bw) and the glycerol test (1.2 g/kg bw). In case of sudden hearing loss, results were compared with hearing gain before and after infusion under treatment with pentoxifylline.

RESULTS

1. Experiments in animals

The hearing loss due to aspirin regresses within seconds after an infusion of prostacyclin. The TTS under noise exposure is biphasic and correlates well with the decline of prostacyclin synthesis.

2. Experiments in man

In case of Menière's disease, Sulproston-administration shows similar results to the glycerol test (Fig. 1). In case of sudden hearing loss, prostacyclin increases the hearing level within 6 hours (Fig. 2).

FIG. 1:

		Pure Tone Audiometry dB hearing gain over all frequencies n patients x 7 frequencies	Speech Audiometry dB hearing gain for numbers n patients
Menière's Disease (n=7)	Glycerol-test	4.1	
	Furosemide-test	1.6	
	PGE_2-test	3.6	
Sudden Hearing Loss (n=4)	Pentoxifylline/days of therapy	2.1 *)	
	PGI_2	8.4	11.75
	Pentoxifylline/days of therapy	-0.6 **)	-0.1

*) before prostacyclin-therapy
**) after prostacyclin-therapy

DISCUSSION

With the animal experiments on the one hand and the first results of the open clinical trial on the other, we think we can speak of prostacyclin as a cochleoprotective hormone, which endogenous deficit causes sensorineural hearing loss and which plays an important role in the still unknown autoregulatory functions of the inner ear.

© 1985 Elsevier Science Publishers B.V. (Biomedical Division)
New dimensions in otorhinolaryngology - head and neck surgery, vol. 2.
E. Myers, editor

STEROID TREATMENT ON IDIOPATHIC SUDDEN SENSORINEURAL HEARING LOSS

MAKETO ODA and YASUYA NOMURA
Department of Oto-Rhino-Laryncology, Faculty of Medicine,
University of Tokyo
Hongo Bunkyo-ku, Tokyo (Japan)

INTRODUCTION

Sudden sensorineural hearing loss may occur due to many causative factors, Higgs[1] clasified these causative factors as follows; infectious, vascular, metabolic, traumatic, neoplastic, post-operative, by pregnancy and idiopathic.

In otological practice, idiopathic sudden sensorineural hearing loss is never uncommon.

Generally speaking, sensorineural hearing loss is considered to be unable to recover decreased hearing. However, sudden deafness is unusual hearing loss which is worthy trying treatment. As having tried steroid treatment for recent eighteen years, we woulk like to report consequence of our treatment.

MATERIAL AND METHOD

Subject

611 cases had treatment in our clinic from 1967 to 1985. Out of these, 251 cases visited within one week. These cases were used as a basic sample.

Method

Evaluation of treatment was based on comparison of an audiogram conducted before treatment with one conducted three months after treatment. From comparison of these two audiograms, effect of treatment was divided into four degree as follows; 1)complete recovery means recovery to within 20 dB of hearing level at each frequency of 250, 500, 1000, 2000, 4000 Hz or recovery to the same level as that of the opposite ear. 2) marked recovery means cases whose hearing gained over 30 dB in average hearing level at above frequencies, 3) recovery means cases where hearing gain was 10 to 29 dB and 4) unchanged.

RESULTS

Recovery of hearing in Group A

More than 50% of patients with hearing levels below 60 dB at first visit showed complete recovery. The rate of complete recovery decreased with deteriorated hearing level at first visit. Only 6% complete recovery was observed in the 49 cases over 1Ø1 dB hearing level. Likewise, a recovery rate of over 5Ø% in each hearing group decreased with hearing level at first visit.

TABLE 3
Averaged Hearing at First Visit

	21-4Ø	41-6Ø	61-8Ø	81-1ØØ	over 1Ø1
2Ø	65.Ø	56.8	4Ø.9	21.2	6.1
3Ø	1ØØ.Ø	75.7	53.8	46.2	8.2
4Ø		91.9	71.Ø	56.8	12.2
5Ø		97.3	81.6	57.3	16.3
6Ø		1ØØ.Ø	9Ø.3	71.2	26.5
7Ø			93.5	88.5	36.7
8Ø			96.8	96.2	57.1
9Ø			1ØØ.Ø	1ØØ.Ø	67.3
1ØØ					75.5
11Ø					81.6
over 11Ø					1ØØ.Ø

In each grade, the statistical difference between steroid therapy and non-steroid therapy was not significant. However, patients who received steroid seemed to show a somewhat better recovery rate than those receiving non-steroid treatment.

REFERENCES

1. Higgs W.A. (1973) In: Sudden dearness as the presenting symptom of acoustic neurinoma. Archiotolaryng 98, 73-76

New dimensions in otorhinolaryngology – head and neck surgery, vol. 2.
E. Myers, editor

DEAFNESS FOLLOWING MUMPS: THE POSSIBLE PATHOGENESIS AND INCIDENCE OF DEAFNESS

YOSHIHIKO MURAKAMI* and NORIO MUZUSHIMA**
*Department of otolaryngology,Yamanashi College of Medicine,Yamanashi,Japan
**Department of Otolaryngology,Nihon University School of Medicine,Tokyo,Japan

INTRODUCTION

Mumps is thought to be the most common cause of unilateral acquired sensorineural deafness in children. It is also well known that mumps deafness is usually sudden in onset, profound or complete, and may be associated with vestibular symptoms. However, the mechanism of onset of the disease and inner ear pathology in connection with this mumps infection have yet to be elucidated because of histopathologic reports on human temporal bone being extremely limited in number. Furthermore, no definite agreement in opinions has been reached yet as to the incidence of this remarkably severe and irreversible inner ear deafness among the patients infected with this virus. From the findings of detailed clinical studies on 53 fresh cases which the authors have encountered in the past 10 years and in which inner ear deafness can reasonably be ascribed to mumps, the authors would like to discuss the possible pathogenesis and the incidence of mump deafness.

STUDIES ON CLINICAL CASES

Since 1974, a definite cause-effect relationship between deafness and mumps has been established by the clinical course, history of the illness and serological or viral examinations in a total of 53 cases. In clinical cases with mumps deafness the age distribution, male-female ratio and presence or not of vestibular symptoms are as presented in Table 1.

Table 1

Age(years)	No.of Cases	Male:Female
--- 5	18 (*5)	10 : 8
6 --- 10	18 (*6)	9 : 9
11 --- 20	6 (*4)	4 : 2
21 --- 30	6 (*4)	2 : 4
31 ---	5 (*5)	1 : 4
total	53 (*24)	26 : 27

(*vestibular involvement = 45.3%)

Age and sex distribution of the patients with mumps deafness(*associated with vestibular symptoms)

The hearing loss in these patients was exclusively unilateral, profound or total and permanent, and more than 45% of the patients developed dysequilibrium of vestibular origin. As for the age, the youngest was a boy aged 1 year and 6 months and the oldest a 38-year old woman. As for the age distribution, those aged under 10 years accounted for the majority with 36 cases(67.9%). The male-female ratio was 26:27, there being little difference between the sexes. No relationship whatsoever is observed between the development of deafness and severity of mumps infection.

PATHOGENESIS AND INCIDENCE OF MUMPS DEAFNESS(LABYRINTHITIS)

In dicussing the mechanism of development of viral labyrinthitis, three routes are generally mentioned for the pathogen to reach the labyrinth; namely, 1) infection via the middle ear(tympanogenic), 2) infection via CSF(meningogenic) and 3) hematogenous infection. As for the infection through the middle ear, this route can be excluded since there are no clinical findings or history of illness that suggests viral otitis media. As to the infection via CSF, this route of invasion could also be ruled out since findings suggestive of meningitis in our present series of mumps deafness were not obtained at all. That mumps meningitis is not associated with deafness as a sequela is also supported by many reports including those of Vuori et al[1)], Azimi et al[2)], Nadol[3)],etc.

As to the mechanism of development or pathogenesis of deafness due to mumps infection, therefore, the hematogenous infection theory is considered most valid. In other words, the viremic state due to mumps reaches the inner ear hematogenously, causes an inflammatory change in the stria vascularis of the cochlea, and then results in severe impairment of the endolymphatic system. Thus, the term "viral endolymphatic labyrinthitis" is proposed as the possible pathogenesis of the deafness. In fact, Lindsay[4)], the first to report on the pathology of human temporal bone in a patient with mumps deafness, also states that the suscepti-bility of the stria vascularis can be explained by its relatively slow blood flow and the intra-epithelial location of its capillary net-work.

As to at what incidence this inner ear deafness develops in mumps patients, references mentioning this point are very limited in number. Some authors have made conjecture that is considerably incorrect. A report of Everberg[5)] would be the only one that gives relatively theoretical values as to the incidence of deafness due to mumps infection. According to his report, inner ear deafness develops at the rate of 0.05 per thousand, that is, 1 out of 20,000 patients with mumps.

CONCLUSION

On the basis of results of a clinical study on 53 cases of inner ear deafness due to mumps, the authors discussed pathogenesis and incidence of the deafness.

Results obtained are summarized as follows: 1) In inner ear deafness found in mumps patients, the viremic state reaches the inner ear hematogenously and brings about an inflammatory change in the stria vascularis of the cochlea to present severe impairment of the endolymphtic system(endolymphatic labyrinthitis) 2) The incidence of deafness in mumps patients is extremely low, and about 0.005% given in the report of Everberg is considered a reasonable numerical value.

References:1)Vuori,M.et al:Acta otolaryngol 55:231,1962 2)Azimi,PH et al:JAMA 206:509,1969 3)Nadol,JB:Laryngoscope 88:739,1978 4)Lindsay,JR:Arch Otolaryng 98: 258,1973 5)Everberg,G:Acta otolaryngol 48:397,1957

New dimensions in otorhinolaryngology - head and neck surgery, vol. 2.
E. Myers, editor

THE CLINICAL USE OF HYPERBARIC OXYGEN THERAPY FOR DISORDERS OF THE INNER EAR

M. Pilgramm, H. Lenders, K. Schumann
Ear Nose & Throat Dept. V of the Federal Army Hospital, Ulm(Medical Director: Prof. Schumann), Oberer Eselsberg 40, 7900 Ulm, West Germany

INTRODUCTION

The use of hyperbaric oxygen as one means of treating anaerobic infections has been known for many years. Gas gangrene, for example, can be managed successfully by increasing the supply of oxygen to the organism. Damaged and non-functioning inner ear sensory sells, which are nontheless still alive, also require an increased supply of nutrients, such as oxygen, of they are to regenerate and recover their functions. Many methods of treatment are known which aim at reactivating the metabolic processes of the damaged inner ear sensory cells and restoring their functions.

Our aim was to investigate whether, by means of a safe increase in the partial oxygen pressure in the inner ear, we could restore hearing and alleviate tinnitus.

MATERIALS AND METHODS

Study groups and patients

Study group I: acute acoustic trauma, 61 patients, average age 23.7 ± 4.3 years.

Study group II: sudden deafness, 37 patients, average age 47.3 ± 12.4 years.

Study group III: non-acute cases of sudden deafness, with unsatisfactory previous treatment, 51 patients, average age 51.3 ± 10.4 years.

Study group IV: non-acute cases of acoustic trauma with associated tinnitus, 58 patients, average age 24.6 ± 3.7 years.

STANDARD THERAPY, HYPERBARIC OXYGEN THERAPY

In all 4 studies, each of which was conducted independently of the others, the patients were randomly assigned to two groups.

1. Group a, Standard Therapy: 500 ml low molecular weight dextran solution intravenously, 600 mg of a vasoactive substance, and 3x2 tablets of a vitamin B complex daily over 14 days. The oral therapy was continued for 4 weeks after release from the hospital.

2. Group b, Standard Therapy plus Hyperbaric Oxygen Therapy:
in addition to the standard therapy above, the patients in this group were given 10 hyperbaric oxygen treatment sessions in the pressure chamber, one sesion daily on 10 consecutive days. Each session lasting 1 hour and using 100% oxygen at 2.5 bar.

INCLUSION CRITERIA

A. Study groups 1 and 2 consisted only of those patients in whom there was virtually no chance whatsoever of spontaneous recovery.

B. In patients of study group 2 a vascular cause hand been positively established

C. In patients of study groups 3 and 4 the medical record included in-patient treatment of the disorder of the inner ear.

D. In all cases, a hyperbaric specialist had no objections to treatment in the pressure chamber.

RESULTS

Study group		N	Hearing gain(dB) after 7 days	SD	P(WK)	Hearing gain(dB) after 42 days	SD	P(WK)
1	a	30	21	4.9	0.001	29	6.3	0.001
	b	31	7	5.6	0.001	16	5.4	0.001
2	a	19	11	6.4	0.001	22	5.7	0.001
	b	18	21	7.2	0.001	30	6.8	0.001
3	a	26	4	3.9	0.01	5	3.2	0.01
	b	25	5	4.2	0.01	4	2.8	0.05
4	a	29	6	2.3	0.001	6	1.7	0.001
	b	29	4	1.9	0.001	3	2.2	0.001

Tab. 1: Development of average hearing recovery by day 7 of treatment and on conclusion of the study on day 42 after admission to the hospital
SD = standard deviation
P(WK) = Wilcoxon test

Study group		N	Initial Tinnitus	Final Tinnitus	% Change
1	a	30	30	24	20
	b	31	30	8	73
2	a	19	9	6	33
	b	18	16	7	56
3	a	26	9	8	10
	b	25	10	8	20
4	a	29	29	28	6
	b	29	29	26	10

Tab. 2: Development of tinnitus in the 4 study groups comparing initial and final data. Figures only include patients with a total absence of tinnitus.

Stabilization of the inner ear in Study Groups 1 and 2

A follow-up examination of all patients from the first two study groups was carried out 1 year after completion of the study. 30% of the patients who had received only standard therapy had experienced a renewed decline in hearing acuity and/or a fresh flare-up of tinnitus. Only 18% of patients treated with oxygen experienced partial relapses.

Side effects:

Of the 113 patients treated with hyperbaric oxygen 6 had to break off the treatment: one because of incipient oxygen poisoning, two because of moderately severe barotrauma and the remaining three because of considerable anxiety experienced in the chamber.

SUMMARY

In the treatment process described above, the partial oxygen pressure physically dissolved in serum can be increased 15 to 18 times. What is still not known is where precisely this increased oxygen supply comes to bear. Based on the statistically significant results of our studies shown above, we have come to the following conclusions:

1. In cases of acute acoustic trauma, hyperbaric oxygen therapy is vastly superior to standard methods of treatment in reducing high-frequency sensorineural hearing loss and tinnitus and for stabilizing the inner ear.

2. In case of sudden deafness, patients treated with oxygen fared better in terms of hearing gain and tinnitus reduction.

3. In the treatment of non-acute inner ear disorders, hyperbaric oxygen therapy has no special advantages compared with standard treatment.

Hyperbaric oxygen therapy therefore represents effective adjunctive therapy in acute inner ear disorders. Serious side effects can be virtually excluded if the patients are under constant supervision by a hyperbaric specialist.

BIBLIOGRAPHY

1.Beck, Chl., Michels H.: Arch. ohr-Nas- u.Kehlk.-H. 174:496(1960)

2.Beck, Chl.: Laryng. Rhinol. 56:350(1977)

3.Davis, H.C., Hunt, T.K.: Undersea Medical Society,USA 1977.

4.Demaertelaere,L., van Opstal, M.:Acto Otorhonolaryng. Belgica,Bruxelles35:3(1981)

5.Lamm,H., Lamm, K., Zimmermann, W.: Arch. Otorhinolaryng. 236:237(1982)

6.Pilgramm, M., Schumann, K.: Hyperbaric Oxygenation for acute acoustic trauma: Arch. Otorhinolaryng. 1985 in press.

7.Pilgramm, M., Lampl, L., Frey, G., Wörner, U.: HNO 33:84(1985).

8.Pottlesch,I.: Anästhesiol. u. Wiederbeleb., Bd. 64: Springer Berlin, Heidelberg, New York (1972).

New dimensions in otorhinolaryngology - head and neck surgery, vol. 2.
E. Myers, editor

ADENOID CYSTIC CARCINOMA OF THE LARYNX - A CASE REPORT

T. WANG and Y.N. LIN

Departments of Otolaryngology and Pathology, Mackay Memorial Hospital, Taipei, Taiwan, R.O.C.

Adenoid cystic carcinoma of the larynx constitutes 1% or less of laryngeal malignancies. It arises almost exclusively in the subglottic and supraglottic regions because of the large number of submucosal minor glands located here. In the 1850's it had been recognized as a distinct clinical-pathological entity that was frequently encountered in the major salivary glands, the lacrimal glands and in the minor salivary glands of the oral cavity and upper respiratory tract. In 1983, Dr. D.T. Donovan was able to find only 69 cases of adenoid cystic carcinoma of the larynx reported in the literature. This paper presents one additional case of adenoid cystic carcinoma originating in the larynx.

The patient, a 54 year old male, visited Mackay Memorial Hospital with symptoms of hoarseness of voice for a long time and progressive dyspnea that began 3 months prior to his first hospital visit. Indirect laryngoscopy revealed a large, smooth tumor mass on the right vocal cord with invasion to the supraglottic region. It was noted that he was a heavy smoker. At this initial visit he refused surgical treatment. Because of the increasing stridor and dysphagia, tracheostomy was performed three months later. Biopsy of the tumor mass through direct laryngoscopy revealed the typical findings of adenoid cystic carcinoma, i.e. nests and columns of cells arranged concentrically in a cribriform pattern around a glandlike space filled with mucinous secretions (Fig. 1). On Oct. 15, 1981, total laryngectomy and T-E shunt formation were performed. The final histopathologic report on the gross laryngectomy specimen reported cancer free margins (Fig. 2). At the most recent follow up 3½ years after the operation, the patient was active with a good T-E shunt voice and free of disease.

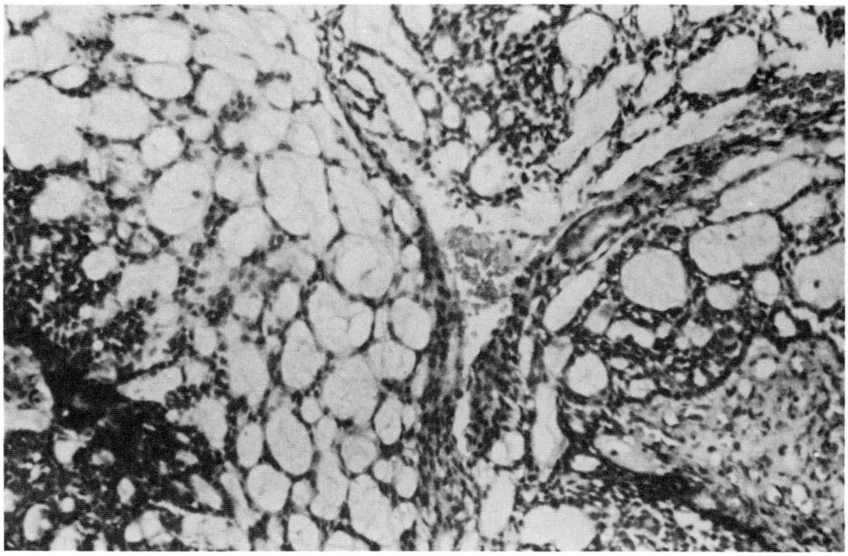

Fig. 1. Histopathology of the biopsy.

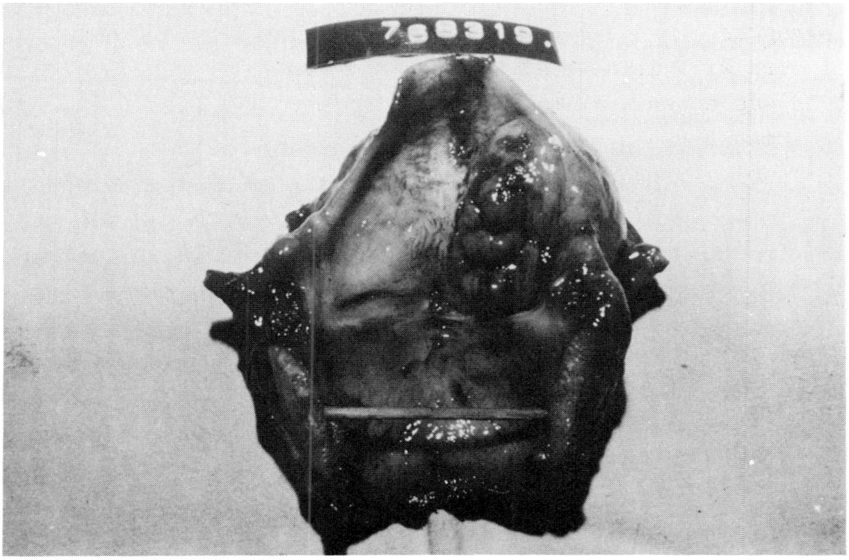

Fig. 2. Gross, total laryngectomy specimen.

© 1985 Elsevier Science Publishers B.V. (Biomedical Division)
New dimensions in otorhinolaryngology - head and neck surgery, vol. 2.
E. Myers, editor

RESULTS OF SURGICAL TREATMENT OF ADVANCED CARCINOMA OF THE LARYNX

W.I. WEI, K.H. LAM, W.F. LAU

INTRODUCTION

In patients suffering from a small carcinoma of the larynx with no lymph nodes in the neck, the results of radiotherapy are comparable to those of surgery. Patients with recurrent tumor after irradiation or having larger tumors should be treated by surgery. When the tumor is localised within the larynx, total laryngectomy is the operation of choice. For those tumors which extend into the hypopharynx, partial or total pharyngectomy should be performed in addition to total laryngectomy.

The present study reviews our experience in the surgical treatment of advanced carcinoma of the larynx.

MATERIAL AND METHOD

A total of 510 patients suffering from carcinoma of the larynx were admitted to the Department of Surgery, University of Hong Kong at the Queen Mary Hospital, Hong Kong, between 1964 and 1984. The UICC classification of 1972 was followed and the pathological findings of the specimen were used in determining the stage of the disease. The present review included 320 patients with T3 or T4 tumors who underwent either total laryngectomy or pharyngolaryngoesophagectomy (P.L.O.) depending on whether the tumor has extended outside the larynx and whether part or whole of the pharynx needed to be removed. Radical neck dissection was carried out for clinically significant lymph nodes.

RESULTS

In this series of 320 patients, the age ranged from 34 to 88 years with a mean value of 59.8 years. There was a marked male preponderance (male : female = 10 : 1). The commonest presenting tumor location was the supraglottic region (173 patient, 54%). It is however more practical to adopt the classification of MacGavran[1]. Of these 320 patients, 174 (54%) had a transglottic lesion. One hundred and eighty-eight patients (59%) had received a full dose of radiotherapy before operation and they were managed surgically as salvage of radiotherapy failures. Respiratory obstruction was present in 135 (42%), so that 104 had preoperative tracheostomy, 18 had endotracheal intubation followed by operation and 13 patients had emergency radical surgery.

Total laryngectomy was the surgical treatment in 206 patients and 16 of them required cutaneous or myocutaneous flaps for repair of the pharynx. Pharyngolaryngoesophagectomy was performed in 114 patients because the tumor had extended to the pyriform fossa or postcricoid area. Transposition of the stomach to the neck via the posterior mediastinum and performing a pharyngogastric anastomosis was the usual form of reconstruction. Radical neck dissection, carried out for clinically significant lymph nodes, was performed on the ipsilateral side in 27% of the patients and on both sides in 22%.

The most frequent complication was the leakage of the repaired pharyngeal wall after laryngectomy in 47 out of 206 (23%), and of the pharyngogastric anastomosis in 31 out of 114 (27%). The majority of them healed with conservative treatment but, when the leakage persisted, these patients usually ended up as hospital mortality. Other complications such as chest infection and cardiac arrythmia occurred in less than 5% of patients.

The overall hospital mortality was 17% in the entire series. The major factors responsible for the mortalities are shown in Table I.

The incidence of local recurrence in this group of patients with advanced carcinoma who underwent surgical treatment was 11%. The overall 5 year actuarial survival was 45%. The results of the improvement of management over the years are shown in Table II.

DISCUSSION

The treatment of advanced and operable carcinoma of the larynx should be surgery combined with radiotherapy[2]. More than half of the patients in the present study were irradiation failures (59%). This was higher than other reports[3]. The rest of our patients had postoperative radiotherapy.

The proportion of patients presenting with evidence of respiratory obstruction in this review is much higher than in other reports[4]. This, together with the high incidence of transglottic tumors, represented the late presentation of patients in our review.

The incidence of recurrence in this review was 11%, this was comparable to other reports, which varied from 11%[5] to 14%[3]. This showed that the surgical procedures in the presented review, was not entirely successful in achieving tumor control. With the introduction of the pectoralis major myocutaneous flaps for reconstruction of the pharynx, more extensive local excision should be carried out and further reduction of local recurrence rate could be expected.

The common causes of hospital death were sepsis, respiratory failure and bleeding from neck vessels. These were related to leakage of the repair of the pharyngeal wall or the pharyngogastric anastomosis. In recent years, with improved patient-care and modified surgical techniques, postoperative complications and hospital mortalities had been reduced. Improved patient-care included pre- and post-operative physiotherapy and availability of intensive care facilities. Modified surgical techniques included the application of 2 layers of interrupted sutures in pharyngogastric anastomosis and also other measures for reducing tension at the anastomotic site as reported elsewhere[6]. In the case of closure of the pharynx after laryngectomy, an extra stitch at the 'T' junction was applied.

All these contributed to a decrease in leakage rate. The 5-year actuarial survival was increased to 54% (Table II), suggesting better tumor control.

Table I : Factors leading to hospital mortality

	P.L.O. n = 114	Total laryngectomy n = 206
Cause of hospital mortality		
sepsis	14	4
respiratory failure	10	3
bleeding	7	6
others	2	7
total	33 (29%)	20 (10%)

Table II : Progress of management over the years

	Overall	1964-1978	1979-1984
leakage rate	24%	31%	17%
hospital mortality	17%	25%	7%
local recurrence	11%	12%	11%
5 year actuarial survival	45%	39%	54%

REFERENCES

1. McGavran MH, Bauer WC, Ogura JH (1961) The incidence of cervical lymph node metastases from epidermoid carcinoma of the larynx and their relationship to certain characteristics of the primary tumor. Cancer, 14:55-66

2. Arriagada R, Eschwege F, Cachin Y, Richard, JM (1983) The value of combining radiotherapy with surgery in the treatment of hypopharyngeal and laryngeal cancers. Cancer, 51:1819-1825

3. Seiden AM, Mantravadi RP, Haas RB, Applebaum EL (1984) Advanced supraglottic carcinoma: A comparative study of sequential treatment policies. Head and Neck Surgery, 7:22-27

4. Baluyot ST, Shumrick DA, Everts EC (1971) 'Emergency laryngectomy'. Arch Otolaryngology, 94:414-417

5. Vikram B, Strong EW, Shah JP, Spiro R (1984) Failure at the primary site following multimodality treatment in advanced head and neck cancer. Head and Neck Surgery, 6:720-723

6. Lam KH, Wong J, Lim STK, Ong GB (1981) Pharyngogastric anastomosis following pharyngolaryngo-esophagectomy, analysis of 157 cases. World J. Surgery, 5:509-516

© 1985 Elsevier Science Publishers B.V. (Biomedical Division)
New dimensions in otorhinolaryngology - head and neck surgery, vol. 2.
E. Myers, editor

COMPLICATIONS OF TOTAL LARYNGOPHARYNGOESOPHAGECTOMY MEDIASTINAL DISSECTION WITH GASTRIC PULL-UP RECONSTRUCTION

CARL F. WURSTER, M.D. AND GEORGE A. SISSON, M.D.

Departments of Otolaryngology Head and Neck Surgery, Medical University of South Carolina, Charleston, South Carolina (USA) and Northwestern University Medical School, Chicago, Illinois (USA)

INTRODUCTION

Although surgical cure of advanced or recurrent tumors of the laryngopharynx and cervical esophagus remains currently uncommon, meaningful operative palliation has become a reality. Following total laryngopharyngoesophagectomy and mediastinal resection, reconstruction of the alimentary tract is problematic. As more experience is gained with the alternative reconstructive methods in several institutions, complications unique and common to each method come to light.

PATIENTS AND METHODS

The post-operative course of thirty patients with a variety of advanced and recurrent tumors of the laryngopharynx and cervical esophagus subjected to total laryngopharyngo-esophagectomy, mediastinal dissection, gastric pull-up reconstruction and pectoralis major myocutaneous flap repair at a single operation was retrospectively reviewed for morbidity and mortality. Two institutions and five different operating surgeons contributed the hospital records of the thirty patients operated on between 1980 and 1984.

RESULTS

The nature of and frequency of major complications appear in Table I. The rate and type of minor complications are summarized in Table II. Finally, the commulative morbidity and mortality rates are presented in Table III.

TABLE I

MAJOR COMPLICATIONS

Type	Number	Percent
Inominate rupture	2	6
Carotid rupture	1	3
Gastric necrosis	1	3
Flap necrosis	1	3

TABLE II

MINOR COMPLICATIONS

Type	Number	Percent
Fistula	5	16
Wound dehiscence	3	10
Ileus	2	6

TABLE III

MORTALITY AND MORBIDITY RATES

Type	Cause	Number	Percent
Mortalities	Vessel rupture (innominate)	2	6
	Renal failure	1	3
	S.M.A. thrombosis	1	3
Total		4	13
Morbidity			
Major Complications		5	16
Minor Complications		10	33
Total		15	50

DISCUSSION

The introduction of single-stage reconstruction of the cervical esophagus and mediastinum with gastric pull-up and the pectoralis major myocutaneous flap by Krespi, Wurster, and Sisson in 1985 offered patients with advanced and recurrent lesions of the laryngopharynx and cervical esophagus a single stage procedure for viable aerodigestive tract reconstruction after radical extirpative surgery[1]. Our results compare favorably with another major study on the complication rate of total laryngopharyngoesophagectomy and gastric pull-up without mediastinal dissection and pectoralis myocutaneous flap reconstruction by Spiro and others[2].

Unquestionably the palliative value of gastric transposition for advanced and recurrent lesions of the larynx, pharynx, and cervical esophagus is being established in centers throughout the world[3].

CONCLUSION

We present the experience of post-operative morbidity and mortality of thirty patients undergoing total laryngopharyngoesophagectomy mediastinal dissection, gastric pull-up and pectoralis major myocutaneous flap reconstruction for advanced and recurrent tumors. The morbidity and mortality rates compare favorably with those of gastric transposition alone.

REFERENCES

1. Krespi YP, Wurster CF, Sisson GA (1985) Immediate reconstruction after total laryngopharyngoesophagectomy and mediastinal dissection Laryngoscope 95: 156-161
2. Spiro RH, Shah JP, Strong EW et al (1983) Gastric transposition in head and neck surgery Am J Surg 146:483-487
3. Davidge-Pitts KJ, Mannel A (1983) Pharyngolaryngectomy with extra thoracic esophagectomy Head Neck Surg 6:571-574

© 1985 Elsevier Science Publishers B.V. (Biomedical Division)
New dimensions in otorhinolaryngology - head and neck surgery, vol. 2.
E. Myers, editor

THE TRIAL FOR SCREENING OF LARYNGEAL CANCER USING COMPUTER

HAJIME YOSHIDA
Yoshida clinic, Nayoro, Hokkaido, Japan 096
SATOSHI EBIHARA
Dept of Head and Neck Surgery, National Cancer Center
5-1-1 Tsukiji, Chuoku,Tokyo,Japan 104
HIDEKI KASUYA
Dept of Electric Engineering,Utsunomiya University
2753 Ishii-machi,Utsunomiya, Japan 321

INTRODUCTION

We have developed the system to distinguish the pathological from the nomal voice,primarily aiming at its application to the first-step clinical screening of laryngeal cancer. We reported the results of its clinical use.

MATERALS AND METHODS

The system employs five acoustic parameters: rate of unvoiced intervals to the whole analysis interval(RUV), three pertubaion parameters(PQ'S),and normalized noise energy(NME).In the system the parameters are automatically computed from the skin vibration in front of the trachea and the speech signals of the sustaind utterance of a vowel /e/,and then subjected to the statiscal analysis in order to decide whether the voce is pathological or normal.

In our study, three evaluations i.e.laryngoscopic and perceptual evaluations and acoustic evaluation with the screening system, were simulaneously carried out for each subject.

RESULTS

We started the study from 1981 and collected 2020 voice samples of the people who live in north part of Hokkaido, Japan. First trial was performed from 1981 to 1982 and 1029 subjects were tested. One laryngeal cancer (Supura glottic T3) was found. In this paper, we will report the results of second trial which was performed from 1983 to 1984, 991 voice samples were collected in this trial. One laryngeal cancer(Glottic T2) was found and treated by radiation.

Table 1 shows the results of laryngoscopic, perceptual and acoustic evaluations. 669 people were normal by all of three evaluations. 86 people were normal by perceptual and acoustic evaluations although laryngoscopy couldn't be performed. It means 755(76.2%)persons were normal and 236(23.8%) were pathological. 10 cases were false negative(laryngoscopic finding was pathologic though acoustic and perceptual exams were normal). Those cases were 4 polypoid degeneration,

2 vorcal cord nodule, 1 chronic laryngitis and recurrent nerve pralysis eacah and 2 others.

47 cases were pathologic by three evaluations, and one laryngeal cancer was included.

Table 2 shows results of re-examination of the subjects who were not diagnosed as pathologic by laryngoscopy but regarded as pathologic by eather perceptual or acoustic evaluation or by both.

CONCLUSION

From the results of three 976 evaluations, we conclude that our system can highly accurately decide under careful recording conditions whether the voice is eather pathologic or normal. It is so easy to handle with and doesn't cause any pain to examinees.

Table 1 Classification of subjicts in terms of three evaluations

Laringo-scopic evaluation	Acoustic evaluation				
	Pathologic		Normal		
	Perceptual evaluation		Perceptual evaluation		
	Pathologic	Normal	Pathologic	Normal	Total
Pathologic	47	3	6	10	66
Normal	109	22	4	669	804
No examination	27	7	1	86	121
Total	183	32	11	765	991

Table 2 Results of reexamination of the subjects who were not diagnosed as pathology by laryngoscopy but regarded as pathologic by either perceptual or acoustic evaluation.

Reexamination	Acoustic evaluation			
	Pathologic	Pathologic	Normal	
	Percetual evaluation			
	Pathologic	Normal	Pathologic	Total
Pathologic	45	8	2	55
Normal	42	13	1	56
Uncertain	49	8	2	59
Tatal	136	29	5	170

Chronic laryngitis 27, Atrophy 12, vorcal cord polyp 5 polypoid degeneration 5, vorcal cord nodule 3.
Recurrent nerve pralysis 1, others2.

© 1985 Elsevier Science Publishers B.V. (Biomedical Division)
New dimensions in otorhinolaryngology - head and neck surgery, vol. 2.
E. Myers, editor

RECONSTRUCTION OF THE CERVICAL ESOPHAGUS WITH THE RIGHT COLON

ROMEO Y. LIM, MD, FACS, CLINICAL ASSOCIATE PROFESSOR OF OTOLARYNGOLOGY, JAMES P. BOLAND, MD, FACS, PROFESSOR OF SURGERY, WEST VIRGINIA MEDICAL CENTER, CHARLESTON WV (U.S.A.)

INTRODUCTION

When Czerny[1] first successfully resected cancer of the esophagus in 1877, esophageal reconstruction had become a surgical challenge. In 1886 Mikulicz[2] reconstructed the cervical esophagus with skin flaps and thereafter various methods of esophageal reconstruction with either skin[3] or gastrointestinal[4] tissues have been reported in the literature.

MATERIALS AND METHODS

Ten patients underwent a cervical esophageal reconstruction in which the right colon was mobilized subcutaneously over the left anterior chest wall to the pharynx at the Charleston Area Medical Center, Charleston, WV. Eight of these patients were men and 2 were women. The youngest was 50 years old; the oldest 90 years old. Four patients had a laryngoesophagectomy for carcinoma and 5 post-laryngectomy patients had a squamous cell carcinoma of the cervical esophagus varying from a 1-3 year interval. One patient had a stenosis of a cervical esophagus previously reconstructed with a Bakamjian flap 4 years prior.

TECHNIQUE

Resection of the esophagus and mobilization of the right colon was performed simultaneously by the head and neck surgical team and the general surgical team. The right colon was mobilized with careful preservation of the marginal arteries and the venous drainage. This includes the ileocolic arteries and a segment of the ileum of approximately 15cm frequently accompanies the right colon. The colon was brought up in a retrogastric fashion over the left costal margin into a subcutaneous position. A wide subcutaneous tunnel was develcped (at least a hand-breadth) up to the cervical incision.

A two-layer closure of the ileocolostomy was done and then the mesenteric approximation was performed. Anastomosis was made between the colon and the lesser curvature of the stomach just at the incisura angularis with no redundant colon to a J-loop. Sutures were then placed between the colon and the rectus fascia so that the colon from the entry point into the abdomen and into the stomach was in a relatively straight line and tension free. The anastomosis between the colon and stomach was made in a two-layer fashion. In addition, a pyloroplasty was performed and closed in a one-layer Gambee (a relatively small Heineke-Mikulicz).

The cervical area was handled in the following fashion; The distal esophagus was oversewn and allowed to retract into the chest cavity. The anastomosis for the hypopharynx and colon was made through the cephalic taenia coli in one layer using a nonabsorbable suture in a Gambee fashion. The colon was suspended by putting a few sutures in the posterior fascia prior to constructing the anastomosis.

RESULTS

All 10 patients had a viable colon conduit. They were swallowing 5 to 7 days after the reconstruction and were all discharged on the 10th postoperative day. A feeding gastrostomy was left in place for one month for supplementary intake. X-ray studies of the esophageal replacement showed rapid passage of the barium into the stomach. Diet was unrestricted and patients were advised to chew their food well. One patient had a ruptured distal esophageal stump on the 15th postoperative day resulting in a fulminating mediastinitis and death. Two patients had a massive gastrocolic anastomotic hemorrage on the 12th postoperative day resulting in death. These 3 patients were in their 8th and 9th decades of life.

DISCUSSION

The colon has advantages not associated with the jejunum or other structures. The mesentery of the right colon is thin and does not cause the colon to be plicated upon a short section of mesentery as is characteristic of the small bowel. The blood supply of the colon is ideal since there is an adequate marginal artery and vein close to the bowel. These marginal vessels communicate with the middle colic, the right colic and in turn the ileocolic vessels. The importance of this vascular pattern is that the colon can be mobilized to a desired distance. The right colon is perferred to other esophageal substitutes because of its ample length, its better blood supply, its isoperistaltic action and its resistance to gastric juice.

The experience with these 10 cases has shown the advantages of performing the procedure without entering the chest cavity and promptly restoring deglutition.

REFERENCES

1. Czerny V: Neu Operationen. Zbl Chir 1877;4:443
2. Mikulicz J: Ein Fall von resection des carcinomatosen oesophagus mit plastichem ersatz des excirdirten Stuckes Prager Med Wschr 1886;11:93
3. Wookey H: The surgical treatment of carcinoma of the pharynx and upper esophagus. Surg Gynec Obstet 1942;75:499
4. Heimlich HJ: Reconstruction of the esophagus with a reversed gastric tube. Surg Gynec Obstet 1962;114:673

New dimensions in otorhinolaryngology - head and neck surgery, vol. 2.
E. Myers, editor

GLOBUS HYSTERICUS: A CLINICO-RADIOLOGICAL STUDY

A.M. TALAAT, M.S. ELWANY, F.M. TALAAT AND M.M. NAHHAS
From The Departments of Otolaryngology, Neuro-Psychiatry and Radiology, Alexandria Faculty of Medicine, EGYPT

INTRODUCTION

A sensation of a lump in the throat for which no organic cause can be established is generally regarded as psychogenic globus hystericus. It has been estimated to account for 3% of adult patients attending the laryngological department[1].

The present report contains the results of an investigation of 173 patients (100 females & 73 males) with globus symptom, aiming at studying its various aspects and to determine the validity of some of the factors that still appear relevant to its etiology.

MATERIAL AND METHODS

All patients were examined clinically and underwent routine laboratory work-up. Roentgenographic examination of paranasal sinuses, cervical region and chest was done. A conventional barium examination of the hypopharynx, esophagus, stomach and small intestine was next performed. Endoscopic examination of the esophagus, stomach and duodenum was performed in patients with positive barium findings.

The therapeutic modalities included psychological treatment e.g. assurance, explanation, suggestion and psychotropic drugs in the form of minor tranquilizers and antidepressants, beside specific treatment of any underlying organic lesion.

RESULTS

Patients were divided into two main groups:

A. The first, or the pure functional group, where no organic lesion could be detected, consisted of 91 patients (73 females & 18 males). Their mean age was 26.3 years. These patients were divided into the following five subgroups according to the psychiatric study:

1. A group of 36 patients (39.5%) were manifesting the globus symptom due to underlying phobic reaction of having cancer throat or cancer thyroid.
2. A group of 21 patients (23%) with anxiety state where the sensation of a lump in the throat was one of the manifestations of the clinical syndrome.
3. A group of 6 patients (6.6%) with mixed anxiety and phobia.
4. A group of 5 patients (5.5%) suffering from endogenous depression, and the sensation of a lump in the throat was one of the hypochondriacal delusions they had.
5. A group of 23 patients (25.3%) with hysterical conversion reaction.

B. The second group, where an underlying organic lesion was found, consisted of

82 patients (55males & 27 females). Their mean age was 35.8 years. The commonest organic lesions encountered in this group were reflux esophagitis (61%), hiatal hernia (11%), sideropenic anemia (9.7%) and gastric and/or duodenal diverticula (10%). Clinical psychiatric assessment of this group revealed that the sensation of the globus was exaggerated when they experience emotional disturbance.

The response to treatment in the first group was on the whole higher than in the second group.

DISCUSSION

Hysterical conversion reactions were present in only 13.3% of the total number of patients. This clearly implies that the connotation hystericus seems inaccurate and unsatisfactory. Primarily, the psychiatric findings tend to suggest that the appearance of the globus syndrome is due to psychic, mainly neurotic, disturbances.

There is a general belief that the globus symptom is produced by increased tone of the pharyngeal constrictor muscles[2]. The intermittent non-peristaltic motor responses in the esophagus may be associated with emotional stress[3]. Some central modification from emotion must have caused a derangement in neural control. It is possible that an identical mechanism underlies cases with an unexpressed fear of cancer "cancer phobia". While we accept unreservedly the theoretical basis for the referred symptoms from the esophagus, stomach and intestine to the neck, we could not find in the present study or in the perusal of literature any evidence that the incidence of reflux esophagitis, hiatal hernia, gastric or duodenal diverticula or iron-deficiency anemia is higher in patients with globus than in normal population[4-6]. In the light of these findings, the importance of all these factors per se remains controversial, and a psychogenic element on top of these organic lesions is imperative for the sensation of the globus to be exaggerated.

We believe that the globus mechanism is a part of the normal human bodily function and that the symptom can be precipitated by strong emotional upset in almost any person with or without any of the above mentioned organic lesions. It is essential that both the somatic and the psychic status of the patient be carefully assessed. When the patient recognizes that his problem is regarded with much attention, as if it were real, then there is a good possibility of successful recovery.

REFERENCES

1. Malcomson KG (1968) J Laryngol Otol 82: 219-230
2. Watson WC, Sullivan SN (1974) Lancet 2:1417-1419
3. Mair IW, Schroder KE, Madalesli B (1974) J Laryngol Otol 88: 1033-1040
4. Nagler R, Spiro HM (1961) Gastroenterology 41:371-379
5. Flores TC, Cross FS, Jones RD (1981) Ann Oto Rhinol Laryngol 90:383-386
6. Maran A, Jacobson I (1971) Laryngoscope 81:412-417

New dimensions in otorhinolaryngology - head and neck surgery, vol. 2.
E. Myers, editor

TREATMENT OF THE LATERAL MIDDLE FACE FRACTURE THROUGH MINIPLATE OSTEOSYNTHESIS: AN ADVANCEMENT?

W.L. MANG
ENT university clinic r. d. Isar, Ismaninger Str. 22,
8ooo München 8o, FRG

INTRODUCTION

Between the years 198o and 1985 at the ENT-Clinic, Clinic r. d. Isar of the Technical University of Munich, 1411 facial skull injuries were operatively treated. 88o of these were Middle Face Fractures. 75,9% of the patients were male. In this lecture we want to discuss lateral middle face fractures in specific: During past years at our Clinic in Munich we have operatively treated 369 lateral middle face fractures. At the same time we have tried to establish a simple fracture classification. The division according to Mang Type I through Type III depends upon the number of fractured area, whereby Type III fractures, which means the so called 3 point impression fractures of cheekbone, are predominat.

RESULTS

With lateral middle face fractures the osteosynthesis of the fractured areas are the most important. Through the attached muscle movements and ligament tension, due to the insufficient fixation of the fragements, a dislocation can occur after repositioning. Therefore it is important to recognize the distinct tendency toward miniplate osteosynthesis by lateral middle face fractures. The techric ist simple, time saving, reliable and signifies an enormous advancement in the treatment of this kind of fracture. By fractures of the jaw cavity wall the additional exploration of the jaw cavity and the insertion of an antral ballon is necessary. The jaw cavity is then opened wide through the "Vestibulum cut" and with the appropriate instruments the damaged soft part of the tissue is repositioned together with the impressed jaw cavity walls and is fixed with an antral ballon. The ballon is then filled with fluid, according to the jaw cavity size, between 8 and 12 ml salt solution. The ballon is slipped through the nase. The antral ballon* has an optimal compatibility with tissue, the placement is simple and gentle and guarantees a good stabilization of the Orbita ground and the remaining jaw cavity walls. The ambulant removal is not problematic and is accomplished on the 21st post operative day. The Figure 1 and 2 show you the operative treatment of lateral middle face fracures with the miniplate osteosynthesis.

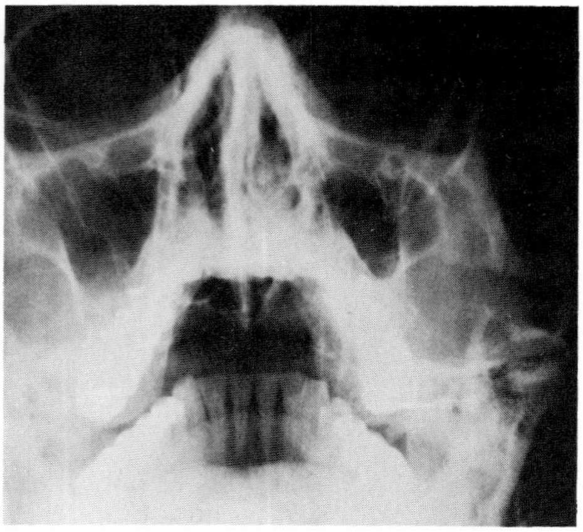

Fig. 1. Lateral middle face fracture (Mang Type III)

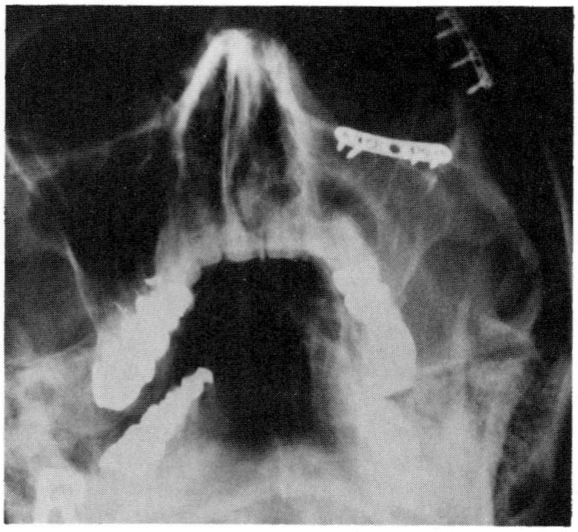

Fig. 2. The operative treatment of this lateral middle face fractures through miniplate osteosynthesis.

The main factor in the treatment of lateral middle face fractures must be the reconstruction of function and aesthetic value. Therefore this concept of the stabile miniplate osteosynthesis offers obvious advantages. The indications for plate osteosynthesis are:
a) fractures with the tendency toward "rotation dislocation" after repositioning due to muscle strain and ligament tension.
b) by cheekbone fractures there is a possibility of individual fixation of the "sutura frontozygomatica". Consequertly a secon osteosynthesisin the area of the orbita ground can be avoided.
c) shattered fractures (jaw cavity fragments, fragments with retraction tendency) offer the possibility for fixation and spanning of bone defects.
With the variation of available miniplates it becomes clear that our instrumentation of the miniplate compression system according to Luhr has been given the advantage because the placement of the plate is fast, unproblematic and provides good compatibility as well optimal stability. The 5 different plate forms, bent and straight with 90° and 110° angles and the T-plate are available in various lengths so that a large selection of combination possibilities exsists in order to justify the anatomical proportion of the operational area. By the all too often thin bone regions of the middle face, the self-cutting characteristics of the screws are a guarantee for a secure hold on the surrounding bone tissue.

SUMMARY

According to our more than 4 years of experience or 369 patients with lateral middle face fractures, we can say that through the application of the miniplate osteosynthesis for the reconstruction of the lateral middle face fracture of the operative possibilities have made an abvious advancement.

REFERENCES

1. Mathog RH (1984) Maxillofacial Trauma. Williams and Wilkins, Baltimore/London
2. Nigst H (1972) Spezielle Frakturen- und Luxationslehre. Band I/1. Thieme, Stuttgart
3. Spiessl B (1976) New Concepts in Maxillofacial Bone Surgery. Springer Verlag, Berlin, Heidelberg, New York

© 1985 Elsevier Science Publishers B.V. (Biomedical Division)
New dimensions in otorhinolaryngology - head and neck surgery, vol. 2.
E. Myers, editor

A NEW HEMIPALATAL APPROACH TO THE NASOPHARYNGEAL CAVITY - EXPERIMENTAL AND CLINICAL STUDY

YANG-GI MIN, JAE HEE KIM

Department of Otolaryngology, College of Medicine, Seoul National University
28 Yeongun-dong, Chongro-gu, Seoul (Korea)

INTRODUCTION

The juvenile nasopharyngeal angiofibroma is an uncommon, highly vascular, locally invasive, non-encapsulated, benign tumor of adolescent males. In its treatment, surgery is considered to be the method of choice. However, the successful excision of the tumor is difficult with high rate of recurrence, due to its relative anatomical inaccessibility, severe extension, and difficulties in controlling the bleeding.

Authors designed an approach that would almost expose the whole extent of the tumor and allow complete resection of the tumor under direct vision.

MATERIAL AND METHOD

Operative Procedures

After routine preparation, mucoperiosteal incision was made as depicted in solid line in figure 1. From this gingival incision, sublabial incision may extended, if needed, for the exposure of the maxillary sinus and pterygopalatine space. The hemipalatal flap including mucoperiosteum was raised. At the junction of the hard and soft palates, mucosa in the nasal side was dissected backwards. To facilitate further exposure, posteromedial wall of the greater palatine canal can be removed, and the hamulus of the pterygoid bone fractured, or the greater palatine neurovascular bundle severed. The flap was reflected laterally. Exposed hard palate was removed in piecemeal as needed. The mucosa of the nasal floor was incised as depicted in dotted line in figure 1. Exposed tumor was removed by sharp and blunt dissection. When the tumor extended to the contralateral nasopharynx, it can be removed easily by spreading

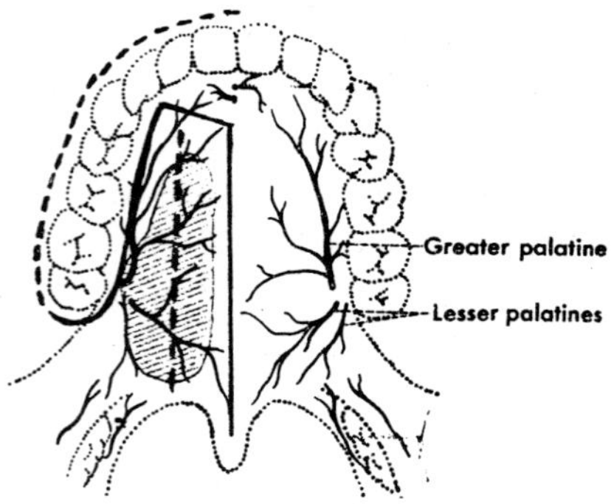

Fig. 1. A new hemipalatal incision

the incised soft palate. Postoperative bleeding was controlled with electrocautery and nasal packing. Nasal mucosa and palatal flap were sutured in 2 or 3 layers.

Experimental study

In 5 cats, the viability of the hemipalatal flap was observed 7 days after above mentioned operation severing the greater palatine neurovascular bundle.

Clinical study

9 patients with nasopharyngeal angiofibroma diagnosed by clinical and radiological studies were managed by above mentioned approach. In 3 patients, the greater palatine artery was cut. In the remaining 6 patients, there were no needs for severing the greater palatine neurovascular bundle.

RESULT

In experimental study, all flap were viable. In 9 patients, the tumor was generally presented unilaterally in the nasopharynx, and extended variably into the paranasal regions and intracranial fossa. The tumor was completely removed by this approach in 8 cases and combined sublabial transantral approach in 1 case in which the tumor extended into the maxillary sinus. Average operation time was 1 hour and 50 minutes, and average operative blood loss was 575cc. There were no wound problem, no flap necrosis, no fistula formation, and no functional deficit until 2 year follow-up.

DISCUSSION

Many surgical approaches and their modifications[1)-3)] were proposed for direct visualization of the nasopharynx and wide exposure of the operative field. Authors designed a hemipalatal flap approach to the nasopharynx. Its major advantages are excellent exposure of the surgical field with more safety, avoidance of unnecessary mutilation of the hard palate with post-operative disturbance of nasal physiology, reduction in intraoperative blood loss by shortening the operation time, and easy extension of the operative field by simple sublabial extension of hemipalatal flap incision. There were no noticeable postoperative complications or morbidities.

REFERENCES

1. Dibble, P.A., and King, J.C. : Juvenile nasopharyngeal angiofibroma. Laryngoscope 72 : 218, 1962
2. Henderson, G.P., and Patterson, C.N. : Further experience in the treatment of juvenile nasopharyngeal angiofibroma. Laryngoscope 79 : 561, 1969
3. Wilson, W.R., Miller, D., Lee, K.J., and Yules, R.B. : Juvenile nasopharyngeal angiofibroma. Laryngoscope 82 : 985, 1972

New dimensions in otorhinolaryngology – head and neck surgery, vol. 2.
E. Myers, editor

INFLUENCE OF DISORDERED NASAL BREATHING ON SLEEP IN CHILDREN

SOICHIRO MIYAZAKI, M.D. and KIYOSHI TOGAWA, M.D.
Dept. of Otolaryngology, Akita Univ. Sch. of Med. (JAPAN)

INTRODUCTION

The purpose of this study was to determine the effect of enlarged adenoids and tonsils on sleep and breathing. While a patient is awake, the influence of disordered nasal breathing is hard to observe because it is compensated by oral breathing. But that influence is notable when he is asleep because there is no conscious compensation. By way of polysomnography, we revealed the fact that disturbances of nasal breathing cause not only serious trouble for the cardio-respiratory function during sleep, but also prevent sound sleep throughout the night.

SUBJECTS AND METHODS

24 children, ages 4 to 7, who had higher than moderate levels of nasal obstructions were studied by polysomnography, including the EEG, EOG, esophageal pressure (EF), tidal volume, transcutaneous PO_2 and PCO_2 (tc PO_2, tc PCO_2), and etc. The examination lasted for one night. No drugs were used.

RESULT

In patients with the severely-obstructed nasal airways, we observed three types of disordered breathing in different sleep stages, i.e., light, deep, and REM sleep. (Figure) During light sleep, obstructive sleep apnea occurred repeatedly. When EP was reduced down to -50 to -60cmH_2O which was significantly lower than that in the waking state, the patients could at last get enough airflow with a loud snoring sound. Apnea lasted as 20 to 50 seconds at times. Tc PO_2 fluctuated within the range of 8 and 15mmHg corresponding with apnea and hyperpnea. During deep sleep, a regular breathing pattern was observed. EP remained between -30 and -40cmH_2O, and regular inspiratory retractions of the anterior chest was observed. Tc PO_2 showed hardly any changes. In other words, the patient must maintain great respiratory effort in order to obtain deep sleep. During REM sleep, Breathing showed rather irregular pattern. EP changed mildly around -30cmH_2O. In spite of relative rapid breathing, tc PO_2 showed a low value. EEG showed characteristic changes. Endeavours for respiration and arousing stimuli from disordered breathing appeared to prevent the patients from passing over into deep sleep. The summary of EEG changes was as follows; 1) The total sleep time was prolonged. 2) Stage 4 latency was also prolonged. 3) The ratio of light sleep was increased and that of deep sleep was decreased. 4) Increased incidence of spontaneous awakenings.

5) Alpha-wave activities in accordance with respiratory effort. 6) Decreased number of spindle-wave activities.

Post adenoid-tonsillectomy, the conditions were improved remarkably. The patients slept well with nasal breathing. EP stayed in the normal range of 5 to 15cmH2O throughout the night, and obstructive apnea disappeared completely. Tc PO2 and PCO2 changed slightly only during REM sleep. Post-operative sleep data showed initial deepening and increased time of deep stages. Alpha-wave activities during light sleep was disappeared and the number of spindle-waves was increased. From the questionnaires to the children who took polysomnography, we knew that the time for falling asleep or waking up became earlier. Also they stopped taking naps after the operation.

CONCLUSION

Children with nasal obstruction suffer from severe disturbance of nocturnal sleep. We must not overlook their respiratory distress.

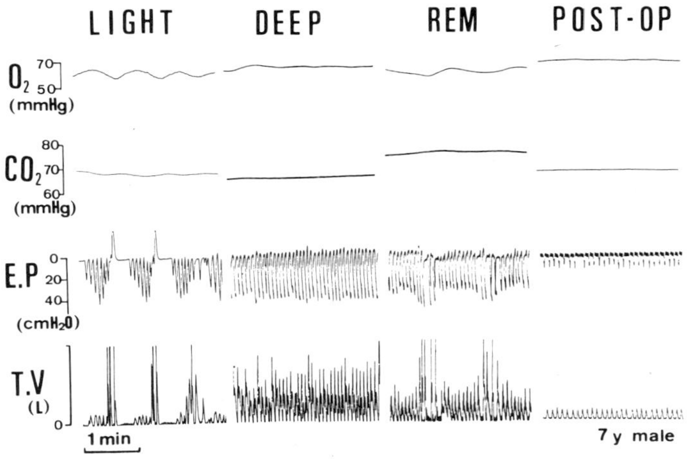

New dimensions in otorhinolaryngology - head and neck surgery, vol. 2.
E. Myers, editor

MALARIA AND OTORHINOLARINGOLOGY IN ENDEMIC COUNTRIES

Dr. KHALIL E.F. MOUSTAFA,D.L.O.

Head of ENT Department,6 October Hospital,Health Insurance Organization, Cairo,Egypt.

INTRODUCTION

Malaria still exists all round the world in the tropics and subtropics inside the so-called " The Malrial Belt" outlined by WHO. It is primarily a blood disease through which the parasitized red cells can reach and affect nearly every organ and tissue causing impairment in their microcirculation,hence disturbance of function. Cerebral malaria, gastrointestinal and malarial nephrosis are well-known examples.

The aim of this paper is to draw the attention of the new fact that the classical,typical clinical picture of malaria characterised by bouts of fevers followed by periods of remissions are now regressng, giving the way instead, to variants of atypical and modified forms in endemic countries.

In a study recently conducted in Egypt, cases presented exclusively with O.R.L. syptoms could be spotted.

MATERIAL AND METHODS

From the years 1979-1984,44 patients, all live in areas known to be malraious*, were referred to ENT clinic whose complaints were either:

A. Relapsing unilateral or bilateral sore throat (31 cases) or,
B. Long standing dry cough with tracheal pain (3 cases) or,
C. Acute frontal afeverish headache (8 cases) or,
D. Unexplained unilateral otalgia (2 cases).

These symptoms were refractory to antibiotics and other lines of treatments. Some could remember a past history of malaira or, malaria-like fever misdiagnosed and passed off as ordinary flu. Their investigation papers included both chest and sinus radiographes,C.S.Scans of both sputum and throat swabs,also hemograms,all, demonstrated nothing of importance in diagnosis. When clinically-examined,objective signs of bacterial or viral infections were never detected. Other diseases of similar symptomatology (e.g. neuralgias) could be easily excluded.

11 cases out of 44(i.e. 25% of the series) were picked at random and had their blood smears been examined for malaria parasite(only once) and reported negative. Serologic test for malaria coundn't be done for technical reasons.

*** Certain parts in Egypt, Sudan, Ughanda and Nigeria.**

The author,then adviced the antimalarial drug " Resochin, in full therapeutic doses.

RESULTS

The Resochin therapeutic response was positive in 40 out of 44 of cases giving 90.9% cure-rate with no recurrence of symptoms. In the failed 4 cases, re-scanning of their throat swabs, revealed agressive types of bacteria.

DISCUSSION

The possibility of the malaria parsite being the causative factor are based on: the type of patient, past history,clinical examination,recurrence of symptoms and the positive Resochin therapeutic test. Negative blood smear doesn't refute this possibility unless* it is been repeated 3 times at least, in different hours night and day because of the variation of the level of parasitemia in the peripheral blood. On the other hand, the appearance of these modified, atypical malaria in endemic countries, could be explained on factors like: low-leveled infection partial immunity or tolerance of the host(acquired/transplacentally transmitted),the inclusion of some antimalarial compounds(e.g. Resochin) in drugs commonly used in treatment of rheumatism in certain pharmacopioe, also the introducion into the field of medicine of some new antibiotics recently claimed to have some antimalarial effect either in the therapeutic or in the prophylactic sides e.g. Minocycline, Clindamycins (Dalacin C),Septrin and similar antifole antibiotics.

CONCLUSION

On the above foundations acute malarial pharyngitis ,and acute malarial tracheo-bronchitis could be justifiablly included in the D.D. of diseases of the pharynx and the upper respiratory tract.

REFERENCES

1. Modern concepts of epicemiology and preventive medicine (Prof. M.OMRAN).
2. Text book of pathology (Boyd).
3. Text book of pathology (Prof. A.M.ELWI).
4. Review of medical pharmacology (6th edition-Meyers).
5. Current medical diagnosis and treatment 1983(Krupp-Chatron).
6. A synopsis of otolaryngology (Ballantyne and Groves).
7. Journal of Laryngology.

*** A rule have been recently laid: One positive test is confirmatory not necessarily so when negative unless repeated.**

New dimensions in otorhinolaryngology – head and neck surgery, vol. 2.
E. Myers, editor

ABOUT UPPER CERVICAL LYMPHADENITIS (UCLA) CAUSED BY MYCOPLASMA INFECTIONS

SUSUMU MUKAI, MD, CHIKAKO MUKAI, MD, KAZUYUKI ASAOKA, MD.
MUKAI Medical Clinic and Mycrobiological Laboratory
Yamatominami 2-8-9, 242 Kanagawa, JAPAN.

INTRODUCTION

UCLA is not a rare disease which followed by epipharyngitis. One of the causative organisms is chlamydia about which we have already reported on.[1)-5)] Next to chlamydia, infection with micoplasma is prevailing.

PATIENTS

CF titers From 1980 to 1984 we examined CF titers of chlamydia and mycoplasma with 743 of UCLA patients. 227 of these patients were sorologicaly diagnosed as having mycoplasma infection by the following criteria. (Table-1)

1) A greater than four fold difference in titers between two or more sera.
2) Over 1:16 at the first examination or during therapy.

(Table-1) Mycoplasma CF titers of the UCLA patients.

CF titers	4≦	8	8*	16	32	64≦
Cases	400	107	23	55	103	41
			227 (positive)			

(* Four folds difference between two or more sera.)

Age distribution (Table-2)

Age	0-5	6-10	11-15	16-20	21-30	31-40	41-
Cases	25	80	27	6	18	23	5

There are much cases in children than in adults.

Patients distribution for month From 51.6% of the patients consulted us between november and february.

CHIEF COMPLAINTS

Cough 104 (45.8%), Otalgia 83 (36.6%), Fever 33 (15.9%), Rhinorrhea 25 (11.0%), Infra-auricular pain 21 (9.35%), Sore throat 15 (6.6%), Infra-auricular swelling 12 (5.3%), next to them were nasal obstruction, epistaxis, cervical pain, headache, abdominal pain, arthralgia and seven had no complaints.

<u>Laboratory finding</u>: WBC increases slightly, their mean cell count were 7,600. CRA (- +), mean CA was 36.7 (standard deviation of 42.13).

THERAPY

Tetracyclinic and/or mocrolides drugs are the remedy of choice. We use MNO and JM. Symptoms and signes are disappear in 1 to 2 weeks following theapy. They are more effective against this infection than chlamydial infection.

DISCUSSION

In UCLA, most common causative organisms are both <u>c.psittaci</u> and <u>mycoplasma</u>. These organisms were mainly thought to cause atypical pneumonia in humans. But by authors experience, UCLA are more common than atypical pneumonias. These organisms drop first in upper respiratory tracts and cause epipharyngitis and UCLA. When they drop in deep, they cause atypical pneumonia.[6] The authers think also the UCLA are missed because of their anatomical difficulty. If you remember UCLA with these infection diagnosis for the grippe will be more accurate.

REFERENCES

1. Mukai S, Mukai C, Suzuki I (1981) 82 cases of cervical lymphadenitis caused by ornithosis. XII World Congress, Budapest.
2. Mukai S, Mukai C, Asaoka K, Suzuki I (1983) Chlamydial infection with main symptoms of upper cervical lymphadenitis. Jap J Otol 86:441-451.
3. Mukai S, Mukai C, Asaoka K, Suzuki I (1985) Chlamydial Infection of head and neck. Ear Nose and Throat J 64:173-179.
4. Mukai S, Mukai C, Asaoka K, Suzuki I (1985) Chlamydial infection with main symptoms of upper cervical lymphadenitis(UCLA)__ isolation of chlamydiae--Jap J Otol:in print.
5. Mukai S (1985) upper-deep cervical lymphadenitis by chlamydial infection. JOHNS 1:129-132.
6. Mukai S, Mukai C, et al (1985) About upper-deep cervical lymphadenitis caused by mycoplasma infection. 17 congress of Kanagawaken infectious disease.

© 1985 Elsevier Science Publishers B.V. (Biomedical Division)
New dimensions in otorhinolaryngology – head and neck surgery, vol. 2.
E. Myers, editor

MACROGLOSSIA IN CHILDREN: AN APPROACH TO DIAGNOSIS AND TREATMENT

CHARLES M. MYER III, ANDREW J. HOTALING, JAMES S. REILLY

Department of Otolaryngology, University of Pittsburgh School of Medicine and Children's Hospital of Pittsburgh, Pittsburgh, PA

Patients with macroglossia exhibit persistent, generally painless, enlargement of the tongue. Although rare, the careful and complete evaluation of macroglossia should be familiar to all physicians who care for children. The ability to classify the varied etiologies of macroglossia into generalized and localized etiologic categories allows the clinician to formulate a differential diagnosis. The factors which must be considered include congenital, inflammatory, traumatic, metabolic and neoplastic causes.[1]

Clinical presentation is marked by tongue hypertrophy with protrusion through the lips. Ulceration and/or necrosis may occur with prolonged exposure. In addition, prolonged hypertrophy of the tongue has been associated with both occlusal abnormalities and airway obstruction. Articulation difficulties may also be observed in addition to significant problems with feeding. Psychological problems are common in patients with macroglossia secondary to their cosmetic deformity.[2]

An organized approach to the evaluation of macroglossia will prove both cost-effective and time-effective. A thorough history and physical examination should be performed in all patients. Chromosome studies may provide essential information and, in a child with multiple birth defects, a dysmorphologist should be consulted. Other diagnostic studies which may be beneficial include thyroid function tests and identification of urinary mucopolysaccharides. Whenever macroglossia appears secondary to localized enlargement of the tongue, neoplastic, granulomatous and infectious disorders must be considered and a biopsy should be performed. Patients with underlying neuromuscular dysfunction (such as cerebral palsy) may exhibit pseudomacroglossia and should be differentiated from patients with true macroglossia.[2,3]

No definitive guidelines have been established for surgical intervention in the treatment of macroglossia.[3] The decision to perform a surgical reduction should be based on several factors, including functional, cosmetic and pathological considerations. An anterior V-shaped wedge resection appears most beneficial in cases of idiopathic tongue enlargement.[4] In spite of adequate surgical therapy, secondary orthodontic care and speech therapy may be necessary in some patients.[5]

REFERENCES

1. Loeffler JR, Duray PH, Sasaki CT (1984) Arch Otolaryngol 110:600-603
2. Shafer AD (1968) Clin Pediatr 7:357-363
3. Behrman RE, Vaughn VC, Nelson WE (1983) Nelson Textbook of Pediatrics (twelfth ed.), W.B. Saunders Co., Philadelphia, p. 885
4. Dinerman WS, Myers EN (1976) Laryngoscope 86:291-296
5. Gupta DP (1971) Arch Otolaryngol 93:378-383

© 1985 Elsevier Science Publishers B.V. (Biomedical Division)
New dimensions in otorhinolaryngology – head and neck surgery, vol. 2.
E. Myers, editor

ISOLATION OF CHLAMYDIAE FROM THE PATIENTS WITH UPPER CERVICAL LYMPHADENITIS (UCLA)

SUSUMU MUKAI, MD, CHIKAKO MUKAI, MD, ISSEI SUZUKI.
MUKAI Medical Clinic and Microbiological Laboratory
Yamatominami 2-8-9, 242 Kanagawa, JAPAN.

INTRODUCTION

We reported a chlamydial disease with main symptoms of upper cervical lymphadenitis (UCLA) associated with chlamydial CF titer. To confirm their relationship we tried to isolate the chlamydiae from the patients with UCLA.

MATERIAL AND METHODS

SPECIMENS (a) Mucous membranes were swabbed from the epipharynx of the UCLA patients. (b) Exudatives were collected from the patients with EOM. These specimens were preserved in the Eagle's MEM(1%FCS), -80°C.
208 of (a) and 35 of (b), total of 243 specimens were examined.

CULTURE 0.5ml of specimen suspended fluid were overlaid on a monolayered HeLa S3 cells which were treated with 30min of DEAE before the inoculations. After centrifugal force of 400g for 1hr, the cells were incubated in 37°C 48hrs with fresh Eagle's MEM(1%FCS).

DETECTION After the incubations chlamydial intracytoplasmic inclusions were microscopically searched by Machiavello and Giemsa stains.

RESULTS

63 out of 208 of the UCLA patients' specimens were detected chlamydial intracytoplasmic inclusions.

The isolated chlamydiae belong to c,psittaci by their morphology. Vacuoles were hardly observed to their intracytoplasmic inclusions.

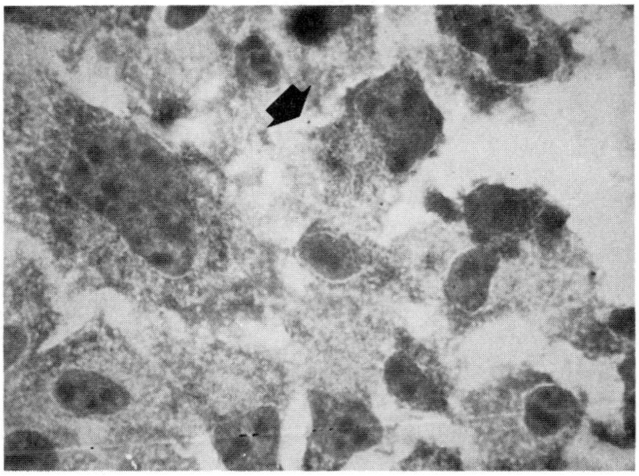

(Photo-1)
Chlamydial intracytoplasmic inclusions.
Female, 9yrs.
Chlamydial CF titer 1:16
(Mechiavello stain;400X)

Their growth rates were faster than the other c.psittaci, such as Meningopneumonitis and Budgerigar strains. Further cultivation of them by tissue culture were difficult.

The relationship between UCLA and chlamydiae became clear by this work.

(Table-1)

Corelation between chlamydial CF titers and isolation of chlamydiae.

Chlamydial CF titers	Cases	Isolation of chlamydia Positive	Negative	Isolation Rate (%)
1: 4	92	21	71	22.8
1: 4	28	11	17	39.3
1: 8	26	10	16	38.5
1: 8*	7	1	6	14.3
1:16	32	14	18	43.8
1:32	18	4	14	22.2
1:64	5	2	3	40.0
UCLA	208	63	145	30.3
EOM	35	0	36	0.0

(* Four fold difference between two sera)

Compare with the isolation rates and CF titers on this disease, we can say that the CF titer of over 1:4 is positive.

Contact with birds

In chlamydia isolated patients, 12 had contact with birds, 24 had no contact with birds and 27 were unknown about their past history with birds.

DISCUSSION

It is said that infection with c.psittaci is contracted by humans through exposure to chlamydia infected birds. But c.psittaci were isolated from the patients who had no contact with birds.

The isolated c.psittaci are different from the other c.psittaci such as Meningopneumonitis and Budgerigar strains with their morphology and biology. So there is a possibility that the isolated chlamydia is a new kind of c.psittaci. Humans can be the host of the isolated c.psittaci.

The relationship between EOM and chlamydia was low.

REFERENCES

1. Mukai S, Mukai C, Asaoka K, Suzuki I (1983) Chlamydial infection with main symptoms of upper cervical lymphadenitis. Jap J Otol 86:441-451.
2. Mukai S (1985) Upper deep cervical lymphadenitis by chlamydial infection. JOHNS 1:129-132.
3. Mukai S, Mukai C, Asaoka K, Suzuki I (1985) Chlamydial infection of head and neck. Ear Nose and Throat J 64:173-179.

© 1985 Elsevier Science Publishers B.V. (Biomedical Division)
New dimensions in otorhinolaryngology - head and neck surgery, vol. 2.
E. Myers, editor

INDICATION OF ELECTRO-COAGULATION USING HIGH FREQUENCY CURRENTS IN OTO-RHINO-LARYNGOLOGY

MIYOJI NIHO, OSAMU SAEKI, NOBUKAZU TADAKI, MAMORU SHIIDA, MINORU ISHIKAWA, JUSEI TOKUNAGA, and KUNIAKI TERAYAMA.
(Society of High Frequency Current Research, Japan.)

In electro-coagulation using high frequency currents, Joule heat generated by the concentrated current on the treatment electrode is utilized. Intense heat is produced when the current is strong or the area between the electrode and tissue is small. On the other hand, mild heat is produced when the current is weak or the contact area is large, enabling mild coagulation without sparks, fumes or a burning odor. Utilizing these characteristics, we have devised various types of electrodes during the last ten years, and have obtained good results in following diseases.

Epistaxis

This technique is applied when there are visible bleeding points. When there is bleeding, the hemorrhage should be controlled with local hemostatics before bringing the electrode into light contact with the bleeding points. If the electrode comes into broad contact with the blood or is pressed strongly against the tissue, bleeding will not be controlled.

Hypertrophic rhinitis with chronic sinusitis

The electro-coagulation is applied to the mucous membrane of the inferior and sometimes the middle turbinates after septomeatal plasty including submucous septum resection, submucous turbinectomy, and intranasal ethmoidectomy is performed when necessary. Because the nasal membrane is adjacent to the bone, the use of a strong current may cause osteitis, and crust formation remains for a long time. It is recommended that a weak current be used after inserting a bipolar needle electrode. When coagulation is adequate, the mucous membrane covered with a jelly-like substance for about 2 weeks. After that, the nasal air passage is improved, and sinusitis is cured in many cases.

Allergic rhinitis

Most cases of allergic rhinitis are classified as Type I according to Gell and Coombs's classification. However, some cases of perennial type show histopathological findings suggesting Type IV without any eosinophilic leucocyte. Surgery may be indicated in such cases.

In cases with septal deviation or hypertrophy of the inferior turbinates, we usually perform mild electro-coagulation of the inferior turbinates after the septomeatal plasty, and have obtained good results.

Nasal Polyps and membranous adhesions

In such cases, bipolar tweezer type electrodes are effective. These affections can be removed without bleeding when a relatively strong current is used pinching the stem of the polyps or the part of adhesions between the two electrodes.

Chronic Tonsillitis

The indication of total tonsillectomy can be summed up as (1) habitual tonsillitis, (2) simple hypertrophy interfering of respiration and food passage, (3) focal tonsillitis, (4) relapsing peritonsillar abscess, and (5) pus plug formation. We have used electro-coagulation in such cases by inserting bipolar electrodes with 5 mm exposed tips and producing mild coagulation. The coagulated tissue disappears spontaneously within 2 weeks, and there is little scar formation after surgery. For focal tonsillitis and relapsing peritonsillar abscesses, the affected tissues in the deeper regions often remain after this procedure, requiring it to be performed several times.

Stomatitis and ranula

Aphthous stomatitis with deep refractory ulcer can be handled by holding a ball electrode in light contact with the tissue delivering a weak current. Pain disappears in a few days and the affected areas quickly heal. Ranula can be handled simply by coagulating the entire surface of the mucous membrane with a relatively strong current.

Otitis media with effusions

Otitis media with effusions is sometimes difficult to cure, and recently, tubing through the tympanic membrane has been performed. While this procedure is very effective, such complications as infection, obliteration, falling off or dropping into the tympanic cavity sometimes occur. We have performed boring of the tympanic membrane using weak current through a knee shaped needle electrode. The perforation lasts for 2 - 4 weeks. Therefore, when the treatment of nasopharyngitis, sinusitis or adenoidectory are performed at the same time, many difficult cases can be cured.

Others

Hypertrophy of the lingual tonsil or small benign neoplasms can be handled through this technique without bleeding.

New dimensions in otorhinolaryngology - head and neck surgery, vol. 2.
E. Myers, editor

CLINICAL SIGNIFICANCE OF ESOPHAGEAL WEB IN PLUMMER-VINSON SYNDROME

HIROSHI OKAMURA, KIYOSADA SUEMITSU AND SHOICHIRO TSUTSUMI
Department of Otolaryngology, School of Medicine, Ehime University
Shizukawa, Shigenobu-cho, Onsen-gun, Ehime 791-02 (Japan)

INTRODUCTION

Plummer-Vinson syndrome is a clinical entity associated with dysphagia, anemia and glossitis. Since a long time ago, it has been well known that an esophageal web is often observed in this syndrome through an esophagography. However, a pathogenesis of the web has not been explained clearly yet.

In this paper, the authors report clinical significances of an esophageal web in this syndrome.

MATERIALS AND METHODS

We observed 19 cases of Plummer-Vinson syndrome associated with an esophageal web in the last eight years. All of the cases were middle-aged females (the range: 38 to 51 y. o.), who had hypochromatic and microcytic anemia with iron deficiency. The chief complaints were dysphagia and soreness when swallowing. Commissular cheilitis and glossitis with atrophy of the papillae were observed in all of the cases.

In the lateral view of the esophgogram, a web projected vertically at the anterior wall of the cervical esophagus just below the level of the cricoid cartilage, and the lengths ranged from two to 12 mm, the mean being 5.6. In the antero-posterior view, a horizontal transparent band corresponding to the site of the web was observed. Endoscopic examinations of the esophagus carried out on 13 of the 19 cases did not reveal the existence of a membranous structure corresponding to the web observed in the esophagogram. However, a diffuse swelling of the anterior wall of the esophagus was observed in seven cases, and atrophy of the mucosa in four cases. Histological examinations showed hyperplasial degenaration of the esophageal mucosa including acanthosis, dyskeratosis and hyperkeratosis.

All of the cases were treated by administrating iron per oral. With the start of treatments, the complaint of dysphagia immediately improved, and the hematological scores were normalized soon after the improvement of dysphagia. The reduction or disappearance of an esophageal web occurred much later than the improvement of dysphagia and the normalization of the hematological scores.

DISCUSSION AND CONCLUSIONS

As mentioned above, a membranous structure, which is corresponding to an esophageal web observed in esophagograms, was not found through endoscopic investigations. Therefore, we need to investigate the mechanism of formation of an esophageal web observed in esophagography in Plummer-Vinson syndrome.

By frame-by-frame analyses of the esophagogram obtained by videotape recording, the esophageal web was visualized when a bolus reached the cervical esophagus and the esophageal wall started dilating. After a bolus passed through the cervical esophagus, the web disappeared, and a dry swallowing of saliva did not cause the formation of a web. On swallowing a solid bolus, a web was not formed by passive dilation of the esophageal wall due to the existence of a solid bolus.

From these observations, we assume that the formation of an esophageal web in esophagogram may be caused by the restriction of dilation of the esophageal wall, which results the repetition of inflamation and its healing process. The histological investigation, which showed the existence of hyperplasial degeneration of the mucosa, supports the above assumption, and iron deficiency anemia may play the main role in the above histological alteration.

From the results mentioned above, it is assumed that the existence of an esophageal web does not cause dysphagia primarily, because the disappearance of dysphagia preceded the reduction of an esophageal web. To clarify the cause of dysphagia, we investigated histologically the inferior pharyngeal constrictors of rabbits with iron dificiency anemia. By staining with NADH hydrogenase, escape of mitochondrias, which is called a "moth-eaton" view, was observed in the Type I muscle fibers. This finding is a morphological change similar to that observed in myasthenia gravis. Therefore, iron deficiency may produce myasthenic change of the inferior pharyngeal constrictor, and this histological alteration may explain the outcome of dysphagia in Plummer-Vinson syndrome.

© 1985 Elsevier Science Publishers B.V. (Biomedical Division)
New dimensions in otorhinolaryngology - head and neck surgery, vol. 2.
E. Myers, editor

SNORING AND OBSTRUCTIVE SLEEP APNEA IN CHILDREN BEFORE AND AFTER ADENOTONSILLECTOMY

J.O. OVESEN, C. SIIM, P. CLEMMESEN, G. WILDSCHIØDTZ and G. KISCHI-NOVSKY
Dept. of Otorhinolaryngology and Sleep Laboratory, Glostrup Hospital, University of Copenhagen, Denmark

The purpose of this study is to determine the nature and frequency of sleep complaints in children referred for operation because of recurrent tonsillitis or hypertrophic tonsils or adenoids.

Parents of 1o5 children between 2 and 12 years were interviewed upon referral to the ENT department for adenotonsillectomy. Mean age was 6 years and there were 38 girls and 67 boys. 1o adenotomies, 24 tonsillectomies and 71 adenotonsillectomies were performed. A questionnaire regarding sleep habits and complaints was filled out prior to as well as 6 weeks after surgery. The questionnaire included questions about respiration during sleep, motor behaviour during sleep, awakening and daytime behaviour.

Before the operation 69% of the children had some sort of breathing complaint. 53% had regular or irregular snoring, 16% had very laborious breathing or apneic events and only 31% had regular breathing without snoring. After the operation only 2 children reported irregular snoring and 2 children reported irregular snoring and snorting. The rest of the children reported quiet regular breathing. 6 boys before the operation reported apneic events. 3 of these were referred for recurrent tonsillitis and the apneic events were undiagnosed by the referring physician and not spontaneously considered unnatural by the parents. All 6 cases were rated by the surgeon as hypertrophic tonsils, 5 of them with insufficient space between the tonsils.

During sleep 28% of the children before the operation were very restless and tossing and turning in bed. 15% had also violent movements of arms and legs and 2% would not lie down. 55% had normal behaviour during sleep. After the operation all except 5 children had normal behaviour during sleep. These 5 children were very restless and tossing and turning in bed and one child also had violent movements during sleep.

21 children were tired upon awakening or difficult to awaken

before the operation. After the operation 4 children were tired upon awakening and one child was difficult to awaken.

14 children before the operation were reported to be very tired during the day and 7 of them had periods with hyperactivity. One child was reported to fall asleep during the day if let alone. After the operation all but 2 children were reported to have normal alert daytime behaviour.

Before the operation more children than after were reported to sleeptalk, have nightmares, awakenings during the night, morning headache, enuresis or bruxism. Many of the children were reported to dream and sleepwalk but no difference was found in the amount reported before and after the operation. The size of the tonsils and the amount of adenoids showed no correlation to the nature of sleep complaint reported before the operation. The surgeon's rating of the amount of space between the tonsils showed some relation to sleep complaints in most of the cases but not in all.

In summary this study shows that in the group of children admitted for adenotonsillectomy breathing complaints are very common. Disturbance of motor behaviour during the night, awakening and daytime behaviour are also reported rather often.

Nature of complaint	Before operation	After operation
Snoring	53%	4%
Breathing difficulties/ apnea	16%	0%
Tossing and turning in bed, violent movements, not lying down	45%	5%
Difficult to awaken or very tired	21%	5%
During daytime very tired, periodically hyperactive or falling asleep	15%	2%

The complaints are often diminised and in most cases relieved by operation. These conditions are not diagnosed if not looked for and consequently they may be very underdiagnosed.

New dimensions in otorhinolaryngology - head and neck surgery, vol. 2.
E. Myers, editor

INDUCTION CHEMOTHERAPY IN HEAD AND NECK CANCER WITH CIS-PLATINUM (C), FLUORO 5 URACILE (F) AND BLEOMYCINE (B)

BASSOT V°*, BRASNU D°, LACAU ST GUILY J°, MENARD°, FABRE A°, DONNADIEU S°, LACCOURREYE H°, JACQUILLAT Cl*
° Department of head and neck surgery, Laennec Hospital, Paris.
* Department of oncololy, Salpetriere hospital, Paris, France

INTRODUCTION

Induction chemotherapy was used since 1970, with a response rate of 30%. In this study, the authors are presenting the preliminary results of a new association (C.F.B) which is used since 1982. The main point is the comparison between clinical and histological (on the specimen) analysis of the response.

MATERIAL AND METHODS

Patients. 344 patients (pts) were treated from 11/82 to 2/85. The percentage of patients included in this protocol is more than 90%. There were 323 men and 21 women. All patients had squamous cell carcinoma and all were previously untreated.

Protocols. First protocol started on 11/82 with : (C) : 100 mg/M2, d1 with hyperhydratation, F : 1g/M2 from d 1 to d 4 by continuous infusion, B : 30 mg d1, 7,5 mg from d2 to d 4 by continuous infusion. Tetracosactide : 2 mg d1, 1 mg from d2 to d 4, Metoclopramide : 60 mg d1 or alizapride : 500 mg d 1.

The second protocol employed started on 9/84 with : C : 15mg/M2 from d1 to d 4 by continous infusion, F : 1g/M2 from d1 to d 4 by continous infusion. Each drug was administred in 1000 ml normal saline. Alizapride : 10 mg each day.

3 courses were initially planed (1 course every 3 weeks).

313 pts were evaluated after 3 Courses. After induction chemotherapy 234 pts underwent a surgical procedure as initially decided. 31 pts didnot received 3 courses : 3 deaths (2 of unknown origin, 1 intravascular coagulation), 3 progressions, 4 septicemias, 4 leukopenias, 3 renal impairments, 2 myocarditis, 4 arterial hypertensias, 3 hepatic toxicities, 1 gastro-intestinal ulcer, 4 patients refused to complete the treatment.

RESULTS. The response rate independently of localisations and stages was good. 191 pts (61%) responded (CR+PR). Response rate by localisation is presented in tables 1 and 2.

TABLE 1	OROPHARYNX					LARYNX				
STAGE	NB	CR	%	CR + PR	%	NB	CR	%	CR + PR	%
1	3	2	67	3	100	6	3	50	5	83
2	5	3	60	4	80	34	9	26	20	59
3	30	14	47	23	76	59	9	15	35	60
4	44	12	27	31	70	30	-	-	14	47
ALL	82	31	38	61	74	129	21	16	74	57

TABLE 2	HYPOPHARYNX					ORAL CAVITY				
STAGE	NB	CR	%	CR + PR		NB	CR	%	CR + PR	%
1	-	-		-	-	2	1	50	2	100
2	8	4	50	7	87	6	1	17	3	50
3	28	6	21	19	68	12	2	17	7	58
4	41	5	12	20	49	5	1	20	3	60
ALL	77	15	20	46	60	25	5	20	15	60

After surgery, tumoral regression on the specimen was analysed in 234 pts. Cf table 3.

TABLE 3	CR (52)		PR (93)		NR (89)		ALL (234)	
	NB	%	NB	%	NB	%	NB	%
. NO TUMOR EVIDENCE	19	37	9	10	3	3	31	13
. RESIDUAL TUMOR	25	48	21	23	1	1	47	20
. TUMOR	8	15	63	67	85	96	156	67

Response rates for these 234 pts were reevaluated according to the histological analysis of the specimen : cf table 4.

TABLE 4

STAGE	NB	P	NR	PR	CR		CR + PR	
					NR	%	NB%	%
1	10	-	2	6	2	20	8	80
2	51	-	23	18	10	20	28	55
3	110	4	53	40	13	12	53	48
4	63	2	36	19	6	10	25	40
ALL	234	6	104	63	31	13	94	40

The nodal response independently of localisations and stages is 61% (83/135). Among patients after surgery (90) 16 pts (18%) had no residual tumor, but 12 pts (75%) were staged as N1b (UICC) at the initial clinical staging. Among clinical NO pts (114) 26% were N+.

TOXICITY.

Toxicities encountered with CFB : gastrointestinal (70%), hematologic (10%), cardiac (aggravation of preexisting disease) (5%), venitis (80%), renal impairment (10%), hypokalemia (45%), pulmonary (infection) (10%).

Toxicities encountered with C.F. : gastrointestinal (30%), hematologic (10%), cardiac (0), veneitis (80%), renal impairment (2%), hypokalemia (5%), pulmonary (10%).

CONCLUSION : Induction chemotherapy with C.F.B. or C.F. is effective. Response rate by clinical evaluation does not always correspond to histological analysis of the specimen. Benefits on locoregional recurrence and survival have to be confirmed.

FURTHER INVESTIGATIONS :

Increase the number of pts to appreciate the efficacity of bleomycin in addition to CDDP and 5FU.

Confirme the decrease of toxicity with continuous infusion of cisplatinum.

Promote home treatment with continuous infusion (Travenol infusor).

© 1985 Elsevier Science Publishers B V. (Biomedical Division)
New dimensions in otorhinolaryngology - head and neck surgery, vol. 2.
E. Myers, editor

INTRA-ARTERIAL CHEMOTHERAPY AND RADIOTHERAPY FOR ADVANCED HEAD AND NECK CANCER: END RESULTS OF 720 CASES.

LUIZ PAULO KOWALSKI, ABRÃO RAPOPORT, JOSIAS DE ANDRADE SOBRINHO, ANTONIO SÉRGIO FAVA, MARCOS BRASILINO DE CARVALHO AND OSWALDO PERES

Head and Neck Service, Heliópolis Hospital, Rua Cônego Xavier 276, São Paulo-SP (Brazil)

INTRODUCTION

The initial treatment of patients with a primary squamous cell carcinoma in the head and neck region has traditionally involved surgery and radiation therapy. Despite advances in surgical technique and improvements in radiotherapy, advanced Stage III and IV unoperable cancer of this area has remained a difficult problem.

Intra-arterial chemotherapy, since its introduction for clinical use, has been proposed as a palliative or adjuvant method in the treatment of patients with advanced head and neck cancer. We will present the end results of 720 cases treated by intra-arterial chemotherapy and radiotherapy.

MATERIAL AND METHODS

From 1971 to 1977, 343 patients were treated at the Head and Neck Service of the A.C. Camargo Hospital-São Paulo-Brazil. Other 377 patients were treated at the Heliópolis Hospital-São Paulo-Brazil from 1978 to 1983.

The majority of patients recieved treatment had histologically proved squamous cell carcinomas (54% of the patients treated until 1977 and 87% of the patients treated since 1978). Ninety three patients of the first group had not a histologically proved recurrent carcinoma and were excluded from the study. The primary tumor sites were: oral cavity, pharynx (mainly the oropharynx) and the maxillary sinus. All patients were advanced Stage III or IV unoperable cancer (226 recurrent tumors after radiotherapy or surgery).

From 1971 to 1977 Methotrexate (0,4mg/kg X 7 days) was used in 30 cases, Triethilenethiophosphoramide (0,4mg/kg X 7 days) was used in 90 patients and a combination of Methotrexate (0,2mg/kg-1st and 3rddays), Bleomycin (7,5mg - 2nd and 4thdays) and Triethilenethiophosphoramide (0,2mg/kg- 5thand 6thdays) in 130 cases. From 1978 to 1983 the schemes were: Bleomycin (15mg/day X 5 days); Methotrexate (10mg/day X 5 days) and Vincristine (1mg -1st and 6thdays); Methotrexate (10mg/day X 5 days), Vincristine (1mg - 1st and 6th days) and Bleomycin(15mg/day X 5 days); Methotrexate (50 mg-1stday), Bleomycin (15 mg/day X 5 days) and Vincristine (1 mg/day -1st and 6th days); Methotrexate, Bleomycin and Vincristine as above plus Cisplatinum (50mg/day at the first day). Other drugs such as Adriamycin and Triethilenethiophosphoramide were used in a few number of patients.

RESULTS

Responses were usually incomplete with remission duration of a few months.More tham fifty per cent of the patients died before one year of follow up. The end results are shown in the following table:

Group	6 mo.	12 mo.	18 mo.	24 mo.	30 mo.	36 mo.
1971-1977	84%	39%	19%	15%	4%	2%
1978-1983	67%	46%	22%	14%	9%	5%

Four hundred and forty two patients treated from 1971 to 1979 were elegible for a 5 year analyses. The best results were seen in previously untreated patients. The five year survival in this group was 10%. Poor results were achieved in patients who had previous radiotherapy or surgery (12% at 1 year and 0% at 5 year).

CONCLUSIONS

1-The frequency of complete remissions after intra-arterial chemotherapy is small and duration brief.

2-Previously untreated patients having squamous cell carcinoma seem to be more sensitive to intra-arterial chemotherapy. A reduced and better oxigenated tumor mass is irradiated more easily and gives a better prognosis.

3-As might be expected, complications are frequent in this type of therapy. Such complications do not imply on enhanced effect against the tumor, on the contrary, a severe toxical effect may prevent the administration of a proper radiation dose.

4-Intra-arterial chemotherapy on the treatment of advanced cancer of the head and neck has been associated to considerable morbidity and limited benefits. Efforts in this area as well as continued programs evaluating new drugs should be encouraged.

© 1985 Elsevier Science Publishers B.V. (Biomedical Division)
New dimensions in otorhinolaryngology - head and neck surgery, vol. 2.
E. Myers, editor

INTERNAL CAROTID ANEURISM OF TRAUMATIC ORIGIN AND OCCURRENCE AS OROPHARNXY TUMOR

J.TRASERRA, A.MORELLO, M.MOLINERO, J.GUEROLA

Servicio de Otorrinolaringología y Servicio de Cirugia Vascular. Hospital Clínico y Provincial. Barcelona. Spain.

Internal Carotid Aneurisms are very rare, only 1% of all peripheral aneurisms (Kaupp,H.A., 1972). The etiology is variable, the most frequent causes being traumatisms and arterioschlerosis, although they can also be of luetic, tuberculous or mycotic origen; or caused by quistic necrosis of the middle layer, radiotherapy, Marfan disease, congenital or some other unkown cause.

The symptomatology consists of tinnitus, hemicrania, vertigo, evolutional dysphagia and in some cases dyspnea. As the aneurism grows, the pain increases and vasculo-cerebral attacks may occur.

The pharingoscopy indicates a protrusion of the lateral wall of the oropharynx as being circumscribed or diffuse according to the type of aneurism. Upon touch this proves to be a soft, beating mass.

We must do the differential diagnosis with all pharynx lateral wall tumorations that are located behind the posterior pillar (Guerrier, Y., 1980): peritonsilar and lateropharinx abscesses, tumors from deep lobes of the parotid gland, neuromas, chemodectomas and tumors originated in the mucous of the pharynx.

In all the tumors of this topography, a vascular exploration should be performed: Retrograde Arteriography, Digital Angiography.

The treatment of these aneurisme is always surgical.

CLINICAL CASE

The case involves a 54 year old male patient who had suffered a knife wound (dagger) in an act of aggression while serving a prison term in a local penitentiary, and who was attended to in this Hospital by one of us. The point of entrance was at the level of the inferior pole of the left parotid gland and showed paresis of the facial nerve, Bernard-Horner syndrome caused by lession of cervical sympathicus, foramen lacerum posterius syndrome with paralysis of soft palate, pharynx, larynx and shoulder which were recuperated, and a left soft palate ecchymosis.

After twelve years had passed, the patient again called for treatment in our Emergency Center, this time complaining of sensing a foreign body, four days' evolution of mild dysphagia and reported to have seen a "lump" on the left side of the pharynx.

Upon examination we found a round tumoration covered with healthy mucous on the left side of the pharynx (Figure 1) which projected the posterior pillar and left tonsil forward and medially. This mass beated upon tactil contact and, when depressing the tongue, its inferior edge could be seen. He also presented residual Bernard-Horner syndrome.

A Digital Angiography was done, observing a voluminous Internal Carotid Aneurism at the level of C2-C3 (Figure 2).

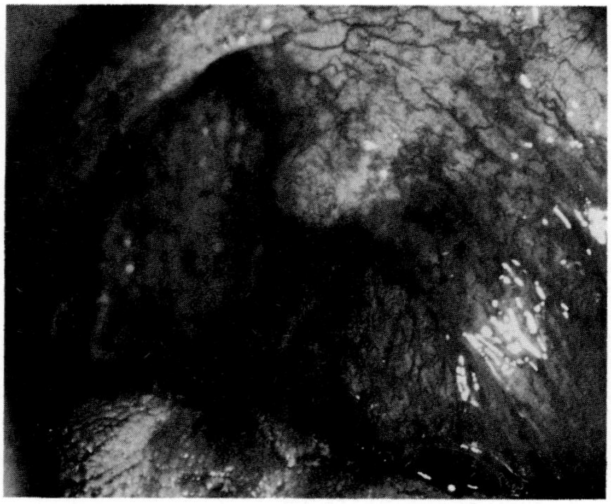

Fig. 1. Oropharynxgoscopy

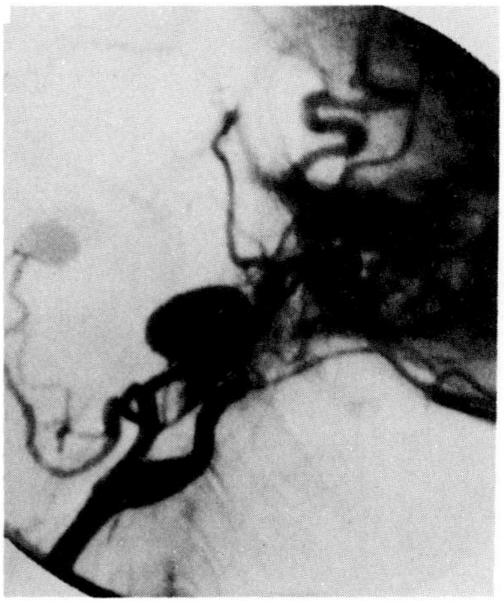

Fig. 2. Digital Angiography

The patient was intervined upon together with the Service of Vascular Surgery, performing the resection of the aneurism with arterial reparation through termino-terminal anastomosis of the Internal Carotid Artery.

Finally, we wish to point out the importance that the diagnosis of these aneurisms has for the E.N.T. specialist and its good surgical prognosis.

REFERENCES

1. Kaupp, H.A. et al.: Aneurisms of the Extracranial Carotid Artery. Surgery. 72: 946. 1972
2. Guerrier, Y.; Portmann, M.: Traité de Technique Chirurgicale O.R.L. et Cervico-Faciale. Tomo 4: 249. Ed. Masson. Paris. 1980

© 1985 Elsevier Science Publishers B.V. (Biomedical Division)
New dimensions in otorhinolaryngology - head and neck surgery, vol. 2.
E. Myers, editor

THREE YEAR SURVIVAL RATES IN ADVANCED HEAD AND NECK CANCER AFTER INDUCTION CHEMOTHERAPY: SIGNIFICANCE OF INITIAL RESPONSE.

W. J. PRIMROSE, C. W. VAUGHAN, W. K. HONG, D. D. KARP, B. WILLETT AND M. S. STRONG.
DEPARTMENTS OF OTOLARYNGOLOGY, MEDICAL ONCOLOGY AND RADIATION THERAPY, BOSTON V.A. MEDICAL CENTER, BOSTON, MASSACHUSETTS 02130

INTRODUCTION

Intense interest in the Head and Neck Oncology literature has been focussed on the initial response to Induction Chemotherapy (IC) in combined modality treatment; few studies however have demonstrated its long term significance.

SUBJECTS AND METHODS

Patients. 100 patients with a variety of Head and Neck cancers (34 oral cavity, 16 oropharynx, 16 larynx, 22 hypopharynx and 12 others) were treated with IC from September 1976 thru December 1981. All were male veterans with ages ranging from 43 to 75 years. Staging and resectability were determined at panendoscopy according to AJC 1977 criteria, and treatment discussed at the inter-disciplinary tumor conference. 2 patients had Stage II (pyriform sinus) tumors, 33 had Stage III and 65 had Stage IV disease.

Selection. Patients with abnormal audiograms, renal and pulmonary function, Karnofsky performance status of <50% and previous treatment were not considered as candidates for IC .

Regimens. 21 patients received a 7 day continuous infusion of Bleomycin and 79 received high dose Cisplatin (100 mg/m^2 or more) followed by Bleomycin in one or more cycles.

Assessment. Response was assessed within 2 weeks of completing IC in 98 patients. A complete response (CR) was defined as clinically complete tumor regression, a partial response (PR) as >50% tumor regression and a minimal response (MR) as <50% regression, stable or progressive disease.

Surgery was performed on 53 patients after IC , depending on resectability and operability, and followed by Radiation Therapy (XRT).

Radiation Therapy alone was administered to 41 patients, following which all patients were re-assessed and followed monthly.

Pathology specimens were examined and correlated with initial stage, treatment response and survival.

RESULTS:

Of the 98 patients assessed after IC , 15 achieved a CR , 48 achieved a PR and 35 achieved an MR . 4 patients received no further treatment, 1 PR , 1 MR and 2

CR's (who refused and ultimately died).

There were 39 patients alive at 3 years from commencement of treatment of whom 30 were clinically disease free. Complete responders have significantly better disease free survival over both partial and minimal responders (p=.02). When patients receiving surgery and XRT are compared to those receiving XRT alone after IC (Table I), there is a significantly better overall disease free survival in the operated group (p=.03). However, patients achieving a CR fare as well or better with XRT alone.

Histological examination of the resection specimens obtained from the 6 CR patients progressing to surgery revealed persistant tumor cells in 4 of the primary sites and 2 of the node dissections.

TABLE I

DISEASE FREE SURVIVAL AT 3 YEARS AND INITIAL RESPONSE TO CHEMOTHERAPY.

Note that only patients completing treatment are compared.

Response	All	Surgery and XRT	XRT Alone
CR	8/13 (62%)	3/6 (50%)	5/7 (71%)
PR	14/47 (30%)	12/29 (41%)	2/18 (11%)
MR	8/34 (24%)	7/18 (39%)	1/16 (6%)
Total	30/94 (32%)	22/53 (42%)	8/41 (20%)

CONCLUSIONS

1. Achieving a CR heralds a significantly enhanced 3 year disease free survival.
2. XRT alone following a CR may be adequate treatment.
3. If a lesser response than a CR is achieved survival is significantly improved by surgery.
4. No significant difference (p=.28) in survival was noted between PR and MR patients, which should make us reconsider the favorable concept of a "major" response (CR + PR).
5. Chemotherapy regimes which improve the number of CR's (up to 54% reported)[1] theoretically should improve 3 year survival and spare some mandibles and larynges.
6. Survival and histologic evidence indicates that despite a CR the tumor is still viable; conventional treatment must follow and if surgery is employed there should be no compromise on resection margins. Similarily if XRT is employed there should be no reduction in field size or dose.

REFERENCES

1. Kish JA, Ensley J, Weaver A, Jacobs JR, Kinzie J, Cummings G, Al-Sarraf M. (1984) Improvement of Complete Response Rate to Induction Adjuvant Chemotherapy for Advanced Squamous Carcinoma of the Head and Neck. Adjuvant Therapy of Cancer IV. Grune and Stratton, pp 107-115

© 1985 Elsevier Science Publishers B.V. (Biomedical Division)
New dimensions in otorhinolaryngology - head and neck surgery, vol. 2.
E. Myers, editor

APPLICATION OF CO_2 LASER IN ORAL AND NASOPHARYNGEAL SURGERY

DANILO RADONJIĆ
Military Medical Academy,ENT Clinic, 11000 Belgrade,Yugoslavia

Classic surgery in the nasopharynx and oral cavity,due to the specificity of these organs and their anatomical relationship, is most often mutilant and hardly approachable for a surgical scalpel,because of which most often very radical and extensive reconstructive surgery are to be performed.Special problems present vascular tumors due to possible abundant bleeding during and after the operation.In all these surgical procedures the postoperative course and care of patients are long lasting and require a special attention.Secondary infections and postoperative bleeding are also very frequent.

Laser surgery in pathology of these regions created new possibilities in successful and faster solving of this complex problem (1,2,3).

At the ENT Clinic of the Military Medical Academy using CO_2 laser the total of 642 patients have been treated with 712 laser interventions performed within the priod 1978-1984.Of this number 41 patient had different pathologic conditions in the nasopharynx and the oral cavity and they are presented in the following table:

Disease	Laser intervention I	II	Total	Postoperative radiotherapy
Choanal atresia	7	2	9	
Hemangioma epipharyngis	5	-	5	
Papilloma oris	6	-	6	
Leucoplakia oris	1	-	1	
Ca linguae	9	2	11	2
Ca arcus alveolaris	5	2	7	4
Ca baseos oris	4	1	5	2
Ca uvulae	1	-	1	
Ca labii inferior	1	-	1	
Ca nasi	2	-	2	
Total:	41	7	48	8

From these regions CO_2 laser was first successfully used by us in choanal atresia by author's original method of epipharyngomicroscopy with the operative microscope and a special epipharyngeal mirror of own construction (4,5).The obtained results were good ,fast and effective without tendency of scar formation and postoperative use of dilatators for maintaining of the lumen.Practically,patients can leave the hospital almost immediately after going out from general anesthesia.

The same method was also used in the treatment of hemangiomas of the nasopharynx and tumors of the oral cavity.In carcinomas of the oral cavity the laser was used in T_1 and T_2.In general,superficial carcinomas were treated by the laser only,while those with deeper infiltrations were treated both by laser and radiotherapy (6).

In tumors of this region of a particular importance is the use of a special epipharyngeal mirror for work in such narrow anatomic regions, so that the laser beam can be directed to the desired area without scaterring of the beam: nasopharynx, the base and posterior parts of the tongue, posterior parts of the soft palate,parts of the alveolar arches, etc.

Our experience and the obtained results in the use of laser surgery in tumors of these regions are encouraging showing laser efficacy in the treatment of this complex problem.All our patients we regularly examined,but critical period of time is still short to state final conclusion.Up to now the only positively sure fact is that the results will be not worse than the classic ones.However, it should be kept in mind that laser in the treatment of malignant tumors,of this region too,is only a new instrument used in solving this problem.Namely,laser surgery in the combination with radio and chemotherapy has broaden possibilities in successful treatment of malignant diseases.

Simplicity,good tolerance,aseptic conditions,rapid recovery of patients are some of advantages of laser over classical surgery in this region.Also,financial effects reffered to shortened hospitalization can not be neglected.It should be particularly emphasized that laser treatment of malignomas of this region enables avoidance of severe and mutilant classic operations which do not provide better results in regard to the final outcome of the treatment.

REFERENCES:

1. Strong M.S.et al : (1979) The Laryngoscope,89,897-905.
2. Healy G.B. et al: (1978) Ann.Otol., 87, 658-662.
3. Mitrović M.et al: (1979) Vojnosanit.Pregled, 36:6,447-450.
4. Radonjić D., et al: (1981) Optoelectronics in Medicine,Laser 81-München,105-107.
5. Radonjić D.,(1984) In: Laser in Medicine,ed SNL Zagreb, 57-59.
6. Radonjić D.,Mitrović M.(1984) In: Laser in Medicine,ed.SNL Zagreb,51-56.

New dimensions in otorhinolaryngology - head and neck surgery, vol. 2.
E. Myers, editor

HIGH FREQUENCY JET VENTILATION DURING LASER MICROLARYNGOSCOPY

L. Signore, M. de Vincentiis, G. Ruoppolo and C. Ungari

ENT Department of the University "La Sapienza" of Rome, ITALY

Although methods for the use of lasers in laryngeal microsurgery have now been sufficiently researched, fewer studies have been made on anaesthesia techniques suitable to the requirements of this new kind of surgery technique.

As is well known during conventional microsurgery, correct ventilation of the patient should not interfere with the needs of the operating surgeon, nor block his view of the operation site. With this in mind, several studies have been made of respiratory equipment capable of functioning with small tracheal catheters, which cause minimum obstruction. In addition to the problems mentioned above, the introduction of lasers has created the need to use endotracheal instruments capapble of resisting the photo-energy released by the laser beam.

Several solutions to this problem have been presented in scientific journals, such as the use of glass orotracheal cannulae, metal tubes, silicone catheters, rubber cannulae covered with muslin, and traditional rubber tubes protected by self adhesive aluminium tape. The last technique appears to most physicians to be the best solution available at the moment. However, the disadvantage of this technique is that it obstructs the view of the operating area, with related complications.

Studies related to the use of H.F.V. in laryngeal microsurgery with lasers owe their origin to the necessity of finding alternative techniques which are more valid than those mentioned so far.

In the last two years (1983-84) at our ENT Department 63 unchosen patients underwent direct therapeutic laryngoscopy by means of CO_2 laser. After the laryngoscopy has been placed in suspensio, the orotracheal tube previously positioned immediately after induction is removed and substituted by the gas mixture injector which is introduced into the patient at high frequency. The injector is positioned according to the guide normally preset for optic fibres, in a location opposite to the operating area. During each operation, the surgeon protects the tracheal mucouse membrane by placing a moistened gauze pad, tied to a recovery thread, next and beneath the operating site, in order to prevent lesions caused by the laser beam.

We have never experienced incidents such as burns on the mucouse membrane, or explosions or combustion of the gas mixture. Certain physicians in circumstances similar to our own, have complained of certain inconveniences, such as vibrations transmitted to the patient's head from the high frequencies produced by the mechanized insufflation process, and the possibility of blood being thrown onto the lens of the microscope. These factors caused no significant problems during our experiments. In fact, any such disadvantages can be minimized by correct suspension of the patient's head; also by the fact that laser surgery involves very little bleeding. As far as the surgeon's field of vision is concerned, results have always proved excellent, obviously owing to the small calibre of the injector. In addition, the possibilities of locating the injector in the anterior commisural position allows the surgeon to operate at the level of the posterior commisure, unlike the usual procedure when conventional catheters are used.

© 1985 Elsevier Science Publishers B V. (Biomedical Division)
New dimensions in otorhinolaryngology - head and neck surgery, vol. 2.
E. Myers, editor

LIP RECONSTRUCTION AFTER MALIGNANT TUMOR SURGERY: METHODS AND RESULTS.

RHEIMS D.M., MEYER R.

Dept. of Otolaryngology, CHUV (Prof.M.SAVARY) Lausanne, Switzerland
Centre de Chirurgie Plastique, Lausanne, Switzerland

INTRODUCTION

The surgical treatment of labial carcinoma must allow the complete excision of the tumor. This must be performed by using an immediate reconstruction procedure without compromising either the lip function or the aesthetic result.

This article presents Rodolphe Meyer's lip reconstruction methods and evaluates the results by a retrospective analysis. These results are based on functional and aesthetic tests.

MATERIAL

From 1973 to 1984 we have operated on 46 patients with lip cancers (87% male, 13% female). The majority of the patients (55%) were between 65 and 85 years of age. There were squamous cell carcinomas in 91% of the cases and basal cell carcinomas in the remaining 9% of cases.

The site of the lesion was the lower lip (80%), the upper lip (18%) and the oral commissure (2%).

METHOD

Partial lip reconstruction (Defect up to 3/4 of the lip)

The Meyer's advancement flap (1964), (3), derived from the methods of Bernard (1) and Ginestet (2), was used, at first, for the lower lip reconstruction.

After performing a wide transfixing cuneiform excision of the lip tumor, the incision is extended on both sides in the labio-chin folds. At the distal points it ends by using a Burow triangle which permits the inferior sliding of the cheek flap on either side.

To permit its superior sliding, we excise two cutaneous Burow triangles along the upper lip vermilion. The base of one of these triangles can achieve a third of the lip length. The superior lip mucosa is undermined so as to release the orbucularis oris muscle. This will be preserved and carefully pushed backward. The new commissure then will take place at the external angle of the excised triangle. (Fig.1 + 2)

The mucosal flap to cover the raw border of the cheek flap, is raised anterior and inferior to Stenson's duct. This mucosal flap is advanced and everted on the cheek flap in order to create the new vermilion border. The advancement also avoids scar retraction (Fig.3). By advancing the cheek flaps, median closure is possible.

Besides the reconstruction of the lower lip and commissure this method can also be used for the reconstruction of the upper lip by reversing the procedure.(5)

Total lip reconstruction.

In these cases we can choose between two methods.

First, if we use the Meyer's advancement flap technique (6), we have to combine it with a reverse Abbe-Estlander flap. This is performed in a two stage procedure to avoid microstomia due to strong tension on the suture line.

Second, Meyer (1980) proposes a one stage procedure utilizing KARAPANDZIC's idea (4) of a local arterial flap.

When reconstructing all of the lower lip, we use two muco-myocutaneous island flaps (7). They are released from each naso-labial region and contain a part of the zygomatic major, the risorius, and the triangularis muscles with their vascular pedicles (Fig.5 + 6). In order to reconstruct the lip, these two flaps are pulled into the defect through a subcutaneous tunnel and sutured one upon the other (Fig.7). The new vermilion border is created by suturing the mucosa to the skin of the upper flap (Fig.8).

RESULTS.

In 6 cases of small excision, a simple closure was all that was necessary.

In 39 cases we used the Meyer's advancement flap technique. In 1 case we used the bilateral muco-myo-cutaneous island flaps.

The results were evaluated by looking at salivary continence, labial mobility, phonation, and the aesthetic appearance.

According to these criteria, we obtained 34 immediate good results(Fig.4). 3 cases demonstrated transitory salivary incontinence all of which spontaneously resolved in less than 8 months. In the one case, using the island flaps, there was moderate salivary incontinence; this was resolved by performing a secondary Z-plasty. 2 cases had a commissural scar string which needed a revision with a final good result. In our series we have no microstomia.

CONCLUSION

The Meyer's lip reconstruction method has been used at the University Clinic of Otolaryngology of Lausanne because of its advantages. First, there is the adaptability to many reconstruction problems wherever the localisation and extension of the tumor. Second, there is the immediate possibility of reconstruction, usually in one stage. Third, there is the good functional result because of the integrity of the orbicularis oris muscle. Finally, there is the acceptable aesthetic result because of the incision chosen.

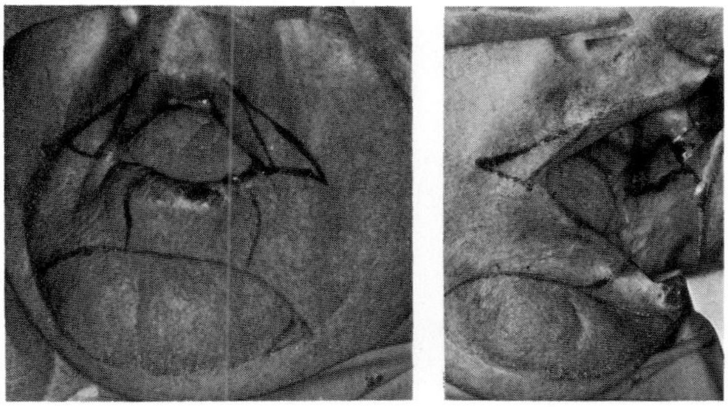

Fig.1+2 Advancement flap outlined

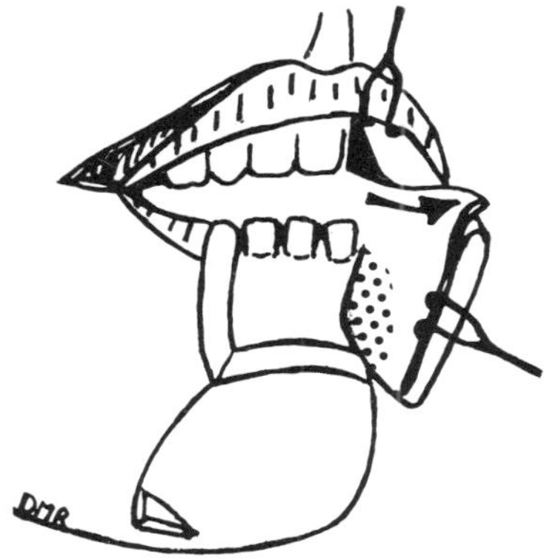

Fig.3: Eversion of mucosal flap

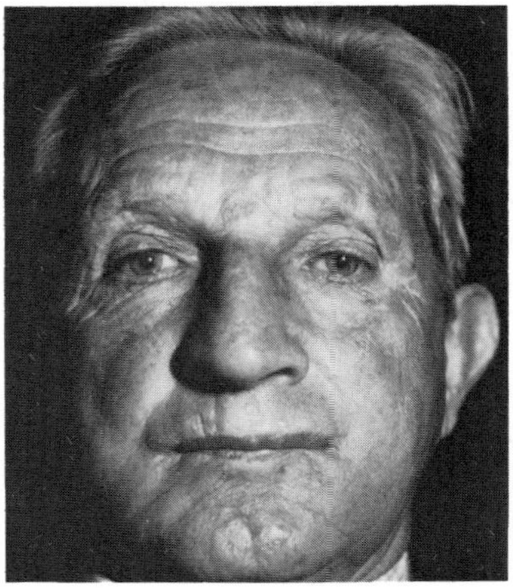

Fig.4: Late result

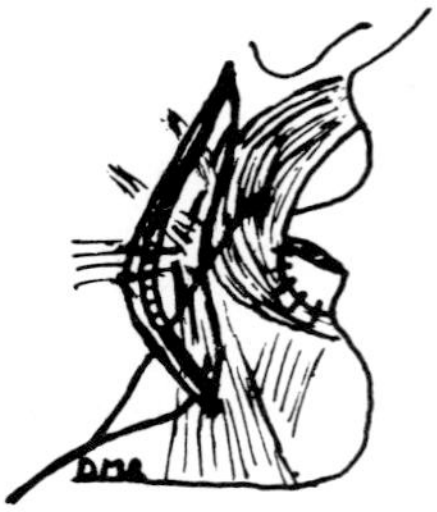

Fig.5:MEYER's muco-myocutan.island flap

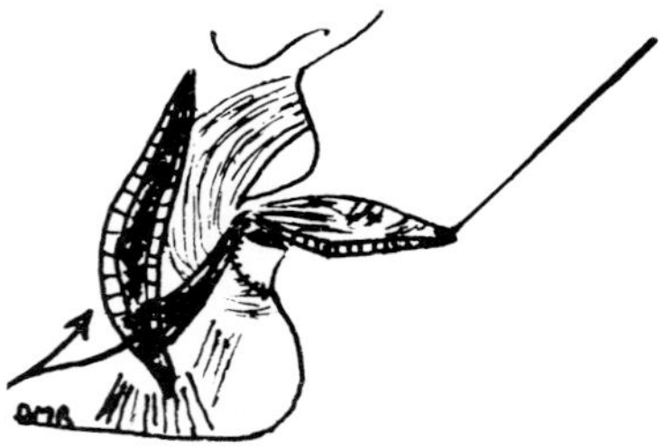

Fig.6:Transfer of the flap

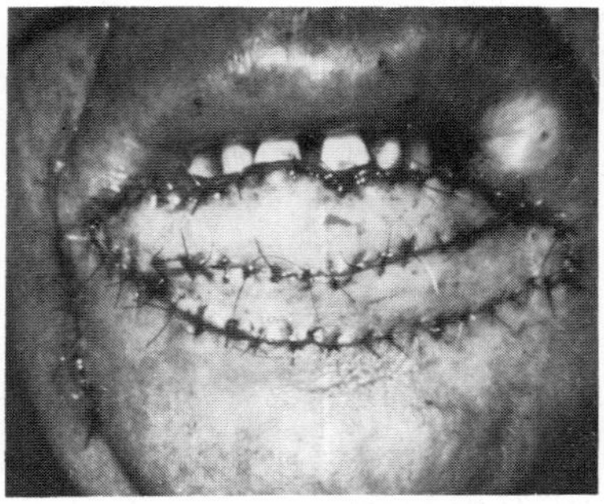

Fig.7: End of the operation

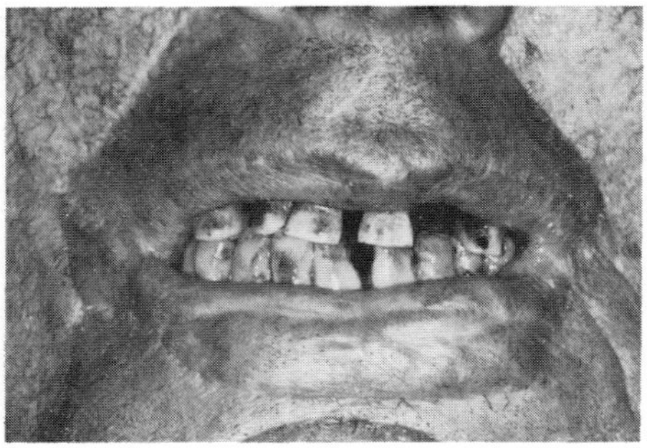

Fig.8: Late result

REFERENCES

1. BERNARD C., Cancer de la lèvre inférieure, opéré par un procédé nouveau. Bulletin M.Soc.Chir. (Paris) 3, 357, 1853.

2. GINESTET G., Reconstruction de toute la lèvre inférieure par les lambeaux nasogeniens totaux - Rev.Odont.Stomat. (Paris) 8, 28, 1946

3. HERTIG P., Une nouvelle technique de reconstruction plastique de la lèvre inférieure. Pract. Otorhinolaryngo. (Basel) 27, 157, 1965.

4. KARAPANDZIC M., Reconstruction of lip defects by local arterial flaps. British Journal of Plastic Surgery, 27, 93-97, 1974.

5. MEYER R., SHAPIRO, D.D., A technique for immediate reconstruction of the lower lip after ablation of tumor. Chir.plast.2,1-16,1973.

6. MEYER R., POGET M., Modification d'une technique de reconstruction après résection totale de la lèvre inférieure. Karger, Basel, ORL, 1,127, 1976.

7. MEYER R, FAILAT A., New concepts in lower lip reconstruction. Head and Neck Surgery, 4, 240-245, 1982.

© 1985 Elsevier Science Publishers B.V. (Biomedical Division)
New dimensions in otorhinolaryngology - head and neck surgery, vol. 2.
E. Myers, editor

COMPARATIVE MEASURES OF VOCAL FUNCTION IN 30 SPEAKERS WITH VOICE DISORDERS

D. M. BLESS, C. F. FORD, H. A. LEEPER, J. H. BRANDENBURG, AND T. W. FRANK
Departments of Otolaryngology and Communicative Disorders
University of Wisconsin-Madison, Madison, Wisconsin, USA

The purpose of the present study was to compare auditory perceptual judgments to visual perceptual judgments based on videostroboscopy, and select acoustic and aerodynamic measurements in three groups of speakers with voice disorders in order to determine if the measures resulted in clinically useful information regarding laryngeal dysfunction.

MATERIALS AND METHODS

Subjects

Thirty adult volunteers with vocal pathologies served as subjects for this study. All subjects included had documented laryngeal abnormalities resulting from vocal nodules, recurrent laryngeal nerve paralysis, or superior and recurrent laryngeal nerve involvement secondary to closed head injury.

Assessment Procedures

The Nagashima PS77 Phonatory Function Analyzer was used to make simultaneous recordings of air flow, air volume, frequency, and intensity during production of several phonatory tasks. Test protocol included conversational speech, reading, maximum phonation time, sustained production of vowels /a/ /i/ and /u/, and total pitch and loudness range of productions. Perceptual judgments were made by two listeners who rated overall severity of the vocal dysfunction using a seven-point scale to assess dimensions of breathy, rough, and strained vocal qualities. Videostroboscopic recordings of laryngeal movements during the sustained production of the vowel /i/ produced during various pitch and loudness maneuvers were viewed for judgments of periodicity, symmetry, glottal closure, hyperfunction of supraglottal structures, amplitude of vibration, and presence of mucosal wave. Examinations were repeated for selected subjects following treatment.

RESULTS AND DISCUSSION

This preliminary study did not support the contention that perceptual judgments of vocal quality are the best measures of vocal function. The perceptual measures used were not sufficiently discrete to detect small changes resulting from treatment. In contrast some of the aerodynamic and acoustic measures provided indices of small changes resulting from therapy, and in some cases even discriminated between pathologies, but only by inference could one interpret what was happening at the level of the laryngeal valve. And like the perceptual judgments any single measure used alone was of questionable significance in interpretion of vocal function. Videostroboscopic images provided information on the specific laryngeal movement pattern exhibited by individual subjects. Since the image was of the vocal folds, movement of the folds, glottal opening, and hyperfunction of the supraglottal structures could be easily visualized in most subjects. Consequently fewer inferences had to be made, and inferences made generally were restricted to the interaction of the respiratory system with the observed vibratory patterns, the effect of the extended tongue and neck flection on sound production, the neurological control, and how typical the observed patterns were of conversational speech. Limitations of this technique were interpreted to provide additional support for the notion of multidimensional testing. Although we were unable to identify a single "best measure of vocal function" the multidimensional testing reported here yielded unique profiles for each subject against which repeated measurements could assess any possible effects from treatment. Because individuals within a specific diagnostic category did not present a homogeneous profile, and because most patients do not have voice testing done prior to the onset of a pathology it is concluded that multiparameter studies are desirable in the evaluation of disordered voice production.

ACKNOWLEDGEMENTS

We gratefully acknowledge the data reduction efforts of Herbert Moore and Maureen Luis in this project.

© 1985 Elsevier Science Publishers B.V. (Biomedical Division)
New dimensions in otorhinolaryngolcgy - head and neck surgery, vol. 2.
E. Myers, editor

MEDICAL PROFILE OF THE LANGUAGE-DELAYED CHILD: OTITIS PRONE VS. OTITIS FREE

PATRICK E. BROOKHOUSER and DAVID E. GOLDGAR

Boys Town National Institute for Communication Disorders in Children,
555 North 30th Street, Omaha, Nebraska 68131 (U.S.A.)

Delay in language development may be associated with an underlying anatomical, neurosensory, or psychological disorder such as: deafness, cerebral palsy, cleft palate, autism, or mental retardation. A condition called specific developmental language delay may occur in children devoid of any other identifiable disorder or developmental delay. Language delay associated with early onset, severe-to-profound hearing impairment has been well documented. Controversial studies have also appeared in the communicative disorders' literature suggesting that fluctuating conductive hearing loss in early childhood can significantly affect the development of language and related academic skills. Some authors have claimed that these deleterious effects can be irreversible.

This study focuses on three groups of preschool children, in whom hearing acuity has been documented: One group with recurrent otitis and language delay; a second group with an equally well documented otitis history but without language delay; and a third group with documented language delay in the absence of any known predisposing conditions, including early-onset, recurrent otitis media. Prenatal, birth and developmental histories of the children in each group were compared in detail to identify any factors which may enhance or ameliorate the effects of fluctuating conductive hearing loss on language development.

In a population of 1,864 children (ages 9-59 months) referred for otolaryngologic and/or communicative evaluation, 480 otherwise normal children (67.6% males; 32.4% females) were found to have a history of early-onset, recurrent otitis media and/or delayed speech and language development on the basis of an extensive evaluation battery. This population was further subdivided into three groups (I = otitis positive/normal language; II = otitis positive/language delay; and III = otitis free/language delay (SDLD).

GROUP	NUMBER	EARLY-ONSET OTITIS	LANGUAGE DELAY
I	114	Yes	No
II	215	Yes	Yes
III	151	No	Yes

Among the 328 children with positive histories for early otitis media (Groups I and II), a significantly higher percentage of those demonstrating language delay were from homes in the lower socioeconomic category. Race and sex showed no significant relationship to language delay among the otitis positive groups, although males were twice as numerous as females in the overall study population. Articulation errors on speech measures and borderline delays in other developmental milestones (standing, walking and toilet training) were also significantly greater in the language delayed group when compared with otitis positive children whose language was age appropriate. Mild dysequilibrium associated with recurrent bouts of otitis media may help to explain an inordinate percentage of walking delay among children with persistent, mostly bilateral middle ear disease.

Persistent borderline conductive hearing loss (15-25dB PTA in the better hearing ear) was associated with significantly depressed performance on speech/language measures. Preliminary longitudinal data suggests that correction of these conductive losses in otherwise normal children will permit language skills to reach age appropriate levels after a relatively short interval in most cases. This finding reiterates the need for prompt and continuous medical/surgical management of children with early-onset, recurrent otitis media. The otitis positive children showed greater improvement in expressive language performance following correction of their conductive losses than did the SDLD group over the same time interval. No objective factors, apart from quantitative differences in speech/language performance, served to identify the SDLD children in the study population. Future studies aimed at assessing the relationship of early-onset, recurrent otitis media to delayed language development must include not only "normal" controls but also a matched control group of children with SDLD who are followed longitudinally.

REFERENCES

Brookhouser, PE, Hixson, PK, Matkin, ND (1979): Early childhood language delay: The Otolaryngologist's Perspective, The Laryngoscope, LXXXIX, 12:1898-1913.

New dimensions in otorhinolaryngology - head and neck surgery, vol. 2.
E. Myers, editor

ANALYSIS OF PRIMARY VERSUS DELAYED TRACHEOESOPHAGEAL PUNCTURE

RR CASIANO, AJ MANIGLIA, AND DS LUNDY

Department of Otolaryngology, University of Miami School of Medicine, Miami, Florida, U.S.A.

INTRODUCTION

Singer and Blom first described their technique for delayed tracheoesophageal puncture (T.E.P.) in 1980 (1). In 1982, Maniglia reported his experience with primary T.E.P. concomitant with total laryngectomy; the main advantage being the avoidance of a second separate surgical procedure and utilizing the stent catheter to provide gastric feedings postoperatively (2). This study attempts to analyze our experience with delayed versus primary T.E.P. with regard to possible short and long-term complications and speech results.

MATERIALS AND METHODS

From 1980 to 1984, 19 patients were selected for primary voice restoration and 28 underwent T.E.P. as a second separate procedure. Patients were divided into two groups: Group A (Primary T.E.P.) and Group B (Delayed T.E.P.). All patients were equally suitable for one or the other procedure.

Charts were reviewed for the usual demographic and medical data. Original cancers were staged according to the American Joint Committee on Cancer guidelines. Postoperative laryngectomy complications within 30 days and any complications after delayed T.E.P. were also noted. Speech prosthesis insertion date was recorded.

Speech parameters were measured by the same full time speech pathologist. The onset of the patient's first phonation after prosthesis insertion and the number of weeks required to achieve best intelligibility was noted. Speech intelligibility was then graded on the following scale: 1 (failure), 2 (poor), 3 (fair), 4 (good), 5 (excellent). Success was defined as fluent, functional and independent tracheoesophageal speech which the patient continued to use for at least three months.

RESULTS

Both groups were comparable for demographic data and average hospitalization. Other than stomal stenosis and improper T.E.P. placement, no significant complication occurred after T.E.P. alone in group B. Table I shows the higher number of unplanned pharyngocutaneous fistula and abscess formation in Group A. All resolved with local wound care and did not affect eventual speech outcome. Preoperative and postoperative radiation or chemotherapy, stage of disease and nutrional status did not influence the higher incidence of fistuli and abscesses.

TABLE I

	GROUP A	GROUP B
PHARYNGOCUTANEOUS FISTULI AND ABSCESSES	41%	22%
PERISTOMAL LOCATION	42%	17%
PREOPERATIVE RADIATION OR CHEMOTHERAPY	14%	50%
STAGE III	71%	83%
STAGE II	19%	17%

TABLE II shows the ease and rapidity that patients developed speech.

TABLE II

	GROUP A	GROUP B
PROSTHESIS INSERTION AFTER SURGERY (days)	14	4
ONSET OF PHONATION (within 1 session)	94%	50%
BEST RATING (4 & 5)	78%	57%
ACHIEVED BEST RATING WITHIN 2 WEEKS	78%	31%
OVERALL SUCCESS RATE	84%	61%

CONCLUSION

The data seems to show a higher complication rate in the primary T.E.P. group. However, the ease and rapidity with which patients can be fitted with a prosthesis and develop intelligible speech may justify the added risk of combining T.E.P. with laryngectomy in selected cases. Nevertheless, further refinements in technique and/or patient selection may be advisable to minimize possibly increased complications related to primary placement of T.E.P.

REFERENCES

1. Singer MI, Blom ED (1980) An Endoscopic Technique for Restoration of Voice after Laryngectomy. ANN Otol; 89: 529-533

2. Maniglia AJ (1982) Vocal Rehabilitation after Total Laryngectomy: A Flexible Fibeoptic Endoscopic Technique for Tracheoesophageal Fistula. Laryngoscope: 92:12, 1437-1439

New dimensions in otorhinolaryngology - head and neck surgery, vol. 2.
E. Myers, editor

THE GRONINGEN BUTTON RESULTS

H.F. MAHIEU and A.A. ANNYAS

E.N.T. Department, University Hospital, P.O. Box 30.001, 9700 RB Groningen (The Netherlands)

INTRODUCTION

Since 1980 more than 100 patients received a Groningen button post-laryngectomy voice prosthesis in the ENT department of the Groningen University Hospital.

The Groningen button is a silicone valve voice prosthesis which is placed in a tracheo-esophageal fistula. Maintenance is not requiered and the prosthesis can easily be changed after several months when neccesary.

PATIENTS

We studied 86 patients who had a follow-up period varying from 6 months to almost 5 years.

In 67 patients the prosthesis was placed as a primary procedure during total laryngectomy. Placement as a secondary procedure was performed in 19 patients, varying from several weeks up to 10 years after total laryngectomy. About one third of our patients decided to have the prosthesis removed, mostly after about a year, when they had mastered a good injection esophageal speech. Almost all of the patients, including those who had the button removed, claim that the button method of speech was louder, more fluent and better intelligible than the injection method.

RESULTS

Voice production

Voice production during the first day of the speech rehabilitation program was achieved in 85% of the patients when the button method was used and less than 20% when the injection method of esophageal speech was used. All patients were taught to use both methods.

Speech proficiency

The speech proficiency was determined using:

1. the judgement of trained speech pathologists
2. maximal vocal intensity
3. speech penetrating capacity measurements
4. Long Term Average Spectral analysis.

More then 80% of the patients using the button method were judged as being good or moderate speakers, who were able to perform all normal communicational activities, including using a telephone and making conversation in a noisy environment.

More than half of the patients using the button method had maximal vocal intensities and speech penetrating capacities which were within the range of normal laryngeal speakers. Whereas only a few patients using the injection method were within the normal range.

The supremacy of the button method over the injection method of esophageal speech can also be seen in the Long-Term-Average-Spectral (L.T.A.S.) analysis of running speech. The spectrograms of the button method much more resemble normal laryngeal speech than the injection method.

Patient satisfaction

Satisfaction of patients is an important factor, often forgotten. In the first few years 35% of our patients was not satisfied, mostly due to poor patient selection for secondary procedures and problems with persisting fistula after button removal. Since we solved these problems by performing preoperative insufflation tests under X-ray examination before secondary procedures and by developing a dermal graft technique for fistula closure, only 3 % of our patients report that they are not satisfied with the prosthesis.

Device life-time

The mean device lifetime is slightly more than 3 months with a range varying from several weeks to 2½ years.

Complications

Complications were few and insignificant. Infection of the tracheo esophageal fistula was observed in 6 patients. Staph. aureus was the prime cause. All patients were succesfully treated with antibiotics

CONCLUSIONS

It is our considered opinion that patients will benefit more from a voice prosthesis if:

- the prosthesis is placed during or shortly after total laryngectomy.
- the indication for a secondary procedure is based on proper pre-operative examination of the pharyngo-esophageal segment.
- a myotomy of the pharyngo-esophageal segment is performed to prevent hypertonicity of the pseudoglottis.
- after removal of the prosthesis, a persisting fistula will be treated effectively.
- treatment is performed by an experienced medical team including a speech pathologist.

New dimensions in otorhinolaryngology - head and neck surgery, vol. 2.
E. Myers, editor

ANALYSIS OF TONGUE DYNAMICS USING THE ULTRASONIC METHOD

SEIJI NIIMI, SHIGERU KIRITANI, HAJIME HIROSE AND ZYN'ICI SIMADA
Research Institute of Logopedics and Phoniatrics, Fucalty of Medicine, University of Tokyo, Hongo, Bunkyo-ku, Tokyo, Japan

INTRODUCTION

Observation of the configuration and dynamics of the tongue during speech is one of the major interests in speech science and speech pathology. Several studies have been conducted on this subject. Methodologically, most of these studies have utilized X-ray techniques. Although these studies have provided data on tongue configuration and dynamics, they have serious limitaions. One of the disadvantages of the X-ray techniques is the fact that excessive X-ray exposure produces unfavorable biological side effects.

In this study, we have utilized ultrasonic technique to avoid biological side effects.

METHOD

In order to visualize tongue configuration and dynamics, an ultrasonic cardiogram system was used. The system was installed with a probe which could emit 3.5MHz ultrasonic pulse train and scan electronically in sector shape. The display modes of the system were B-mode and M-mode. The probe was held against the subject's submandibular skin. The tongue configuration and its dynamic patterns were analysed by using a VTR system and a mini-computer. A normal male and two dysarthric patients served as subjects of this study.

In order to get the indication of the vocal tract shape, the palatal configuration gotten by the prosthesis of the palate was superimposed onto the ultrasonic image of the tongue by aid of image memory and mini-computer.

RESULTS

Ultrasonic images of the tongue during five Japanese vowels production were agreeable with the prevous observation of the ordinary X-ray technique.

The movement patterns taken by the M-mode display were corresponding well to some parameters of the acoustic signals.

By observing the tongue movement during bilabial stop consonants, it can be concluded that the tongue gesture was not influenced by the articulatory movements of the lips and the tongue started to articulate following vowel during this closure period.

Up and down movement of the tongue were analysed on the dysarthric patients as well as a normal speaker. Comparing the normal subject, ataxic patient (spino-cerebellar degeneration) showed arrythmic repetition of the syllables and the excursion of the tongue movement were irregular. For a amyotrophic lateral sclerosis case, speed of the tongue movement was slow and the excursion was small. In either case, the alternative maovements of different parts of the tongue were maintained as well as the normal case. These findings were compatible with their speech output.

DISCUSSION

Ultrasonic technique provide compatible data with the ordinary X-ray technique without any unfavorable side effects. Since the ultrasonic beam was radiated from beneath the mandible, the palatal configuration could not be visualized. When we want to correspond movement of the tongue and acoustic output, it is desirable to know the vocal tract shape or at least palatal shape. For this purpose, we have used the palatal prosthesis and a VTR image processing system to get the numerical data of the position of the probe by aid of the mini-computer. Using the numerical data gotten from this system, we could visualize and analyse the tongue shape and its dynamics with satisifactory consistency.

© 1985 Elsevier Science Publishers B.V. (Biomedical Division)
New dimensions in otorhinolaryngology - head and neck surgery, vol. 2.
E. Myers, editor

T-CELLS LYMPHOPROLIFERATIVE DISORDERS IN THE PATHOGENESIS OF MIDLINE GRANULOMA AND WEGENER's GRANULOMATOSIS

V.RICCI and V.COLLETTI

Department of Otolaryngology, University of Verona, Italy.

The present study deals with 3 patients (two men and one women, aged 36, 41 and 23 years respectively) suffering from ulcerative-necrotizing granulomatous lesions in the nose associated with elevated ESR and fever.

Symptoms and midface lesions temporarily improved after the immunosoppressive treatment. As the clinical features included also the development of granulomatous conditions affecting kidney, liver and lung, a Wegener's granulomatosis was diagnosed.

Worsening of the disease process led to death in one patient 6 to 11 month from onset.

The histopathological investigation demonstrated widespread dense infiltration of the tissues by lymphoid cells of different size: the smaller ones showed scarce cytoplasm and irregular and hyperchromic nucleus devoid of nucleoli;the larger ones showed more abundant cytoplasm and small and sometimes multiple nucleoli.

Vascular walls were infiltrated by these lymphoid cells.

The immuno-cyto-chemical investigation of midface specimen showed helper and suppressore T-lymphocites proliferation (see Table). This different functional pattern is a new and important feature.

Despite various clinical aspects, T-cell lymphoproliferative disorders show similar hystopathogenetical characteristics to reticulosis polimorpha and to reticulosis polimorpha and to lymphogranulomatosis. These are: diffuse cells proliferation, polimorphous lymphoid population due to their size and unusual cellular shape, vascular coats infiltration with ischemic necrosis, presence of reacting cells like plasmacells, macrophages, granulocytes, and skin involvement (Collins et al.,1979).

All these features are also present in Wegener's granulomatosis and in granuloma gangrenescens.(Liebow et al., 1981)

The T-cell different functional pattern, characterizing these lymphoproliferative disorders, shold be confirmed and evaluated. (Table 1)

TABLE I

CYTO-IMMUNO-CHEMICAL INVESTIGATION

Specimen: nasal mucosa

CP = proliferative cells

AcP	CP: negative. Presence of several macrofages
ATPase	Presence of several positive elements
DAP IV	CP: prevalently positive
OKT 3	CP: positive (pan-T)
OKT 4	CP: partially positive (helper)
OKT 8	CO partially positive (suppressor)

Conclusions: presence of several cells with cyto-chemical and cyto-immunolo gical properties of functionally heterogeneous T-cells.

Legend: AcP = Acid phosphatase (specific of mácrofages)
ATP = Adenosintriphosphatase (in T-cells)
DAP IV = Dipeptidylaminopeptidase IV (in T-cells)
OKT 3 = T-cells specific monoclonal antiserum
OKT 4 = T-helper specific monoclanal antiserum
OKT 8 = T-suppressor specific monoclonal antiserum

The lymphomatoid cells have been hypothesized to sometimes retain their immunological functions (Brondin et al., 1979).

In this contest, it is significant to point out in one of our patient a skin reaction to PPD. This reaction has been found in previously published cases (1960) with midface lesions. Moreover, some Authors (Boumsell et al.,1981;King et al.,1981) demonstrated delayed hypersensitivity skin reaction and serum Ig increased in some patients with T-cell skin lymphoma. These data confirm the clinical course of these necrotizing midface granulomatous lesions, suggesting a new pathogenetic classification for these disorders, different from until now proposed in Literature.

REFERENCES

1. Boumsell L. et al.(1981) Blood 57:526-530
2. Collins R.D. et al. (1979) Am.J.Clin.Pathol. 72:699-707
3. Ishii Y. et al.(1982) Cancer 50:2336-2344
4. Liebow A.A. et al. (1972) Hum. Pathol. 3:457-536
5. Ricci V. (1959) Omnia Medica, Pisa Ed.

© 1985 Elsevier Science Publishers B.V. (Biomedical Division)
New dimensions in otorhinolaryngolcgy - head and neck surgery, vol. 2.
E. Myers, editor

BURNS AND TRACHEOTOMY

DAHLIA M. SATALOFF, ROBERT THAYER SATALOFF

Although the role of tracheotomy in the management of burn patients appears controversial at first, a careful review of the literature reveals fairly widespread agreement. Indications have included upper airway obstruction, inability to handle secretions, respiratory tract irritation, as an aid to anesthesia in patients with facial burns, prophylaxis against respiratory obstruction in patients with deep facial burns, prophylaxis against aspiration of vomitis, and associated injuries. Most of the "prophylactic" indications have been dropped.

The complication that has provoked the greatest interest is its possible relationship to pulmonary infections.

From the available literature, one can conclude that patients whose injury is severe enough to require tracheotomy have a higher mortality and morbidity than those who do not require tracheotomy. However, there is no good evidence for a cause-and-effect relationship. The extent of injuries in the two groups is generally not comparable, and there have been no random controlled studies. It would be better to compare patients with tracheotomy to patients treated with prolonged intubation, but fortunately prolonged intubation is rarely used. One might also compare patients with no artificial airway with a group of comparable patients with elective tracheotomy. However, elective trachectomy is also not performed routinely in responsible hands. In fact, even in the older literature, tracheotomy was generally performed only on the most severely injured patients who already had the highest mortality and morbidity on the basis of their injuries. Thus, most authors have either compared unlike groups or reported anecdotal observations; and their conclusions are suspect.

Our recommended indications are:

1. Upper airway obstruction: As in all cases of upper airway obstruction, endotrachial or nasotrachial intubation should be used initially whenever possible. When edema or facial burns are so severe as to preclude intubation, tracheotomy is necessary.
2. Prolonged intubation.
3. Children: As in epiglottitis, intubation to manage a compromised upper airway in children under approximately two years of age should be considered only in the most skilled intensive care units. Otherwise, tracheotomy is safer.

Two other situations in which further clarification of the role of tracheotomy is needed have not been adequately investigated.

1. Laryngeal burn: Because of the life-threatening severity of burns with inhalation injury, relatively little attention has been paid to the burned

larynx itself. As burn treatment improves and more patients survive, the otolaryngologist will probably be called upon more often to treat the sequelae of laryngeal injury. Since the best treatment of a scarred larynx is prevention, the otolaryngologist should be involved early in burn management and tracheotomy should be considered.

2. Severe Oropharyngeal and Facial Burns: The relative merits of *nasotracheal* intubation, *orotracheal* intubation and tracheotomy in severe burns of the nasal, oral and pharyngeal surfaces, have not been evaluated adequately. While concerns about trachial infection and erosion have been widely discussed in literature, very little attention has been paid to the hazards of passing a tube through a nasal, oral or supraglottic burn. It seems possible that this foreign body might not only predispose to stricture, but it might also result in posterior pharyngeal injury or erosion. Infection or abscess in this location is also potentially lethal in a debilitated burn patient. The relative merits of the various treatment modalities warrant closer scrutiny than they have had.

Tracheotomy Technique

The hazards of high tracheotomy have been widely recognized for many years, particularly the propensity for subglottic stenosis. Complications of excessively low tracheotomy have also been reported in burn patients, although these were apparently due to failure to modify the tracheotomy tube so that the tip was situated in proper position. As in other patients, the tracheotomy in burn patients should be performed below the second trachial ring. An inferior based flap between the second and third *tracheal* rings, extending through the third and fourth rings is recommended.

Conclusion

Increased involvement of otolaryngologist with burn management teams is recommended to improve patient assessment acutely and after recovery and to optimize therapy.

New dimensions in otorhinolaryngology – head and neck surgery, vol. 2.
E. Myers, editor

ULTRASONOGRAPHICAL DIAGNOSIS OF THYROID TUMOR WITH NEW METHOD AND CRITERIA

KAZUHIKO SHOJI M.D., HIROYUKI KITAMURA M.D., ATSUKO NISHIKAWA M.D.,
KENSUKE NOSE M.D., SHINICHI TAKAGITA M.D., KEISUKE TABUCHI M.D.
Dept. of Otholaryngology, Tenri Hospital, Nara Pref., Japan

INTRODUCTION

Ultrasound examination has become general and important as a diagnostic imaging of thyroid tumors and this owes much a great advance in the apparatus for ultrasonic diagnosis, especially introduction of the electronic linear scanner with a high frequency transducer. This apparatus permits excellent visualization of thyroid tumor in real time, and provides a great deal of diagnostic information that was previously unobtainable. But even if information have become more because of development of the hard ware, this does not directly lead to improvement of the diagnostic rate. It is essential for us to select the information of diagnostic importance. We analysed 90 thyroid tumors with multivariate analysis and propose new mehtod and criteria for ultrasonographical diagnosis of thyroid tumor.

MATERIALS AND METHODS

Eighty eight patients of thyroid tumor were operated at our department in 1982. Among them 86 patients received ultrasonic examination preoperatively. The newest apparatus — Toshiba SAL-50A with 5 MHz transducer was used. They had 90 nodules pathologically diagnosed postoperatively which consisted of 23 cancers and 67 benign nodules. Following five items were set as factors showing differences between benign and malignant tumor. 1. Margin 2. Shape 3. Internal Echo 4. Cystic component 5. Calcification.

RESULTS

Table 1 shows frequency of each category of five items in benign group and malignant group and category weights which were calculated with multivariate analysis-theory of quantification II in order to know how important each category of each item is.

When partial correlation coefficients were calculated, the two times of Margin and Internal echo were not significant and also figure below the decimal point were not practical. Therefore the new diagnostic method and criteria were devised on the basis of these category weights. (Table 2)

Application of this method to the original population shows the predicative values of 80.6% in benign group and of 78.3% in malignant group, and totally of 80.0%. Next in order to decide whether or not this diagnostic method is applicable to clinical practice, it must be applied to groups other than the analysed population for evaluation. We applied it to 44 cases operated at our department from January to July, 1983 which consisted of 17 cancers and 27 benign tumors. The diagnostic accuracy was 88.2% in cancers and 88.9% in benign tumors, and 88.6% totally. Based on this result, this new method seems to have the possibility to serve as a standard for ultrasonography of thyroid tumor.

TABLE 1

Item	Category	Benign Group	Malignant Group	Category Weight
Margine	clear	52 (78%)	14 (61%)	-0.8785
	unclear	15 (22%)	9 (39%)	0.0000
Shape	regular	45 (67%)	8 (35%)	2.5195
	irregular	22 (33%)	15 (65%)	0.0000
Internal Echo	homogeneous	11 (16%)	2 (9%)	1.4670
	heterogeneous	56 (84%)	21 (91%)	0.0000
Cystic Component	(+)	41 (61%)	4 (17%)	3.3444
	(-)	26 (39%)	19 (83%)	0.0000
Calcification	(+)	7 (10%)	12 (52%)	-5.5614
	(-)	60 (90%)	11 (48%)	-1.9171

TABLE 2

METHOD OF SCORING FOR THYROID ULTRASONOGRAPHY

Item	Category	Score
1 Shape	regular	2
	irregular	0
2 Cystic Component	(+)	3
	(-)	0
3 Calcification	(+)	-5
	(-)	0

Criteria total score ≧ 2 : benign

total score ≦ 0 : malignant

New dimensions in otorhinolaryngology - head and neck surgery, vol. 2.
E. Myers, editor

TREATMENT OF KELOIDS WITH THE CO_2 LASER

F J STUCKER, MD
Department of Otolaryngology/Head and Neck Surgery, LSU School of Medicine, P.O. Box 33932, Shreveport, Louisiana 71130-3932

INTRODUCTION

Histologically a keloid is indistinguishable from a hypertrophic scar.[1] All wounds are characterized by an inflammatory phase followed by fibroplasia. Fibroblasts migrate into the wound from perivascular spaces and manufactured collagen. This collagen synthesis increases and with it a corresponding increase in the wounds tensile strength. The acceleration of collagen plateaus at approximately three weeks but the tensile strength continues to increase. The so-called maturation phase is marked by the stabilization of synthesis and degradation of collagen and is also noted for the alignment of the collagen fibers from an initial haphazard orientation. Embryonic Type III collagen is replaced by Type I collagen.

CLINICAL CHARACTERISTICS

The abnormal accumulation of fibrous tissue of keloids represents an aberration in a complex biological equilibrium between collagen synthesis and collagen lysis. Keloids are rare in non-Caucasians and there is evidence of a familial incidence. Our patients have been remarkably free of symptoms in the absence of infection or when the keloid is located where it interferes with normal activities.

TREATMENT

Much exciting work is in progress utilizing agents which affect the exaggerated accumulation of scar tissue. Lathyrogenic agents and colchicine are currently being investigated by Peacock[1] for use in the treatment of keloids. Although these pharmacologic agents have a theoretical basis for their use but as yet no controlled reports corroborate their adjunctive.

For our clinical evaluation, we have separated our patients into four groups. The first are those with involvement limited to one or both ear lobes and these represent the largest group. Single neck keloids, single body keloids and multiple keloids are the other three groups.

Our treatment includes CO_2 laser excision and closure if this can be done without tension. All lesions are excised with the CO_2 laser, but if a tensionless closure is not possible, the wounds are allowed to contract and re-epithelize. The patients are followed closely and intralesional triamcinolone commenced with evidence of recurrence. If the keloid is not controlled adequately the keloid is re-excised with the CO_2 laser and followed and recurrence managed in the same manner.

More than half our keloid patients presented with ear lobe lesions. Our success rate with the described technique is universally good. Recurrence is about 15% and all have been controlled with interlesional triamcinolone.

Single body and neck keloids also yield excellent results; however, several have required a second CO_2 laser resection for control.

The fourth group, and by every measure the most disappointing, are those with multiple lesions. We have several patients with over 20 large keloids. We have some promising results with laser resections in this group, but on balance the results are disappointing.

SUMMARY

Although there are exciting pharmacologic potentials in the treatment of keloids, current treatment continues to require surgical resection. We present our recommended treatment which consists of resection with the CO_2 laser and tensionless closure or re-epithelization.

REFERENCES

1. Peacock EE (1984) Wound Repair (3rd ed) WB Saunders Co, Philadelphia, Pennsylvania, pp 485-503

New dimensions in otorhinolaryngology - head and neck surgery, vol. 2.
E. Myers, editor

ETIOLOGICAL STUDY ON ISOLATED ESOPHAGEAL ATRESIA

TÜNDE SZENDREY

Department of Otorhinolaryngology and Bronchology, Apáthy István Children's Hospital, Bethesda u. 3, H-1146 (Hungary)

INTRODUCTION

In Hungary the birth prevalence of isolated esophageal atresia (EA) with or without tracheo-esophageal fistula is 0.18 per 1000 total births (1). The birth prevalence of esophageal atresia with other congenital abnormalities is 0.14 per 1000 total births. The etiology of EA is largely unknown. In this paper we report the results of our etiological study in 160 EA cases.

MATERIAL AND METHODS

The Hungarian Congenital Malformation Register includes 230 isolated EA cases born between 1970 and 1977. We were finally able to evaluate the etiological data of 160 index patients (69.6%) and 160 controls. The control group included healthy children matched for year of birth, sex and residence of their parents. Personal interviews with parents of index patients and controls enabled us to fill out specific data sheets designed for this purpose.

RESULTS

Epidemiology

The annual birth prevalence of EA did not show any significant change in the period studied. The monthly distribution of births does not indicate a significant seasonality, although the difference between the maximum (October: 0.24) and the minimum (February: 0.12) is considerable. Onehalf of the 160 EA cases were males. The lack of an excess of males our study may be due to the homogenity of our material, because there is a predominance of males in cases of EA associated with other malformations. The distribution of birth weight and gestational week groups of EA cases showed a significant difference from those of the controls. The shift in gestational weeks is more pronounced (Fig.1). EA was twice as frequent in mothers giving birth under 19 years of age and mothers over 30 again showed a surplus of EA births (Fig.2). This U-shaped distribution of maternal age differed significantly from that of the controls.

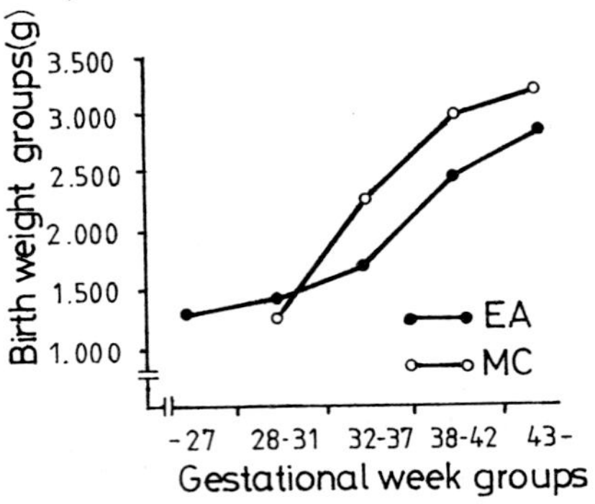

Fig. 1. Gestational week groups plotted against birth weight groups

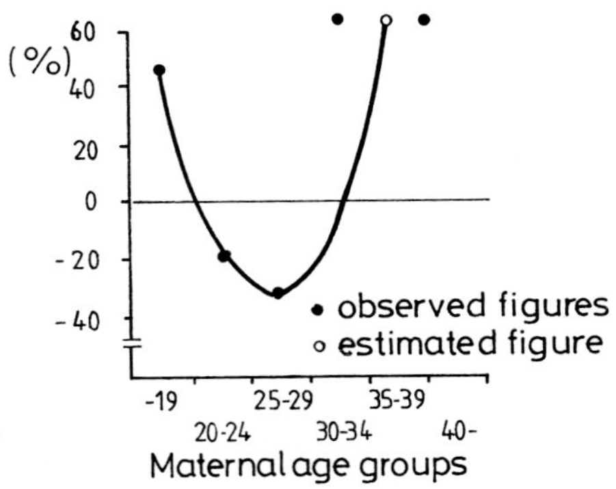

Fig. 2. U-shaped distribution of maternal age groups in the study group of EA

Family planning and teratology

There were more extramarital conceptions, more pregnancies in spite of contraceptiv pills and more delayed conception in index patients mothers. The teratogens studied did not have an obvious pathological effect here.

Genetics

We could examine 527 first-degree relatives of index patients. One brother had isolated EA. Thus the specific sib-occurence was 0.43 ± 0.40. Among the nonspecific CAs, high frequencies of spina bifida occulta and anencephaly are worth mentioning (3). We recorded information about 747 second- and 669 third-degree relatives of index patients based of parents' information, but these data are not reliable enough to draw conclusion about the familial occurence of EAs and CAs. Mendelian monogenic inheritance and chromosome aberrations do not seem to play a role either. Polygenic inheritance could not be excluded. However, the frequent association of EA with other CAs, e.g., VACTERL-type CAs, is an established fact (2). Many experts consider EA to be a manifestation of a wide spectrum of developmental anomalies. Some epidemiological data and the caracteristics of family planning may act as maternal triggering factors.

REFERENCES

1. Czeizel A, Vitéz M (1981) Acta Paediatr Acad Sci Hung 22: 172-176
2. David TJ, O Callaghan SE (1975) J Med Genet 12: 1-11
3. Fraser FC, Czeizel A (1982) Lancet 11: 144-145

© 1985 Elsevier Science Publishers B.V. (Biomedical Division)
New dimensions in otorhinolaryngology - head and neck surgery, vol. 2.
E. Myers, editor

LIMITATIONS OF RADIONUCLIDE SCANS IN PAROTID TUMORS

VISHWAS D. TADWALKAR, VLADIMIR B. SANTOS
Dept. of Otolaryngology, The Long Island College Hospital, Brooklyn, N.Y.

INTRODUCTION

Certain benign tumors like Warthin's tumor and oncoytoma have the ability to concentrate sodium pertechnetate Tc99m and thus, they show up as 'hot' or 'functioning' nodules. The other parotid tumors are not able to accumulate this material. This has been well documented in various reports by McGuirt and McCabe[1], Schall[2] Ausband et al[3], and Siddiqui and Weisberger[4].

CASE REPORTS

Case I - E.B. A 37 year old oriental female with a history of a painless, slow-growing mass over the left parotid region. Physical examination revealed the presence of a firm, fairly mobile, non-tender, well delineated mass, measuring about 2.5 cm in its greatest diameter, over the left parotid area. There was no evidence of facial paralysis. There were no palpable lymph nodes in the neck. A parotid scan revealed the presence of a 'hot' nodule on the left side in the area of the palpable mass. Patient underwent a left superficial parotidectomy with facial nerve preservation. Histopathological examination revealed a carcinoma ex-pleomorphic adenoma of the left parotid gland. Post-operative radiation therapy was given.

Case II - A.H. A 57 year old hispanic male with the history of a mass behind the angle of the jaw on the right side for 4 to 6 months prior to admission. The mass was essentially asymptomatic. Physical examination revealed a firm, non-tender mass in the right retromandibular area about 1 cm in diameter. There were no palpable lymph nodes in the neck. There was no involvement of the facial nerve on that side. A radionuclide scan showed a 'cold' nodule in the area of the palpable mass on the right side. Patient underwent a right superficial parotidectomy with facial nerve preservation. Pathology report showed a Warthin's tumor.

DISCUSSION

The oncocyte is derived from the ductal epithelium and has the ability to concentrate Tc99m and secrete it in the central lumen. In the case of the Warthin's tumor and oncocytoma, this is not in communication with the ductal system. Thus, it is trapped within the tumor and gives rise to a radio-opaque appearance. Oncocytic carcinoma has been rarely reported and may understandably give rise to a positive scan, having its origin in the oncocyte.

McGuirt and McCabe[1] reported a case of epidermoid carcinoma with a positive salivary scan. They felt that the location of the tumor in the gland and its size may influence its appearance on the scan.

A mucous producing papillary adenocarcinoma in the presence of a positive scan has been reported by Noyek et al[5] in an elderly female patient. The reason for the accumulation of Tc99m is uncertain according to them. However, they proposed that the pertechnetate is presumably actively secreted in the tumor as the intracellular and extracellular mucin production, possibly in the same manner that it is actively excreted in the saliva.

The appearance of a Warthin's tumor showing a cold nodule on the scan in our case could not be explained, though three similar cases have been reported after a review of worldwide literature by Schall[6].

The malignant mixed tumor in our case may have given rise to a 'hot' nodule on the scan because it was a carcinoma ex-pleomorphic adenoma and the benign mixed tumor that it started from, may have shown a 'hot' nodule. Twenty five percent of benign mixed tumors have been reported to give radiopositive scans by Grove and DiChiro[7] and up to fifty percent by Gates[8]. This appearance may also be explained by possible trapped excretion of Tc99m enhanced in the scan after the sialogogue was given with the excretion of saliva from the normal glandular parenchyma into the ductal system and then into oral cavity.

In conclusion, information gained from radionuclide scans of the parotid gland could sometimes be misleading and should not be used as criterion for selection of patients for surgical treatment. In addition, an intraoperative frozen section examination is highly recommended so that a definite histopathological diagnosis can be reached and appropriate surgical therapy can be carried out at the same time depending on the histology of the tumor.

REFERENCES

1. McGuirt WF, McCabe BF, Limitations of Parotid Scans, Am. Otol. 86, 247-277-1977
2. Schall GL, DiChiro G, Clinical Usefulness of Salivary Gland Scanning-Sem. Nuclear Med. 2, 270-277-1972
3. Ausband JR, Kittrell BJ, Cowan RJ, Radioisotope Scanning for Parotid Oncocytoma Arch. Otolaryng. 93-628-629-1971
4. Siddiqui AR, Weisberger EC, Possible Explanation of Appearance of Warthin's tumor on I-123 and Tc99m Pertechnetate Scans. Clin, Nuclear Med. 6, 258-259, 1981
5. Noyek AM, Greyson ND, Fernandes BJ, Chapwick JS, Radionuclide Salivary Scan Imaging of a 'functioning' Malignant Parotid Tumor (mucous producing papillary adenocarcinoma) - J. of Otol. II (2) 83-85-1982
6. Schall GL, Role of Radionuclide Scanning in the Evaluatioon of Neoplasms of The Salivary Glands: A review, J. Surg. Oncl. 3,699-714, 1971
7. Grove AS, DiChiro G. Salivary Gland Scanning with Technicium 99m Pertechnetate AJR 120 (Z) 109-116, 1968
8. Gates GA, Sialography and Scanning of the Salivary Glands, Otol. Clinics of North America 10, 379-390, 1977

© 1985 Elsevier Science Publishers B.V. (Biomedical Division)
New dimensions in otorhinolaryngology - head and neck surgery, vol. 2.
E. Myers, editor

SURGICAL TREATMENT FOR DYSPHAGIA

TEIJI TANAHASHI AND KIYOKO KATSUMI

Department of Otolaryngology, Nagoya University Branch Hospital,
I-I-20, Daikominami, Higashi-ku, Nagoya 458 (Japan)

INTRODUCTION

The treatment of dysphagia is complicated by aspiration. Following our basic reasearch on dysphagia and aspiration using rabbits we have acquired some knowledge that in spite of normal laryngeal closure function aspiration had occurred in the rabbit in which motion of the larynx was severely restricted but after having fixed the larynx in a swallowing position aspiration disappeared all together. By clinical observation using cineradiography, spacio-temporal relationship between bolus, motion of the hyoid bone and the larynx and pharyngo-esophageal junction of the patients who had suffered from dysphagia became disarranged. We have utilized two methods and in the past decade applied a surgical treatment of dysphagia.

MATERIAL AND METHODS

Subjects in the present study were 22 patients. Of the patients with dysphagia I7 were men and 5 were women. Aged ranged from 26 to 77 years. Medical diagnoses were brain stem lesion in 5 patients, neck trauma or surgery in IO patients, cerebellar infarction in I patient and others in 6 patients. The method is consisting of 2 types of surgery named type I and type II. Type I is applied on severe dysphagia with aspiration that follows disruption of the movement of swallowing, especially that of the hyoid bone and the larynx. Type II applied nearly the same status except hyoid bone motion of which is within normal limit.

RESULTS

In I3 patients we performed type I operation. Results were shown in table I. Of these patients, 9 have obtained complete recovery of swallowing function and could return to their normal routine business. Of another 4 patients one was incomplete and 2 were partial recovery but in one patieht his swallowing function did not improve. He had expansive jaw and neck resection and beside that a retitive tumor. Type II operation was performed on 9 patients. Complete recovery was obtained in 5 patients but in 4 other patients it was incomplete. In 3 of these patients we found it necessary to perform type I operation. After type I operatin these patients all have regained complete swallowing function.

TABLE I

Results of type I operation.

Nr	Name	Age	Sex	CP Myotomy	Result	Medical Diagnoses
I	Y.W.	29	f	L&R	CR	Bulbar Palsy
2	S.Y.	66	m	L&R	CR	Multiple Cranial Neurophaty
3	A.I.	67	m	L&R	CR	Brain Stem Infarction
4	I.I.	66	m	L&R	CR	Wallenberg's Syndrom
5	K.K.	67	m	L&R	CR	Wallenberg's Syndrom
6	K.T.	7I	f	L&R	PR	Brain Stem Infarction
7	T.M.	77	f	L&R	PR	Myositis
8	Y.H.	40	m	L	CR	Surgery
9	S.N.	60	m	R	NC	Surgery
I0	K.S.	60	m	L	CR	Surgery
II	M.S.	60	m	L	CR	Surgery
I2	I.M.	6I	m	L&R	CR	Trauma
I3	G.M.	54	m	-	IR	Trauma

*CR : Complete recovery, IR : Incomplete recovery, PR : Pertial recovery and NC : No change. CP Myotomy : Cricopharyngeal muscle myotomy.

Table 2

Results of type II operation

Nr	Name	Age	Sex	CP Myotomy	Result	Medical Diagnoses
I	T.H.	3I	m	L	CR	Trauma
2	H.O.	26	m	L	CR	Trauma
3	S.S.	46	m	R	CR	Surgery
4	K.S.	60	m	L	CR	Surgery
5	K.A.	74	m	L	PR	CNS Disorders
6	M.S.	57	f	L	CR	Cerebellum Inferction
7	T.I.	75	m	L&R	PR	CNS Disorders
8	S.Y.	66	m	L&R	PR	Multiple Cranial Neurophathy
9	T.M.	77	f	L&R	PR	Myositis

REFERENCES

I. Kaplan S and Hills B (I957) Paralysis of the swallowing mechanism following bulbar poliomyelitis. Arch Otolaryngol 65:495-498

2 Olson NR (I976) Laryngeal suspension and epiglottic flap in laryngopharyngeal trauma. Ann Otol 85:533-537

© 1985 Elsevier Science Publishers B.V. (Biomedical Division)
New dimensions in otorhinolaryngology - head and neck surgery, vol. 2.
E. Myers, editor

TRANSORAL RESECTION OF SUBMAXILLARY GLAND

ALEJANDRO ERNESTO TERZIAN
From the 1st. Chair Otolaryngology-Chairman Profesor Dr. Juan Carlos Arauz. Buenos Aire's University-ARGENTINA.

The technique of oral resection of the submaxillaris glard was described in 1954 by Bourghet and Le Branchu. Our experience and that of other surgical team (Yoel,1961) was not satisfactory enough to widely recommend this technique due to inadequate and deep exposure of the anatomic elements.

Now with the introduction of surgical microscope, we approach the gland through a longitudinal incision of the free portion of the floor of the oral cavity. As soon as the sublingual compartment is exposed a clear identification of it's anatomy is possible and it can be adequately dissected with microsurgical instruments.

The Warthon duct, the lingual nerve with it's classical plexus and the arteries goin to the submaxillary gland very specially can be clearly identified and regarding these arteries ligation becomes an easy task, as well as the total remotion of the Wharton cuct in one piece with the gland.

The postoperative period was smooth with highly satisfactory aesthetic results thus we consider this technique to be specially useful in young patients and more so in females.

We employed the above mentioned technique in 4 cases (one a malignant tumor), and a complete remotion of the gland was achieved, avoiding external skin scars, depression of the area or the so feared section of Jaffe's mandibularis nerve.

Regarding the operative difficulties, we believe that this procedures is not adequate in large glands with firm adhesions to sorrounding anatomic structures.

Reprints: Dr. ALEJANDRO ERNESTO TERZIAN
ECUADOR 1428- 4°
1425-BUENOS AIRES-ARGENTINA

New dimensions in otorhinolaryngology – head and neck surgery, vol. 2.
E. Myers, editor

POLYSOMNOGRAPHIC STUDY OF SNORE --PATHOPHYSIOLOGY AND THERAPEUTIC EFFECT--

KIYOSHI TOGAWA, SOICHIRO MIYAZAKI & AKIYOSHI KONNO
Department of Otolaryngology, Akita University School of Medicine
1-1-1, Hondo, Akita 010 (JAPAN)

INTRODUCTION

Snore is no doubt one of the signs indicating the existence of upper airway obstruction during sleep. While asleep, the upper airway becoms narrower than that while awake because of relaxation of pharyngeal muscles and falling back of the soft palate. If the stenosis of any character exists either in the nose or the pharynx, the respiratory airstream passing through the narrowed airway vibrates these mucosa, creating snorrs.

SUBJECTS AND METHODS

Polysomnographic studies were performed all night through on 30 adult snorers with various causes. Parameters such as EEG, EOG, tidal volume, intraesophageal pressure-change(Pes), transcutaneous PO_2 and PCO_2($tcPO_2$, $tcPCO_2$), expiratory FO_2 and FCO_2 etc were recorded on a data-recorder and analyzed later.

RESULTS

Corresponding to the grade of upper airway obstruction, normal breathing through the nose was disturbed and accompanied with snores of various loudness and types, periodic or continued.

Breathing pattern showed two types; an alternate pattern consisted of apnea and hyperpnea, and a constant pattern. In the former, apnea caused marked decrease in $tcPO_2$ and increase in $tcPCO_2$. For the relief of hypoxia developed, great increase in Pes appeared reflexively until it prevailed over the stenosis. This pressure initiated hyperpnea and large snores correspondingly. Enough ventilation recovered the blood gas levels. Then, Pes decreased, which resulted in apnea again. Such phenomena were repeated during sleep. EEG showed disturbed sleep condition with stages 1 and 2 predominance. In the latter, deep and slow breaths continued and were accompanied with snores of constant tone, though the pitch and loudness of which varied case to case. Pes kept considerably larger value than that of the normals fairly constantly. Blood gas levels of low PO_2 and high PCO_2 were not so fluctuated.

Majority of the obese more than 120% of the normal weight have snoring. Their breathing pattern tended to be irregular and periodic, which created worse influence on cardio-respiratory and sleep conditions than the regular breathing did.

Flexible fiberscopic examination of the pharynx while the patients were asleep visualized the vibration of the soft palate and the lateral pharyngeal wall mucosa, which were approximated each other by inspiratory flow created with large negative pressure, and pushed up by expiratory flow with positive pressure. Secretions on the surface of the mucosa also joined into vibration.

Based on the polysomnographic data, 22 cases with surgical indication underwent surgeries such as uvulopalatopharyngoplasty, intranasal corrective surgery, sinusectomy or these combinaticn.

In general, the results were satisfactory, both subjectively and objectively. Surgical removal of obstruction in the upper airway resulted ir sound sleep with regular breathing pattern. Polysomnography showed normal EEG pattern of stage-variation with initial deepening and stepwise depth-change.$TcPC_2$ and $tcPCO_2$ showed minimal fluctuations within the normal range. Pes decreased markedly from 40 to around 10 cmH_2O. Recovery of sound sleep and good rest resulted in refreshing and active lives all the day.

CONCLUSION

Snoring, the disturbed nasal breathing during sleep caused not only serious troubles on their circulo-respiratory functions, but also the failure of sound sleep all the night. Polysomnography provides us the most useful information on these respects including the surgical indication and the effects.

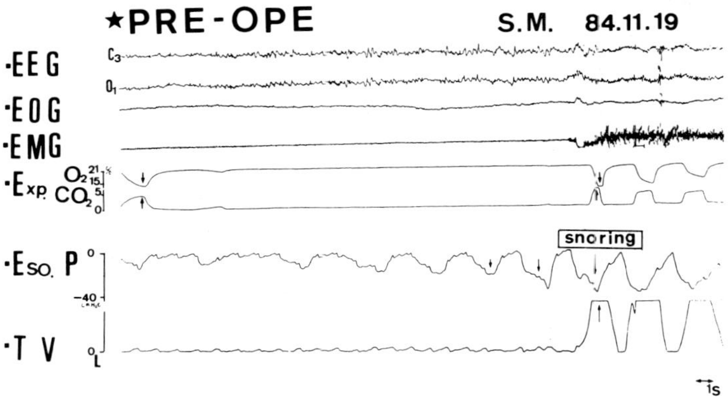

New dimensions in otorhinolaryngology - head and neck surgery, vol. 2.
E. Myers, editor

ELECTROCOCHLEOGRAPHIC STUDY OF NON-HUMAN PRIMATES WITH COLLAGEN-INDUCED EAR DISEASE

T. TAKEDA[1], D. ORCHIK[2], R. A. FLOYD[1], T. ISHIBE[3], N. SUDO[1], Y. YAZAWA[4], G. OLSON[1], J. J. SHEA[2], T. J. YOO[1]

[1]University of Tennessee, Memphis, Tennessee, USA; [2]Shea Clinic, Memphis, Tennessee, USA; [3]Kansai Medical University, Osaka, Japan; [4]Shiga University of Medical Science, Shiga, Japan

INTRODUCTION

The concept of autoimmune ear disease, first proposed by B. F. McCabe (1), is relatively new in the otologic field. Recently, T. J. Yoo et al (2) have suggested that an immunity to type II collagen may be a major factor in autoimmune sensorineural hearing loss. The present study was performed to examine this hypothesis in non-human primates, that is, to examine whether or not type II collagen-immunized monkeys develop auditory disorders.

MATERIALS AND METHOD

Five monkeys were used for this study. One non-immunized monkey and one monkey immunized with native bovine type I collagen (BIn) served as controls. The remaining three monkeys were immunized with native bovine type II collagen (BIIn). The auditory function of these monkeys was followed by the measurement of E. Coch. G and ABR. Both E. Coch. G and ABR were evoked by monoaural presentation of 0.1 msec to the right ear at a rate of 10 /sec, and 1000 responses to these acoustic stimuli were amplified and summed with Amplaid Medelec ERA Mark III. In addition, blood samples were collected on the sacrifice of animals to examine antibody titers to type II collagen. Antibody assay was carried out by an ELISA method.

RESULTS AND CONCLUSIONS

The follow-up of E. Coch. G and ABR was conducted for 16 months except for one animal which was sacrificed three months after the first immunization. The threshold of pre-immunized and control monkeys was between 45 and 55 dB p.e. SPL. Furthermore, the threshold did not fluctuate over 10 dB during this experimental period for the control monkeys. Thus, the threshold of normal monkeys was determined to be within 55 dB p.e. SPL.

Two out of 3 monkeys immunized with BIIn showed a distinct elevation of threshold. Further, this elevation of threshold was associated with a remarkable decrease of APs-amplitude, but without a broad waveform that is characteristic of an enhanced negative summating potential. These auditory disorders were confirmed by the marked decrease of wave I and III-V in ABR. Moreover, these monkeys showed temporally prolongation of the interpeak latency between waves I and II, which is suggestive of disorders of the primary cochlear nerve including the spiral ganglion.

On the other hand, the BIIn-immunized monkey which had no distinct trend in elevation of threshold showed a decrease of APs-amplitude in E. Coch. G. All BIIn-immunized monkeys showed high antibody titers to type II collagen. (Table I) Since the BIIn-immunized monkeys showed autoimmune sensorineural hearing loss, immunity to type II collagen is thought to play a major role in these auditory disorders.

TABLE I

ANTIBODY TITER TO TYPE II COLLAGEN

Dilution of Serum	Non-Immunized	BIn	BIIn	BIIn	BIIn
1/100	0.048	0.028	>1.500	0.591	0.522
1/1000	0.010	0.001	1.216	0.129	0.166

ACKNOWLEDGEMENTS

This research was supported by grants from the Deafness Research Foundation, National Hearing Association, American Otological Society, and Veterans Administration

REFERENCES

1. McCabe BF (1979) Autoimmune Sensorineural Hearing Loss Ann Otl 88:585-589

2. Yoo TJ, Tomoda K, Stuart JM, Cremer MA, Townes AS, Kang AH (1983) Type II Collagen-Induced Autoimmune Sensorineural Hearing Loss and Vestibular Dysfunction in Rats. Ann Otl Rhino Laryn 92:267-271

© 1985 Elsevier Science Publishers B.V. (Biomedical Division)
New dimensions in otorhinolaryngology - head and neck surgery, vol. 2.
E. Myers, editor

PRACTICAL USE OF HRP FOR DEFINING IMMUNE MECHANISMS OF TONSIL

KOICHI TOMODA, TAKEO MITANI, NORIO MAEDA, TADAMI KUMAZAWA

Department of Otolaryngology, Kansai Medical University, Fumizonocho, Moriguchi, Osaka, Japan

INTRODUCTION

It is widely accepted that the tonsils, being located in the first gate of both digestive and respiratory systems, have the primary immunological defense activity against bacteria and other exogenous antigens. On the other hand, the tonsil is often the site of secondary diseases, such as focal infections.

We have investigated how the tonsil responds to the horseradish peroxidase (HRP) injected as an antigen and the effects to the regional lymphnode and distant organ (Kidney). We wish to report the results of human and animal study.

MATERIAL AND METHODS

Human study. We used 20 subjects of human palatine tonsil and Horseradish peroxidase (HRP) Type VI (Sigma) as an antigen and tracer. Under general anesthesia, HRP (8mg/ml) was injected into tonsillar crypts, and 10 to 15 min later, tonsillectomy was performed. Tissue samples were incubated in Hanks solution containing HRP (3mg/ml) for 30 min, then fixed in glutaraldehyde and picric acid-paraformaldehyde solution for 24 hours and frozen sections were made. After staining with 3,3'-diaminobenzidine (DAB) for 5 min, light and electronmicroscopic observations were carried out.

Animal study. 12 rabbits, weighing 3.2-3.8 kg, were immunized with 0.2 mg of HRP solution containing HRP (type VI), 10 mg/ml, emulsifying with an equal volume of complete Freund's adjuvant, which was injected into tonsillar crypts, once weekly for 2, 4, and 8 weeks. One week after the last immunization, tonsils, regional lymphnodes and kidney were all removed and observed immunohistochemically or electronmicroscopically. As a control, saline or only adjuvant were injected with an identical method.

RESULTS

In human palatine tonsils, HRP injected was largely seen in the crypts and microcrypts, and in the cytoplasm of phagocytes that infiltrated in the interfollicular space and near the capsule. These phagocytes were often seen around the blood vessels. Some epithelial cells also contained HRP.

Silver staining sections showed trabecular-like mesh work of lymph capillary and particular arrengement with forming one line of lymphocytes in the fine pod-like tubes at the interfollicular space. Lymphocytes were migrating into the vessel through such mesh work resembling the seeds of green peas, as in the report of Hamashima[1].

In the animal study, rabbit's tonsils showed the findings similar to those seen in the humans. When sections were incubated with HRP solution to detect antibody specific to HRP, the cytoplasm of plasma cells was positively stained. These plasma cells also responded to rabbit IgG antibody. In the regional lymphnodes, phagocytes injesting HRP and plasma cells producing antibody specific to HRP were also well observed.

Electronmicroscopically, the cytoplasm of such plasma cells had largely dilated cisternae of rough endoplasmic reticulum that indicate an active production of antibodies. These plasma cells were often seen around the vessels and stained positively with rabbit IgG.

The severity of phagocyte and plasma cell reaction in the tonsil and lymphnode were increased with repeating immunization. However, no reactions were found in the kidney.

DISCUSSION

HRP as an exogenous antigen entered the tonsil mostly from the microcrypt and less entered through the epithelial layer. Maeda[2] in 1979 reported that microcrypt is the most important part to receive the exogenous antigens. In the interfollicular space, phagocytes, plasma cells and lymphocytes migrated and reponded to HRP. These immuno competent cells reacted and HRP itself may emigrate through the lymph-capillary nets beside the capsule or septum into the lymph or blood stream, and may react in the regional lymphnodes or kidney. Pabst[3] 1984 reported that the tonsils participate in the exchange of lymphocytes between lymohoid organs at a high rate and probably many lymphocytes primed within the tonsils migrate to different part of the lymphoid system. In this study, however, we could not detected any immune reactions in the kidney. Rearrengement of immunization and further study of immune complex should be considered to discuss.

REFERENCES

1. Hamashima Y (1970) Jan J Tonsil 9 : 118-127
2. Maeda S, Mogi G, Oh M (1982) Ann Otol Rhinol Laryngol 91; suppl 94: 1-8
3. Pabst R, Nowara E (1984) Arch otorhinolaryngol 240: 7-13

New dimensions in otorhinolaryngology - head and neck surgery, vol. 2.
E. Myers, editor

THE FEASIBILITY OF SERUM. VZV-SPECIFIC IgA ANTIBODIES IN ZOSTER OF THE HEAD AND NECK

FERIT TOVI[1], TUVIA HADAR[1], JACQUES SIDI[1], BATYA SAROV[2] AND ISRAEL SAROV[3].
[1]E.N.T. Dept., Units of [3]Virology and [2]Epidemiology, Soroka Medical Center, P.O.Box 151, Beer Sheva, Israel

INTRODUCTION

Early treatment by antiviral drugs prevents the development of life threatening conditions in immunocompromised zoster patients (1). Early initiation of steroids may alter the course of postherpetic neuralgia (2), or may avoid motor sequela in neuropathies associated with zoster (3). Since some of the cases of zoster of the head and neck present with unusual clinical patterns posing diagnostic difficulties, and skin manifestations of bacterial or other viral infections may mimic a zosteriform eruption, the definitive and early diagnosis of the zoster by a simple and rapid serologic assay must be of clinical value.

Serum VZV-specific IgA responses in herpesviruses infections were recently reported (4,5). In the present study we examined the possibility whether the serum VZV-specific IgA antibodies may be an early signal of VZV infection reactivation.

PATIENTS AND METHOD

This study is based on 26 patients with zoster of the head and neck, and age and sex matched healthy controls, ranging in age from 6 to 67 years. Serial blood samples were collected at intervals of approximately 10 days and tested by indirect immunoperoxidase assay (IPA) for VZV-specific IgA and IgG antibodies (5,6).

SEROLOGY

Specific VZV-IgG antibodies were found in the first serum sample of all the patients who showed fourfold rises or decreases in titer in subsequent samples, indicating the diagnosis of zoster. In 17 (80.9%) of 21 patients from whom a serum sample was available as early as 1-5 days after onset of illness, VZV specific IgA antibodies were detected. The second serum sample, taken in the convalescence period was VZV-specific IgA positive in all of the patients and showed marked rises in the titer (see Fig. 1). While all the matched controls had VZV specific IgG antibodies, VZV specific IgA antibodies were detected in low titer in only 3 (10.4%) of the subjects (see Fig. 1). These three subjects were middle aged adults (43, 45 and 50 years of age) who might have been affected by a silent reactivation of VZV that occurs with aging (7). By using a VZV-

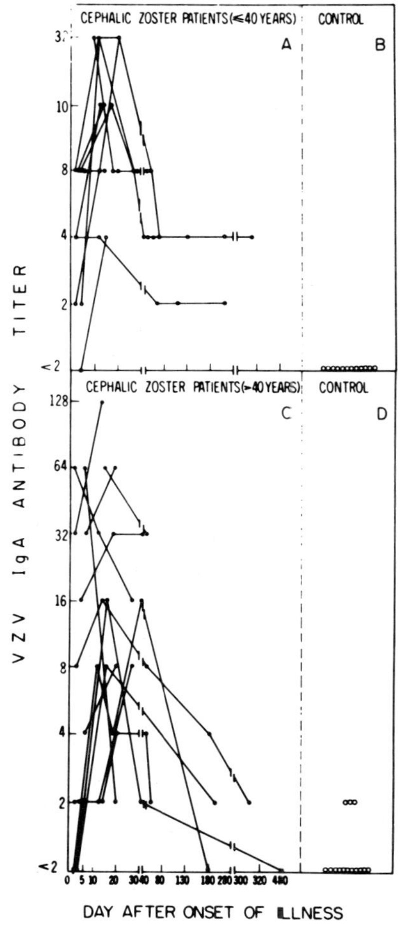

Fig. 1. VZV-specific IgA titers in zoster patients according to days after onset of illness.

specific IgA antibody titer of ≥2 and ≥4 by IPA as a "cut-off" for young and adult patients with zoster, respectively, one can obtain an early diagnosis of VZV-infection in 83% of the young group ($P < 0.001$) and 50% of the adult ($P < 0.02$) patients with a single serum determination of VZV-specific IgA antibody titer. Accordingly, determination of VZV-specific IgA antibodies by IPA technique might be a helpful adjunct in early serodiagnosis of patients with zoster.

REFERENCES

1. Bean B, Bracin C, Balfour HH (1982) Lancet ii 118-121
2. Eaglstein WH, Katz R, Brown JA (1970) JAMA 211:1681-1683
3. Harner SG, Heiny BA, Nervell RC (1970) Arch Otolaryngol 92:632-635
4. Brunell PA, Gershon AA, Uduman SA, Steinberg S (1975) J Inf Dis 132:49-54
5. Haikin H, Sarov I (1982) J Clin Pathol 35:645-649
6. Haikin H, Leventon-Kriss S, Sarov I (1979) J Inf Dis 140:601-604
7. Gershon A, Steinberg S, Borkowsky W, Lenette D, Lenette E (1981) Pediat Res 15:610

New dimensions in otorhinolaryngology – head and neck surgery, vol. 2.
E. Myers, editor

TYPE II COLLAGEN-INDUCED AUTOIMMUNE ENDOLYMPHATIC HYDROPS

T. J. YOO[1], N. SUDO[1], Y. YAZAWA[2], R. A. FLOYD[1], T. ISHIBE[3], T. TAKEDA[1]

[1]University of Tennessee and VAMC, Memphis, TN, USA; [2]Shiga University of Medical Science, Otsu, Japan; [3]Kansai Medical University, Osaka, Japan

INTRODUCTION

Since we first reported our original observation on the production of type II collagen-induced endolymphatic hydrops in guinea pigs (1,2), we have extended our observations further by changing the duration between the final immunization, the sacrifice dates and the cell transfer experiments. This study was designed to define how these factors influence the production of type II collagen-induced endolymphatic hydrops.

MATERIALS AND METHODS

Sixty-seven guinea pigs (Hartly, strain 13, strain 2) were employed in this study. The guinea pigs were immunized with 400ug of native bovine type II collagen in incomplete Freund's adjuvant and boosted 1 week later. The guinea pigs were sacrificed 3, 5, 7, 14, 21 and 28 days and 6 months post-immunization.

For cell transfer study, 20 guinea pigs received 1×10^7, 2×10^7, or 2×10^8, spleen or lymph node cells intravenously from guinea pigs sensitized with type II collagen. These recipient guinea pigs were sacrificed one month later. The temporal bones were immediately fixed in 10% buffered Formalin, decalcified, and embedded in paraffin and celloidin. Sections were cut at 8μ horizontally and stained with hematoxylin and eosin.

RESULTS AND CONCLUSION

The results of the relationship between hydrops incidence and time sequence are shown in Table I. A high incidence of hydrops was observed in immunized animals sacrificed 14 days and 6 months post-immunization. Other histopathological findings in the immunized guinea pigs are as follows: spiral ganglion degeneration, atrophied organ of Corti, cystic lesions of the stria vascularis, mild atrophy of surface epithelium of endolymphatic duct, and macrophages and precipitates in the endolymph.

Five out of 20 cell transferred guinea pigs showed mild to severe hydrops and the degree and the incidence of hydrops seemed to depend on the cell dosage.

The results of these experiments show that the production of collagen-induced hydrops depends on the mode of immunization, antigen dosage and post-immunization sacrifice date. Furthermore, the results of the cell transfer experiment indicate that autoimmune hydrops is transferable by immune cells. Thus, hydrops appears to be another manifestation of immunologic injury resulting in an accummulation of mediator rather than any specific pathological entity.

TABLE I

HYDROPS INCIDENCES VS DURATION AFTER THE ANTIGEN CHALLENGE

Degree of Hydrops	3d	5d	7d	14d	21d	28d	6mo
++	0	0	0	1	0	0	0
+	2	0	1	8	0	2	2
±	0	0	0	3	0	1	2
0	2	4	3	15	0	16	1
Ears used	4	4	4	27	4	19	5

ACKNOWLEDGEMENTS

This research was supported by grants from the Deafness Research Foundation, National Hearing Association, American Otological Sciety, and Veterans Administration

REFERENCES

1. Yoo TJ, Yazawa Y, Tomoda K, Floyd R (1983) Type II Collagen-Induced Autoimmune Endolymphatic Hydrops in Guinea Pig. Science 222:65-67

2. Yoo TJ, Tomoda K, Hernandez AD (1984) Type II Collagen-Induced Autoimmune Inner Ear Lesions in Guinea Pigs. Ann Oto Rhino Laryn (supplement 113)93:3-5

New dimensions in otorhinolaryngology – head and neck surgery, vol. 2.
E. Myers, editor

TYPE II COLLAGEN-INDUCED TYMPANOSCLEROSIS MODEL IN GUINEA PIGS

Y. YAZAWA[1], T. J. YOO[2], T. ISHIBE[3], K. TOMODA[3], R. FLOYD[2], N. SUDO[2], T. TAKEDA[2], S. HA[2]

[1]Shiga University of Medical Science, Otsu, Japan; [2]University of Tennessee, Memphis, TN USA; [3]Kansai Medical University, Osaka, Japan

INTRODUCTION

The first tympanosclerosis model in animals was developed by passively sensitizing guinea pigs with anti-guinea pig tympanic membrane serum and tympanic membrane trauma such as acid treatment (1). The chemical nature of the agent(s) responsible for the induction of their tympanosclerosis model remain unidentified. This present communication describes a tympanosclerosis model in guinea pigs which was developed by immunizing them with type II collagen, one of the main components of the tympanic membrane (2), followed by tympanic membrane trauma from surgical incision.

MATERIALS AND METHODS

Strain 13 guinea pigs were immunized with 400μg of chemically purified bovine type II collagen in complete Freund's adjuvant and boosted 3 or 4 times. One month after the last booster, a surgical incision was made in the left tympanic membrane and the right ear was kept intact. Non-immunized control guinea pigs also received surgical trauma to the left tympanic membrane. Animals were sacrificed 35 days after the surgical incision. For histopathological examination, the temporal bones were removed and fixed in 10% buffered Formalin, decalcified in 5% trichloroacetic acid, embedded in celloidin-paraffin, cut in sections and stained with hematoxylin and eosin. For the immunofluorescence study, the temporal bones were fixed in cold 95% alcohol, decalcified in EDTA, embedded in paraffin, cut in sections and stained first with goat anti-guinea pig IgG or C3, followed with rabbit anti-goat IgG labeled with FITC.

RESULTS AND CONCLUSION

Six of the 11 tympanic membranes from the immunized guinea pigs with incisions in their tympanic membranes showed hyperplasia with calcium deposition which occurred sporadically in the fibrous layer and IgG and C3 deposits in the lamina propria (Table 1). Only 1 of the 11 tympanic membranes from the immunized guinea pigs without incisions showed hyperplasia without calcium deposition. No pathological changes were observed in the tympanic membranes from the non-immunized guinea pigs without incisions.

These results suggest that tympanosclerosis could result from autoimmune responses to type II collagen which was stimulated by trauma to the tympanic membrane.

TABLE 1

HISTOPATHOLOGICAL CHANGES IN THE TYMPANIC MEMBRANE

	Number of Animals	Hyperplasia	Calcification	IgG & C3 Deposition
No Immunization:				
No incision	8	0	0	0
Incision	8	1	0	0
Type II Collagen Immunization				
No incision	1[illegible]	1	0	2
Incision	1[illegible]	8	6	6

ACKNOWLEDGEMENTS

This research was supported by grants from the Deafness Research Foundation, National Hearing Association, American Otological Society, and Veterans Administration

REFERENCES

1. Shiff M, Poliquin JF, Catanzaro A, Ryan AF (1980) Tympanosclerosis: A Theory of Pathogenesis. Ann Otol 89(suppl 70):1-16

2. Yoo TJ, Tomoda K, Ishibe T, Kang AH, Cremer MA (1985) Type II Distribution in the Ear Tissue. (Submitted)

New dimensions in otorhinolaryngology – head and neck surgery, vol. 2
E. Myers, editor

LYOPHILISED PLEURAL CARTILAGE IN RHINOPLASTY

A.SKEVAS, TH.TSOULIAS, K.MPLIOURAS, G.EXARCHAKOS, N.PAPADOPOULOS.
E.N.T. Clinic., University of Ioannina. IOANNINA - GREECE

INTRODUCTION

For the surgeon who operates on a nose with deformity of its shape, it is many times nesseccery to use different grafts in order to have a good as functional as cosmetic result.

The grafts which can be used are cartilage, bone, composite graft, fascia, lyfilished dura meninge or skin.

MATERIAL AND METHOD

We use lyfilished pleural cartilage in rhinoplasty for more than eight years. The reasons we prefer them are:

1. We take them ready from the Research center.
2. They are easy in proccessing, well accepted in humman organism without absorption and they are flexible and soft.
3. There is no need of special conditions to keep them and can be used up to six months after lyphilitation.

These grafts can be a)lyphilished and radiated, or sterilised with ethilenoxide under N_2 pressure or vacum.
b) Without lyphilization, radiated of sterilized with ethilenoxide into water for injection.

The grafts which will be transplanted must be put into normal saline under sterilize conditions two hours before use will stay into an antibiotic solution for half an hour and then it is ready for use.
Three main types of grafts.

1. A straight graft which is put into dorsum to eliminate a sadle nose or into colummela to elevate the tip of nose.
2. A complex graft with two separate pieces, one for dorsum and one for colummela.
3. A angular graft like the capital letter L for both colummela and tip.

The first graft is usually atractoid in order to fit and stabilize well on dorsum with no possibility of moving.
In second case the two parts of the graft have a notch on them, meeting each other on the tip of the nose where, one insert to the other, so they are kept in place. The base of vertical part is wide enough having a notch too so it can fit well on antirior nasal spine. To prevent dorsum´s graft moving we have to make a groove into nasal bones, in which the graft will be put, or we can

restrain graft using sutures.

The third case is a combination of the two previous cases.

Operation is done under local or general anesthesia. After repairing the malposition of colummela or septum's diviation, in case we want to transplant cartilage into dorsum we make a sheath in it, where the graft is put. Some times we are obliged to make a groove on nasal bones and septum, to be sure that cartilage will stabilize and no moving of it will happen. We rarely use suture to hold on the graft.

When we transplant cartilage into colummela we make a sheath between the two petals of a septum mucus at the anterior part of nose and in front of anterior nasal spine where we put the graft.

If tip of nose needs small elevation, we do an incision of skin in front of inner part of great alar cartilage where we put a small graft. In case we use the L shape cartilage there is a combination of the techniques above.

CONCLUSION

We believe that lyphilized cartilage is a graft easy in use and preservation with no problems of absorptions or rejection, which can help a lot in cosmetic and functional rhinoplasty.

© 1985 Elsevier Science Publishers B.V. (Biomedical Division)
New dimensions in otorhinolaryngology - head and neck surgery, vol. 2.
E. Myers, editor

THE HISTOLOGICAL BEHAVIOR OF LYOPHILISED PLEURAL BONE

A.SKEVAS, TH.TSOULIAS, N.PAPADOPOULOS, G.PAPACHRISTOU, K.MPLIOURAS.
E.N.T. Clinic., University of Ioannina. IOANNINA - GREECE

MATERIAL AND METHODS

In this experimental study we examined the histological behavior of lyphilished pleural bone which was transplanted subcutaneous into rabbit albinons back. The specimens was examined under light microscope after forty days, four and seven months.

RESULTS

The first graft was examined 40 days after transplantation.
In this graft the main portion of bone tissue consisted of normal cancelous bone. The bone marrow which filled up the trabeculae appeared in many places a high depree of cellularity. The cells of the myeloid tissue which composed from leukocytes and erythrocytes of mature shape, mantain their natural ratio.(2:1)

The most mature neutrophils were recognized by their small size and darkly stained multiple nuclear lobes.

The cytoplasm of these most mature cells might not appear to stain or might be very light pink.

Karyolysis was observed in a quite small number of cells which belonged to the white serie. A small number of cells appeared to lie in a syncytial mass with indiastinct cytoplasmic borders. The cytoplasm was weakly to moderately eosinophilic and generally homegeneously stained. These cells obviously were degenerated precursors shapes. Between these cells small collections of mature lymphocytes and plasma cells could be seen. Among the myeloid cells were vacuolated spaces which corrisponded in depenerated fat cells. Fig. 1.

The second graft which was examined 4 months after transplantation consisted of small parts of cancelous bone tissue, among which, bone marrow cellularity often could be seen.

The ratio of white and red series was found in normal levels (2:1)-
Karyolysis was seen in a great number of leykocytes as well as groups of cells in syncytial mass appearance.
Between the above cells a small number of lynphocytes and plasmacells could be seen. Fig.2.
The third graft which was examined 7 months after transplantation, consisted of small parts of cancelous bone tissue, which characterised, of myeloid tissue cellularity in different places.

The ratio of white and red cells series, as well as karyolysis and degenerated cells in syncytial mass, was found to be at the same level as in second case. Fig. 3.

Our conclutions from this experimental study are:

1. In all cases we found the normal myeloid : erythroid (M:E) ratio 2:1.
2. The grafts in all three cases were surrounded by fibrous connective tissue.
3. There was a gradual reduction of lymphocytes and plasma cells from first to third case, whille in the same time, was a gradual increase of leukocytes having karyolysis, as well as degenerated cells, in syncytial mass.
4. The cellularity of myeloid tissue appeared a mild degree reduction from first to second and third case.

As general conclusion we believe that first graft has, an almost normal bone marrow tissue, whille the second and third grafts have mild degree degenerated lesions, without important desturbance of normal architecture.

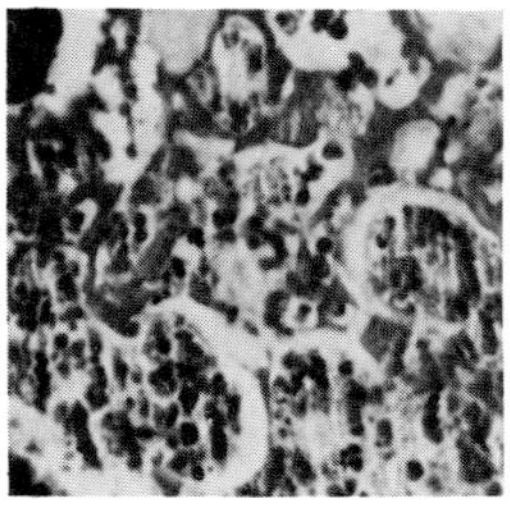

Fig. 1.

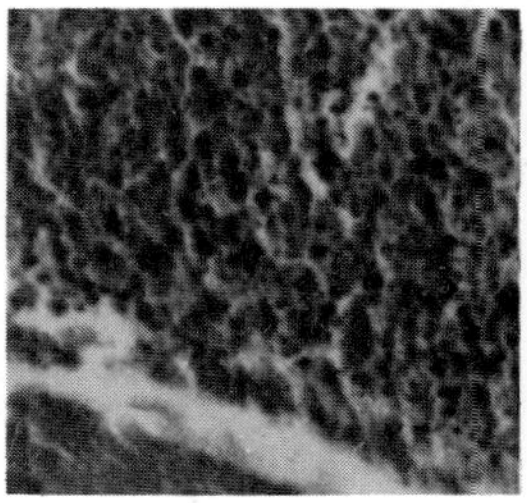

Fig. 2.

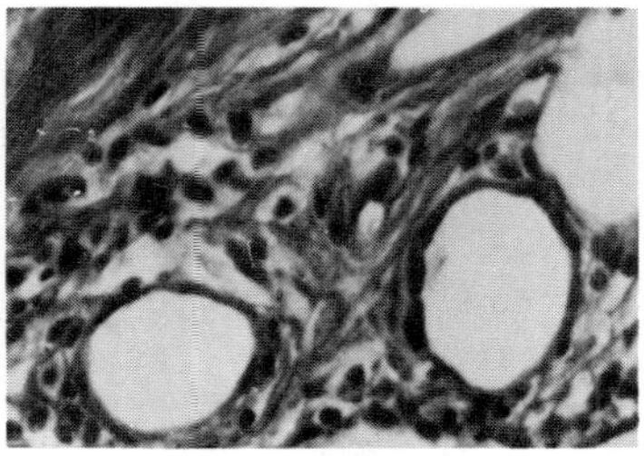

Fig. 3.

© 1985 Elsevier Science Publishers B.V. (Biomedical Division)
New dimensions in otorhinolaryngology – head and neck surgery, vol. 2.
E. Myers, editor

SLEEP APNEA INDUCED BY TONSILLAR HYPERTROPHY

J Udaka, K Takeichi, T Ishida, Y Koike
Department of Otorhinolaryngology, the University of Tokushima School of Medicine, Tokushima (Japan)

Recently tonsillar hypertrophy has drawn attention as a cause of infant's sleep apnea. That is, adenoids and/or palatine tonsillar hypertrophy bring a mechanical obstruction of the upper respiratory tract, and then result in sleep apnea accompanied by some changes in the physiological condition in sleep. But the relationship between tonsillar hypertrophy and sleep apnea still leaves quite a few obscure points. So we measured the mesopharyngeal pressure using a high quality miniaturized pressure transducer[1] and got some interesting findings.

SUBJECTS AND METHODS

The subjects were 2-10 years old, 50 infants who had admitted to our hospital to undergo adenotonsillectomy from July 1983 to June 1984. They were classified into three groups according to the symptoms in sleep. Group A were 9 cases who complained of frequent sleep apneic episodes. Group B consisted of 23 cases who did not complain sleep apneic episodes, but had some symptoms of the upper respiratory obstruction in sleep. Group C were 18 cases who had no symptom of the upper respiratory obstruction. According to Ishida method[2] we put the Gaeltec pressure transducer just under the palatine tonsils through the nostril and fixed it. In about half of the subjects, we put another transducer under the adenoids. We waited until the subject fell in sleep and recorded the change in the upper respiratory pressure usually for 7 hours on end.

RESULTS

Fig.1-a indicates the maximum amplitude of the mesopharyngeal pressure between the inspiratory and the expiratory phase of all 50 cases in sleep before operation. The pressure of groups A and B were higher than that of group C. Especially the amplitude was notably high for the group A which had apnea. Adenotonsillectomy dissolved obstructive sleep apnea completely and the obstructive symptoms of groups A and B almost disappeared. Fig.1-b indicates the post-operative mesopharyngeal pressure amplitude. The amplitude for these three groups were less than about 10 cm H_2O without exception. Fig.2 indicates the pressure data from 20 cases, which were measured under adenoids at the same time. Only limited cases have a high amplitude of the pressure under adenoids. So the obstructive portion was thought to be chiefly about palatine tonsils.

CONCLUSIONS

1) The mesopharyngeal pressure is closely related to obstructive symptoms. 2) The upper respiratory obstruction is chiefly brought about by the palatine tonsils, and rarely by the aderoids. 3) Adenotonsillectomy reduces sleep apnea and other obstructive symptoms. 4) The measurement of the mesopharyngeal pressure with a miniaturized transducer is thought to be simple, harmless and useful in deciding the stenotic portion and the degree of stenosis in the upper respiratory tracts.

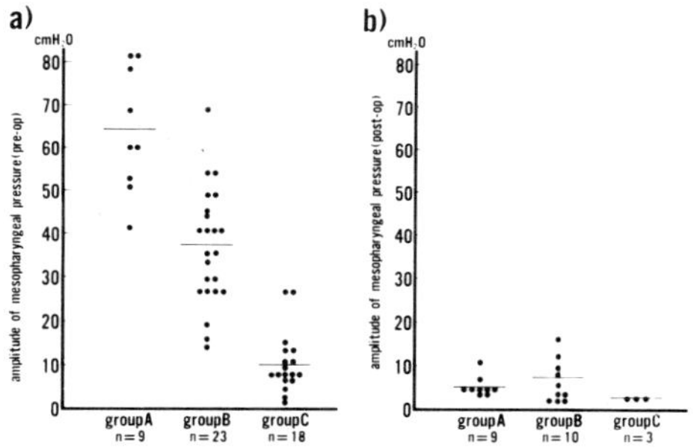

Fig.1 The maximum amplitudes of pre- and post-operative mesopharyngeal pressure.

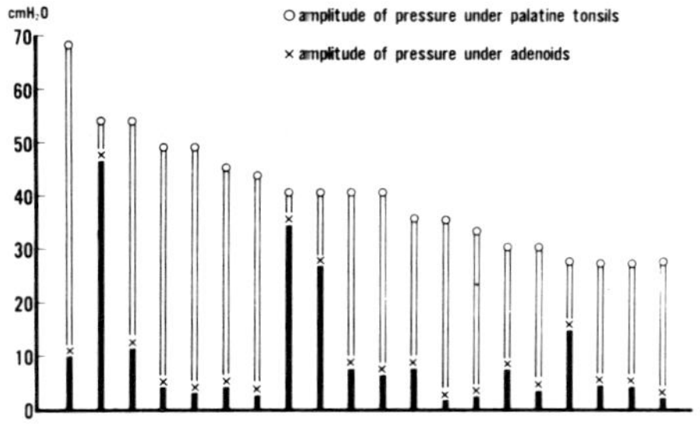

Fig.2 The pressure amplitudes under palatine tonsils and adenoids.

REFERENCES

1. Koike Y, Perkins W (1968) Foria phoniat 20:360-368
2. Ishida T (1985) Practica otologica (Kyoto) 78:411-432

New dimensions in otorhinolaryngology – head and neck surgery, vol. 2.
E. Myers, editor

SIMULTANEOUS MANOMETRY AND ELECTROMYOGRAPHY IN THE PHARYNGO-ESOPHAGEAL SEGMENT.

R.H.L. PAPING, J.J.M. VAN OVERBEEK AND H.P. WIT

ENT-Department, University Hospital Groningen, P.O. Box 30.001,
9700 RB Groningen (The Netherlands)

Whether the occlusion between hypopharynx and esophagus is established by anatomical relations and tissue elasticity or by a functional resting tone of the muscle fibers is not quite clear. This study describes simultaneous electromanometry and electromyography in the pharyngo-esophageal segment to solve this problem.

To register the EMG from the hypopharyngeal constrictor muscle and the upper esophageal sphincter, two copper wire electrode pairs with hooked bare ends were used. These electrodes were introduced in the muscle through a rigid esophagoscope with the aid of a specially designed instrument. By means of this method we demonstrated at rest the existence of a continuous muscle tone in the upper esophageal sphincter, disappearing during the relaxation period in deglutition. The period of electrical silence is followed by an increase of activity due to postrelaxation contraction (Fig. 1.).

The technique of simultaneous manometry and EMG will supplement diagnostic procedures in dysphagia patients and will strongly support to indicate myotomy of the upper esophageal sphincter.

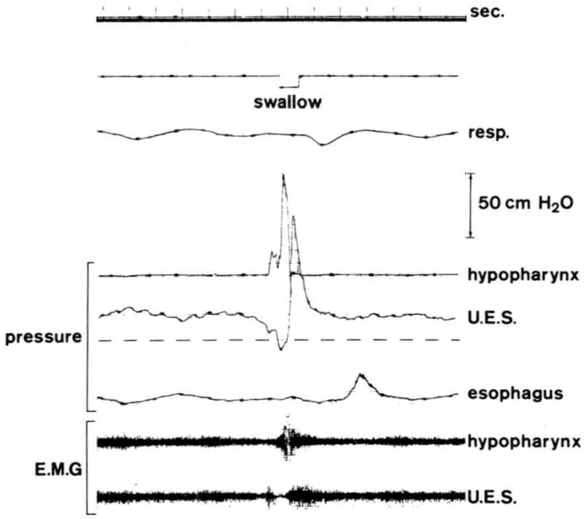

Fig. 1. Example of simultaneous manometry and EMG recordings in the pharyngoesophageal segment at rest and during swallowing.

REFERENCE

1. Overbeek JJM van, Wit HP, Paping RHL (1985) Laryngoscope 95:582-584.

© 1985 Elsevier Science Publishers B.V. (Biomedical Division)
New dimensions in otorhinolaryngology - head and neck surgery, vol. 2.
E. Myers, editor

PRESERVATION OF THE SPINAL ACCESSORY NERVE IN RADICAL NECK DISSECTION, IS IT WORTHWHILE?

W.I. WEI, K.H. LAM, W.F. LAU, T.K. CHOI

Department of Surgery, University of Hong Kong, Queen Mary Hospital, Hong Kong

INTRODUCTION

First described by Crile in 1906, the radical neck dissection aims at removing completely all lymph nodes and channels which represent the primary drainage area of malignancies arising in the head and neck region[1]. In the classical radical neck dissection, the spinal accessory nerve, the sternomastoid muscle and the internal jugular vein are all removed. With the spinal accessory nerve sacrificed, the patient usually experiences a dull ache in the shoulder which is exacerbated by motion. In addition there is also reduced shoulder abduction[2]. To ameliorate these functional disabilities, various modifications of the classical radical neck dissection have been suggested, such as preservation of the spinal accessory nerve with the sternomastoid muscle and the internal jugular vein, or preservation of the nerve alone. Studies regarding functional aspects of the shoulder in these patients revealed that the functional scoring was highest when the least amount of tissue was removed[4].

The removal of the spinal accessory nerve in radical neck dissection was claimed to be essential for tumour clearance, because the frequency of tumour involvement of the spinal accessory lymph nodes was not less than other lymph nodes in the neck[3]. Other study however showed that the incidence of local tumour recurrence with the preservation of the spinal accessory nerve alone was not increased[5].

In the past years, we have preserved the spinal accessory nerve in patients suffering from tumours of the head and neck region with no clinical palpable lymph nodes, by dissecting free the nerve from the base of the skull to its entry into the trapezius muscle. Contributions to the accessory nerve from the cervical plexus were all severed and the sternomastoid muscle was removed. The present review aims to study the functional aspects of the shoulder in these patients, to demonstrate that in fact significant shoulder function is maintained with preservation of the spinal accessory nerve.

MATERIAL AND METHODS

Surviving patients who had radical neck dissection in the Department of Surgery, University of Hong Kong, Queen Mary Hospital since 1974, were included in the study.

As a first step the patients were questioned directly on the following 3 aspects, pain in the operated side of shoulder, the ability to raise the arm above their head, such as combing hair or reaching out for objects on a shelf, and finally, whether they can handle their preoperative jobs equally well. Then a physical examination was carried out regarding their shoulder form and the ability to shrug their shoulder and to abduct the arm. For each of these assessments, a scoring system ranging from 1 to 5 was given (Table I).

In addition electromyographic study of the trapezius by stimulating the accessory nerve on both sides of the neck were performed on 10 patients who had unilateral radical neck dissection with preservation of the accessory nerve.

RESULTS AND DISCUSSION

A total of 41 patients were included in the study. Two of them had bilateral radical neck dissection. Thus there were 17 sides of neck with preservation of the accessory nerve and 26 sides of neck with accessory nerve removed. The results of functional evaluation are shown in Table II.

In the group of patients where the accessory nerve were preserved, the functional abilities were close to normal. In the other group, wasting of the trapezius muscle may be responsible for the loss of the suspension effects on the shoulder, thus leading to the complaint of pain. The scoring of the ability to return to work is close to normal, this may be that the patient is using the opposite arm at the time of work or his job does not require the movement of his shoulder joint.

When the scorings are analysed, the difference between the groups is statistically significant (Mann Whitney's test, $p < 0.001$), showing the advantageous results of preserving the accessory nerve.

In the 10 patients where the electromyography was performed on the operated side, the peak motor action potiential was similar to that of the normal side suggesting that the muscle contraction is not weakened. Analysis of latency however showed delay. This may be due to the displacement of the nerve or the formation of fibrous tissue around the nerve.

From the present study, the preservation of the accessory nerve during radical neck dissection has helped to reduce post-operative shoulder dysfunction by preservation of muscle function.

Table I : Assessment score system

	Score 1	→	Score 5
pain in shoulder	severe pain	→	no pain
ability to raise arm	cannot raise arm	→	can raise arm easily
ability to work	have to give up job	→	return to job
shoulder form	loss of shape	→	normal form
shrugging of shoulder	loss of function	→	normal function
abduction	loss of function	→	normal function

Table II : Results of assessement

	Mean score					
	pain	ability to raise arm	work ability	shoulder form	shoulder shrugging	abduction
accessory nerve preserved	4.7	4.8	4.8	4.7	4.8	4.7
accessory nerve excised	3.4	3.8	4.1	3.1	4.2	3.8

REFERENCES

1. Crile GW (1906) Excision of cancer of the head and neck. JAMA 47:1780-6

2. Nahum AM, Mullally W, Marmor L (1961) A syndrome resulting from radical neck dissection. Archives of Otolaryngology 74:424-428

3. Schuller DE, Platz CE, Krause CJ (1978) Spinal accessory lymph nodes: A prospective study of metastatic involvement. Laryngoscope 88:439-508

4. Leipzig B, Suen JY, English JL, Barnes J, Hooper M (1983) Functional evaluation of the spinal accessory nerve after neck dissection. Am J Surg 146:526-530

5. Roy PH, Beahrs OH (1969) Spinal accessory nerve in radical neck dissection. Am J Surg 118:800-804

New dimensions in otorhinolaryngology - head and neck surgery, vol. 2.
E. Myers, editor

ISOLATION OF AN AUTOLOGOUS FIBRINOGEN ADHESIVE FOR MICROSURGERY

ROBERT A. WEISMAN, M.D. AND GORDON H. EPSTEIN, M.D.

Department of Otorhinolaryngology and Human Communication, University of Pennsylvania School of Medicine, 3400 Spruce St., Philadelphia, PA 19104, USA

INTRODUCTION

Many microsurgical reconstructive procedures would be facilitated by a safe surgical adhesive. A fibrinogen based adhesive (Tisseel) has been effective in a variety of microsurgical procedures in Europe, but because it is derived from pooled human blood, it carries a risk of transmitting hepatitis, AIDS and other illnesses. This report details a newly developed procedure for creating an autologous fibrinogen based adhesive, obviating these risks.

MATERIALS AND METHODS

A prodedure for obtaining concentrated fibrinogen and Factor XIII from human blood was developed, modifying the technique of Masri (1). Forty-five ml of blood was drawn into a syringe containing five ml of 3.8% sodium citrate, pH 7.4. The entire isolation procedure was then performed at room temperature. The citrated blood was spun in a centrifuge at 2000 rpm, and the cell-free supernatant was saved. Barium sulfate (2.25gm) and magnesium sulfate (0.01235gm) were added to 20 ml of plasma to absorb out prothrombin. The prothrombin-thrombin free plasma was decanted, and enough 30% polyethylene glycol (PEG) MW 1000, in sodium citrate solution, pH 7.4, was added to make a 10% w/v PEG mixture. This mixture was spun in a centrifuge at 10,000 x g for 20 minutes to form a precipitate rich in fibrinogen and Factor XIII. The supernatant was discarded and the precipitate was resuspended in sodium citrate, pH 7.4, to a final volume of 1 ml. This product was then divided into 0.1 ml aliquots, which were either used immediately, or stored at -20°C for later use.

RESULTS

Isolations of concentrated fibrinogen and Factor XIII have been performed in our laboratory on blood from over 40 human donors and 20 rabbits. The yield of fibrinogen from plasma ranges from 42-91%, and can be varied by changing the concentration of PEG. With 10% PEG, up to 90% of the total protein precipitated is fibrinogen. The concentration of fibrinogen in the final product volume of 1 ml is 50-60 mg/ml, similar to that found in Tisseel. The concentration of prekallekrein, an important cofactor in the fibrinolytic system, was reduced to 1% or less of its concentration in plasma. When combined with calcium chloride and bovine thrombin, a firm coagulum is produced in 1-3 minutes. The time required for coagulation could be controlled by varying the concentration of thrombin from 4 to 500 IU/ml.

This adhesive system has been evaluated in animal models. In a preliminary study, the PEG derived adhesive was compared to Tisseel and normal saline (control) for potential toxicity in the middle ear of chinchillas. No mucosal necrosis or inflammation was seen histologically 30 days after any of these substances were placed on the oval and round windows and the promontory. The cochleas of the animals treated with PEG derived adhesive and Tisseel were identical to the normal saline control subjects. Auditory brainstem response thresholds and acoustic reflexes remained stable in all three groups for thirty days after surgery.

Bonding of a bone chip to the malleus with the PEG adhesive derived from single human donors has been achieved in 10 consecutive chinchillas. The bond consists of fibrous tissue, with occasional foreign body giant cells, covered with normal mucosa. In rabbits, enough blood can be drawn to produce a volume of autologous adhesive sufficient for surgery in the same animal. Preliminary studies have shown good bonding of autologous cartilage grafts to the rabbit ear. No significant inflammation or tissue reaction was seen 3, 7, 14, 21, or 28 days after grafting, compared to controls in which no adhesive was used. No significant reaction was seen over similar time intervals to 0.1 ml of autologous PEG derived adhesive implanted subcutaneously, based on light microscopic examination.

DISCUSSION

The technique described for isolating autologous fibrinogen (and Factor XIII) could make it possible to use a patient's own blood as the source of an adhesive for microsurgery. Because this material is autologous, it would be free of the risks associated with the administration of products derived from pooled plasma. The technique of isolation is simple, fast (about 2 hr), and could be performed with equipment available in most blood banks. The autologous fibrinogen component could be isolated from a blood sample drawn from a patient at the time of preoperative blood testing, and frozen until the time of surgery, or could be prepared on the day of surgery. Preliminary data from animal studies suggest that a durable bond, adequate for most microsurgical procedures, is formed. Based on these studies, autologous fibrinogen adhesive derived by PEG precipitation, holds great promise as a safe and effective adhesive for many applications in microsurgery.

REFERENCES

1. Masri NA, Masri SA, Boyd (1983) Thromb Haemostas (Stuttgart) 42(2): 116-119

© 1985 Elsevier Science Publishers B.V. (Biomedical Division)
New dimensions in otorhinolaryngology - head and neck surgery, vol. 2.
E. Myers, editor

HEAD AND NECK MANIFESTATIONS OF GOLTZ'S SYNDROME

JAN ZEMPLENYI, M.D. AND JEROME W. THOMPSON, M.D.

Dept. Head/Neck Surgery, Univ. Calif., Los Angeles and Dept. of Otolaryngology, Childrens Hospital, Los Angeles, California (USA)

INTRODUCTION

Focal dermal hypoplasia is an uncommon syndrome described by Goltz in 1962. It is characterized by focal, linear areas of skin hypoplasia with herniation of nodules of subcutaneous fat. Numerous other anomalies of both ectodermal and mesodermal origin are frequently associated. This syndrome has manifestations of importance to the head and neck surgeon.

CASE REPORT

A seven year old Caucasian female was seen because of loud snoring and dysphagia. Past medical history revealed her to be a product of an uncomplicated pregnancy. At birth areas of dermal hypoplasia were noted. Other anomalies included a severe deformity of right leg, syndactyly of 3rd and 4th digits of both hands, dystrophic nails and an omphalocele. Work-up included a normal karyotype, and a biopsy of the skin lesions revealed normal epidermis with markedly attenuated dermal layer replaced by normal-appearing adipocytes. Subsequently the patient underwent several operations to repair her omphalocele and skeletal deformities. At the age of 5 she was seen with complaints of dysphagia and loud snoring. Markedly hypertrophied tonsils and adenoids were excised. After 1½ symptom-free years she presented to the ENT clinic with a recurrence of dysphagia, loud snoring and intermittent stridor.

On exam she was a thin child of normal intelligence. Loud exertional stridor was heard. Scalp hair was thin and sparse. Skin revealed focal hypoplasia on the back, axillae and the extremities (Fig. 1). A warty lesion of about 1 cm in diameter was located on the lower lip. The teeth were hypoplastic and irregularly spaced. A fleshy mass was obscuring the right faucial arch (Fig. 2). The skeletal exam showed anomalies as above, and evidence of past surgical procedures.

Routine laboratory tests including an audiogram were normal. In the operating room the lip lesion was excised, and the base was vaporized with a CO_2 laser. The base-of-tongue lesion was exposed using a mouth gag and tongue-traction sutures. The lesion was dissected off, and the base was oversewn. Airway-obstructive symptoms subsided. Histological examination of the lip revealed a squamous papilloma. The tongue lesion showed a hyperplastic lingual tonsil with polypoid and reactive changes.

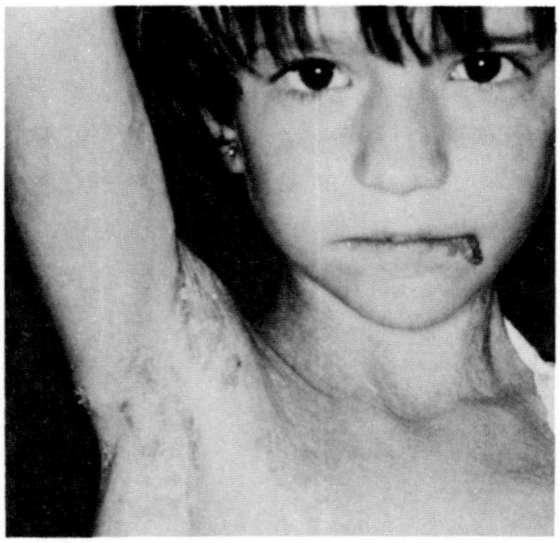

Fig. 1. Dermal hypoplasia is seen in the axilla. Also note the sparse hair and verrucous lesion of the lip.

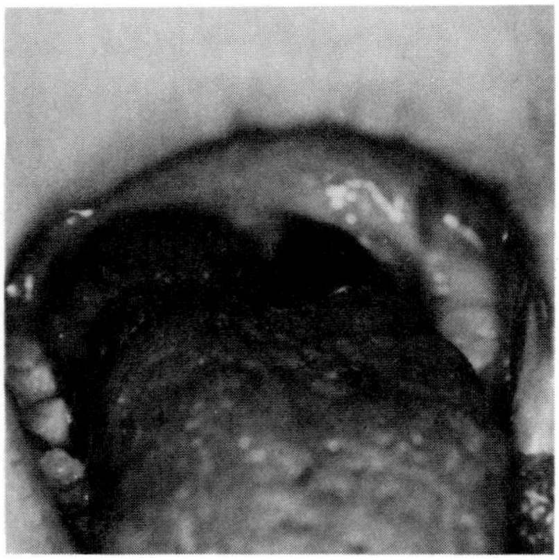

Fig. 2. Note the massive lesion at the base of tongue obscuring the faucial arch.

DISCUSSION

The present case demonstrates many of the features of the Goltz's syndrome. It presents with focal dermal hypoplasia and constellation of mesoectodermal defects. Histologically the pathognomonic skin lesion shows an attenuated dermis and adipose layer abutting the epidermis. Of the approximately 100 cases reported thus far, 90% are females. The syndrome may be due to a sex-linked chromosomal defect usually lethal in a male fetus or a x-autosomal translocation. Karyotypes are normal. Various skeletal defects are present in 80% of cases. Oral and dental anomalies are found in about 50% of patients. Papillomas of gingivae, tongue, palate, tonsil and buccal mucosa have been reported, although secondary airway-obstructive symptoms due to a polypoid mass have not been described. The dental defects include enamel and dental hypoplasia, notching, irregular spacing, etc. Forty percent of cases have ocular anomalies including defects of iris, retina, optic nerve and microphthalmia. This is only the second reported case in the Otolaryngologic literature.

REFERENCES

1. Goltz RW, Peterson WC, Gorlin RJ, et al: Focal dermal hypoplasia. Arch Dermatology 86:52-61, 1962.
2. Mair IWS, Hoy C: Focal dermal hypoplasia. J. Laryngol Otol 85:853-856, 1971.
3. Hall EH, Terezhalmy GT: Focal dermal hypoplasia syndrome. J. Am. Acad. Dermatol 9:443-451, 1983.

INDEX OF AUTHORS